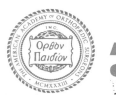

**American Academy of
Orthopaedic Surgeons**

Orthopaedic
Knowledge
Update

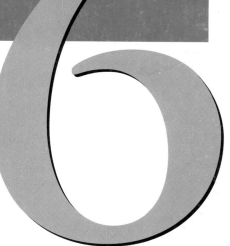

Home Study
Syllabus

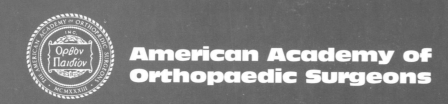

**American Academy of
Orthopaedic Surgeons**

Orthopaedic
Knowledge
Update

Home Study
Syllabus

6

James H. Beaty, MD
Editor

Published 1999
by the American Academy of Orthopaedic Surgeons®
6300 North River Road
Rosemont, Illinois 60018
1-800-626-6726

Copyright ©1999
by the American Academy of Orthopaedic Surgeons®

The material presented in *Orthopaedic Knowledge Update 6: Home Study Syllabus* has been made available by the American Academy of Orthopaedic Surgeons® for educational purposes only. This material is not intended to present the only, or necessarily best, methods or procedures for the medical situations discussed, but rather is intended to represent an approach, view, statement, or opinion of the author(s) or producer(s), which may be helpful to others who face similar situations.

Some drugs or medical devices demonstrated in Academy courses or described in Academy print or electronic publications have not been cleared by the Food and Drug Administration (FDA) or have been cleared for specific uses only. The FDA has stated that it is the responsibility of the physician to determine the FDA clearance status of each drug or device he or she wishes to use in clinical practice.

At the time of this writing, bone screws placed posteriorly into vertebral elements have been cleared for use in this specific manner by the Food and Drug Administration (FDA) to provide immobilization and stabilization as an adjunct to fusion in the treatment of the following acute and chronic instability or deformities of the thoracic, lumbar and sacral spine: degenerative spondylolisthesis with objective evidence of neurological impairment; fracture; dislocation; scoliosis; kyphosis; spinal tumor and failed previous fusion (pseudoarthrosis). In addition, anterior vertebral body screws (cervical, thoracic, and lumbar) are Class II devices and can be used as labeled in vertebral bodies.

Furthermore, any statements about commercial products are solely the opinion(s) of the author(s) and do not represent an Academy endorsement or evaluation of these products. These statements may not be used in advertising or for any commercial purpose.

ISBN 0-89203-211-1

Editorial Board

Contributors

Michael D. Aiona, MD
Assistant Chief of Staff
Shriners Hospitals-Portland Unit
Portland, Oregon

Edward Akelman, MD
Vice Chairman
Department of Orthopedics
Brown University
Providence, Rhode Island

Todd J. Albert, MD
Associate Professor of Orthopaedic Surgery
Co-Director, Division of Reconstructive
  Spine Surgery
Rothman Institute
Thomas Jefferson University
Philadelphia, Pennsylvania

Jeffreys C. Albright, MD
Instructor in Orthopaedic Surgery
New England Medical Center
Tufts University School of Medicine
Boston, Massachusetts

Howard S. An, MD
The Morton International Professor
  of Orthopaedic Surgery
Department of Orthopaedics
Rush Medical College
Rush-Presbyterian St. Luke's Medical Center
Chicago, Illinois

Robert B. Anderson, MD
Chief, Foot and Ankle Service
Department of Orthopaedic Surgery
Carolinas Medical Center
Miller Orthopaedic Clinic
Charlotte, North Carolina

Gunnar B.J. Andersson, MD, PhD
Professor and Chairman
Department of Orthopaedic Surgery
Rush-Presbyterian St. Luke's Medical Center
Chicago, Illinois

John L. Andreshak, MD, Major, USAF
Assistant Chief, Orthopaedic Spine Surgery
Department of Orthopaedic Surgery
Wilford Hall Medical Center
Lackland Air Force Base, Texas

Thomas P. Andriacchi, PhD
Professor
Department of Mechanical Engineering
  and Functional Restoration
Stanford University
Stanford, California

James Aronson, MD
Professor and Chief
Pediatric Orthopaedics
University of Arkansas for Medical Sciences
Arkansas Children's Hospital
Little Rock, Arkansas

Lauren Sutula Bargmann, MS
Research Engineer
Dartmouth Biomedical Engineering Center
Thayer School of Engineering
Dartmouth College
Hanover, New Hampshire

C. Lowry Barnes, MD
Orthopaedic Specialists
Little Rock, Arkansas

viii

Robert L. Barrack, MD
Professor of Orthopaedic Surgery
Director of Adult Reconstructive Surgery
Department of Orthopaedic Surgery
Tulane University School of Medicine
New Orleans, Louisiana

Douglas N. Beaman, MD
Director, Foot and Ankle Services
Portland Orthopedic Clinic
Portland, Oregon

James H. Beaty, MD
Professor of Orthopaedics
Department of Orthopaedics
University of Tennessee-Campbell Clinic
Memphis, Tennessee

Daniel J. Berry, MD
Assistant Professor of Orthopaedics
Mayo Medical School
Consultant in Orthopaedic Surgery
Mayo Clinic
Rochester, Minnesota

John G. Birch, MD, FRCSC
Assistant Chief of Staff
Department of Orthopedics
Texas Scottish Rite Hospital for Children
Dallas, Texas

Nancy J.O. Birkmeyer, PhD
Research Assistant Professor
Department of Surgery
Dartmouth Medical School
Lebanon, New Hampshire

Ralph B. Blasier, MD
Associate Professor
Department of Orthopaedic Surgery
Wayne State University
Detroit, Michigan

R. Dale Blasier, MD, FRCSC
Associate Professor of Orthopaedic Surgery
Division of Pediatric Orthopaedics
Arkansas Children's Hospital
University of Arkansas for Medical Sciences
Little Rock, Arkansas

Neil Blumberg, MD
Professor and Director, Transfusion Medicine
Department of Pathology and
  Laboratory Medicine
University of Rochester
Rochester, New York

Scott D. Boden, MD
Associate Professor of Orthopaedic Surgery
Director, The Emory Spine Center
Department of Orthopaedic Surgery
The Emory University School of Medicine
Atlanta, Georgia

Michael E. Brage, MD
Assistant Professor of
  Clinical Orthopaedic Surgery
Department of Orthopaedics
University of California, San Diego
San Diego, California

James H. Calandruccio, MD
Orthopaedic Surgeon
Campbell Clinic
Memphis, Tennessee

John J. Callaghan, MD
Professor
Department of Orthopaedics
University of Iowa College of Medicine
Iowa City, Iowa

James E. Carpenter, MD
Assistant Professor
Department of Surgery
Section of Orthopaedic Surgery
University of Michigan
Ann Arbor, Michigan

Anthony J. Checroun, MD
Shoulder Fellow
Department of Orthopaedics
Shoulder Service
Hospital for Joint Diseases Orthopaedic Institute
New York, New York

John P. Collier, DE
Myron Tribus Chair in Innovation
Professor of Engineering
Director
Dartmouth Biomedical Engineering Center
Thayer School of Engineering
Dartmouth College
Hanover, New Hamphsire

Evan D. Collins, MD
Assistant Professor
Department of Orthopaedic Surgery
Baylor College of Medicine
Houston, Texas

Mark R. Colville, MD
Clinical Associate Professor
Department of Orthopaedic Surgery
Oregon Health Sciences University
Portland, Oregon

Patrick M. Connor, MD
Associate
The Shoulder and Elbow Center
Miller Orthopaedic Clinic
Charlotte, North Carolina

Charles N. Cornell, MD
Director
Department of Orthopaedics
New York Hospital Medical Center, Queens
Flushing, New York

R. Jay Cummings, MD
Chairman
Department of Orthopaedics
Nemours Children's Clinic
Jacksonville, Florida

Frances Cuomo, MD
Chief, Shoulder Service
New York University-Hospital for Joint Diseases
Department of Orthopaedics
Hospital for Joint Diseases
New York, New York

Bradford L. Currier, MD
Consultant, Department of Orthopaedics
Mayo Clinic and Mayo Foundation
Assistant Professor of Orthopaedics
Mayo Medical School
Rochester, Minnesota

Donald F. D'Alessandro, MD
Director
The Shoulder and Elbow Center
Miller Orthopaedic Clinic
Charlotte, North Carolina

Douglas A. Dennis, MD
Professor, Colorado School of Mines
Director, Rose Institute for Joint Replacement
Director, Rose Musculoskeletal Research
  Laboratory
Denver, Colorado

Frederick R. Dietz, MD
Professor
Department of Orthopaedic Surgery
University of Iowa
Iowa City, Iowa

John P. Dormans, MD
Chief of Orthopaedic Surgery
Children's Hospital of Philadelphia
Associate Professor of Orthopaedic Surgery
University of Pennsylvania School of Medicine
Philadelphia, Pennsylvania

John S. Early, MD
Assistant Professor
Department of Orthopaedics
University of Texas Southwestern Medical School
Dallas, Texas

x

Thomas A. Einhorn, MD
Professor and Chairman
Department of Orthopaedic Surgery
Boston University School of Medicine
Boston, Massachusetts

Evan F. Ekman, MD
Assistant Professor of Orthopaedic Surgery
Director, University of South Carolina
  Sports Medicine Center
Department of Orthopaedic Surgery
University of South Carolina
Columbia, South Carolina

Neal S. Elattrache, MD
Associate, Kerlan Jobe Orthopaedic Clinic
Associate Clinical Professor
Department of Orthopaedics
University of Southern California
  School of Medicine
Los Angeles, California

Sanford E. Emery, MD
Associate Professor
Department of Orthopaedics
University Hospitals of Cleveland
Case Western Reserve University
Cleveland, Ohio

Marybeth Ezaki, MD
Assistant Professor of Orthopaedic Surgery
University of Texas Southwestern Medical School
Texas Scottish Rite Hospital
Dallas, Texas

Anthony B. Fiorillo, MD
Assistant Professor of Medicine
Department of Internal Medicine
University of Pittsburgh School of Medicine
Pittsburgh, Pennsylvania

Thomas J. Fischer, MD
Clinical Associate Professor
Department of Orthopaedic Surgery
Indiana University School of Medicine
Indianapolis, Indiana

Evan L. Flatow, MD
Professor of Orthopaedic Surgery
Associate Chief, The Shoulder Service
New York Orthopaedic Hospital
Columbia-Presbyterian Medical Center
New York, New York

Kevin L. Garvin, MD
Professor
Department of Orthopaedic Surgery
University of Nebraska Medical Center
Omaha, Nebraska

Sanjitpal S. Gill, MD
Resident
Department of Orthopaedic Surgery
University of Virginia Health Sciences Center
Charlottesville, Virginia

Victor M. Goldberg, MD
Professor
Department of Orthopaedics
Case Western Reserve University
Cleveland, Ohio

Ben K. Graf, MD
Associate Professor
Department of Surgery
Divison of Orthopedic Surgery
University of Wisconsin Hospital
Madison, Wisconsin

Thomas J. Graham, MD
Chief of Hand and Elbow Surgery
Department of Orthopaedic Surgery
The Cleveland Clinic Foundation
Cleveland, Ohio

Gregory P. Graziano, MD
Associate Professor of Surgery
Section of Orthopaedic Surgery
  and Neurosurgery
University of Michigan Medical Center
Ann Arbor, Michigan

Kenneth J. Guidera, MD
Assistant Chief of Staff
Shriners Hospitals for Children
Tampa, Florida

Gregory P. Guyton, MD
Department of Orthopaedics
University of North Carolina
Chapel Hill, North Carolina

Douglas P. Hanel, MD
Associate Professor
Department of Orthopaedics
University of Washington
Seattle, Washington

Arlen D. Hanssen, MD
Associate Professor of Orthopedics
Mayo Medical School
Mayo Clinic and Mayo Foundation
Rochester, Minnesota

Christopher D. Harner, MD
Professor of Orthopedic Surgery
University of Pittsburgh School of Medicine
Pittsburgh, Pennsylvania

Stephen D. Heinrich, MS, MD
Associate Professor
Section of Pediatric Orthopedics
Department of Orthopedic Surgery
Louisiana State Medical Center
Department of Orthopedics
Children's Hospital
New Orleans, Louisiana

Laurence D. Higgins, MD
Assistant Professor
Department of Surgery
Division of Orthopaedics
Duke University Medical Center
Durham, North Carolina

G. Brian Holloway, MD
Knoxville Orthopaedic Clinic
Knoxville, Tennessee

Thomas R. Hunt, MD
Head, Section of Hand Surgery
Department of Surgery
The Virginia Mason Clinic
Seattle, Washington

Debra E. Hurwitz, PhD
Assistant Professor
Department of Orthopaedic Surgery
Rush-Presbyterian St. Luke's Medical Center
Chicago, Illinois

John Hwang, MD
Department of Orthopaedic Surgery
Washington University School of Medicine
St. Louis, Missouri

Joseph P. Iannotti, MD, PhD
Professor of Orthopaedic Surgery
Chief of Shoulder and Elbow Service
Department of Orthopaedic Surgery
University of Pennsylvania
Philadelphia, Pennsylvania

Louis G. Jenis, MD
Attending Surgeon
Department of Orthopaedic Surgery
New England Baptist Hospital
Boston, Massachusetts

xii

Darren L. Johnson, MD
Chief, Section of Sports Medicine
Assistant Professor and Residency Director
Team Physician, University of Kentucky
Division of Orthopaedic Surgery
University of Kentucky School of Medicine
Lexington, Kentucky

James D. Kang, MD
Assistant Professor
Department of Orthopaedic Surgery
Division of Spine Surgery
University of Pittsburgh
Pittsburgh, Pennsylvania

Lori A. Karol, MD
Assistant Professor
University of Texas Southwestern Medical School
Staff Orthopaedist
Texas Scottish Rite Hospital for Children
Dallas, Texas

Michael W. Keith, MD
Professor
Orthopaedic Surgery and
  Biomedical Engineering
Case Western Reserve University
Cleveland, Ohio

Michael A. Kelly, MD
Director
Insall Scott Kelly Institute for
  Orthopaedics and Sports Medicine
Department of Orthopaedic Surgery
Beth Israel Hospital-North Division
New York, New York

Scott A. Kirkley, MD
Assistant Director
Blood Bank and Transfusion Medicine Unit
Associate Professor
Department of Pathology
  and Laboratory Medicine
University of Rochester Medical Center
Rochester, New York

Kenneth J. Koval, MD
Associate Professor
Department of Orthopaedics
New York University-School of Medicine
New York, New York

Matthew J. Kraay, MS, MD
Assistant Professor of Orthopaedic Surgery
Case Western Reserve University
  School of Medicine
University Hospitals of Cleveland
Cleveland, Ohio

Michael L. Lee, MD
R.E. Carroll Hand Fellow
Department of Orthopaedic Surgery
Columbia University-New York
  Orthopaedic Hospital
New York, New York

Sang-Hong Lee, MD, PhD
Associate Professor
Department of Orthopaedic Surgery
Chosun University School of Medicine
Kwang-Ju, South Korea

Lawrence G. Lenke, MD
Assistant Professor
Pediatric and Adult Scoliosis and
  Spinal Reconstructive Surgery
Department of Orthopaedic Surgery
Washington University School of Medicine
St. Louis, Missouri

David M. Lichtman, MD
Chairman and Director
Fort Worth Affiliated Hospitals
Orthopedic Residency Program
John Peter Smith Hospital
Fort Worth, Texas

Jay R. Lieberman, MD
Associate Professor
Department of Orthopaedic Surgery
UCLA School of Medicine
Los Angeles, California

Randall T. Loder, MD
Associate Professor
Department of Surgery-Orthopaedic Section
University of Michigan
Ann Arbor, Michigan

Gary M. Lourie, MD
Assistant Clinical Professor
Department of Orthopaedics
Emory University School of Medicine
Atlanta, Georgia

John P. Lubicky, MD
Professor of Orthopaedic Surgery
Rush Medical College
Shriners Hospitals for Children
Chicago, Illinois

William J. Maloney, MD
Associate Professor
Chief of Service
Department of Orthopaedic Surgery
Washington University School of Medicine
St. Louis, Missouri

Peter D. McCann, MD
Assistant Chairman
Department of Orthopaedic Surgery
Beth Israel Medical Center
New York, New York

Robert F. McLain, MD
Staff Surgeon, Section of Spine Surgery
Director, Spine Research
Department of Orthopaedic Surgery
The Cleveland Clinic Foundation
Cleveland, Ohio

Gregory A. Mencio, MD
Assistant Professor
Department of Orthopaedics and Rehabilitation
Vanderbilt University Medical Center
Nashville, Tennessee

Alexander D. Mih, MD
Associate Professor of Orthopaedic Surgery
Department of Orthopaedic Surgery
Indiana University
Indianapolis, Indiana

Mark D. Miller, MD, Lt Col, USAF, MC
Clinical Associate Professor,
  Uniformed Services University
Deputy Chairman, Chief of Sports Medicine
Department of Orthopaedic Surgery
Wilford Hall USAF Medical Center
Lackland Air Force Base, Texas

Berton R. Moed, MD
Professor
Department of Orthopaedic Surgery
Wayne State University
Detroit, Michigan

James F. Mooney III, MD
Assistant Professor
Department of Orthopaedic Surgery
Bowman Gray School of Medicine
Winston-Salem, North Carolina

Vincent S. Mosca, MD
Associate Professor
  and Chief of Pediatric Orthopaedics
Department of Orthopaedics
University of Washington School of Medicine
Seattle, Washington

Regis J. O'Keefe, MD
Associate Professor of Orthopaedics
Department of Orthopaedics
University of Rochester, School of Medicine
Rochester, New York

Wayne G. Paprosky, MD
Associate Professor
Department of Adult Joint Reconstruction
Rush Medical College
Chicago, Illinois

Ira M. Parsons IV, MD
Resident, Orthopaedic Surgery
Department of Orthopaedic Surgery
University of Pittsburgh
Pittsburgh, Pennsylvania

Vincent D. Pellegrini, Jr, MD
Michael and Myrtle Baker Professor
Chair, Department of Orthopaedics
  and Rehabilitation
Milton S. Hershey Medical Center
Pennsylvania State University
  College of Medicine
Penn State Geisinger Health System
Hershey, Pennsylvania

Michael S. Pinzur, MD
Professor of Orthopaedic Surgery
Department of Orthopaedic Surgery
Loyola University Stritch School of Medicine
Maywood, Illinois

Roger G. Pollock, MD
Assistant Professor of Orthopaedic Surgery
Columbia University
The Shoulder Service
Columbia-Presbyterian Medical Center
New York, New York

Hollis G. Potter, MD
Chief, Magnetic Resonance Imaging
Hospital for Special Surgery
Assistant Professor of Radiology
Department of Radiology
Cornell University Medical College
New York, New York

George T. Rab, MD
Professor of Orthopaedic Surgery
Chief of Pediatric Orthopaedics
University of California Davis
Sacramento, California

Matthew L. Ramsey, MD
Assistant Professor of Orthopaedic Surgery
University of Pennsylvania School of Medicine
Penn Musculoskeletal Institute
Presbyterian Medical Center
Philadelphia, Pennsylvania

Keith B. Raskin, MD, FACS
Clinical Associate Professor
Director of Hand Surgery
Department of Orthopaedic Surgery
New York University Medical Center
New York, New York

Mitchell F. Reiter, MD
Instructor
The Emory Spine Center
Department of Orthopaedic Surgery
The Emory University School of Medicine
Atlanta, Georgia

John J. Regan, MD
Associate Clinical Professor
Department of Orthopaedics
University of Texas Southwestern Medical School
Texas Back Institute
Plano, Texas

Robert S. Richards, MD, FRCSC
Associate Professor, Division of Plastic Surgery
Division of Orthopaedic Surgery
University of Western Ontario
London, Ontario, Canada

John C. Richmond, MD
Associate Professor of Orthopaedic Surgery
New England Medical Center
Tufts University School of Medicine
Boston, Massachusetts

Aaron G. Rosenberg, MD, FACS
Professor of Orthopaedic Surgery
Arthritis and Orthopaedic Institute
Rush-Presbyterian St. Luke's Medical Center
Rush Medical College
Chicago, Illinois

Melvin P. Rosenwasser, MD
Professor of Orthopaedic Surgery
Columbia University
Department of Orthopaedic Surgery
Columbia Presbyterian Medical Center
New York, New York

Randy N. Rosier, MD, PhD
Professor of Orthopaedics
Department of Orthopaedics
The University of Rochester
Rochester, New York

James H. Roth, MD, FRCSC
Professor, Division of Orthopaedic Surgery
Director, Hand and Upper Limb Centre
University of Western Ontario
St. Joseph's Health Centre
London, Ontario, Canada

Richard Rozencwaig, MD
Acting Instructor
Department of Orthopaedics
University of Washington
Seattle, Washington

Harry E. Rubash, MD
Chief, Orthopaedic Surgery
Massachusetts General Hospital
Boston, Massachusetts

Charles L. Saltzman, MD
Associate Professor
Departments of Orthopaedic Surgery
 and Biomedical Engineering
University of Iowa
Iowa City, Iowa

Andrew K. Sands, MD
Section Chief, Foot and Ankle Surgery
Department of Orthopaedic Surgery
Beth Israel Medical Center-Petrie Division
New York, New York

Bruce J. Sangeorzan, MD
Professor and Chief of Orthopaedics
Harborview Medical Center
Department of Orthopaedics
University of Washington
Seattle, Washington

John F. Sarwark, MD
Associate Professor of Orthopaedics
Department of Orthopaedics
Acting Division Head
Division of Pediatric Orthopaedic Surgery
Children's Memorial Hospital
Chicago, Illinois

Thomas P. Schmalzried, MD
Associate Director,
Joint Replacement Institute
 at Orthopaedic Hospital
Los Angeles, California

D. Hal Silcox III, MD
Assistant Professor
Department of Orthopaedic Surgery
The Emory Spine Center
Emory University School of Medicine
Atlanta, Georgia

J. Michael Simpson, MD
Director of Spine Surgery
Tuckahoe Orthopaedics Ltd
Richmond, Virginia

Kevin L. Smith, MD
Assistant Director
Department of Orthopaedics
University of Washington
Seattle, Washington

Michael D. Smith, MD
Staff Surgeon
Twin City Spine Center
Minneapolis, Minnesota

Paul D. Sponseller, MD
Associate Professor
Chief of Pediatric Orthopaedics
Johns Hopkins University
Baltimore, Maryland

Marvin E. Steinberg, MD
Professor and Vice Chairman
Department of Orthopaedic Surgery
University of Pennsylvania School of Medicine
Philadelphia, Pennsylvania

Robert J. Strauch, MD
Assistant Professor of Orthopaedic Surgery
Columbia-Presbyterian Medical Center
Columbia University
New York, New York

Jeffrey A. Sum, BSE
Department of Orthopaedic Surgery
Rush-Presbyterian St. Luke's Medical Center
Chicago, Illinois

Michael D. Sussman, MD
Chief of Staff
Director, Pediatric Orthopedic Surgery
Shriners Hospital for Children
Portland, Oregon

Marc F. Swiontkowski, MD
Professor and Chairman
Department of Orthopaedics
University of Minnesota
Minneapolis, Minnesota

David C. Templeman, MD
Assistant Professor of Orthopaedic Surgery
University of Minnesota
Department of Orthopaedic Surgery
Hennepin County Medical Center
Minneapolis, Minnesota

Richard M. Terek, MD
Assistant Professor of Orthopaedic Surgery
University Orthopaedics
Brown University
Providence, Rhode Island

Andrew L. Terrono, MD
Assistant Clinical Professor
Department of Orthopaedics
Tufts University School of Medicine
New England Baptist Bone and Joint Institute
Boston, Massachusetts

Kevin D. Tetsworth, MD
Assistant Professor
Division of Orthopaedic Surgery
University of Maryland Medical System
Baltimore, Maryland

John G. Thometz, MD
Associate Professor
Department of Orthopaedic Surgery
Medical College of Wisconsin
Milwaukee, Wisconsin

George H. Thompson, MD
Professor, Orthopaedic Surgery and Pediatrics
Director, Pediatric Orthopaedics
Rainbow Babies and Children's Hospital
Case Western Reserve University
Cleveland, Ohio

Jonathan B. Ticker, MD
Island Orthopaedics and Sports Medicine, PC
Massapequa, New York

Paul Tornetta III, MD
Associate Professor
Director of Orthopaedic Trauma
Department of Orthopaedic Surgery
University Hospital of Brooklyn
Brooklyn, New York

Laura L. Tosi, MD
Associate Professor of Orthopaedics
Department of Orthopaedics
George Washington University Medical Center
Washington, District of Columbia

Alexander R. Vaccaro, MD
Associate Professor
Thomas Jefferson Medical College
Rothman Institute
Philadelphia, Pennsylvania

Jon J.P. Warner, MD
Director, Shoulder Service
Associate Professor
Department of Orthopaedic Surgery
University of Pittsburgh
Pittsburgh, Pennsylvania

William C. Warner Jr, MD
Associate Professor
Department of Orthopaedics
University of Tennessee
Memphis, Tennessee

Ray C. Wasielewski, MD
Assistant Professor of Orthopaedic Surgery
Director, Resident Research
Division of Orthopaedics
Department of Surgery
Ohio State University
Columbus, Ohio

Peter M. Waters, MD
Assistant Professor
Harvard Medical School
Department of Orthopaedic Surgery
Children's Hospital
Boston, Massachusetts

J. Tracy Watson, MD
Professor of Orthopaedic Surgery
Department of Orthopaedic Surgery
Division of Orthopaedic Traumatology
Wayne State University School of Medicine
Detroit, Michigan

James N. Weinstein, DO, MS
Professor of Surgery and Community
 and Family Medicine
Medical Director, Spine Center
 and Patient Preference Laboratory
Dartmouth and The Dartmouth Hitchcock
 Medical Center
Hanover, New Hampshire

Arnold-Peter C. Weiss, MD
Professor, Department of Orthopaedics
Brown University School of Medicine
Rhode Island Hospital
Providence, Rhode Island

James G. Wright, MD, MPH, FRCSC
Associate Professor of Surgery
 and Public Health Sciences
Division of Orthopaedic Surgery
Clinical Epidemiology and Health Care Research
The Hospital for Sick Children
University of Toronto
Toronto, Ontario, Canada

Ken Yamaguchi, MD
Assistant Professor
Chief, Shoulder and Elbow Service
Department of Orthopaedic Surgery
Washington University School of Medicine
St. Louis, Missouri

Joseph P. Zeppieri, MD
Eastern Shore Special Surgery
Groton, Connecticut

Table of Contents

Section 2
Systemic Disorders

Editors and authors are listed alphabetically

Section Editors

Randall T. Loder, MD

Randy N. Rosier, MD

Section 3
Upper Extremity

Editors and authors are listed alphabetically

Section Editors

Evan L. Flatow, MD

Thomas J. Graham, MD

Randall T. Loder, MD

Section 4
Lower Extremity

Editors and authors are listed alphabetically

Section Editors

John J. Callaghan, MD

Christopher D. Harner, MD

Kenneth J. Koval, MD

Randall T. Loder, MD

Bruce J. Sangeorzan, MD

Section 5
Spine

Editors and authors are listed alphabetically

Section Editors

Howard S. An, MD

Randall T. Loder, MD

Preface

Fifteen years ago, in response to a demand for more learner-centered educational material, the first Orthopaedic Knowledge Update was produced to provide a "useful, comprehensive, and accessible synthesis of the latest information and knowledge available..." Through 5 subsequent editions, this goal has remained constant.

Advances in basic science fields, such as genetic and cellular, and an increasing awareness of the effects of systemic conditions on the musculoskeletal system have resulted in innovative diagnostic and treatment methods, so that orthopaedics today is a much more sophisticated specialty than in the "cast and buckle" era. To provide optimal patient care, orthopaedists must be familiar with a wide variety of medical specialties. To reflect this broad spectrum of knowledge, sections are presented on topics such as bone metabolism, soft-tissue physiology, bone healing, perioperative medicine, and genetic disorders. Information concerning clinical epidemiology, practice guidelines, and workers' compensation issues emphasize the integration of orthopaedics into the overall healthcare system and the impact of healthcare reforms. These newer areas of focus are added to more traditional areas of orthopaedics, such as trauma, joint reconstruction, spinal surgery, sports medicine, and pediatric orthopaedics. These topics have been enhanced by descriptions of new techniques and advances in knowledge that may have an impact on treatment methods.

Some technical changes were made in this edition to make it easier to use. A second color was added to highlight topics, more tables were added to summarize information and provide a quick synopsis of information in the text, a number of original illustrations were drawn and others were redrawn, and the type style is easier to read.

Such an undertaking would not have been possible without the cooperation of the many authors and section editors who contributed their time and expertise to this project. Most of the chapters in this edition of OKU are multiauthored, with each author contributing a special-ized section or sections to the chapter. The Editorial Board had the daunting task of reviewing and combining hundreds of manuscripts to compile chapters that presented the current concepts of orthopaedic knowledge and treatment recommendations. My thanks to all contributors and board members who worked so diligently to make this project successful. I am grateful to Bob Poss and Jim Kasser, editors of earlier editions of Orthopaedic Knowledge Update, for their advice and encouragement.

I also am indebted to a number of other people who worked so hard to make this edition a reality. Mark W. Wieting, Marilyn L. Fox, PhD, Joan Abern, Lisa Moore, Pamela Erickson, Sophie Tosta, David Stanley, and all of the Academy publications staff put in long hours organizing and managing stacks of manuscripts and illustrations. Campbell Foundation staff members Kay Daugherty, Linda Jones, Joan Crowson, and Barry Burns provided invaluable editorial, research, and graphics assistance. I owe a special thanks to my wife, Terry, and my children, Eric and Meredith, for their patience and support. As always, such a publication is the culmination of many hours of work by many people, and I am grateful for the assistance I received from all of them.

The authors and editors have attempted to put into perspective the large amount of information generated since the last edition. Orthopaedic Knowledge Update is not intended to be a comprehensive text covering all aspects of orthopaedics, but rather a compilation of core information and updated information from the orthopaedic literature (1994 through early 1998). We hope this book is indeed a "useful, comprehensive, and accessible synthesis of the latest information and knowledge available..." and that it provides information in a concise, "user-friendly" fashion that makes it useful in daily practice and helps physicians provide the best possible patient care.

James H. Beaty, MD
Editor

Section 1
General Knowledge

American Academy of Orthopaedic Surgeons

Chapter 1
Soft-Tissue Physiology and Repair

Articular Cartilage

Structure and Function

Similar to other connective tissues, articular cartilage consists of cells (chondrocytes), water, and an extracellular matrix (ECM) framework from which it derives its form and mechanical properties. Despite its lack of blood vessels, lymphatic vessels, and nerves, detailed study of the morphology and biology of articular cartilage shows that it has an elaborate, highly ordered structure and that multiple complex interactions between the chondrocytes and the matrices actively maintain tissue balance.

Chondrocytes from different cartilage zones differ in size, shape, and metabolic activity, but all cells contain the requirements for matrix synthesis. They frequently contain intracytoplasmic filaments as well as short cilia extending from the cell into the matrix. These structures may have a role in sensing mechanical changes in the immediate surrounding environment. Individual chondrocytes are very active metabolically in the homeostasis of their surrounding matrix. They derive their nutrition from nutrients in the synovial fluid, which must pass through a double diffusion barrier: first the tissue and synovial fluid, and then the cartilage matrix.

The ECM consists primarily of water (65% to 80% of its total wet weight), proteoglycans, and collagen. The predominant collagen is type II (95%), but smaller amounts of other collagens (types IV, VI, IX, X, XI) also have been identified. The functions of the remaining types of collagen are under investigation. Types IX and XI may help form and stabilize the collagen fibrils assembled primarily from type II collagen. Type VI may form an important part of the matrix immediately surrounding the chondrocyte and assist with matrix attachment. The interaction of these substances gives articular cartilage its mechanical properties. The aggrecan proteoglycan molecule comprises many glycosaminoglycan chains (keratan sulfate and chondroitin sulfate) that contain numerous charged carboxyl and sulfate groups. The organization of these aggrecans within the collagen framework produces a strong, cohesive collagen-proteoglycan solid matrix. The proteoglycans with their predominate negative charge and counterions are responsible for the water content of the articular cartilage, which has a direct influence on its deformational properties.

Articular cartilage has a highly organized tissue structure and can be divided into 4 distinct zones (Fig. 1). It is arranged in layers of differing morphology and biochemical composi-

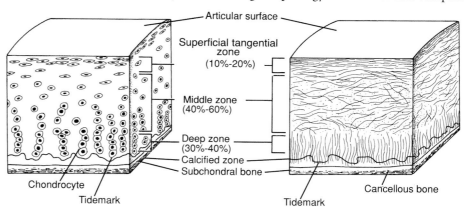

Figure 1

Structure of articular cartilage. (Reproduced with permission from Buckwalter JA, Mow VC, Ratcliffe A: Restoration of injured and degenerated articular cartilage. *J Am Acad Orthop Surg* 1994;2:192–201.)

The Articular Cartilage section of this chapter has been adapted from Buckwalter JA, Mankin HJ: Articular cartilage: Tissue design and chrondrocyte matrix interactions, in Cannon WD Jr (ed): *Instructional Course Lectures 47*. Rosemont, IL, American Academy of Orthopaedic Surgeons, 1998, p 477–486.

tion, with mechanical properties varying according to the distance of the layer from the joint surface. The homeostasis between chondrocytes, water, collagen, ultrastructural architecture, and proteoglycans dictates the tensile stiffness and strengths of each zone. From the superficial to deep zones, sheer stress increases while tensile stiffness decreases. The superficial zone contains chondrocytes that synthesize a matrix that has a high concentration of collagen and a low concentration of proteoglycan. The parallel arrangement of the collagen fibrils in this zone provides greater tensile stiffness and strength than in the deeper zones, and this may help resist shear forces generated during use of the joint. The middle (transition) zone has a morphologic and matrix composition in between that of the superficial and deep zones and comprises the largest part (40% to 60%) of the articular cartilage. The deep (radial) zone has the largest-diameter collagen fibrils, the highest concentration of proteoglycans, and the lowest concentration of water. The collagen fibrils pass into the tidemark, a thin basophilic line seen on light microscopy sections of decalcified articular cartilage that roughly corresponds to the boundary between calcified and uncalcified cartilage. Shear stresses are greatest at the tidemark. A zone of calcified cartilage separates the radial zone from the subchondral bone. The cells of this zone have a very small volume and appear to be surrounded completely by calcified cartilage. Recent work suggests that they may have a role in the development and progression of osteoarthrosis.

Biomechanics and Physiology

Articular cartilage exhibits a time-dependent behavior (viscoelastic) when subjected to a constant load or constant deformation. When a constant compressive stress (load/area) is applied to the tissue, its deformation will increase with time, that is, it will creep until an equilibrium value is reached. Similarly, when the tissue is deformed and held at a constant strain, the stress will rise to a peak, followed by a slow stress-relaxation process until an equilibrium value is reached. Two mechanisms are responsible for viscoelasticity: a flow-independent and a flow-dependent mechanism.

During walking or running, articular cartilage is subjected to compressive forces that rise to several times body weight within a very short period of time. Under this dynamic loading environment, interstitial fluid trapped within the cartilage matrix enables the tissue to resist these high compressive forces without mechanical damage. The instantaneous increased hydrostatic pressure will be sustained within the tissue matrix for an extended period of time. When the interstitial fluid flows through the dense matrix, a frictional interaction between the fluid and the matrix is created, providing a mechanism for energy dissipation. This phenomenon, the

flow-dependent biphasic viscoelasticity of articular cartilage, provides additional protection of the tissue matrix from mechanical damage. Independent of the interstitial fluid flow, the proteoglycan molecules and the collagen fibers themselves have shown significant viscoelastic characteristics. Thus, the cartilage matrix constitutes the intrinsic viscoelasticity in shear deformation. This second phenomenon is called flow-independent intrinsic viscoelasticity, and has been shown to significantly govern the short-term behavior of articular cartilage immediately after a mechanical load is applied to the tissue, such as in running or walking.

Joint loading and motion are required to maintain normal adult articular cartilage. Immobilization of a joint will cause a rapid loss of proteoglycans from the cartilage matrix. Proteoglycan content is affected to a greater extent than collagen composition. Because proteoglycan is lost, fluid flux and deformation in response to compression will increase. Tensile properties, which depend primarily on collagen, are maintained. These biochemical and biomechanical changes are, at least in part, reversible with the restoration of motion. The extent of recovery decreases with increasing periods of immobilization.

Increased joint loading, either through excessive use or increased magnitudes of loading, will also affect articular cartilage. Disruption of the intra-articular structures, such as menisci or ligaments, will alter forces acting on the articular surface. In experimental animal models, responses to transection of the anterior cruciate ligament (ACL) or meniscectomy have included fibrillation of the cartilage surface, increased hydration, and changes in proteoglycan content. Significant and progressive decreases in the tensile and shear modulus have been observed in response to transection of the ACL.

While the overall metabolic activity of articular cartilage is low, the activity surrounding each individual chondrocyte and surrounding ECM is quite dynamic. This activity is determined by a cellular response to soluble mediators (nutrients, growth factors, cytokines), mechanical loads, matrix composition, hydrostatic pressure changes, and electric fields. Growth factors, such as insulin-like growth factor-I and transforming growth factor-β (TFG-β), may stimulate matrix synthesis and cell proliferation. Chondrocytes synthesize and release these growth factors, which further enhance the metabolic activity of chondrocytes and matrix production. Matrix catabolism is mediated by enzymes, including stromelysin, aggrecanase, and collagenase, which are regulated in a complex manner by local factors such as interleukin-1 (IL-1), prostaglandins, TFG-β, tumor necrosis factor, and other molecules.

The ECM is known to act as a signal transducer for the

chondrocytes and may transmit signals that result from mechanical loading of the articular surface to the chondrocytes. The chondrocytes respond to these signals by altering the matrix, possibly through the expression of cytokines that act through local factors. It has been shown that a persistent abnormal change in joint loading or immobilization of a joint may change the concentration of proteoglycans in articular cartilage and the degree of proteoglycan aggregation that alters the mechanical properties of cartilage. The exact details of how the mechanical loading of joints influences the functions of chondrocytes remains investigational, but deformation of the matrix produces mechanical, electrical, and physiochemical signals that may have major roles in stimulating chondrocytes.

Articular Cartilage Injury

Mechanical injuries to articular cartilage can be separated into 3 distinct types: (1) microscopic damage to the chondrocytes and ECM without visible disruption of the articular cartilage surface, (2) macrodisruption of the articular cartilage alone (chondral fracture), and (3) osteochondral fracture or disruption of the articular cartilage and subchondral bone.

Microscopic injury may result from a single traumatic event or multiple repetitive loads. A reliable method of detecting damage to articular cartilage in the absence of surface disruption (ie, chondral fracture) has yet to be developed. This microscopic mechanism most likely results in damage to the chondrocytes and affects their ability to produce collagen and proteoglycans. The point at which the accumulated microdamage becomes irreversible is unknown. Chondrocytes have the ability to restore lost proteoglycans if the rate of loss does not exceed the rate of production. If there is concomitant damage to the collagen ultrastructural architecture or if a sufficient number of chondrocytes have been damaged, an irreversible degeneration process may ensue. Although the exact natural history of this type of damage is still being defined, the decrease in proteoglycan concentration, the increase in tissue hydration, and disorganization of the articular cartilage is worrisome.

Clinically, this scenario has been observed in conjunction with knee ligament injuries. After an ACL injury to the knee, an occult osteochondral lesion or "bone bruise" may be detected in up to 80% of patients by magnetic resonance imaging (MRI). The most common location of these lesions is within the lateral compartment of the knee, on the lateral femoral condyle at the sulcus terminalis, and the posterolateral tibial plateau. Although the area may appear normal during arthroscopic examination, recent in vivo histologic studies have shown a significant disruption of the articular

cartilage. The reversiblity of these chondral injuries is still being debated. It is hoped that ongoing clinical and basic science studies will provide the clinician with new scientific information on the natural history and optimal treatment of these injuries.

Isolated partial and full-thickness articular cartilage injuries (chondral fractures) are often problematic because of the limited blood supply. This relatively poor blood supply (in comparison to bony injuries where a vascular response is robust) combined with the isolated environment of the chondrocyte makes the potential healing of articular cartilage poor. For smaller lesions (< 1 cm in size), overall joint homeostasis may not be affected; however, as the lesion increases in size, overall joint congruity is affected, resulting in increased loading of the immediately adjacent articular cartilage and subchondral bone. Over time, the remaining healthy articular cartilage may be affected, eventually leading to more incongruity and damage.

With increasing force, the depth of the injury may extend beyond the articular cartilage into the subchondral bone, resulting in an osteochondral injury. These injuries, which cross the tidemark, cause hemorrhage and clot formation, thereby activating the inflammatory cascade. This type of injury has many biologic differences from a pure chondral injury. Blood products within the fibrin clot release vasoactive mediators and growth factors or cytokines. These factors may stimulate vascular invasion and migration of undifferentiated cells, which may play an important role in stimulating repair of this injury. The undifferentiated mesenchymal cells that migrate into the chondral portion of the defect produce a repair cartilage that has a combination of types II and I collagen. The cells in the osseous portion of the defect eventually produce immature bone that is gradually replaced by mature bone.

The composition of this repair tissue rarely replicates the structure of the normal articular cartilage and subchondral bone. The subchondral portion of the defect is filled with regions of fibrous tissue and hyaline cartilage. The composition and structure of the chondral repair tissue are intermediate between those of hyaline cartilage and fibrocartilage. The inferior material properties of this repair tissue within the defect make it more susceptible to injury under physiologic loading conditions.

Repair/Regeneration

Numerous methods exist to replace or regenerate articular cartilage. The efficacy of all current techniques is still being evaluated by basic science research and clinical trials. Depending on the location and depth of the lesion (Fig. 2), different techniques may be used. Pure chondral injuries can

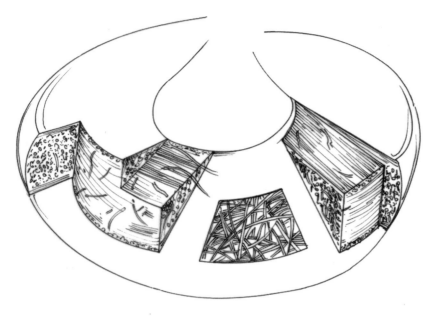

Figure 2

Meniscus showing complex orientation of collagen fibers of the meniscus. (Reproduced with permission from Bullough PG, Munuera L, Murphy J, et al: The strength of the menisci of the knee as it relates to their fine structure. *J Bone Joint Surg* 1970;52B:564–570.)

be treated by either chondral or osteochondral replacement techniques. Osteochondral injuries (traumatic or congenital) require the replacement of both bone and cartilage.

Procedures that penetrate the subchondral bone (abrasion arthroplasty or microfracture technique) are designed to allow bone marrow cells to fill the defect. A clot forms, and these cells have the ability to form fibrocartilage with predominantly type I cartilage. This, however, is different from hyaline cartilage (type II), and the resulting mechanical properties are inferior.

The limited ability of host cells to restore articular surfaces has led investigators to seek methods of transplanting cells that form cartilage into chondral and osteochondral defects. Studies have shown that both chondrocytes and undifferentiated mesenchymal cells placed in articular cartilage defects survive and produce a new cartilage matrix. The use of transplants of autogenous chondrocytes to treat localized cartilage defects of the femoral condyle or the patella has been reported. These early reports suggest that the transplantation of chondrocytes combined with the use of periosteal grafts can promote the restoration of articular surface. More work is needed to assess the function and durability of the new tissue, to determine if it improves joint function and delays or prevents joint degeneration, and to ascertain if this approach will

be beneficial in the treatment of osteoarthritic joints.

Pure chondral defects also can be surgically treated by autograft or allograft osteochondral techniques. The use of osteochondral grafts for articular cartilage defects of the knee is not new. Numerous authors have reported various techniques, but to date no "large" series with even moderate (> 2 years) follow-up has been published. The use of autogenous osteochondral plugs (2.5 to 10 mm in diameter) for condylar and patellar defects has gained much interest. The procedure can be done open, or arthroscopically in the case of smaller lesions (usually < 1.5 cm^2), with commercially available instruments. Much debate continues as to the size of the defect that can be safely treated with this technique. Donor site morbidity has not been defined. A cadaveric study showed that no donor site in the knee is free from contact pressures, but whether or not articular contact at these sites will lead to degenerative changes or any other problems is unknown. Extreme caution is recommended when using this technique for lesions > 2.5 cm^2. For symptomatic lesions of this size allografts should be considered. This technique seems to offer a viable option for osteochondral lesions < 2.5 cm^2 (eg, irreparable osteochondritis dissecans). For pure chondral defects < 2.5 cm^2, it is unclear if autologous osteochondral plugs are superior to procedures that penetrate subchondral bone (eg, abrasion and microfracture). There is no question, however, that the harvesting and transplantation of autologous plugs is more complex and invasive.

Articular cartilage allografts (fresh and fresh frozen) have been used for traumatic and pathologic (tumor, degenerative arthritis) defects since the early part of the century. To date long-term success of these grafts has not been determined. The patients most successfully treated appear to be those with large traumatic femoral osteochondral defects.

Ninety-two fresh osteochondral allografts were used in transplantation procedures in a group of patients with post-traumatic osteochondral defects of the knee joint. Success rates were reported to be 75% at 5 years and 63% at 14 years. In another series, 37 patients with large femoral condylar defects were treated with fresh osteochondral (shell) allografts. Excellent or good results were seen in 8 of the 9 patients followed up at 5 years after surgery.

Many factors affect the fate of allograft and autograft articular cartilage transplants, including depth, size, and location of the lesion; limb alignment; status of meniscal cartilage; and ligament stability. All of these factors must be taken into account in the evaluation and management of articular cartilage defects.

Growth factors influence a variety of cell activities, including proliferation, migration, matrix synthesis, and differentiation. Many have been shown to affect chondrocyte metabolism and chondrogenesis. Bone matrix has been found to contain a variety of these molecules as well. The osteochondral injury and exposure of bone as a result of loss of articular cartilage may release agents that affect the formation of cartilage repair tissue. These agents probably have an important role in the formation of new articular surfaces after currently used surgical procedures, including resection arthroplasty, penetration of subchondral bone, soft-tissue grafts, and possible osteotomy.

The treatment of chondral defects with growth factors or cell transplants requires a method of delivery for the growth factors or cells in the defect. The success, therefore, depends on the use of an artificial matrix. Investigators have reported that implants formed from a variety of biologic and nonbiologic materials may facilitate the restoration of an articular surface. It is difficult at this time to make any comparison between the relative merits of different types of artificial matrixes.

Meniscal Cartilage

Structure and Function

The meniscus is a specialized fibrocartilaginous structure capable of load transmission, shock absorption, stability, articular cartilage nutrition, and proprioception. It is composed of a complex 3-dimensional (3-D) interlacing network of collagen fibers, proteoglycan, glycoproteins, and interspersed cells of fibrochondrocytes that are responsible for synthesis and maintenance of the ECM. The ECM is composed of primarily type I collagen. Most of these fibers are oriented circumferentially to resist tension. The complex 3-D collagen architectural arrangements explain this unique function (Fig. 2). The meniscal cartilage, like articular cartilage, possesses viscoelastic properties. The ECM is a biphasic structure composed of a solid phase (eg, collagen, proteoglycan), which acts as a fiber reinforced porous-permeable composite, and a fluid phase, which may be forced through the solid matrix by a hydraulic pressure gradient. Although these properties are shared with articular cartilage, the meniscus is more elastic and less permeable than articular cartilage.

The outer aspect of each meniscus obtains its blood supply from a circumferentially arranged perimeniscal capillary plexus from the superior and inferior geniculate arteries. This capillary plexus penetrates up to 30% of the medial and up to 25% of the lateral meniscus. A vascular synovial fringe extends 1 to 3 mm over the femoral and tibial surfaces of the peripheral aspect of each meniscus. The inner two thirds of the meniscus is essentially avascular and receives its nutrition from the synovial fluid. Menisci have been found to contain both free nerve endings and corpuscular mechanoreceptors concentrated at the meniscal root insertion sites as well as the periphery. The menisci may act as a source of proprioceptive information for muscular coordination about the extremity.

Kinematic analysis of the knee has demonstrated that the menisci are dynamic structures that move anterior with extension and posterior with flexion. The lateral meniscus is more mobile than the medial, and the anterior portion of the lateral meniscus has the greatest mobility. The relative immobility of the medial meniscus may help explain why there is a higher prevalence of medial meniscal lesions. Menisci, through their shape and structure, provide several very important functions in the knee joint. The shapes of the medial and lateral menisci improve the congruency of the articulating surfaces and increase the surface area of joint contact, thus adding load transmission across the knee joint. The menisci are responsible for transmission of 50% of knee joint force when the knee is in extension, and 88% to 90% of the joint force with knee flexion. Their viscoelastic properties allow their stiffness to increase with higher deformation rates. The medial meniscus also provides a very important secondary restraint to anterior translation of the tibia. This function has not been seen with the lateral meniscus.

With weightbearing, centrifugal radial forces are resisted by the firm attachments of the anterior and posterior horns of the menisci to the tibia. This situation produces large circumferentially oriented hoop tensile stresses, which are countered by the circumferential arrangement of most collagen fibers in the meniscus. Proteoglycans contribute to the compressive properties of the menisci through their ionic repulsive forces, which increase matrix stiffness, and by contributing to the osmotic pressure within the meniscus.

Compressive forces in the knee generate tensile stresses in the meniscus. There are significant regional variations in the tensile strength and stiffness of differing anatomic portions of the menisci that appear to be a result of differences in collagen ultrastructure rather than of biochemical variations. The presence of radial fibers in a particular portion of the meniscus may increase tensile stiffness and strength under radially applied tension.

Meniscal Injury

The detrimental effects of both complete and partial menis-cectomy have been demonstrated in numerous experimental and clinical studies. Loss of the meniscus alters the pattern of load transmission in the knee and results in accelerated artic-ular cartilage degeneration. Experimental studies have shown that higher peak stresses and greater stress concentration in the articular cartilage, decreased shock-absorbing capability, and alterations in the pattern of strain distribution in the proximal tibia occur with meniscal deficiency. In vitro stud-ies demonstrated that removal of 16% to 34% of the posteri-or horn of the medial meniscus may result in a 350% increase in contact forces. The degree of degenerative knee joint changes has been shown to be directly proportional to the amount of meniscus removed. The removal of any meniscal tissue should not be viewed as a benign procedure.

The menisci play an important role in knee stability and proprioception. Individuals who underwent complete meniscectomy before anterior cruciate ligament (ACL) reconstruction reported subjective complaints and activity limitations more commonly than those whose menisci were intact at the time of ACL reconstruction. Significant correla-tions were found with pain, swelling, partial giving way, full giving way, and reduced activity status after surgery.

Meniscal Repair

The importance of blood supply for meniscal healing has been demonstrated. An injury in the vascular zone of the meniscus (outer third) results in the formation of a fibrin clot at the site of injury. This fibrin clot acts as a scaffold for ves-sel ingrowth from the perimeniscal capillary plexus and vas-cular synovial fringe. The lesion may heal by fibrovascular scar tissue in 10 to 12 weeks. The inability of lesions in the avascular portion of the meniscus (inner two thirds) to heal has led to investigation of methods to provide a blood supply to the injured region. These methods include creation of vas-cular access channels, pedicle grafts of synovium placed over the injured meniscus, and abrasion of the synovial fringe to produce a vascular pannus. Study results support the use of an exogenous fibrin clot in meniscal tears in the avascular zone to enhance healing. The clot provides chemotactic and mitogenic factors, such as platelet-derived growth factor and fibronectin, which stimulate the cells involved in wound repair. The clot also provides a scaffold for the support of the reparative response. In the intra-articular environment, a naturally-occurring fibrin clot from surgical bleeding may be rendered ineffective by synovial fluid dilution. An exogenous clot theoretically concentrates the chemotactic and mitogenic factors to overcome this dilution.

Meniscal Replacement

Meniscal regeneration or replacement has been developed in an attempt to interrupt or retard the progressive joint deteri-oration in patients in whom the meniscus has been removed or completely destroyed. Approaches to meniscal replace-ment currently include autograft, bovine collagen implants, and allograft.

Autograft material used has included fascia lata, fat pad, and ligaments that have been rolled into tubes and sewn into the knee joint. All of these tissues have failed to restore the nor-mal properties of the meniscus. Meniscal regeneration using an implanted absorbable copolymeric collagen-based menis-cal scaffold is currently being investigated in clinical trials. Scaffolds are created by reconstituting enzymatically purified collagen from bovine Achilles tendons. Human studies of the collagen meniscal implant have shown that at 2 years after implantation, the defects filled generally represented segmen-tal defects in the middle and posterior aspects of the menis-cus cartilage. These data seem to demonstrate the successful replacement of at least a portion of each meniscus cartilage. Histologically, progressive resorption of the implant material and replacement by collagen fibers in healthy meniscal fibro-chondrocytes appears to occur. Clinically, the patients improved their activity levels and had near-complete relief of pain. How well these regenerated menisci will protect the joint surfaces will be determined with further study. The definitive success of collagen meniscus implants awaits the results of prospective clinical trials that are now being done.

Meniscal Allografts

The use of meniscal allograft tissue continues to receive a great deal of attention in orthopaedics. Allograft menisci, if sized correctly, remain the only way available to replace an entire meniscus. Unfortunately, most meniscal reconstruc-tions have been performed on patients who have either com-plex problems of joint deterioration with meniscal deficien-cy, ligamentous instability, or combinations requiring both ligamentous, osteochondral, and meniscal reconstruction. Determining the outcome of the isolated meniscal recon-struction in these combined cases is difficult. This lack of uniformity between patient selection, surgical technique, and follow-up criteria makes the clinical results between different groups difficult to interpret.

Basic science animal studies as well as clinical studies have shown promising results using fresh frozen allograft menisci for transplantation. However, complete cellular repopulation of the allograft with reconstitution of the normal 3-D colla-gen ultrastructural architecture has yet to be scientifically proven. Although it is clear that the meniscal allograft heals to the peripheral tissue, biopsy specimens have revealed persistent changes within the cellular makeup, cellular content, collagen architecture, and proteoglycan content, raising questions about the long-term viability and the predisposition for further injury.

Ligament

Structure and Function

Optimal joint function depends on the complex interaction around the joint of ligaments as static restraints and muscle-tendon units as dynamic restraints, as well as other factors, including articular geometry. Ligaments are dense connective tissues that link bone to bone. The gross structure varies with the location (ie, intra-articular, capsular, and extra-articular) and function. Geometric variations within different regions of a ligament, such as the anterior and posterior cruciate and inferior glenohumeral ligaments, are frequently observed. Under microscopic examination, the collagen fibers are relatively parallel and aligned along the axis of tension, but they have a more interwoven arrangement than that found in tendon. Characteristic sinusoidal patterns within the bundles, or crimp (Fig. 3), are routinely observed. Two distinct regions within a ligament may also demonstrate different patterns of collagen alignment or crimping, as well as variations in fiber diameters.

Fibroblasts, which are relatively low in number, are responsible for producing and maintaining the extracellular components. Growth factors have been shown to stimulate fibroblast cell division in vitro for both the ACL and medial collateral ligament (MCL). The response varies by the particular growth factor and differs between the two ligaments. Matrix synthesis also is affected, in particular by transforming growth factor-β (TGF-β), as well as epidermal growth factor (EGF) at the higher doses studied. This response appears to be dose-dependent for TGF-β in both ligaments, and for EGF in the ACL. Furthermore, when the responses of cultured explants from ligament and tendon were compared, the ACL was more sensitive to TGF-β, whereas platelet-derived growth factor resulted in a proliferative response in the patellar tendon that was not observed in the ACL. In addition, combinations of growth factors may have a synergistic effect at the cellular level.

The major biochemical component of ligaments is water, about 60% to 80%. Collagen constitutes approximately 70% to 80% of the dry weight, with type I collagen accounting for approximately 90% of the collagen content and type III and others making up the remainder. An important component to the strength characteristics of the collagen fibers is the formation of cross-links. The ground substance includes proteoglycans, which have the capacity to contain water molecules and to affect the viscoelastic properties of soft tissues. The protein elastin assists with the tissue's ability to lengthen under an applied load by storing energy and returning the tissue to its original length when the load is removed. Other noncollagenous proteins are found in very low concentrations.

Structural and mechanical (material) properties have been demonstrated for a variety of ligaments. Differences in these properties have been reported among various ligaments, but also between different regions of the same ligament, including the inferior glenohumeral ligament and posterior cruciate ligament. The structural properties, expressed by the load-elongation curve (Fig. 4, *A*), reflect the behavior of the tissue as a whole, being influenced by its geometry, insertion sites, and material characteristics. The mechanical properties, expressed by the stress-strain curve (Fig. 4, *B*), depend on the ligament substance, molecular bonds, and composition, without influence from the geometry or the insertion sites. Stress is defined as force per unit area, and strain describes the change in length relative to the original length. When a ligament is placed under tension, it deforms in a nonlinear fashion. In the initial stages, or toe region, the coiled nature of the collagen and the crimping are recruited to be more aligned along the axis of tension. Once this is complete, with continued tension, the collagen fibers become taut and then stretch; this is defined as the linear region. The slope of the linear region for the load-elongation curve

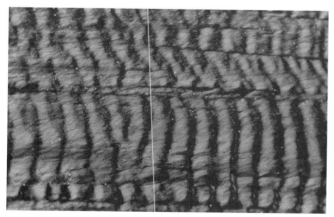

Figure 3

Uniform alignment and crimping of collagen fiber bundles in the anterior axillary pouch of the inferior glenohumeral ligament. (Hematoxylin-eosin, polarized, × 50). (Reproduced with permission from Ticker JB, Bigliani LU, Soslowsky LJ, Pawluk RJ, Flatow EL, Mow VC: Inferior glenohumeral ligament: Geometric and strain-rate dependent properties. *J Shoulder Elbow Surg* 1996;5:269–279.)

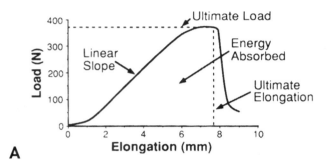

Structural Properties of FMT Complex
(Load-Elongation Curve)

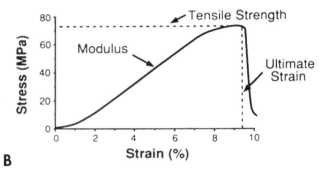

Mechanical Properties of Ligament Substance
(Stress-Strain Curve)

Figure 4

A, Load-elongation curve demonstrating the structural properties of a bone-ligament-bone specimen and B, stress-strain curve demonstrating the mechanical properties of the ligament substance. (Reproduced with permission from Woo SL-Y, Weiss JA, MacKenna DA: Biomechanics and morphology of the medial collateral and anterior cruciate ligaments, in Mow VC, Ratcliffe A, Woo SL-Y (eds): *Biomechanics of Diarthrodial Joints*. New York, NY, Springer-Verlag, 1990, pp 63–104.)

describes the stiffness of the tissue, and the slope of the stress-strain curve denotes the tensile modulus. Overload occurs at the yield point, where tissue failure is observed. The ultimate load and elongation are defined at this point for the structural properties. The ultimate tensile stress and strain are defined at this point for the mechanical properties. These sinusoidal curves demonstrate the nonlinear nature of soft connective tissues. In addition, ligament and tendon biomechanical characteristics demonstrate time-dependent viscoelastic behavior.

The properties of the insertion sites differ from those of the ligament midsubstance, with greater strain found in these areas when tested under uniaxial tension. The failure patterns of bone-ligament-bone complexes change under a variety of circumstances. Age has been shown to be the predominant factor in the rabbit MCL. The skeletally-immature specimens failed at the tibial insertion site, whereas in the mature specimens, failure occurred in the midsubstance. Ligament substance appears to mature earlier than the insertion sites. Strain rate, or rate of elongation, has been shown to affect the failure pattern of both the ACL and the inferior glenohumeral ligament. At higher strain rates, the strength and tensile modulus increased, and failures occurred more in the ligament substance than at the insertion sites, as seen with slower strain rates.

The axis of loading has been shown to affect failure patterns. When the ACL was loaded along the axis of the tibia and not the ligament, the femur-ACL-tibia complex demonstrated decreasing load at failure with increasing flexion angle, and failure was more likely to occur in the ligament substance. Recent investigations with clinical implications have drawn attention to sex differences in the rate of ACL injuries among women and men. It has been theorized that this difference may be a result of the estrogen and progesterone receptors in cells of the ACL. In an animal model, the ACL failure loads were significantly less in an estrogen-treated group. As ligaments age, the structural and material properties change in response to loading conditions. The load at failure of the human ACL from older specimens was 33% to 50% of that found in younger bone-ligament-bone specimens. Reduced properties with aging also have been reported for the anterior portion of the inferior glenohumeral ligament from humans. However, only slight decreases in the structural properties of the MCL bone complexes were noted when skeletally mature specimens were compared with specimens from rabbits at the onset of senescence. Biochemical changes that occur include a decrease in water and collagen content. In addition, there is a change from a higher concentration of the immature, more labile, cross-links to a higher concentration of the mature, more stable, forms. Fibroblasts are less metabolically active with aging and assume a more elongated shape. The effect of growth factors on fibroblast proliferation seems to be diminished with age, and fibroblasts in the ACL appear more sensitive than fibroblasts in the MCL. It would appear that whereas maturation influences the insertion sites of ligaments as demonstrated in the failure patterns, aging and senescence have a detrimental effect on the ligament substance.

Response to Exercise and Loading
Under conditions in which loading is enhanced for a long period of time, the properties of ligaments demonstrate a

modest, yet positive, response. Overall mass increases, and stiffness and load at failure increase. In addition to these changes in structural properties, the material properties are affected with an increase in ultimate stress and strain at failure. Similar changes have been shown in the experimental setting when the MCL in rabbits was placed under increased tension for a sustained period.

Response to Immobilization and Disuse

Immobilization and disuse lead to a much more dramatic effect on ligaments and compromise the structural and material properties. The load at failure decreased by 25% after 4 weeks of immobilization for the cruciate ligaments in rats, although in a rabbit model, only the strain at failure, which increased, was altered significantly. In addition, immobilization in two different knee flexion angles did not cause a difference. The load at failure decreased by 66% after 9 weeks of immobilization for the rabbit MCL, with a corresponding decrease in the stiffness and tensile modulus observed. Thus, changes in both the ligament substance and insertion sites are evident after immobilization. Subperiosteal bone resorption at the insertion sites from increased osteoclastic activity has been observed to affect failure patterns. With even longer periods of immobilization, degradation of collagen increases as collagen synthesis decreases, resulting in less total collagen. A decrease in water and proteoglycan content contributes to an overall decrease in ligament mass. A smaller cross-sectional area was noted in the ACL, and ultrastructural changes in fibroblasts have been observed after immobilization.

The recovery period after immobilization is more rapid in the ligament substance than at the insertion sites. It may take up to 1 year for the insertion sites to return to a level approaching that of controls. However, after 9 weeks of immobilization and 9 weeks of remobilization, the material properties were similar to controls, confirming the more rapid recovery of the ligament substance when motion and loading are permitted.

Response to Injury and Mechanisms of Repair

The MCL in the knee has been studied most extensively after injury. After a rupture in the ligament substance, healing occurs in 3 histologic phases: inflammatory, reparative, and remodeling. After healing is complete, collagen fibrils have a greater diameter and are more densely packed, with an increase in total collagen content. The collagen alignment remains at a less organized level compared with controls. An overall increase in cross-sectional area persists and contributes to the return of the structural properties, which approach normal values. However, after remodeling, the material properties that are not affected by tissue geometry

do not return completely to preinjury levels.

Various factors that influence ligament healing include degree of injury, location of the ligament, and modes of treatment. A more severe injury will result in greater damage to the tissue and a larger gap, prolonging and possibly impairing healing. In the case of the rabbit MCL, injuries near the insertions heal more slowly. Associated injury to the ACL has an unfavorable effect compared with an isolated MCL injury. Reconstruction of the ACL may counteract this effect. In addition, 1 year after reconstruction of the ACL, MCL repair was not necessary for successful healing. Controlled passive motion leads to a more rapid repair and enhances the collagen alignment and the biomechanical properties of the healing MCL. Immobilization after injury has the opposite effect.

The MCL has an intrinsic healing response not observed in the ACL, and this difference may be the result of a number of biologic factors. Intra-articular ligaments, such as the cruciates, have a limited blood supply and are in an environment that does not promote the initial phase of healing, unlike the extra-articular and possibly intracapsular ligaments. Fibroblast adhesion and migration appears to be different between the MCL and ACL in an inflammatory environment. Growth factors have been detected at the site of ligament injury and have been shown to enhance tissue healing. Recent investigations have studied their effects in the early healing phase. Platelet-derived growth factor (PDGF) and TGF-β are increased in healing MCL, whereas the opposite is found in healing ACL in an animal model. The healing response in MCL also is affected by PDGF, which enhances the structural properties. The timing when growth factors are administered and their doses also have been shown to influence healing. In a study of PDGF in a healing rat MCL, early administration of this factor, less than 24 hours after injury, was most effective. In addition, a plateau effect was noted with the increasing doses used. Others have reported that much higher doses of growth factors studied in vitro may, in fact, be detrimental to the material properties. As the effect of growth factors and other cytokines is further studied, their role in normal development and healing for both intra- and extra-articular ligaments, as well as after ligament reconstruction, will be further defined with possible clinical applications delineated.

Grafts for Reconstruction

Ligament reconstruction using a graft substitute, particularly of the anterior and posterior cruciate ligaments, is performed to restore joint stability. Choices for autografts include patellar tendon, semitendinosus and gracilis tendons, quadriceps tendon, fascia lata, and iliotibial band. The central third of the patellar tendon is a commonly used graft, and early studies using a 14-mm wide graft demonstrated a higher load at failure than the ACL itself, while other grafts had lower failure loads. More recent studies have shown that the patellar tendon had greater stiffness, and, therefore, greater structural properties that are affected by size, compared with hamstring tendons. However, the hamstring tendons had higher tensile modulus, or higher material properties, compared with patellar tendon. These findings suggest that a larger size for the hamstring grafts, such as a quadrupled graft that would improve its structural properties, offers a good alternative autograft for ACL reconstruction when compared with the patellar tendon autograft. However, a hamstring graft with 4 bundles does not necessarily offer a construct that is 4 times as strong as a single tendon. Furthermore, after implantation, no graft substitute has ever demonstrated biomechanical properties near to that of the ACL when studied as long as 3 years after reconstruction. In addition, neither the patellar tendon graft nor the hamstring graft used for reconstruction fully restores the kinematics of the intact knee.

Graft incorporation involves an initial phase of ischemic necrosis, followed by revascularization. Remodeling and maturation include a transition of cellularity, distribution of collagen types, fiber size and alignment, and biochemical characteristics that are more ligament-like. This process appears to be affected by the initial tension placed on the graft. In addition, different levels of growth factors have been detected in early remodeling, suggesting a role in this process. The insertion sites and incorporation have been studied for patellar tendon and hamstring grafts, both with and without detachment of the tibial insertion. Initial failure after replacement surgery is at the fixation sites. As these attachments heal, either bone-to-bone or tendon-to-bone failure is more likely to occur within the graft substance. Tibial fixation closer to the anatomic origin of the ACL, investigated using robotic testing, improved initial stability. Allograft tissue, particularly in the settings of multiple ligament injuries and revision ligament surgery of the knee, offers a reliable alternative. Final allograft incorporation in ACL surgery is similar to that seen in autografts, but occurs at a slower rate, with inferior properties found at 6 months compared with autografts in the animal model.

Response of Collagenous Tissue to Thermal Energy

Whereas laser and other electrosurgical devices usually have been used to incise and ablate soft tissues, these instruments have more recently been used to deliver thermal energy to selectively shrink capsular tissue during arthroscopic procedures, in particular in the glenohumeral joint. Experimental and clinical evidence has demonstrated that collagenous tissues can be shortened after the application of thermal energy, but the amount of shortening reported has been variable. Studies designed to assess the temperature level necessary to cause shortening of collagen using heated fluid baths at controlled levels demonstrated more dramatic effects at 65°C and above. A threshold to shrinkage of 60°C after 3 to 5 minutes' duration in the fluid bath was noted in one study. As temperatures increased, the shrinkage was greater and occurred more rapidly, along the dominant alignment of the collagen fibers. Furthermore, with increasing temperatures, greater alteration in the collagen structure was noted histologically. At temperatures above 80°C, collagen tissue was grossly observed to fall apart in one study, whereas others reported an amorphous histologic appearance of the collagen, with loss of fibrillar structure, at 80°C.

In vitro animal studies with increasing laser energy using the holmium:yttrium-aluminum-garnet (Ho:YAG) laser on capsular and tendinous tissue lead to increasing tissue shrinkage, up to 45% to 50% in some studies, but also decreased stiffness at higher energy levels. Ultimate failure loads were decreased, with tissue failure occurring in the region of the lased tissue. A clear change in the collagen fiber structure has been observed histologically, with denaturation of the tissue and increasing size of the area affected as increasing energy was used. The biomechanical properties of human inferior glenohumeral ligament-bone complexes were studied after laser application to shorten the tissue 10%. Although no difference was found for ultimate stress or elastic modulus between lased and nonlased specimens, the ultimate strain was higher and the energy absorbed during cyclic loading was lower in the laser-treated specimens. Tissue failure was not observed through the laser-treated region.

In vivo studies in rabbit patellar tendon treated with the Ho:YAG laser demonstrated tissue shortening initially, with localized, although severe, changes in the collagen found on histology. However, after 8 weeks of unrestricted activity, the tissue was lengthened (Fig. 5) compared with the controls, and stiffness decreased despite an increase in cross-sectional area after the laser procedure. In addition, a more generalized fibroblastic response throughout the entire tissue was noted, with small diameter collagen fibers replacing the normal distribution of both large and small fibers. Others have noted thickened synovium, with inflammation, tissue necrosis, and decreased cellularity in the glenohumeral capsular tissue in dogs at 6 weeks after a laser procedure. Because of the amount of tissue alteration reported as well as observations of tissue lengthening and altered biomechanical properties in animal and human studies, these factors must be carefully considered and further studied before general application of procedures using thermal energy to shrink capsular tissue is

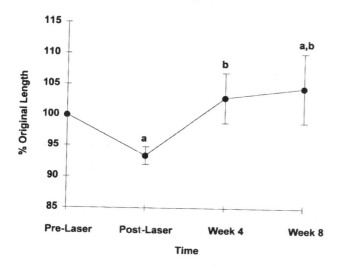

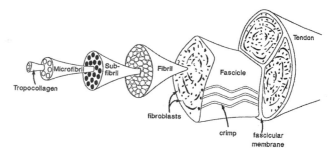

Figure 6

Schematic representation of the microarchitecture of a tendon. (Adapted with permission from Kastelic J, Baer E: Deformation in tendon collagen, in Vincent JFV, Currey JD (eds): *The Mechanical Properties of Biologic Materials.* Cambridge, Cambridge University Press, 1980, pp 397–435.)

Figure 5

Length changes following laser treatment of rabbit patellar tendon demonstrating initial shrinkage with subsequent elongation, after unrestricted activity (a = significantly different from prelaser, b = significantly different from postlaser). (Adapted with permission from Schaefer SL, Ciarelli MJ, Arnoczky SP, Ross HE: Tissue shrinkage using a holmium:yttrium aluminum garnet laser: A postoperative assessment of tissue length, stiffness, and structure. *Am J Sports Med* 1997;25:841–848.)

attempted in a clinical setting. To date, the difference between the use of laser and other electrosurgical devices to effectively shrink collagenous tissue has not been defined.

Tendon

Structure and Function

Tendons are dense, primarily collagenous tissues that link muscle to bone. As a highly specialized tissue with parallel-oriented bundles of collagen, the tendon's primary function is to transmit the load generated by muscle to bone. Synovial sheaths surround some tendons, such as flexor tendons of the hand, to facilitate excursion and gliding. Histology reveals crimping and low cellular density in addition to the highly uniform, parallel alignment of the fibers (Fig. 6). Collagen content of the dry weight is slightly greater than that found in ligaments and is predominantly type I, approximately 95%. Type III collagen, which is a more immature form and often found in greater concentrations in healing tissue, constitutes approximately 5% of the total collagen content.

Proteoglycans have a very small concentration in tendons, but serve to support the structure and function of collagenous tissues. Regions of tendons that are subjected to compressive loads are more fibrocartilaginous and have a higher glycosaminoglycan, aggrecan, and biglycan content, which approaches that found in articular cartilage. A lower glycosaminoglycan content is associated with smaller proteoglycans, including decorin, in tendons undergoing primarily tensile loads. Cyclic compressive loading of tendon has been shown to stimulate production of aggrecan and biglycan, and this appears to be further enhanced by TGF-β. Removal of compression in a zone of fibrocartilaginous tendon in an in vivo animal model results in a decrease in glycosaminoglycan content, cellular density, cross-sectional area, and compressive stiffness.

The organization and composition of tendon make it ideally suited to resist high tensile forces. Tendons deform less than ligaments under an applied load and are able to transmit the load from muscle to bone. It has been demonstrated that under tension the fibrocartilaginous zone of tendon, which experiences both tensile and compressive forces, has decreased material properties compared with regions of tendon primarily exposed to tensile forces. However, the greater cross-sectional area observed in the fibrocartilaginous zone may represent a response by the tissue to enhance its structural properties under tension. Structural and degenerative changes as a result of aging have been reported. The overall diameter of the Achilles tendon decreases. The mean collagen fibril diameter decreases with increasing age, as do total cell count and the amount of crimp. A decrease in the endoplasmic reticulum within the fibroblast suggests diminished cellular metabolic activity. The biochemical composition changes with an increase in collagen content and amount of cross-links and a decrease in glycosaminoglycans. Biomechanically, an increase in stress at failure and in stiffness during maturation and then a decrease with senescence has been noted. The effects of decreased activity, or relative disuse, play a role in the changes seen with aging tendon.

Response to Exercise and Loading

Controlled increases in training appear to have differential effects on tendons. The biomechanical properties of swine flexor tendons did not change after exercise, although a beneficial effect was noted at the bony insertion sites. However, swine extensor tendons subjected to a long-term exercise regimen responded by developing increased cross-sectional area and tensile strength. This suggests that extensor tendons have the capacity to respond to a training regimen, whereas flexor tendons function on a regular basis at their peak. Investigators have reported an increase in the number and density of smaller diameter fibrils in response to exercise. Although further investigations are warranted, it may be that the muscle and the tendon-bone insertion sites have a greater capability to adapt to an environment of sustained increases in loading than the tendon itself.

Response to Immobilization and Disuse

Restriction of motion to protect injured tissue or aid in the repair process can affect tendons. Without stress as a stimulus, both the midsubstance of tendons and the insertion sites appear to be affected, demonstrating diminished biomechanical properties. After immobilization, stiffness decreases within the tendon. Presumably, other biomechanical as well as biochemical and histologic changes occur, but these have yet to be demonstrated specifically for tendon. Whether or not such changes are reversible also is unknown.

Response to Injury and Mechanisms of Repair

Injury or damage to tendons can result from 1 of 3 mechanisms: (1) transection within the substance (direct injury), (2) avulsion from bone at the insertion (indirect injury), or (3) intrasubstance damage from intrinsic or extrinsic factors and subsequent failure (Fig. 7). Transections or partial lacerations are associated with trauma and are most common in the flexor tendons of the hand. Bone avulsions can occur after overwhelming tensile loads, as seen in the flexor digitorum profundus insertion into the base of the distal phalanx of the ring finger. Degenerative changes within tendon can arise from repetitive tensile loading during the life of an individual; however, impingement of tendon by a rigid surface, such as with the rotator cuff beneath the acromion, is an important factor leading to tendon failure. At the point where the tendon is overloaded, individual fibers can fail, with the load transferred to adjacent collagen fibers. Continued loading will lead to further failure until the applied force ceases or the tendon ruptures. If the injury is incomplete and the healing

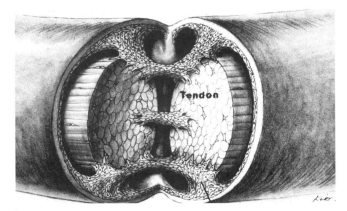

Figure 7

Drawing of an immobilized tendon illustrating extrinsic and intrinsic repair. (Courtesy of Richard H. Gelberman, MD, Boston, MA.)

process is interrupted, episodes of microtrauma will result in a weakened tendon structure. Repetitive microtrauma to the tissue is seen in overuse injuries. The bone-tendon junction also may be involved in the injury process.

Tendon healing after an acute injury follows similar phases to other soft-tissue healing. The inflammatory response provides an extrinsic source for cellular invasion to begin the repair process. For injury to avascular tendons within a synovial sheath (eg, flexor tendons of the hand), an intrinsic mechanism for tendon healing has been proposed that appears to be modulated by the stress of passive motion, thereby questioning the role of the extrinsic inflammatory response. Cells from within the tendon proliferate at the wound site along with increased vascularity leading to collagen synthesis and further tissue maturation with time. Although evidence for both intrinsic and extrinsic mechanisms of healing has been supported, other factors may determine which is the primary mechanism for healing, such as the local environment, vascularity, or stress.

In the initial phase of healing after tendon repair, the tensile strength is significantly less than for controls. At 3 weeks, the tensile strength increases more progressively. Controlled passive motion has been shown to decrease adhesions, lead to a stronger repair, and accelerate gains in tensile strength. Collagen reorganization and alignment, as well as maturation, appear to benefit from controlled application of stress. In vitro experiments using cyclic tension have demonstrated an enhanced intrinsic response, with proliferation and migration of fibroblasts in the line of tension and increased collagen synthesis, resulting in a thickened epitenon. In vivo experiments on partial flexor tendon lacerations support the role of tension, in addition to motion, which leads to increased tensile strength as well as increased cellular activity in the epitenon and well-developed collagen fiber formation by 4 weeks. With improved suture techniques for flexor tendon repairs, such as a 6-strand repair and modified epitendinous suturing, early active motion may now be possible while avoiding gap formation at the suture repair site. Such advances also may have a positive effect on the biomechanical characteristics and adhesion formation without significantly increasing resistance to gliding. Understanding of the role of growth factors and cytokines in connective tissue healing is evolving. In animal models of tendon transection, PDGF, produced at the site of tendon injury as a result gene therapy, and insulin-like growth factor I, introduced directly into the site of tendon injury, have been shown to enhance the healing process.

Rotator Cuff Tendons

Several aspects of the anatomy and biology of the tendons of the rotator cuff suggest that they have slightly different properties than other tendons, such as the flexor tendons. The supraspinatus, infraspinatus, teres minor, and subscapularis tendons do not have separate insertions, but rather interdigitate with the adjacent tendon to form a continuous insertion on the greater and lesser tuberosities of the humerus. Particularly in the supraspinatus and infraspinatus, a complex, 5-layered structure has been observed, composed of tendon fibers, loose connective tissue, and capsule, as well as the coracohumeral ligament in the anterior portion of the supraspinatus. The varied orientation of the tendinous fibers and the interwoven fiber patterns observed suggest an important role in the mechanical response to an applied load, but also may account for pathologic conditions, such as intratendinous tears. In addition, this normal anatomy of the tendon insertion does not appear to be altered by increasing age, although tendon degeneration may occur.

The biomechanics of the rotator cuff tendons has not been as well studied as that of other tendons, in part because of its more complex structure. However, variations in geometry and mechanical properties have been observed within the supraspinatus tendon, with its posterior third noted to be thinner and the anterior third found to be mechanically stronger than the middle or posterior portions. In addition, mechanical testing of the articular and bursal sides of the supraspinatus tendon suggests that the articular side may be at greater risk for failure under tension.

Other characteristics unique to rotator cuff tendons include the presence of the coracoacromial arch and the variation of acromial morphology. The observation of greater amounts of glycosaminoglycans and the proteoglycans, aggrecan and biglycan, are associated with the more fibrocartilaginous tissue found in areas of tendon undergoing compressive loads compared with tendon undergoing tensile loads. The function of these proteoglycans in tendon was thought to be analogous to their function in articular cartilage, to resist compression. Increased glycosaminoglycan content and proteoglycans also have been noted in the rotator cuff tendons, as well as variations in proteoglycan gene expression between different portions of the rotator cuff tendon. Although the presence of proteoglycans in the rotator cuff may indicate a pathologic response to compression, such as that proposed by the impingement theory, their distribution found within the tendon substance may be a normal adaptive response to its structure and function. In addition, it would appear that rotator cuff pathology results not only from extrinsic causes, such as impingement beneath the coracoacromial arch, but may result in part from intrinsic causes, including tensile overload and degeneration, or a combination of processes. This has recently been investigated using in vivo animal models. The reported hypovascularity of the supraspinatus tendon also may be involved in the pathologic process; however, its role is now less clear. More recently, attention has been drawn to the potential for injury to the articular surface of the rotator cuff tendon from repetitive compression on the posterior superior glenoid rim.

The potential for healing in the unrepaired rotator cuff tendon appears to be limited, despite evidence of granulation tissue formation at the tendon edge and a vascular response. Tendon has been shown to heal well to bone, and in the repaired rotator cuff tendon studied in an animal model, there appears to be no advantage in the healing process to repairing the tendon edge to a cancellous trough because similar properties were noted with rotator cuff tendon healing to cortical bone. Biomechanical testing has demonstrated that the strength of a suture repair through transosseous tunnels is enhanced by using a braided suture material in a locking fashion, such as the modified Mason-Allen technique, and it would seem preferable to use a nonabsorbable material to maintain its properties during the healing process. In a transosseous repair, having a cortical bone bridge of 1 cm rather than 0.5 cm located 2 cm from the tip of the greater tuberosity is advantageous because there is thicker cortical bone in this more distal location.

Muscle

Structure and Function

Skeletal muscle originates from bone and adjacent connective tissue surfaces and inserts into bone via tendon. The myotendinous junction is a highly specialized region for load transmission, with an increased surface area from membrane infolding. When the muscle fiber shortens, it is referred to as a concentric contraction. In an eccentric contraction, the muscle generates a force greater in magnitude than a concentric contraction, while the muscle fiber lengthens. An important effect of an eccentric contraction is deceleration of the portion of the limb the muscle acts upon, while acceleration occurs from a concentric contraction.

The characteristics of the muscle contraction depend on the muscle fiber types. Most muscles in the body comprise equal amounts of 2 types of fibers, type I and type II (Table 1). Type I, or slow-twitch oxidative fibers, predominate in postural muscles and are well suited for endurance by an aerobic metabolism, an ability to sustain tension, and relative fatigue resistance, with higher amounts of mitochondria and myoglobin. In addition to the slow rate of contraction, slow oxidative muscle fibers also have a relatively low strength of contraction. On the other hand, type II fibers, or fast-twitch fibers, have a fast rate of contraction with a relatively high strength of contraction. The type IIB, or fast-twitch glycolytic fibers, are more common in muscles that rapidly generate power but have a greater dependence on anaerobic metabolism and are less capable of sustaining activity for prolonged periods due to buildup of lactic acid. The characteristics and composition of the type IIA, or fast-twitch oxidative glycolytic fibers, which have aerobic capacity, are intermediate between type I and type IIB.

Like other tissues in the body, skeletal muscle undergoes changes with aging. Muscle mass decreases slowly between 25 and 50 years of age. From this point, the rate of muscle atrophy increases, but the loss of muscle size and strength can be diminished with strength training. With aging, the total number of muscle fibers decreases and muscle stiffness increases, which may be related to the increase in collagen content seen with aging. Furthermore, muscle fiber diameter decreases with aging, primarily in type II fibers. These effects also may be the result, in part, of decreased activity and mobility with increasing age.

Response to Exercise and Loading

Training and exercise can stimulate alterations in skeletal muscle if the activity is sustained and there is sufficient load. Under an appropriate program of exercise and loading, muscle can increase its functional capacity to respond. For example, "low tension, high repetition" training of a relatively long duration results in greater endurance, which is to the advantage of the long-distance runner. An increase in capillary density and mitochondria concentration is associated with

Table 1
Characteristics of human skeletal muscle fiber types

	Type I	Type IIA	Type IIB
Other names	Red, slow twitch (ST) Slow oxidative (SO)	White, fast twitch (FT) Fast oxidative glycolytic (FOG)	Fast glycolytic (FG)
Speed of contraction	Slow	Fast	Fast
Strength of contraction	Low	High	High
Fatigability	Fatigue-resistant	Fatigable	Most fatigable
Aerobic capacity	High	Medium	Low
Anaerobic capacity	Low	Medium	High
Motor unit size	Small	Larger	Largest
Capillary density	High	High	Low

(Reproduced with permission from Garrett WE Jr, Best TM: Anatomy, physiology, and mechanics of skeletal muscle, in Simon SR (ed): *Orthopaedic Basic Science*. Rosemont, IL, American Academy of Orthopaedic Surgeons, 1994, pp 89–125.)

greater capability for oxidative metabolism, primarily affecting type I, slow-oxidative fibers. Furthermore, resistance to fatigue is increased by these adaptations (Fig. 8). Muscle flexibility can be enhanced by warming or stretching of muscles. Conversely, application of cold to a muscle group will decrease its flexibility. Together, heat and stretching have a combined beneficial effect on muscle flexibility. In addition, the risk for muscle strain injury appears to be diminished by these factors.

"High tension, low repetition" training emphasizes development of greater muscle strength and power. When loads are progressively increased, muscle size increases, mostly from muscle hypertrophy of primarily type II fibers. This mode of training benefits the sprinter, who requires short and powerful bursts of speed to achieve higher performance. Unlike endurance training, which can be performed more frequently, strength training requires a period of rest or recovery for the muscle tissue and should not be performed daily. Under this regimen, anaerobic metabolism is maximized and tissue injury avoided.

Response to Immobilization and Disuse

When stimulation to the muscle fibers is withdrawn, the adaptations in skeletal muscle can be reversed. If muscles are further unloaded, either by disuse or immobilization, the effect on skeletal muscle is magnified. Loss of endurance and strength is observed in the muscle groups affected. As muscle atrophies, changes are observed at both the macro- and microstructural levels, with decreasing fiber size and number, as well as changes in the sarcomere length-tension relationship. Changes at the cellular and biochemical level occur, and these may affect the aerobic and anaerobic pathways of energy production.

Immobilization of muscle in a lengthened position has a less deleterious affect. This is a result of the relatively greater tension that is placed on these muscle fibers and their physiologic response to the load, compared with muscles immobilized in a shortened position. In addition to the effects on muscle, immobilization has an effect on the bone and motor end plates. With remobilization after a similar period of immobilization (4 weeks), the detrimental changes in muscle cross-sectional area and receptors in the motor end plate can be reversed, but the bone density is not completely restored. In an animal model of remobilization after immobilization, growth hormone stimulation as measured by levels of insulin-like growth factor (IGF-1) resulted in greater return of muscle size and strength during the period of remobilization compared with controls.

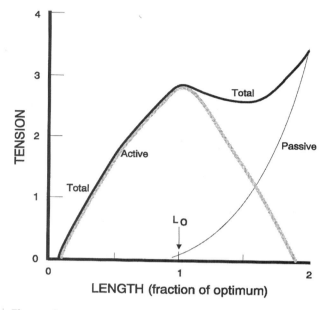

Figure 8

Representative isometric tension-length curve of skeletal muscle. (Reproduced with permission from Garrett WE Jr, Best TM: Anatomy, physiology, and mechanics of skeletal muscle, in Simon SR (ed): *Orthopaedic Basic Science*. Rosemont, IL, American Academy of Orthopaedic Surgeons, 1994, pp 89–125.)

Response to Injury and Mechanisms of Repair

Muscle injury can result from an indirect overload that overwhelms the muscle's ability to respond normally or a direct injury, such as a contusion or laceration. The indirect mechanism of injury includes muscle strains and delayed-onset muscle soreness. Injury from muscle strains in which muscles are unable to accommodate the stretch during eccentric contractions is commonly reported in sports activity. Muscles that function across 2 or more joints, such as the hamstrings, are at greater risk for strain injury. In addition, fatigue has been associated with increased rates of strain injury when muscle has a diminished ability to perform and act as an energy or "shock" absorber. Fatigued muscles have been shown to absorb less energy than muscles that are not fatigued.

The spectrum of muscle strain injury can range from microscopic damage or partial tears to complete tears and disruption with a palpable defect within the muscle. The degree of injury from a tensile overload will dictate the potential of the host response and the time course for repair. The status of muscle contraction at the time of overload usually is eccentric, and failure most often occurs at or near the myotendinous junction unless there is previous injury to the muscle. Although muscle strain injury may predominantly affect fast glycolytic fibers, this does not appear to be the result of the low oxidative capacity of these fibers.

After muscle injury, healing is initiated in the inflammatory phase. The repair process includes fibroblast proliferation and collagen production leading to scar formation, with muscle regeneration resulting from myoblasts stemming from satellite cells. Both of these processes occur at the same time; however, motion during healing has been shown to limit scar size. It also has been demonstrated that muscles in the process of healing are at an increased risk for reinjury, suggesting that return to strenuous activity should be delayed until satisfactory healing has taken place. The role of growth hormones in the healing process is evolving. Nonsteroidal anti-inflammatory medications may enhance recovery initially, as shown in an animal model, up to 7 days after muscle injury. However, these medications have a deleterious effect on the functional recovery of muscle when studied at 28 days, possibly because the inflammatory response is suppressed.

Delayed-onset muscle soreness (within 24 to 72 hours) is another form of indirect injury to the muscle. However, this occurs within the muscle fibers as a result of intense training or exercise to which the muscle is unaccustomed. The cellular and microstructural changes that occur and the weakness that is present are reversible. Muscle contusions result from a direct blow, usually to the muscle belly. The degree of hematoma formation, subsequent inflammation, and delay in healing is directly proportional to the compressive force absorbed, and it will also affect the amount of scar formation and muscle regeneration. However, when muscle is contracted, it is less vulnerable to this type of injury. A more rapid recovery is observed under conditions that promote increased vascularity, as seen in limbs that undergo early motion, and, possibly, in a younger age group. Heterotopic bone, or myositis ossificans, is not an infrequent finding after a more severe contusion injury, but this finding should not be treated surgically until healing is complete and the resulting bone is fully matured. Repair and recovery after muscle laceration depends on regeneration across the site and reinnervation. Muscle distal to the site of injury that regenerates but is incompletely reinnervated has diminished function.

The use of a tourniquet during arthroscopic knee procedures and its effect on thigh musculature have been investigated. When applied for an average duration of less than 50 minutes, it did not affect quadriceps or hamstring recovery at 4 weeks when compared with procedures performed without a tourniquet. Tourniquet pressure in this study was determined from thigh circumference and systolic blood pressure. The effect of tourniquet use was also studied after arthroscopic ACL reconstructions averaging 87 minutes, with the tourniquet set to 150 mm Hg over systolic blood pressure. At 1 month, diminished thigh girth and a greater incidence of abnormal electromyographic studies were suggested but not shown statistically. At 6 and 12 months postoperatively, all muscle parameters studied were similar in the groups treated with and without a tourniquet. In another study, an animal model had a greater loss from direct compression on the underlying tissue than from muscle ischemia distal to the tourniquet when studied 2 days later. It would appear that tourniquet use, as studied thus far, does not have any harmful effects on muscle functional recovery in the clinical setting.

Nerve

Structure and Function

The nerve cell body gives rise to a single axon, the extension that conveys the signal of information as a graded or action potential within the peripheral nervous system. A sensory axon carries this signal as an electrical impulse from the periphery to its cell body in the dorsal root ganglion (afferent), whereas a motor axon carries information from the cell body in the anterior horn in the spinal cord (efferent) to the end organ. Cell bodies in the autonomic nervous system are in paravertebral ganglia. Although all axons have a surrounding Schwann cell, an axon that is insulated with a myelin sheath from many Schwann cells aligned longitudinally has a higher conduction velocity than an unmyelinated axon. This rate is further enhanced by a small interruption in the myelin sheath called the node of Ranvier (Fig. 9).

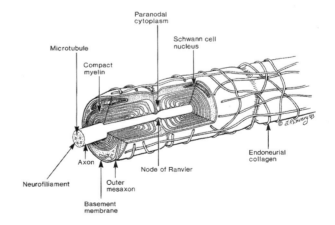

Figure 9

The Schwann cell tube and its contents. (Reproduced with permission from Brushart TM: Peripheral nerve biology, in Manske PR (ed): *Hand Surgery Update.* Englewood, CO, American Society for Surgery of the Hand, 1994, pp 1–14.)

Materials, such as proteins, that support the structure and function of the axon are produced within the cell body and travel along the axon via slow and fast antegrade transport systems. Materials, including waste products, return to the cell body via a fast retrograde transport system. The rate of transport is diminished with decreasing temperature; transport stops at 11°C as well as after a period of anoxia.

The ultrastructure of a peripheral nerve begins with the axon and myelin sheath, which make up the nerve fiber, and is enclosed within a basement membrane and connective tissue layer, the endoneurium (Fig. 10). These fibers are grouped into a bundle called a fascicle, which is surrounded by the perineurium. The perineurium serves as a barrier to diffusion of fluid. A variable number of fascicles together form the peripheral nerve. The peripheral nerve is enclosed by the outer epineurium, which has an interstitial or inner component between the fascicles to protect and support the nerve. Intra- and interfascicular connections are typical. Blood vessels travel within the epineurium and have a system of branches around and within the fascicles, extending to capillaries at the endoneurium. Peripheral nerves demonstrate viscoelastic properties typical of other connective tissues; however, low levels of strain can lead to alterations in peripheral nerve conduction. Strain around 12% can result in permanent changes, including impairment of blood flow, which may result in further changes in conduction.

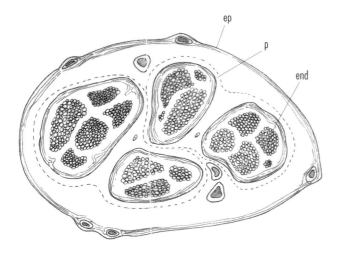

Figure 10

Schema of peripheral nerve trunk shows epineurium (ep), perineurium (p), and endoneurium (end). (Reproduced with permission from Lundborg G, Rydevik B, Manthorpe M, Varon S, Lewis J: Peripheral nerve: The physiology of injury and repair, in Woo SL-Y, Buckwalter JA (eds): *Injury and Repair of the Musculoskeletal Soft Tissues.* Park Ridge, IL, American Academy of Orthopaedic Surgeons, 1988, pp 297–352.)

Injury, Degeneration, and Regeneration

Different types of injury patterns occur after traumatic insult to a peripheral nerve. First-degree injury, or neurapraxia, involves loss of conduction across the injured segment of nerve without wallerian degeneration or degradation. Because the axon is not disrupted, recovery is complete. A second-degree injury, or axonotmesis, is damaging because the axon is disrupted. The remaining axon distal to the site of injury and a small portion of the proximal axon degenerate. The Schwann cell layer, termed the endoneurial sheath, remains intact and serves to guide the regenerating axon during recovery.

Neurotmesis is more severe because the nerve itself is disrupted. In a third-degree injury, the structures within the perineurium, the nerve fibers of the fascicle, are damaged. Because the endoneurial tubes are disrupted, regeneration occurs in a disorderly fashion. A nerve with fibers that serve a similar function and a distally located nerve injury have a more favorable prognosis. The interfascicular structure is lost, but the outer epineurium remains intact in a fourth-degree injury. The chances for an effective regeneration process are minimal; surgery usually is indicated. The most severe damage occurs in a fifth-degree injury. The nerve is completely disrupted and scar is likely to form between the severed ends; surgical repair is necessary for recovery.

The process of wallerian degeneration begins immediately after transection of a nerve fiber. A neuron is more likely to survive when the injury is further distal, away from the cell body. The neuron appears to change from its usual functions to removal of cellular debris and production of the proteins necessary for regeneration. Within hours, changes are noted in the cell body, and the process of regeneration begins as growth cones project from the proximal stump of the axon and the nearest intact node of Ranvier. Schwann cells that accompany axonal growth (bands of Bungner) guide the process of regeneration and synthesize nerve growth factor, but also are the limiting factor to the rate of growth. The zone of injury must be crossed and contact made with the endoneurial tubes of the distal stump for regeneration to proceed. Greater damage, further distance, and increased scar in this zone have an adverse effect. Surgical repair counteracts these problems. Following nerve repair, regeneration occurs at an average rate of 1 mm/day in humans and is faster and better in children. Reinnervation to a muscle is more time-dependent than reinnervation to a sensory end organ.

Several factors applied locally or systemically enhance regeneration; these factors include hormones, proteins, and growth factors. Insulin-like growth factor (IGF), which is present in regenerating nerves and nerve targets, has neurotropic activity. Anti-IGF serum causes a sustained decrease in the rate of axon regeneration. Systemic administration of IGF has shown a small but significant improvement in regeneration after a nerve crush injury. Acidic fibroblast growth factor enhances regeneration distances when administered locally or systemically. Direct current electrical fields and hyperbaric oxygen also promote regeneration. In an animal study, collection of axoplasmic fluid and its reinjection proximal and distal to the repair site resulted in increased axon count and better return of limb function compared with controls. Local environmental factors also can influence axonal growth and direction.

Nerve Repair

Peripheral nerve repair is used to reestablish continuity of the nerve; results are best when repair is done tension-free soon after nerve transection. A primary repair is preferable to the alternative techniques of nerve grafting but repair under tension requires the latter. Mobilization of the nerve stump and tension should be limited because diminished perfusion and ischemia can result. Primary repair is less likely in more severe trauma, such as crush injuries in which a larger amount of damaged tissue at the ends of the 2 stumps requires resection before nerve repair. Younger patients and more distal locations of injury have better prognoses.

Of the 2 types of nerve repair, a fascicular suture repair, theoretically, has a better chance to correctly restore nerve function than does an epineurial suture. However, the only prospective comparison of fascicular and epineurial digital nerve repairs in humans showed no difference between the 2 groups. Regardless of the technique used for nerve repair, an atraumatic technique under magnification and without tension is beneficial. Fascicular repair necessitates identification of matching fascicles of the proximal and distal stumps, which provides improved alignment, although greater scarring can result from the intraneural dissection. In addition to direct observations, intraoperative awake stimulation and staining techniques aid with alignment of the fascicles. When fascicular matching is not possible, based on the internal topography of the peripheral nerve at the level of transection, epineurial suture repair is preferable.

Nerve Grafting

Nerve injuries with gaps that are not reparable or would result in undue tension after repair are considered for nerve grafting. The standard for management of these problems is an autogenous graft; the most common sources are the sural nerve or medial and lateral antebrachial cutaneous nerves. The proximal-to-distal direction is reversed when a graft is placed in the bed between the 2 stumps. When possible, fascicular groups from stumps on both sides are matched. A sin-

gle segment typically is used for grafting smaller nerves, whereas a few segments of graft may be used with larger nerves. Alternatives include conduits, such as a vein or synthetic tube, and allografts, which avoid donor-site nerve loss and morbidity. The best results occur in younger individuals. Shorter grafts in more distal locations have greater recovery. Tension at the graft repair site must be avoided.

Annotated Bibliography

General Reference

Simon SR (ed): *Orthopaedic Basic Science*. Rosemont, IL, American Academy of Orthopaedic Surgeons, 1994.

This text offers the most comprehensive review for basic science of soft tissues, as well as the entire neuromusculoskeletal system.

Articular Cartilage

Breinan HA, Minas T, Hsu HP, Nehrer S, Sledge CB, Spector M: Effect of cultured autologous chondrocytes on repair of chondral defects in a canine model. *J Bone Joint Surg* 1997;79A: 1439–1451.

Using a canine model, the authors studied 3 treatment groups of cartilage repair (12 to 18 months follow-up): cultured autologous chondrocytes implanted under subperiosteal flap, periosteal flap without chondrocytes, chondral defect without either. They could detect no significant difference among the 3 groups.

Brittberg M, Lindahl A, Nilsson A, Ohlsson C, Isaksson O, Peterson L: Treatment of deep cartilage defects in the knee with autologous chondrocyte transplantation. *N Engl J Med* 1994;331:889–895.

Two-year clinical results of patients undergoing chondrocyte transplantation combined with a periosteal flap are presented. Fourteen of 16 patients with femoral condyle defects had good to excellent results, but patients with patellar lesions did poorly.

Buckwalter JA, Mankin HJ: Articular cartilage: Tissue design and chondrocyte-matrix interactions, in Cannon WD Jr (ed): *Instructional Course Lectures 47*. Rosemont, IL, American Academy of Orthopaedic Surgeons, 1998, pp 477–486.

Buckwalter JA, Mankin HJ: Articular cartilage: Degeneration and osteoarthritis, repair, regeneration, and transplantation, in Cannon WD Jr (ed): *Instructional Course Lectures 47*. Rosemont, IL, American Academy of Orthopaedic Surgeons, 1998, pp 487–504.

These 2 chapters review the current understanding of the design of articular cartilage, interactions between chondrocytes and their matrices, degeneration of articular cartilage, relationships between degeneration of articular cartilage and osteoarthrosis and joint use, and restoration of the composition, structure, and function of articular cartilage.

Coutts RD, Sah RL, Amiel D: Effect of growth factors on cartilage repair, in Springfield DS (ed): *Instructional Course Lectures 46.* Rosemont, IL, American Academy of Orthopaedic Surgeons, 1997, pp 487–504.

This chapter offers an excellent review on the current understanding of growth factors involved in cartilage injury and repair. Substances reviewed include insulin-like growth factor, basic fibroblast growth factor, and transforming growth factor beta. Growth factor carriers reviewed include bovine dermal collagen, fibrin, fibrinogen, and hyaluronic acid.

Hangody L, Kish G, Karpati Z, Szerb I, Udvarhel I: Arthroscopic autogenous osteochondral mosaicplasty for treatment of femoral condylar articular defects: A preliminary report. *Knee Surg Sports Traumatol Arthrosc* 1997;5:262–267.

The authors present a preliminary report on their experiences with mosaicplasty of the knee. They used both open and arthroscopic techniques. Retrospective results on select cases with variable follow-up are given.

Johnson DL, Urban WP Jr, Caborn DN, Vanarthos WJ, Carlson CS: Articular cartilage changes seen with magnetic resonance imaging-detected bone bruises associated with acute anterior cruciate ligament rupture. *Am J Sports Med* 1998;26:409–414.

The authors have shown that a geographic bone bruise (continuous with subchondral bone plate) found on MRI indicates substantial damage to normal articular cartilage. Histologic biopsies confirmed chondrocyte degeneration, proteoglycan loss, and collagen architectural changes.

Sellers RS, Peluso D, Morris EA: The effect of recombinant human bone morphogenetic protein-2 (rhBMP-2) on the healing of full-thickness defects of articular cartilage. *J Bone Joint Surg* 1997;79A:1452–1463.

Using a rabbit model, the authors have shown the capacity of rhBMP-2 to accelerate the healing of full-thickness defects of articular cartilage and improve the histologic appearances and biochemical characteristics.

Simonian PT, Sussmann PS, Wickiewicz TL, Paletta GA, Warren RF: Contact pressures at osteochondral donor sites in the knee. *Am J Sports Med* 1998;26:491–494.

Using cadaveric knees the authors showed that all recommended donor sites used for osteochondral transplantation experienced contact forces during functional knee motion. Four of the 10 sites tested showed decreased contact pressures over the other sites.

Meniscus

Burks RT, Metcalf MH, Metcalf RW: Fifteen-year follow-up of arthroscopic partial meniscectomy. *Arthroscopy* 1997;13:673–679.

The authors present a review of 146 patients who have undergone partial meniscectomy. Age and medial/lateral meniscus was not shown to be a factor in outcome. ACL-deficient knees with partial meniscectomy had significantly poorer results than stable knees with partial meniscectomy.

Cameron JC, Saha S: Meniscal allograft transplantation for unicompartmental arthritis of the knee. *Clin Orthop* 1997;337:164–171.

The authors present 67 fresh meniscal transplants in 63 patients with 1- to 5-year follow-up. Over 80% of patients had good results, with the most frequent complication being unsuccessful healing of the posterior horn of the medial meniscus.

Johnson DL, Swenson TM, Livesay GA, Aizawa H, Fu FH, Harner CD: Insertion-site anatomy of the human menisci: Gross, arthroscopic, and topographical anatomy as a basis for meniscal transplantation. *Arthroscopy* 1995;11:386–394.

Using cadaveric knees the authors have described in great detail the bony insertion sites of each meniscal root. The authors have shown their "three dimensional topographical" orientation as well as identified arthroscopic landmarks for observation.

van Arkel ER, de Boer HH: Human meniscal transplantation: Preliminary results at 2 to 5-year follow-up. *J Bone Joint Surg* 1995;77B:589–595.

The authors present 23 cases of meniscal transplantation using cryopreserved allograft with 2- to 5-year follow-up. Twenty patients had satisfactory results.

Ligament

Schaefer SL, Ciarelli MJ, Arnoczky SP, Ross HE: Tissue shrinkage with the holmium:yttrium aluminum garnet laser: A postoperative assessment of tissue length, stiffness, and structure. *Am J Sports Med* 1997;25:841–848.

The authors observed structural and biomechanical changes in patellar tendons of rabbits after a laser procedure that resulted in immediate tissue shortening. The relative lengthening of the treated tissue, demonstrated after 8 weeks of unrestricted activity in the postoperative period, requires further clinical consideration.

Schmidt CC, Georgescu HI, Kwoh CK, et al: Effect of growth factors on the proliferation of fibroblasts from the medial collateral and ACLs. *J Orthop Res* 1995;13:184–190.

This, and other studies, shed light on a growing area of interest, the role of growth factors and cytokines in normal tissue and their effect on healing tissues. In this study, 8 growth factors administered into the culture medium at varying doses had different effects, which appear to be dose-dependent, on fibroblast proliferation for the anterior cruciate and MCLs.

Ticker JB, Bigliani LU, Soslowsky LJ, Pawluk RJ, Flatow EL, Mow VC: Inferior glenohumeral ligament: Geometric and strain-rate dependent properties. *J Shoulder Elbow Surg* 1996;5:269–279.

The geometry of the inferior glenohumeral ligament, thicker anteriorly and medially, and its material properties, when tested at varying strain rates, support the role of the more anterior structures, the superior band as well as the anterior axillary pouch, as important static restraints to anterior glenohumeral instability.

Tendon

Blevins FT, Djurasovic M, Flatow EL, Vogel KG: Biology of the rotator cuff tendon. *Orthop Clin North Am* 1997;28:1–16.

The current state of knowledge of the biology and biochemistry of tendons is reviewed, highlighting the rotator cuff. Alterations induced in tendons by different mechanical stresses, in particular, compression, are discussed.

Kubota H, Manske PR, Aoki M, Pruitt DL, Larson BJ: Effect of motion and tension on injured flexor tendons in chickens. *J Hand Surg* 1996;21A;456–463.

In addition to motion, application of tension to a partial flexor tendon laceration increased the breaking strength of the healing tendon. The combination of motion and tension further enhanced the biomechanical properties of the healing tendon, as well as demonstrated the highest cellular activity on histology.

St. Pierre P, Olson EJ, Elliott JJ, O'Hair KC, McKinney LA, Ryan J: Tendon-healing to cortical bone compared with healing to a cancellous trough: A biomechanical and histological evaluation in goats. *J Bone Joint Surg* 1995;77A:1858–1866.

In an animal model, tendon healing to cortical bone and to a cancellous trough were not significantly different histologically or structurally at 6 and 12 weeks after surgical repair. Of note, the load to failure, energy to failure, and stiffness in the treated groups at 12 weeks were approximately one third that of the controls.

Muscle

Cooper LW, Lohnes J, Smith SC, Rolf TD, Garrett WE: The effect of passive cooling and heating on muscle flexibility. *Trans Orthop Res Soc* 1996;21:137.

Heat or stretching resulted in increased muscle flexibility, and when combined, these factors had a greater effect.

Mair SD, Seaber AV, Glisson RR, Garrett WE Jr: The role of fatigue in susceptibility to acute muscle strain injury. *Am J Sports Med* 1996;24:137–143.

Fatigued muscles stretched to the same length at failure as nonfatigued muscles when tested biomechanically, but had significantly less energy absorbed at failure at all rates of stretch studied. This more clearly defines fatigue as a factor in muscle injury.

Mishra DK, Friden J, Schmitz MC, Lieber RL: Anti-inflammatory medication after muscle injury: A treatment resulting in short-term improvement but subsequent loss of muscle function. *J Bone Joint Surg* 1995;77A:1510–1519.

The nonsteroidal anti-inflammatory medication flurbiprofen enhanced recovery initially from a muscle strain injury up to 7 days after injury, as shown in a rabbit model. However, this medication had a deleterious effect on the functional recovery of muscle when studied at 28 days.

Nerve

Watchmaker GP, Mackinnon SE: Advances in peripheral nerve repair. *Clin Plast Surg* 1997;24:63–73.

This article presents the recent advances in understanding the basic science of neural regeneration and their application to the management of primary repairs and nerve gaps.

Watchmaker GP, Mackinnon SE: Nerve injury and repair, in Peimer C (ed): *Surgery of the Hand and Upper Extremity*. New York, NY, McGraw-Hill, 1996, pp 1251–1275.

This chapter offers a comprehensive review of the past and present understanding of nerve anatomy and nerve injury. Treatment options for nerve injuries are clearly delineated.

Son YJ, Thompson WJ: Schwann cell processes guide regeneration of peripheral axons. *Neuron* 1995;14:125–132.

Using a rat model, the authors have shown that Schwann cell processes lead and guide peripheral regeneration, thus functioning as leaders rather than followers during the regenerative process.

Classic Bibliography

Armstrong CG, Mow VC: Variations in the intrinsic mechanical properties of human articular cartilage with age, degeneration, and water content. *J Bone Joint Surg* 1982;64A:88–94.

Arnoczky SP, Warren RF, Spivak JM: Meniscal repair using an exogenous fibrin clot: An experimental study in dogs. *J Bone Joint Surg* 1988;70A:1209–1217.

Arnoczky SP, Warren RF: Microvasculature of the human meniscus. *Am J Sports Med* 1982;10:90–95.

Bodine SC, Lieber RL: Peripheral nerve physiology, anatomy, and pathology, in Simon SR (ed): *Orthopaedic Basic Science*. Rosemont, IL, American Academy of Orthopaedic Surgeons, 1994, pp 325–396.

Buckwalter JA, Mow VC, Ratcliffe A: Restoration of injured or degenerated articular cartilage. *J Am Acad Orthop Surg* 1994; 2:192–201.

Clark JM, Harryman DT II: Tendons, ligaments, and capsule of the rotator cuff: Gross and microscopic anatomy. *J Bone Joint Surg* 1992;74A:713–725.

Convery FR, Meyers MH, Akeson WH: Fresh osteochondral allografting of the femoral condyle. *Clin Orthop* 1991;273: 139–145.

Fairbank TJ: Knee joint changes after meniscectomy. *J Bone Joint Surg* 1948;30B:664–670.

Fowler PJ: Bone injuries associated with anterior cruciate ligament disruption. *Arthroscopy* 1994;10:453–460.

Fu FH, Harner CD, Johnson DL, Miller MD, Woo SL-Y: Biomechanics of knee ligaments: Basic concepts and clinical application. *J Bone Joint Surg* 1993;75A:1716–1727.

Gelberman RH, Manske PR, Akeson WH, Woo SL-Y, Lundborg G, Amiel D: Flexor tendon repair. *J Orthop Res* 1986;4: 119–128.

Jackson DW, McDevitt CA, Simon TM, Arnoczky SP, Atwell EA, Silvino NJ: Meniscal transplantation using fresh and cryopreserved allografts: An experimental study in goats. *Am J Sports Med* 1992;20:644–656.

Jackson DW, Whelan J, Simon TM: Cell survival after transplantation of fresh meniscal allografts: DNA probe analysis in a goat model. *Am J Sports Med* 1993;21:540–550.

Levy I, M, Torzilli PA, Warren RF: The effect of medial meniscectomy on anterior-posterior motion of the knee. *J Bone Joint Surg* 1982;64A:883–888.

Lundborg G (ed): *Nerve Injury and Repair*. Edinburgh, Scotland, Churchill Livingstone, 1988.

Mahomed MN, Beaver RJ, Gross AE: The long-term success of fresh, small fragment osteochondral allografts used for intraarticular post-traumatic defects in the knee joint. *Orthopedics* 1992;15:1191–1199.

McConville OR, Kipnis JM, Richmond JC, Rockett SE, Michaud MJ: The effect of meniscal status on knee stability and function after anterior cruciate ligament reconstruction. *Arthroscopy* 1993;9:431–439.

Mankin HJ, Mow VC, Buckwalter JA, Iannotti JP, Ratcliffe A: Form and function of articular cartilage, in Simon SR (ed): *Orthopaedic Basic Science*. Rosemont, IL, American Academy of Orthopaedic Surgeons 1994, pp 1–44.

Mow VC, Bigliani LU, Flatow EL, Ticker JB, Ratcliffe A, Soslowsky LJ: Material properties of the inferior glenohumeral ligament and the glenohumeral articular cartilage, in Matsen FA III, Fu FH, Hawkins RJ (eds): *The Shoulder: A Balance of Mobility and Stability*. Rosemont, IL, American Academy of Orthopaedic Surgeons, 1993, pp 29–67.

Mow VC, Kuei SC, Lai WM, Armstrong CG: Biphasic creep and stress relaxation of articular cartilage in compression: Theory and experiments. *J Biomech Eng* 1980;102:73–84.

Newton PM, Mow VC, Gardner TR, Buckwalter JA, Albright JP: The effect of lifelong exercise on canine articular cartilage. *Am J Sports Med* 1997;25:282–287.

Noonan TJ, Best TM, Seaber AV, Garrett WE Jr: Thermal effects on skeletal muscle tensile behavior. *Am J Sports Med* 1993;21:517–522.

Oegema TR Jr, Thompson RC Jr: Histopathology and pathobiochemistry of the cartilage-bone interface in osteoarthritis, in Kuettner KE, Goldberg VM (eds): *Osteoarthritic Disorders*. Rosemont, IL, American Academy of Orthopaedic Surgeons, 1995, pp 205–217.

Rodeo SA, Arnoczky SP, Torzilli PA, Hidaka C, Warren RF: Tendon-healing in a bone tunnel: A biomechanical and histological study in the dog. *J Bone Joint Surg* 1993;75A:1795–1803.

Shapiro F, Koide S, Glimcher MJ: Cell orgin and differentiation in the repair of full-thickness defects of articular cartilage. *J Bone Joint Surg* 1993;75A:532–553.

Stein LN, Fischer DA, Fritts HM, Quick DC: Occult osseous lesions associated with anterior cruciate ligament tears. *Clin Orthop* 1995;313:187–193.

Sunderland S (ed): *Nerve Injuries and Their Repair: A Critical Appraisal*. Edinburgh, Scotland, Churchill Livingstone, 1991.

Taylor DC, Dalton JD JR, Seaber AV, Garrett WE Jr: Experimental muscle strain injury: Early functional and structural deficits and the increased risk for reinjury. *Am J Sports Med* 1993;21: 190–194.

Thompson RC, Oegema TR Jr, Lewis JL, Wallace L: Osteoarthritic changes after acute transarticular load: An animal model. *J Bone Joint Surg* 1991;73A:990–1001.

Thompson WO, Thaete FL, Fu FH, Dye SF: Tibial meniscal dynamics using three-dimensional reconstruction of magnetic resonance imaging. *Am J Sports Med* 1991;19:210–215.

Veltri DM, Warren RF, Wickiewicz TL, OiBrien SJ: Current status of allograft meniscal transplantation. *Clin Orthop* 1994;303: 44–55.

Bone Healing and Grafting

Fracture Healing Biology

Fracture repair is unique in that healing is completed without formation of a scar. In contrast to the healing of other tissues such as skin only mature bone remains in the fracture site at the end of the repair process. Fracture healing has two fundamental prerequisites: a biologically adequate blood supply and a mechanically stable environment for bone deposition. Fracture repair requires restoration of mechanical stability, which can be achieved by a natural process of healing or by means in which the fractured bone ends are partially or completely stabilized. Each of these processes has unique histologic characteristics, and each can occur in isolation or in concert with the other to achieve union.

Spontaneous fracture healing begins with formation of a hematoma within the fracture site. The hematoma is replaced by ingrowth of fibrovascular tissue. The fibrocartilage that then develops stabilizes the bone ends (Fig. 1). This step is followed by restoration of bony continuity as the cartilage and fibrous tissue are replaced through endochondral and intramembranous bone formation. Necrotic bone fragments are initially enveloped and stabilized by the mineralizing callus and are later remodeled. Secondary remodeling can lead to correction of residual malalignment while woven bone is replaced by lamellar bone.

Tissue differentiation in the fracture gap is strongly influenced by the mechanical forces acting on the various cell populations and by the vascularity of the surrounding soft-tissue envelope. The presence of a fracture gap, motion of the fracture fragments, and an intact soft-tissue envelope encourage periosteal callus formation. In several studies, investigators have attempted to correlate tissue differentiation within the fracture to the mechanical loading environment of the fracture site. The findings from these studies indicate that increasing the stability and rigidity of the early fracture fixation decreases interfragmentary motion, thereby leading to decreased callus formation after early healing. Mechanical loading of fractures stimulates revascularization and callus formation with optimal restoration of strength after healing if loading of the fracture occurs after the early stages of tissue differentiation within the callus. This finding suggests that fracture healing is benefited by early stability, which allows revascularization to occur. Following the early stages of healing, which occur within the first month after injury, loading

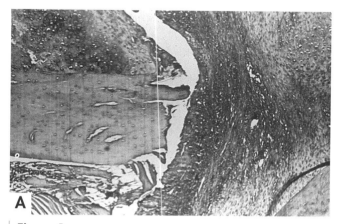 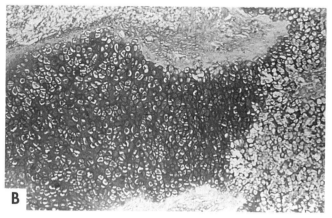

Figure 1

A, Photomicrographs of the development of fibrovascular stroma with inflammatory cells, which replaces the initial fracture hematoma. This stage is histologically described as the stage of inflammation and occurs from day 3 to 21 following injury. B, Cartilage has replaced the fibrovascular stroma heralding the stage of soft callus. Clinically, this development is indicated by reduction of fracture fragment instability and resolution of pain. Complete healing occurs by replacement of the cartilage with a woven bone by the process of endochondral ossification. (Reproduced with permission from Ostrum RF, Chao EYS, Bassett CAL, et al: Bone injury, regeneration, and repair, in Simon SR (ed): *Orthopaedic Basic Science*. Rosemont, IL, American Academy of Orthopaedic Surgeons, 1994, pp 277–323.)

and interfragmentary motion stimulate a more exuberant callus, which ultimately leads to greater strength of the healed bone.

Prolonged, rigid stabilization of fractures leads to healing without significant periosteal callus. This type of healing is observed in fractures stabilized by rigid fracture plates. In regions of the fracture where there is anatomic cortical contact, healing occurs by direct haversian remodeling. In regions where there is a fracture gap, healing occurs by intramembranous bone formation (Fig. 2). Gap healing in regions rigidly stabilized by bone plates occurs by filling in of the gap by a woven bone matrix that subsequently is remodeled into lamellar cortex. As in spontaneous fracture repair, the differentiation of tissue within immobilized fracture gaps is influenced by local, mechanical strains applied to the healing tissue. In regions of low strain, osseous tissue ingrowth occurs. In regions with micromotion resulting in higher strain, osseous tissue differentiation is discouraged.

The vascularity of the fracture site also influences tissue differentiation and the course of healing. The early stages of fracture healing essentially represent the ingrowth of a vascular stroma that replaces the avascular fracture hematoma. Fracture healing is often impaired in bones with a poor blood supply, such as the femoral neck, talar neck, and carpal scaphoid. Internal fixation devices may cause varying degrees of damage to either the endosteal or periosteal circulation and alter the course of spontaneous healing. Plates may compromise periosteal vessels. Screws create small localized areas

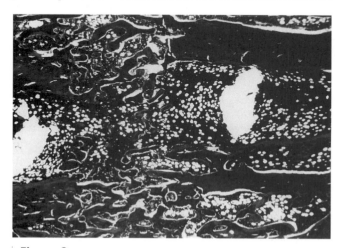

Figure 2

Gap healing is illustrated in this photomicrograph. An experimental osteotomy has been stabilized by a rigid plate. The inferior cortex was intimately apposed across the osteotomy and has healed by direct cortical healing. The superior cortices were separated by a gap which has healed by direct intramembranous type bone formation. The woven bone at the top of the osteotomy illustrates the histologic appearance of the gap healing process.

of cortical necrosis, and intramedullary devices disrupt blood supply to the endosteal cortex. Methods of fixation that preserve blood supply interfere the least with the healing process. The healing of oblique osteotomies has been compared between cohorts treated with compression plates, intramedullary nails, and external fixation. When an external fixator is used, it causes the least disturbance to the fracture vascularity.

Recent studies have demonstrated the advantage of using an indirect fixation method that reduces and stabilizes complex fractures. For example, in treatment of femoral shaft fractures, plate fixation techniques that only expose the lateral femoral cortex by subperiosteal or submuscular dissection, preserve medial soft tissues, and minimize the number of screws placed allow exuberant healing in the medial cortex opposite the plate.

Regulation of Fracture Healing

Fracture healing involves a specific cascade of cellular events that begin with inflammation followed by fibrous tissue then cartilage differentiation terminating through endochondral ossification with bone formation. These events are influenced by the presence of undifferentiated cells in the region of the fracture and may involve regulation by signaling growth factors released into the fracture environment. Osteoinduction is a term used to describe this key step in fracture repair. It is the process that encourages mitogenesis of undifferentiated mesenchymal cells, leading to formation of osteoprogenitor cells that have the capacity to form new bone. Osteoinductive growth factors can lead to bone formation in extraskeletal sites. The roles of numerous growth factors in fracture repair have been investigated, but, to date, the exact mechanisms and influence of any of these factors remains poorly understood. Current understanding of the regulatory role of growth factors in fracture healing recently has been extensively reviewed. The factors influencing fracture repair can be divided into 2 groups. The first are those that promote peptide signaling including transforming growth factor-beta (TGF-β), bone morphogenetic proteins (BMPs), fibroblast growth factors (FGF), and platelet derived growth factor (PDGF). The second group contains the immunoregulatory cytokines including interleukin-1 and interleukin-6.

TGF-β is a multifunctional growth factor that participates in a variety of responses to injury, inflammation, and tissue repair. The largest source of TGF-β is the extracellular bone matrix. Chondrocytes and osteoblasts synthesize TGF-β, and it has been shown to accumulate in extracellular matrix produced during endochondral ossification. Genetic expression of TGF-β in fracture callus occurs in the early and late stages of repair, suggesting a role as a director of tissue differentiation in fracture repair.

BMPs are potent osteoinductive agents. This family of proteins was characterized after investigating the potent healing potential of demineralized bone matrix. Monoclonal antibodies assays have been used to demonstrate that BMP-2 and BMP-4 are actively produced during the early stages of fracture repair that lead to endochondral ossification with decreasing production after bone formation occurs. FGFs (acidic and basic) increase proliferation of osteoblasts and chondrocytes and FGF-2 stimulates angiogenesis.

Although the role of these factors in normal fracture repair remains only poorly understood, many experimental attempts have been made to use them as exogenously applied agents to enhance fracture repair. It has been demonstrated that BMP-2 enhances healing of femoral defects in the rat model. The efficacy of human osteogenic protein-1 on healing of segmental defects in nonhuman primates has been demonstrated in some studies. In other studies, investigators have been unable to demonstrate influence of FGF-1 and FGF-2 on normal fracture healing in rats. Demineralized bone matrix is a potent agent that improves healing of bone segmental defects. Although early work in this field is promising, the role of growth factors in the enhancement of healing and as substitutes for traditional bone grafting of poorly healing fractures requires further study. This field remains in a stage of experimental infancy.

Delayed Union, Nonunion: Fractures at Risk

Delayed union is defined as the failure of a fractured bone to heal within an expected time course while maintaining the potential to heal. Delayed union is a clinical diagnosis. Gross motion or pain at the fracture site and radiographic evidence of persistent radiolucency are factors suggesting failure of healing. Nonunion is defined as a state in which all healing processes have ceased before complete healing has occurred. Nonunions lack the potential to heal without intervention.

Fractures at risk are those commonly associated with problematic healing. The incidence and, therefore, risk of nonunion varies with the site of bone involvement and the mechanism and energy of injury. When nonunion sites are tabulated by bone, the tibia accounts for 45% of nonunions, the femur 16%, the humerus 9%, and the ulna, radius, and carpal scaphoid 5% each.

Nonunions can be classified as hypertrophic/vascular versus atrophic/avascular by radiographic and histologic appearance. Hypertrophic nonunions demonstrate excessive vascularity and callus formation, and they maintain healing potential. In hypertrophic nonunions, excessive motion prevents endochondral and intramembranous bone formation across the fracture gap. Stabilization of hypertrophic nonunions predictably leads to healing.

Atrophic nonunions radiographically show little callus surrounding a fibrous tissue filled fracture gap. Atrophic nonunions are devoid of osteogenic substrate and lack the potential to heal. Treatment requires debridement of intervening fibrous tissue, implantation of an osteoconductive matrix with osteoinductive or osteogenic agents or bone graft, and surgical stabilization of the fracture fragments.

Treatment of Nonunions and Fractures at Risk

Fractures at risk of nonunion commonly result from high-energy trauma in which the initial fracture displacement has damaged the surrounding soft tissues, leading to profound changes in the medullary and periosteal blood supply, eg, open fractures of the tibia. Union is further delayed by the extensive debridement required in severe open fractures or if infection occurs. Other factors implicated in designating fractures at risk include comminution, fracture fragment distraction, bone loss, inadequate immobilization, and a history of smoking. Fractures that fail to progress in healing over a 3- to 5-month period of observation represent delayed unions with a poor prognosis for healing, indicating that a change in treatment is necessary to avoid the long-term morbidity associated with nonunion. For example, if delayed healing of the tibia is encountered after unreamed intramedullary nailing, exchange to a reamed intramedullary nail can achieve union without need for autogenous bone graft. Another commonly used intervention, posterolateral bone grafting, is a useful alternative. Several studies suggest that a combination of internal fixation and aggressive bone grafting provides the best results in severe open fractures with bone loss. Protocols developed for management of severe open fractures include aggressive debridement to avoid infection, early microvascular tissue transfer, and direct bone grafting beneath vascularized flaps.

Nonunion represents a state in which the healing process has ceased and the potential for continued healing does not exist. An intervention is necessary to restart the healing process to achieve union. That intervention has two aspects: first, the mechanical stability must be obtained generally by some form of fracture fixation; and second, the biologic environment must be enhanced to restart the cascade of healing. The variety of options for surgical management have been carefully reviewed. In general, diaphyseal nonunions of most long bones, especially hypertrophic nonunions, are amenable to reamed, intramedullary nailing. Atrophic nonunions, metaphyseal nonunions, and nonunions with significant deformity usually require open reduction and internal fixation. Infected nonunions that require extensive sequestrectomy should be considered for initial treatment using external fixation.

A review of the treatment of tibial nonunion using a variety of methods has led to the identification of risk factors for failure of treatment of a given nonunion. The 6 factors are described in Outline 1. Failures due to prior bone grafting and failures treated previously with electrical stimulation are combined and designated as failures of prior attempt at treatment.

When no risk factors are present in simple nonunions, most nonunion treatment methods including bone grafting, electrical stimulation, or closed management with capacitance coupling are equally effective in achieving union. As risk factors appear, the prognosis for healing worsens. Nonunions with durations greater than 10 months and reattempts of failed methods are associated with a high risk of failure. Electrical stimulation and capacitance coupling are not successful for atrophic nonunions, nonunions with gross instability, or an established synovial pseudoarthrosis. Active infection is a contraindication to the use of electrical stimulation without additional intervention. For nonunions of greater than 70 months duration with 4 or more risk factors, only aggressive treatment plans combining surgery and bone grafting have a potential for success.

Bone Grafts in Fracture Healing

Autogenous Bone Grafts

Currently, autogenous bone grafting is considered the best method and material for enhancement of the fracture repair process. Autogenous cancellous grafts are the most effective graft material because they provide the 3 elements required for bone regeneration: osteoconduction, osteoinduction, and osteogenic cells. Osteoconduction in cancellous grafts occurs because of the porous, 3-dimensional architecture of cancellous bone that allows for rapid ingrowth of fibrovascular tissues in the host bed. In its matrix, cancellous bone contains growth factors, especially BMPs, which by osteoinduction encourage the growth and differentiation of mesenchymal cells to osteoblastic lineages. Finally, living periosteal and other osteoblasts transplanted with the graft are osteogenic, producing new bone directly. After implantation, cancellous grafts are invaded by surrounding tissues. New bone forma-

Outline 1
Risk factors in treatment of nonunions

Duration of nonunion

Open fracture

Presence of infection

Comminuted or oblique fracture

Atrophic nonunion

Failed prior treatment

tion occurs on the cancellous trabeculae, and the graft integrates with preexisting osseous structures. The graft is then remodeled under the influence of local mechanical stresses and gains structural strength and integrity.

Cortical grafts undergo a similar process of incorporation but, as a result of the density of the cortex and its relative lack of porosity, the process is slowed. For cortical bone to incorporate, it must undergo a period of resorption that increases its porosity, allowing vascular invasion and subsequent osseous integration. Cortical grafts are often chosen for the initial structural support they provide in bridging large defects. However, the surgeon must be aware that cortical grafts rapidly loose their structural strength as integration develops. The process of graft incorporation results in a 30% reduction in strength over 6 to 18 months.

Vascularized cortical grafts maintain viability and avoid some of the problems of large nonvascularized grafts. The vascularized fibula graft is most commonly used but ribs and iliac crest can also be transplanted. Vascularized fibula is considered superior to nonvascularized grafts when bridging gaps or areas more than 12 cm in length. The major drawback to vascularized fibula grafts is the morbidity associated with their harvest and the extensive surgical procedure involved. It is proposed that after 6 months of incorporation nonvascularized grafts have similar strength to that of vascularized grafts. Cortical fibular autografts can be used to improve local bone quality, thereby enhancing the stability of internal fixation of certain nonunions, particularly of the humerus. This approach demonstrates how creative applications of bone grafts can enhance the surgeon's ability to address significant loss of bone stock in reconstruction of complicated nonunions.

Disadvantages of autogenous bone grafts include donor site morbidity, limited supply, and occasionally inferior biomechanical strength of the graft.

Allogeneic Bone Grafts

Allogeneic bone provided as fresh frozen, freeze-dried, and demineralized bone has been used extensively for skeletal reconstruction. The major experience in use of allograft bone has been in bulk replacements for skeletal loss. Little has been published on use of allografts in fracture care. It is clear that allografts generate an intense immune response that interferes with graft incorporation. Studies have demonstrated that immune-mismatch significantly interferes with allograft incorporation. Although freezing decreases the rejection of mismatched grafts, frozen allograft incorporates less well than fresh autograft. Allograft incorporation is also much slower than that of autografts, prompting the need for rigid internal fixation to provide optimal support during allograft incorporation. Any form of allograft has less ability to incorporate than autograft due to decreased osteogenic and osteoinductive capacities.

The major concern regarding use of allografts remains the potential for disease transmission. Allograft bone readily transmits retrovirus infection in spite of routine processing and removal of bone marrow. The major defense against such disease transmission is careful screening of donors, but the potential for human error in the screening process will always remain. This unsolved problem as well as the expense of providing processed allograft contributes to the continued interest in developing engineered bone graft substitutes.

Synthetic Engineered Bone Graft Substitute

Synthetic or engineered bone graft substitutes present the opportunity to provide materials that enhance fracture healing without concerns of disease transmission or availability. Synthetic graft substitutes consist of an osteoconductive matrix to which may be added osteoinductive proteins and/or osteoprogenitor cells.

Several clinically available osteoconductive substances use calcium-phosphate ceramics. Calcium phosphate ceramics are available as porous or nonporous dense implants, or porous granules. The optimal porosity of hydroxyapatite materials appears to be between 200 and 600 μm with a high degree of interconnectivity. This optimal porosity is characteristic of coraline hydroxyapatites, which have well documented clinical usefulness. Although hydroxyapatite implants do not resorb, they cause little inflammation and are well tolerated in metaphyseal sites. However, because they are brittle and have limited potential for remodeling, the use of hydroxyapatite implants as graft substitutes for diaphyseal defects of long bones is less successful.

Composite osteoconductive grafts that combine porous hydroxyapatite-tricalcium phosphate ceramics with type I collagen have been shown to be as effective as autogenous cancellous bone graft in the treatment of long-bone fractures. Composite graft substitutes of this type have been evaluated in a multicenter study and have been shown to be as effective as cancellous graft while avoiding the morbidity of iliac crest harvest. In this study, use of the composite graft substitute also led to a shorter time in surgery and a lower overall infection rate. This composite graft substitute is currently approved by the Food and Drug Administration for use in treatment of long-bone fractures.

The use of osteoinductive agents has not yet been reported in a human series. Demineralized bone matrix (DBM) prepared by acid extraction of allograft bone is osteoconductive and somewhat osteoinductive and has been made available as a commercial product. The results of use of DBM in clinical trials have been excellent. To date this is the only available source of an osteoinductive material other than autogenous bone.

Autogenous bone marrow can provide a source of osteoprogenitor cells. Autogenous marrow is an efficacious addition to artificial bone grafts in experimental models. Development of recombinant BMP and grafts composed of artificially enhanced osteoprogentor cells in combination with synthetic osteoconductive carriers show promise but are still early in their investigative development.

Biophysical Stimulation of Healing

Implantation of direct current cathode and inductive coupling pulsed electromagnetic fields have been used for electric stimulation of fracture healing for many years. In spite of relatively convincing basic science research, prospective randomized clinical trials that demonstrate the effectiveness of treating delayed unions with capacitance coupling are fairly recent. Although these studies are recent and involve small numbers, they have been performed as placebo controlled, prospective randomized trials. The benefit of capacitance coupling can only be demonstrated in properly selected cases of hypertrophic nonunion with no gap or gross motion at the fracture site.

Low intensity ultrasound also has been found to stimulate healing of fractures and nonunions in animal experiments. Two carefully controlled prospective clinical trials have clearly documented that ultrasound stimulation shortens the time to healing and insures a higher union rate in low energy, stable, tibial fractures and fractures of the distal radius.

Distraction Osteogenesis

Distraction osteogenesis (DO) can be defined as a gradual mechanical process of stretching two vascularized bone surfaces apart at a critical rate and rhythm such that new bone forms within the expanding gap, reliably bridges the gap, and ultimately remodels to normal structure. Distraction of a low-energy osteotomy, early fracture callus, or even a hypertrophic nonunion can stimulate DO, thus avoiding the need for autograft, allograft, bone substitute, or prosthetic implant. DO allows for most soft tissues (eg, skin, fascia, nerves, vessels, and possibly muscle) to accommodate by gradual stretching.

DO has been useful in the treatment of challenging skeletal problems in both children and adults. These problems include congenital limb deficiencies (eg, hemimelias), acquired limb shortening (eg, growth arrests, posttraumatic leg-length discrepancy), deformities (eg, Blount disease or malunions), intercalary bone defects (eg, open fractures, osteomyelitis, or tumor resections), and nonunions (eg, posttraumatic or congenital tibial pseudarthrosis).

This innovative technique was introduced by Ilizarov who used a modular, ring external fixation system with tensioned transosseous wires to mechanically shift bone segments in all spatial planes (lengthening, angulation, rotation, and translation). Based on biologic principles of DO, Ilizarov used (1) percutaneous surgical techniques; (2) 3-dimensional correction of deformity; (3) simultaneous, multifocal treatment (eg, lengthening at two or more sites within a limb or spanning an adjacent joint to prevent muscle contracture or hyaline cartilage compression during lengthening); (4) noninvasive approaches for nonunion treatment; and (5) bone transportation to regenerate intercalary defects.

The method requires analysis of one or multiple sites of deformity and deficiency of bone, soft tissue, or both. Mechanical and anatomic axes are identified and a treatment plan formulated that includes a strategy for managing the biologic and mechanical requirements at each site (Fig. 3). Multiple transosseous wires or half-pins may be inserted via anatomic safe zones within the limb. Most commonly, the bone is separated by a low-energy osteotomy (to maximize local vascularity) and then distracted at a rate of 1 mm per day divided into a rhythm of 0.25 mm 4 times per day following a latency. The latency period is the time following an osteotomy when callus bridges the cut bone surfaces prior to initiating distraction. After the distraction phase, the external fixator stabilizes the limb until bony consolidation occurs. The latency, usually 5 days, varies up to 21 days depending on the age of the patient and the type of osteotomy. The healing index, the number of months from operation to fixator

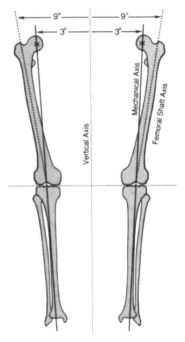

Figure 3

Mechanical axis and femoral shaft (anatomic) axis. (Adapted with permission from Beaty JH: Congenital anomalies of lower extremity, in Crenshaw AH (ed): *Campbell's Operative Orthopaedics*, ed 8. St. Louis, MO, Mosby Year Book, 1992, pp 2061–2158.)

removal (distraction plus consolidation), for each centimeter of new bone length is usually 1.0 in children and increases with patient age.

The choice of an external fixator is generally determined by the surgeon's experience and preference, the complexity of the problem, and the number of sites requiring treatment (Fig. 4). Monolateral fixators are most successful for simple lengthenings, while ring fixators are capable of mechanical correction of complex deformites with angulation and rotation or of those requiring more than 2 sites of treatment. Intramedullary nails have been used for both bone transportation and lengthening without disturbing periosteal bone formation. In conjunction with external fixation to drive the bone separation, the nail can be interlocked at the end of distraction for early removal of the external fixator, particularly in femoral lengthenings. Currently, intramedullary nails with internal driving devices are being developed to avoid external fixation altogether.

Many studies indicate that the periosteum is the major contributor to osteogenesis during distraction. Consequently, methods of bone separation that disrupt the periosteum, such as a widely displaced osteotomy, can inhibit osteogenesis. Alternatively, any vascularized bone surface, whether

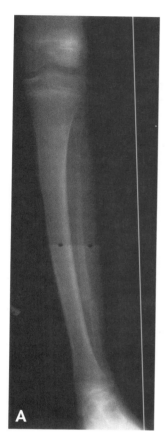 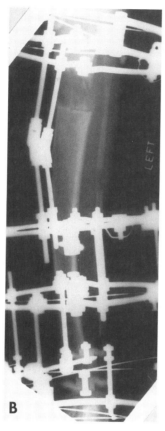 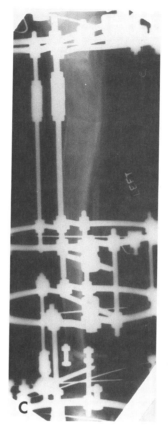 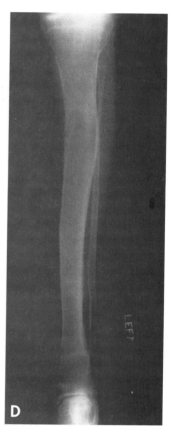

Figure 4

Radiographs of a child with a 6-cm limb-length discrepancy due to fibular hemimelia. A, Anteroposterior radiograph depicts proximal and distal tibial valgus, as well as ball-and-socket ankle and hypoplasia of the fibula. Patient previously underwent tibial lengthening with a monolateral fixator. B, Acute correction of distal tibial valgus deformity was performed. Frame was constructed to first lengthen the proximal tibia and then achieve angular correction. Note hinge application at apex of proximal tibial valgus deformity distal to site of corticotomy. Frame extends to foot to prevent subluxation or contracture. C, Radiographic appearance after desired lengthening. Progressive correction of proximal tibial valgus was then sequentially performed, with desired bending of regenerate. D, End result, with equalization of limb length and mechanical-axis realignment. (Reproduced with permission from Murray JH, Fitch RD: Distraction histiogenesis: Principles and indications. *J Am Acad Orthop Surg* 1996;4:317–327.)

periosteal, endosteal, cortical, or trabecular, can promote osteogenesis when gradually distracted from a similarly vital vascular surface.

Most histologic investigations of DO have confirmed that bone forms from pure intramembranous ossification occurring in uniform zones. The central zone made of type I collagen bridges adjacent zones of vascular ingrowth where proliferating and differentiating osteoblasts deposit osteoid along the collagen bundles that consolidate into longitudinal bone columns. These bone columns parallel the distraction force imparted by the external fixator and eventually bridge the host bone surfaces after distraction is discontinued. During consolidation the columns are remodeled into cortical and trabecular bone.

DO has expanded the treatment options in several clinical areas: limb lengthening, nonunion repair, deformity correction, and regeneration of intercalary defects. Lengthening by DO is limited primarily by the surrounding soft tissues. Bone formation by DO can be perpetuated for well over 10 cm with a normal cross-sectional area. Angular lengthening necessitates a range of distraction rates from 0.5 to 2.0 mm per day for DO to bridge the gap. Multifocal sites of distraction can expedite the overall treatment time for bone healing but increase the complications from soft tissues, such as muscle contractures and stiff or subluxed joints.

Deformity correction necessitates the measurement of both anatomic and mechanical axes (Fig. 3), length, rotation, and joint alignment. Weightbearing, full length radiographs of both lower extremities and careful clinical examination are critical to plan this treatment. Special modifications of the external fixator can focus the mechanical forces around fulcrum-hinges constructed at the apex of the deformity for gradual correction. Alternatively, acute corrections via an osteotomy can be mechanically stabilized until callus bridges the site and then is distracted to regain length.

Nonunions also require preoperative analysis. The type of nonunion dictates the choice of mechanical force. A hypertrophic nonunion can be distracted primarily to stimulate DO and then compressed to obtain union if necessary. Atrophic nonunion must be gradually compressed, then distracted and finally recompressed to unite. An adjacent osteotomy for length restoration can accelerate the healing of an atrophic nonunion. Associated shortening, angulation, translation, and rotation deformities can also be corrected during nonunion treatment. Conversion of a fibrous nonunion or synovial pseudarthrosis to a solid bone bridge by compression and distraction forces has been called transformation osteogenesis (TO).

Bone transportation (BT) is a unique innovation, derived from both DO and TO. During BT, a vascularized segment of bone is separated surgically and then mechanically pulled by wires or half-pins across a preexisting bone gap. The trailing end regenerates bone by DO and the leading end fuses to the other surface by TO. BT has been used successfully to regenerate intercalary gaps from resected chronic osteomyelitis, acute posttraumatic bone loss, and after failed allograft or successful tumor resection.

Independent of the method and etiology, any extended lengthening routinely encounters a plethora of complications. Complications have been categorized as (1) pin tract (acute mechanical or thermal damage or late inflammation to frank infection of the underlying bone or scar formation); (2) bone (premature consolidation, delayed consolidation, nonunion, axial deviation, late bending or fracture); (3) joint (subluxation or contracture); (4) neurovascular (acute or delayed nerve or vessel injury, local edema, systemic hypertension, reflex sympathetic dystrophy, or compartment syndromes); and (5) psychological problems.

Despite a lower complication rate than that reported for the traditional Wagner technique, experience with DO for limb lengthening still reveals higher complication rates than those reported by Ilizarov. Quite a disparity exists when comparing the complication rates of Wagner (45%), DeBastiani (14%), and Ilizarov (5%), and an even greater disparity (1% to 225%) exists when comparing all series, related to differing definitions of "complication."

In 2 independent reports, major complication rates were carefully compared to the surgeon's experience. It was found that complications dropped significantly with experience, from 72% to 25% after the first 30 cases and from 69% to 35% after the first year of using the Ilizarov method on a regular basis. The incidence of minor complications remained relatively constant, independent of surgeon experience and fixator type.

Generally, the number of complications and failed lengthenings increases proportional to the length of the distraction. The number of complications was correlated to the severity of the preoperative problem and not the type of external fixator used. The immediate postoperative pain of an Ilizarov procedure was found to be similar in magnitude to that of a standard orthopaedic operation (osteotomy), but pain of some degree persisted throughout the entire period of external fixation. Pin site inflammation has been reported to occur in 95% of the patients and 10% of the total number of pins, with the majority (97% of patients and 99.7% of pins) resolved by local pin care and/or a short course (5 days) of oral antibiotics. Joint subluxation and contracture are 2 of the more serious complications that can be minimized by special preoperative planning and therapy during fixation.

Annotated Bibliography

Fracture Healing

Augat P, Merk J, Ignatius A, et al: Early, full weightbearing with flexible fixation delays fracture healing. *Clin Orthop* 1996;328:194–202.

In this experimental study using sheep, the effect of early weightbearing on healing was evaluated. Early weightbearing resulted in greater abundance of callus but a slower development of flexural rigidity within the callus. This suggests that early protection from weightbearing may be advantageous in fractures fixed with flexible fixation systems.

Bland YS, Critchlow MA, Ashhurst DE: Exogenous fibroblast growth factors-1 and -2 do not accelerate fracture healing in the rabbit. *Acta Orthop Scand* 1995;66:543–548.

FGF-1 and FGF-2 were not found to have a significant effect on the natural healing process in a rabbit tibial fracture model.

Bostrom MP, Lane JM, Berberian WS, et al: Immunolocalization and expression of bone morphogenetic proteins 2 and 4 in fracture healing. *J Orthop Res* 1995;13:357–367.

In this experimental study using a rat femoral fracture model, monoclonal antibodies to BMP-2 and BMP-4 were used to determine the expression or presence of these 2 growth factors in the fracture callus.

The investigators found abundant staining for both BMP-2 and BMP-4 during early stages of healing when chondrogensis and osteogenesis were actively occurring. Their presence disappeared when remodeling phases began.

Brighton CT, Shaman P, Heppenstall RB, Esterhai JL Jr, Pollack SR, Friedenberg ZB: Tibial nonunion treated with direct current, capacitive coupling, or bone graft. Clin Orthop 1995;321: 223–234.

The authors reviewed 271 nonunions of the tibia. Three treatment methods were compared, and 7 risk factors for failure of treatment were identified.

Chapman MW, Bucholz R, Cornell C: Treatment of acute fractures with a collagen-calcium phosphate graft material: A randomized clinical trial. J Bone Joint Surg 1997;79A:495–502.

The authors present the results of a multicenter, prospective study of a composite bone graft substitute used as an alternative to autogenous grafting of acute long-bone fractures. The study was randomized assigning patients to either an autogenous graft or a graft substitute. Follow-up evaluation radiographically and clinically showed no difference in outcome. Infection rate was lower in the graft substitute group. The authors concluded that this composited bone graft substitute was effective when used to graft acute long-bone fractures.

Cook SD, Ryaby JP, McCabe J, Frey JJ, Heckman JD, Kristiansen TK: Acceleration of tibia and distal radius fracture healing in patients who smoke. Clin Orthop 1997;337:198–207.

Ultrasound stimulation of tibial and distal radial fractures was found to mitigate the delayed healing effect of smoking and to reduce the incidence of delayed union in a smoking population compared to non-smokers.

Cook SD, Wolfe MW, Salkeld SL, Rueger DC: Effect of recombinant human osteogenic protein-1 on healing of segmental defects in non-human primates. J Bone Joint Surg 1995;77A:734–750.

The effect of recombinant human osteogenic protein-1 (OP-1) on the healing of segmental bone defects was studied in monkeys. An ulnar defect model was used. Human OP-1 elicited healing that was superior to healing elicited by autogenous bone graft.

Court-Brown CM, Keating JF, Christie J, McQueen MM: Exchange intramedullary nailing: Its use in aseptic tibial nonunion. J Bone Joint Surg 1995;77B:407–411.

The authors' experience with exchange nailing for aseptic tibial nonunions is presented. The authors found the technique useful for all closed fractures and for grade I, II, and IIIA open fractures. The technique failed in grade IIIB fractures with segmental bone loss. A protocol is presented.

Einhorn TA: Enhancement of fracture-healing. J Bone Joint Surg 1995;77A:940–956.

This is a review of the current understanding of the physiology of fracture healing and the status of experimental efforts to enhance it.

Gazdag AR, Lane JM, Glaser D, Forster RA: Alternatives to autogenous bone graft: Efficacy and indications. J Am Acad Orthop Surg 1995;3:1–8.

This is a scholarly review of the status of bone grafting and the indications for use of various substitutes for autogenous grafts in management of acute fractures.

Goodship AE, Watkins PE, Rigby HS, Kenwright J: The role of fixator frame stiffness in the control of fracture healing: An experimental study. J Biomech 1993;26:1027–1035.

The effects of adjustments in the stiffness of external fixation on the healing of transverse osteotomies in ovine tibia were studied. Increased stiffness of the external fixator slowed the rate of healing. A technique useful in testing the degree of healing by instrumenting the external fixator is reviewed.

Green SA: Skeletal defects: A comparison of bone grafting and bone transport for segmental skeletal defects. Clin Orthop 1994;301:111–117.

Two techniques for management of severe bone loss associated with tibial nonunion were studied. The author presents a protocol which combines aspects of both techniques.

Heckman JD, Ryaby JP, McCabe J, Frey JJ, Kilcoyne RF: Acceleration of tibial fracture-healing by non-invasive low-intensity pulsed ultrasound. J Bone Joint Surg 1994;76A:26–34.

A prospective, randomized clinical trial is reported in which effect of ultrasound on fracture healing was tested in 77 closed, stable tibial fractures treated by long leg cast. Ultrasound conclusively accelerated the time to union.

Kristiansen TK, Ryaby JP, McCabe J, Frey JJ, Roe LR: Accelerated healing of distal radial fractures with the use of specific, low-intensity ultrasound: A multicenter prospective, randomized, double-blind, placebo-controlled study. J Bone Joint Surg 1997;79A:961–973.

Ultrasound was found to be an effect accelerator of fracture healing in a prospective, double-blind, placebo-controlled trial of distal tibial fractures amenable to closed reduction and casting.

Nemzek JA, Arnoczky SP, Swenson CL: Retroviral transmission in bone allotransplantation: The effects of tissue processing. Clin Orthop 1996;324:275–282.

The authors demonstrate that routine processing of bone allografts does not eliminate the transmission of retroviral infection to recipients.

Noordeen MH, Lavy CB, Shergill NS, Tuite JD, Jackson AM: Cyclical micromovement and fracture healing. J Bone Joint Surg 1995;77B:645–648.

The authors report a prospective, randomized trial in 56 patients with tibial shaft fractures stabilized with three different external fixation systems. Group I was dynamized at 4 weeks; group II was dynamized at 4 weeks but the fixator caused a cyclical movement; and group III allowed cyclical movement from the start. Cyclical movement delayed fracture healing compared with simple dynamization.

34   General Knowledge

Patzakis MJ, Scilaris TA, Chon J, Holtom P, Sherman R: Results of bone grafting for infected tibial nonunion. *Clin Orthop* 1995;315:192–198.

The authors' results with management of infected tibial nonunions are reviewed. Autogenous bone grafting combined with infection control methods was successful in 29 of 32 patients.

Schenck RK, Hunziker E: Histologic and ultrastructural features of fracture healing, in Brighton CT, Friedlaender GE, Lane JM (eds): *Bone Formation and Repair*. Rosemont, IL, American Academy of Orthopaedic Surgeons, 1994, pp 117–146.

The influence of blood supply and mechanical influences is carefully reviewed in this up-to-date and scholarly review of the current knowledge of the biology of fracture repair.

Scott G, King JB: A prospective, double-blind trial of electrical capacitive coupling in the treatment of non-union of long bones. *J Bone Joint Surg* 1994;76A:820–826.

A prospective, randomized, placebo-controlled trial of capacitive coupling in the treatment of stable, hypertrophic nonunions is described. Capacitive coupling yielded significantly better results.

Seibold R, Schlegel U, Kessler SB, Cordey J, Perren SM, Schweiberer L: Healing of spiral fractures in the sheep tibia comparing different methods: Osteosynthesis with internal fixation, interlocking nailing and dynamic compression plate. *Unfallchirurg* 1995;98:620–626.

The authors report a histologic and biomechanical study of healing of sheep osteotomies stabilized by differing methods of fixation.

Stevenson S, Li XQ, Davy DT, Klein L, Goldberg VM: Critical biological determinants of incorporation of non-vascularized cortical bone grafts: Quantification of a complex process and structure. *J Bone Joint Surg* 1997;79A:1–16.

The authors studied the incorporation of bone grafts of varying degrees of immunohistocompatibility. They found that incorporation of grafts is profoundly affected by histocompatibility.

Vander Griend RA: The effect of internal fixation on the healing of large allografts. *J Bone Joint Surg* 1994;76A:657–663.

The author has reviewed his experience with bulk allografts. Stable fixation was found to be critical for healing with the host bone. No difference between plate fixation and intramedullary fixation was noted as long as stable fixation in all planes was achieved.

Wallace AL, Draper ER, Strachan RK, McCarthy ID, Hughes S: The vascular response to fracture micromovement. *Clin Orthop* 1994;301:281–290.

This experimental study using ovine tibial osteotomies demonstrates the influence of the initial mechanical environment on the revascularization of the fracture site. Greater initial stiffness was associated with earlier return of blood flow to the fracture.

Watson JT, Anders M, Moed BR: Management strategies for bone loss in tibial shaft fractures. *Clin Orthop* 1995;315:138–152.

The authors review their experience with tibial reconstruction following severe open fractures with bone loss. They have developed a protocol that calls for free tissue transfer to cover open wounds and bone grafting beneath the flap directly into the skeletal defect. Direct grafting was found to be superior to posterolateral graft placement.

Weitzel PP, Esterhai JL Jr: Delayed union, nonunion, and synovial pseudarthrosis, in Brighton CT, Friedlaender GE, Lane JM (eds): *Bone Formation and Repair*. Rosemont, IL, American Academy of Orthopaedic Surgeons, 1994, pp 505–527.

The authors review the classification and management of nonunions.

Wenda K, Degreif J, Runkel M, Ritter G: Technique of plate osteosynthesis of the femur. *Unfallchirurg* 1994;97:13–18.

In this clinical study, 39 patients with complex femoral fractures were treated by plating without grafting. The authors describe the technique of biologic plating, which minimizes vascular injury to the bone. All 39 fractures healed without infection. Excellent healing of the medial cortex was noted in 37 patients; 8 subsequently required bone grafts to achieve union.

Wiss DA, Stetson WB: Tibial nonunion: Treatment alternatives. *J Am Acad Orthop Surg* 1996;4:249–257.

In this thorough review of the etiology of tibial nonunion, a detailed approach to management is presented. The results of various approaches to treatment are reviewed.

Wright TW, Miller GJ, Vander Griend RA, Wheeler D, Dell PC: Reconstruction of the humerus with an intramedullary fibular graft: A clinical and biomechanical study. *J Bone Joint Surg* 1993;75B:804–807.

In this series of 8 patients, repair of the humerus was augmented by an intramedullary fibula autograft. The authors refer to this as quadricortical fixation. The biomechanical study demonstrates that the quadricortical fixation is as strong as augmentation with methylmethacrylate.

Distraction Osteogenesis

Aronson J: Limb-lengthening, skeletal reconstruction, and bone transport with the Ilizarov method. *J Bone Joint Surg* 1997;79A:1243–1258.

This article is a comprehensive review of the basic science and clinical applications of this method; it has extensive references.

Aronson J: Experimental and clinical experience with distraction osteogenesis. *Cleft Palate Craniofac J* 1994;31:473–481.

A single surgeon reviews his first 100 cases of the Ilizarov method, including types of applications, results, and complications.

Coglianese DB, Herzenberg JE, Goulet JA: Physical therapy management of patients undergoing limb lengthening by distraction osteogenesis. *J Orthop Sports Phys Ther* 1993;17: 124–132.

The authors describe regimens of physical therapy used for these patients.

Dahl MT, Gulli B, Berg T: Complications of limb lengthening: A learning curve. *Clin Orthop* 1994;301:10–18.

Experience with the Ilizarov method is compared to the Wagner and Debastianni techniques with respect to complications, and a learning curve is plotted.

Paley D, Herzenberg JE, Paremain G, Bhave A: Femoral lengthening over an intramedullary nail: A matched-case comparison with Ilizarov femoral lengthening. *J Bone Joint Surg* 1997;79A:1464–1480.

The authors introduce the lengthening-over-a-nail method with follow-up results.

Young N, Bell DF, Anthony A: Pediatric pain patterns during Ilizarov treatment of limb length discrepancy and angular deformity. *J Pediatr Orthop* 1994;14:352–357.

Methods for grading pediatric pain are presented and correlated to the Ilizarov treatment.

Classic Bibliography

Bucholz RW, Carlton A, Holmes RB: Interporous hydroxyapatite as a bone graft substitute in tibial plateau fractures. *Clin Orthop* 1989;240:53–62.

Cheal EJ, Mansmann KA, DiGioia AM III, Hayes WC, Perren SM: Role of interfragmentary strain in fracture healing: Ovine model of healing osteotomy. *J Orthop Res* 1991;9:131–142.

Cierny G III, Mader JT, Penninck JJ: A clinical staging system for adult osteomyelitis. *Contemp Orthop* 1985;10:17–37.

Enneking WF, Burchardt H, Puhl JJ, Piotrowski G: Physical and biological aspects of repair in dog cortical-bone transplants. *J Bone Joint Surg* 1975;57A:237–252.

Green SA: Ilizarov method. *Clin Orthop* 1992;280:2–6.

Green SA: Postoperative management during limb lengthening. *Orthop Clin North Am* 1991;22:723–734.

Ilizarov GA: Clinical application of the tension-stress effect for limb lengthening. *Clin Orthop* 1990;250:8–26.

Joyce ME, Roberts AB, Sporn MD, Bolander ME: Transforming growth factor-beta and the initiation of chondrogensis and oseogenesis in the rat femur. *J Cell Biol* 1990;110:2195–2207.

Mast J, Jakob R, Ganz R (eds): *Planning and Reduction Technique in Fracture Surgery*. Berlin, Germany, Springer-Verlag, 1989.

May JW Jr, Jupiter JB, Weiland AJ, Byrd HS: Clinical classification of post-traumatic tibial osteomyelitis. *J Bone Joint Surg* 1989;71A:1422–1428.

Meister K, Segal D, Whitelaw GP: The role of bone grafting in the treatment of delayed unions and nonunions of the tibia. *Orthop Rev* 1990;19:260–271.

Paley D: Current techniques of limb lengthening. *J Pediatr Orthop* 1988;8:73–92.

Paley D: Problems, obstacles, and complications of limb lengthening by the Ilizarov technique. *Clin Orthop* 1990;250:81–104.

Paley D, Chaudray M, Pirone AM, Lentz P, Kautz D: Treatment of malunions and mal-nonunions of the femur and tibia by detailed preoperative planning and the Ilizarov techniques. *Orthop Clin North Am* 1990;21:667–691.

Pals SD, Wilkins RM: Giant cell tumor of bone treated by curettage, cementation, and bone grafting. *Orthopedics* 1992;15:703–708.

Tiedeman JJ, Connolly JF, Strates BS, Lippiello L: Treatment of nonunion by percutaneous injection of bone marrow and demineralized bone matrix: An experimental study in dogs. *Clin Orthop* 1991;268:294–302.

Velazquez RJ, Bell DF, Armstrong PF, Babyn P, Tibshirani R: Complications of use of the Ilizarov technique in the correction of limb deformities in children. *J Bone Joint Surg* 1993;75A: 1148–1156.

Wagner H: Operative lengthening of the femur. *Clin Orthop* 1978;136:125–142.

Yasko AW, Lane JM, Fellinger EJ, Rosen V, Wozney JM, Wang EA: The healing of segmental bone defects, induced by recombinant human bone morphogenetic protein (rhBMP-2): A radiographic, histological, and biomechanical study in rats. *J. Bone Joint Surg* 1992;74A:659–670.

Younger EM, Chapman MW: Morbidity at bone graft donor sites. *J Orthop Trauma* 1989;3:192–195.

Chapter 3
Biomechanics and Gait

Introduction

Objective measurements of human movement are becoming an important component in the treatment of musculoskeletal conditions. The primary measures of human movement include descriptors of motion (kinematics) and force (kinetics). These kinematic and kinetic parameters are particularly relevant to understanding the pathomechanics of human movement. This chapter will focus on the description of these kinematic and kinetic parameters and identify clinically relevant applications.

Human Movement

Description

Human locomotion is often described by the relative angles between adjacent limb segments. In general, limb motion takes place in 3 dimensions, although in practice, sagittal plane motion of adjacent lower extremity segments (flexion-extension) is primarily used in the analysis of locomotion. The complexity of kinematic analysis substantially increases when going from a sagittal plane analysis to a complete 3-dimensional (3-D) analysis. Overall, the relative motion of 1 limb segment with respect to an adjacent limb segment can be described by 6 independent parameters. In mechanical terms, this means there are 6 independent degrees of freedom (3 translational and 3 rotational) that describe the motion of a segment in 3 dimensions. Recent studies have used fluoroscopic techniques to study 3-D knee movement from planar images. Although these methods show promise, they are still limited by a small field of view and technical concerns regarding the ability to dissolve a 3-D motion from 2-D images.

Normal patterns of flexion-extension motion are surprisingly reproducible and consistent among the normal population. Given the complexity of normal human locomotion, a much greater degree of variability in the patterns of flexion-extension motion among normal subjects would be expected. It is useful to examine these kinematic parameters in terms of the subdivisions of the gait cycle because the timing of deviations from the normal patterns often indicate specific pathology.

The stance phase of gait is typically described in terms of 5 segments: initial contact, loading response, midstance, terminal stance, and preswing. Swing phase has been described in terms of initial swing, midswing, and terminal swing. At initial contact, the hip joint is in a flexed position (approximately 30°), the knee joint is near full extension, and the ankle is slightly plantarflexed (Fig. 1). As the limb moves into the loading response phase, the hip joint extends, the knee joint flexes, and the ankle joint dorsiflexes. At midstance phase, the hip joint continues to extend from its initially flexed position, the knee joint reaches a relative maximum, and the ankle remains in a dorsiflexed position. As the limb goes into terminal stance, the hip reaches an extended position, the knee flexes in preparation for swing phase, and the ankle plantarflexes. During initial swing phase, the hip and knee flex while the ankle moves toward dorsiflexion from an initially plantarflexed position. In terminal swing, the hip reaches maximum flexion, the knee extends for heelstrike, and the ankle plantarflexes.

The relatively small standard deviation of the motion curves (Fig. 1) at the hip, knee, and ankle suggests that the characteristics of these patterns do not vary substantially during normal gait. However, care must be taken in measuring certain peak amplitudes, because it has been shown that these values are related to walking speed. For example, the maximum stance phase flexion during midstance increases linearly with walking speed and, thus, in attempting to evaluate this parameter between normal controls and patients with walking abnormalities, controlling for walking speed is important. The influence of walking speed is an important consideration for almost all aspects of gait analysis.

Clinical Example: Hip Osteoarthritis

Kinematic measurements can help quantify specific joint involvement associated with a particular type of walking disability. Often patients will adapt their patterns of locomotion to stimuli such as pain, instability, neuromuscular disability, or muscular weakness. Biomechanical analysis of the adaptation provides more information that can reveal the nature of the underlying abnormality.

For example, patients with hip pain and flexion contractions caused by osteoarthritis adopt an abnormal gait pattern. Studies have shown that patients with hip osteoarthritis

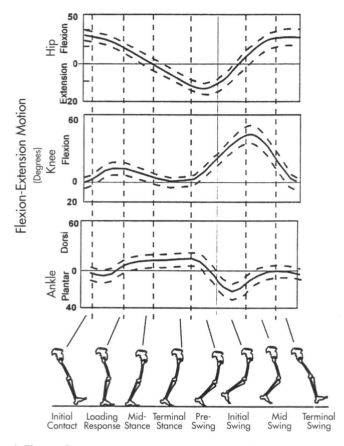

Figure 1

In this figure the stance phase is divided into 5 segments and the swing phase into 3. The curves represent the normal patterns of motion for the hip, knee, and ankle. The limb below the curves illustrates the position of the pelvis, thigh, and tibia as they would be observed during each of these segments of the gait cycle. The normal sequence of events is reproducible as indicated by the relatively narrow standard deviation (dashed-line segments) for the group of normal subjects.

walked with a decreased dynamic hip range of motion (17° + 4°) (Fig. 2). The majority (74%) of osteoarthritic patients displayed a similar abnormality on the affected side that consisted of a hesitation or reversal in the flexion-extension motion as they reached the limit of their hip extension motion during stance. This hesitation or reversal in motion was evident in only 5% of the normal subjects. Patients with a hesitation or reversal in hip motion had a greater loss in hip range of motion during gait and a greater passive flexion contracture than patients with a smooth pattern of hip motion. The reversal or hesitation in the hip motion may be reflective of a mechanism to increase hip extension during gait. One possible mechanism to compensate for inadequate hip exten-

sion would be to increase lumbar lordosis and flex the pelvis forward.

Loads on the Musculoskeletal System

Many gait adaptations are associated with changes in muscle and joint loading. These loads substantially influence the progression and treatment of musculoskeletal problems. The motion of the musculoskeletal system is the result of a balance between external and internal forces. The external forces on the skeletal system include gravity, inertia, and foot-ground reaction forces during walking. Internal forces are created by muscle contraction, passive soft-tissue stretching, and bony contact at joint articulations. At any instant during walking or any activity of daily living, the external forces and moments must be balanced by internal forces and moments. Joint moments can be used to interpret internal forces within the muscles and on the joint surfaces. For example, a flexion moment at the knee is generated when the ground reaction force vector passes posterior to the knee (Fig. 3). This moment is balanced internally by contraction of the quadriceps muscles. Similarly, as the ground reaction force vector passes anterior to the knee joint, an external extension moment is generated. This moment is balanced internally by the knee flexor muscles.

Thus, the moments measured in the gait laboratory (external moments) can be used to infer the net balance between joint flexor and extensor muscles, because these muscles generate most of the internal moment producing flexion or extension at the joint. Similarly, in the frontal plane, the abduction-adduction moments can be directly related to internal forces. When the appropriate care is taken in the interpretation of joint moments, they can be extremely valuable in identifying changes in patterns of muscle activity in joint loading because they are very sensitive to abnormal functional changes.

Characteristics of Flexion-Extension Moments

Normal patterns of net flexion and extension moments at the hip, knee, and ankle are illustrated in Figure 4. It is useful to examine the characteristics of the moment curves during the 5 segments of stance phase. These curves are quite reproducible in a normal population. Typically, at initial contact the loads acting on the lower extremity require net hip extension moments, net knee flexion moments, and net ankle dorsiflexion moments for equilibrium. Moving into the loading response phase, there is still a net hip extension moment, the knee moment reverses to a net extension moment, and the

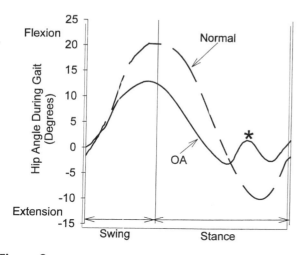

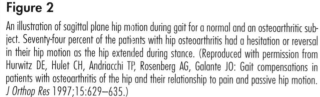

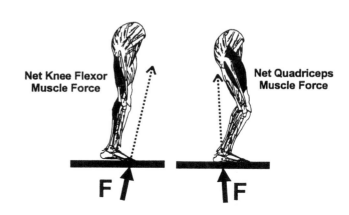

Figure 2

An illustration of sagittal plane hip motion during gait for a normal and an osteoarthritic subject. Seventy-four percent of the patients with hip osteoarthritis had a hesitation or reversal in their hip motion as the hip extended during stance. (Reproduced with permission from Hurwitz DE, Hulet CH, Andriacchi TP, Rosenberg AG, Galante JO: Gait compensations in patients with osteoarthritis of the hip and their relationship to pain and passive hip motion. *J Orthop Res* 1997;15:629–635.)

Figure 3

As the ground reaction force passes anterior to the knee joint an external moment tending to extend the knee is generated. This moment is balanced by a net moment created by knee flexor muscle contraction. Similarly, a ground reaction force posterior to the knee is balance by net quadriceps muscle contraction. (Reproduced with permission from Andriacchi TP, Hurwitz DE, Bush-Joseph CA, Bach BR Jr: Clinical implications of functional adaptations in patients with ACL deficient knees. *Sportorthopadie-Sporttraumatologie* 1997;13: 153–160.)

ankle becomes a net plantarflexion moment. In midstance, the net hip extension moment reduces to zero, the knee moment reverses again to a net flexion moment, and the ankle moment continues as a net plantarflexion moment. During terminal stance, the hip moment reverses to a net flexion moment, the knee moment remains a flexion moment, and the ankle remains a plantarflexion moment. During preswing, only the knee moment changes direction from flexor to a net extensor muscle moment. The muscle moments depicted in Figure 4 are the net balance between the flexors and extensors. Electromyographic (EMG) activity shows that at heel strikes, both flexors and extensors are active at both the hip and knee joint. The presence of antagonistic muscle activity at this phase of the gait cycle is probably the result of the need to stabilize the limb for initial contact. It should be emphasized that the gait laboratory measurements provide external measures of moments acting at the limb. The internal net moments described here are inferred from these external measurements.

The component of the joint moment tending to flex and extend the joint is very important in the analysis of gait. The flexion-extension component is associated with propulsion during walking as well as lowering and raising the body against gravity. Examining the factors that influence the magnitude of the flexion-extension moments is useful, because these parameters can be related to the muscle and joint forces.

Clinical Example: Anterior Cruciate Deficient Knee

Most studies have shown that the flexion-extension moment at the knee is quite sensitive to subtle changes in motion. For example, in a study of patients with ruptured anterior cruciate ligaments (ACLs), it has been shown that a substantial change in the pattern of flexion-extension moment can be seen during level walking. Patients with ACL-deficient knees tested in the gait laboratory have a significantly lower than normal net quadriceps moment during the middle portion of stance phase. Commonly, the net moment reverses from one demanding net quadriceps activity to one demanding net hamstrings activity. This type of gait has been interpreted as a tendency to avoid or reduce the demand on the quadriceps muscle and has been called a "quadriceps avoidance." This quadriceps avoidance gait in chronic ACL-deficient patients may seem surprising because the demand on the quadriceps muscles is relatively low during walking. However, despite the relatively low demands on the knee that occur during level walking, 75% of the patients in a recent report had the quadriceps avoidance gait and 25% had a normal biphasic flexion-extension moment (Fig. 5). This quadriceps avoidance gait can be associated with the loss of the ACL. Near full extension, the patellar ligament at the knee tends to place an anterior pull on the tibia. The quadriceps avoidance gait seen

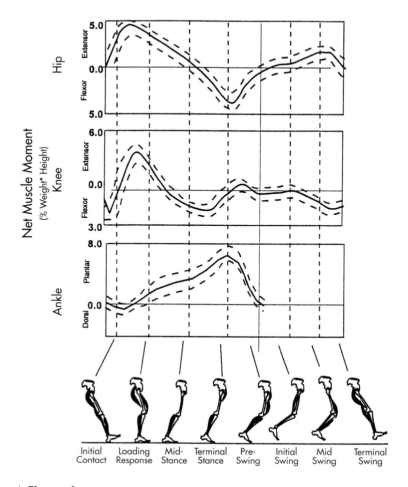

Figure 4

The typical net moments required to balance external loads acting on the limb during walking. The moments are expressed as net muscle moments because they are the minimum internal moments required to balance the externally acting moments in the absence of antagonistic muscle activity. These patterns are typical of a normal gait at an average walking speed.

knee (depending on walking speed). The magnitude and cyclic nature of the compressive force in the tibiofemoral joint are important considerations in the design of a total joint replacement. Failure due to cyclic fatigue of both interfaces and implant materials must be considered.

Another important loading factor that comes from studies of knee joint forces is related to a substantial asymmetry in the total load across the knee joint. Approximately 70% of the load across the knee joint is sustained by the medial compartment of the knee. The adduction moment is the primary reason for a larger joint reaction force on the medial side of the knee than on the lateral side of the knee. An increase in the adduction moment during walking has been related to an increase in the medial compartment loading on the knee. This information has been generated from basic modeling approaches. Thus, the dynamic adduction moment measured in the gait laboratory can be used as a measure of medial compartment loading. This moment can be applied directly to studies of patients with medial compartment gonarthrosis.

Clinical Example: High Tibial Osteotomy

The clinical outcome of treatment of patients with medial compartment arthritis with high tibial osteotomy has been related to the magnitude of the adduction moment (Fig. 6). The patients were considered to have a high adduction moment if it was higher than 4% body weight times height when walking at a speed of approximately 1 m/s. All other patients were classified as having "low adduction moments." Approximately 50% of the patients with medial compartment gonarthrosis had low adduction moments (lower than 4% body weight times height). Thus, it was possible for approximately 50% of the patients to adapt their gait dynamically to reduce the normal loading across the knee. It has been shown that patients with this adaptive gait tend to have better results than patients with high adduction moments. The patients who had low preoperative adduction moments maintained a better clinical result than did patients in the high adduction moment group at an average of 6 years.

in patients with ACL deficiencies can be associated with a functional adaptation to avoid this anterior pull on the tibia when the knee is near full extension. The anterior pull on the tibia from the patellar mechanism is reduced as the knee approaches 45° and, thus, the adaptation would be greatest near full extension and most apparent during walking.

Forces at the Knee Joint

Studies of forces on the articular surface of the knee joint during gait have used analytical methods to study loading at the knee joint during gait. The general characteristics of the forces at the knee joint show 3 peaks during stance phase. Maximum forces from 4 to 7 body weights can occur at the

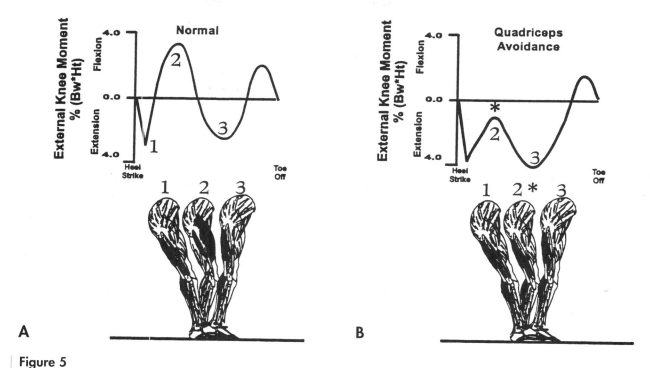

Figure 5

A, The normal flexion-extension moment during the stance phase of gait tended to oscillate between flexion and extension. B, In patients with anterior cruciate ligament deficient knees, the magnitude of the quadriceps demand (2*) was reduced or avoided during stance phase. (Reproduced with permission from Andriacchi TP, Hurwitz DE, Bush-Joseph CA, Bach BR Jr: Clinical implications of functional adaptations in patients with ACL deficient knees. *Sportorthopadie-Sporttraumatologie* 1997;13:153–160.)

Further, 79% of the knees in the low adduction moment group had maintained valgus correction, whereas only 20% of the knees in the high adduction moment group remained in valgus alignment. The adaptive mechanism used by some patients to reduce the adduction moment has been related to a shorter stride length and an increased external rotation (toe-out) of the foot position during stance phase. The adaptation using the toe-out mechanism greatly affected the reduction of the adduction moment during gait. Gait analysis can be used as an additional means of selecting patients who have a higher probability of good results with high tibial osteotomy. It also potentially is used as a basis for training patients to lower the loads at the knee joint.

Forces at the Hip Joint

Hip joint forces have been estimated indirectly using analytical methods and measured directly in vivo with implanted transducers. It is useful to examine and compare information obtained from both approaches. In general, the force at the hip joint reaches an initial peak in early stance phase and a second peak in late stance phase. Although the majority of the information on hip joint forces comes from analytical

prediction, several studies have used direct force measurement using an instrumented prosthesis. The most recent studies have the longest postoperative follow-up of any of the instrumented devices. The peak magnitudes for level walking at normal speeds ranged between approximately 2 and 5 body weights.

The transducer studies showed a similar double-peak pattern to that first obtained using analytical methods. This information is extremely relevant to the analysis of total hip replacement, because it provides not only a description of the magnitude but also the cyclic nature of the load. Many of the failure mechanisms in total joint replacements are not only affected by load magnitude, but by the cyclic nature of the loads. During a single cycle of the support phase of gait, 2 cycles of joint reaction loading occur. Thus, in evaluating cyclic fatigue, 2 cycles of load variation must be considered for every step taken. The studies using instrumented hip joints also raised some important issues regarding the rotational torques generated by the out-of-plane loads at the hip joint. These rotational torques have been related to fixation failure of the femoral component of a total hip replacement. The consistency of the characteristics of the loads reported

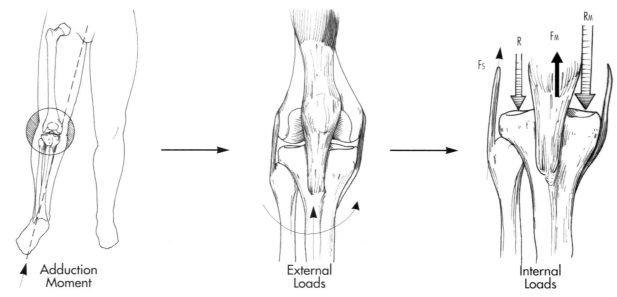

Figure 6

Knee adduction moment during gait. The ground reaction force acting through a lever arm to the center of the knee joint produces the major portion of the adduction moment during gait. Limb segment inertia properties have minimal effect on this calculation. The adduction moment during gait is an external load tending to thrust the knee into varus.

from the various studies is also quite important. The initial analytical work compares favorably with measurements of forces obtained directly from in vivo devices. It is likely that the variations seen between the different studies are more a result of variations in component positioning and walking speed. In addition, the transducer studies are often reported in the early postoperative period when the gait of patients probably is not comparable to normal.

Studies using instrumented implantable devices provide invaluable information that can be used to gain an understanding of the biomechanics of function. This information is useful for comparison to indirect external measurements as described in the early sections of this chapter. The limitations of direct in vivo measurements are, of course, the cost and invasive nature of the test.

Stair Climbing

Description
Stair climbing is a common activity of daily living. The biomechanics of stair climbing provides a basis for analyzing lower extremity joint pathology. Stair climbing requires increased ranges of joint motion, higher muscular demands, and higher joint forces than during level walking. Several events during the climbing cycle are particularly important to the evaluation of knee function. The pattern of knee flexion

motion combined with the flexion moments at the knee joint illustrate the fundamental mechanics of knee function while stair climbing (Fig. 7). At the initiation of the stair climbing cycle the knee is fully extended (preswing). The knee flexes to approximately 90° during swing phase while the foot is clearing the next step. Thus maximum knee flexion occurs during swing phase. The next important event occurs when the foot is planted on the step and the knee begins to extend (extension phase). During this extension phase, the maximum demand is placed on the quadriceps muscles while the knee is at approximately 60° of flexion (Fig. 7). But as the body moves forward, the moment reverses direction, requiring the knee flexor muscles to decelerate forward momentum (deceleration phase).

Clinical Example: Total Knee Replacement
Stair climbing tests have been used to differentiate the functional characteristics of different types of designs during stair climbing. Data from several studies have suggested that patients with cruciate-retaining knee replacements have more normal function while ascending stairs than patients with cruciate-sacrificing replacements. One of the key features of the functional abnormality while ascending stairs was a reduction in the moment sustained by the net quadriceps contraction. Patients with cruciate-sacrificing knee replacements had a tendency to reduce the moment sustained by the quadriceps by leaning forward during the por-

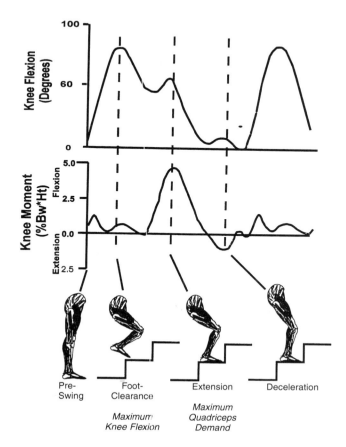

Figure 7

The sagittal plane mechanics of the knee during stair climbing. The knee reaches maximum flexion (approximately 90°) during swing phase as the foot clears the next step. The flexion moment curve demonstrates that the maximum demand on the quadriceps muscles occurs at approximately 60° of knee flexion.

tion of the support phase of ascending stairs when the quadriceps moment would reach a peak value (Fig. 7). The peak moment occurs at 60° of knee flexion. This finding was also consistent with findings in a study in which EMG activity was measured during stair climbing. In that study, maximum quadriceps activity was found in patients with posterior cruciate ligament (PCL)-sparing and substituting designs. However, patients with PCL-sacrificing designs required increased use of the soleus muscle while stair climbing. The increased soleus activity suggested a forward lean, similar to that described in other studies, was occurring in the PCL-sacrificing designs.

The functional differences between the PCL-retaining and PCL-sacrificing designs were associated with the normal posterior movement of the femur on the tibia (rollback) with flexion. This finding has been explained by the dynamic interaction between the PCL and tibiofemoral rollback with flexion and the changing lever arm of the quadriceps. The functional adaptations seen in patients with cruciate-sacrificing designs were likely associated with the need to compensate for the lack of normal femoral rollback in knees where the cruciate ligament is removed. Thus, rollback must occur in the early phases of flexion to have an appropriate quadriceps lever arm to sustain normal stair climbing.

Annotated Bibliography

Sports Medicine

Hurwitz DE, Andriacchi TP, Bush-Joseph CA, Bach BR Jr: Functional adaptations in patients with ACL-deficient knees. *Exerc Sport Sci Rev* 1997;25:1–20.

The identification of gait adaptations over time provides further information on the natural history of ACL deficiency and may have implications regarding conservative rehabilitation, evaluation of outcomes, progression of meniscal injury, and the development of degenerative arthritis of the knee.

Ounpuu S: The biomechanics of walking and running. *Clin Sports Med* 1994;13:843–863.

An increased knowledge of the biomechanics of normal walking and running, through the use of modern computerized gait analysis techniques, will improve understanding of the mechanisms of pathology and ultimately improve the treatment of pathology and injury.

Joint Arthroplasty/Osteoarthritis

Andriacchi TP, Yoder D, Conley A, Rosenberg A, Sum J, Galante JO: Patellofemoral design influences function following total knee arthroplasty. *J Arthroplasty* 1997;12:243–249.

The functional influence of patellofemoral design was evaluated by testing 2 cohorts of patients with total knee arthroplasty during daily activities. The results suggest a relationship between a nonanatomic trochlea and abnormal function during stair climbing, whereas the group with the anatomic trochlea did not have abnormal function.

Bergmann G, Graichen F, Rohlmann A, Linke H: Hip joint forces during load carrying. *Clin Orthop* 1997;335:190–201.

This study determined by instrumented implants how the forces in both hip joints are influenced by the magnitude of the load and the manner in which it is carried.

Bergmann G, Kniggendorf H, Graichen F, Rohlmann A: Influence of shoes and heel strike on the loading of the hip joint. *J Biomech* 1995;28:817–827.

The forces and moments acting at the hip joint influence the long-term stability of the fixation of endoprostheses and the course of coxarthrosis. These loads may depend on the kind of footwear and the walking or running style. These factors were investigated in a patient with instrumented hip implants.

Bryan JM, Sumner DR, Hurwitz DE, Tompkins GS, Andriacchi TP, Galante JO: Altered load history affects periprosthetic bone loss following cementless total hip arthroplasty. *J Orthop Res* 1996; 14:762–768.

Dual energy X-ray absorptiometry and gait analysis were used to measure bone mass and joint loading bilaterally in 8 patients 10 years after unilateral total hip arthroplasty. Asymmetries in bone mass were related to the asymmetries in hip joint loading and demonstrate that reduction in loading after hip arthroplasty can result in a reduction of bone mass.

Chassin EP, Mikosz RP, Andriacchi TP, Rosenberg AG: Functional analysis of cemented medial unicompartmental knee arthroplasty. *J Arthroplasty* 1996;11:553–559.

Gait analysis was used to study patients who underwent cemented medial unicompartmental knee arthroplasty. The results imply that preservation of the ACL during unicompartmental knee arthroplasty allows patients to maintain normal quadriceps mechanics, and that residual varus alignment results in higher loads.

Fisher NM, White SC, Yack HJ, Smolinski RJ, Pendergast DR: Muscle function and gait in patients with knee osteoarthritis before and after muscle rehabilitation. *Disabil Rehabil* 1997; 19:47–55.

This study examined the effects of knee osteoarthritis on gait before and after quantitative progressive exercise rehabilitation. Although clinical measures improved, no significant changes in gait variables were observed after rehabilitation.

Hilding MB, Lanshammar H, Ryd L: A relationship between dynamic and static assessments of knee joint load: Gait analysis and radiography before and after knee replacement in 45 patients. *Acta Orthop Scand* 1995;66:317–320.

An evaluation was made of the relationship between dynamic measurements of knee joint load and static and radiographic measurements of alignment. Correlations were found between the knee joint moments in the frontal plane and the hip-knee-ankle angles as well as between preoperative and postoperative changes in moments and angles.

Hilding MB, Lanshammar H, Ryd L: Knee joint loading and tibial component loosening: RSA and gait analysis in 45 osteoarthritic patients before and after. *J Bone Joint Surg* 1996;78B:66–73.

This study reported a prospective study of gait and tibial component migration in 45 patients with osteoarthritis treated by total knee arthroplasty. A relationship was found between gait with increased flexion moments and risk of tibial component loosening.

Kramers-de Quervain IA, Stussi E, Muller R, Drobny T, Munzinger U, Gschwend N: Quantitative gait analysis after bilateral total knee arthroplasty with two different systems within each subject. *J Arthroplasty* 1997;12:168–179.

The functional behavior of two kinematically different knee arthroplasty systems within each subject was studied after bilateral surgery by gait analysis. Asymmetry seen in the knee motion patterns may be related to other factors such as the patella-extensor mechanism and ligament balancing rather than kinematic design of the implant.

Loizeau J, Allard P, Duhaime M, Landjerit B: Bilateral gait patterns in subjects fitted with a total hip prosthesis. *Arch Phys Med Rehabil* 1995;76:552–557.

This report examined the muscle powers and the mechanical energies developed during gait of patients with a total hip prosthesis. The results demonstrate asymmetry in the powers and energies at the hip and knee between the prosthetic and normal limb. Powers and energies developed bilaterally were reduced compared to those of a control population.

Wilson SA, McCann PD, Gotlin RS, Ramakrishnan HK, Wootten ME, Insall JN: Comprehensive gait analysis in posterior-stabilized knee arthroplasty. *J Arthroplasty* 1996;11:359–367.

Sixteen patients implanted with a posterior stabilized prosthesis were evaluated by isokinetic muscle testing and comprehensive gait analysis. The range of motion during level walking and stair descent was significantly decreased in the study group compared to normal. The external knee flexion moment (net quadriceps moment) was substantially reduced from normal values during stair ascent, although these differences were not statistically significant in this study.

Wimmer MA, Andriacchi TP: Tractive forces during rolling motion of the knee: Implications for wear in total knee replacement. *J Biomech* 1997;30:131–137.

The results of the study suggest that there are feasible conditions following total knee replacement, which can lead to tractive forces during rolling motion at the tibiofemoral articulation, that should be considered in the analysis of factors leading to polyethylene damage in total knee replacement.

Basic Concepts

Andrews M, Noyes FR, Hewett TE, Andriacchi TP: Lower limb alignment and foot angle are related to stance phase knee adduction in normal subjects: A critical analysis of the reliability of gait analysis data. *J Orthop Res* 1996;14:289–295.

Gait analysis and complete radiographic evaluation of the lower extremity were performed on 11 healthy subjects. The results suggest that the alignment of the lower extremity and the foot progress in angle and serve as predictors of knee joint loading. Tests performed on 2 separate days for each subject were compared.

Kerrigan DC, Deming LC, Holden MK: Knee recurvatum in gait: A study of associated knee biomechanics. *Arch Phys Med Rehabil* 1996;77:645–650.

The objective was to quantitatively evaluate peak knee extensor torque values imparted to the posterior knee structures during gait in patients with knee recurvatum. Knowledge of knee hyperextension angle and other clinical factors were only partially useful in predicting peak knee extensor torque imparted to the posterior knee structures.

Shiomi T: Effects of different patterns of stairclimbing on physiological cost and motor efficiency. *J Hum Ergol* (Tokyo) 1994; 23:111–120.

This study investigated the effects of different motion patterns of ascending and descending stairs on oxygen consumption, heart rate, and efficiency. The results suggested that normal climbing has the advantages of lower physiologic cost and higher efficiency than the stepping climb with increased stepping rate.

Simonsen EB, Dyhre-Poulsen P, Voigt M, Aagaard P, Sjogaard G, Bojsen-Moller F: Bone-on-bone forces during loaded and unloaded walking. *Acta Anat* (Basel) 1995;152:133–142.

Joint moments and bone-on-bone forces in the ankle, knee, and hip joint were studied in 7 healthy male subjects during unloaded and loaded walking. The peak joint moments were the most dominant contributor to the peak bone-on-bone forces.

Classic Bibliography

Andriacchi TP, Birac D: Functional testing in the anterior cruciate ligament-deficient knee. *Clin Orthop* 1993;288:40–47.

Andriacchi TP, Galante JO, Fermier RW: The influence of total knee-replacement design on walking and stair-climbing. *J Bone Joint Surg* 1982;64A:1328–1335.

Bergmann G, Graichen F, Rohlmann A: Hip joint loading during walking and running: Measured in two patients. *J Biomech* 1993;26:969–990.

Berman AT, Quinn RH, Zarro VJ: Quantitative gait analysis in unilateral and bilateral total hip replacements. *Arch Phys Med Rehabil* 1991;72:190–194.

Gage JR: An overview of normal walking, in Greene WB (ed): *Instructional Course Lectures XXXIX*. Park Ridge, IL, American Academy of Orthopaedic Surgeons, 1990, pp 291–303.

Inman VT, Ralston HJ, Todd F (eds): *Human Walking*. Baltimore, MD, Williams & Wilkins, 1981.

Lamoreux LW: Kinematic measurements in the study of human walking. *Bull Prosthet Res* 1971;10:3–84

Morrison JB: The mechanics of the knee joint in relation to normal walking. *J Biomech* 1970;3:51–61.

Noyes FR, Schipplein OD, Andriacchi TP, Saddemi SR, Weise M: The anterior cruciate ligament-deficient knee with varus alignment: An analysis of gait adaptations and dynamic joint loadings. *Am J Sports Med* 1992;20:707–716.

Paul JP, McGrouther DA: Forces transmitted at the hip and knee joint of normal and disabled persons during a range of activities. *Acta Orthop Belg* 1975;41(suppl 1):78–88.

Perry J (ed): *Gait Analysis: Normal and Pathological Function.* Thorofare, NJ, Slack, Inc 1992.

Perry J: Determinants of muscle function in the spastic lower extremity. *Clin Orthop* 1993;288:10–26.

Prodromos CC, Andriacchi TP, Galante JO: A relationship between gait and clinical changes following high tibial osteotomy. *J Bone Joint Surg* 1985;67A:1188–1194.

Sutherland DH (ed): *Gait Disorders in Childhood and Adolescence.* Baltimore, MD, Williams & Wilkins, 1984.

Chapter 4
Biomaterials in Total Joint Arthroplasty

Current Issues

Ultra-high molecular weight polyethylene (hereafter called polyethylene) has performed well as a bearing surface in most total joint replacements. However, research efforts continue to make improvements in the material. A prominent issue during the past few years has been the sterilization of polyethylene components. Recent research has shed light on poor fatigue resistance of the material and traced it back to sterilization using gamma radiation in air. Researchers determined that this previous standard sterilization method was initiating a degradative process in the material that was found to be directly correlated to cracking and delamination of the components in service (Fig. 1). As a result of this, the manufacturers have modified their sterilization methods to reduce the potential for fatigue failure in polyethylene.

The current focus has shifted to better understanding the wear of polyethylene and how to reduce wear rates. Wear of the polyethylene typically occurs through 3 mechanisms: abrasion, adhesion, or third body wear. Third body debris has contributed to the wear in a high percentage of retrievals. However, the mechanisms for reducing this factor are primarily through modification of implant designs and surgical techniques. Abrasion and adhesion may be partially addressed by changes in the polyethylene.

Wear in the hip appears to be dominated by adhesive and abrasive mechanisms, whereas in the knee fatigue contributes significantly (Figs. 2 and 3). Therefore, new materials for the hip and knee may be different from each other in the emphasis being placed on fatigue resistance versus maximum reduction in surface wear. Reduction of wear, through altering and enhancing material processing, may increase longevity of the bearings and decrease the incidence of osteolysis and fatigue. The next section describes the fabrication and processing steps of polyethylene, all of which can greatly impact the material and its performance. Special attention is given to enhanced polyethylenes that are currently being introduced.

Powder Fabrication

Polyethylene bearings used in total joint replacements are formed from polyethylene powder, generally using 1 of 3 techniques: direct compression molding of the powder into components, compression molding of powder into sheet, or ram extrusion of the powder into bar stock. In the case of bar and sheet fabrication, these materials are subsequently machined into components.

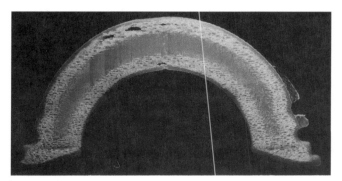

Figure 1
Cross section of an acetabular liner showing a degraded region caused by gamma sterilization in air.

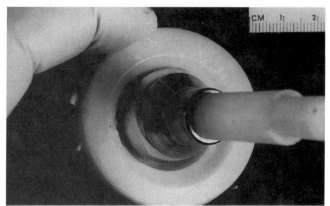

Figure 2
Retrieved acetabular liner showing wear generated by adhesive and abrasive mechanisms.

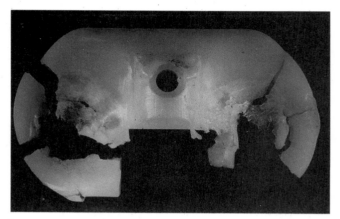

Figure 3

Retrieved tibial tray showing fatigue damage manifest as cracking and delamination.

The polyethylene powder is produced using titanium chloride and an aluminum alkyl catalyst and a co-catalyst. A different co-catalyst, the identity of which is proprietary, is used by each company. This difference results in subtle variations in the powder including trace element levels and particle morphology. The resin is generated via a polymerization process whereby ethylene monomers are linked together and transformed into a polymer chain, which sustains growth provided necessary reactants are supplied.

Physical properties and molecular weight are largely determined by the polymerization process, which can be affected by conditions including temperature and pressure, and by chemicals including the catalyst. Therefore, it is imperative that the reaction be closely monitored and controlled. The powder must pass the standards indicated in the *ASTM Annual Book of Standards*. According to one guideline (F648), if the resulting polyethylene powder has a relative solution viscosity of 2.30 or greater and certain trace element levels, it can be used in medical grade applications, such as total joint replacement.

Powder Grades

There are 3 different types of polyethylene powder typically used in medical grade applications: Hostalen GUR 1150 (previously labeled GUR 415) and Hostalen GUR 1120 (previously labeled 412) (Hoechst Celanese and Hoechst Germany), and Himont 1900. Each type is available both with and without the addition of calcium stearate (in the case of GUR products, 1120 without stearate is 1020; 1150 with-

out stearate is 1050). This metal stearate was historically added to the resin (0.05% of the total volume) to act as a lubricant, anticorrosive agent, and whitener. However, recent questions about the possible contribution of calcium stearate to the wear of polyethylene have led to use of calcium-free materials by many manufacturers.

Slight differences in properties, due to differing molecular weights, account for some differences between the aforementioned resins. Other important differences between Himont 1900 and the GUR powders include the particle morphology (1900 is flake-like and the GUR powders more spherical) and the ability to mold the powder. Several manufacturers have reported that 1900 resin is easier to mold, although both powders have been used in some applications.

Polyethylene Stock and Component Fabrication

Polyethylene components used in total joint replacement are typically made using 1 of 2 processes. Components are either formed by machining or compression molding. In the first case, components are machined directly from either polyethylene sheet or bar stock supplied from a converter (Perplas, Lancaster, England; Poly Hi Solidur, Fort Wayne, IN; Westlake Plastics, Lenni, PA; Hoechst, Germany) using one of the powders described above. Compression molded components are made by molding powder directly into the required geometry. In both stock formation and direct compression molding, control of the consolidation parameters including temperature, pressure, atmosphere, time, heating rate, and cooling rate are necessary to ensure a homogeneous and defect-free material (Fig. 4).

Component Packaging and Sterilization

Fully fabricated components are packaged in materials selected by the manufacturer and then sterilized. Most polyethylene components are sealed in plastic containers that are nested within an outer plastic container and a box. The protection that the packaging provides from oxygen infiltration varies depending on the manufacturer and type of sterilization used.

Current methods of sterilization are gamma irradiation, gas plasma, or ethylene oxide gassing. Gamma irradiation of components is the most common method for sterilization and, because the radiation penetrates entirely through the

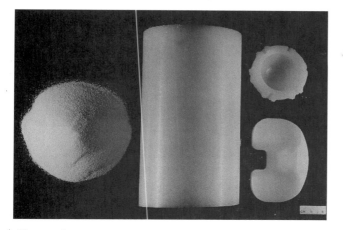

Figure 4

Polyethylene fabrication stages: resin, stock, and final component. (Reproduced with permission from Sutula LC, Collier JP, Wrona M: The role of polyethylene quality in wear, in Callaghan JJ, Dennis OA, Paprosky WG, Rosenberg AG (eds): *Orthopaedic Knowledge Update: Hip and Knee Reconstruction*. Rosemont, IL, American Academy of Orthopaedic Surgeons, 1995, pp 35–41.)

component, is suitable for factory assembled, multipiece designs as well as monoblock components. Components are prepackaged, historically in air, but currently in an inert atmosphere, such as argon or nitrogen, or in vacuum. The dose, measured by dosimeters that change color according to absorbed dosage, typically ranges from 2.5 to 4.5 Mrads.

The second method for component sterilization is surface sterilization using either ethylene oxide (EtO) or gas plasma. In both techniques, the sterilizing media does not penetrate through the material. As a result, they are suitable for individually packaged components but are not typically used for multipiece designs.

Effects of Sterilization on Polyethylene

Gamma sterilization has long been recognized as having an effect on polymers by causing chain scission, cross-linking, and/or oxidation. The radiation dissociates molecular bonds and generates free radicals in the polymer, which can result in 1 of 3 outcomes: the chains can reattach at the scission points; reattach to other chains causing cross-linking; or combine with oxygen, resulting in oxidation that deteriorates the polyethylene. The process whereby radicals react with oxygen is time dependent and increases with time after irradiation.

This oxidation, which occurs both in storage and in vivo, has been linked to the fatigue failure of joint replacement bearings. Oxidation causes embrittlement of the material and an associated loss of mechanical properties. Long preimplantation shelf lives, which allow oxidation to occur prior to implantation, may leave the polyethylene more vulnerable to in vivo oxidation. The oxidation level of an implant, prior to implantation, may influence the rate of further oxidation in vivo, and thus mechanical properties and clinical performance of the bearings.

Conversely, nonradiation, surface sterilization techniques, such as EtO or gas plasma, do not alter the polymer. Over time, polyethylene sterilized with these methods should resemble and maintain the properties of never-sterilized stock.

Enhanced Polyethylene For Improved Performance

Recently several companies have introduced "enhanced" polyethylenes, which are termed such because of special processing conditions thought to beneficially alter the material. It is suggested by the manufacturers that these conditions may enhance resistance to wear and oxidation. To date, it is unclear whether such changes have a beneficial impact in the clinical arena. One such product is the Hylamer product produced by DuPont (Wilmington, DE). Hylamer and Hylamer M are made from GUR 415 bar stock, which has been isostatically compressed to increase the material crystallinity.

ArCom, produced by Biomet (Warsaw, IN) is another "enhanced" product. ArCom begins with 1900 resin and is compression molded at high pressure, in an argon environment, into bar stock from which components can be made. The ArCom products are also barrier packaged (barrier packaging is airtight) and sterilized in an argon environment. ArCom's manufacturer claims that the material has a higher ultimate tensile strength and a lower wear rate than standard polyethylene.

Duration (Howmedica, Rutherford, NJ) is a product designed to be chemically stable over time following gamma sterilization. Components are machined from bar stock, barrier packaged in an inert environment, and gamma sterilized using standard dosages. Subsequent to sterilization, the implants are heated for some period of time with the goal of increasing the activity of the chains to promote recombination and cross-linking. This action would reduce the number of free radicals, thereby reducing the potential for later oxidation in vivo. The manufacturer also claims improved wear resistance.

The newest approach to increasing the wear resistance of polyethylene involves a focused approach to increasing the amount of cross-linking (currently in the investigational state). Cross-linking of polyethylene changes the properties of the material, resulting in decreased ultimate tensile strength and decreased elongation to failure. Methods for controlled cross-linking include chemical means (peroxide), variable dose gamma irradiation, and electron beam irradiation. Studies indicate substantial reduction in wear associated with cross-linked polyethylene. Recent wear simulator studies indicate that with optimal cross-linking, the type of wear that occurs in acetabular cups can be reduced by greater than 95%. The benefits of cross-linking may not carry over to the types of wear that occur in total knee replacement.

Chemically cross-linked material has been produced in large-scale batches for use in tubing and other commercial applications. However, a concern with this material is that peroxides are still present in the material after cross-linking and could reduce the long-term oxidation resistance of the material in vivo.

Gamma radiation cross-linking involves the use of dosages that are typically greater than standard sterilization doses. Studies of the wear resistance of materials subjected to dosages of up to 100 Mrad have been reported. These higher radiation dosages generate greater numbers of free radicals that, if left in the material, have the potential to cause high rates of oxidation. To prevent this, the irradiated material is heated to near its melting point, which is thought to quench and eliminate many of the free radicals. Finished components require terminal sterilization just as any other orthopaedic prosthesis. Nonradiation methods for terminal sterilization appear to be the preferred option.

In summary, research has led the orthopaedic community to recognize that long-term success with polyethylene joint replacements requires consistent material properties that do not deteriorate in service. The historic use of gamma sterilization in air has been associated with the subsequent oxidation of some retrieved polyethylene components and has resulted in the development of a variety of strategies to reduce the potential for oxidation. All orthopaedic manufacturers have undertaken this effort. Techniques to increase crystallinity and extent of consolidation have been associated with slight improvements in wear as measured by simulators, but there are limited clinical data to support these findings. The recent development of highly cross-linked polyethylene appears to have the potential (as determined by wear simulators) of dramatically improving the wear resistance, but the associated reduction in mechanical properties reported by some researchers indicates that considerable thought about appropriate applications will be required.

Metal-on-Metal Bearings

Despite generally inferior clinical results with metal-on-metal total hip replacements implanted in the 1960s and 1970s, many metal-on-metal implants lasted over 2 decades or are still functioning in patients who received the implant at a young age. The clinical failure of early metal-on-metal prostheses is currently thought to be multifactorial. As has been seen with metal-on-polyethylene hips, loosening can occur as a result of nonbearing factors, such as suboptimal stem and/or cup design, manufacturing, or implantation technique.

Alloys of cobalt and chromium have traditionally been preferred for metal-on-metal bearings in total hip replacement. High chromium content provides good corrosion resistance. Because of their hardness, dispersed carbides improve wear resistance. The size and distribution of the carbides depends on the manufacturing process. The wear resistance and clinical performance of a hard-on-hard bearing are more sensitive to macrogeometry than a metal-on-polyethylene bearing. Clearance is the size of the gap between the surfaces at the equator of the bearing and is a function of the difference in the diameters of the surfaces of the ball and socket. Contact area can be increased by increasing the size (diameter) of the bearing surfaces and/or by decreasing the clearance. Contact stresses are a function of material properties and are inversely proportional to contact area. Clearance also influences lubrication, because the size of the gap has implications for the amount and mechanism of lubrication. The location of the contact area is important. Equatorial contact produces higher frictional torques, and it may have been a factor in the failure of some early designs. Relatively polar contact is preferred.

In a hip simulator study, calculated linear wear rates ranged from 1.3 to 100 μm per million cycles with the corresponding wear volumes ranging from 0.09 to 61 mm^3 per million cycles. For most pairs, the wear rate decreased substantially after the first 0.1 to 0.5 million cycles. The greatest variability among designs and/or alloys was seen during this initial "running in" period after which 14 of 17 pairs demonstrated very low long-term wear rates (0.12 to 0.72 mm^3 per million cycles). The poorest performance was associated with a very high clearance of 630 μm.

The strength of the conclusions of retrieval analyses is limited because of the relatively small number of specimens in each report and the large number of variables. Metal-on-metal bearings have demonstrated combined average femoral and acetabular linear wear rates ranging from less than 4 up to about 12 μm per year and volumetric wear rates from less than 0.5 up to about 25 mm^3 per year. This is about 20 to 100 times lower than that of metal-on-polyethylene. Radial clearances should be on the order of about 50 to 150 μm. Radial clearances exceeding 300 μm have been associated with higher wear. The initial in vivo wear rate of a metal-on-metal bearing (running-in) may be comparatively high but is followed by a lower steady-state wear rate. It is thought that as wear proceeds, the contact area at asperity tips increases and produces a more favorable microgeometry and macrogeometry for lubricant films to separate the surfaces and reduce wear.

Since 1988, a second-generation metal-on-metal bearing has been implanted in Europe. In contrast to early designs, which mated specific ball and cup pairs, improved manufacturing allows any head to be mated to any cup. There have been short-term retrievals for infection, heterotopic ossification, instability, and aseptic loosening. Hips revised for dislocation demonstrated higher wear, likely caused by damage of the head from the dislocations. There appeared to be an initial higher wear rate of 15 to 20 μm per year per component, consistent with running-in of the bearing, followed by a lower long-term rate of about 2 to 5 μm per year per component. In the United States, with up to 4 years' follow-up, the results in a series of 74 hips with this bearing have been good to excellent. Twenty-seven of these patients have a contralateral metal-on-polyethylene bearing hip of similar design, and none of them could detect a difference between the 2 hips. It is likely that a larger number of patients with follow-up on the order of 10 years will be needed to demonstrate any differences between the clinical performance of hips with metal-on-metal bearings and established standards.

The volume of periprosthetic inflammatory tissue associated with metal-on-metal bearings appears to be less than with metal-on-polyethylene; however, osteolysis does occur in hips with metal-on-metal bearings. The metal wear particles are even smaller than the submicron polyethylene wear particles. Little is known about the rates of metallic particle production in vivo, lymphatic transport of metallic particles from the joint, and systemic dissemination. The levels of metal ions in blood and urine are elevated in patients with metal-on-metal bearings. The levels are generally higher in patients with recently implanted joints (< 2 years) compared to those with longer-term implants (> 20 years), which is consistent with a reduction in wear after running-in. The toxicologic significance of these trace metal elevations has not been established, and available data do not answer questions regarding the risks of ion toxicity and carcinogenesis. Rigorous long-term studies are needed. Metal-on-metal bearings currently have investigational status and do not have FDA approval.

Ceramic-on-Ceramic Bearings

Ceramic bearings, made of alumina, have demonstrated the lowest in vivo wear rates to date of any bearing combination. Because of the high modulus and hardness of the material, the wear characteristics are sensitive to design, manufacturing, and implantation variables, and rapid wear has been observed in some cases. Bulk ceramic materials are more biologically inert than metal alloys but the relative size, shape, number, reactivity, and local versus systemic distribution of the respective wear particles has not been determined.

The United States experience with ceramic-on-ceramic has essentially been limited to the Autophor/Xenophor prosthesis that was conceived and initially implanted in Europe by Mittlemeier. The clinical results with the Autophor were generally less satisfactory than those with established metal-on-polyethylene designs. Similar to the interpretation of metal-on-metal bearings based on the clinical performance of the McKee-Farrar prosthesis, interpretation of the performance of the ceramic-on-ceramic bearing has been complicated by the fact that both the cementless femoral stem and the nonarticular portion of the cementless Autophor acetabular component had features that are now recognized as suboptimal. Clinical failure associated with dislocation, neck-socket impingement, and aseptic loosening appears to have been more a function of design features of the stem, the neck, and the outer surface of the cup than of the ceramic-on-ceramic bearing. Performance of the ceramic bearing does appear to be sensitive to implant position. Hips with a lateral opening less than 30° or greater than 55° and/or a high neck-shaft angle (greater than about 140°) are at risk for neck-socket impingement and/or high wear as a result of stress concentration in the very stiff ceramic material.

In a 10-year experience of hips reconstructed with a cemented ceramic-on-ceramic prosthesis, wear of the bearings could not be detected radiographically. The major problem, however, was aseptic loosening of the socket, which occurred not only at the cement-bone interface but also at the ceramic-cement interface. Finite element analysis indicates that the shear stresses at the cement-prosthesis interface are greatly increased with the very stiff alumina socket compared to polyethylene. The 10 to 14 year experience with 77 of 100 hips implanted with a ceramic-on-ceramic bearing include 25 hips revised for loosening associated with gross wear on both sides of the ceramic bearing couple. Similar to other particulates, the ceramic particles appeared to induce granulation tissue along the implant-bone interface. The inconsistent performance of the ceramic-on-ceramic bearings in this series was thought to be due to inhomogeneity of the ceramic material and batch to batch variation in grain composition.

Improvements in the manufacturing of ceramics and ceramic components will minimize or eliminate mechanical problems such as fracture and accelerated wear. It is anticipated that improved ceramic-on-ceramic bearings will be marketed in the United States with established femoral components. To address issues of acetabular component fixation, modular ceramic bearings will be combined with established cementless acetabular shells. Such ceramic-on-ceramic bearings currently have investigational status and do not have FDA approval.

Annotated Bibliography

Amstutz HC: Metal on metal hip prostheses: Past performance and future directions. Association of Bone and Joint Surgeons workshop. *Clin Orthop* 1996;329(suppl):S2–S303.

Clinical success and failure are multifactorial. Loosening can occur as a result of nonbearing factors, such as suboptimal stem and/or cup design, manufacturing, or implantation technique. The wear resistance and clinical performance of a hard-on-hard bearing are more sensitive to macrogeometry than those of a metal-on-polyethylene bearing. The toxicologic significance of metal particles and metal ions has not been established, and available data do not answer questions regarding the risks of ion toxicity and carcinogenesis.

Currier BH, Currier JH, Collier JP, Mayor MB, Scott RD: Shelf life and in vivo duration: Impacts on performance of tibial bearings. *Clin Orthop* 1997;342:111–122.

Not all retrieved bearings that are gamma sterilized in air exhibit elevated oxidation and mechanical property degradation that lead to early failure. This article investigates why this may not occur in some components and concludes that the preimplantation shelf life of the bearing is a key factor. Bearings with less than 1 year of shelf life after gamma sterilization in air had less degradation and performed better than those with longer shelf lives.

Hoechst Celanese: Hostalen GUR UHMW polymer technical literature. Houston, TX, Hoechst Celanese, 1994.

Material literature contains description of all of the GUR ultra-high molecular weight polyethylene resin available. The chemical and mechanical properties of each grade are documented along with recommended processing conditions.

Jasty M, Bragdon CR, O'Connor DO, et al: Marked improvement in the wear resistance of a new form of UHMWPE in a physiologic hip simulator. *Trans Orthop Res Soc* 1997;22:785.

A new form of polyethylene, created by irradiating polyethylene while melted, is discussed. The new polyethylene had increased cross-linking with minimal oxidation. Cross-linked material was tested in wear stimulator studies; it was found to have an order of magnitude less wear than conventional polyethylene, and was said to show no detectable wear at 3 million cycles.

Livingston BJ, Chmell MJ, Spector M, Poss R: Complications of total hip arthroplasty associated with the use of an acetabular component with a Hylamer liner. *J Bone Joint Surg* 1997; 79A:1529–1538.

The authors observed failure and signs of accelerated wear of Hylamer. Hylamer components wore more than the polyethylene liners in the study. The wear rate for Hylamer liners was greater when the cup was mated with a femoral head that was not from DePuy. The authors suggest that Hylamer performance should be monitored.

Shen FW, McKellop HA, Salovey R: Irradiation of chemically crosslinked ultrahigh molecular weight polyethylene. *J Polymer Sci* 1996;34:1063–1077.

Polyethylene was cross-linked in the presence of peroxide and was subsequently gamma irradiated in air. The irradiation produced further cross-linking and increased crystallinity. The authors indicate that peroxide cross-linking reduces the effect of irradiation on the cross-linked network. Wear rates were found to be lower for the chemically cross-linked cups, which showed about one fifth of the wear of control cups in the range of 0.5 to 1 million cycles.

Sun DC, Stark CF: Non-oxidizing polymeric medical implant. International Patent PCT/IB94/00083. 1994.

The patent involves 2 basic technologies for altering ultra-high molecular weight polyethylene (or other polymers) and for producing superior oxidation resistance on irradiation. Postirradiation annealing to quench free radicals is included, as well as inert atmosphere consolidation and annealing of raw material.

Sutula LC, Collier JP, Saum KA, et al: Impact of gamma sterilization on clinical performance of polyethylene in the hip. *Clin Orthop* 1995;319:28–40.

Gamma sterilization of polyethylene acetabular liners in an air environment was found to cause high subsurface oxidation and reduced strength and ductility in many polyethylene retrievals. The presence of cracking and delamination in retrievals was correlated with the oxidized, embrittled region.

Wroblewski BM, Siney PD, Dowson D, Collins SN: Prospective clinical and joint simulator studies of a new total hip arthroplasty using alumina ceramic heads and cross-linked polyethylene cups. *J Bone Joint Surg* 1996;78B:280–285.

The authors report on findings from a prospective clinical trial and stimulator study of ceramic femoral heads articulation with cross-linked polyethylene. Ceramic-cross-linking combinations had lower average penetration rates than metal-polyethylene couplings. The authors claim excellent tribologic features of ceramic/cross-linked implants.

Classic Bibliography

Boutin P, Christel P, Dorlot JM, et al: The use of dense alumina-alumina ceramic combination in total hip replacement. *J Biomed Mater Res* 1988;22:1203–1232.

Clarke IC: Role of ceramic implants: Design and clinical success with total hip prosthetic ceramic-to-ceramic bearings. *Clin Orthop* 1992;282:19–30.

Ellis JR: Packaging/sterilization: EtO Does it have a future? *Medical Device & Diagnostic Industry* 1990;50–51.

Mahoney OM, Dimon JH III: Unsatisfactory results with a ceramic total hip prosthesis. *J Bone Joint Surg* 1990;72A:663–671.

Mittelmeier H, Heisel J: Sixteen-years' experience with ceramic hip prostheses. *Clin Orthop* 1992;282:64–72.

Nizard RS, Sedel L, Christel P, Meunier A, Soudry M, Witvoet J: Ten-year survivorship of cemented ceramic-ceramic total hip prosthesis. *Clin Orthop* 1992;282:53–63.

Oonishi H, Takayama Y, Tsuji E: Improvement of polyethylene by irradiation in artificial joints. *Radiat Phys Chem* 1992;39:495–504.

Walker PS, Gold BL: The tribology (friction, lubrication and wear) of all-metal artificial hip joints. *Wear* 1971;17:285–299.

Walter A: On the material and the tribology of alumina-alumina couplings for hip joint prostheses. *Clin Orthop* 1992;282:31–46.

Winter M, Griss P, Scheller G, Moser T: Ten- to 14-year results of a ceramic hip prosthesis. Clin Orthop 1992;282:73–80.

Chapter 5
Blood Transfusion

Improved Screening Tests for the Nation's Blood Supply

Risks of transfusion transmitted diseases, especially human immunodeficiency virus (HIV), continue to be the overwhelming concern of patients faced with the possibility of transfusion during surgery. While the risk of previously identified transfusion transmitted diseases continues to decline, new infectious disease risks are being identified or postulated. In March 1996, the United States Food and Drug Administration (FDA) licensed a new HIV screening test for blood products that detects the p24 capsular antigen of the virus. This HIV antigen is detectable about 6 days earlier in the course of an HIV infection than are anti-HIV antibodies, thereby shortening the "window period" of infectivity without positive testing from about 22 days to about 16 days. This test should be considered supplementary to previous HIV testing methods because the presence of p 24 antigen in the circulation is transient early in the disease, requiring the anti-HIV antibody tests for detection in the later course of the disease. Although this test sounds as if it would result in a large reduction in risk, because of the already low incidence of HIV in the 12 million units of blood collected per year, the new test is expected to prevent only 4 to 6 of the estimated 18 to 27 potentially infectious units per year released using the antibody test alone.

Other test modalities, which are presently being studied, include RNA and DNA polymerase chain reaction methods to detect viral genetic material. These molecular biology techniques are still too cumbersome and expensive for donor screening, but they are being evaluated for bulk screening of products such as plasma pools for fractionation into albumin or clotting factor concentrates. The overall risk, nationwide, of HIV infection from a unit of blood is presently considered to be between 1 in 450,000 and 1 in 660,000.

Screening for hepatitis C has also improved since its inception in May 1990. The latest version was approved in May 1996 and detects antibodies directed against the viral core, the RNA polymerase, and nonstructural proteins, shortening the interval between infection and detection of antibody, and has reduced the number of false positive tests. The present

estimate of the chance of a unit transmitting hepatitis C is about 1 in 121,000 units transfused.

Two diseases have recently generated interest as potential transfusion transmitted diseases here in the United States. The first is Creutzfeldt-Jakob disease (CJD). This disease, with an incidence worldwide of about 1 per million, is a transmissible spongiform encephalopathy, which causes rapidly progressive ataxia, dementia, and myoclonus, eventually leading to death. The apparent infective agent for the disease is purported to be an infectious proteinaceous particle, or prion, which has no reproductive capacity itself (no DNA or RNA) but induces a conformational change in native cell proteins that leads to aggregation of these proteins. This disease has gained recent notoriety because of a number of cases of an apparent variant strain of CJD in England, associated with eating beef from cattle with suspected bovine spongiform encephalitis or "mad cow disease." The disease has been transmitted by donor tissue transplants, such as dura mater, corneal transplants, and growth hormone derived from human pituitary glands. There has been no record of transmission of CJD by blood components, and studies have shown no increase in the incidence of CJD when compared to nontransfused controls. Lookback studies involving the recipients of blood components from individuals who later developed CJD show no evidence for transmission. Despite the lack of evidence for transmission by blood components, the FDA has required deferral of all donors with a history of receiving pituitary derived human growth hormone since 1987, and since 1995 has extended its deferral to include any persons having a family history of CJD or a dura mater transplant.

Trypanosoma cruzi, the causative agent of Chagas' disease, has been known for some time to be transmitted by blood components, but only recently has this threat been of concern in the United States and Canada. Transmission by transfusion is common in endemic areas of Central and South America, where the problem has been addressed by a combination of donor screening tests in minimally affected areas and by addition of gentian violet and ascorbate to all blood collections in heavily affected areas. In the United States and Canada there have been only 3 documented cases of Chagas' disease transmitted by transfusion, all from donors who had lived in endemic regions. With increasing immigration to the United States from Middle and South America, this may become a more severe problem. No FDA approved test is presently available.

Recent Additions to the "Alphabet Soup" of Hepatitis

Presently our viral hepatitis alphabet goes from hepatitis A to E for fairly well characterized viral disease, hepatitis F and G/GB for not so well characterized disease, and non-A to G hepatitis for the remaining uncharacterized viral hepatitis (Table 1).

Hepatitis A (HAV) and hepatitis E (HEV) are enterically

transmitted viruses; HAV has rarely been documented to be transmitted by blood components or serum, with occasional outbreaks among intravenous drug users. Fecal-oral contamination accounts for the vast majority of HAV and HEV, with HEV being found outside the United States and Canada, mostly in third-world countries in which it is associated with a high (~20%) mortality rate among pregnant women. Acute disease with these viruses may be fulminant and life threatening, but neither is associated with chronic liver disease. A vaccine is available for prevention of HAV but not HEV. A virus causing enterically transmitted hepatitis has tentatively been labeled as hepatitis F, but its naming was probably a bit hasty because the uniqueness of this virus has not been substantiated.

Hepatitis B (HBV), hepatitis C (HCV), and hepatitis D

Table 1
Hepatitis and blood transfusion in the United States

Type	Approximate Risk of Transmission per Unit Transfused	Other Known Modes of Transmission	Vaccine Available
A	Very rare	Enteric	Yes
B	1 in 66,000 to 1 in 200,000	Intravenous drug use Intimate contact Needlestick Perinatal	Yes
C	1 in 121,000	Intravenous drug use Intimate contact Needlestick	No
D	Very rare	Intravenous drug use Intimate contact Needlestick	No
E	Unknown	Enteric	No
G/GB*	Unknown	Intravenous drug use Perinatal	No

* G/GB has not been shown to be an etiologic agent of non-A-E hepatitis and infection with G/GB alone does not appear to cause chronic liver disease

(HDV) are the viruses closely associated with transmission by intravenous drug use, needlestick or sharps injury, or blood components. They are also spread by sexual contact and perinatally, although HCV appears to be spread much less effectively via these routes. With the advent of a vaccine against HBV and its increasing usage, especially among children, it is hoped that physicians will see less and less of the sequelae of chronic HBV infection. Because HBV is transmitted effectively via needlesticks and sharps injuries, all health care workers should be vaccinated. The duration of protection from the vaccine is unknown, but protection from acute disease continues even after the antibody levels become undetectable. Presently, booster vaccination is not routinely recommended except after needlestick or sharps injury from an HBsAg positive source.

HCV accounts for the majority of non-A, non-B viral hepatitis in the United States. Although it is less effectively transmitted by needlestick or sharps injury, these routes continue to be a risk for health care personnel and encourage the adherence to universal precautions against infectious diseases. There is no vaccine or effective postexposure prophylaxis at this time. No neutralizing antibodies are formed against the virus because patients who are anti-HCV positive still harbor virus and transmit the disease.

HDV is a "defective" virus that requires the presence of another hepatitis virus for replication and transmission. This second virus is almost universally HBV. HDV can infect a person concurrently with acute HBV infection or can infect a person who is a chronic carrier or who has chronic HBV disease. The disease is endemic in the Mediterranean region but outbreaks occur in the United States, primarily among intravenous drug users. Acute HDV infection is clinically indistinguishable from HBV infection although it may be more likely to have a fulminant course. HDV coinfection in chronic HBV infection often leads to more rapid disease progression. There is no vaccine for HDV, but vaccination against HBV will prevent transmission because the presence of HBV virions is required.

Hepatitis G (HGV) is a recently described RNA virus; its RNA has been found in a number of patients who have hepatitis serologically and are polymerase chain reaction (PCR) negative for hepatitis A through E. The virus, which appears to be closely related to the family of hepatitis viruses, was first isolated in 1967 from a surgeon with acute hepatitis. This virus family is referred to as the GB viruses. The hepatitis G/GB virus appears to be a distant relation to HCV. Oddly, the virus is rather prevalent, according to the initial screening studies looking for HGV RNA in normal blood donors. An incidence of 1.7% has been reported in normal donors, and about the same percentage in donors who tested high for ala-

nine aminotransferase levels. Patients infected with HGV alone may not exhibit symptoms and do not progress to a chronic disease state. Severe disease appears to be associated with coinfection with HCV. In fact, most HGV RNA positive people show no evidence of any liver dysfunction. The extent of the problem for transfusion recipients, health care workers, and the general public cannot be accurately assessed until more rapid, sensitive, and specific serologic tests become available.

Update on Blood Substitutes

With the advent of the acquired immunodeficiency syndrome (AIDS) era, there has been a renewed push to come up with a reasonable substitute for human red blood cells. Whereas blood transfusion is a relatively safe procedure as far as medical therapies go, there are a number of potential advantages to a successful blood substitute. An ideal blood substitute would be cheap to manufacture, easy to store, and have a long shelf life. It would also be nontoxic, sterile or easily sterilized, easily excreted or metabolized, and it would deliver adequate amounts of oxygen to the patient's tissues. Unfortunately, very few of these parameters have been met by the recent generations of blood substitutes.

The first substitute used in humans was the perfluorocarbon Fluosol®, which showed poor efficacy and numerous side effects. Newer formulations have been developed with greater oxygen-carrying capacity than Fluosol®, but they still cannot be given in adequate doses to significantly replace the oxygen-carrying capacity of blood, and they have been associated with reduced pulmonary compliance.

A number of obstacles limit usefulness of cell-free hemoglobin as a red cell replacement. Problems include poor stability, inability to release oxygen, vasoconstriction, hypertension, inhibition of macrophage function, enhancement of endotoxin effects, potential promotion of bacterial growth, and interference with a large number of spectrophotometry-based laboratory tests.

The problems with hemoglobin solutions have been approached by chemically modifying the hemoglobin to help reduce the O_2 affinity and prevent dissociation of the tetramer, using a variety of cross-linking agents. Methods have been developed to encapsulate the hemoglobin in liposomes or conjugate it to large polymers such as dextran or hydroxyethyl starch. A number of these hemoglobin-based oxygen carriers are now in phase III clinical trials, but it appears that banked human blood will still be used for quite a while.

Indications for Red Blood Cell Transfusions

Over the last decade or so, a major push has been made to reduce the hematocrit at which transfusions are given. Some hospital transfusion committees require written justification for all transfusions to nonbleeding patients with a hematocrit over the 21 to 24 level. The older "transfusion trigger" had been a hematocrit of 30, which was based on work from many decades ago. Randomized studies assessing the risks and benefits of transfusion in various clinical settings have not been performed. These issues are clouded by controversy over relatively newly described adverse effects of transfusion that come under the broad title of "transfusion immuno-modulation," which is discussed later in this chapter.

Patients who are severely anemic clearly have a decreased quality of life and more difficulty with the intensive rehabilitation programs that accompany orthopaedic surgery. Orthopaedic patients are often older and frail. There is general agreement that severely anemic, symptomatic patients should be transfused. That having been said, is asymptomatic severe anemia an indication for transfusion pre-, intra-, or postoperatively? No definitive answers are possible. However, in patients without cardiovascular disease who refuse transfusions for religious reasons, mortality is not strikingly increased, at least down to hematocrits in the range of 18 to 20 (hemoglobin of about 6 to 7) when blood loss is less than about 2 units (about 1 liter). A study was conducted in 2,000 Jehovah's Witnesses, a group that refuses transfusion, who were undergoing a wide variety of surgical procedures. The mortality in the month after surgery was 1.3% in patients with preoperative hemoglobins of >12 g/dl, which increased to 33% in patients with levels of < 6 g/dl. The odds of death increased only from 1.1 at hemoglobins of about 11 to 12, to 1.4 at hemoglobins of 6 to 7 in patients without histories of cardiac or vascular disease who experienced blood loss of 1 liter or less. In contrast, the mortality odds increased from 1.5 to 12.3 for those with similar anemias and blood loss who had a history of cardiovascular disease. Patients with cardiac disease also have a slightly greater mortality even if not severely anemic, but this difference in mortality between those with and without cardiac disease increases dramatically if blood loss is large or preexisting anemia is severe.

The remaining question is whether transfusion would modify these outcomes and, if so, how much. No randomized trial exists comparing clinical outcomes with different transfusion triggers, so clinicians must resort to clinical experience. Patients with angina, heart failure, histories of myocardial infarction, or vascular disease who have hematocrits of < 30 (hemoglobins < 10 g/dl) and are bleeding should proba-

bly be transfused with red blood cells before their anemia becomes more severe. Patients without suspicion of cardiovascular disease who are hemodynamically stable can easily tolerate severe anemia if they are not bleeding rapidly. The problem is that many patients do not fit neatly into these 2 extremes. Randomized trials to test different transfusion triggers would be very helpful to clinicians weighing the risks and benefits of this powerful but potentially dangerous therapy. In the interim, clinical judgment and experience at the bedside will remain the primary tools for making transfusion decisions.

Indications for Specially Processed Blood Components

Leukodepleted, irradiated, or washed blood components are often indicated for patients with certain diagnoses or clinical conditions. The increased use and combination of these processes have led to some confusion as to the clinical benefits of these modifications and when such products are appropriate. Components with a total leukocyte count of less than 5×10^6, achieved by filtration or apheresis are considered leukodepleted. Leukodepleted components are used to reduce alloimmunization to HLA antigens, prevent cytomegalovirus (CMV) transmission to immunosuppressed patients, and prevent febrile, nonhemolytic transfusion reactions in patients previously having such reactions. Indications for leukoreduced components include CMV negative immunosuppressed patients, premature infants, candidates for bone marrow or solid organ transplants, pregnant women prior to delivery, and patients with repeated or severe febrile, nonhemolytic transfusion reactions.

Irradiating blood components prevents proliferation of donor lymphocytes in the recipient, thereby preventing graft versus host disease. This is only a problem in severely immunosuppressed individuals, patients with some hematologic malignancies, fetuses, premature infants, and, potentially, in patients receiving blood from close relatives. Irradiated components should be given to bone marrow transplant candidates and recipients, patients with congenital immune deficiencies, patients with hematologic malignancies, premature infants, and fetuses. All directed blood donations from relatives should be irradiated.

Washed products, which are depleted of plasma proteins, are used in patients who have had repeated allergic type nonhemolytic transfusion reactions to plasma proteins. In sensitized immunoglobulin A deficient patients, anaphylactic reactions may be prevented by repeatedly washing cellular components. Combinations of these processes, especially leukodepletion and irradiation, are often required. Correct product selection may require consultation with a transfusion medicine specialist.

Coagulopathy During Massive Transfusion

Massive transfusion is usually defined as blood replacement exceeding the patient's total blood volume within a 24-hour period. In a previously normal patient, massive transfusion may be accompanied by disorders of coagulation, which often can have multiple causes. Most often this coagulopathy is attributed to dilution of platelets or plasma coagulation factors by plasma- and platelet-poor red cell units. Adequate platelet numbers and coagulation factors are usually maintained until more than a blood volume (> 5,000 ml for a 70-kg patient) of fluid and red cells are given. Still, the development of coagulopathy is unpredictable, and clinical assessment of abnormal bleeding is critical. Other clinical factors causing or contributing to coagulopathy include acidosis, hypothermia, and hypotension. Coagulation factor and platelet replacement should be guided by abnormal laboratory test results and clinical evidence of abnormal bleeding or oozing. Replacement formulas, such as ratios of red cells to fresh frozen plasma (FFP), should not be used. At lower blood usage levels these ratios lead to overuse of FFP and at high blood usage levels, where there is profound dilution of platelets and coagulation factors, such formulas may lead to undertreatment of the patient.

Alternatives to Allogeneic Transfusions

Experience over the last few years confirms that use of autologous blood donated before surgery and preoperative normovolemic hemodilution are effective strategies for reducing the need for allogeneic donor blood, and one or both modalities are used widely throughout the United States. Normovolemic hemodilution immediately preoperatively is more convenient for the patient, cheaper, and probably safer because it is performed by experienced anesthesiologists with careful monitoring. However, not all anesthesiologists are experienced or comfortable with this procedure, nor are all operating theaters provided with equipment for this relatively simple and rapid procedure. Thus, predonation of autologous blood is the more common approach. Although questions have been raised as to whether autologous predonation is cost-effective, most such analyses have dramatically under-

estimated the morbidity and costs of allogeneic transfusions. Data from colorectal and hip replacement surgeries in several institutions have documented that each allogeneic transfusion is associated with approximately $1,000 to $2,000 in additional hospital costs. These costs are due primarily to an increased incidence of postoperative infection in patients receiving allogeneic blood. These costs are compared with the additional costs of perhaps $50 to $200 per unit of transfused autologous blood, a cost that includes the fact that 50% of such blood is discarded unused.

The operational reality of autologous donation is that slightly more blood is collected than the average need at surgery, so that most of the patients donating do not require allogeneic blood. Discard rates of 30% to 60% are therefore appropriate for autologous blood programs and are not problematic, as would be equally high discard rates for volunteer donor blood. Autologous blood is not "crossed over" to the general blood supply in most hospitals because the donors are not truly volunteers and usually do not meet the criteria required for such donors.

Erythropoietin (EPO), the growth factor primarily responsible for red cell production, has recently been approved for perisurgical use based on data obtained in patients undergoing joint replacement surgery. Patients who are mildly to moderately anemic (hemoglobin between 10 and 13 g/dl) receiving regimens of 300 U/kg daily for 10 days prior to surgery and for 4 days afterward, or of 600 U/kg weekly for 3 weeks prior to surgery and on the day of surgery can reduce their exposure to allogeneic blood by about 1 unit per patient on average. The vast majority of patients receiving EPO required no allogeneic blood. At such high doses, iron balance becomes an issue, and some patients may require intravenous iron supplementation to achieve maximal hemoglobin gains. The cost of the 600 U/kg dose is about $1,700, compared with about $3,150 for the daily regimen of 300 U/kg. Clinical results appear identical. The dose of EPO is usually given subcutaneously or intravenously. Patients with hematocrits above 40, patients with severe or uncontrolled hypertension, or patients with histories of embolic or thrombotic disease should probably not receive the drug except under careful observation and after carefully weighing the risks and benefits. There is some general concern that patients with preexisting vascular/cardiac disease may be at greater risk of thrombotic events if their hematocrit is raised fairly rapidly. In the surgical trials, such events were not seen significantly more frequently in the EPO group than the control group, but such events have been reported in patients receiving EPO for chronic renal failure. The drug has not been FDA approved as yet for use in conjunction with autologous blood donation or normovolemic hemodilution, but such multimodal approaches may be worth trying in selected patients with large anticipated blood needs during surgery.

Two other frequently used alternatives to allogeneic transfusion are intraoperative and postoperative blood salvage. Intraoperative salvage using a semiautomated centrifugal cell washer is usually warranted only when blood losses exceed 1,000 ml, and its use should be avoided in surgeries involving potential bacterial contamination of the surgical site and in cancer surgery. Recently, there have been some encouraging in vitro experiments involving the use of leukodepletion filters to eliminate contaminating tumor cells in salvaged red cells. Postoperative salvage continues to be a controversial area. These products are given unwashed and often contain fibrin degradation products, free hemoglobin, plasmin, and activated clotting factors. Although these appear to be tolerated by most patients, reinfusion of larger volumes of shed blood has been associated with hypotension, respiratory distress, and possibly disseminated intravascular coagulation. Also at issue is the volume of red cells actually saved by these procedures. Whereas volumes reinfused in most studies range up to 1,000 ml of drainage, the hematocrit in these collections is low. A number of studies have been done supporting or opposing the idea that postoperative salvage is cost-effective and saves on the use of allogeneic red cells, and this issue remains controversial.

Transfusion Immunomodulation and Postoperative Infection

Over the last 15 years it has become increasingly apparent that blood transfusion has generalized effects on immune function. These effects have been postulated to underlie the clinical observations that transfused patients have more rapid or frequent return of malignant tumors, decreased allograft rejection, decreased incidence of repetitive spontaneous abortions, increases in severity of viral infection, and increases in postoperative bacterial infections. The immunologic findings include decreases in natural killer cell, macrophage,

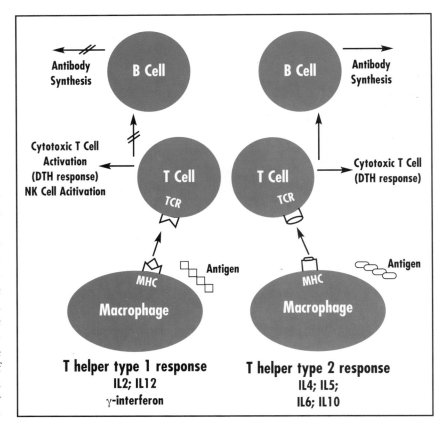

Figure 1

The T helper type 1/T helper type 2 paradigm is shown in schematic, simplified form. Immunologic responses sometimes become polarized so that primarily cellular immunity or humoral immunity is favored. Allogeneic transfusion favors T helper type 2 responses. DTH, delayed-type hypersensitivity; NK, natural killer; IL, interleukin; TCR, T cell reactivity; MHC, major histocompatibility complex.

and T cell function. Recently, it has been shown that these decreases in cellular immunity are probably caused in part by a shift in peripheral blood cell cytokine secretion toward a T helper lymphocyte type 2 (Th2) phenotype. The Th2 phenotype is characterized by secretion of interleukin-4 (IL-4) and IL-10 and impaired secretion of T helper type 1 (Th1) cytokines, such as IL-12, IL-2, and gamma-interferon. "Immune deviation" toward Th2 cytokine secretion leads to upregulation of immunoglobulin E and some immunoglobulin G secretion (ie, humoral immunity), and down regulation of Th1 cytokines that support such functions as antigen processing, macrophage activation, T lymphocyte cytotoxic function, and neutrophil and monocyte cidal activity (ie, cellular immunity) (Fig. 1). That allogeneic (but not autologous) transfusion causes immune deviation toward Th2 cytokine secretion has now been demonstrated in surgical patients, medical patients, and experimental animals. Surgery alone also causes a Th2 immune deviation, which probably accounts for the anergy sometimes seen in surgical patients postoperatively. The delayed type hypersensitivity reactions, which are measured by the skin test reactions used to measure anergy, are mediated by Th1 cytokines, and these are suppressed in additive fashion by both surgical trauma and allogeneic transfusion. Thus, transfusion appears to add to the suppression of cellular immunity caused by surgery.

The decreases in cellular immunity seen in allogeneic transfusion recipients after surgery may be a contributing cause of the twofold to fivefold increase in postoperative infections seen in such patients. In 40 cohort studies, transfusion was often observed to be the single best predictor of postoperative infection, postoperative antibiotic use, and hospital length of stay. Because the immunomodulatory properties of allogeneic blood in animal models have been linked to transfused white blood cells, clinical trials of leukocyte-reduced blood have been performed in 3 centers. Two studies in patients undergoing colorectal surgery demonstrated dramatic reductions in postoperative morbidity and infections in patients receiving leukocyte-reduced transfusions. One multicenter study found no advantage to use of leukocyte-reduced transfusions. However, a subsequent single-center study in cardiac surgery demonstrated a threefold reduction in morbidity and mortality in recipients of leukocyte-reduced transfusions. Whether leukocyte-reduced transfusions would have comparable benefits to patients undergoing major orthopaedic procedures is unknown.

The time may have come to consider the use of leukocyte-reduced transfusions for all surgical patients. Many have been reluctant to advocate this action given the $20 to $40 per unit additional costs of leukocyte-reduced red blood cells. However, in colorectal surgery, the additional costs of complications prevented (upward of $2,000 per unit transfused) more than compensate for the costs of the filters used to perform leukoreduction.

Several case control studies have demonstrated that recipients of autologous blood have no greater morbidity and no more infections after surgery than patients receiving no transfusions at all. However, there was a reduction in infections with use of autologous transfusions in 1 of the 2 randomized trials and no reduction in infections in the other. Both studies were carried out in colorectal surgery. In the study with decreased infections, there also was a probable reduction in the incidence of tumor recurrence with autologous transfusions. Both studies were hampered by the fact that patients donated only 2 units of blood in the experimental arm, and thus up to 30% of patients in the autologous transfusion arm also received some allogeneic blood.

Current advice to prevent the complications of immunomodulation in the surgical setting is to use conservative transfusion practices, employ autologous transfusion and/or hemodilution to reduce the need for allogeneic blood, and consider use of erythropoietin in selected anemic patients. Use of leukocyte-reduced blood in orthopaedic patients at high risk of postoperative infection has not been tested, but the data from chest and abdominal surgery and animal models suggest that this product may have the potential to reduce morbidity postoperatively.

Annotated Bibliography

General

Lemos MJ, Healy WL: Blood transfusion in orthopaedic operations. *J Bone Joint Surg* 1996;78A:1260–1270.

This is an excellent general overview with particular emphasis on issues of interest to orthopaedists.

Viral Transmission and Transfusion

Alter MJ, Gallagher M, Morris TT, et al: Acute non-A-E hepatitis in the United States and the role of hepatitis G virus infection: Sentinel Counties Viral Hepatitis Study Team. *N Engl J Med* 1997;336:741–746.

In this surveillance study of the incidence and clinical course of acute and chronic hepatitis G infection in patients with acute hepatitis, it was concluded that hepatitis G was unlikely to be responsible for morbidity associated with non-A-E hepatitis.

Menitove JE. Transfusion-transmitted infections: Update. *Semin Hematol* 1996;33:290–301.

This is a review of recent developments and potential concerns in transfusion-transmitted infections of various etiologies.

Schreiber GB, Busch MP, Kleinman SH, Korelitz JJ: The risk of transfusion-transmitted viral infections. *N Engl J Med* 1996;334:1685–1690.

This recent estimate of the risks of transfusion-transmitted viral infections based on repeat blood donation and testing involves more than half a million volunteer blood donors. In this surveillance study of the incidence and clinical course of acute and chronic hepatitis G infection in patients with acute hepatitis, it was concluded that hepatitis G was unlikely to be responsible for morbidity associated with non-A-E hepatitis.

Update on Blood Substitutes

Hess JR: Blood substitutes. *Semin Hematol* 1996;33:369–378.

The author examines both hemoglobin-based and perfluorocarbon oxygen carriers with review of efficacy, toxicities, and preliminary results of clinical trials.

Erythropoietin

Faris PM, Ritter MA, Abels RI: The American Erythropoietin Study Group: The effects of recombinant human erythropoietin on perioperative transfusion requirements in patients having a major orthopaedic operation. *J Bone Joint Surg* 1996;78A:62–72.

The authors present the data that were largely responsible for the licensure of EPO for use in moderately to mildly anemic orthopaedic patients who cannot or do not wish to donate autologous blood.

Coagulopathy During Massive Transfusion

Hiippala ST, Myllya GJ, Vahtera EM: Hemostatic factors and replacement of major blood loss with plasma-poor red cell concentrates. *Anesth Analg* 1995;81:360–365.

This is an assessment of changes in coagulation factors and platelets during massive transfusion.

Indications for Red Blood Cell Transfusions

Carson JL, Duff A, Poses RM, et al: Effect of anaemia and cardiovascular disease on surgical mortality and morbidity. *Lancet* 1996;348:1055–1060.

This is the report of a soon-to-be classic epidemiologic study of the effects of anemia and blood loss on perioperative mortality.

Transfusion Immunomodulation and Postoperative Infection

Blumberg N, Heal JM: Immunomodulation by blood transfusion: An evolving scientific and clinical challenge. *Am J Med* 1996;101:299–308.

This current general overview includes the public health and cost impacts of transfusion immunomodulation in surgical patients.

Jensen LS, Kissmeyer-Nielsen P, Wolff B, Qvist N: Randomised comparison of leucocyte-depleted versus buffy-coat-poor blood transfusion and complications after colorectal surgery. *Lancet* 1996;348:841–845.

Data from this definitive study show the benefits of leukocyte-depleted transfusions in surgical patients.

Chapter 6
Coagulation and Thromboembolism in Orthopaedic Surgery

Review of the Thrombotic Process

Thrombosis occurs secondary to a disturbance in the equilibrium between the prothrombotic and antithrombotic factors that are normally present within the bloodstream. Three factors associated with thrombosis—venous stasis, hypercoagulability, and endothelial trauma—have been described. Venous thrombi generally form in regions of stasis composed of red blood cells enmeshed in an extensive network of fibrin strands with few platelets present. In contrast, arterial thrombi usually are associated with high shear forces and high flow in vessels in which blood flow has been altered by atherosclerotic plaques. Arterial thrombi are composed mainly of platelet aggregates with only a few fibrin strands. In general, arterial thrombosis occurs as a result of platelet reaction to a vessel wall injury, whereas venous thrombosis is often secondary to venous stasis and the development of a hypercoagulable state.

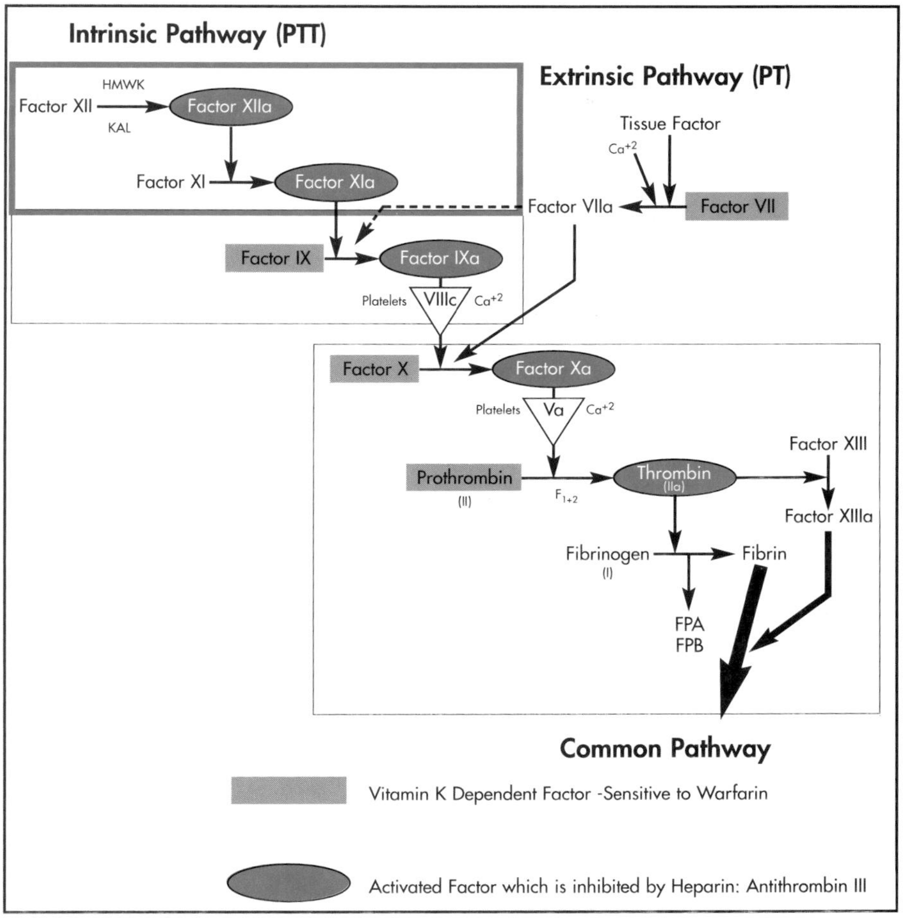

The Coagulation Mechanism

The coagulation cascade consists of relatively inactive zymogens or cofactors that, when activated, lead to fibrin clot formation. These reactions occur on or near phospholipid surfaces on platelets, endothelial cells, and white blood cells.

The coagulation cascade consists of 2 pathways. The intrin-

Figure 1

The coagulation pathways. Important features include the contact activation phase, vitamin K-dependent factors (affected by warfarin), and the activated serine proteases that are inhibited by heparin-antithrombin III. Prothrombin time measures the function of the extrinsic and common pathways; the partial thromboplastin time measures the function of the intrinsic and common pathways. (Adapted with permission from Stead RB: Regulation of hemostasis, in Goldhaber SZ (ed): *Pulmonary Embolism and Deep Venous Thromboembolism.* Philadelphia, PA, WB Saunders, 1985, p 32.)

sic pathway involves components normally found in blood, and the extrinsic pathway is activated by tissue lipoprotein. Both pathways converge, leading to activated factor X, which activates prothrombin to form thrombin. The formation of thrombin is the essential step in thrombus formation and activates the conversion of fibrinogen to fibrin, which eventually results in fibrin clot formation (Fig. 1).

Fibrinolysis, which is initiated at the same time as the clotting mechanism, acts to maintain blood vessel patency by removing fibrin deposits. Plasmin readily digests fibrin and inactivates other coagulation factors including factors V and VIII and fibrinogen. Finally, the thrombotic process is also regulated by 3 natural anticoagulant pathways: the heparin-antithrombin III pathway, the protein C-thrombomodulin-protein S pathway, and the tissue factor inhibitor pathway.

Epidemiology of Venous Thromboembolic Disease

A number of different risk factors have been identified as predisposing patients to the development of venous thromboembolic disease (VTED). Hypercoagulable states can be classified as either primary (inherited) or secondary (acquired). Inherited disorders involve quantitative or qualitative deficiencies in one of the natural anticoagulant mechanisms. The secondary hypercoagulable states include a variety of clinical conditions that predispose patients to developing VTED. Patients undergoing major hip or knee surgery, multiple trauma patients, and spinal cord injury patients are at high risk for having a venous thromboembolic event. If these patients also have either a primary or anoth-

er secondary hypercoagulable state (eg, malignancy or lupus anticoagulant), the risk increases (Table 1).

Deep vein thrombosis (DVT) usually develops in an area of reduced blood flow, such as a valve cusp in a deep calf vein. Most of these thrombi are small, clinically silent, and have no adverse consequences. However, there is a strong association between proximal DVT and pulmonary embolism (PE). In one study, approximately 50% of patients with documented DVT demonstrated objective evidence of PE at the time of diagnosis.

Prophylaxis

Patients who undergo total hip (THA) or knee (TKA) arthroplasty are at highest risk for venous thromboembolism. The ultimate goal of prophylaxis in thromboembolic disease is to prevent the fatal pulmonary embolism; the prevention of PE, proximal DVT, and chronic venous stasis contribute to this end. There is general agreement that patients undergoing THA and TKA, patients with multiple trauma, and those with spinal cord injury are at high risk for developing DVT. If prophylaxis is not used, DVT develops in 40% to 80% of these patients, proximal DVT in 15% to 50%, and fatal PE in 0.3% to 0.5%. PE is the most common cause of death after a total joint arthroplasty when thromboprophylaxis is not used.

A variety of pharmacologic and mechanical approaches have been used to decrease the risk of venous thromboembolism. The pharmacologic approaches have included warfarin, fixed- or adjusted-dose heparin, low-molecular-weight heparins (LMWHs) and heparinoids, aspirin, and dextran. Mechanical approaches have included early immobilization, graded compression stockings, sequential intermittent pneumatic compression boots, and intermittent plantar compression. In addition, there is evidence to suggest that the use of hypotensive epidural anesthesia may reduce the risk of formation of DVT after THA and TKA.

Influence of Anesthesia on Thromboembolic Disease

A number of studies have documented decreased rates of DVT in patients who have THA with the use of epidural or spinal anesthesia compared with DVT rates in patients in whom general anesthesia was used. This decrease in thrombus formation has been attributed to the sympathetic blockade with subsequent vasodilatation and increased blood flow to the lower extremity that occur with regional anesthesia. Hypotensive epidural anesthesia further reduces blood loss,

Table 1
Hypercoagulable states

Primary	Secondary
Antithrombin II deficiency	Trauma
Protein C deficiency	Surgery (orthopaedic, gynecologic)
Protein S deficiency	Immobilization
APC (activated protein C) resistance	Advanced age
	Malignancy, cancer
	Chronic venous stasis
	Congestive heart failure
	Pregnancy
	Oral contraceptives
	Nephrotic syndrome
	Lupus anticoagulant

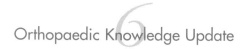
preserves blood volume, and increases blood flow to the lower extremities. This leads to a reduction in venous stasis and a more normal coagulation profile as exemplified by a decrease in the depletion of antithrombin III (ATIII) that usually occurs when total joint arthroplasty is performed with the patient under general anesthesia. Therefore, it is hypothesized that hypotensive epidural anesthesia minimizes activation of the clotting cascade, thereby leading to the low DVT rates reported in a number of series using this anesthetic technique in total joint arthroplasty patients.

There is evidence that without prophylaxis, patients with regional anesthesia have a lower rate of DVT than those who have general anesthesia. However, it has not been demonstrated whether regional anesthesia further reduces DVT rates in patients who also receive effective prophylaxis.

Pharmacologic Intervention

Warfarin

Warfarin blocks transformation of vitamin K in the liver, thereby inhibiting the production of vitamin K-dependent clotting factors II, VII, IX, and X (Table 2). Warfarin has been demonstrated to decrease the prevalence of DVT by 60% to 80% and of proximal vein thrombosis by 70% compared with no prophylaxis.

Traditionally, warfarin prophylaxis has been initiated with a 5- or a 10-mg dose either the evening before or the evening of the surgical procedure. Subsequent doses have been determined by the measurement of the prothrombin time (PT). According to the low-dose warfarin protocol, the target PT is maintained between 1.3 and 1.5 times the control value. Because the anticoagulant effect associated with a particular PT has varied considerably among different institutions, depending on the thromboplastin sensitivity, the international normalized ratio (INR) was developed. The INR is defined as the observed prothrombin ratio[ISI] (ISI = international sensitivity index of thromboplastin). The INR represents the prothrombin ratio that would be obtained if the international reference thromboplastin had been used instead of local reagent at a particular laboratory. Therefore, the INR represents the same degree of anticoagulation from center to center. The INR should be maintained between 1.8 and 2.5 for DVT prophylaxis.

The advantages of low-dose warfarin prophylaxis are oral administration and low cost. Major disadvantages include monitoring of the INR, interactions with a large number of medications, delayed onset of action, and the potential for bleeding. The low rates of symptomatic PE associated with low-dose warfarin prophylaxis suggest that warfarin may prevent proximal clot migration of early clinically silent thrombi and the development of a symptomatic PE.

Table 2
Pharmacologic agents administered for prevention of deep venous thrombosis

Agent*	Mechanism of Action†	Monitoring Test§	Complications
Warfarin	Blocks transformation of vitamin K in the liver, thereby inhibiting production of clotting factors II, VII, IX, and X	INR	Potential for bleeding
Heparin	Enhances ability of ATIII to inhibit coagulation factors thrombin (IIa), IXa, and Xa	aPTT	Potential for bleeding
LMWHs	Inhibit factors Xa and IIa		Potential for bleeding
Aspirin	Inhibits cyclo-oxygenase		Gastrointestinal symptoms
Dextran			Volume overloading, hypersensitivity reactions, bleeding

* LMWH, low-molecular-weight heparin
† ATIII, antithrombin III
§ INR, international normalized ratio; aPTT, activated partial thromboplastin time

Heparin

Standard unfractionated heparin is a heterogeneous mixture of glycosaminoglycans with an average molecular weight between 12,000 and 15,000 daltons (range, 5,000 to 30,000 d). The major anticoagulant effect of heparin occurs through its interaction with ATIII (Table 2). This interaction enhances the ability of ATIII to inhibit the coagulation factors thrombin (IIa), Xa, and IXa. Heparin binds thrombin more rapidly than factor Xa and inactivates thrombin by forming a ternary complex of heparin, ATIII, and thrombin.

Standard fixed low-dose heparin (5,000 units subcutaneous twice daily) has not been shown to be effective in preventing proximal DVT after hip surgery. Adjusted-dose heparin was developed to have a mild but measurable effect on the coagulation cascade. The heparin dose is adjusted daily to attain an activated partial thromboplastin time (aPTT) of 1 to 5 seconds greater than the upper limit of normal. Daily monitoring of the aPTT is necessary.

Low-Molecular-Weight Heparin

Low-molecular-weight fractions of standard heparin generally are prepared by chemical or enzymatic depolymerization. LMWHs vary in size between 1,000 and 10,000 d. The LMWHs retain the unique pentasaccharide required for binding to ATIII, but in a lower proportion than seen in standard heparin. Because the inactivation of thrombin (IIa) by heparin depends on molecular size, the LMWHs have greater anti-Xa activity than anti-IIa activity (Table 2). When compared to standard heparin, the LMWHs are less likely to cause bleeding because inhibition of platelet function is reduced and there is less microvascular permeability. The LMWHs have a bioavailability of 90%, and the reduced binding of LMWHs to plasma protein prolongs the half-life of these drugs. These properties limit variations of the antithrombotic effect of each LMWH and allow for once- or twice-daily dosing without laboratory monitoring. The dosages used for DVT prophylaxis do not increase either the PT or the aPTT. Because the molecular weights of the LMWHs differ, the efficacy of these agents varies from drug to drug. Potential limitations of the LMWHs include cost and parenteral administration, which makes it more difficult to administer the drug after hospital discharge.

Other Pharmacologic Agents

Aspirin would seem to be an ideal prophylaxis agent because of its antiplatelet action by inhibition of cyclo-oxygenase (Table 2). Although aspirin has been associated with low symptomatic PE rates in a few nonrandomized studies, its role as a prophylaxis agent remains controversial. In a number of randomized orthopaedic trials, aspirin did not reduce the rate of DVT. Furthermore, in one study aspirin was found to be significantly less effective than pneumatic compression boots in reducing proximal clot formation in TKA patients. Dextran has moderate efficacy in reduction of DVT after total joint arthroplasty, but the use of this agent is limited because of the concerns with volume overloading, hypersensitivity reactions, bleeding, and cost and because other agents provide better protection (Table 2).

Mechanical Methods

Mechanical methods of prophylaxis have gained increased popularity over the past decade because they do not require laboratory monitoring, there is no risk of bleeding, and they have almost no side effects. Compression stockings alone have not been demonstrated to decrease the risk of thromboembolic disease and must be used in conjunction with an effective prophylactic agent. Continuous passive motion machines have not been shown to reduce the rate of DVT formation after major knee surgery.

External pneumatic compression boots reduce stasis in the lower extremity by increasing the velocity of venous blood flow and by enhancing endogenous fibrinolytic activity. Intermittent plantar compression in the foot works by mimicking the hemodynamic effect that occurs during normal walking when a physiologic pump in the foot is activated by flattening of the plantar arch. Phlebographic studies have confirmed that a large plantar venous system is rapidly emptied when weightbearing flattens the plantar arch. Intermittent plantar compression is intended to increase venous return and prevent venous stasis without the risk of bleeding associated with pharmacologic prophylaxis.

Current Status of Prophylaxis

Routine prophylaxis has been the standard of care since the National Institutes of Health Consensus Conference in 1986, and low intensity warfarin has been the agent most often used by orthopaedic surgeons for the past 2 decades. Nonetheless, while the prevalence of DVT is considerably reduced, it remains between 15% and 25% after THA and 35% and 50% after TKA. Clinically significant bleeding events with warfarin have been reduced to 1% to 2% with acceptance of low intensity anticoagulation to maintain the INR between 1.8 and 2.5 (formerly a prothrombin time index of 1.3 to 1.5). Although the numbers indicate that VTED is more refractory to standard prophylaxis after TKA, most (85% to 90%) thrombi occur below the venous trifurcation in the deep calf veins and, therefore, carry less immediate risk of embolization. In contrast, the distribution after THA was historically a nearly equal split between proximal (40%) and distal (60%) thrombi, but more recent trials with contemporary prophylaxis agents report less than 10% proximal thrombi with the remainder occurring in the calf. Therefore, under the influence of current prophylaxis, 85% to 90% of all DVT after both THA and TKA occur in the calf.

Unresolved issues that are central to a current discussion of VTED include the role of routine surveillance and the type and optimal duration of prophylaxis in the face of abbreviated hospitalization.

Low-Molecular-Weight Heparin

Although warfarin is the time-honored popular pharmacologic agent for prophylaxis, LMWHs offer a more selective antithrombotic inhibition of activated factor X by interaction with ATIII. No monitoring of coagulation parameters is necessary, but these agents are only administered parenterally. Increased efficacy in prevention of DVT has been demonstrated primarily in controlled trials against unfractionated heparin in both THA and TKA. A few recent studies demonstrated a reduced prevalence of DVT in patients given LMWHs when compared with warfarin, especially after TKA. An overall frequency of DVT as low as 6% after THA and 25% after TKA both represent significant reductions in prevalence over that provided by warfarin. However, there were no significant differences in symptomatic PE or proximal clot rates between patients given LMWHs and those given warfarin. Bleeding complications, especially related to the surgical site with major and overall bleeding rates of 4% and 12%, respectively, have been as much as 2 to 4 times more frequent with LMWHs than with warfarin. Rare cases of thrombocytopenia have also been documented. Published results to date clearly suggest a dose-response relationship with LMWHs, with increased efficacy in DVT prevention obtained at the expense of an increase in hemorrhagic events when compared with the warfarin experience. Further clinical study is necessary to determine the risk-benefit profile of this family of agents and their ultimate role in joint replacement surgery. The rapid onset of action, relatively short half-life, and ease of use in the intensive care unit has already established a place for LMWHs in the management of VTED in high-risk polytrauma patients with long bone and pelvic fractures. Market-driven establishment of drug cost and identification of true bleeding rates with further clinical trials will be the major determinants of cost efficacy of these agents.

Mechanical Modalities

When compared with warfarin, external pneumatic compression boots have been associated with a reduction in calf DVT but a greater prevalence of high-risk proximal DVT after THA. External pneumatic compression boots alone and the combination of plantar foot compression and aspirin reduce the prevalence of proximal DVT after TKA more than does aspirin alone. External pneumatic devices may offer some advantage when used in combination with pharmacologic agents but this combination of modalities requires further study. Although the value of elastic compression stockings is widely accepted, a recent study suggests their influence after THA was only to shift the distribution of DVT from distal to proximal with no effect in reducing the absolute prevalence of DVT.

Anesthetic

With the exception of a few centers, anesthetic type has received limited attention for its role in modifying expression of VTED; regional epidural anesthesia has been associated with a reduction in overall, proximal, and distal DVT. The role of the anesthetic method deserves further study. More importantly, it must be acknowledged as a variable and controlled in future trials comparing efficacy of different methods of prophylaxis.

Diagnosis

Deep Venous Thrombosis

The clinician cannot rely solely on the physical examination and clinical findings, such as swelling, pain in the calf, palpable cords, or a positive Homan's sign, to reliably diagnose DVT. Unfortunately, fatal PE may be the presenting manifestation of VTED, which underscores the importance of early and accurate diagnosis. A number of diagnostic tools are available to recognize DVT, but at the present time only contrast venography and ultrasonography are widely used in practice.

Ascending contrast venography remains the most reliable and sensitive method for detection of asymptomatic and nonocclusive venous thrombi in high-risk postoperative arthroplasty patients. It is equally effective in identification of proximal and distal thrombi. The disadvantages of venography include local discomfort at the injection site, hypersensitivity reaction, and thrombosis secondary to the contrast agent. The recent introduction of more expensive nonionic iso-osmolar contrast agents has reduced the risk of iatrogenic venous thrombosis to acceptable rates well below 1%. The use of venography as a routine surveillance tool has been suggested, but its cost-benefit ratio remains to be definitively established.

Ultrasound is a noninvasive diagnostic imaging technique that allows visualization of venous channels and graphic presentation of blood flow; the addition of Doppler technology allows determination of flow directionally. Duplex ultrasound and color flow Doppler ultrasound have been sensitive in identifying spontaneous onset thrombi in symptomatic patients but have had variable sensitivity in asymptomatic patients. The sensitivity of color Doppler ultrasound compared with that of venography ranges from 38% to 100% in detecting silent postoperative proximal DVT and from 10% to 88% for calf DVT. It has been shown in a number of studies that ultrasonography can be used reliably as a screening device, but the efficacy of this diagnostic tool is highly dependent on the skill of the operator.

Pulmonary Embolism

The clinical signs of PE are often nonspecific and include pleuritic chest pain, tachycardia, pleural rub, tachypnea, and dyspnea. Patients with proximal DVT may complain of pain or swelling in the thigh. In general, as with the diagnosis of DVT, these clinical signs are unreliable. Objective testing is necessary to establish the diagnosis of PE. Ventilation-perfusion (V/Q) scanning, when used with a preoperative baseline scan as in clinical trials, is a reliable screening test for PE. However, in the absence of a comparison study, a single V/Q scan incorrectly predicts PE in 15% of "high probability" scans and incorrectly rules out PE in 15% of "low probability" scans. A normal perfusion scan essentially rules out the possibility of meaningful PE. Pulmonary angiography remains the best method to positively establish the diagnosis of PE.

Surgeons are concerned about instituting unnecessary heparin therapy because of the consequences for the patient and concerns about bleeding in the early postoperative period. Therefore, a rational diagnostic protocol is necessary when PE is suspected. The initial investigation has traditionally been a V/Q scan. If the V/Q scan reading is a "low probability" for a PE, then a duplex ultrasound (US) should be obtained to rule out the presence of a proximal clot. If the duplex US is negative, prophylaxis should be continued but heparinization is not necessary. If the V/Q scan is a "high probability" for PE, then immediate management depends on the surgeon's index of clinical suspicion for PE. If there is a high index of clinical suspicion, then heparin therapy (intravenous heparin or LMWH) is begun. If the surgeon doubts the diagnosis of PE, a pulmonary angiogram can be obtained to confirm the diagnosis and heparin therapy can be instituted if the angiogram is positive. Approximately 75% of patients have a "moderate probability" scan and the presence or absence of PE remains uncertain. If a patient has a moderate probability scan, some authors suggest a duplex US

should be obtained. If the duplex US is positive, then the patient should be treated with heparin. If the duplex US is negative, then a pulmonary angiogram can be obtained to rule out a PE or a repeat duplex US can be obtained within 5 days, depending on the degree of clinical suspicion.

There remains an unfulfilled need to reliably establish the diagnosis of DVT and PE by reproducible noninvasive means. Magnetic resonance (MR) venography has shown promise in the study of pelvic venous thrombosis and MR angiography may prove equally valuable in the evaluation of PE. Helical or spiral computed tomography allows direct visualization of all but small peripheral lung emboli and also allows evaluation of the mediastinum and pulmonary parenchyma. Before either of these modalities is adopted as standard practice, more extensive clinical trials are necessary to establish efficacy.

Treatment

The principal objective in treatment of VTED is to prevent occurrence of fatal PE, with secondary goals to reduce the morbidity of acute and recurrent DVT and to minimize the risk of late postphlebitic syndrome.

Established Deep Venous Thrombosis

Treatment of proximal DVT begins with full intensity intravenous heparin, which has an immediate effect on the intrinsic cascade of the coagulation system. The goal is to prolong the activated partial thromboplastin time (aPTT) to 2.0 times control. The purpose of heparinization is to prevent an extension of clots and recurrence of PE. However, full heparinization within 5 days of joint replacement was accompanied by major bleeding events in more than one third of patients in one study. Avoidance of a heparin bolus to initiate therapy should be considered. Alternatively, subcutaneous LMWH has been shown to be effective in the treatment of proximal DVT and PE; LMWH appears to be equally safe and may be more cost-effective than traditional intravenous heparin therapy.

An inferior vena cava filter is reserved for specific circumstances when full anticoagulation is absolutely contraindicated or in the event of recurrent pulmonary emboli despite intravenous heparin and a therapeutic aPTT.

Warfarin is instituted simultaneously with the heparin therapy; an INR of 2.0 to 3.0 is recommended for 3 to 6 months for proximal DVT and PE. Contraindications to the use of extended warfarin therapy include pregnancy, liver insufficiency, noncompliance, severe alcoholism, uncontrolled hypertension, active major hemorrhage, and inability to return for monitoring.

Recent studies suggest that more protracted oral anticoagulant therapy of established DVT reduces risk of thromboembolic complications and late recurrence; during a 2-year follow-up, 6 months of warfarin reduced second events by 50% (9.5% versus 18.1%) compared with the conventional 6-week therapy, with an identical frequency of bleeding complications. Similarly, management of isolated calf DVT in the postoperative setting is controversial. Newer data demonstrate that untreated calf DVT after THA was a precursor of proximal clot propagation in 17% to 23% of patients; oral anticoagulant (warfarin) therapy or serial surveillance for this condition is reasonable.

Managing Extended Risk of Thromboembolic Disease

The risk of late postoperative DVT after total joint arthroplasty continues for 3 months, long beyond the usual 5-day hospital stay. Two viable strategies include extended outpatient thromboembolic prophylaxis for all patients or routine surveillance and selective treatment of identifiable DVT. LMWH therapy compared with placebo in patients with normal venograms at hospital discharge reduced the prevalence of new asymptomatic DVT (7.1% versus 19.3%) identified by venogram 3 weeks later. In several other studies in which LMWH prophylaxis was extended beyond hospital discharge after joint replacement, the incidence of new venogram-positive DVT was 12% to 20% in the absence of continued anticoagulation. The clinical significance of these data is unclear in the context of readmission rates of less than 1% for symptomatic VTED in venogram-negative patients discharged without further anticoagulation. Alternatively, a strategy of routine postoperative surveillance and selective treatment of DVT reduces outpatient anticoagulation and is accompanied by similar frequency of 0.8% readmission for VTED, but requires a reliable screening test. Although current opinion in North America supports continued prophylaxis beyond the acute hospitalization, specific guidelines for this practice are not yet established.

Annotated Bibliography

Bergqvist D, Benoni G, Bjorgell O, et al: Low-molecular-weight heparin (enoxaparin) as prophylaxis against venous thromboembolism after total hip replacement. N Engl J Med 1996;335:696–700.

Continuation of enoxaparin for 3 weeks after discharge reduced DVT rates from 39% (placebo after discharge) to 18%; proximal DVT was reduced from 24% to 7%, and PE occurred in 2 placebo and no enoxaparin patients.

Clarke MT, Green JS, Harper WM, Gregg PJ: Screening for deep-venous thrombosis after hip and knee replacement without prophylaxis. J Bone Joint Surg 1997;79B:787–791.

With unilateral venography on postoperative day 5 to 7 in 252 THA and TKA patients having general anesthesia, the prevalence of DVT was 32% after THA (half proximal and half distal) and 66% after TKA (one fourth distal and three fourths proximal).

Colwell CW Jr, Spiro TE, Trowbridge AA, et al: Enoxaparin Clinical Trial Troup: Use of enoxaparin, a low-molecular-weight heparin, and unfractionated heparin for the prevention of deep venous thrombosis after elective hip replacement. A clinical trial comparing efficacy and safety. J Bone Joint Surg 1994; 76A:3–14.

Among 604 patients who were evaluated, the prevalence of DVT was 6% with twice daily dosing compared with 15% with daily dosing and 12% for unfractionated heparin. Major bleeding occurred in 4%, 1%, and 6%, respectively, in these same groups.

Francis CW, Pellegrini VD Jr, Totterman S, et al: Prevention of deep-vein thrombosis after total hip arthroplasty: Comparison of warfarin and dalteparin. J Bone Joint Surg 1997;79A: 1365–1372.

Greater efficacy in prevention of DVT with dalteparin (15% versus 26%) was at the expense of greater wound-related bleeding complications (4% versus 1%; $p = 0.03$) and more frequent need for postoperative transfusion (48% versus 31%; $p = 0.001$).

Geerts WH, Code KI, Jay RM, Chen E, Szalai JP: A prospective study of venous thromboembolism after major trauma. N Engl J Med 1994;331:1601–1606.

Venographic prevalence of DVT in polytrauma patients was 58% with 18% proximal thrombi; nearly all were asymptomatic. Skeletal injury predicted the greatest DVT risk: pelvic fracture 61%, tibia fracture 77%, femur fracture 80%.

Geerts WH, Jay RM, Code KI, et al: A comparison of low-dose heparin with low-molecular-weight heparin as prophylaxis against venous thromboembolism after major trauma. N Engl J Med 1996;335:701–707.

Enoxaparin reduced overall DVT from 44% to 31% and proximal DVT from 15% to 6% compared with unfractionated heparin. Major bleeding was 5 times more frequent with enoxaparin (3.9% versus 0.7%).

Gefter WB, Hatabu H, Holland GA, Gupta KB, Henschke CI, Palevsky HI: Pulmonary thromboembolism: Recent developments in diagnosis with CT and MR imaging. *Radiology* 1995; 197:561–574.

This is an excellent review of newer radiographic techniques for diagnosing pulmonary embolism.

Hull R, Raskob G, Pineo G, et al: A comparison of subcutaneous low-molecular-weight heparin with warfarin sodium for prophylaxis against deep-vein thrombosis after hip or knee implantation. *N Engl J Med* 1993;329:1370–1376.

In a large venogram endpoint trial of 1,207 patients, the benefit of reduced relative risk of DVT with fractionated heparin (31% versus 37%; $p = 0.03$) was offset by an increased frequency of major bleeding (2.8% versus 1.2%; $p = 0.04$).

Hull RD, Raskob GE, Pineo GF, et al: Subcutaneous low-molecular-weight heparin vs warfarin for prophylaxis of deep vein thrombosis after hip or knee implantation: An economic perspective. *Arch Intern Med* 1997;157:298–303.

Cost of drug, INR monitoring, and bleeding are the most important determinants of cost-efficacy of TED prophylaxis. In the United States, the established price of fractionated heparin preparations will determine their cost-benefit balance.

Imperiale TF, Speroff T: A meta-analysis of methods to prevent venous thromboembolism following total hip replacement. *JAMA* 1994;271:1780–1785.

All prophylaxis types except aspirin reduced both overall and proximal DVT rates; aspirin reduced neither. Clinically important bleeding on fractionated heparin was sixfold greater than controls and 50% greater than with warfarin.

Kalodiki E, Nicolaides AN, al-Kutoubi A, Cunningham DA, Crofton M: Duplex scanning in the postoperative surveillance of patients undergoing total hip arthroplasty. *J Arthroplasty* 1997;12:310–316.

Duplex scanning in 78 THA patients had a sensitivity of 56% (5/9) for proximal thrombi compared with 93% (13/14) with color flow Doppler; color flow identified only 79% (15/19) of thrombi in the calf.

Leclerc JR, Geerts WH, Desjardins L, et al: Prevention of venous thromboembolism after knee arthroplasty: A randomized, double-blind trial comparing enoxaparin with warfarin. *Ann Intern Med* 1996;124:619–626.

Among 417 patients, enoxaparin reduced overall DVT from 51.7% to 36.9% compared with warfarin. There was no difference in proximal DVT; 10.4% versus 11.7%. Major bleeding occurred in 1.8% on warfarin and 2.1% on enoxaparin.

Lensing AW, Doris CI, McGrath FP, et al: A comparison of compression ultrasound with color Doppler ultrasound for the diagnosis of symptomless postoperative deep vein thrombosis. *Arch Intern Med* 1997;157:765–768.

For asymptomatic nonocclusive DVT after hip or knee replacement, the addition of color Doppler technology added no increased sensitivity to screening with compression ultrasound (sensitivity 60% proximal, 33% distal DVT).

Lieberman JR, Geerts WH: Prevention of venous thromboembolism after total hip and knee arthroplasty. *J Bone Joint Surg* 1994;76A:1239–1250.

This is a current review of measures for DVT prophylaxis.

Lieberman JR, Huo MM, Hanway J, Salvati EA, Sculco TP, Sharrock NE: The prevalence of deep venous thrombosis after total hip arthroplasty with hypotensive epidural anesthesia. *J Bone Joint Surg* 1994;76A:341–348.

Hypotensive epidural anesthesia and aspirin were associated with low proximal (1%) and distal (6%) DVT rates.

Lieberman JR, Wollaeger J, Dorey F, et al: The efficacy of prophylaxis with low-dose warfarin for prevention of pulmonary embolism following total hip arthroplasty. *J Bone Joint Surg* 1997;79A:319–325.

In 1,099 THA patients receiving low intensity warfarin (PT index 1.3 to 1.5) an average of 15 days, there were 12 (1.1%) symptomatic PE and major bleeding events, associated with a PT over 17 seconds, after 32 (2.9%) procedures.

Lotke PA, Steinberg ME, Ecker ML: Significance of deep venous thrombosis in the lower extremity after total joint arthroplasty. *Clin Orthop* 1994;299:25–30.

Increasing size of venographically identified thrombosis was associated with an increased risk of PE as determined by ventilation perfusion scanning. PE rate following THA and TKA was similar.

Millenson MM, Bauer KA: Pathogenesis of venous thromboembolism, in Hull R, Pineo GF (eds): *Disorders of Thrombosis.* Philadelphia, PA, WB Saunders, 1996, pp 175–190.

This is a current review of the factors operative in venous thromboembolism.

Oishi CS, Grady-Benson JC, Otis SM, Colwell CW Jr, Walker RH: The clinical course of distal deep venous thrombosis after total hip and total knee arthroplasty, as determined with duplex ultrasonography. *J Bone Joint Surg* 1994;76A:1658–1663.

Of 41 patients with distal DVT, 7 (17%) evidenced asymptomatic extension to proximal veins on serial duplex ultrasonography at 14 days postoperatively; 1 patient (3%) manifested symptomatic proximal DVT 11 months after THA.

Pellegrini VD Jr: Prevention of thromboembolic disease in patients after total joint arthroplasty by selective posthospitalization treatment. *Semin Arthroplasty* 1997;8:248–257.

Current practice must reconcile short hospital stays with a 3-month risk period for VTED. Routine surveillance with venograms and selective treatment provide acceptable protection while minimizing outpatient anticoagulant exposure and bleeding risk. However, the cost-effectiveness of this regimen requires further study.

Pellegrini VD Jr, Clement D, Lush-Ehmann C, Keller GS, Evarts CM: Natural history of thromboembolic disease after total hip arthroplasty. *Clin Orthop* 1996;333:27–40.

Six-month readmission rate for VTED was 0% in 55 patients treated for a positive venogram, 1.1% in 269 patients with a negative venogram and no further prophylaxis, 1.6% in 732 patients without screening venography, and 17.4% in 23 patients with a false negative venogram who received no warfarin therapy.

Planes A, Vochelle N, Darmon JY, Fagola M, Bellaud M, Huet Y: Risk of deep-venous thrombosis after hospital discharge in patients having undergone total hip replacement: Double-blind randomised comparison of enoxaparin versus placebo. *Lancet* 1996;348:224–228.

Venogram negative patients at hospital discharge received enoxaparin or placebo for 3 weeks; overall DVT was reduced by continued prophylaxis (7% versus 19%), nearly entirely by decrease in calf DVT. No PE occurred in either group.

RD Heparin Arthroplasty Group: RD heparin compared with warfarin for prevention of venous thromboembolic disease following total hip or knee arthroplasty. *J Bone Joint Surg* 1994; 76A:1174–1185.

Fifty anti-factor Xa units/kg body weight given twice daily reduced VTED rates from 27% to 16% compared with warfarin. Blood loss index and clinically important bleeding events occurred more often (7% versus 5%) with RD heparin.

Robinson KS, Anderson DR, Gross M, et al: Ultrasonographic screening before hospital discharge for deep venous thrombosis after arthroplasty: The post-arthroplasty screening study. A randomized controlled trial. *Ann Intern Med* 1997;127:439–445.

Patients were randomized to undergo either bilateral compression ultrasonography or a sham procedure prior to hospital discharge. In the screening group the total outcome event rate (symptomatic DVT [4] and major bleeding [1]) was 1.0% (5 of 518 patients). In the placebo group, the total outcome event rate (symptomatic DVT [3] and nonfatal PE [2]) was 1.0% (5 of 506 patients). The use of screening with ultrasonography at discharge did not reduce symptomatic thromboembolic complications and, therefore, screening does not appear to be justified.

Schulman S, Rhedin AS, Lindmarker P, et al: A comparison of six weeks with six months of oral anticoagulant therapy after a first episode of venous thromboembolism: Duration of Anti-coagulation Trial Study Group. *N Engl J Med* 1995;332: 1661–1665.

During a 2-year follow-up period of 897 patients, the recurrence rate of VTED was 18.1% with 6 weeks and 9.5% with 6 months of coumadin therapy for established DVT; mortality and major hemorrhage were the same in both groups.

Warwick DJ, Whitehouse S: Symptomatic venous thromboembolism after total knee replacement. *J Bone Joint Surg* 1997; 79B:780–786.

The 3-month readmission rate from symptomatic TED after 1,000 consecutive TKA was 1.1% with no differences observed in prophylaxis as compared with no prophylaxis groups.

Warwick D, Williams MH, Bannister GC: Death and thromboembolic disease after total hip replacement: A series of 1162 cases with no routine chemical prophylaxis. *J Bone Joint Surg* 1995;77B:6–10.

Among 1,152 consecutive THA the total VTED morbidity in 6 months was 3.4%; 0.34% fatal PE, 1.2% clinically apparent PE (0.7% readmission), and 1.89% venographically confirmed clinically apparent DVT (1.13% readmission). The authors consider evidence insufficient to recommend postdischarge prophylaxis.

Wells PS, Lensing AW, Davidson BL, Prins MH, Hirsh J: Accuracy of ultrasound for the diagnosis of deep venous thrombosis in asymptomatic patients after orthopedic surgery: A meta-analysis. *Ann Intern Med* 1995;122:47–53.

In the 17 studies reviewed, the sensitivity for detection of asymptomatic proximal vein thrombosis ranged from 38% to 100%; only 2 had adequate venogram control for analysis of distal DVT and sensitivity ranged from 20% to 88%.

Westrich GH, Sculco TP: Prophylaxis against deep venous thrombosis after total knee arthroplasty: Pneumatic plantar compression and aspirin compared with aspirin alone. *J Bone Joint Surg* 1996;78A:826–834.

Plantar compression and aspirin reduced DVT rates from 59% to 27% compared with aspirin alone; no proximal thrombi were observed with compression contrasted with 12 (14%) in the aspirin group.

Classic Bibliography

Amstutz HC, Friscia DA, Dorey F, Carney BT: Warfarin prophylaxis to prevent mortality from pulmonary embolism after total hip replacement. *J Bone Joint Surg* 1989;71A:321–326.

Haas SB, Insall JN, Scuderi GR, Windsor RE, Ghelman B: Pneumatic sequential-compression boots compared with aspirin prophylaxis of deep-vein thrombosis after total knee arthroplasty. *J Bone Joint Surg* 1990;72A:27–31.

Hirsh J: Oral anticoagulant drugs. *N Engl J Med* 1991;324: 1865–1875.

Hirsh J, Levine MN: The optimal intensity of oral anticoagulant therapy. *JAMA* 1987;258:2723–2726.

Hirsh J, Levine MN: Low molecular weight heparin. *Blood* 1992;79:1–17.

72   General Knowledge

Hull RD, Raskob GE, Hirsh J, et al: Continuous intravenous heparin compared with intermittent subcutaneous heparin in the initial treatment of proximal-vein thrombosis. *N Engl J Med* 1986;315:1109–1114.

Johnson R, Green JR, Charnley J: Pulmonary embolism and its prophylaxis following the Charnley total hip replacement. *Clin Orthop* 1977;127:123–132.

NIH Consensus Development Conference Statement: Prevention of venous thrombosis and pulmonary embolism. Bethesda, MD, U.S. Department of Health and Human Services, Office of Medical Applications of Research, 1986, vol 6, no 2.

Patterson BM, Marchand R, Ranawat C: Complications of heparin therapy after total joint arthroplasty. *J Bone Joint Surg* 1989;71A:1130–1134.

Sikorski JM, Hampson WG, Staddon GE: The natural history and aetiology of deep vein thrombosis after total hip replacement. *J Bone Joint Surg* 1981;63B:171–177.

Chapter 7
Perioperative Medicine

Introduction

With an aging population, elective and emergency ortho-paedic surgery is being performed on patients with more complex problems, necessitating evaluation by both the operating surgeon and medical consultants. The preoperative assessment goals are to identify (1) treatable comorbid conditions, (2) comorbid conditions that are not reversible yet may impact the surgical outcome, and (3) previously unrecognized conditions and allow for correction of these problems. Ideally, preoperative consultation should be done in the outpatient setting approximately 2 weeks before the proposed surgery. With such knowledge the surgeon can anticipate postoperative problems unique to the underlying conditions as well as prepare for common postoperative problems: fever, atelectasis, volume overload, and deep vein thrombosis prophylaxis.

Patients requiring emergency surgery should be assessed quickly by the surgical team, anesthesiologists, and medical consultants. This assessment team should establish a problem list, correct medical problems when possible (ie, hyper-glycemia, metabolic acidosis, etc), and confer as to the risk and benefit of immediate surgery or delaying surgery. The decision to delay in the elderly population may result in additional complications (pneumonia, deep vein thrombosis, fever, decubitus), thereby further diminishing the patient's chance of a functional recovery.

Use of Preoperative Laboratory Data

There have been many studies addressing the utility of routine laboratory testing for elective surgery. These laboratory data add a new diagnosis in only 0.7% of patients. When laboratory data define normal as a bell-shaped curve (Gaussian distribution), then 5% of normal patients on a given test will fall outside the reference range. With a chemistry 20 profile, 64% of patients in a healthy population will have at least 1 abnormality.

These laboratory abnormalities often have little impact on overall surgical outcome. The chance of finding a significant laboratory abnormality that will affect the surgical outcome is much less than 1%. Most clinicians are now using selective testing based on age, sex and comorbid conditions. Table 1 is a guide, although not a substitute for clinical judgment.

The complete blood count is important in orthopaedic patients because many of these patients have been on non-steroidal anti-inflammatory agents, which can predispose to iron deficiency anemia secondary to indolent gastrointestinal bleeding. Patients with inflammatory arthritis can have anemia of chronic disease. Both situations can result in severe anemia (less than 8 gm hemoglobin) that will impact surgical risk. Many orthopaedic procedures can be associated with significant blood loss so a baseline value is beneficial. Studies on the preoperative value of the white blood cell count have demonstrated an abnormality rate in the range of 0 to 9.5%. Severe abnormalities are uncommon (< 0.7%). Abnormal platelet counts are seen in 0 to 11.8% of patients. Severe abnormalities contributing to an increased risk of bleeding are uncommon. In elective orthopaedic surgery it is uncommon to encounter consumptive thrombocytopenia requiring platelet transfusion. In contrast, trauma patients often develop mild to severe consumptive thrombocytopenia. It is therefore reasonable to obtain a baseline platelet count for these patients.

Chemistry studies to assess renal function (creatinine and blood urea nitrogen), hepatic enzyme abnormalities (transaminases: SGOT, SGPT, GGTP), serum glucose, and electrolyte abnormalities also demonstrate a low utility in screening for asymptomatic disease. Coagulation studies (prothrombin time, partial thromboplastin time) are not helpful in identifying asymptomatic patients who will have bleeding problems. A history and physical examination are the best tools to assess hemostasis. The bleeding time has little use in predicting postoperative hemorrhage, except in those patients taking aspirin or nonsteroidal anti-inflammatory agents.

In general surgery, the urinalysis has very low utility in identifying patients at risk for perioperative infectious complications. However, treating asymptomatic bacteriuria preoperatively in orthopaedic patients may be beneficial to reduce secondary infection of surgical implants, especially total hip and knee. Perioperative urologic instrumentation of these asymptomatic patients may lead to transient bacteremia and, in turn, infection of implants. Preoperative bacteriuria can be cured over 80% of the time with a simple 1-dose regimen of 3 g of amoxicillin (six 500-mg tablets) or 2 sulfamethoxazole/trimethoprim DS (800 mg/160 mg) tablets.

Table 1
Preoperative laboratory testing guide

Disease/Condition	Hct/Hgb	PT/INR	PTT	Test* E-Lytes	Cr/BUN	Glu	CXR	EKG
Age < 40 years								
40 to 49 years								yes:male
> 50 years								yes
Hypertension					yes			yes
Coronary artery disease							yes	yes
Vascular disease							yes	yes
Pulmonary diseases							yes	yes
Hepatic disease	yes			yes	yes			
Renal disease	yes			yes	yes			
Diabetes				yes	yes	yes > 40 years	yes	
Medications								
Digoxin				yes	yes			
Diuretics				yes	yes			
Steroids	yes			yes				
Warfarin/heparin	yes	yes	yes					

*Hct/Hgb, hematocrit/hemoglobin; PT, prothrombin time; PTT, partial thromboplastin time; INR, International Normalized Ratio; E-Lytes, electrolytes; Cr/BUN, creatinine/blood urea nitrogen; Glu, glucose; CXR, chest radiograph; EKG, electrocardiograph

Chest radiograph abnormalities are very common in patients older than 60 years of age. The influence of a preoperative abnormality on outcome is small. While chronic obstructive lung disease changes and abnormalities consistent with heart failure may influence management decisions, the history and physical examination remain more important in assessing pulmonary or cardiac risk than the radiograph.

The abnormal electrocardiogram (EKG) probably generates the most attention in the preoperative setting. Up to 52.7% of patients older than 45 years may have an abnormality on routine EKG. Goldman has demonstrated the poor predictive value of ST-segment and T-wave changes in predicting cardiac events. Detecting a "silent" myocardial infarction based on EKG is a rare event (0.3%) but may have some validity in risk stratification. Patients with recent myocardial infarction appear to be at highest risk for perioperative myocardial infarction. Bifascicular block rarely progresses to complete heart block during surgery and is not an indication for temporary pacemaker placement.

In summary, laboratory testing should be selective rather than routine in patients undergoing surgery. Testing should be done based on symptoms, underlying disease, and to a lesser extent on age and sex.

Cardiovascular Assessment

Preoperative cardiac risk assessment is of prime importance in any surgery. Over the last 20 years studies have validated Detsky's and Goldman's criteria for assigning risk of perioperative cardiac complication (myocardial infarction, congestive heart failure, or death) based on history, physical examination, and laboratory data (Table 2). Patients with the highest points carry the greatest risk. Patients with a myocardial infarction less than 6 months before surgery, pulmonary edema within 6 months, unstable angina or angina with minimum exertion, aortic stenosis, or patients with multiple risk factors identified in the table are at greatest risk.

Table 2
Detsky's modified multifactorial index

Factor*	Points
Coronary artery disease	
MI within 6 months	10
MI after 6 months	5
CSS angina class 3	10
CSS angina class 4	20
Unstable angina within 3 months	10
Alveolar pulmonary edema	
Within 6 months	10
Ever	5
Valvular disease	
Suspected hemodynamically significant aortic stenosis	20
Electrocardiogram	
Nonsinus rhythm or sinus with frequent PACs on preoperative test	5
More than 5 PVCs	5
Poor medical status	5
Age > 70 years	5
Emergency operations	10
Total maximum points	**125**

(Reproduced with permission from Detsky AS, Abrams HB, McLaughlin JR, et al: Predicting cardiac complications in patients undergoing noncardiac surgery. *J Gen Intern Med* 1986;1:212.)

* MI, myocardial infarction; CSS, carotid sinus stimulation; PAC, premature atrial contraction; PVC, premature ventrical contraction

Stable angina, controlled hypertension, left ventricular hypertrophy, bifascicular block, or nonspecific ST changes on EKG do not increase cardiovascular risk. Nor does recent coronary artery bypass grafting appear to increase risk.

At times the history alone may not be sufficient to establish cardiac risk because many elderly patients with joint disease do not exercise enough to cause angina. In this case, noninvasive pharmacologic stress testing using intravenous persantine or adenosine to cause redistribution of blood flow coupled with thallium imaging can stratify patients' risk for myocardial ischemia. An abnormal thallium stress test with fixed defects or an abnormal test with reversible ischemia in 1 coronary territory is not an indication for catheterization or revascularization. These patients can be treated medically and have an acceptable surgical risk. Patients with global ischemia or ischemia in 2 or more areas of myocardium are at perioperative risk and should be studied with coronary arteriography. As in all risk assessment, the risk of revascularization (angioplasty, vascular stent, atherectomy, or coronary artery bypass grafts) and orthopaedic surgery must be weighed against the risk of the orthopaedic surgery itself.

Congestive heart failure (CHF) can be the consequence of many forms of cardiac (myocardial ischemia, aortic or mitral valvular disease, arrhythmias) and noncardiac (hypertension, anemia, hemochromatosis) disease. The underlying disease and cardiac function should be optimally managed before surgery. Patients who have a history of CHF have a 6% risk of recurrent CHF and a 5% mortality. Those patients with an S3 gallop, jugular venous distention, or rales have a 20% mortality. It is important to identify the cause and reverse CHF if possible. Echocardiography to assess left ventricular function and the presence of significant valvular disease can be helpful preoperatively. Patients with poor exercise capacity and severe impairment of left ventricular function (ejection fraction < 25%) are at increased risk for CHF, dysrhythmia, and death. These patients should be monitored with Swan Ganz catheter and arterial lines. If available, a transesophageal echocardiogram can be used to facilitate management of fluid balance as well.

Aortic stenosis and mitral stenosis are associated with increased preoperative myocardial ischemia and pulmonary edema. Clinical recognition of these murmurs and preoperative assessment by echocardiography are necessary.

Patients with mechanical valves need to be heparinized preoperatively and their coumadin should be stopped 3 to 5 days in advance of surgery. Generally these patients can stop the heparin 4 to 6 hours prior to surgery and it can be resumed within 24 hours of surgery. These patients should also receive antibiotic endocarditis prophylaxis if a bladder catheter is inserted.

Patients with atrial fibrillation with controlled ventricular rates pose no special problems. The surgeon must always be concerned about the etiology of the atrial fibrillation in terms of how it impacts risk. Patients who have significant ventricular arrhythmias are maintained on their usual medication. If they have atrial or ventricular ectopy perioperatively with normal left ventricular function and no hemodynamic compromise these arrhythmias are not treated.

Pulmonary Assessment

Pulmonary complications after surgery remain a leading cause of surgical morbidity. Thoracic and upper abdominal procedures pose the highest risk. In patients undergoing orthopaedic surgery other than spine surgery there are negligible changes in vital capacity and functional residual capacity. An ileus can occur postoperatively that can compromise pulmonary function. Atelectasis, aspiration, pneumonia, pulmonary edema, pleural effusion, and pulmonary embolism remain the major problems seen postoperatively.

Patients with restrictive lung disease secondary to pleural or pulmonary parenchymal disease in general do well because respiratory drive is preserved. Patients with morbid obesity, or skeletal or neuromuscular disorders that result in restrictive lung disease are at risk for pulmonary complications.

Surgery can be done on patients with reversible airway disease (chronic obstructive pulmonary disease, asthma) without fear of respiratory distress when these patients are free of a bronchospasm. Metered-dose inhalers of beta 2 agonist (albuterol), intermediate acting steroid (beclomethasone), and anticholinergic bronchodilator (ipratropium bromide) have become standard therapies for these patients. They should be used 2 weeks preoperatively to assure stable pulmonary function, and continued through the postoperative period. Theophylline preparations should be used in this same manner. Patients should refrain from smoking several weeks in advance of surgery. Although PFTs (pulmonary function tests) are commonly done there is no clear cut level of forced expiratory volume in 1 second, forced vital capacity, and forced expiratory flow midexpiratory phase that can predict pulmonary complications. The patient's prehospitalization functional capacity, assessed through a history and physical examination, is the best indicator of postoperative complications.

Antibiotics should be used if evidence is present for bacterial airway infection; ie, abnormal chest radiograph or a change in sputum. Preoperative and postoperative respiratory therapy instruction in the use of incentive spirometry, coughing, and deep breathing exercises should be implemented. Early ambulation after surgery should also be encouraged.

Renal Disease

Patients with chronic renal insufficiency (CRI), creatinine clearance < 20 ml/min, and end-stage renal disease are at higher risk for postoperative complication. With careful preoperative evaluation these risks can be minimized.

Creatinine clearance can be estimated by the following formula: creatinine clearance = (140 – age) × weight in kg/serum creatinine × 72. Patients with low creatinine clearance need adjustments in most medications and are susceptible to rapid volume shifts. Patients may present with dehy-

dration and hyperkalemia, or volume overloaded with severe hyponatremia. Both conditions may result in cardiac arrhythmia. Chronic metabolic acidosis is often present with respiratory hyperventilation. Well compensated patients should maintain serum bicarbonate above 18 meq/liter. Preoperatively the physician should try to correct the acidosis with bicarbonate therapy. Hypocalcemia and hyperphosphatemia are hallmarks of CRI and may lead to cardiac dysrhythmia during general anesthesia. Anemia is normal in patients with CRI, and uremia leads to platelet dysfunction and excessive bleeding.

Acute renal failure can occur in the postoperative setting. Renal failure occurring in the first 24 hours after surgery often is a result of hypotension during surgery, unrecognized preoperative volume depletion, or the nephrotoxicity of dye during preoperative testing. Late postoperative renal failure (> 3 days) is usually due to nephrotoxic medications (aminoglycosides) or volume depletions caused by poor oral intake. The elderly are more susceptible to renal failure resulting from multiple comorbid conditions, medications that alter renal function, and age-related decline in glomerular filtration rate. Trauma may lead to rhabdomyolysis, myoglobinuria, and acute tubular necrosis.

Liver Disease

Mild abnormalities of 1 or more liver function tests are common during screening of asymptomatic individuals. This is also true following anesthesia and surgery. These are generally nonspecific changes that spontaneously resolve. Patients with asymptomatic chronic hepatitis tolerate surgery well. In acute viral hepatitis or alcoholic hepatitis, surgery should be postponed until resolution of inflammation and evidence of improved hepatic synthesis (near normal prothrombin time, < 15 sec). Preexisting liver disease, such as viral hepatitis, alcoholic hepatitis, or cirrhosis, in the postoperative period can lead to a more profound change in serum transaminases, transient hepatic decompensation, poor wound healing, excessive bleeding, or death.

Diabetes

Diabetes mellitus affects approximately 5% of the population. Type I diabetes (juvenile diabetes) is a state of insulin deficiency associated with ketoacidosis, which commonly is seen in the young but can present as late as the third decade of life. By definition, insulin is necessary for management. Type II diabetes is a resistance to endogenous insulin and or disturbance of the glucose/insulin coupling; it is not associated with ketoacidosis. Type II diabetes is managed by diet, oral hypoglycemic agents, insulin, or combinations of the 3.

Diabetes mellitus is a risk for preoperative cardiac complications. Symptomatic or asymptomatic cardiac disease is commonly seen in patients who have been diabetic for over 15 years. A preoperative EKG is required in all diabetics. The finding of the loss of R-R variation on a resting EKG may indicate autonomic neuropathy. The presence of Q waves may identify an old transmural myocardial infarction. Compared with the general population, the incidence of silent ischemia is higher in the diabetic population, thus in assessing these patients prior to surgery, cardiac testing (stress test, echocardiography) may be helpful.

Renal function assessment should include a physical examination, serum electrolytes, blood urea nitrogen, and creatinine. A urine analysis for protein is also essential. Knowledge of the presence of renal dysfunction is necessary when choosing perioperative medication such as antibiotics or the use of radiographic contrast dyes. Because asymptomatic bacteriuria is common, a urine culture should be obtained prior to arthroplasty.

The presence of autonomic neuropathy may complicate the postoperative course with blood pressure and pulse variation and asymptomatic hypoglycemia. Postoperative nausea with gastroparesis is frequent in the diabetic and is successfully treated with intravenous metoclopramide, 10 to 30 mg every 6 to 8 hours.

Glucose Management

The goal in management is to keep blood glucose levels at or below 240 mg/dl yet avoid perioperative hypoglycemia, < 80 mg/dl. This range is chosen because it decreases glycosuria, reducing the risk of dehydration and, experimentally, phagocytosis and wound healing are improved.

The diabetic on oral agents should hold the medication the day of surgery. The blood glucose should be checked the morning of surgery or preoperatively and then every 4 to 6 hours intra- and postoperatively. Human synthetic regular insulin can be administered on a sliding scale for any blood glucose over 200 mg/dl. An intravenous solution of 5% dextrose should be administered to avoid starvation ketosis. On the morning after surgery, an 1,800-calorie American Diabetes Association (ADA) diet can be started along with the oral hypoglycemic if the patient is taking food well.

The type II diabetic on insulin can be managed in a similar fashion to that outlined above. The use of a long acting insulin on the morning of surgery is a clinical judgment and should be individualized.

Many protocols for insulin management have been suggested for diabetes mellitus type I. No regimen is superior to any other in preventing postoperative complications. Good control of blood glucose should begin weeks before surgery. The type I diabetic, with the guidance of his or her physician, should strive to attain stable blood glucose (100 to 160 mg/dl) for at least 7 days prior to the operation. Dietary adherence with control of glucose should replete hepatic glycogen stores, thereby reducing the risk of intraoperative hypoglycemia.

The well-controlled type I diabetic can be managed with a half dose of the morning insulin and frequent serum glucose monitoring (every 4 hours). A sliding scale with short-acting insulin should be used throughout the first 24 hours after surgery. The following morning the patient can return to a standard insulin dose only if able to consume a full ADA diet.

In those type I diabetics who demonstrate a wide variation in preoperative glucose or a history of poor control, ie, "the brittle diabetic," an insulin drip is most appropriate. While simultaneously administering 5% dextrose in water, a maintenance insulin drip is begun at 2 units per hour. Serum glucoses should be checked hourly and insulin adjusted accordingly. The morning after surgery, the insulin infusion can be stopped 3 hours after administering subcutaneously two thirds of the patient's usual morning insulin. Coverage with a sliding scale of regular insulin is then appropriate.

Rheumatoid Arthritis

Patients with rheumatoid arthritis (RA) commonly are candidates for total joint replacement as well as other surgeries. RA is associated with anatomic and physiologic changes, including cervical spine disease, anemia, and pulmonary and cardiac involvement, that must be evaluated prior to general anesthesia.

Studies have shown 30% to 40% of patients with RA admitted to the hospital have radiographic evidence of cervical spine subluxation. This commonly involves the first and second cervical vertebrae. Between 2% and 5% have demonstrable long-tract findings. Subluxation of a diseased atlantoaxial joint during endotracheal intubation may compromise the respiratory center of the medulla. A careful history for symptoms of pain in the C1 and C2 nerve roots during routine daily activity is necessary. Dynamic flexion and extension radiographs can identify this problem. If there is any question, a computed tomography scan of the upper cervical spine is obtained.

Lung disease in RA has many manifestations: pleuritis, interstitial fibrosis, and pleural based nodules that can result in restrictive lung disease. A history of exertional dyspnea or rales on examination should be evaluated by a chest radiograph and spirometry with or without carbon monoxide diffusion capacity.

The heart may also be involved in the form of pericarditis, myocarditis, noninfective vegetation on the valves, conduction defects, and, rarely, coronary arteritis. A history, physical examination, and an EKG are sufficient screening for RA patients. If a murmur exists, antibiotic prophylaxis is necessary.

The use of corticosteroids is common in this patient population. The patient's use of chronic steroid within 9 months of surgery requires steroid prophylaxis preoperatively. A common protocol is intravenous (IV) hydrocortisone, 100 mg 30 to 60 minutes prior to the procedure followed by 100 mg IV every 8 hours for 2 doses, then 50 mg IV every 8 hours for 24 hours, and finally, on postoperative day 2, return to preoperative daily dose.

Postoperative Complications

Delirium and confusional states are common in the postoperative period. Elderly patients and those with multiple medical problems are more susceptible to confusion. Preoperative baseline assessment of mental status is important. Elderly patients become adept at hiding cognitive deficits, thus Folstein's mini mental status examination offers a good tool to assess cognitive impairment. The mini mental status examination is a standardized test of short-term memory, mathematic and language capability, abstract thought, the processing of a simple direction, and spatial orientation that detects deficits in particular cognitive areas. Postoperative confusion increases the risk for postoperative complication: higher mortality, longer length of stay, aspiration, combative behavior leading to trauma, and so forth.

Evaluation of the confused patient should include a history and physical examination, a neurologic examination and simple laboratory evaluation. A previous episode of delirium and/or memory decline may suggest Alzheimer's type or vascular dementia. A history of drug or alcohol abuse may present postoperatively as acute withdrawal, delirium tremens, or Wernicke's encephalopathy. The presence of fever and delirium suggest pneumonia, sepsis, or pulmonary emboli. Congestive heart failure may first present as delirium. A focal deficit with delirium may suggest a stroke or intracerebral bleed. Laboratory assessment should include oxygen saturation, serum electrolytes, calcium, magnesium, creatinine, and urea nitrogen. A review of medications is paramount. Narcotics and their metabolites, short acting benzodiazepam, antidepressant, antiemetics, and even antibiotics (ie, sulfa/

trimethoprim) can cause a confusional state. Confusion is often multifactorial. Treatment is directed to the underlying disease, correcting any metabolic derangement, and stopping psychoactive medications.

Postoperative tachycardia is often multifactorial: anemia, hypovolemia, pain, anxiety, and the humoral-hyperadrenergic response to surgery. A careful examination including orthostatic blood pressure, skin turgor, and mucosal moisture is necessary. Electrolytes, hemoglobin and hematocrit, and an EKG are necessary. Atrial fibrillation is common postoperatively in the elderly and may be a clue to underlying heart disease. Cardiac consultation with monitoring is necessary. Treatment of tachycardia is directed at the underlying heart disease.

Annotated Bibliography

General

Iannotti J, Spindler KP, Kelly J, Brown FH: Evaluation of the patient undergoing orthopaedic surgery, in Goldmann DR, Brown FH, Guarnieri DM (eds): *Perioperative Medicine: The Medical Care of the Surgical Patient*, ed 2. New York, NY, McGraw Hill, 1994, pp 139–151.

This chapter presents issues unique to the orthopaedic patient. The entire book is an exhaustive evaluation of perioperative medicine in many types of surgery.

Assessment of Cardiac Disease

Fleisher LA, Eagle KA: Screening for cardiac disease in patients having noncardiac surgery. *Ann Intern Med* 1996;124: 767–772.

This is the most up-to-date single source review of cardiac assessment tools.

Mangano DT, Goldman L: Preoperative assessment of patients with known or suspected coronary disease. *N Engl J Med* 1995; 333:1750–1756.

This is an extension of the classic study 20 years later with new insights to cardiac assessment.

Patients With Diabetes Mellitus

Schiff RL, Emanuele MA: The surgical patient with diabetes mellitus: Guidelines for management. *J Gen Intern Med* 1995;10: 154–161.

The authors provide a succinct review of protocols to manage blood sugars during and after surgery. The authors also discuss the rationale behind their management.

Patients with Renal Disease

Kellerman PS: Perioperative care of the renal patient. *Arch Intern Med* 1994;154:1674–1688.

This is an overview of issues pertaining to acute perioperative renal failure and the management issues of chronic renal disease at time of surgery.

Postoperative Delirium and Confusion

Marcantonio ER, Goldman L, Mangione CM, et al: A clinical prediction rule for delirium after elective noncardiac surgery. *JAMA* 1994;271:134–139.

In addition to clinical guidelines for assessment of delirium, the authors also discuss the differential in acute postoperative confusion.

Classic Bibliography

Detsky AS, Abrams HB, McLaughlin JR, et al: Predicting cardiac complications in patients undergoing non-cardiac surgery. *J Gen Intern Med* 1986;1:211–219.

Goldman L: Cardiac risks and complications of noncardiac surgery. *Ann Intern Med* 1983;98:504–513.

Gustafson Y, Berggren D, Brannstrom B, et al: Acute confusional states in elderly patients treated for femoral neck fracture. *J Am Geriatr Soc* 1988;36:525–530.

Jackson CV: Preoperative pulmonary evaluation. *Arch Intern Med* 1988;148:2120–2127.

Macpherson DS, Snow R, Lofgren RP: Preoperative screening: Value of previous tests. *Ann InternMed* 1990;113:969–973.

Merli GJ, Weitz HH: The medical consultant. *Med Clin North Am* 1987;71:353–355.

White RH: Preoperative evaluation of patients with rheumatoid arthritis. *Semin Arthritis Rheum* 1985;14:287–299.

Chapter 8
Imaging Beyond Conventional Radiology

Magnetic Resonance Imaging

General Principles

Given its lack of ionizing radiation, direct multiplanar capabilities, and superior soft-tissue contrast, magnetic resonance (MR) imaging has replaced many conventional imaging techniques in the detection of musculoskeletal pathology. When the patient is placed in a high-strength external magnetic field, a vector of hydrogen ions within the body aligns with the axis of the external field. A series of imparted radiofrequency (RF) pulses alters the energy state of the protons, causing them to move from the axis of the external magnetic field, known as longitudinal magnetization, to the plane of transverse magnetization. Once the disturbing pulse is turned off, thermal equilibrium is regained, and electromagnetic energy is released, which induces a current in the receiver imaging coil. This electrical current is the MR signal, and when spatially encoded through a mathematical process known as Fourier transformation, it generates an MR image. Although clinically useful information may be obtained on a variety of field strengths (0.2 to 1.5 Tesla), superior image quality is achieved by recruiting more protons on a high strength "closed" MR unit (1.5 T). Open MR units are ideally suited for patients whose size or weight precludes traditional imaging. However, open MR units are of a lower magnetic field strength and, in general, are not able to reproduce the image quality of closed systems. Specially designed open units exist that permit interventional MR imaging, including MR-guided biopsies and real-time joint kinematic and weightbearing evaluation, but these units are currently limited to largely research applications.

Differential tissue contrast is achieved by altering the time between successive RF pulses (repetition time or TR) and the time between the imparted RF pulse and the recording of generated signal (echo time or TE) (Table 1). The rate of recovery of longitudinal magnetization (back to the axis of the external magnet) is known as T1 relaxation time. The decay of transverse magnetization, when protons have been "flipped" from the longitudinal to the transverse plane, is known as T2 relaxation time.

Spin Echo Imaging

A typical T1-weighted MR image uses short TR and TE to accentuate differences in longitudinal recovery, or release of energy from the excited protons to the surrounding environment. With increasing TE, sequences become more T2 weighted, resulting in image degradation due to the rapid decay of signal that occurs in the transverse plane. This is a function of inherent field inhomogeneities, as well as the interaction between the protons in the imaging sample. More rapid T2 decay of signal is promoted by the presence of paramagnetic substances (hemosiderin), as well as ferromagnetic substances (orthopaedic instrumentation). It should be noted that cortical bone and normal tendons and ligaments

Table 1

Basic magnetic resonance (MR) signal characteristics of tissue

Tissue	MR Pulse Sequence	
	T1-Weighted (short TR/short TE)*	T2-Weighted (long TR/long TE)*
Fat	High	Intermediate to High
Articular Cartilage	Intermediate	High
Fluid (Joint, CSF)†	Low	High
Cortical Bone	Low	Low
Tendon/Ligament /Fibrocartilage	Low	Low
Hemosiderin	Low	Very Low

* TR, repetition time; TE, echo time

† CSF, cerebrospinal fluid

of type I collagen appear low signal on all pulse sequences because of their highly ordered cellular structure, with a relatively small number of free hydrogen atoms, and restriction of water molecules in type I collagen.

Gradient Echo Imaging

Gradient echo MR imaging is an MR pulse sequence that uses short repetition times with rapid successive RF pulses, with flip angles typically less than 90°, yielding multiple images within a relatively short scan time. Gradient echo images are recognized by small TE values but high signal from fluid (similar to T2-weighted images), a coarse appearance of trabecular bone, poor contrast between fat and muscle, and flow-related enhancement or high signal from flowing protons in blood. Such techniques have been used to study joint kinematics, where rapid successive images are obtained and displayed on a cine computer program, simulating real time joint assessment. In the shoulder this technique allows visualization of the capsular labral complex in internal and external rotation, and in the wrist, detection of subtle carpal instability patterns.

Fast Spin Echo and High Resolution Imaging

Although gradient echo sequences allow for rapid acquisition of MR data, they are severely degraded in the presence of orthopaedic instrumentation because of susceptibility artifact. Fortunately, fast spin echo techniques permit assessment of adjacent soft-tissue structures surrounding orthopaedic instrumentation. Such techniques have been used to assess meniscal allografts despite adjacent instrumentation from concomitant osteotomies and ligament reconstruction, correlating well with second-look arthroscopy. Similarly, the posterior soft-tissue envelope surrounding hip arthroplasty in patients with repeated dislocations may be assessed. Following screw fixation of femoral fractures, these techniques may be used to assess articular cartilage and to detect early osteonecrosis before changes are evident on plain radiographs.

MR Contrast Agents

Intravenous administration of the MR contrast agent gadolinium is useful in distinguishing vascularized scar from recurrent disk material in the postoperative spine patient (particularly after the initial 6 months following surgery). Gadolinium is also used frequently to help distinguish "reactive" marrow edema from frank osteomyelitis, and contrast-enhanced MR imaging has a reported specificity equivalent to or greater than that of combined technetium 99 bone and indium 111 white blood cell scans. In addition, malignant tumors and many benign tumors exhibit gadolinium enhancement.

Articular Cartilage and Labral Imaging

The superior soft-tissue contrast of MR imaging makes it ideally suited for assessing articular cartilage. The recent advent of autologous cartilage implantation and mosaicplasty has stimulated demand for accurate, reproducible, and ideally noninvasive methods to detect and monitor articular cartilage lesions. Using arthroscopy as a standard, accuracies of 97% have been reported in the patellofemoral joint, and 92% in all knee compartments. Vigilant attention to proper MR technique is crucial, however, because differential contrast must be achieved between synovial fluid, articular cartilage, and fibrocartilage. MR imaging has replaced conventional tomography in the detection and surface mapping of physeal bars in the skeletally immature patient. Specialized software programs can volumetrically quantify cartilage in arthritic joints, enabling noninvasive monitoring of disease progression and response to treatment.

Superior surface coils have enabled assessment of articular cartilage in joints other than the knee, including the shoulder and the hip. "Phased-array" coil design implies several coils working in concert to increase signal to noise. Such coils are commercially available, but may be site specific. MR imaging may be used preoperatively to define articular cartilage or labral hip lesions suitable for arthroscopic debridement, thus reserving hip arthroscopy for therapeutic applications. MR arthrography has been used in such patients, requiring intra-articular injection of MR contrast medium, most commonly gadolinium chelates diluted with saline. While MR arthrography of the hip has been shown to accurately detect labral lesions, it removes the noninvasive advantage of MR imaging, is typically more expensive, and is not currently FDA approved, requiring, in most cases, informed consent and approval by an institutional review board. High resolution imaging using surface coils to decrease the field of view permits accurate assessment of chondral and labral hip lesions (Fig. 1) without contrast agents, even in the absence of joint effusion.

Recent studies have also reported the variable MR appearance of the acetabular labrum, triangular fibrocartilage complex, lumbar spine, and menisci in asymptomatic patients. The magnetic properties of soft tissues are a reflection of their histopathologic state, and clearly these changes may exist in the absence of clinical symptoms.

Diagnostic evaluation of the unstable shoulder is challenging, because it must provide accurate assessment of both the dynamic and static restraints of the glenohumeral joint to assist in surgical planning. There has been some contention in the imaging literature that MR arthrography is superior to noncontrast MR in the evaluation of the glenohumeral capsular-labral complex. However, cases of capsular laxity in the

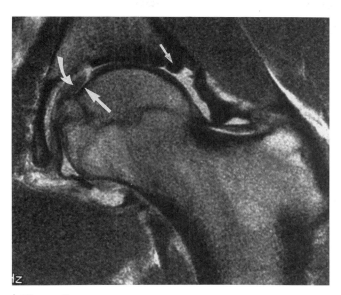

Figure 1

Coronal surface coil high resolution magnetic resonance image of the hip in a professional football player following a posterior translational episode. There is a chondral shearing injury with a displaced fragment of articular cartilage (curved arrow) in the suprafoveal portion of the femoral head. Note the differential contrast between the articular cartilage (curved arrow), subchondral plate (long straight arrow), and the fibrocartilaginous labrum (short straight arrow).

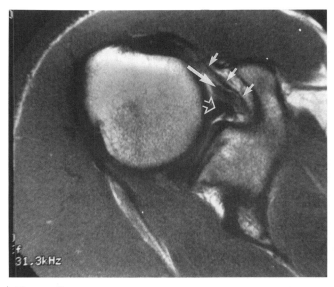

Figure 2

Noncontrast magnetic resonance image demonstrating surgically confirmed anterosuperior glenoid labral tear. Note the displaced low signal anterosuperior labrum (open arrow), adjacent to the thickened but intact superior fibers of the middle glenohumeral ligament (long straight arrow), and the intact anterior capsule (short straight arrows).

absence of discrete Bankart lesions have been overlooked despite the use of intra-articular contrast agent. With strict attention to proper MR technique, noncontrast high resolution MR imaging has been noted to be 95% accurate compared with arthroscopy in the detection and localization of labral lesions. In the setting of an acute dislocation, early recognition and distinction of a primary labral detachment from a pure capsular injury may be made and has prognostic significance regarding recurring dislocation, thereby allowing for prompt stabilization of true Bankart lesions.

Superior labral lesions have recently come into recognition as an important cause of shoulder pain, often presenting without clinically demonstrable instability. MR assessment of the superior labrum requires careful review of axial and oblique coronal images as well as a knowledge of normal variants (Fig. 2). These lesions are made more conspicuous in the presence of paralabral ganglion cysts, which can preferentially decompress into the spinoglenoid notch, thereby causing compressive suprascapular neuropathy. Recognition of MR patterns of muscle denervation is important to account for rotator cuff weakness in the face of an intact muscle tendon unit. Acutely denervated muscle (less than 6 months) typically appears hyperintense on T2-weighted images because of increased water content. The subacute

phase (approximately 6 to 12 months) manifests as edema in the muscle as well as increased fatty infiltration, and chronically denervated muscle (greater than 12 months) is noted as a diminution in muscle bulk and increased fatty content.

Small Joint Imaging

Software advances have enabled thin section, high resolution images of small joints, including the wrist, fingers, and elbow. Thin section (1 mm) MR images obtained with high resolution techniques permit detection and localization of tears of the triangular fibrocartilage complex, with a reported accuracy of 97% when compared to arthroscopy (Fig. 3). Advantages of MR imaging, as opposed to triple compartment conventional contrast arthrography, include visualization of the morphology of the disc, discriminating degenerative tears from peripheral detachments, which may be treated with primary arthroscopic repair, as well as disclosing tendinopathy and chondral lesions that may also account for ulnar sided wrist pain. Such techniques may also be used to evaluate the radial and ulnar collateral ligaments and flexor and extensor tendons of the elbow.

MR Angiography

MR angiography is a noninvasive technique that depicts vascular structures based on the magnetic properties of flow.

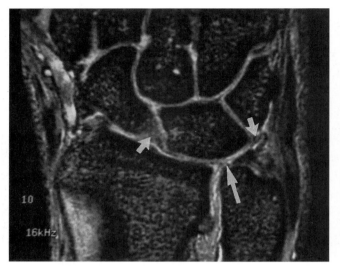

Figure 3

Thin (1 mm) section magnetic resonance image of the wrist demonstrating a surgically confirmed radial side tear of the triangular fibrocartilage (long arrow). Note the intact interosseous scapholunate and lunotriquetral ligaments (short arrows).

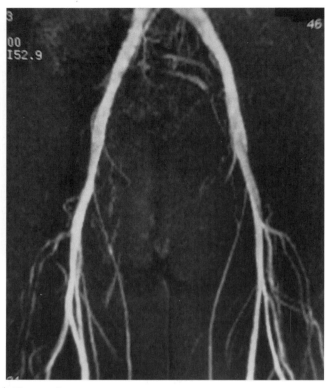

Figure 4

Projection image of an magnetic resonance venogram obtained in a patient with an acetabular fracture. Normal flow is maintained in the iliac veins of the pelvis, as well as in the veins of the proximal thighs. Superior visualization of the deep femoral veins is achieved when compared to traditional contrast venography, obtained via dorsal foot vein cannulation.

Selective MR venograms or arteriograms may be obtained. Differential contrast is achieved between increased signal intensity in flowing blood, representing fully magnetized but unsaturated protons, versus stationary background tissue that becomes saturated by repetitive RF pulses. MR venography has been used to assess the deep venous system of the pelvis and thighs in patients with acetabular and pelvic fractures (Fig. 4). MR venography is the most reliable way to detect deep venous thrombosis in the pelvis, particularly in the internal iliac veins, because these vessels cannot be reliably seen on color Doppler ultrasound or conventional contrast venography. Contrast-enhanced MR angiography has also been used to assess the pulmonary vasculature, yielding high sensitivity and specificity in the detection of pulmonary emboli. Although conventional contrast angiography remains the gold standard, MR angiography may eventually supplant conventional techniques. Finally, MR angiography may be used in planning free tissue transfer, and in patients in whom conventional contrast angiography is not possible as a result of impaired renal function.

MR Spectroscopy

MR spectroscopy is used to obtain resonance signal from biochemical compounds in the body, yielding a frequency-based spectrum. Clinical applications of MR spectroscopy include evaluation of metabolic disorders and inflammatory myopathies with phosphorus (^{31}P) spectroscopy. Combined hydrogen and ^{31}P spectroscopic determinations have been used as indicators of prognosis in human and animal soft-tissue sarcomas, helping to identify those patients most likely to respond to hyperthermia and radiation therapy. Hydrogen spectroscopy has been used to provide a noninvasive method to quantify total creatinine in human muscle, helping to elucidate the role of altered creatinine metabolism in diseased muscle, thereby assisting in treatment regimens. To date, however, these techniques remain experimental, with no broad-based clinical implementation.

Nuclear Medicine

Traditional bone scintigraphy with technetium 99m diphosphonate compounds is quite sensitive in detecting areas of increased bone turnover, because these compounds are incorporated into the hydroxyapatite matrix of bone. Routine bone scans are helpful in assessing distribution of metastatic disease and in the diagnosis of stress or insufficiency fracture. Incremental rotation of the gamma camera permits tomographic assessment (single photon emission computed tomography, [SPECT] imaging) of emitted radiotracer, which helps to localize subtle fractures, particularly of the pars interarticularis of the spine. Whereas bone scans are sensitive in detecting bone turnover, they are often nonspecific, which has been problematic in detection of bone and joint infection. Gallium 67 citrate imaging yields slightly increased specificity, but may show increased uptake in healing surgical wounds and noninfectious inflammatory processes. While combined technetium and indium-111-labeled white cell scanning increases specificity, a relatively high prevalence of false positive scans (positive predictive value 28%) has been reported following traumatic injuries. Indium-111-labeled polyclonal human immunoglobulin G (IgG) has been used more commonly outside of the United States, because it has not yet been approved for routine clinical use. While these techniques may impart increased specificity for detecting infection, the potential induction of anti-IgG antibodies may preclude serial IgG scanning.

In addition, functional radionuclide testing has been used with positron emission tomography (PET). Absorption patterns of 2-[fluorine 18]-fluoro-2 deoxy-D-glucose (FDG) have been used to assess primary and metastatic neuroblastoma, Ewing's sarcoma, malignant melanoma, and lymphoma. FDG PET in conjunction with MR imaging has been used to quantify the degree of wrist inflammation in patients with inflammatory arthritis, correlating with standardized clinical assessment.

Computed Tomography

The advent of helical (spiral) computed tomography (CT) has enabled more rapid data acquisition in diminished scan time, minimizing motion artifact. A true volumetric data set yields small reconstruction increments (1 to 2 mm) and superior three-dimensional (3D) image reformation, which is helpful in assessing fractures of the pelvis, acetabulum, and glenohumeral joint, as well as quantifying the residual limb soft-tissue envelope for prosthetic planning. Postprocessing

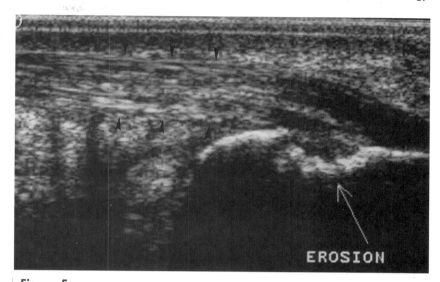

Figure 5

Longitudinal sonogram of the Achilles tendon (arrowheads) insertion. The tendon is inhomogeneous and widened distally, with an erosion at the calcaneal insertion (arrow). This appearance is seen with the enthesopathy associated with Reiter's disease. (Courtesy of Ronald S. Adler, MD)

of 3D acquired images permits subtraction of components of the image; for example, the femur from an acetabular fracture, as well as rotation of the pelvis when planning osteotomy. Use of a thicker collimation acquisition with helical CT has been shown to impair fracture detection in a cadaveric model, when compared to conventional CT. Attention to technique is necessary in trauma patients, where a higher exposure dose and thinner collimation improves diagnostic fracture detection when using helical techniques.

Ultrasound

Although used extensively outside of the United States, routine use of musculoskeletal ultrasound within this country has been hampered by operator dependency and poor reproducibility of results. Recent development of improved transducers, yielding increased spatial resolution, has prompted an increased interest that is further enhanced by the comparatively lower cost of ultrasound when compared to MR imaging, as well as its lack of ionizing radiation compared to CT. The "traditional" use of musculoskeletal ultrasound in the United States has been in the noninvasive assessment of developmental hip dysplasia, lesions of the rotator cuff, and soft-tissue masses, where it helps to distinguish cystic from solid content. With proper attention to scanning technique, good accuracy may be achieved in detecting partial and complete tears of the rotator cuff and biceps tendons, further augmented by dynamic imaging during shoulder rotation. Application to the unstable shoulder is, however, limited by poor penetrance to deep structures, including the anterior capsular labral complex.

The use of ultrasound has also been expanded to evaluate additional tendinopathy, including the patella, ankle (Fig. 5), and the hand. Ultrasound is considered the initial procedure of choice for localizing superficial foreign bodies.

As the cortex of bone appears echogenic, the proximity of fluid collections adjacent to cortex may be evaluated. Ultrasound has been used to evaluate normal and abnormal pseudocapsules surrounding loosened hip arthroplasty. Periprosthetic fluid collections can also be detected in cases of infected total joint arthroplasty. Ultrasound has also been used to assess fracture healing over areas of intramedullary instrumentation, as well as to evaluate osseous continuity following Ilizarov-type lengthening procedures.

Because of its ability to depict blood flow, power Doppler sonography may assess alterations in muscle blood volume following exercise, quantitating the degree of fractional moving blood volume through muscle placed under stress. Such quantitative changes may provide new insight in the dynamic assessment of patients with compartment syndrome. Power Doppler, unlike conventional color Doppler imaging, is essentially angle independent and extends the dynamic range of vascular flow in soft tissue, rather than limiting evaluation to the mean or maximal velocity. Finally, ultrasound has been used to assess subtle surface fibrillations in an in vitro osteoarthritic model, providing a noninvasive model to assess response to individual treatment regimens.

Summary

Because multiple imaging tests are available, the cost versus benefit of the individual test must be weighed with regard to the specific patient and the clinically suspected diagnosis. Although superior soft-tissue contrast may be achieved with MR imaging, superficial soft-tissue structures may be well delineated by ultrasound, and occult fractures may be detected with the use of radionuclide examinations. In certain circumstances (eg, pediatric patients), sedation may be necessary for lengthier examinations such as MR imaging, and depending on the area of clinical concern, diagnostic questions may be answered with more conventional imaging tests that do not require sedation. Above all, diagnostic imaging tests reflect the anatomy of the tissue studied. They are but one component of a comprehensive diagnostic assessment, and must be correlated with a complete physical examination and patient history, in order to provide an effective and accurate diagnosis.

Annotated Bibliography

Disler DG, McCauley TR, Kelman CG, et al: Fat-suppressed three-dimensional spoiled gradient-echo MR imaging of hyaline cartilage defects in the knee: Comparison with standard MR imaging and arthroscopy. *Am J Roentgenol* 1996;167: 127–132.

The authors compared MR imaging with arthroscopy in 48 patients in the detection of cartilage defects of the knee, using both standard and specialized cartilage pulse sequences, reporting 86% sensitivity and 97% specificity in the prospective evaluation of all articular surfaces.

Gusmer PB, Potter HG, Schatz JA, et al: Labral injuries: Accuracy of detection with unenhanced MR imaging of the shoulder. *Radiology* 1996;200:519–524.

The authors prospectively compared high resolution noncontrast MR imaging to arthrography in 103 patients, finding 95% accuracy in the detection and localization of tears. The results of this study suggest that MR arthrography may not be necessary to detect labral tears.

Meaney JF, Weg JG, Chenevert TL, Stafford-Johnson D, Hamilton BH, Prince MR: Diagnosis of pulmonary embolism with magnetic resonance angiography. *N Engl J Med* 1997;336: 1422–1427.

The authors compared gadolinium-enhanced noninvasive MR of the pulmonary arteries to standard pulmonary angiography in 30 patients, noting high MR sensitivity and specificity for detection of pulmonary emboli. Although conventional pulmonary angiography remains the standard, MR angiography may eventually replace traditional techniques.

Montgomery KD, Potter HG, Helfet DL: Magnetic resonance venography to evaluate the deep venous system of the pelvis in patients who have an acetabular fracture. *J Bone Joint Surg* 1995;77A:1639–1649.

The authors performed a prospective blinded assessment of preoperative MR versus conventional venography in the detection of deep venous thrombosis in 45 patients with displaced acetabular fracture. MR venography was superior to contrast venography in detecting pelvic thrombi, particularly in the internal iliac veins.

Palmer WE, Caslowitz PL: Anterior shoulder instability: Diagnostic criteria determined from prospective analysis of 121 MR arthrograms. *Radiology* 1995;197:819–825.

The authors prospectively evaluated 121 patients with MR arthrography and arthroscopy, noting that MR arthrography was highly accurate in detecting inferior labral ligamentous lesions, but missed cases of capsular laxity in the absence of an inferior labral tear. The authors noted no correlation between the site of capsular insertion and clinical instability.

Potter HG, Asnis-Ernberg L, Weiland AJ, Hotchkiss RN, Peterson MG, McCormack RR Jr: The utility of high resolution magnetic resonance imaging in the evaluation of the triangular fibrocartilage complex of the wrist. *J Bone Joint Surg* 1997;79A: 1675–1684.

The authors prospectively assessed 77 patients with high resolution MR imaging of the triangular fibrocartilage complex compared to arthroscopy. MR imaging yielded high sensitivity and specificity for the detection and localization of tears, as well as distinction between complete and partial tears.

Peterfy CG, van Dijke CF, Janzen DL, et al: Quantification of articular cartilage in the knee with pulsed saturation transfer subtraction and fat-suppressed MR imaging: Optimization and validation. *Radiology* 1994;192:485–491.

The authors provide a method to reproduce volumetric quantification of articular cartilage in the knee using commercially available MR pulse sequences.

Shulkin BL, Mitchell DS, Ungar DR, et al: Neoplasms in a pediatric population: 2-[F-18]-fluoro-2-deoxy-D-glucose PET studies. *Radiology* 1995;194:495–500.

The authors evaluated the use of FDG PET in pediatric neoplasms, reporting increased sensitivity of PET compared with routine scintigraphy.

van Holsbeeck MT, Eyler WR, Sherman LS, et al: Detection of infection in loosened hip prostheses: Efficacy of sonography. *Am J Roentgenol* 1994;163:381–384.

This study is among the first to use ultrasound to assess bone, specifically to contrast the normal and infected pseudocapsules following total hip arthroplasty.

Chapter 9
Clinical Epidemiology

Introduction

Epidemiology has been defined as the study of the distribution and determinants of human diseases. Clinical epidemiology is the use of epidemiologic principles and methods to improve clinical observation and interpretation and to assess the impact of clinical interventions on the course of disease. As such, clinical epidemiology applies epidemiologic methods to the clinical activities of physicians, including diagnosis, risk and prognostic assessment, treatment, and prevention.

Modern epidemiologic research has tended to focus on disorders with high mortality rates, such as cardiovascular disease and cancer, rather than conditions primarily affecting quality of life. As the concept of health has evolved from the "absence of infirmity or disease" to "physical, mental, and social well-being" so too has epidemiology changed from focusing primarily on fatal diseases and their risk factors to the evaluation of the spectrum of health outcomes that people experience. These outcomes, in addition to morbidity and mortality, include functional status, health-related quality of life, and satisfaction. This shift in the focus of epidemiology has led to the development of a wide range of instruments designed to measure these aspects of health.

Despite the societal and individual impacts of orthopaedic disorders, relatively little is known about the epidemiology of many of these diseases or about the relative effectiveness of therapies used to treat them. The lack of widely agreed upon diagnostic criteria for many orthopaedic conditions, barriers to the use of functional status and health-related quality of life measures in patient care and clinical investigation, and the paucity of secondary sources for this type of data have likely contributed to limiting these lines of inquiry. The purpose of this chapter is to introduce the basic concepts of clinical epidemiology.

Considerations for Assessing the Validity of Epidemiologic Evidence

Chance

By necessity, observations about disease are ordinarily made on a sample of patients from the relevant population rather than on the relevant population as a whole. Even if the sample is randomly chosen from the relevant population, inference drawn from data from a sample may be wrong because of variation resulting from measurement or sampling error. Measurement error results from inaccuracies in the instrument used to measure something or in the interpretation of the information by the person recording the measurement. Sampling error results if the sample chosen for study is not large enough or representative enough of the biologic variation in the measurement. Statistics can be used to assess the probability that measurement error or random variation is a likely explanation for observations made in a sample.

Bias

Bias refers to any systematic error in the assessment of exposures or outcomes among patients under study that results in an incorrect estimate of the association between the factors under study. Bias can take many forms, but selection and measurement biases are frequent concerns. Selection bias refers to comparisons of groups of patients that differ systematically with respect to determinants of outcome other than those under study. It can result from a number of circumstances related to the way in which individuals are verified and chosen for study, including referral of individuals into the study, diagnosis, and follow-up. Measurement bias refers to differential methods of measurement of exposure among compared groups of patients. Specific biases are of particular concern for different study designs and will be covered more thoroughly in the relevant sections on study design (Table 1).

Confounding

Confounding is a mixing of the effect of the exposure under study on the outcome with that of a third factor. In order to confound the relationship, the third factor must be independently related to the outcome under study and differentially distributed among the groups being compared. For example, patients undergoing surgery for lumbar spinal stenosis (SpS) have higher rates of postoperative complications and death than those undergoing surgery for lumbar disk herniation (LDH). However, assessment of this association must account for the 20-year difference in mean age of patients undergoing surgery for lumbar SpS and LDH. In this example, age is a confounder of the relationship between diagno-

Table 1
Strengths and limitations of the observational study designs

	Cohort Study*	Case-control Study*	Cross-sectional Study*
Selective survival	+	–	–
Recall bias	+	–	–
Loss to follow-up	–	+	+
Time sequence of events	+	–	–
Time to complete	–	+	+
Expense	–	+	+/–

* + = Strength; – = Limitation

(Reproduced with permission from Kasser JR (ed): *Orthopaedic Knowledge Update 5*. Rosemont, IL, American Academy of Orthopaedic Surgeons, 1996, pp 71–80.)

sis and surgical complications with lumbar surgical procedures because it is differentially distributed among the diagnostic categories and independently related to risk of postoperative complications. Confounding can be controlled in the study design by using matching or randomization techniques, or it can be controlled in the analysis of the data by using stratification, standardization, or multivariate modeling techniques.

Effect Modification
Effect modification, also known as interaction, occurs when the association between the exposure and the outcome under study differs for varying levels of another factor. In contrast to confounding, which is a distortion of the true effect, effect modification reflects biologic variation in the effects that an exposure has on an outcome for some groups of people. For example, if it was observed that the magnitude or even direction of the effect of age on risk of postoperative complications with lumbar surgical procedures differed by sex (eg, if risk of postoperative complications were 3 times greater for male patients over the age of 80 but only 2 times greater for female patients over the age of 80), sex would be considered an effect modifier of the relationship between age and risk of postoperative complications.

Causal Relationships
Once an epidemiologic association has been deemed valid and statistically significant, the possibility that the relationship is causal may be considered. The criteria for assessing whether an epidemiologic relationship is causal include the strength of the association, the biologic plausibility of the association, consistency with other investigations, establishment of the time sequence of exposure preceding outcome, and whether there is a dose-response relationship between the exposure and the outcome.

Study Design

Descriptive Epidemiology
Descriptive epidemiology concerns general characteristics about the distribution of diseases or health outcomes. Descriptive studies are most useful for hypothesis generation and less useful for hypothesis-testing because of various limitations in the design of descriptive studies.

A case report is a careful, detailed report of the course of disease for a single patient. Case series are similar but include a small group of like patients. New diseases or epidemics may be detected by similarities noted among case reports. For example, the relationship between epidural bleeding and the combination of low molecular weight heparins and heparinoids with epidural anesthesia was recognized after the publication of case reports of patients who had epidural bleeding after total hip replacement. The United States Food and Drug Administration issued a public health advisory on the health risks of using these drugs in combination following the publication of more than 30 case reports.

Correlational studies use data from entire populations to compare disease or health outcome frequencies between different groups during the same time period or in the same population at different points in time. For example, rates of osteoporosis have been compared internationally. These studies have suggested many hypotheses about contributing causes of osteoporosis, including dietary and genetic differences. Although these studies raise the hypothesis that these factors are associated with rates of osteoporosis, they are limited in their ability to test these hypotheses. This is because in correlational studies it is not possible to link exposures to risks of disease or occurrence of particular health outcomes in individuals. For example, in a correlational study design it is not possible to discern whether women who develop osteoporosis in any particular country are those with the lowest calcium intakes, only that on average, countries with the lowest levels of calcium consumption have the highest rates of osteoporosis. There may be other differences between countries in factors that are associated with the consumption of calcium (ie, nutrition in general, socioeconomic status, etc) that might be associated with consumption of calcium but that actually account for the observed differences in rates of osteoporosis.

Small area analysis, also known as "medical care epidemiology" refers to the use of epidemiologic methods to study the use of health services and the allocation of resources within the health care system. Small area analysis can be used to assess population-based rates of the use of health care services, to measure variation in provider-specific use rates, to provide comprehensive descriptions of the health care delivery system (ie, to measure the types and quantities of health resources, per capita expenditures on health care, health services provided, and resulting health outcomes), and finally to answer questions relevant to health policy. Small area analysis has been used to assess population-based rates of hospitalization for hip fracture, variations in rates of surgery and surgical complications for low back pain and joint replacement, and treatment and use of services for limb and cervical spine fractures.

Observational Epidemiology

The cross-sectional study is a type of observational study in which exposure and disease status are measured simultaneously among individuals of a population. These types of studies are used to assess the prevalence of various health conditions, the distribution of various physiologic and biochemical measurements, and the impact (ie, as measured by hospitalizations, physician visits, or days lost from work or school) of various health problems. Among the most well known cross-sectional studies is the National Health and Nutrition Examination Survey (NHANES), which has been conducted periodically since the United States Congress passed the National Health Survey Act in 1956. These surveys of a random sample of the U.S. population provide data on the prevalence of acute and chronic diseases, disabilities, use of health care resources, and relevant demographic and personal characteristics for use in health care planning, administration, and research. These surveys have provided a great deal of information about the epidemiology of musculoskeletal disorders, including their prevalence and health impacts relative to other common health problems.

A case-control study is a type of observational study in which people are selected for study on the basis of disease or health outcome status. A sample of people with the disease or health outcome (cases) are compared to a sample of people without the disease or health outcome (controls) with respect to exposure to a characteristic or characteristics thought to

contribute to risk of the disease or health outcome in question. This type of study design has obvious advantages for certain circumstances, including the study of rare diseases or outcomes or those with long asymptomatic phases. This study design is also useful in the early stages of an epidemic to generate hypotheses about possible contributing exposures. These studies are relatively inexpensive and time efficient. On the other hand, because both exposure and disease have already occurred at the time of entry into the study, this design is particularly susceptible to various biases, especially in the selection of study participants and in the assessment of exposures.

A cohort study is a type of observational study in which people are selected for study on the basis of exposure status and then followed forward in time to assess the occurrence of a disease or health outcome of interest. Because all participants must be free of the disease or outcome in question at the time of entry into the study, the temporal sequence of exposure preceding disease is established. A retrospective cohort study is a type of cohort study in which the exposures took place in the past and outcome status is assessed at the time that the study is initiated. The cohort study design is especially useful when studying rare exposures (such as occupational or genetic factors) and can be used to assess a variety of health effects of a single exposure. The drawbacks of this study design are that these studies are time-consuming and expensive. In addition, they are susceptible to biases resulting from differential losses to follow-up.

Interventional (Experimental) Studies: Clinical Trials

A clinical trial is a type of cohort study in which the investigators allocate an exposure to study participants and then keep track of them to assess the effect (either preventive or therapeutic) of that exposure on some health outcome of interest. When a clinical trial is "controlled" that means that an alternative agent (either a placebo or some standard treatment) is allocated to some of the patients for comparison with the exposure of interest. Controls are used to avoid the "placebo effect" whereby individuals tend to report a favorable response to any therapy, perhaps because of the belief that the treatment will work. When a clinical trial is "blinded," either the participants or the investigators, or both, are unaware of which exposure any particular study participant has received. The use of blinding is a method for minimizing bias in the ascertainment of subjective outcomes or side-effects of the exposure. When a clinical trial is "randomized" that means the exposures are allocated to the participants by chance, using a method of random allocation (Fig. 1). Randomization prevents confounding of the study results, by

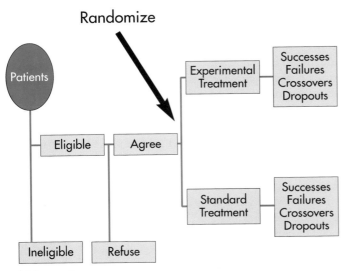

Figure 1

Randomized controlled trial. (Reproduced with permission from Kasser JR (ed): *Orthopaedic Knowledge Update 5.* Rosemont, IL, American Academy of Orthopaedic Surgeons, 1996, pp 71–80.)

factors known or unknown, because when applied to a large enough group of subjects, it (usually) ensures comparability of the patients in each of the treatment arms of the trial.

Special Topics

Sample Size and Power

In epidemiologic research, it is almost always the case that studies are based on data that are drawn from a sample of a relevant population. Therefore, measurements of the characteristics of a sample are used to estimate the same characteristics of the associated population. The degree to which this is successful depends on the amount of variation resulting from errors in measurement and on random variation. One of the major determinants of the degree to which chance affects the findings in any particular study is sample size. The possible results when using a sample to estimate true population characteristics can be illustrated using a 2 × 2 table (Table 2). Errors that result in the conclusion that a difference exists when it really does not are called type I or alpha errors. On the other hand, errors that result in the conclusion that no difference or relationship exists when one really does, are called type II or beta errors. The probability of finding a specified difference or relationship when one truly exists is called statistical power.

Power is related to sample size; the larger the sample size,

the greater the power. If a study finds no statistically significant difference it may be because there is no difference or it may be because the study lacked sufficient power to detect a difference because the sample was too small. When calculating the required sample size for a study, power is usually set at 0.8 or 0.9. In addition, sample size calculations require an estimate of the effect size or magnitude of the difference to be detected. Finally, sample size calculations depend on characteristics of the data. For studies in which the outcome is expressed as a count or proportion, statistical power depends on the rate of events. The larger the number of events, the greater the statistical power for a given number of people at risk. If the outcome measure is continuous, statistical power depends on the amount of random variation in measurement of that variable.

Diagnostic Testing

Regardless of the kind of data produced by diagnostic tests, they are usually reduced to simpler forms for use in clinical practice. Frequently, tests are said to be positive or negative based on some chosen cutoff point for the measurement. Table 3 summarizes the relationship between the results of a diagnostic test and the actual presence of disease. Patients may either be classified correctly as having the disease (true positive) or not having the disease (true negative) or incorrectly classified as having the disease (false positive) or not having the disease (false negative). Sensitivity and specificity are 2 measures of the validity of a diagnostic test. Sensitivity is defined as the probability of a positive test given that the patient actually has the disease. Specificity is defined as the probability of a negative test given that the patient does not have the disease.

Because the definition of positive and negative test results usually depends on a chosen cutoff point to discriminate the range of normal from a range of abnormal results, there is

Table 2

2 by 2 table for illustrating type I and type II sampling errors reality

	Reality	
Results of Study	**Different**	**Not Different**
Different	Correct	Type I (α)
Not Different	Type II (β)	Correct

Power = $1 - \beta$

frequently a trade-off between the sensitivity and specificity of diagnostic tests. In such cases, setting the cut off point to assure a high sensitivity (such that everyone who had the disease would test positive) is usually accomplished at the expense of specificity (because many who did not have the disease would also test positive). The Receiver Operating Characteristic (ROC) is a graphic representation of this trade-off that plots the true positive rate versus the false positive rate over the range of possible cutoff points. The area beneath the ROC curve is a frequently reported measure of test performance that ranges from 0.5 (indicative of a useless test) to 1.0 (indicative of a perfect test). For many orthopaedic conditions there are no objective standards for disease. Diagnosis is usually made using some combination of physical examination, history, and imaging test results.

Table 3
2 by 2 table for illustrating diagnostic test characteristics

	Gold Standard Result		
Diagnostic Test Result	Positive	Negative	
Positive	True positive (TP)	False positive (FP)	TP + FP
Negative	False negative (FN)	True negative (TN)	FN + TN
	TP + FN	FP + TN	

Sensitivity, proportion of persons with the disease who test positive, TP/(TP + FN)
Specificity, proportion of persons without the disease who test negative, TN/(FP + TN)
Positive predictive value,* probability that disease is present given a positive test, TN/(FP + TN)
Negative predictive value,* probability that disease is absent given a negative test, TN/(FN + TN)
*Sensitive to the prior probability or prevalence of the disease in the population (TP + FN)/(TP + FP + FN + TN)

Screening

A sometimes controversial use of diagnostic tests is for screening of asymptomatic patients to identify patients at risk for, or with early stages of, disease. There are several important considerations in the decision to screen for a disease. First among these is the effectiveness of early treatment. Assessing the effectiveness of early treatment is fraught with difficulty because of biases inherent to such investigations. Lead time bias refers to the fact that people who are diagnosed by screening for a deadly disease will, on average, live longer from the time of diagnosis than people who are diagnosed after they get symptoms, even if there is no effective treatment. Length bias refers to the fact that screening is more likely to detect less severe forms of disease whereas regular care finds those with worse prognoses, even if the prognosis of each is unchanged by treatment. In either case, the bias has the effect of making the prognosis of those detected by screening appear better than the prognosis of those diagnosed by other means. In addition to the effectiveness of early treatment, the accuracy, safety, and cost of the test must be considered in decisions about whether or not to screen for early disease.

Meta-Analysis

Meta-analysis goes by many names including statistical/quantitative overview, data pooling, and research synthesis. It is a method of statistically combining the results of multiple independent studies (usually clinical trials) on a specific topic. The reasons for doing meta-analysis include increasing statistical power by increasing sample size, resolving inconsistencies in the evidence derived from different studies, and improving estimates of effect size. Although there are several different methods, meta-analyses all combine data to arrive at a summary estimate of the effect size, a measure of its variance and 95% confidence interval, and a test for homogeneity of effect size. The methods can be classified broadly by their underlying assumptions of either fixed or random effects. The Mantel-Haenszel, Peto, general variance, and confidence interval methods assume fixed effects, or that inference is conditional on the studies actually done. The DerSimonian and Laird method assumes random effects, or that the studies are a random sample of some hypothetical population of studies. In general, the random-effects method is considered more conservative; however, the methods yield similar results so long as there is not much heterogeneity or variation between studies. In the presence of significant heterogeneity, the between-study variance terms will dominate the weights assigned to the studies using the random-effects model, and large and small studies will tend to be weighted equally. In this situation, the results gleaned from random and fixed effects models, which weight studies based on the sample size only, may differ significantly.

Most criticisms of meta-analysis relate to criticisms of the source literature rather than meta-analytic methods themselves. Publication bias refers to a preference for nonnull (supporting the hypothesis) results that makes the published literature biased toward significant, nonnull effects. This bias is well-documented in studies of the published literature. It is common to attribute this tendency to editorial preferences; however, this hypothesis was not supported by a study that found that over 90% of institutional review board approved, but unpublished, studies had never been submitted. The fact that some published studies are of higher quality than others has lead to methods for weighting studies to be included in a meta-analysis on the basis of quality. These methods include blinding of the quality raters such that quality is assessed independently of the outcome or of other information that might bias the rater. Differing variable definitions and study entry criteria are substantial barriers to meta-analysis. Such concerns have led to the development of standardized reporting standards for many areas of medical research.

Decision Analysis

Decision analysis is a systematic, quantitative method for assessing the relative value of different options. It can be used in clinical decision making for individual patients or for developing policy for management of groups of patients based on an analysis of information about the relative risks and benefits of the different approaches to clinical management. Decision analyses are usually organized in 5 steps. The first step is to identify and focus the question or problem to be addressed by listing the alternative courses of action as well as the relevant potential outcomes. The second step involves structuring the problem. Frequently this is accomplished by constructing a diagram known as a decision tree.

By convention, branches indicating the different options are usually connected by square-shaped decision "nodes," and branches indicating chance events are connected by circle-shaped chance "nodes." The possible outcomes are at the end of the right most or "terminal" branches and are often rectangular shaped. The third step in decision analysis is to assign probabilities to the chance events and numeric values or "utilities" to the outcome events. Frequently, probabilities and utility values are derived from some combination of raw data, the literature, and expert consensus. Specialized methods known as "utility assessment" are used to collect primary data on the value or preferences of individuals or society for the full spectrum of possible health outcomes. The fourth step in a decision analysis is to calculate the expected value of each strategy by multiplying the probability of each outcome by the utility for that outcome and summing the relevant products for each strategy. The final step in a decision analy-

sis, called sensitivity analysis, assesses stability of the results to varying estimates of the included probabilities and utilities.

Cost-effectiveness analysis is a type of decision analysis that compares the outcome of various strategies in terms of their ratio of cost to unit of effectiveness. For example, a cost effectiveness analysis might have as its outcome measure cost per year of life saved. Cost-effectiveness is used to guide policy by setting priorities for resource allocation and to decide among alternative treatments or interventions.

Conclusion

This chapter has attempted to introduce some of the basic concepts, strengths, and limitations of clinical epidemiology. Although clinical medicine and epidemiology both concern scientific approaches to the causes and consequences of disease in humans, they have until recently remained largely separate disciplines. Clinical medicine has traditionally been based on the belief that through understanding the mechanisms of disease, it is possible to predict its course and select appropriate therapies. For this reason, medical training has focused on basic sciences, including biochemistry, anatomy, and physiology. Epidemiology has traditionally been concerned with describing and statistically analyzing patterns of disease in human populations. The combination of clinical medicine and epidemiology is believed to enrich both disciplines. Epidemiology benefits from the incorporation of clinical judgments about the important questions to be answered regarding the clinical course disease and effectiveness of treatment. Clinical medicine is improved by the application to the practice of medicine of scientific methods designed specifically for the study of disease in humans.

Annotated Bibliography

Ingelfinger JA, Mosteller F, Thibodeau LA, Ware JH (eds): *Biostatistics in Clinical Medicine*, ed 3. New York, NY, McGraw-Hill, 1994.

This book was written to help physicians understand statistics and the application of probabilistic theory to patient care. The use of statistics and probability in diagnosis, treatment, and follow-up are emphasized. Topics covered include: probabilistic approaches to diagnosis and treatment, the application of statistical inference to clinical practice, and the evaluation and application of data from clinical trials.

Petitti DB (ed): *Meta-Analysis, Decision Analysis, and Cost-Effectiveness Analysis: Methods for Quantitative Synthesis in Medicine.* New York, NY, Oxford University Press, 1994.

This book describes how to design, conduct, analyze, and interpret the results from 3 types of studies that involve the synthesis of data from other studies: meta-analysis, decision-analysis, and cost-effectiveness analysis. It is meant as an introductory overview that focuses on the practical application of these methods rather than the quantitative underpinnings.

Classic Bibliography

Dawson-Saunders B, Trapp RG (eds): *Basic and Clinical Biostatistics.* Norwalk, CT, Appleton & Lange, 1990.

Feinstein AR (ed): *Clinical Epidemiology: The Architecture of Clinical Research.* Philadelphia, PA, WB Saunders, 1985.

Fletcher RH, Fletcher SW, Wagner EH (eds): *Clinical Epidemiology: The Essentials,* ed 2. Baltimore, MD, Williams & Wilkins, 1988.

Hennekens CH, Buring JE, Mayrent SL (eds): *Epidemiology in Medicine.* Boston, MA, Little Brown & Co, 1987.

Kelsey JL (ed): *Epidemiology of Musculoskeletal Disorders.* New York, NY, Oxford University Press, 1982.

Maggi S, Kelsey JL, Litvak J, Heyse SP: Incidence of hip fractures in the elderly: A cross-national analysis. *Osteoporo Int* 1991;1:232–241.

Thornbury JR, Fryback DG, Turski PA, et al: Disk-caused nerve compression in patients with acute low-back pain: Diagnosis with MR, CT myelography, and plain CT. *Radiology* 1993;186:731–738.

Chapter 10
Practice Guidelines

Introduction

Standardized approaches to patient management have become increasingly commonplace. Although informal guidelines for the treatment of patients are ancient, more modern attempts to codify knowledge have taken place as part of attempts to improve health care by identifying "best practices" and evaluating cost effectiveness. Under the rubric of Clinical Pathways or Standardized Plans of Care, many orthopaedic surgeons have become familiar with the concept of using a guideline in managing patients. Guideline is a relatively nonspecific term, which in many cases is used interchangeably with clinical policies, practice parameters, clinical algorithms (Fig. 1), clinical pathways, and so forth. The plethora of terms used to characterize practice guidelines is somewhat confusing; however, there are few specifically defined differences among the terms commonly used.

The term selected by the American Medical Association (AMA) is Practice Parameters, and this remains one of the most generic terms used to describe working tools for patient management developed by formal processes. The AMA has developed parameter attributes that provide a basis for determining guideline quality.

According to this standard, guidelines should: (1) be developed by or with physicians' organizations that have appropriate scientific and clinical expertise; (2) be based on reliable methodologies, including the integration of appropriate clinical expertise and research findings; (3) include the description of the methods used to gather evidence as well as the evidence used and the methods used to reach consensus; (4) include the qualifications of experts; (5) be specific regarding clinical management strategies; and (6) be based on current information, disseminated in peer-reviewed journals or other appropriate publications and reviewed within 3 years of its original writing.

Three fundamental issues are of concern in the development of guidelines: (1) methods used for topic selection and guideline development, dissemination, and testing; (2) usefulness, value, or worth of a guideline; and (3) medicolegal implications of guidelines.

Guideline Development

Methodologic issues in guideline development are significant. Three basic approaches that can be used (and combined in various ways) include: literature review, expert opinion consensus, and large scale clinical trials.

Literature review may be more or less "scientific." It can range from the review of a biased selection of literature, promoting a specific viewpoint, by experts with common training, background, and prejudices, to meta-analysis, involving a specifically defined literature search, inclusion of only methodologically appropriate studies, and statistical compilation of results. Although meta-analysis helps to decrease individual reviewer bias and explicitly lists criteria for the literature search and study inclusion, it may suffer by leaving out important studies that do not fit the rigid criteria established for the meta-analysis. Moreover, many important clinical issues are not addressed in the "scientific" literature.

Expert opinion consensus has the advantage of incorporating clinical experience with the expert's individual understanding of the literature. However, bias in selection of panel members and in the deliberative group processes remains a significant issue in this method. Specific methods in the selection of experts as well as the use of formal rating scales and other group processing techniques may be useful in minimizing bias in this setting.

Performance of large-scale prospective clinical trials has the potential to be the most scientifically valid; however, it is incapable of exploring more than 1 or 2 issues of significance in what is most commonly a more complex constellation of clinical issues. In addition, the performance of such trials is expensive and time consuming, making this method the least frequently used.

Most guidelines can be categorized as being developed through a standard structure, the specific implementation of which provides for the differences in the actual guideline development process. These include: topic selection, panel member selection criteria, scope and perspective of the guideline, processes used to extract information from various sources, the sources considered, the group processes

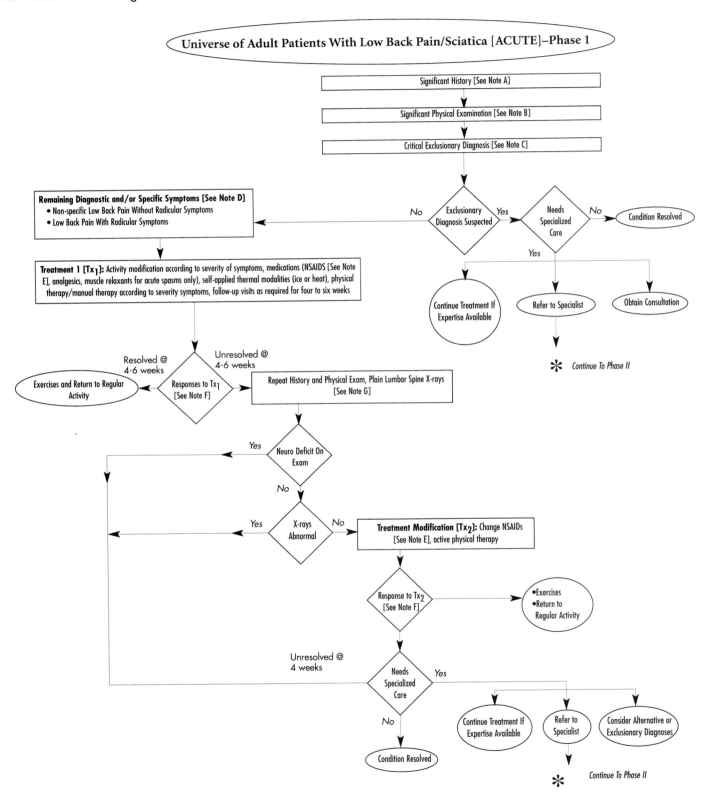

Universe of Adult Patients With Low Back Pain/Sciatica [ACUTE]–Phase 1

Significant History [See Note A]

Significant Physical Examination [See Note B]

Critical Exclusionary Diagnosis [See Note C]

Remaining Diagnostic and/or Specific Symptoms [See Note D]
- Non-specific Low Back Pain Without Radicular Symptoms
- Low Back Pain With Radicular Symptoms

No ← Exclusionary Diagnosis Suspected → Yes → Needs Specialized Care → No → Condition Resolved

Yes

Continue Treatment If Expertise Available

Refer to Specialist

Obtain Consultation

✱ *Continue To Phase II*

Treatment 1 [Tx₁]: Activity modification according to severity of symptoms, medications (NSAIDS [See Note E], analgesics, muscle relaxants for acute spasms only), self-applied thermal modalities (ice or heat), physical therapy/manual therapy according to severity symptoms, follow-up visits as required for four to six weeks

Resolved @ 4-6 weeks ← Responses to Tx₁ [See Note F] → Unresolved @ 4-6 weeks

Exercises and Return to Regular Activity

Repeat History and Physical Exam, Plain Lumbar Spine X-rays [See Note G]

Yes ← Neuro Deficit On Exam

No

Yes ← X-rays Abnormal → No → **Treatment Modification [Tx₂]:** Change NSAIDs [See Note E], active physical therapy

Response to Tx₂ [See Note F] → • Exercises • Return to Regular Activity

Unresolved @ 4 weeks

Needs Specialized Care → Yes

No

Condition Resolved

Continue Treatment If Expertise Available

Refer to Specialist

Consider Alternative or Exclusionary Diagnoses

✱ *Continue To Phase II*

Algorithm Notes

A. Significant History

- Location of symptoms: % low back or leg
- Duration: acute (<6 weeks) or chronic
- Mechanism of onset: insidious or specific (trauma)
- Character or description of pain: mechanical, radicular, claudicant, non-specific
- Neurologic history: distribution, bowel and bladder symptoms, weakness, numbness (saddle)
- Constitutional (ie, fever or weight loss)
- Previous spinal surgery with persistent pain

B. Significant Physical Examination

- Inspection of posture, stance, and gait
- ROM testing of spine, hip, and lower extremity
- Specific tests (straight leg raise and reverse straight leg raise)
- Neurological (motor strength, muscle wasting, sensation, deep tendon reflexes, specific reflexes such as Babinski and Clonus)
- Directed medical exam

C. Critical Exclusionary Diagnoses

- Cauda Equina Syndrome (CES)

  1-Acute, severe low back pain
  2-Saddle anesthesia
  3-Profound/progressive neurologic deficit
  4-Loss of bowel and bladder control

- Progressive neurologic changes and/or severe progressive symptomatology
- Neurologic deficit (muscle weakness and/or reflex loss)
- Fracture
- Neoplasm
- Infection
- Previous spinal surgery with persistent pain
- Chronic pain syndrome

D. Remaining Diagnostic and/or Specific Symptoms

Consider diagnosis and symptoms such as:

- Low Back Strain
- Herniated Nucleus Pulposus
- Spondylolisthesis
- Osteoarthritis DJD
- Spinal Stenosis
- Instability

E. NSAIDs

NSAIDs are relatively contraindicated in patients with renal insufficiency or pregnancy. Administer cautiously in individuals with hypertension or gastrointestinal intolerance. Side effects and toxicity should be monitored during administration.

There is no evidence that administration of NSAIDs are more efficacious than simple analgesics or acetaminophen in relieving symptoms in non-inflammatory conditions.

F. Response Criteria

Good:

- Patient satisfied with outcome
- Patient function improved

Poor or Partial:

- Patient dissatisfied with outcome
- Patient function unimproved or worsened
- Persistent sequelae or complications

G. Imaging

- AP lateral
- Spot lateral

American Academy of Orthopaedic Surgeons and North American Spine Society

Low Back Pain/Sciatica [Acute]—Phase I Version 1.0–©1996

Cannot be reproduced without permission.   **DRAFT**

This orthopaedic clinical algorithim should not be construed as including all proper methods of care or excluding other acceptable methods of care reasonably directed to obtaining the same results. The ultimate judgement regarding any specific procedure or treatment must be made by the physician in light of all circumstances presented by the patient and the needs and resources particular to the locality or institution.

Figure 1

American Academy of Orthopaedic Surgeons/North American Spine Society draft clinical algorithm on diagnosis and treatment of low back pain.

used to consider and decide on evidence, the extent to which the guideline is linked to "scientific" evidence, and the degree to which the methods used are explicit, documented, and available.

Guideline topics can be chosen by a variety of means and from differing perspectives. Election of topics may be by survey of interested parties or by fiat, such as governmental or administrative. Criteria that have been used to determine topic appropriateness, including public health impact; disease prevalence, incidence, and severity as well as the potential for prevention or treatment; variation in clinical practice; and availability of evidence, are important characteristics. These factors may determine whether or nor valid guideline formation is feasible in a given area. The prevalence of large regional discrepancies or variations in patterns of practice is one of the fundamental forces driving the creation of practice guidelines. Thus, well established variations may represent an ideal focus for guideline development. Additional criteria are cost (particularly when an intervention may become part of a widely available and used screening tool), controversy (when clinicians disagree on subjects of sufficient demographic or economic importance), and new technology subject to potentially inappropriate use.

The creation of panels to evaluate available data or to select topics for guideline development are also subject to bias. All surgical panels tend to establish indications for surgery at a much higher rate than mixed groups of surgeons and other health care experts. The magnitude of this effect may be large; one group of surgeons assessing carotid endarterectomy found 70% of cases to be appropriate for surgery, whereas a multidisciplinary group found 38% to be appropriate. Cultural bias has been shown in some studies to be related to nationality and experience with differing health delivery systems. In addition, there is a tendency to appoint clinicians whose practice patterns are most likely to be affected by the guideline. This tendency frequently leads to panels containing "enthusiasts" or panels that of necessity contain a high proportion of users with similar bias. The importance of incorporating nonphysicians, such as nurses, epidemiologists, health care economists, and experts in the psychosocial aspects of a given health concern, is readily apparent.

Defining the scope of a guideline is of great importance both before and during its development. Resource usage issues may play an important role in the implementation of any guideline. In addition, failure to consider health system constraints and patient preference may result in a guideline with unrealistic or even undesirable recommendations. Thus, guideline developers must consider patient preferences, as well as important aspects of patient health status and functioning in determining specific recommendations.

Evidence Gathering and Decision Making

High quality guidelines can be produced only within the context of appropriately gathered, screened, and evaluated medical evidence. Thus, a systematic approach to literature review is required. The likelihood of post-hoc adjustments in the review process and the introduction of bias can be reduced by defining (1) the questions to be addressed; (2) the way in which the literature will be searched; (3) the type of studies included in the analysis; (4) the type of outcomes; (5) how variations in outcome will be evaluated; and (6) variations in study parameters.

Analysis of data to determine appropriate clinical choices requires ranking of evidence quality. Many such systems have been proposed and implemented, and different guidelines within a single agency have used different ranking systems. Although most ranking systems are quite similar, the only consensus is that the randomized controlled trial (RCT) remains the best standard of medical evidence. Thus, a typical ranking system (from the Canadian Task Force on Periodic Health Examination) ranks the RCT as grade I evidence; a well-designed, controlled but not randomized study as grade II-1; a well-designed case control or cohort study preferably from more than 1 center or research group as grade II-2; evidence compared across time or place with and without the intervention under investigation as grade II-3; and opinions of respected authorities, based on clinical experience, descriptive study, or expert committee reports as grade III.

Quantitative synthesis of data may take place by appropriate statistical methodology (so-called meta-analysis) if sufficient high-quality data are available for combining similar studies. Because of the lack of such studies in most areas, some type of qualitative synthesis is commonly required. Unfortunately, there is less guidance in the area of qualitative data synthesis. However, guidelines for the qualitative synthesis of data include consideration of (1) the study population; (2) the intervention delivered and indications for its delivery; (3) factors such as the skill level of the delivery team; (4) psychosocial implications of the delivery setting and the patient population as they relate to compliance and outcome reporting issues; and (5) the outcome measures used, including robustness, relative importance, and comparability.

In a similar fashion, the process by which group decisions are reached regarding the meaning or implications of the evidence can be either informal or formal. Informal group methods can be suboptimal as a result of lack of focus in the discussion or domination by more prominent, aggressive, or vocal members of the group. Formal methods, such as the

Nominal Group and the Delphi techniques have been shown to be superior to informal group methods in generating new ideas and have been shown to ensure member participation and to improve decisions.

Formatting Guidelines

The format in which guidelines are presented has serious implications for use. Evidence tables are a useful method of summarizing important data and have been used in guidelines developed by the Agency for Health Care Policy and Research. They are less useful for actual clinical management decisions. Algorithmic decision trees require clear cut, well-described decision nodes and treatment branch points. This format seems to be preferred by clinicians over prose descriptions of appropriate treatment decision making, and has been shown to be more easily assimilated by medical students as well as junior and senior level residents. However, algorithms may be complicated and lengthy and, subsequently, unwieldy and confusing when evaluated on paper. Eventually these clinical tools will be more easily incorporated into clinical practice as part of an electronic patient record and management system.

A more rigorous approach to clinical decision making has been gained by the application of mathematical modeling principles. Using multivariate analysis of clinical signs and symptoms to determine the probability of disease or of a particular outcome, clinical prediction rules have proven highly accurate in determining the need for radiography of the injured knee and ankle in the emergency department setting.

Dissemination and Evaluation

The ultimate goal of guidelines is to change physician behavior. The first step in so doing is dissemination of the guideline in a way that will lead to changes in health care outcomes.

The sources of influence on physician practice are numerous and varied, interacting in a complex manner that is not completely understood. However, certain implications for the design of strategies to influence practice behavior are well known. Evidence is one of many inputs into decision making and may be overwhelmed by other factors. Simple dissemination of information is ineffective in changing behavior. Information flows through multiple channels, and the likelihood of information acceptance is increased if larger numbers of channels are used.

At the current time, multiple methods are used to evaluate alterations in outcome and little consensus exists, but there is certainly a growing trend toward the use of self-assessment, economic considerations, and standardized instruments. In general, because economic and financial incentives drive this type of research into guideline effectiveness, the earliest reports available on guideline effectiveness are from settings where cost reduction is an important outcome. A common example is practice of occupational medicine, in which there is a strong incentive to reduce wide variations in practice and desire to standardize diagnostic and therapeutic decisions while moving outcome statistics to acceptable levels and reducing costs.

A recent study of rates of lumbar spine surgery in a workers' compensation cohort in which those patients treated without guidelines were compared to those with reimbursement linked to following guidelines showed a distinct reduction in surgery rates in the guidelines group. No attempt was made to measure clinically relevant outcomes. The study also found that involvement of the physician groups in the development and dissemination of the guidelines may have substantially contributed to the decline in surgical rates. There is a growing body of literature, which demonstrates that musculoskeletal surgical patients may be treated with standard postoperative protocols (guidelines frequently called clinical pathways) that decrease length of stay and reduce treatment costs, while not diminishing and, in some cases even improving, the quality of care. Literature in several areas of medical practice now support guidelines as reducing costs by standardizing the use of pharmaceutical products in multiple settings and reducing the frequency of certain diagnostic studies in multiple disease states with no diminution in the quality of care of patients studied.

Legal Implications

Despite the apparent advantages to guideline development and usage in medicine, there are multiple hurdles to both development and acceptance. Not the least of these are medicolegal. A number of potential legal issues are raised when standardized guidelines are applied to patient populations. These issues can be divided into several different categories, including (1) issues of development, dissemination, and implementation; (2) the creation of standards; (3) the physician's fiduciary responsibility as regards malpractice and other patient related issues; (4) fraud, abuse, and the concepts of credentialling via guideline adherence; (5) effects on cost containment, payment policies, and access to care; and (6) influences on quality of care for individual patients along with ethical issues related to implementation.

The guidelines process will continue to use an increasing amount of the health care policy research dollar. Although they are not the only avenue for improving health care outcomes, these attempts to standardize processes, to establish minimal standards, and to improve overall quality will continue as they have in most other fields of human endeavor.

Annotated Bibliography

Auleley GR, Ravaud P, Giraudeau B, et al: Implementation of the Ottawa ankle rules in France: A multicenter randomized controlled trial. JAMA 1997;277:1935–1939.

This is an evaluation of the implementation of an orthopaedic prediction rule.

Colloquium Report on Legal Issues Related To Clinical Practice Guidelines. Washington DC, National Health Lawyers Association, 1995.

This is a thorough discussion of legal issues related to guideline development.

Elam K, Taylor V, Ciol MA, Franklin GM, Deyo RA: Impact of a workers' compensation practice guideline on lumbar spine fusion in Washington state. Med Care 1997;35:417–424.

This study documents the effectiveness of guidelines in maintaining quality and reducing costs in the workers' compensation arena.

Ellrodt G, Cook DJ, Lee J, Cho M, Hunt D, Weingarten S: Evidence-based disease management. JAMA 1997;278:1687–1692.

The authors review evidence-based medicine principles, including their relationship to the guidelines development and utilization process.

International Journal of Technology Assessment in Health Care 1997:13(2).

This issue is a review of principles in guideline development, dissemination, and evaluation. It includes a glossary of terms describing evidence based medical principles.

Laupacis A, Sekar N, Stiell IG: Clinical prediction rules: A review and suggested modifications of methodological standards. JAMA 1997;277:488–494.

This is an evaluation of clinical prediction rules and methodologic attributes.

Mozena JP, Emerick CE, Black SC (eds): Clinical Guideline Development: An Algorithm Approach. Gaithersburg, MD, Aspen Publishers, 1996.

This monograph is an excellent description (in workbook fashion) of the practical techniques required to develop and implement a guidelines process for patient care.

U.S. Congress Office of Technology Assessment: Identifying Health Technologies That Work: Searching for Evidence, OTA-H-608. Washington, DC, U.S. Congress, 1994.

This is a complete review of technology assessment in health care with an excellent section on the guidelines process.

Chapter 11
Outcomes Assessment

Introduction

Outcomes research has been used to describe many different types of research including area variation research, investigations of treatment effectiveness, and the development of outcome measures. Outcomes research has investigated many orthopaedic conditions, focusing extensively on the treatment of low back pain and the use of total joint replacement. This section will (1) review the phenomenon of area variation and discuss recent research in this area, (2) briefly review the principles and types of outcomes research used to investigate treatment effectiveness, and (3) discuss the different types of measures that may be used to evaluate the outcome after orthopaedic intervention.

Small Area Analysis

The rates of many surgical procedures vary according to geographic area, a phenomenon called area variation (other names include regional variation, geographic area variation, small or large area variation). Said another way, the probability of receiving many surgical procedures differs according to where people live. (This definition highlights an important methodologic aspect of this research, which is that geographic area variation analyzes where patients live rather than where patients received their procedure.)

Surgeons usually are not surprised to learn of variation in the rates of procedures in different areas. However, some procedures, such as hip fracture repair, have low rates of regional variation, whereas the rates of other elective surgical procedures, such as total joint replacement, may vary six- to eightfold between low and high usage areas. Moreover, this phenomenon is found in both small and large geographic areas (small areas refer to counties or market areas, whereas large areas refer to states or Health Care Finance Administration regions), across different time periods (areas with high or low usage year after year tend to remain as high or low usage areas, respectively), and in different countries. The phenomenon of area variation raises 2 important questions: (1) what is the "correct" rate for a surgical procedure, and (2) what is/are the explanation(s) for area variation?

The question of what is the correct rate for a surgical pro-

cedure has important policy implications. If the correct rate is close to the mean (or median) rate, then patients in areas below this rate may not be receiving enough of a potentially beneficial procedure, such as total joint replacement. Furthermore, and of great interest to health policy makers, patients in high usage areas may be receiving too much or "inappropriate" care. Although no research has determined the "correct" rate for a surgical procedure, several studies have compared the rates of inappropriate surgery in high and low usage areas. Appropriateness of the surgical procedure is based on reviews of patients' charts with explicit criteria for surgery. Research to date has not found high rates of inappropriate care in high usage areas. Furthermore, one research study found that many people with severe arthritis have not received total joint replacement, suggesting that the correct rate (at least for total joint replacement) may be closer to higher rates of usage. Determination of the correct rate is essential to plan appropriate health policy. If inappropriate overuse is occurring, then efforts need to be directed toward reducing surgical rates. Alternatively, if inappropriate underuse is occurring, then efforts need to be directed toward ensuring patients have unimpeded access to beneficial procedures. The determination of the correct rate for surgical procedures is critical to efforts to reduce area variation, but will await future research.

Different reasons have been offered to explain area variation. One obvious explanation for area variation has been that the differences in regional variation could be due to limitations in the quality of data or limitations in the types of data available in databases used to perform this type of research (usually administrative claims database). Although databases do have some limitations in the quality of the data and the types of data, this would not appear to explain area variation.

Explanations for area variation can occur at all stages of the patient's course from the onset of disease until surgery. First, disease prevalence or disease severity may differ according to geographic areas. Patients in high usage areas could either have more prevalent disease or a more severe disease. Several studies, however, would suggest this is not a major explanation for area variation. Second, patients may differ when they present with a particular disease, such as knee osteoarthritis (or may differ when they decide to proceed with surgical treatment). Thus, for discretionary procedures, such as total joint replacement, patients with the same symptoms may have very different expectations of surgery. This possible explanation has not been investigated for orthopaedic procedures. In other surgical areas, such as urology, differing patient preferences may partially account for area variation. Interactive videodisk is one way of providing patients with all the necessary information to make informed decisions about surgery. Third, for patients who present to primary care clinicians, the ease and skill with which the correct diagnosis is made may explain area variation. Difficulty with diagnosis is an unlikely explanation for regional variation in most orthopaedic conditions. However, several studies have shown that referring clinicians differ substantially in their opinions about indications for and perceptions of the outcomes of the procedure. These differences probably affect how the patients are treated and the likelihood of patients being referred to an orthopaedic surgeon. Fourth, access to an orthopaedic surgeon (or access to the hospital or procedure) may also affect regional variation. This factor may account for some regional variation for orthopaedic procedures. Finally, the opinions of orthopaedic surgeons about the indications for and outcomes of surgery do vary and also may partially explain regional variation in the rates of surgical procedures.

In conclusion, although further research is necessary, it appears that the characteristics and opinions of patients and doctors are the most likely causes for regional variation in orthopaedic procedures.

Conduct of Outcomes Research

Surgeons have always been interested in determining and comparing the outcome of different surgical treatments. Outcomes research, when used to evaluate treatment effectiveness, describes a number of different research strategies including literature review (meta-analysis), large database analyses, and decision analyses. Outcomes research has 4 characteristics that distinguish it from other forms of evaluative research: (1) a focus on patient-based assessments, (2) an assessment of care occurring in the community (not just in referral or academic centers), (3) the use of large databases (to get a more complete view of patterns and the scope of care), and (4) a hope that research findings would lead to changes in clinical practice, and, thereby, a continuous loop of improvement.

Meta-analyses are used to systematically review and combine previously performed studies. The primary use of meta-analysis is combining randomized clinical trials. One practical difficulty of meta-analysis is the identification of all appropriate articles, including non-English and unpublished studies. The main methodologic concern of meta-analysis is the questionable validity of combining multiple studies performed in different populations, at different times, with slightly different interventions.

Outcomes research, when using large databases, has certain methodologic weaknesses that relate primarily to the limitations of the data available in large databases, including (1) imprecise information on diagnoses and procedures, (2) lack of information on severity of disease or severity of coexisting disease (called comorbidity), (3) limitation to in-hospital information, (4) difficulty differentiating between preexisting disease and complications, (5) lack of patient-based outcomes, and (6) numerous potential coding problems, such as determining the side of a surgical procedure, identifying individual surgeons versus institutions, and differentiating primary from secondary surgery. Another limitation of outcomes research is that the interventions are usually not randomly allocated, leading to potential bias. Despite these limitations, outcomes research has been used to investigate several important orthopaedic problems, including the results with lumbar spine fusion and disk surgery and evaluating the relationship between volume of procedures performed by institutions and complication rates.

Future outcomes studies will overcome some of the deficiencies of databases by surveying patients to obtain more complete outcome information and collating database information with information from the medical record.

Health Assessment Measures

The aims of orthopaedic surgery are to prevent death (as in orthopaedic oncology), to restore function (as in trauma patients), to prevent future decline in function (as in pediatric orthopaedics), and most often, to relieve pain and improve function. Differences in outcome between patient groups when comparing 2 or more treatments, provided patients are similar in every way other than treatment they received, are used to make inferences about treatment effectiveness. Thus, the outcome used to assess therapeutic efficacy is of critical importance.

Many different outcomes of treatment can be used to evaluate therapeutic interventions and each provides different information. The World Health Organization has classified the consequences of disease as impairments, disabilities, and handicaps. Impairments are restrictions or abnormalities in physiologic or anatomic structures or function, disabilities are restrictions of abilities to perform activities within the range considered normal, and handicaps are disadvantages that limit fulfillment of usual role. Orthopaedic evaluations in the past have focused primarily on impairment measures, such as range of joint motion, muscle strength, or radiographic measures. Impairment measures have the advantage of being objective and often are easily measured by the surgeon. The main disadvantage of impairment measures is that they may bear little relevance to the reasons patients had the procedure or to how patients evaluate the outcome. Thus, impairments are one important outcome of treatment, but because they do not provide a complete picture, they need to be supplemented by other outcome measures. Because of limitations of impairment measures, the focus of outcomes assessment has shifted to patient-based subjective assessments of outcome. These assessment scales focus on patients' health status, quality of life, or satisfaction with care. Satisfaction with care is an important outcome because it evaluates directly what the patients think of their treatment. However, because patients may have unreasonable expectations of their surgery and because many factors, other than the outcome of surgery, affect patients' satisfaction with care, other measures, such as health status, should probably be the primary outcome of interest.

Measures of health status have been classified as either generic or disease-specific. Generic instruments, such as the SF-36, measure a broad perspective of health status (including not only physical function but also role limitations due to physical and emotional health, vitality, mental health, social functioning, bodily pain, and general health). Disease- (or condition- or region-) specific instruments focus on those complaints resulting from the conditions that are most relevant to clinicians and patients. The main disadvantage of generic measures, such as the SF-36, is that they may not focus on those concerns that are most relevant to patients, and thus, disease-specific measures tend to show greater change compared with generic measures after treatment (a characteristic of measurement called "responsiveness" to change).

The American Academy of Orthopaedic Surgeons™ (AAOS) in conjunction with the Committee of Musculoskeletal Specialty Societies and the Council of Spine Societies has developed region-specific outcome instruments appropriate for spine, lower extremity, upper extremity, and pediatrics. The instruments are intended to be used as standardized methods of assessment useful in multiple contexts, including routine office-based assessment.

The current 4 AAOS instruments provide a common and standardized current health assessment that includes patient demographics, comorbidity, self-assessment of patients' overall health, and expectations of surgery. Each scale has an initial and a follow-up assessment form. The 4 scales are self-administered by the patient. The content of the scales includes symptoms and functional disability relevant to the particular region. Several of the scales have subscales. The spine instrument has cervical, lumbar, and scoliosis subscales; the upper extremity instrument has a sports/musical instrument/work module; the pediatrics instrument has an adolescent and parent form; and the lower extremity instrument includes sports knee, lower limb, hip/knee, and foot/ankle subscales. The instruments have undergone testing for reliability, validity, and responsiveness, although not all instruments have completed all stages of all testing. The Musculoskeletal Function Assessment (MFA) is another instrument designed to assess patients with musculoskeletal disorders, except those with spinal disorders.

One problem in assessing patients with traumatic injuries is the lack of pretreatment/preinjury scores. Having patients rate their preinjury function is unsatisfactory because of the practical difficulty of having patients who are intubated or those with head injuries complete the instruments and the concern that the types of injuries or issues of litigation will affect reporting of preinjury scores. When assessing or comparing therapeutic interventions (and without baseline scores), randomization has an important role in minimizing bias. In absence of randomization, investigators will have to rely on other patient characteristics to determine if treatment groups are similar prior to treatment.

The Musculoskeletal Outcomes Data Evaluation and Management System (MODEMS™) is an office-based computerized system that allows "physicians to collect data on patients' demographics, general health status, musculoskeletal function, and resource utilization." In addition to demographic information and the AAOS outcomes instrument, included are an employment module, hip and knee surgery forms, a physical examination form, a discharge form, a postdischarge complication form, and a physician form that includes clinicians' ratings for disease severity, pain, and functional information. This service is subscribed through the AAOS and allows physicians to collect information in an office-based practice. MODEMS™ also provides patient outcomes of individual practitioners compared with national norms.

Annotated Bibliography

Atlas SJ, Deyo RA, Keller RB, et al: The Maine Lumbar Spine Study, Part II: 1-year outcomes of surgical and nonsurgical management of sciatica. *Spine* 1996;21:1777–1786.

This prospective cohort study found the outcomes of surgically treated spinal stenosis to be better than those of nonsurgical treatment.

Atlas SJ, Deyo RA, Keller RB, et al: The Maine Lumbar Spine Study, Part III: 1-year outcomes of surgical and nonsurgical management of lumbar spinal stenosis. *Spine* 1996;21:1787–1794.

A prospective cohort study found symptomatic relief for patients with sciatica was better for surgical compared with nonsurgical treatment. There was no difference for compensation or employment.

Callahan CM, Drake BG, Heck DA, Dittus RS: Patient outcomes following tricompartmental total knee replacement: A meta-analysis. *JAMA* 1994;271:1349–1357.

This meta-analysis demonstrated safety and efficacy of total knee replacement.

Coyte PC, Hawker G, Wright JG: Variations in knee replacement utilization rates and the supply of health professionals in Ontario, Canada. *J Rheumatol* 1996;23:1214–1220.

This study found no relationship between regional variation and density of orthopaedic surgeons.

Engelberg R, Martin DP, Agel J, Obremsky W, Coronado G, Swiontkowski MF: Musculoskeletal Function Assessment instrument: Criterion and construct validity. *J Orthop Res* 1996;14:182–192.

The validation of the MFA is described.

Fear J, Hillman M, Chamberlain MA, Tennant A: Prevalence of hip problems in the population aged 55 years and over: Access to specialist care and future demand for hip arthroplasty. *Br J Rheumatol* 1997;36:74–76.

This population survey found that many patients with hip arthritis had not received joint arthroplasty.

Kreder HJ, Deyo RA, Koepsell T, Swiontkowski MF, Kreuter W: Relationship between the volume of total hip replacements performed by providers and the rates of postoperative complications in the state of Washington. *J Bone Joint Surg* 1997;79A:485–494.

This study found that centers with low volume hip replacement surgeries have higher complication rates.

Kreder HJ, Wright JG, McLeod R: Outcome studies in surgical research. *Surgery* 1997;121:223–225.

This is an overview of types of outcomes research.

Martin DP, Engelberg R, Agel J, Snapp D, Swiontkowski MF: Development of a musculoskeletal extremity health status instrument: The Musculoskeletal Function Assessment instrument. *J. Orthop Res* 1996;14:173–181.

The development of the MFA is described.

van Walraven CV, Peterson JM, Kapral M, et al: Appropriateness of primary total hip and knee replacements in regions of Ontario with high and low utilization rates. *CMAJ* 1996;155:697–706.

This study found that rates of inappropriate surgeries were similar in high and low usage areas.

Wright JG, Coyte P, Hawker G, et al: Variation in orthopedic surgeons' perceptions of the indications for and outcomes of knee replacement. *CMAJ* 1995;152:687–697.

This study showed significant variation in orthopaedic surgeons' perceptions about knee replacement surgery.

Wright JG, McLeod RS, Lossing A, Walters BC, Hu X: Measurement in surgical clinical research. *Surgery* 1996; 119: 241–244.

This is an overview of methods for development and evaluation of outcomes measurements.

Classic Bibliography

Ellwood PM: Shattuck lecture: Outcomes management. A technology of patient experience. *N Engl J Med* 1988;318: 1549–1556.

Epstein AM: The outcomes movement: Will it get us where we want to go? *N Engl J Med* 1990;323:266–270.

Gartland JJ: Orthopaedic clinical research: Deficiencies in experimental design and determinations of outcome. *J Bone Joint Surg* 1988;70A:1357–1364.

Turner JA, Ersek M, Herron L, et al: Patient outcomes after lumbar spinal fusions. *JAMA* 1992;268:907–911.

Wennberg J, Gittelsohn A: Small area variations in health care delivery. *Science* 1973;182:1102-1108.

Wennberg JE, Freeman JL, Culp WJ: Are hospital services rationed in New Haven or over-utilised in Boston? *Lancet* 1987;1:1185–1189.

Chapter 12
The Medical Care of Athletes

Introduction

It is essential that the orthopaedic surgeon be familiar with other systems and medical issues of concern to the athlete. It is important to take a leadership role in the education and development of patients, trainers, therapists, athletes, and parents alike.

Ideally, the orthopaedic surgeon should be the leader as team physician of an organized sports medicine program composed of an athletic director, coaches, athletic trainers, and other physicians. Close involvement with the team (ie, attending practices and parent meetings and giving lectures) will enhance the athletes' and coaches' confidence in the physician. This relationship will foster a team concept, which will ultimately assist the physician with on-the-field evaluations and decisions under fire. Emergency care should be provided on a regular basis. Prior planning will ensure the availability of all necessary equipment (Outline 1).

This chapter offers an update on current issues involving the medical care of athletes. By necessity, this includes consideration of injury incidence and prevention; care of the athlete pre-, mid-, and postseason; and a discussion of medical issues and overuse injuries in sports. These issues may not be as popular and appealing as an update on the latest surgical techniques, but are just as critical for all orthopaedic surgeons who treat athletes and call themselves team physicians.

Injury Incidence and Prevention

Fitness Profiles

A dramatic increase in sports-related injuries has accompanied the overwhelming interest in fitness that has swept across the country in recent years. To characterize these injuries and look at risk factors, it is often helpful to establish fitness profiles for various sports. Such factors as age, fitness history, body habitus, flexibility, training environments, and intensity of training are important considerations in developing these profiles. Studies have shown that in football, for example, as the level of competition increases, so do height, weight, and fat-free weight of the players. Football players at all levels are becoming stronger, and strength training pro-

---

Outline 1
Equipment that should be available

The Team Physician's Bag

Oral airway	Stethoscope
Thermometer	Eyepatches
14-gauge catheters	Scissors (blunt)
Tape (1/2", 1", 2")	Penlight
Ace bandages	Slings
Tongue depressors	Cotton (Q-tip) applicators
Xeroform/Vaseline gauze	Gauze pads (sterile/non-sterile)
Betadyne swabs	
Betadyne scrub	Antiseptic ointment (Bacitracin)
Near-vision-card	
Suture kit	Adhesive strips (Band-aid, Steri-strip)
Hydrogen peroxide/saline irrigating solution	Albuterol inhaler
Epi-pen (self-injectable epinephrine)	Plaster of paris/fiberglass
Aluminum splints	Home care head injury forms
Latex gloves (Sterile and non-sterile)	Scalpel

Sideline/Fieldhouse Equipment

Spine board	Stretcher
Crutches	Splints (board type)
Sand bags/Philadelphia collar	Bolt cutter/screwdriver
Intravenous/D5 Ringer's lactate, sterile irrigant (saline)	Oxygen tank with mask
	Telephone

---

grams are largely responsible for improved strength and performance profiles of these players. Exposure time and a history of previous injury remain the most important predictors for sports injuries.

Sex-Specific Injuries

As more women participate in sports, it has become apparent that different injuries, injury rates, and physiologic differences are important considerations in these athletes. Anterior

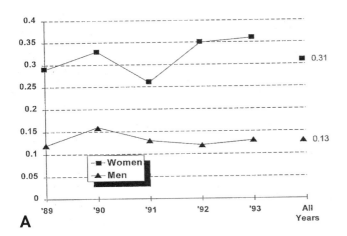

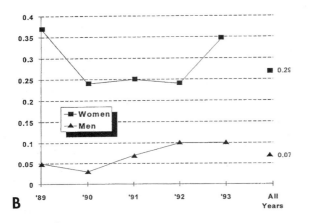

Figure 1

Anterior cruciate ligament injury rate among men and women in soccer (A) and basketball (B). (Reproduced with permission from Arendt E, Dick R: Knee injury patterns among men and women in collegiate basketball and soccer: NCAA data and review of literature. *Am J Sports Med* 1995;23:694–701.)

injuries include smaller muscle fiber size, hamstring torque differences, and differences in body composition. It is important to understand these physiologic differences when designing training programs.

The female athlete triad, consisting of menstrual dysfunction, disordered eating, and decreased bone mineral density, is well known to most sports medicine physicians. Menstrual dysfunction, including oligomenorrhea (irregular menstrual cycle length from 35 to 90 days) and amenorrhea (absence of menstrual bleeding), can often be treated with progesterone or oral contraceptives. Disordered eating can include anorexia nervosa, bulimia nervosa, or poor nutritional habits. Treatment requires a multidisciplinary approach. Decreased bone mineral density, which occurs more frequently in female athletes, can lead to stress fractures. Modification of training and nutritional practices are important considerations. Gymnastics and other impact loading sports have a positive effect on bone mineral density.

Recent research has revealed that the 3 arms of the triad are often closely related. In one study, it was found that the age of onset of amenorrhea had a greater influence on bone loss than the age of onset of anorexia nervosa. It also was found that recovery of bone mineral density required both weight gain and restoration of menses. Estrogen and progesterone administration alone may not reverse the profound osteopenia seen in many young females.

Age-Specific Injuries

Adolescent upper extremity injuries about the shoulder and elbow are common in baseball players, especially pitchers. Rule changes that limit the amount of competition for these players have helped reduce the frequency of these injuries. As a general rule, young athletes should not progress more than 10% per week in the amount and frequency of training. Strength, flexibility, and technique training, and proper coaching are essential. Early recognition and treatment of injuries are critical and can help prevent long-term disability.

Because the emphasis on health and fitness has extended to the older population, it is important to recognize the special needs and injuries of older athletes. Exertional and overuse injuries are common in this population. The physician must use care in prescribing nonsteroidal anti-inflammatory drugs (NSAIDs) for this population because of the increased gastrointestinal side effects and their different metabolism. In general, long-term immobilization should be avoided in older athletes.

Lifestyle Changes

Evidence continues to mount supporting the beneficial effects of exercise. Studies have shown a positive effect on

cruciate ligament (ACL) injury rates are significantly higher in women's basketball, soccer, rugby, and other sports (Fig. 1). Although there may be no single explanation for this, factors such as muscular strength, limb alignment, skill level, notch dimensions, and ligament size are important considerations. Female athletes have more anterior tibial laxity and less muscle strength and endurance than males. They also take significantly longer to generate maximum hamstring muscle torque during isokinetic testing. Female athletes appear to rely more on their quadriceps muscles in response to anterior tibial translation than males. Recent studies have suggested that ligament size may also be a critical intrinsic factor associated with ACL injury risk.

Other differences between the sexes that may contribute to

cholesterol values; cardiovascular fitness; osteoporosis; the incidence of colon, breast, and testicular cancer; pulmonary disease; hypertension; and mental well-being. These positive effects extend into the elderly population. Running, brisk walking, water aerobics, and other forms of moderate exercise are all beneficial. Cardiovascular benefits appear to be at least partially related to enhanced fibrinolysis. Hypertension appears to be controlled by exercise mediated changes in urinary kallikrein, which reduces sympathetic nervous system activity.

Sports-Specific Injuries

An understanding of injury incidence in specific sports can assist the physician in treatment and prevention of these injuries. Table 1, created after a thorough review of the recent literature, represents a summary of common injuries in different sports. Although it is not all-inclusive, this represents some of the more important injuries seen in athletes in the sports listed.

Anatomic-Specific Injuries

Ankle ligament injuries have been found to be significantly greater in patients with an eversion to inversion strength imbalance. There is also an increased risk of ankle injuries in patients with greater plantarflexion strength and an associated muscle strength imbalance. This increase may occur because there is a loss of protective reflexes with increasing plantarflexion. Another recent study demonstrated that both a peripheral reflex reaction of the peroneal muscles and a centrally mediated reaction of the muscles and joints occur as a result of sudden inversion. Unfortunately, both of these reactions are too slow to prevent lateral ligament overloading unless the inversion is anticipated.

The incidence of ankle injuries may also be reduced by rule changes in certain sports. One recent study demonstrated that volleyball players frequently injure their ankles when landing on other players' feet after blocking or attacking in the net zone. Rule changes that would create a "safety zone" under the net and better technical skills training may reduce the incidence of these injuries.

Recurrent ankle sprains are unfortunately too common. A recent epidemiologic survey revealed that recurrence rates were higher in athletes who still had residual symptoms and if they believed that their performance was affected.

Knee ligament injuries are known to occur most commonly as a result of pivoting injuries (ACL) or valgus injuries (medial collateral ligaments). Articular cartilage damage does not appear to occur as a result of a lifetime of regular weight-bearing exercise, at least in an animal model.

Hamstring strains are complex multifactorial injuries that involve strength imbalances, lack of flexibility, muscle fatigue, and insufficient warm-up. Rehabilitation of these injuries should focus on these factors. Return to play should only be allowed following complete recovery to avoid reinjury.

Cervical spine abnormalities associated with a risk for quadriplegia in contact sports include cervical stenosis, axial loading, and equipment considerations. Fortunately, the rate of these catastrophic injuries in American football has dramatically declined with new rule changes that were a result of careful epidemiologic study.

In the lumbar spine, spondylolysis associated with dysplastic changes at the lower edge of L-5 or the upper level of S-1 in juvenile athletes may indicate a high risk of progression to spondylolisthesis. Computed tomography (CT) scan can play a key role in diagnosis, assessment of defects, monitoring healing, and determining prognosis in spondylolysis.

Prophylactic Bracing

A great deal of attention has been paid to the role of prophylactic ankle bracing in the recent literature. Cadaveric studies have demonstrated a combined effect of braces and high-top shoes. Prospective studies have also demonstrated the efficacy of braces in reducing the incidence of ankle sprains in basketball, soccer, and other sports. Further, these braces do not appear to inhibit athletic performance.

Although there continues to be controversy regarding the efficacy of prophylactic knee bracing in football, recent studies have suggested that there is a slight decrease in medial collateral ligament injury rates with prophylactic bracing, especially for linemen and linebackers. The prophylactic use of knee braces for anterior knee pain is equally controversial, yet a recent study suggests that they may be effective.

Cadaver studies have demonstrated that in-line skating wrist guards do not appear to be effective in preventing wrist fractures; however, they may reduce the severity of injuries. Doweled hand guards, used in gymnastics, can lead to increased tensile forces across the wrist, which may actually contribute to growth plate injuries in young gymnasts.

Shoewear

Shoe height has been shown to not significantly affect an individual's ability to actively resist *eversion* moments; however, it can increase the maximal resistance to an *inversion* moment in moderate ankle plantarflexion. Newer footwear with thick, soft soles may have a destabilizing effect. Increasing heel height in running shoes did not affect Achilles tendon forces in a recent biomechanical study.

Hot temperatures and long cleat length are important factors in football knee injury risk considerations on artificial turf. Only the flat-soled basketball-style shoe, with no cleats

Table 1
Sports-specific injuries

Sport	Common Injuries*	Prevention/Treatment*
Baseball/softball	Ankle sprains Shoulder subluxation/cuff injury	Break-away/impact bases Modify mechanics/rehabilitation
Basketball	ACL injury Finger injuries Ankle sprains	Females at risk Early diagnosis important High top shoes/bracing
Bicycling	Abrasion, contusion, AC injury Concussions Neck and back pain Numbness (hand, perineum)	Safety concerns Helmet use Limit exposure Padding/positioning
Dance/ballet	Hallux valgus, os trigonum Ankle sprain	Overuse related Proprioception training
Diving	Foot injuries Spondylolysis	Technique related Limit exposure
Football	Spondylolysis Pneumothorax Cervical injury Shoulder injury Ankle sprain Knee MCL sprain	Technique (interior linemen) Catheter/chest tube Screening, technique, equipment Cuff rehabilitation/reconstruction Rule out syndesmotic injury Prophylatic bracing
Golf	Back pain Hamate fracture Medial epicondylitis	Rehabilitation - trunk muscles Technique dependent Symptomatic treatment
Gymnastics	Wrist injuries	Training intensity/ulnar positive
Hockey	Facial lacerations ACL injury	Face masks Shoulder pads/technique
Horse riding	Neck injury, fractures	Safety
Hurling	Finger injury, hamstring strain	Conditioning, protection, rules
Luge	Hand contusion, neck strain	Conditioning, sled design
Martial arts	Lower extremity strain/sprain	Equipment, rules, technique

Table 1
Sports-specific injuries (continued)

Sport	Common Injuries*	Prevention/Treatment*
Rock climbing	Upper extremity tendinitis "Climbers finger"	Overuse PIP/digital pulley injury
Rowing	Back and knee overuse injury	Conditioning
Rugby	Cervical spine injury Knee injury	Technique related (tackle/scrum) Technique
Running	Iliotibial band syndrome Lower extremity stress fractures	Rest/avoid running hills Activity modification
Skiing	ACL injury Knee chondral injury (trochlea) Thumb UCL injury	Patient education Arthroscopy Wrist strap on ski pole
Snowboarding	Upper extremity injury	Technique related
Soccer	Ankle sprain, knee ligament Knee chondral injury Head injury	Symptomatic Arthroscopic treatment Padded goal post
Swimming	Shoulder subluxation	Rotator cuff rehabilitation
Tennis	Shoulder instability Lateral epicondylitis	Rotator cuff rehabilitation Symptomatic treatment
Trampoline	Fractures, sprains, head injury	Limit recreational use
Volleyball	Shoulder instability Ankle sprains Patellar tendinitis	Rotator cuff rehabilitation Training/bracing Symptomatic
Water skiing	Hamstring injury Boating injury	Technique related Boating safety
Weight lifting	Spondylolysis Distal clavical osteolysis, pec inj	Technique
Wrestling	Spondylolysis	Limit exposure

* ACL, anterior cruciate ligament; AC, acromioclavicular; MCL, medial collateral ligament; PIP, proximal interphalangeal; UCL, ulnar collateral ligament; pec inj, pectoral injury

can be considered "probably safe" at all temperatures studied in one report. Another study of football cleat design suggests that players who wore "Edge" cleats, with longer irregular cleats placed at the peripheral margin of the sole with smaller pointed cleats interiorly, were at higher risk for ACL injuries on natural turf. Additional considerations include the effect of taping over or "spatting" of the shoes, and wetness of the field.

Therapeutic Bracing

It is now well recognized that ACL functional bracing has not been proved to be efficacious at high functional levels of force that occur in most sport settings. Recent studies have demonstrated that these braces can lead to premature muscle fatigue (because of increased muscle relaxation pressures) and are associated with slow hamstring muscle reaction times. The efficacy of "sleeves" in patients with anterior knee pain continues to be controversial, with some studies suggesting that they may have a beneficial effect on proprioception, and other reports suggesting that they may not be helpful in a clinical setting. There appears to be a beneficial effect of pneumatic leg braces in athletes with tibial stress fractures, with a quicker return to full unrestricted sports participation.

Protective Equipment

The mandatory use of helmets in hockey has resulted in a reduction in the number of facial injuries, but there is some concern that the style of play has changed as well with an increased risk of cervical spine injury. Other recent studies have demonstrated that in football players with potential cervical spine injuries, the helmet and shoulder pads should not be removed, if at all possible, when immobilizing the head and neck on the field.

Although anecdotal reports have suggested that the incidence of football injuries (including to the knee) is higher on artificial surfaces, there have not yet been any well-designed studies reported in the literature.

Preparticipation Examination

In order to reduce the incidence of sudden death in young athletes, renewed emphasis has been placed on the preparticipation physical examination (PPE). What follows is a summary of the purpose and focus of the examination, and new concepts.

Purpose and Focus of the Examination

In addition to fulfilling legal requirements of states, leagues, and schools, the PPE can provide information regarding the fitness level and predisposition to injury, create a baseline for later comparison, identify conditions that may limit participation, and allow better cooperation between medical personnel and coaches and athletes. The overall goal is to ensure the athlete's health and safety.

Components of the examination include medical history (especially a family or individual history of cardiovascular disease), vital signs, general medical examination, musculoskeletal examination (with a focus on prior injuries and surgeries), performance testing, body composition, maturity determination (for adolescent athletes), and other special considerations. Current recommendations suggest that a complete examination should be done at least 6 weeks before the season for athletes entering a new program, followed by a limited history and physical on an annual basis, and a complete examination biannually.

Disqualifying Criteria

There are 5 considerations for clearing the athlete for sports participation: (1) Does the problem place the athlete at risk of injury? (2) Is any other participant at risk of injury because of the problem? (3) Can the athlete safely participate with treatment? (4) Can limited participation be allowed while treatment is underway? (5) Can the athlete safely participate in limited activities?

Important items that may result in sports disqualification can often be identified in the PPE. Of particular concern are a history of dizziness with exercise, asthma, body mass index, systolic blood pressure, visual acuity, heart murmur, and abnormalities on musculoskeletal examination. Other conditions that are "disqualifiers" for sports participation include carditis (associated with sudden cardiac death), diarrhea (associated dehydration risk), and fever (increased risk for cardiac and heat-related illness). Systolic murmurs are common in athletes, but accentuation of the murmur with Valsalva should alert the physician to the possibility of asymmetric septal hypertrophy and obstructive hypertrophic cardiomyopathy. Unexplained ventricular ectopia should raise the possibility of cocaine abuse. The upper limits of blood pressure accepted as not requiring further evaluation are 130/75 for children 11 years of age and younger and 140/85 for children 12 years and above. Providers may not legally be able to prevent athletes from participating. In these cases, the athlete and/or their parents may be asked to sign an exculpatory waiver, thereby assuming the risk and relieving the physician from liability.

Exercise induced asthma can often not be diagnosed from history and examination alone. Pulmonary function testing following a submaximal exercise challenge may help identify more of these individuals during the examination.

Hypertrophic cardiomyopathy is the most common cause of sudden death in young competitive athletes. If this condition can be identified during the examination, then patients should be restricted from competition if they have a ventricular wall thickness > 20 mm, outflow obstructions > 50 mm, rhythm disturbances occurring on a 24-hour electrocardiogram, or a history of sudden death in a family member with this condition. Patients with a proven single coronary artery should also be restricted from competitive sports. Athletes with symptomatic arrhythmias, mitral valve prolapse, and other cardiovascular conditions should also be restricted until a thorough evaluation is made. Unfortunately, the PPE is of limited value in identification of underlying cardiovascular abnormalities that can result in sudden death. Nevertheless, athletes should be informed about early warning signs of cardiovascular-associated sudden death (Outline 2). Interestingly, sudden cardiac death is extremely rare in female athletes.

On-the-Field Evaluation

The orthopaedic surgeon needs to be prepared to treat any athlete who is "down" no matter what the etiology. An important preseason consideration is to understand what needs to be included in the medical bag and what is available on the sidelines. Such items as oral airways, a stethoscope, large bore catheters, injectable anticonvulsants and epinephrine, a

Outline 2
Early warning signs of cardiovascular-associated sudden death

Heart rate over 120 beats/minute

Resting blood pressure over 140/90 mm Hg

Absent or large discrepancy between femoral and brachial pulses

Angina during exercise

Nausea or abdominal discomfort

Dizziness

Generalized fatigue

(Adapted from the NATA and AOSSM palm card "The Preparticipation Physical Examination and Non-Traumatic Cardiovascular Sudden Death in Athletes.")

scalpel, and other items should be immediately available on the sidelines.

Perhaps of most concern to team physicians is sudden cardiac death (SCD). Fortunately, the incidence of SCD is low, but all physicians who "cover" sporting events need to be prepared to resuscitate athletes and spectators alike. Recognition of cardiac symptoms is critical in the prevention of SCD. First aid, basic life support, and advanced cardiac life support intervention must be readily available. Unexpected blows to the chest can result in SCD from cardiac contusion or commotio cordis. Despite immediate CPR administered on the scene, ventricular fibrillation that often results from this condition may be irreversible.

Syncope can be caused by cerebral ischemia, resulting from inadequate oxygen or glucose delivery to the brain. It is usually caused by a benign problem (vasovagal, hyperventilation, or orthostatic hypotension); however, it may be a prelude to sudden death. A thorough workup of athletes with syncope, with a focus on the cardiac and neurologic examination, is critical.

"Stingers" or "burners" occur commonly in American football as a result of a blow to the head and shoulder. Players should be restricted from play until all symptoms resolve. Burner syndrome is characterized by immediate, sharp, burning pain radiating from the supraclavicular area down the arm. Often, the athlete will try to shake the arm to "get the feeling back" or walk off the field holding the involved arm. The symptoms frequently resolve in minutes, and transient weakness, most commonly of the deltoid, biceps, and spinatus muscles (winging scapula), may follow the pain. However, the motor deficit may not present at all or it may present several hours or days following the initial injury. It is critical that the team physician perform a thorough on-site examination of the neck and upper extremities (with all equipment removed). Burner syndrome is most commonly an injury to the upper trunk of the brachial plexus involving the C5 and C6 roots. An athlete who has sustained a burner may return to play the same day if he can demonstrate a normal range of painless cervical motion without any residual neurologic deficit. The athlete who has suffered a recurrent burner should not be allowed to play until cervical spine pathology has been excluded.

Spinal stenosis, or narrowing of the anteroposterieor (AP) diameter of the cervical spine, has been observed in athletes who play collision sports such as football. Stenosis can be congenital or developmental. The ratio of the spinal canal to the vertebral body, as measured on lateral radiographs (normally > 0.8), can be helpful in the initial evaluation of this condition. Patients with stenosis and recurrent symptoms, progressive radiographic changes, and other findings ("spear-tackler's spine") should not continue in collision sports.

Abdominal injuries, which usually occur as a result of blunt trauma, may not be recognized immediately. An athlete who is complaining of continuous and persistent abdominal pain requires serial abdominal examinations and determination of vital signs. Solid organs are most often injured, with the spleen (football) and kidneys (boxing) most commonly involved. Symptoms, such as pallor, increased pulse, shortness of breath, abdominal pain and guarding, and faintness, necessitate emergency referral to the nearest medical center.

Chest trauma can also occur in contact sports. Rib fractures are the most common chest injury and usually involve the middle ribs. Radiographs are important to rule out associated pneumothorax; however, special rib series may not be necessary because the treatment of rib fractures and rib contusions is basically the same. The team physician should always be concerned about the possibility of a tension pneumothorax, which can be life threatening. The findings of absent or diminished breath sounds, hypotension, and a possible shift of the trachea to the contralateral side, requires immediate decompression with a chest tube, or if this is not available, then a large bore catheter placed into the second intercostal space in the midclavicular line.

Eye injuries in sports are often preventable. The proper use of eye protection should be emphasized. Soccer, basketball, and racket sports have a high incidence of ocular injuries. Open eyeguards are not recommended for racquetball because these glasses may actually increase eye injuries by "funneling" a compressible ball into the orbit. Hyphema, or the presence of blood in the eye, can be associated with vitreous and/or retinal lesions over half of the time. In the presence of a serious eye injury, a firm patch should be applied and the athlete should be referred to the closest emergency room. Associated fractures to the facial bones can often accompany orbital injuries. Regular gonioscopy and peripheral retinal examination by a specialist should be considered following blunt trauma to the eye.

Head injuries are also common in contact sports. The most common athletic head injury is a concussion. While concussions vary widely in severity, team physicians should be knowledgeable of the Colorado Medical Society guidelines for concussions (Table 2), which match the NCAA guidelines. No player should be allowed to return to competition if symptoms (headache, nausea, blurred vision, confusion, etc) persist, because of the risk of second impact syndrome. This syndrome, in which a second, often minor, injury occurs, carries a mortality risk of up to 50%. Concussion with amnesia requires removal from contact for at least 1 week.

Long-term effects of head injury are becoming increasingly recognized. Perhaps this is most evident in boxers. Even mild head injuries, however, can result in visuospatial deficits that persist at least 1 year after the injury. Neuropsychological testing is being used on a more frequent basis in the evaluation of professional athletes.

Intracranial hemorrhage is the leading cause of head injury death in sports. The use of helmets and protective gear is critical. This includes horseback riding, bicycling, in line skating, skateboarding, winter sports, and other high risk activities. Recent studies have documented a decrease in head injury rates with helmet use.

Adjunctive Treatments/Rehabilitation

Rehabilitation can be defined as any measure used to restore an injured patient to normal activity as quickly and safely as possible. Physical therapy includes the use of physical modalities, therapeutic exercise, and functional exercise. Physical modalities include heat, cold, and electricity designed to effect soft-tissue healing; reduce pain, swelling, and spasm; and reduce or increase blood flow. Therapeutic exercises are movements designed to restore or improve range of motion, flexibility, and muscle performance. Functional exercises are movements designed to restore strength and agility.

More aggressive, "accelerated" rehabilitation has become commonplace. Other trends, such as closed chain rehabilitation, cryotherapy, proprioception and other aspects of postoperative management, have also emerged. New recommendations on rehabilitation for specific injuries and postoperative protocols will be discussed in anatomic-specific sections.

Physical Modalities

Although physical modalities are frequently prescribed to promote healing and recovery after injury, very little has appeared in the recent literature that recommends expanding their use.

Cryotherapy has been shown to decrease soft-tissue blood flow up to 30%. New studies have demonstrated that at least in the shoulder, surface applied cryotherapy does not penetrate into the joint. Recent investigations suggest that its effect may be related to a localized decrease in blood flow. Other studies, however, suggest that cold therapy offered no advantage following ACL reconstruction. Ice immersion of the foot and ankle does not appear to affect performance on agility testing.

Thermotherapy, or heat application, produces vasodilation, and at least in theory, increases enzymatic activity, collagen

Table 2
Grading concussions in sports and guidelines for return to play

| | Grading | Guidelines | | |
Severity	Signs/symptoms	First Concussion	Second Concussion	Third Concussion
Grade I (mild)	Confusion without amnesia; no loss of consciousness	May return to play if asymptomatic[††] for at least 20 minutes	Terminate contest/practice; may return to play if asymptomatic[††] for at least 1 week	Terminate season, may return to play in 3 months if asymptomatic[††]
Grade II (moderate)	Confusion with amnesia*; no loss of consciousness[†]	Terminate contest/practice; may return to play if asymptomatic[††] for at least 1 week	Consider terminating season; may return to play if asymptomatic[††] for 1 month	Terminate season; may return to play next season if asymptomatic[††]
Grade III (severe)	Loss of consciousness[†]	Terminate contest/practice and transport to hospital; may return to play 1 month after 2 consecutive asymptomatic[††] weeks; conditioning allowed after 1 asymptomatic week[††]	Terminate season; may return to play next season if asymptomatic[††]	Terminate season; strongly discourage return to contact/collision sports

* Posttraumatic amnesia (amnesia for events following the impact) or more severe retrograde amnesia (amnesia for events preceding the impact)

[†] Some clinicians include "brief" loss of consciousness in grade II and reserve "prolonged" loss of consciousness for grade III. However, the definitions of "brief" and "prolonged" are not universally accepted

[††] No headache, confusion, dizziness, impaired orientation, impaired concentration, or memory dysfunction during rest or exertion

(Adapted with permission from the Colorado Medical Society: *Report of the Sports Medicine Committee: Guidelines for the Management of Concussion in Sports.* Denver, CO, Colorado Medical Society, 1991, revised.)

synthesis, and tissue extensibility. Although controversial, most authorities recommend its use for chronic soft-tissue injuries.

Therapeutic ultrasound and diathermy use energy to heat deep tissues. Although there are few clinical studies, animal studies suggest that there may be some limited beneficial effect of this treatment in wound healing.

High voltage pulse galvanic stimulation (HVPGS) has also been advocated for the treatment of soft-tissue injuries. Electrical stimulation with a short pulse and high voltage allows deep soft-tissue penetration. It has been proposed that alterations in ion, amino acid, and protein flow provides a beneficial effect.

Hyperbaric Oxygen
Hyperbaric oxygen therapy has been proposed as a method to allow more rapid healing of injuries. It has been used to help return professional athletes to competition sooner. A recent double-blind, randomized study failed to show any benefit in the treatment of ankle sprains. Its efficacy for use in the treatment of other injuries will have to await further clinical studies.

Local Steroid Use
Steroid injections have been demonstrated to significantly impair the healing process in acutely injured ligaments. Local injections of steroid have been found to be efficacious in the treatment of osteitis pubis and some other conditions. Excessive steroid injections may actually have detrimental effects, including corticosteroid-induced arthropathy, inhibited ligament healing, and tendon injury. Fat atrophy and localized skin pigment changes commonly occur as a side effect of these injections.

Steroids can also be delivered transcutaneously via ultrasound (phonophoresis) or electrically (iontophoresis). Iontophoresis with dexamethasone was shown to be helpful in the immediate treatment of plantar faciitis in athletes in one study, but the effect did not persist.

Therapeutic Exercise
Therapeutic exercise is designed to promote flexibility and muscular performance. It is also used to counter the response of tissues to injury or immobilization. These responses include contracture, decreased ligament strength, muscle atrophy and strength loss, and decreased bone density.

Flexibility Flexibility can be defined as the full range of motion possible at or in a joint or series of joints. Flexibility training encompasses a variety of techniques for different sports. Controversy exists as to whether flexibility does, in fact, decrease the chance of injury. Nevertheless, it has been incorporated into the exercise regimes for many sports.

Flexibility training encompasses static stretching, ballistic stretching, and proprioceptive neuromuscular facilitation (PNF). The static method places the muscle tendon unit under a slow gentle stretch for 20 to 60 seconds. This method reduces the intensity of the stretch reflex and the muscle tone of the involved group. Ballistic stretching involves quick, repetitive, and more forceful movements to overcome the muscles to be stretched. Ballistic techniques can, in fact, initiate the stretch reflex, thus countering the stretch.

PNF aims to stimulate Golgi tendon organs to decrease muscle tone. A slow stretch takes the muscle tendon unit (MTU) to its end range and is held for several seconds. A maximal isometric contraction against a partner's resistance is then performed for 5 to 10 seconds. The MTU is then relaxed and slowly stretched by the partner. It is felt that isometric contraction with the MTU at its greatest length will maximally stimulate the Golgi apparatus. Reciprocal inhibition of the muscle under tension will result and allow further stretch upon relaxation.

Controversy exists as to which method of flexibility training is most effective. Static and ballistic techniques have yielded equal results, but injury risk increases with ballistic stretching. PNF has been found to be superior in some studies but not in others. The partner requirement is another disadvantage. Because pain may increase due to increased muscle activity, PNF must be done in a supervised setting.

Enhancement of Muscle Performance Clearly, muscles are involved in any athletic endeavor. There are various parameters of muscular performance (Table 3). Although one or more of these variables may be enhanced by training, the generic term covering all types of such exercise is strength training (Table 4).

Isometric exercise is inexpensive and unlikely to cause injury. If immobilization is required, isometrics can decrease muscle atrophy. This form of exercise can be very useful in the early postinjury/postsurgery period. However, isometrics have serious drawbacks. Strength gains are specific to the joint angle used for the exercise. Because athletic performance requires motion, applicability to functional performance is limited. Multiangle isometrics can be used when exercise through range is limited by pain.

Isotonic exercise can be done with manual resistance, free weights, or machines. Free weights carry a potential for

| Table 3 | |
| Parameters of muscle performance | |

Parameter	Definition
Strength	Maximum force generated by a muscle
Work	Force x distance
Torque	Rotation measurement of work: force x lever arm
Power	Work/unit time
Endurance	Ability to generate force over time without fatigue

(Reproduced with permission from Kasser JR (ed): *Orthopaedic Knowledge Update 5*. Rosemont, IL, American Academy of Orthopaedic Surgeons, 1996, pp 89-101.)

| Table 4 | |
| Types of strength | |

Type	Definition
Isometric	Muscle contraction against resistance without changing length
Isotonic	Muscle contraction against constant resistance through an arc
Isokinetic	Dynamic muscle exercise at a constant velocity
Eccentric	Contraction occurs while muscle lengthens

(Reproduced with permission from Kasser JR (ed): *Orthopaedic Knowledge Update 5*. Rosemont, IL, American Academy of Orthopaedic Surgeons, 1996, pp 89-101.)

injury. Machines have limited availability and adaptability to smaller individuals. Isotonic training can produce strength gains throughout at least part of a range of motion. However, the specific applicability to sports in which explosive strength is required is at issue because most isotonic training occurs at relatively slow speeds.

Isokinetic machines allow exercise and/or testing up to 300°/s. Studies have established normative data for isokinetic output in athletes, mostly in the upper extremity. These data can be used to measure a patient's progress through rehabilitation. An experienced tester must monitor the patient's position and effort during testing. Isokinetics do have some disadvantages. First is the expense of the machine and the requirement for therapist/athletic trainer monitoring. Second is the limited availability and sturdiness of these machines. Most importantly, there are few if any data that correlate isokinetic exercise performance to athletic performance. Shoulder internal rotation velocity in throwing, for example, is approximately 7,000°/s.

Concentric muscle contraction occurs as the muscle shortens, while lengthening of a contracting muscle is an eccentric contraction. Eccentric exercise can be done isotonically or isokinetically. Sport-related tasks requiring rapid deceleration, such as changing direction, jumping, and throwing, all involve eccentric activity. The basic science of eccentric exercise may not be well understood at present, but strength gains from concentric and eccentric exercises probably occur independently. If needed, eccentric exercises should be added to the overall strength program and can be incorporated in functional exercise. The development of muscle soreness is common. Close monitoring is needed to be sure eccentric exercises are done correctly.

Closed chain exercises are those in which the foot is on the ground and the athlete squats and then straightens. An alternative technique is the leg press. The technique strengthens multiple muscle groups, including the flexors and extensors of the hip, knee, and ankle. It includes eccentric and concentric contractions. The shear forces across the joints are minimized as a result of cocontraction of opposing muscle groups (eg, anterior shear on the knee by the quadriceps is minimized by coactivation of the hamstrings).

Functional Exercise
Functional exercise aims to restore strength and agility through various techniques that do not require standard strength training equipment. Examples include the improvement of proprioception using tilt boards, core strength by use of the Swiss ball, agility by carioca or single leg diagonal jumps, leap by box jumping, and throwing by high speed elastic tubing exercise. Such exercises have recently gained popularity in places where the need for individual, sport-specific activity is oftentimes counterbalanced by the necessity for cost containment. The role of the athletic trainer/physical therapist in patient instruction and monitoring should be emphasized for good outcomes.

Plyometrics and Proprioception
Plyometric training has become a popular preseason conditioning technique, especially in sports that require explosive muscular power. Plyometrics are performed by having the athlete repeatedly jump from and land on surfaces of different heights. This training reportedly enhances the myotactic (muscle stretch) reflex.

Plyometric training can be effective in decreasing impact forces and increasing hamstring torques in female athletes. This may have a positive effect on knee stabilization and prevention of serious knee injuries in this population.

Proprioception, or the sensation of joint position and movement, is becoming a major focus of research, and rehabilitation programs in the future will likely incorporate this training. Proprioception is impaired following ACL injury. Unfortunately, in at least one study, this effect did not improve following ACL reconstruction. Perhaps newer rehabilitation programs may improve this ability.

Sport-Specific Conditioning
Conditioning programs should focus on preparing athletes for individual sports. The concept of "periodization," or scheduling the frequency, duration, and intensity of work an athlete does during various periods of an athletic season, is an integral part of this program. Five phases have been described in this program (Fig. 2): (1) active rest (brief period of total rest followed by cross-training); (2) off season

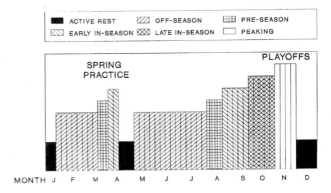

Figure 2
Sample conditioning plan for football. The phases are indicated in the key. During active rest, the athlete does cross training and activities that are noncompetitive; off-season activities emphasizes general fitness and flexibility with heavy weight training and aerobics. Preseason activities concentrate on high-intensity and sport-specific work. Early in-season activities continue high but submaximal frequent conditioning. Late in-season work has less emphasis on conditioning and light weight training with tapering of conditioning before competition. (Reproduced with permission from Kibler WB, Chandler TJ: Current concepts: Sport-specific conditioning. *Am J Sports Med* 1994;22:424–432.)

(emphasizes general athletic fitness, flexibility, and weight training); (3) preseason (sports-specific skills are practiced and refined); (4) early in-season (maintenance of condition with recovery periods after competition); and (5) late in-season (maximize efficiency of performance).

Medical Issues

Human Immunodeficiency Virus

The American Medical Society for Sports Medicine and the American Orthopaedic Society for Sports Medicine recently issued a joint position statement concerning athletes with human immunodeficiency virus (HIV). This statement concludes that HIV infection alone is insufficient grounds to prohibit athletic competition. Educating athletes on limiting their exposure to blood on the field and, more importantly, to the risks of transmission through sexual contact and contaminated needles is an important duty of physicians. When counseling athletes with known HIV, the physician should consider the athletes' general health, the type of sport they are involved in, the potential impact of stress from competition, and the potential risk of HIV transmission. Blood exposure must be minimized, and universal precautions used at all times.

Ergogenic Drugs and Supplements

As competition continues to intensify, athletes continue to seek a competitive edge. This is not a new phenomenon; athletes in the first Olympics in ancient Greece reportedly used strychnine for this purpose. The use of anabolic steroids, which are derivatives of testosterone, has declined in part because of strict testing of athletes and perhaps as a result of better efforts to educate athletes on the side effects of their use. Known side effects of steroids involve cardiac, hepatic, renal, neurologic, and psychological problems. Recent studies have also demonstrated stiffer, more easily injured tendons with anabolic steroid use.

Unfortunately, the use of growth hormone, which is undetectable, has increased among athletes. Side effects can include acromegaly, myopathy, osteoporosis, and diabetes. Creatine, a nutritional supplement that may affect muscle function by increasing myosin synthesis and increasing water content in muscle cells, has been popular in football players in recent years. Many potential side effects are still unknown; however, muscle cramping, a 30% nonresponse rate, and heat intolerance can be seen. There appear to be no positive or adverse effects from aspirin or sodium bicarbonate. Other abused drugs include clenbuterol, ephedrine, and numerous nutritional supplements. Anti-oxidants may be beneficial for

athletes. Proper nutrition, using the food guide pyramid, should be emphasized.

Other Medical Issues

Exercise induced hematuria and/or proteinuria will usually resolve within 48 hours. This is a benign condition, in contrast to more serious conditions that persist for longer periods. Most anemia in athletes is from a dilutional effect. Suspected true anemia should be evaluated with a complete blood cell count, reticulocyte count, and ferritin level in order to determine the etiology and treatment. Similarly, abnormal liver function tests can occur in endurance athletes. If levels remain persistently elevated after 3 days of cessation of exercise, then additional workup is indicated. Hypertension and its treatment usually are not contraindications to sports participation. Antihypertensive drugs that are *not* recommended for competitive athletes in endurance sports include verapamil, all beta-blockers, and diuretics. Asthma, in and of itself, does not disqualify athletes from sport. Asthmatics should consider sports with short bursts rather than continuous movement (eg, tennis) and sports that allow them to breathe warm, moist air (eg, swimming), should warm up intensely before competition, and should use medications as directed. Inhalers can be useful before competition and should be available on the sidelines.

Muscle Injury

Hamstring injuries are common and often debilitating. One recent study identified hamstring weakness (versus the opposite side and/or the ipsilateral quadriceps) with isokinetic testing, as an injury risk factor. Another study demonstrated a positive effect with repeated muscle stretch. This effect returned to normal, however, within 1 hour. Stretching and strengthening of the hamstring muscles after injury continues to be the mainstay of treatment. Isokinetic testing can be a helpful tool in determining when an athlete can return to play. A goal of 85% of the strength of the opposite hamstrings during testing has been proposed. Recent studies have pointed out that isokinetic testing may not correlate with functional performance. Functional testing, to include a 1-leg hop, shuttle run, cutting drills, and long jump, can also help in making the return-to-play decision. Both tests should be considered together.

Animal studies have demonstrated a threshold for injury that appears to be between 20% and 30% of muscle length. Additionally, a threshold for injury of 60% to 70% of the failure rate for that muscle tendon unit was demonstrated. These same investigators demonstrated the effect of fatigue in susceptibility to acute muscle strain injury. According to other studies that they have conducted, there is an early beneficial effect of NSAID treatment of muscle injury. This effect, however, did not persist past 2 days. In both anatomic and clinical studies, these investigators also described the anatomy of the proximal rectus femoris and suggest that some patients may actually benefit from surgical resection of scar mass in this area. These researchers also found that fatigued muscles were injured at the same length as rested muscles; however, they were able to absorb less energy before reaching the degree of stretch that causes injuries. Muscle fatigue is also believed to play a role in the pathomechanics of knee injury (especially ACL injury) in sports due to an altered neuromuscular response to anterior tibial translation.

Immobilization is known to adversely effect the vascular density at the myotendinous junction. One recent study has demonstrated that this effect will return to normal after 8 weeks and will actually increase with progressively increasing physical training. This may have a positive effect in reducing the rate of reinjury. Immobilization is also associated with long recovery times for muscle strength. One study demonstrated that even at 6 months following immobilization, concentric and eccentric Achilles tendon strength was not equal to that of the opposite side.

Overuse Injuries

Soft-Tissue Overuse Injuries
Chronic soft-tissue overuse injuries are common in sports. These include tendon injuries (tendinitis, tendinosis, paratenonitis), bursitis, strains, sprains, synovitis, and inflammation. With the exception of knee injuries, most of these patients will improve with time and therapy. Activity modification, exercise, and NSAIDs appear to have little effect on long-term outcome.

Stress Fractures
Femoral shaft stress fractures may be more common than once believed. A new clinical test, the fulcrum test, has been described which can help in the diagnosis of this injury. In this test, the examiner places his own forearm (fulcrum) under the sitting patient's affected femur, directly under the area of a suspected stress fracture. Gentle pressure is applied to the dorsum of the knee. Pain at the area of the fulcrum suggests a stress fracture.

Anterior tibial stress fractures can be particularly difficult to treat. Once lateral radiographs demonstrate a "dreaded black line," seen as a linear lucency on the anterior cortex, then nonsurgical management has usually failed. Surgical treat-

Table 5	
Sports-specific stress fractures	
Sport	**Injury**
Running	Tibia, navicular, fibula, hip/femur
Marching	Second metatarsal
Golfing	Rib
Bowling	Ulna
Weight lifting	Ribs, clavicle
Gymnastics	Foot, acromion, distal radius, spine (pars interarticularis)
Basketball	Fibula, foot (fifth metatarsal, navicular), proximal tibia
Football	Metatarsals
Dancing	Metatarsals, midshaft tibia
Rowing	Rib

ment options include bone grafting and intramedullary rodding. Interestingly, one recent MRI investigation suggests that "shin splints" may actually be part of a continuum of stress response in bone.

Recently, MRI has been proposed as an alternative to bone scans for imaging of stress fractures. MRI may be more accurate in correlating the degree of bone involvement, lacks exposure to ionizing radiation, and requires less time; however, these advantages must be weighed against the added expense for this imaging modality.

Athletes will often develop stress fractures following an increase in their training length, time, and/or intensity. Risk factors for stress fractures in men are not clear. In women, lower bone density, a history of menstrual disturbance, less lean mass in the lower limb, leg length discrepancy, and a lower fat diet are all significant risk fractures in runners.

Many stress fractures are sports-specific. Table 5 outlines some more common stress fractures associated with specific sports. In general, successful treatment of stress fractures includes early diagnosis, modified activities, and a carefully monitored rehabilitation and training program.

Conclusion

The orthopaedic surgeon must accept the challenge of remaining current with not only the most recent advances in surgical techniques, but also with the most current nonsurgical treatment plans. Proper practice of sports medicine requires an understanding of the many factors affecting the health of the athlete. Prevention, preseason evaluation, on the field evaluation, medical issues, and overuse injuries are important issues for the orthopaedic sports medicine physician of today.

Annotated Bibliography

Introduction

Boland AL: Presidential Address of the American Orthopaedic Society for Sports Medicine: Our qualifications as orthopaedic surgeons to be team physicians. *Am J Sports Med* 1996; 24:712–715.

This article represents an appeal to orthopaedic surgeons to remain in the lead as team physicians.

Injury Incidence and Prevention

Arendt E, Dick R: Knee injury patterns among men and women in collegiate basketball and soccer: NCAA data and review of literature. *Am J Sports Med* 1995;23:694–701.

Review of data from the National Collegiate Athletic Association (NCAA) Injury Surveillance System identified a disturbing trend in the incidence of ACL injuries among female athletes. The authors outline a training and rehabilitation program based on age and preinjury pitch speed.

Congeni J, McCullouch J, Swanson K: Lumbar spondylolysis: A study of natural progression in athletes. *Am J Sports Med* 1997;25:248–253.

This article highlights the usefulness of CT in evaluating athletes with spondylolysis.

Gill TJ IV, Micheli LJ: The immature athlete: Common injuries and overuse syndromes of the elbow and wrist. *Clin Sports Med* 1996;15:401–423.

This article focuses on common injuries in the adolescent throwing athlete. This entire issue of the journal focuses on the adolescent athlete.

Kallinen M, Markku A: Aging, physical activity and sports injuries: An overview of common sports injuries in the elderly. *Sports Med* 1995;20:41–52.

This article focuses on the special needs and injuries of the aging athlete.

Newton PM, Mow VC, Gardner TR, Buckwalter JA, Albright JP: The effect of lifelong exercise on canine articular cartilage. *Am J Sports Med* 1997;25:282–287.

This paper demonstrated that a lifetime of weightbearing exercise did not increase dog articular cartilage injury or arthritis.

Pate RR, Pratt M, Blair SN, et al: Physical activity and public health: A recommendation from the Centers for Disease Control and Prevention and the American College of Sports Medicine. *JAMA* 1995;273:402–407.

This article reviews the epidemiologic research on the benefits of exercise. It also issues a "call to action" for all health care professionals.

Teitz CC (ed): *The Female Athlete.* Rosemont, IL, American Academy of Orthopaedic Surgeons, 1997.

This monograph summarizes several important issues concerning the female athlete, but also has a section on the preparticipation examination and other items that involve all athletes.

Torg JS, Stilwell G, Rogers K: The effect of ambient temperature on the shoe-surface interface release coefficient. *Am J Sports Med* 1996;24:79–82.

These physicians have investigated the important considerations of cleat design and artificial turf injuries. They recommend the flat, no-cleat design of basketball shoes for various temperatures and caution that soft rubber sole shoes on warm artificial turf creates an increased risk for knee injury.

Van Mechelen W, Twisk J, Molendijk A, Blom B, Snel J, Kemper HC: Subject-related risk factors for sports injuries: A 1-yr prospective study in young adults. *Med Sci Sports Exerc* 1996; 28:1171–1179.

These researchers identified risk factors in adolescent injuries.

Williford HN, Kirkpatrick J, Scharff-Olson M, Blessing DL, Wang NZ: Physical and performance characteristics of successful high school football players. *Am J Sports Med* 1994;22:859–862.

Athletes from a successful high school football program were thoroughly evaluated at a human performance laboratory. Their results were similar to previously evaluated college players.

Preparticipation Physical Examinations

Sanders B, Nemeth WC: Preparticipation physical examinations. *J Orthop Sports Phys Ther* 1996;23:149–163.

This article reviews the purpose of the examination, organizational considerations, components of the examination, and special considerations.

Smith DM, Kovan JR, Rich BSE, Tanner SM (eds): *Preparticipation Physical Evaluation,* ed 2. Minneapolis, MN, McGraw-Hill Healthcare, The Physician and Sports Medicine, 1997.

This monograph, endorsed by 5 major medical societies (including the American Orthopaedic Society for Sports Medicine), outlines the key features of the preparticipation examination.

Rifat SF, Ruffin MT IV, Gorenflo DW: Disqualifying criteria in a preparticipation sports evaluation. *J Fam Pract* 1995;41:42–50.

This article identifies 7 disqualifying criteria that occur in relative frequency in a study of over 2,500 preparticipation physical evaluations.

On The Field Evaluation

Filipe JA, Barros H, Castro-Correia J: Sports-related ocular injuries: A three-year follow-up study. *Ophthalmology* 1997; 104:313–318.

This is a good overview of eye injuries and their incidence.

Maron BJ, Shirani J, Poliac LC, Mathenge R, Roberts WC, Mueller FO: Sudden death in young competitive athletes: Clinical, demographic, and pathological profiles *JAMA* 1996;276:199–204.

In a thorough review of 158 cases of sudden deaths among athletes, the authors identify the major causes. Preparticipation screening was found to be of limited value in identification of underlying cardiovascular abnormalities

Rehabilitation

Edwards DJ, Rimmer M, Keene GC: The use of cold therapy in the postoperative management of patients undergoing arthroscopic anterior cruciate ligament reconstruction. *Am J Sports Med* 1996;24:193–195.

In a prospective, randomized study comparing cryocuff with ice water, cryocuff with room temperature water, and no cryocuff, the authors could not determine any difference between the 3 groups in visual analog pain scores, amount of analgesic required, or range of motion.

Eriksson E: The scientific basis of rehabilitation. *Am J Sports Med* 1996;24(suppl 6):S25–S27.

This article reviews new advances in rehabilitation with an emphasis on the need for scientific study.

Fadale PD, Wiggins ME: Corticosteroid injections: Their use and abuse. *J Am Acad Orthop Surg* 1994;2:133–140.

This is an excellent review of the mechanism of action, solutions, tissue effects, and other issues concerning the use of injectable steroids. The paper points out that despite frequent use, few studies exist regarding the efficacy of corticosteroid use.

Hewett TE, Stroupe AL, Nance TA, Noyes FR: Plyometric training in female athletes: Decreased impact forces and increased hamstring torques. *Am J Sports Med* 1996;24:765–773.

This article showed a beneficial effect of plyometrics in female athletes.

Kibler WB, Chandler TJ: Sport-specific conditioning. *Am J Sports Med* 1994;22:424–432.

The authors describe this program and introduce the concept of periodization. They also provide a sample program for football.

Lephart SM, Pincivero DM, Giraldo JL, Fu FH: The role of proprioception in the management and rehabilitation of athletic injuries. *Am J Sports Med* 1997;25:130–137.

This article provides an overview of the emerging science of proprioception.

Swenson TM, Lauerman WC, Blanc RD, et al: Cervical spine alignment in the immobilized football player. *Am J Sports Med* 1997;25:226–230.

Angular sagittal alignment of the cervical spine significantly increased when the helmet was removed with the shoulder pads in place.

Wiggins ME, Fadale PD, Barrach H, Ehrlich MG, Walsh WR: Healing characteristics of a type I collagenous structure treated with corticosteroids. *Am J Sports Med* 1994;22:279–288.

This article demonstrated that steroid injections, given to rabbits with medial collateral ligament injury, impaired the healing of the ligament when studied at 10 days and 3 weeks postinjury.

Medical Issues

Selected Papers from the Third IOC World Congress On Sport Sciences. *Am J Sports Med* 1996;24(suppl):S1–S106.

This supplement includes articles on nutrition, drugs, and medical aspects involving the care of athletes.

Overuse Injuries

Selected Papers from the Third IOC World Congress On Sport Sciences. *Am J Sports Med* 1996;24(suppl).

This issue contains 3 excellent review articles on muscle strain, muscle fatigue, and muscle function.

Classic Bibliography

Akeson WH, Amiel D, Abel MF, Garfin SR, Woo SL: Effects of immobilization on joints. *Clin Orthop* 1987;219:28–37.

American College of Sports Medicine: Position stand on the use of anabolic-androgenic steroids in sports. *Med Sci Sports Exerc* 1987;19:534–539.

The American Medical Society for Sports Medicine (AMSSM) and the American Academy of Sports Medicine (AASM): Joint position statement: Human immunodeficiency virus (HIV) and other blood-borne pathogens in sports. *Am J Sports Med* 1995;23:510–514.

Cantu RC: Guidelines for return to contact sports after a cerebral concussion. *Phys Sportsmed* 1986;14:75–83.

122   General Knowledge

Eisele SA, Sammarco GJ: Fatigue fractures of the foot and ankle in the athlete, in Heckman JD (ed): *Instructional Course Lectures 42*. Rosemont, IL, American Academy of Orthopaedic Surgeons, 1993, pp 175–183.

Epstein SE, Maron BJ: Sudden death and the competitive athlete: Perspectives on preparticipation screening studies. *J Am Coll Cardiol* 1986;7:220–230.

Green NE, Rogers RA, Lipscomb AB: Nonunions of stress fractures of the tibia. *Am J Sports Med* 1985;13:171–176.

Saunders RL, Harbaugh RE: The second impact in catastrophic contact-sports head trauma. *JAMA* 1984;252:538–539.

Sitler M, Ryan J, Hopkinson W, et al: The efficacy of prophylactic knee brace to reduce knee injuries in football: A prospective, randomized study at West Point. *Am J Sports Med* 1990;18: 310–315.

Torg JS, Pavlov H, Genuario SE, et al: Neurapraxia of the cervical spinal cord with transient quadriplegia. *J Bone Joint Surg* 1986;68A:1354–1370.

Torg JS, Vegso JJ, O'Neill MJ, Sennett B: The epidemiologic, pathologic, biomechanical, and cinematographic analysis of football-induced cervical spine trauma. *Am J Sports Med* 1990; 18:50–57.

Chapter 13
The Multiply Injured Patient

Injury is the leading cause of death in the first 4 decades of life. The cost to society from hospitalization and lost productivity approaches $100 billion per year. The Committee on Trauma of the American College of Surgeons (ACS) has developed criteria by which a hospital and its personnel could demonstrate differing levels of trauma care in order to be recognized as a trauma center. These trauma systems, when implemented, have been shown to improve the quality of care and to reduce the number of preventable deaths due to injury. These systems are also capable of improving the outcome of the most severely injured patients.

Although the value of comprehensive trauma systems has been verified, few states have organized trauma care systems. It has been documented that 90 trauma centers have closed in the recent past. Only an estimated 25% of the population in the United States has access to organized trauma care.

Acute trauma care comprises between 1% and 2% of US health care expenditures. The economic status of trauma centers, levels of automobile insurance reimbursement, cost containment activities, and physician support exhibit a wide variation among different geographic locations. It seems likely that these complex and varied financial problems will remain a challenge for trauma centers.

Injuries from gunshots have increased at an alarming rate over the last decade. In 1994, there were an estimated 38,500 deaths and 90,000 to 100,000 nonfatal injuries in the United States related to firearms. Gunshot wounds occur 90 times more frequently in the United States than in any other industrialized country in the world. In urban hospitals, as many as 24% of orthopaedic admissions are the result of gunshots. Reported costs range from $7,000 to $20,000 per patient depending on the inclusion criteria. These high costs are underscored by the fact that as many as 60% of these patients are not insured.

The use of 3-point restraints (seat and shoulder belts) combined with air bags has been shown to be effective in reducing the morbidity and mortality associated with motor vehicle accidents. However, these devices were designed to protect against frontal impact and are less effective in reducing injuries from lateral impact. A recent study of lateral impact accidents noted an association of traumatic aortic ruptures and pelvic fractures. The recent increase in sales of large recreational urban vehicles has created a physical mis-match between these vehicles and the more standard-sized US cars. Sport utility vehicles have a greater mass and higher bumpers, which result in increased intrusion into the passenger compartment of standard cars during collisions.

The use of seat belts and air bags reduces the severity of brain injury, decreases the incidence of facial injuries, and may offer some protection against lower extremity injuries. However, a substantial number of pelvic and lower extremity fractures occur despite the use of both air bags and seat belts.

Injury Recognition

Injury recognition is important to separate a physiologically unstable multiple trauma victim from a stable trauma patient with a single-system or minor injury. Injury severity scores can be used to assist in the triage of patients, to evaluate outcomes, and to compare different systems of care. Scoring systems are based on anatomic and/or physiologic parameters. Approximately 50 different scores have been developed in attempts to study the complexities and variabilities of injuries sustained by polytraumatized patients.

Several scoring systems, including the Revised Trauma Score (RTS) and the Glasgow Coma Scale (GCS), are used in the initial assessment of the injured patient (Tables 1 and 2). These systems, which determine the degree of injury and the resulting physiologic impairment, are used in organized trauma systems to triage patients to comprehensive trauma care facilities. Data suggest that if the GCS score is less than 13 or the RTS is less than 11, patients should be transported to comprehensive facilities.

The immediate care of unstable, multiply injured patients has been outlined by the ACS Advanced Trauma Life Support course. This course divides the care of the patient into 4 stages, which provide a template for trauma management. The initial care stage is the primary survey phase, in which immediately life-threatening injuries are identified and treated. The resuscitation phase, which includes placement of various lines and tubes for monitoring and resuscitation, begins simultaneously. The third phase includes the secondary survey or history and physical evaluation of the patient, which are used to identify any other, non life-threatening injuries that the patient has incurred as a result of the accident. The

Table 1
Revised Trauma Score

Parameter	Measurement	Score
Respiratory rate*	10–29	4
	≥ 30	3
	6–9	2
	1–5	1
	None	0
Systolic blood pressure*	≥ 90	4
	76–89	3
	50–75	2
	1–49	1
	No pulse	0
Add Glasgow Coma converted score	13–15	4
	9–12	3
	6–8	2
	4–5	1
	1	0
	Total	—

Table 2
Glasgow Coma Scale

Level of Consciousness*		Score
Eye opening arousability	Opens spontaneously	4
	Open to voice	3
	Open to painful stimuli	2
	No eye response	1
Best verbal response	Oriented conversation	5
	Confused conversation	4
	Inappropriate words	3
	Incomprehensible sounds	2
	No verbal response	1
Best motor response	Obeys simple commands	6
	Localizes–painful stimuli	5
	Withdraws–painful stimuli	4
	Decorticate (flexion)	3
	Decerebrate (extension)	2
	No motor response	1

Totals (Glasgow Coma Scale Range: 3–15[†])

*record point value corresponding to patient's ability
[†]< 8, Severe head injury; ≤ 7, intubate

final phase is the definitive care, consisting of surgical intervention or chronic monitoring.

The first priority in management of a multiply injured patient is to establish a clear airway, followed by ventilation and circulation. Standard radiographs of the chest, pelvis, and lateral cervical spine are obtained early in the course of care. The physician should determine the patient's level of neurologic function, followed by physical examination of the patient's entire body to detect all areas of potential injury. Fluid resuscitation is guided by the patient's vital signs and by estimates of fluid loss. A rectal and vaginal examination should be performed; a Foley catheter is placed after assessing the possibility of urethral injury. Abdominal peritoneal lavage or abdominal computed tomography (CT) are used to detect intra-abdominal injury. A head CT is indicated in patients who have evidence of a head, midface, or cervical spine injury.

Despite adherence to ACS protocols, the incidence of missed injuries approaches 10% in the blunt injury patient population. Patients who are unable to cooperate or respond because of head injuries, alcohol intoxication, or intubation, are more likely to have undiagnosed injuries. Musculoskeletal injuries are the most frequent undiagnosed injuries. Commonly missed injuries include spinal fractures, fractures of the feet, and carpal injuries. The missed diagnosis of cervical spine injuries may lead to neurologic deficits. A tertiary examination or routine follow-up in-hospital assessment is recommended to reduce the risk of missing injuries in multiply injured patients. The tertiary musculoskeletal examina-

tion is ideally performed with a responsive and cooperative patient who can alert the physician to areas of pain or tenderness.

Trauma Injury Management

Closed Head Injury
The classic approach to the management of the multiply injured patient with significant head trauma has been stabilization using appropriate fluid management and rapid CT scan to define the extent of injury. Treatment is designed to reduce cerebral hypertension and includes hyperventilation ($PaCO_2$ of 26 to 28 mm Hg), head elevation, and osmotic diuresis. However, lowering $PaCO_2$ to these levels may contribute to cerebral ischemia. Similarly, controlling the arterial blood pressure and reducing cerebral hypertension may injure the patient. Some neurosurgeons are now suggesting that $PaCO_2$ be maintained between 32 and 35 mm Hg. Osmotic diuresis, using mannitol or urea, remains helpful in treating patients with acute cerebral edema. The role of agents that reduce cerebral activity (such as phenobarbital) has been studied, but few data exist as to the benefits of reducing cerebral metabolism in patients with acute brain injury.

A standard of care regarding the timing of fracture fixation in patients with brain injuries has not been established, partly because of a lack of prospective studies evaluating this injury combination. Retrospective studies have led to conflicting conclusions regarding the appropriate timing of fracture fixation in patients with closed head injuries. Proponents of early fixation are concerned that pulmonary complications will occur when stabilization of femoral shaft fractures is delayed. Another group argues that a delay of approximately 48 hours will benefit the patient by allowing the brain injury to stabilize without placing the patient at undue risk for pulmonary failure. A nonrandomized study indicated that patients with closed head injuries who underwent fracture fixation within 24 hours of injury experienced more hypoxia and hypotension than a group of patients who had fracture fixation after 24 hours. The late fixation group left the hospital with higher mean GCS score (15.0), compared to the early fixation group (13.5). This retrospective study did not establish that delays are appropriate for the fixation of fractures in patients with head injuries, but it does highlight the controversy regarding the timing of fixation. Another series, which emphasized that patients with closed head injuries undergo early fracture fixation for pulmonary care, did not find evidence to support the worsening of the neurologic status by early fracture fixation. At this time, a definitive recommendation regarding the timing of major fracture fixation in patients with severe head injuries cannot be made.

Chest

In a multiple-trauma patient with thoracic injury, a major concern is lung damage with resulting hypoxia. Pulmonary contusion, hemothorax, pulmonary laceration, and pneumothorax all can result in significant hypoxia. Usually these problems can be treated by airway maneuvers such as intubation, mechanical ventilation, or tube thoracostomy. Historically, this type of patient has not been a good candidate for open reduction and internal fixation (ORIF) of long-bone injuries. However, early ORIF of long-bone fractures may improve pulmonary status and should make nursing care easier.

Controversy remains regarding the best way to evaluate a patient with suspected injury to the thoracic aorta. Several studies have confirmed aortography as the standard against which other diagnostic modalities (such as dynamic CT) should be compared. A patient with a wide mediastinum must be evaluated before repair of long bone injuries to rule out serious aortic injury.

The ventilation management of the critically injured patient in the intensive care unit includes refinements of technique such as pressure support and permissive hypercapnia. These modifications lower energy use by the patient and reduce the potential for barotrauma.

Abdomen

Evaluation of acutely injured multiple-trauma victims includes peritoneal lavage for unstable patients suspected of having intra-abdominal injury; however, reasonably stable patients with suspected abdominal injuries are more often evaluated with CT scanning. Several large series have demonstrated that this is appropriate and appears to be much more specific than diagnostic peritoneal lavage. The use of CT has reduced the number of patients requiring urgent laparotomy secondary to positive lavage. A number of patients revealed by CT to have injured livers and spleens and who are stable are now observed. The one injury that CT appears to miss is small perforations of the gastrointestinal tract. Close observation and serial examinations are, therefore, mandatory when diagnostic peritoneal lavage is not used and CT scan is the primary mode of evaluation of the abdomen.

The use of ultrasound as a screening tool is gaining wider acceptance. Abdominal ultrasound can be performed with a high degree of accuracy by the surgical team in the emergency room. This study does not require the transport of critically ill patients to other areas of the hospital, and can easily be repeated as a follow-up examination.

Spine

Cervical spine radiographs are routinely obtained during the evaluation of trauma patients. The consequence of missing a fracture of the cervical spine justifies this radiography, despite a very low true positive rate. Thoracolumbar spinal fractures are associated with a neurologic deficit in approximately 45% of patients. Because of the consequence of a missed fracture of the thoracic or lumbar spine, surveillance radiographs are now recommended for trauma patients with multisystem blunt injuries, a fall equal to or greater than 10 ft, ejection from a motor vehicle or motorcycle, a GCS score ≤ 8, a neurologic deficit, or back pain or tenderness on physical examination.

The initial (field) care and stabilization of patients with spinal injuries is outlined for prehospital personnel in *Emergency Care and Transportation of the Sick and Injured* (American Academy of Orthopaedic Surgeons, 1995). With 14,000 new spinal cord injuries occurring each year, the initial care is important to prevent further injury and functional loss.

High-dose methylprednisolone is recommended in the care of acute injury to the spinal cord. A multicenter national acute spinal cord injury study reported improvement in motor scores in patients with incomplete spinal cord injuries after treatment with high-dose methylprednisolone within 8 hours of injury. These results were compared to those of a similar group of patients treated with naloxone (opiate receptor antagonist) or with a placebo. There was no significant difference between groups when treatment was begun later than the initial 8 hours after injury. One year after the injury, the group treated with high-dose methylprednisolone had a higher probability of improved motor function.

The current recommendation is to give methylprednisolone by intravenous administration to all acute spinal cord injury patients. The recommended dose is 30 mg/kg of body weight over 15 minutes followed by an infusion of 5.4 mg/kg/hr for 23 hours.

Pelvis and Lower Extremities

An improved mortality rate is noted when major pelvic and long bone fractures are stabilized early in the care of the multiply injured patient. All long bone and pelvic fractures should be stabilized within 48 hours in this patient group. However, data from recent laboratory and clinical studies have suggested that intramedullary (IM) nailing with reaming may be detrimental to patients with preexisting lung injuries. Intraoperative transesophageal echocardiography has confirmed that multiple embolic particles, some large, pass through the right atrium and ventricle during IM reaming. The passage of emboli to the left ventricle can occur in a patient with a patent foramen ovale, a condition present in approximately 20% of adults.

Pulmonary damage from reaming may be caused by either the mechanical effects of the emboli or by the biochemical effects of the emboli on the lung parenchyma. The reamer design and the diameter of the shaft of the reamer are important variables that affect IM pressures. Smaller diameter shafts and reamers with deeper cutting flutes significantly reduce IM pressures.

IM nailing increases pulmonary triglyceride levels, pulmonary artery pressures, and pulmonary capillary resistance. However, in a well-designed animal study, there were no significant differences in pulmonary function between animals that had reaming and those that did not. Pulmonary function was not worsened by the presence of a pulmonary contusion.

Techniques for stabilizing femoral fractures have been compared in several studies. Because plating does not have an effect on IM pressures and does not generate emboli, it provides a "control" to study the effect of IM nailing with reaming. In a study of patients with femoral fractures and pulmonary injuries, plate fixation was compared with IM nailing with reaming. Both groups of patients experienced similar rates of adult respiratory distress syndrome. Direct comparisons of IM nailing with and without reaming in prospective and randomized studies have found that IM nailing without reaming requires less surgical time and has a lower blood loss, but is associated with a higher rate of tech-

nical complications, including delayed union. There was no difference in pulmonary function between the 2 groups of patients. It appears that most femoral fractures in patients who have sustained multiple trauma can be safely stabilized with an interlocked IM nail inserted after reaming. Some patients, however, such as those who have an associated severe pulmonary injury, may benefit from an alternative method of fracture fixation; the specific characteristics of this patient population are presently unknown.

Health Care Worker Risk

The number of patients at many urban trauma centers who use drugs or are involved in violent acts continues to increase. The high incidence of human immunodeficiency virus (HIV) and hepatitis infections in these patients poses a hazard to health care workers. The most critically ill patients tend to have a higher incidence of HIV and hepatitis. In providing care for these patients, the following should be recognized: (1) these high-risk patients require emergent care, and invasive procedures are often required under emergent situations; (2) these severely injured patients are an important educational component for young physicians in training, but also place these physicians at increased risk; and (3) the presence of these infections (HIV, hepatitis C) may worsen the prognosis of these patients. All of these factors underscore the need for universal precautions and hepatitis virus vaccination of health care workers. The estimated risk of transmission of HIV after percutaneous exposure to infected blood is estimated to be 0.3%. Postexposure prophylaxis with zidovudine may be protective.

The Pathophysiology of Multiple Injuries

The degree of response to injury is related to the severity of the injury and the number of organ systems involved. Major mechanical or thermal injuries result in tremendous increases in caloric requirements (as much as 150% of normal in severely burned patients). Provision of adequate nutrition to support this requirement has been a major advance in the field of trauma care. Similarly, major injuries resulting in tissue damage and shock have been shown to markedly stimulate the stress response and alter the endocrine balance of the patient. There is an increased secretion of the hormones related to mobilization of fats and glucose. Insulin secretion appears to be elevated during the stress response.

Cytokines are a generic term for proteins that mediate cell function by binding to specific cell-surface receptors. This term is used to replace both lymphokines and monokines.

Significant concentrations of these substances have been found associated with the soft-tissue injury and fracture hematoma that accompany major fractures. The systemic circulation of cytokines from the site of soft-tissue injury is an area of interest for understanding systemic inflammation and occasional immune suppression observed in patients with multiple injuries.

Multiple system organ failure occurs at 2 different times after the initial injuries. The early presentation occurs without sepsis and is thought to be a result of the initial posttraumatic inflammatory response. The late presentation of multiple system organ failure is associated with sepsis and is thought to be related to uncontrolled infection or sepsis. In addition to sepsis, surgery performed in the posttraumatic period may increase the high level of inflammation and cause multiple system organ failure.

The concept that surgery performed after the initial resuscitation may act as a "second hit" to the multiply injured patient is of interest to orthopaedic surgeons. In one study, 38% of secondary surgeries performed on multiply injured patients preceded a deterioration in organ function. Markers of inflammation such as C-reactive protein, neutrophil elastase, and platelet counts may offer a means of assessing the patient's level of inflammation. In the future, it may be possible to use different measures of inflammation to help predict which patients are at risk for developing multiple system organ failure. This information could then help orthopaedic surgeons to determine the appropriate timing of fracture fixation in severely injured patients.

Prophylaxis Against Complications

The immediate care of multiply injured patients consists of determining what is injured and repairing those injuries in the correct order of importance and in a timely fashion. The subsequent care involves monitoring the patient and preventing complications. Prophylactic therapies indicated in the care of acutely injured patients include: (1) determining nutritional needs; (2) preventing stress bleeding, venous thrombosis, and pressure sores; and (3) assessing antibiotic coverage.

Early nutrition is a critical part of the care of multiply injured patients. Ideas concerning surgical nutrition have actually come full circle. Following the development of the techniques of parenteral nutrition, surgeons advised early institution of parenteral alimentation in the care of these patients. This concept has gradually been revised. The current recommendation is to provide early enteral nutrition to patients who have a functional gastrointestinal tract. Several

new immune-enhancing formulations have shown great promise by increasing the number of calories provided to acutely injured patients and decreasing the complications associated with immune suppression, which may occur with parenteral nutrition or no nutrition at all. Support of the early hypermetabolism associated with injury and prevention of the protein calorie malnutrition that occurs within a day or 2 of injury are the goals. The data suggest that many septic complications can be minimized by early enteral nutrition. Even after abdominal procedures, feeding directly into the small bowel (by nasoduodenal or jejunostomy tubes) is tolerated without significant ileus. Similarly, it appears that early enteral nutrition (using the newer formulations) does not result in significant diarrhea. This diarrhea appears to be more related to the prolonged absence of enteral feeding, and early feeding appears to limit its subsequent development.

Severely injured patients exhibit a stress response that includes the release of hormones that stimulate gastric acid production. The introduction of agents to decrease acid secretion has decreased the number of patients requiring treatment of stress bleeding. Prevention of stress bleeding by the use of histamine blockade or mucosal barrier protection is required in any significantly injured patient and is especially required in those not being fed enterally.

Deep venous thrombosis and pulmonary embolism are major concerns in patients with multiple trauma. Some form of prophylaxis or treatment is required. The best form of therapy remains full anticoagulation; however, anticoagulation frequently is not indicated because of the multiple sites of injury and the potential for bleeding, especially in the central nervous system. Appropriate forms of prophylaxis, which depend on the types of injury, should include 1 or a combination of the following: (1) passive motion of lower extremities, (2) segmental compression devices for the extremities, (3) vitamin K antagonist (warfarin, Coumadin), (4) low dose or minidose heparin, (5) early ambulation, or (6) placement of a vena cava filter. These have been shown to be effective in reducing the incidence of pulmonary embolism. The indications for insertion of prophylactic inferior vena cava filters are currently being debated.

The development of pressure sores frequently adds $50,000 or more to the cost of caring for injured patients. Therefore, interventions to reduce the incidence of decubital pressure sores are vital. In multiply injured patients (especially patients with interference of movement secondary to paralysis or prolonged procedures), attention is directed to preventing prolonged pressure on dependent areas. Preventive measures include obtaining the appropriate bed, removing the patient from rigid spine boards as rapidly as possible, and mobilizing the patient as early as is feasible. It is unfortunate that preventing decubitus ulcers often is a low priority item in critically ill or injured patients and frequently these measures are begun only after the problem is noted.

The final prophylactic regimen that is important early in patient care is the choice of antibiotics. The care of multiply injured patients frequently includes the neurosurgery, plastic surgery, general surgery, and orthopaedic surgery services. Prophylactic antibiotics are chosen based on the needs of each of the individual services. Fortunately, most studies indicate that for closed injuries to many different organ systems, prophylaxis against surface organisms requires only a first generation cephalosporin. The choice of prophylactic antibiotics becomes more challenging when open injuries exist. Coverage against gram-negative and anaerobic organisms may be suggested by the type of wound and the patient's location when the injury occurred.

Outcome of Multiply Injured Patients

Improvements in critical care have reduced the mortality associated with multiple system organ failure from 90% to 50%. Patients who survive multiple system organ failure usually exhibit normal pulmonary, hepatic, and renal function at long-term follow-up. Of equal importance is that many of these severely injured patients will return to work within 1 year of their injuries. The prognosis for return to a productive lifestyle is difficult to predict and may be related as much to social factors as to the pattern of injuries. Important social factors include professional versus manual labor, degree of education, and level of compensation.

The relative morbidity of different fractures of the lower extremity appears to be time dependent. In the hours after injury, long bone fractures must be stabilized to prevent pulmonary complications. Although severe fractures of the ankle and foot do not pose a risk to survival in the early phases of an injury, late disability from pilon fractures, calcaneal fractures, and other foot injuries has been well documented. Fractures of the foot become the major determinants of lifelong impairment often after the other multiple fractures have healed.

Annotated Bibliography

Bosse MJ, MacKenzie EJ, Riemer BL, et al: Adult respiratory distress syndrome, pneumonia, and mortality following thoracic injury and a femoral fracture treated either with intramedullary nailing with reaming or with a plate: A comparative study. *J Bone Joint Surg* 1997;79A:799–809.

Multiply injured patients with fractures of the femoral shaft with and without a thoracic injury were studied at 2 different trauma centers. One center used IM nailing with reaming in 95% of patients treated and the other used open reduction and internal fixation with plating in 92% of patients studied. The overall occurrence of adult respiratory distress syndrome (ARDS) in the 453 patients with a femoral fracture was only 2%. Patients with a thoracic injury, but no femoral fracture, developed ARDS in 6% of patients at one center and 8% of patients at the other. The incidence of the problems studied for the patients who had a femoral fracture and a thoracic injury was similar regardless of which fracture treatment had been used.

Cardo DM, Culver DH, Ciesielski CA, Srivastava PU, et al: A case-control study of HIV seroconversion in health care workers after percutaneous exposure: Centers for Disease Control and Prevention Needlestick Surveillance Group. *New Engl J Med* 1997;31:1485–1543.

This study of 33 patients who seroconverted after HIV exposure and 665 who did not showed that significant risk factors for seroconversion were: deep injury, injury with a visibly contaminated device, procedures involving placing a needle in the source patient's vein or artery, and exposure to a source patient who died of acquired immunodeficiency syndrome within 2 months afterward. Patients who seroconverted were significantly less likely to have taken zidovudine after exposure.

Duwelius PJ, Huckfeldt R, Mullins RJ, et al: The effects of femoral intramedullary reaming on pulmonary function in a sheep lung model. *J Bone Joint Surg* 1997;79A:194–202.

In this study, the relationship between embolization and pulmonary dysfunction with IM nailing performed with and without reaming was evaluated using a sheep model. There was a transient increase in pulmonary vascular resistance in the reamed group and a significant increase in the amount of fat emboli in both groups. Opening of the intramedullary canal by an awl was associated with the greatest number of emboli.

Grotz M, Hohensee A, Remmers D, Wagner TO, Regel G: Rehabilitation results of patients with multiple injuries and multiple organ failure and long-term intensive care. *J Trauma* 1997;42:919–926.

Results of functional and occupational rehabilitation of 50 patients 4.9 ± 0.3 years after injury are presented. Range of motion of the elbow, hip, knee, or ankle was limited in 25% of patients; permanent motor nerve lesions were found in 40%; and permanent sensory nerve lesions in 50%. However, 60% returned to work.

Kropfl A, Berger U, Neureiter H, Hertz H, Schlag G: Intramedullary pressure and bone marrow fat intravasation in unreamed femoral nailing. *J Trauma* 1997;42:946–954.

IM pressure and bone marrow fat intravasation were monitored in 31 unreamed and 8 reamed IM femoral nailing procedures. IM pressure increased more in the reamed than in the unreamed group. Bone marrow fat intravasation depended on the rise in IM pressure and occurred less frequently in the unreamed group.

McKee MD, Schemitsch EH, Vincent LO, Sullivan I, Yoo D: The effect of a femoral fracture on concomitant closed head injury in patients with multiple injuries. *J Trauma* 1997;42:1041–1045.

This retrospective study examined patients with multiple injuries and mean Glasgow Coma Scale scores of 7.8 with matched controls of patients with multiple injuries with head injuries, but without femur fractures. Results suggested that a femoral fracture in a patient with a concomitant head injury did not increase mortality or neurologic disability and supported early IM nailing of femoral fractures in these patients.

Poole GV, Tinsley M, Tsao AK, Thomae KR, Martin RW, Hauser CJ: Abbreviated Injury Scale does not reflect the added morbidity of multiple lower extremity fractures. *J Trauma* 1996;40: 951–954.

It was found that the abbreviated injury score and the severity score reflected the impact of extraskeletal injuries in patients with femur fractures, but did not adequately reflect the increased morbidity associated with multiple lower extremity fractures.

Quigley MR, Vidovich D, Cantella D, Wilberger JE, Maroon JC, Diamond D: Defining the limits of survivorship after very severe head injury. *J Trauma* 1997;42:7–10.

The authors retrospectively reviewed the outcomes of 380 patients admitted to a level 1 trauma center with a Glasgow Coma Score of 3 to 5. Outcome a minimum of 6 months after injury was determined for all but 5 patients. Overall nonvegetative survival was 12.5%, with no survivors in the advanced age decades.

Schemitsch EH, Jain R, Turchin DC, et al: Pulmonary effects of fixation of a fracture with a plate compared with intramedullary nailing: A canine model of fat embolism and fracture fixation. *J Bone Joint Surg* 1997;9A:984–996.

A canine model was used to examine the pulmonary effects of the timing and method of fixation of a fracture. The amount of intravascular fat in the lungs, kidneys, and brain after pressurization of the IM canal was not affected by the method of fixation of the fracture. The development of pulmonary dysfunction from fat emboli appears to depend on other factors than the presence of fat in pulmonary vessels.

Sloan EP, McGill BA, Zalenski R, et al: Human immunodeficiency virus and hepatitis B virus seroprevalence in an urban trauma population. *J Trauma* 1995;38:736–741.

The authors found that young urban trauma patients were 15.3 to 17.6 times more likely to be HIV infected and 3.9 to 7.9 times more likely to be infectious for HIV and hepatitis B virus than the trauma population overall.

Tornetta P III, Olson SA: Amputation versus limb salvage, in Springfield DS (ed): *Instructional Course Lectures 46*. Rosemont, IL, American Academy of Orthopaedic Surgeons, 1997, pp 511–518.

This is an in-depth discussion of scoring systems, rating criteria, and other criteria to help a surgeon decide between amputation and salvage of a severely injured limb.

Classic Bibliography

Bonanni F, Rhodes M, Lucke JF: The futility of predictive scoring of mangled lower extremities. *J Trauma* 1993;34:99–104.

Bone LB, McNamara K, Shine B, Border J: Mortality in multiple trauma patients with fractures. *J Trauma* 1994;37:262–264.

Bostman O, Pihlajamaki H: Routine implant removal after fracture surgery: A potentially reducible consumer of hospital resources in trauma units. *J Trauma* 1996;41:846–849.

Brumback RJ, Jones AL: Interobserver agreement in the classification of open fractures of the tibia: The results of a survey of two hundred and forty-five orthopaedic surgeons. *J Bone Joint Surg* 1994;76A:1162–1166.

Burgess AR, Dischinger PC, OíQuinn TD, Schmidhauser CB: Lower extremity injuries in drivers of airbag-equipped automobiles: Clinical and crash reconstruction correlations. *J Trauma* 1995;38:509–516.

Georgiadis GM, Behrens FF, Joyce MJ, Earle AS, Simmons AL: Open tibial fractures with severe soft-tissue loss: Limb salvage compared with below-the-knee amputation. *J Bone Joint Surg* 1993;75A:14311441.

Loo GT, Siegel JH, Dischinger PC, et al: Airbag protection versus compartment intrusion effect determines the pattern of injuries in multiple trauma motor vehicle crashes. *J Trauma* 1996;41: 935–951.

Napolitano LM, Koruda MJ, Meyer AA, Baker CC: The impact of femur fracture with associated soft tissue injury on immune function and intestinal permeability. *Shock* 1996;5:202–207.

Regel G, Lobenhoffer P, Grotz M, Pape HC, Lehmann U, Tscherne H: Treatment results of patients with multiple trauma: An analysis of 3,406 cases treated between 1972 and 1991 at a German Level 1 Trauma Center. *J Trauma* 1995;38:70–78.

Roessler MS, Wisner DH, Holcroft JW: The mangled extremity: When to amputate. *Arch Surg* 1991;126:1243–1248.

130   General Knowledge

The Violence Prevention Task Force of the Eastern Association for the Surgery of Trauma: Violence in America: A public health crisis. The role of firearms. *J Trauma* 1995;38:163–168.

van der Sluis CK, ten Duis HJ, Geertzen JH: Multiple injuries: An overview of the outcome. *J Trauma* 1995;38:681–686.

Chapter 14

The Physician, the Illness, and the Workers' Compensation System

Workers' Compensation: A Clinical Problem

Treatment outcomes shift more toward fair and poor levels of recovery with longer disability when patients come into the workers' compensation system. The negative shift in outcome indicates that workers' compensation introduces additional factors, which influence patients and frustrate treatment efforts. Orthopaedists must understand and address those factors to recover the more favorable outcome ratios that are seen in nonworkers' compensation injuries.

Medical education is heavily weighted to the scientific study of biologic systems of health and disease to the exclusion of other factors. Physicians who provide care for diseased and injured people are often inadequately prepared to deal with the psychological, social, and economic issues that influence the outcomes of treatment. This chapter attempts to outline and assist in management of these issues.

Impairment versus Disability, Injury versus Illness

The differences between impairment and disability, and between disease and illness are crucial concepts. The World Health Organization defines impairment as the "Loss of, or abnormality of psychological, physiologic or anatomic structure or function..." Disability is "Any restriction or lack of ability to perform an activity in the manner or within the range considered normal for a human being." Disease is a pathologic condition of a body part. Illness is the total effect of an injury or disease on the entire individual. Disease and impairment are purely biologic issues concerned with the anatomy and physiology of the organ or organ system affected. Illness and disability are the total manifestation of disease and impairment on the individual. Illness and disability

include the subjective affectation influenced by the psychological, social, and economic environment in which the diseased or impaired individual lives.

Once, at a cocktail party, entertainment was provided by a piano player who performed beautifully. He was a little man with a short left upper extremity. His left hand was about half the size of the right hand. The fingers were short and the interphalangeal joints appeared to be stiff. If this man had presented to an orthopaedist's office and said, "Doctor they want me to play the piano, and I just can't," the physician would have said, "Of course you can't. You have a disease, the congenital failure of development of your left upper extremity. This disease has left you with an impairment of your left upper extremity so that it would be unreasonable to expect you to play the piano. Therefore you are disabled insofar as piano playing is concerned." The rationale would be correct. The conclusion could not be more wrong.

There is no correlation between impairment and disability except in cases of the most extreme injuries. Patients assume the ill and disabled roles because of the influence of other factors in their lives. Symptom magnification is the rule, but true malingering is rare. Physicians dealing with minor back aches and strains must recognize and address the psychological, social, and economic factors that have more effect on the recovery of patients than the physical problem (Fig. 1).

Physicians can work exclusively within the scientific arena that is well known to all, properly diagnosing and technically treating diseases with all the available scientific and technical knowledge. However, simultaneously ignoring the illness and the psychological, social, and economic factors that contribute to that illness may lead to failure. It is important to treat the illness. The pain drawing and the Minnesota Multiphasic Personality Inventory Test (MMPI) are 2 tools that help to define some of these additional sources of illness. In practicing the art of medicine, physicians intuitively sense the presence of these other factors. Patients describe their anger as a primary feature in giving a history. Depressed

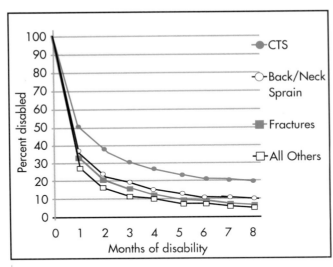

Figure 1

The similarity of disability duration curves for vastly different types of injuries suggest a common nonbiological group of forces driving the period of disability. CTS, carpal tunnel syndrome. (Reproduced with permission from Cheadle A, Franklin G, Wolfhagen C, et al: Factors influencing the duration of work-related disability: A population-based study of Washington State workers' compensation. *Am J Pub Health* 1994;84:190–196.)

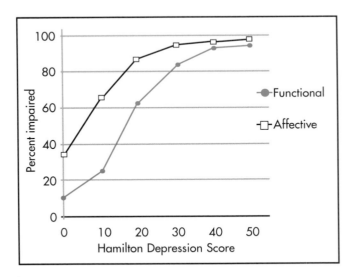

Figure 2

The functional curve indicates the percent of patients with the correlating Hamilton Depression Score who actually are disabled from their employment. The affective curve indicates the percent of patients with the correlating Hamilton Depression Score who feel that they are disabled because of their depression, but who continue to work nonetheless. The area between the curves represents millions of Americans who go to work each day while thinking they can't. (Reproduced with permission from Fawcett J: The morbidity and mortality of clinical depression. *Int Clin Psychopharmacol* 1993;8:217–220.)

patients can depress their physicians. Exaggerated, dramatic, and confusing descriptions of symptoms give strong clues of these additional factors that contribute to the illness.

Social, Psychological, and Economic Factors

Social and economic conditions can also predispose patients to prolonged periods of disability. The duration of disability increases with age. This is caused partially by slower healing rates and partially by increasing comorbidity, including depression, as aging increases. It may also be a result of the proximity of normal retirement. Marital status correlates with protracted disabilities. Those who never have married have the shortest periods of disability following injury. Married persons have shorter disability periods than those who are divorced; and widowed individuals have the longest periods of disability. Males have higher disability rates than females. However, females tend to have longer periods of disability than males once injured.

The family can influence the attitude of an injured worker. Disability can become a conditioned illness because it can be a means of obtaining support from family members. On the other hand, the family may react angrily forcing the injured worker to justify the sick role by exaggerating his or her illness. Finally, the disability of a major provider may compel another family member to assume the position of the primary provider, thus affecting his or her response to the disability of the patient. The newly empowered spouse may support the patient's assumption of the sick role and the continued disability.

Physicians can make a fair estimate of the time to healing and recovery for most injuries based on knowledge of the process of wound healing and empiric knowledge of specific injuries (Table 1). Comorbidity with diseases such as diabetes, anemia, and emphysema is expected to prolong the recovery period. Comorbidity with psychological disorders predisposes patients to longer periods of disability than diabetes, anemia, and emphysema. The comorbidity of psychiatric illness and back pain can make the diagnosis difficult, the problem recalcitrant to treatment, and the disability longer. In one study at least one psychiatric disorder was found in 54% of patients with low back pain and in 77% of patients with carpal tunnel syndrome.

Depression

Depression is the most common of the primarily disabling psychiatric disorders. Five percent to 10% of the adult population experience an episode of depression each year. The

Table 1
Guidelines for tasks in job categories

Job Category	Job Description	Weight Lifted, lbs*	Weight Pushed or Pulled, lbs*	Weight Carrier, lbs*	Climbing†	Body Motion‡	Sitting-Standing Transition§	Walking, % of day
1	Sedentary	10/0	150/0	≤ 10/0	Ramp/none	< 10	30 min	10
2	Sedentary to light	15/≤ 5	200/100-125	15/≤ 5	None/ramp	< 10	30 min	20
3	Light	20/≤ 10	250/125-150	20/10-15	Stairs/none	10-15	30-45 min	30
4	Light to medium	35/≤ 20	300/200-250	35/20	None/stairs	15-20	45 min to 1 hr	40
5	Medium	50/≤ 20	350/250-300	50/25-30	Ladder/stairs	20-30	1-1.5 hr	50
6	Medium to heavy	75/≤ 35	400/300-350	75/30-40	Scaffold/ladder	30-40	1.5-2 hr	60
7	Heavy	100/ ≤ 50	450/350-400	100/40-50	Poles/scaffold	40-60	2-2.5 hr	70
8	Very heavy	> 100/> 50	> 450/> 400	> 100/> 60	Rope/poles	> 60	> 2.5 hr	80

* Values are expressed as weight infrequently involved/weight frequently involved

† Descriptions are expressed as type of climbing infrequently performed/type of climbing frequently performed

‡ Values are number of instances of body motion (bending, kneeling, squatting, or reaching) engaged in per hour

§ Values are time spent in continuous transition between sitting and standing positions

(Reproduced with permission from Millender LH, Conlon M: An approach to work-related disorders of the upper extremity. *J Am Acad Orthop Surg* 1996;4:134-142.)

overall 30-day prevalence of depression in the United States is 4.9%. Depression accounts for nearly two thirds of the absent days resulting from mental health diagnoses. Depression may be the result of protracted disability with an injury. However, consideration of its prevalence in the general population leads to the recognition that depression is an important predisposing factor for protracted disability following a work injury. The effects of depression are additive with any other disabling condition. Depression itself is more disabling than most back injuries, and the rate of recurrence is higher. Depressed patients have more physical illness and greater disability from those illnesses than nondepressed people. The depressed person perceives himself or herself as more disabled than he or she is. When an individual with depression is disabled by a minor back injury, the disability will be protracted (Fig. 2). Physicians who do not simultaneously provide care for the underlying psychiatric problem cannot expect success in treatment of the injury.

Other Disturbances

The habitual use of alcohol is associated with prolonged disability. The combination of drug or alcohol abuse with depression or anxiety neurosis is a major risk factor for suicide. A somatic complaint may be the only acceptable way for a patient with a psychiatric disturbance to present his or her problem. Individuals unable to cope with emotional and psychological stresses within their lives resort to the sick role. This may provide a mechanism to keep them from becoming more depressed. A patient with a factitious disorder has a psychological need to assume the role of sick person without regard to secondary gain. The somatic presentation of psychiatric disorders may be more common than a psychiatric complaint. Somatizers overreport both physical and psychological symptoms. These patients change doctors frequently and demand multiple tests and consultations. Thus, a minor injury in one of these patients will be exaggerated and will lead to extended disability. Somatization is considered a major problem in all areas of medicine.

Comorbidity with psychiatric problems, somatification, influence of the family, aging, marital status, and gender can affect the outcome of treatment in the noncompensation population. However, these factors are major considerations for the workers' compensation population.

Secondary Gain

The term "secondary gain" implies that the patient derives a benefit from continuing in the illness role. Many oversimplify the issue by attributing failures in treatment entirely to secondary financial gain. The predominance of psychological issues in secondary gain has been clearly articulated. The desire for compensation on the part of the injured person may be a substitute for other issues. In some instances, the patient may enjoy being cared for or the attention gained. In other situations, the injury provides a means of retaliation against the patient's employer, a way to avoid an unhappy work situation, or a perceived solution to a family problem. Unfortunately the gains are not real, and the patient can continue them only by continuing the disability. While the financial support provided by the workers' compensation system usually is not the motivating factor for assuming the sick role, it is the enabling factor.

Disability Causes Additional Illness

Disability itself is pathogenic for additional morbidity beyond that produced by the original injury. Feelings of displacement, depression, and suicide increase as disability is protracted. There is a higher incidence of drug and alcohol abuse and of family disruption and divorce among disabled workers. Therefore, return to employment must be a goal of treatment when the injury recovery has progressed to a point that work is possible.

Doctor and patient must establish return to work as a goal of treatment. This goal should be an explicit agreement between the doctor and the patient at the beginning of treatment. The physician must keep his or her patients focused on their recovery. If the physician allows illness behavior to control the patient, he or she contributes to protracted disability. Disability can be iatrogenic in extreme cases.

Know the Language and Use it

The terms *temporary total disability, temporary partial disability, maximum medical improvement, permanent total disability, permanent partial disability, apportionment, and reasonable medical certainty,* are the basis that the other members of the system require to fulfill their obligations to the patient. Temporary total disability means that the patient is not capable of any gainful employment, but he or she may improve. He or she should receive full compensation benefits during the period of temporary total disability. Temporary partial disability means that the patient can do some work, but is not expected to return to his or her previous level of employment yet. The attending physician should describe the impairment and just how it limits the patient. Individuals who lack a medical background at the personnel department of the patient's work place, the claims management department of the insurer, and the workers' compensation commission should use that physician's assigned limits to direct the injured worker to appropriate work within his or her capabilities. The patient may receive reduced benefits during this time, and he or she may be required to show evidence of a diligent attempt to find work within his or her abilities.

Maximum medical improvement means that the patient has recovered to the highest level that can be expected for the specific injury in the specific patient. Any disability at that point is permanent, either total or partial. When a physician decides that the patient has reached maximum medical improvement, he or she should describe the impairment and, using appropriate guides, assign a permanent impairment rating. The insurer and compensation commission use that rating to assign a "disability" percentage and compute the compensation for the loss according to the statutes covering that jurisdiction.

Apportionment is sometimes used to distribute liability to more than one employer and more than one insurer. If there are 2 separate injuries to 1 body part at 2 separate times, both may have left permanency. It is appropriate to apportion the permanency to the separate injuries. For example, a man may fall from a ladder and sustain a fracture of a transverse process of a lumbar vertebra while painting his house. He recovers from that and later lifts a heavy load at work suffering a disk herniation. Table 75, I of chapter 3 of the American Medical Association (AMA) Guidelines allows a permanent impairment of 5% of the whole person for the transverse process fracture and Table 75, II, D allows 8% for the lumbar disk herniation. The total impairment is the sum of 5% plus 8%, but the physician should apportion only 8% to the work related injury.

The awards given for permanent impairment are arbitrary. There is no way to adequately compensate a patient with money for a loss of function of his or her body. Because the awards are arbitrary, they seem to vary greatly from physician to physician and case to case. The only way that physicians can impact any fairness to this system is to be consistent with impairment ratings. The only way to be consistent in an arbitrary system is to use an impairment rating guide. The AMA Guidelines are the most widely accepted.

When offering opinions for impairment or causation, the physician should use his or her best judgment and common sense and offer his or her opinion authoritatively and unequivocally. This is no time for humility. If a new point of view is presented that changes the opinion later, the physician can acknowledge the new information and revise the opinion. However, humble opinions with various disclaimers offer conflicting parties points for contention. Contention engenders litigation. Litigation prolongs disability. Disability delays recovery and introduces new illness. "Reasonable medical certainty" means that the opinion is more probably right than wrong. That means a 51% probability of being right. The system requires that the physician offer his or her best opinion with reasonable medical certainty. Offer opinions without ambivalence.

Recognize that there are other parties who can affect a patient's recovery. The physician must communicate with them in terms that they can understand and can use to fill their respective missions. Use their language. Define the diagnosis, the impairment, the reasonable function that the individual can undertake, and establish a date of maximum medical improvement at every visit.

The Other Parties and a Different Agenda

The employer, the employer's compensation insurance carrier, the workers' compensation commission, the union, the physician, the predisposition of the injured worker and his family, and the injured worker's attorney all influence the attitude of the injured worker. Without returning to work the patient must assume and continue the illness role to justify continued disability. Each of the other parties has a unique viewpoint and interest. Each of them can affect the rate at which physicians return patients to work. Each party acts independently, often with a minimum of communication with the others. The treating physician learns of actions of the employer, commission, and insurer only through the patient and the patient's attorney.

Disability Costs

Employers and insurers are most concerned by the rapid rise in disability costs. The workers' compensation system experienced double digit increases in costs during the 1970s and 1980s. The total cost of workers' compensation was approximately 5.2 billion dollars in 1971 and 57.3 billion dollars in 1993. Back injuries were a leading force in driving up medical and indemnity expenses. The exact amount of workers' compensation expense for back pain is uncertain but estimates vary between 16 and 56 billion dollars per year. In 1986, more than 11 million patients had low back impairments and 5.6 million patients were disabled by low back pain in the United States. Fourteen percent of all health care dollars for back pain came from workers' compensation in 1987, while only 1.25% of the costs of all medical problems came from workers' compensation. The most significant observation is that 10% of back injuries account for 90% of the losses. The same observation can be made for all injuries covered by workers' compensation. It is the 10% who have protracted disabilities who account for 90% of the expense throughout the spectrum of workers' compensation injuries.

Society changes the criteria for entitlement to compensation because disability cannot be determined with certainty. Insurers, employers, and legislatures have responded to the rapid escalation in costs by reducing payments and denying access to benefits for all injured workers instead of responding to the 10% of the workers' compensation recipients who overutilize the system.

Insurer Responses

The rate of increase of workers' compensation losses has decreased since 1990. The overall health cost in the United States rose by 8.3%, but the health care expenditure for workers' compensation rose by only 4.9% from 1990 to 1993. Workers' compensation insurers realized record profits with lowest loss ratio and highest return on net worth in 1994 and 1995. The average period of disability is down by almost 20% following workers' compensation injuries.

The trend is expected to continue. State legislatures, competing for new industries to locate within their state, will limit employers' liability for injuries. Cuts will focus on injuries that have significant causal connection to factors outside the workplace. Because repetitive motion and cumulative trauma injuries are the fastest growing type of workers' compensation claim, attempts to restrict compensability to "single event" injuries will continue. There will be attempts to apportion impairment ratings so that only the impairment resulting from the work injury is compensated. There will be attempts to introduce thresholds so that the injured employee will have to prove that the work injury was the major cause of his or her disability. Managed care in workers' compensation will continue to increase with fee schedules and medical treatment protocols being increasingly prevalent. Trends of concern are to deny access to treatment and compensation, to reduce the level of benefits, and artificially to cap costs for medical treatment for all injured workers.

Employee Responses

When insurers delay paying benefits and may deny medical treatment, the injured worker is forced to either accept the financial losses that come with the injury or to seek legal assistance to contest the insurer's action. Once an attorney is involved, the injured worker may be coached in ways to demonstrate the most severe aspects of the injury. Disability is protracted. The patient cannot give up his or her disability and illness behavior until the case passes through a long legal process to settlement. The underlying injury goes untreated and the illness behavior establishes a pattern. The probability for return to work diminishes as time progresses. If the patient is out of work for 2 years, there is virtually no chance of his or her ever returning to work. If the patient returns to work early, he or she gives evidence that the injury was not all that bad. Not only do indemnity costs for a protracted disability go up, but the medical expenses of multiple tests, consultations, and independent medical examinations also rise.

Disincentives to Returning to Work

The individual employer has the greatest opportunity to reduce losses in the workers' compensation system. Injury prevention is key to reducing losses. However, once a disabling injury has occurred, there are many factors within the control of management that will alter the course of a worker's disability. Job satisfaction is the foremost factor correlating with an early return to work. Persons with high levels of discretion are more than 2 times as likely to be working as those with less autonomy. Those with high demands and little discretion to deal with them are far less likely to return to work after a disabling injury. An unpleasant and stressful work environment will greatly reduce the probability for return to work. A single supportive phone call from the employer to the injured worker would be a strong force in motivating the patient to return to work, especially if the patient is experiencing depression or has a need for emotional support.

Some employers respond angrily to the injured worker and refuse to file an initial report of injury. Thus, not even the insurer has the opportunity to deal with the injured worker. Occasionally, the employer is simply happy to be rid of the injured worker and does as little as possible to promote his or her return to work. Considering the prevalence of psychiatric comorbidity, it is possible to understand that attitude. Depressed, anxious, or substance abusing people do not make the most desirable and productive employees.

Unions with rigid seniority policies may assign the easier jobs to workers with more seniority instead of to those with limited abilities. This also hampers return to work efforts. Unions with strict rules prohibiting a worker from crossing trades can also hinder return to work. Unions can also promote safety and return to work as specific contract issues in negotiating a labor contract.

There is a minimum of communication from insurers, unions, and employers to physicians about the availability of limited work for any given patient. The only source of information to the physician regarding the work place is the patient. The patient who is disposed to assume the illness role can produce a multitude of obstacles to his or her return to work.

Treating physicians should understand the system, establish return to work as priority in the treatment plan, and report the diagnosis, treatment plan, disability status, and expected period of disability following each patient encounter. The treating physician should recognize that disability itself is pathogenic and make return to work a goal of treatment and, therefore, should try to engage the employer in helping to return the patient to work. The treating physician must provide consistent permanency ratings. Most importantly, the treating physician should expand his or her view beyond the diagnosed injury to the whole patient and all of the factors affecting that patient, and then beyond to the societal impact of the patient's disability.

Change the Focus from Antagonism to Cooperation

When patients are disabled for longer periods of time they suffer more because of the morbidity associated with disability. The insurer, employer, and society suffer the economic losses of that disability. The key to turning a lose-lose situation to win-win lies in prompt treatment and return to work. Physicians must end the antagonism between payers and providers and begin to communicate and cooperate. The best interest of the injured worker, the financial interests of the employer and the insurer, and the intended fairness of the system would be served best by a joint effort of all parties to reduce the period of disability and promote return to work. Across the board cuts in benefits, restriction of access to the system, and delaying medical treatment all promote conflict between patient, employer, physician, and insurer. Conflicts may lead to litigation, prolonged disability, greater illness, and greater expense. The physician should focus on the problem, the 10% of the injured workers who account for 90% of the losses, the prolonged illness behavior and disability. Then there will be a basis for cooperation among all of the parties concerned.

Annotated Bibliography

Amadio PC: Pain dysfunction syndromes. *J Bone Joint Surg* 1988;70A:944–949.

This is an excellent review article discussing the distinctions between somatiform disorders, somatization, factitious disorders, malingering, and reflex sympathetic dystrophy. Amadio also discusses their interaction with triggering physical events.

American Academy of Orthopaedic Surgeons. Working it out. Report of workshop sponsored by American Academy of Orthopaedic Surgeons 1990–1992.

Using the Delphi method for consensus building, this report identifies major problems in delivery of health care to workers' compensation patients. Participants included representatives from employers, insurers, physicians, and government.

Barsky AJ, Borus JF: Somatization and medicalization in the era of managed care. *JAMA* 1995;274:1931–1934.

This article demonstrates the prevalence of psychiatric disorders as a basis for physical complaints, and discusses these problems in terms of economic impact.

Hadler NM: The disabling backache: An international perspective. *Spine* 1995;20:640–649.

The author discusses historical background of workers' compensation in various parts of the world.

Mayer TG, Gatchel RJ, Kishino N, et al: Objective assessment of spine function following industrial injury: A prospective study with comparison group and one-year follow-up. *Spine* 1985;10:482–493.

The authors introduce functional restoration as a successful rehabilitation program for patients disabled with low back pain. Similar results have been reproduced in subsequent reports and studies from other centers.

Norris CR: Understanding Workers' Compensation Law. *Hand Clin* 1993;9:231–239.

This is an excellent discussion of United States workers' compensation laws, their evolution, and relevance to the practicing physician.

Waddell G: A new clinical model for the treatment of low back pain. *Spine* 1987;12:632–644.

This article recognizes the fallacy of the traditional medical model for disease in cases of low back pain. The author promotes active exercises instead of the traditional rest model in treating chronic back pain.

Waddell G, McCulloch JA, Kummel E, Venner RM: Nonorganic physical signs in low-back pain. *Spine* 1980;5:117–125.

This paper documents the validity of 5 tests which indicate a nonorganic basis for patients' low back pain.

Chapter 15
Amputations and Prosthetics

Amputation

Amputation of all or part of a limb is performed for peripheral vascular disease, trauma, infection, tumor, or congenital anomaly. It should be viewed as the first step in the rehabilitation of a patient with a nonreconstructible limb and not the final step in treatment. Regardless of etiology, the following questions should be asked when considering amputation versus limb salvage. (1) Will a salvaged limb functionally outperform amputation and prosthetic fitting? (2) What are the patient-specific relative outcome expectations for limb salvage and amputation? (3) Is the resource and time commitment needed for limb salvage justified to both the patient and health care system? (4) What are the relative costs of each option?

Metabolic Cost of Walking

The metabolic energy cost of walking with an amputated limb is inversely proportional to the length of the residual limb and the number of functioning joints preserved. Patients have decreased self-selected and maximum walking speeds and a corresponding increased oxygen consumption with more proximal amputation. Functional independence measure (FIM) scores also correspond well with the length of the residual limb. Young amputees have a large energy reserve, but the metabolic cost of walking may be so severe in vascular transfemoral amputees that it precludes walking outside of the home.

Load Transfer (Weightbearing)

The soft-tissue envelope acts as the interface between the bone of the residual limb (stump) and the prosthetic socket. Weightbearing is accomplished by either direct or indirect load transfer. An example of direct load transfer is end bearing impact, through the expanded distal surface of a disarticulation. In diaphyseal amputations, where the terminal bearing surface is small, distribution of forces by hydraulic mechanisms represents the indirect load transfer option. To compensate for these weight transfer limitations, the residual limb must be flexed 7° to 10° in transtibial levels and adducted in transfemoral levels to allow dissipation of the load over an expanded surface about the shafts of the tibia and femur, respectively. Dynamic bony positioning is accomplished by securing muscles at functional lengths by myodesis (direct suture to bone through drill holes) or myoplasty (securing muscle to periosteum or compartment fascia). Because a true intimate prosthetic socket fit is rarely achieved, the soft-tissue envelope in these residual limbs should ideally be composed of a nonadherent muscle mass and full-thickness skin capable of tolerating shear forces. Skin grafts are best reserved for areas of decreased load or shear application.

Amputation Wound Healing

Wound healing requires an environment with adequate tissue oxygenation, nutrition, and immunocompetence. Amputation wound healing is often supported by collateral blood flow; therefore, the arteriogram is rarely a useful preoperative test. The ultrasound Doppler has historically been used as the measurement tool to determine adequate perfusion to support amputation wound healing. An absolute Doppler pressure of 70 mm Hg or an ischemic index (ratio of Doppler pressure at the proposed amputation level to the brachial pressure) of 0.5 reflects adequate perfusion. The most commonly used parameter is the ankle-brachial index (ABI), which is used as a measure of perfusion of the foot. The ultrasound Doppler measures arterial pressure directly and blood flow indirectly. This measure is adequate in patients without peripheral vascular disease, but not optimal in the presence of peripheral vascular disease where calcified arteries produce falsely elevated Doppler pressures in at least 15% of patients. Transcutaneous oximetry measures the partial pressure of oxygen at the skin level. The threshold transcutaneous oxygen ($TcpO_2$) capable of supporting amputation wound healing is between 20 and 30 mm Hg. These values are more predictable than ultrasound Doppler, except in the presence of localized soft-tissue infection, where the values may be falsely depressed.

Patients are considered malnourished when their serum albumin is below 3.5 g/dl, and immunodeficient when their total (absolute) lymphocyte count is below 1,500. Wound healing rates can be increased from 40% to 90% when adequate inflow, serum albumin of 3.0 g/dl, and total lymphocyte count of 1,500 are achieved prior to definitive amputation. In the presence of sepsis, incision and drainage or open distal amputation can be performed in conjunction with oral nutritional support prior to definitive amputation.

Technical Considerations

Handling of soft tissues is critical to achieving optimal functional outcomes. The skin is often fragile as a result of impaired circulation or recent trauma. Surgical technique must be meticulous. Flap thickness should be maximized. In adults, periosteal elevation should be limited to 1 cm proximal to the bony transection level to prevent bony overgrowth. Overgrowth is common in children. Epiphyseal or Silastic capping, or excessive periosteal excision have been used, with limited success, in children.

Muscles should be secured at dynamic lengths to bone (myodesis) or overlying periosteum (myoplasty) to achieve dynamic control within the prosthetic socket for optimal prosthetic biomechanics. A stable soft-tissue envelope with adequate dynamic control of the bone functions far more efficiently than a residual limb with an adherent, insufficient soft-tissue envelope, or one with excessive muscle or redundant skin.

All transected nerves form neuromas. To prevent sensitive, painful neuromas, nerves should be mobilized, transected with a fresh scalpel, and allowed to retract between muscle masses, where the neuroma will be cushioned from direct pressure. Crushing the nerve with a clamp prior to transection should be avoided, because crush may predispose the nerve to a painful causalgia/reflex sympathetic dystrophy type of syndrome. Ligation, cauterization, crushing, capping, perineural closure, and end-loop anastomoses have not been shown to be more effective than gentle distal traction and proximal transection.

Split-thickness skin grafting is best avoided in areas where end bearing or shear forces are applied to the residual limb. When essential to salvage residual limb length in young patients, free tissue transfer or tissue expanders can be used to improve the soft-tissue envelope. The prosthetic socket can be lined with Silastic gel materials to accommodate a poor soft-tissue envelope.

Pediatric Amputation

Pediatric amputations are performed for congenital limb deficiencies, trauma, or tumors. Congenital limb deficiency is based on the concept of failure of formation. The present classification system of limb deficiency was developed at a 1991 Consensus Conference of the International Society for Prosthetics and Orthotics (ISPO). Deficiencies are either longitudinal, transverse, or intercalary. Preaxial refers to the radial or tibial side, and postaxial to the ulnar or fibular side. Amputation is rarely indicated for congenital upper limb deficiency, because sensate, even rudimentary appendages will generally outperform an insensate prosthesis. Amputation of an unstable lower extremity segment may enhance functional walking with a prosthesis. Residual limbs

in growing children should be as long as possible to enhance prosthetic suspension and leverage as the child grows. Disarticulation is favored in the child because it retains the growth potential, and allows direct load transfer. Disarticulation also eliminates terminal bony overgrowth, which commonly occurs in transosseous amputations of the humerus, fibula, tibia, and femur. Symptomatic terminal bony overgrowth is best treated with surgical revision.

Amputation in Trauma

The only absolute indication for amputation in trauma is an ischemic limb with nonreconstructible vascular injury. In the lower extremity, severe open fracture (Gustilo-Anderson grade IIIC) combined with an insensate foot plantar surface is generally best treated with immediate amputation. The grading scales for evaluating mangled extremities are not absolute predictors for amputation, but act as reasonable guidelines for determining whether salvage is appropriate. Although these limbs can often be salvaged, the risk of sepsis, late tissue breakdown, and limited recovery of function makes immediate amputation a sound option. Poor functional outcomes in grade IIIA and IIIB fractures of the tibia and fibula suggest that a careful assessment of bony injury, soft-tissue envelope, sensibility, and motor function should be made before deciding in favor of limb salvage. Outcome expectations should drive decision-making in the evaluation and treatment of mangled extremities. The population of patients sustaining grade III tibial fractures is predominantly young, male, and employed in heavy labor occupations. These individuals are much more likely to return to their work following amputation and prosthetic fitting. The surgeon must consider the patient's employment capacities, rehabilitation potentials, resource availability, and psychological support systems before embarking on a prolonged course of limb salvage, which will require multiple surgeries, expense, and pain.

Salvage of the upper limb should be attempted whenever there is a reasonable potential to retain some sensation and prehension, because the primary role of the upper extremity is prehension, a task modulated by sensibility. Prosthetic replacement of the lower extremity approximates functional task performance, as opposed to the upper limb where sensation critical to optimal function is absent with the prosthesis.

When amputation of the upper extremity is performed for trauma, salvage of length is even more crucial than in the lower extremity. When more than one joint needs to be replaced, the prosthesis becomes increasingly heavy and cumbersome to operate. Joints have to be activated sequentially as opposed to the simultaneous activity in able-bodied individuals.

Amputation in Peripheral Vascular Disease

Peripheral vascular disease of sufficient magnitude to require limb amputation is not limited to the extremities. These patients have concomitant multiple organ system disease; therefore, they must possess the cognitive capacities of memory, attention, concentration, and organization to enable them to learn to walk with a prosthesis and care for their residual limbs. Patients with cognitive deficits or psychiatric disorders are unlikely to achieve prosthetic walking independence. A reasonable expectation of rehabilitation potential should be obtained prior to amputation.

Approximately half of lower extremity amputations are performed in diabetics. The most significant risk factor for amputation in diabetics is peripheral neuropathy. Diabetics become at-risk when they have peripheral neuropathy, as measured by insensitivity to the Semmes-Weinstein 5.07 monofilament (Fig. 1). Other risk factors are peripheral vascular disease, ipsilateral or contralateral partial or total foot amputation, presence or history of diabetic foot ulcer, or previous hospital admission for diabetic foot infection. Diabetics at risk should have ongoing foot examination, prophylactic nail and callus care, and use soft leather, inlay-depth shoes with pressure-dissipating foot orthoses.

The biologic amputation level is the most distal functional amputation level with a reasonable probability (90%) of supporting wound healing. This level is determined by assessing vascular inflow and biologic wound healing capacity. A realistic assessment of rehabilitation potential can then be used to select the rehabilitation amputation level, ie, the surgical amputation level that will optimize functional rehabilitation with a reasonable downside risk of wound failure.

Musculoskeletal Tumors

Current techniques in chemotherapy and radiation, combined with the surgical creation of adequate surgical margins and intercalary allograft or prosthetic reconstruction, have made amputation an infrequent surgical choice for the musculoskeletal oncologic surgeon. This choice is somewhat dependent on level. A transtibial amputee will generally outperform those with intercalary reconstructions below the knee, whereas even complex reconstructions above the knee generally fare better functionally than transfemoral amputations. This is true even when surgical margins require removal of sciatic or posterior tibial nerves. Protective orthotic strategies generally protect these individuals, although they are not as successful following trauma or in the presence of severe diabetic peripheral neuropathy. Although controversial in the adult, knee disarticulation is considered to functionally perform better than transfemoral amputation, because of its end bearing prosthetic capacity.

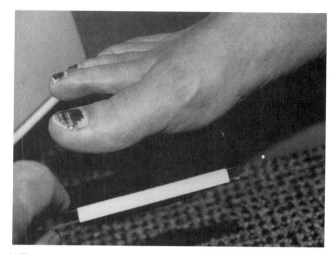

Figure 1

Semmes-Weinstein 5.07 monofilament. Diabetic patients insensate to plantar pricking with this nylon monofilament are at risk to develop foot ulcers eventually leading to amputation.

The role of surgery is to provide adequate margins regardless of the method. Presently, survival rates, measurements of the metabolic cost of walking, and lifestyle outcome analyses have shown that results of both limb salvage and amputation are similar.

Gas Gangrene

There are 3 types of bacterial gas-forming infections that lead to amputation. Patients with classic clostridial gas gangrene become critically ill immediately following an open injury. The classic syndrome is rapid onset sepsis (fever is often over 40°C), pain, and disorientation. They have a typical brownish discharge from the wound with crepitus in the extremity along the involved tissue planes. This is an infection of the muscles contiguous with the open wound, so treatment requires emergent open amputation at a level 1 joint above all involved muscle compartments, combined with high-dose penicillin therapy and adjuvant hyperbaric oxygen therapy.

Streptococcal myonecrosis is a tissue-plane infection. The clinical evolution is slower, and patients are not as critically ill as those with clostridial infection. Treatment requires excision of all involved muscle compartments combined with open wound management and penicillin therapy.

Anaerobic gas-forming infections caused by gram-negative bacilli are common in diabetics with open ulcers. Frequently, these infections are polymicrobial. Treatment requires open debridement combined with broad-spectrum antibiotics until surgical tissue cultures provide identification of the causative organisms.

Postoperative Care

Postoperative care encompasses tissue and wound management, as well as the overall rehabilitation of the patient. Tissue care is dictated by the disease process as well as the goals in treatment. When amputation is performed secondary to trauma, the zone of injury should be managed as a Gustilo-Anderson grade III open fracture. Wounds should be treated open at the most distal viable level. Bones are not shortened until the time of secondary wound closure. Neither skin traction nor sutures under tension should be used, because the traction/tension will only add further trauma to already traumatized tissue. Because of the elasticity of the skin and muscle, length can easily be regained at the time of secondary wound closure, typically at 5 to 7 days following the injury. Foot and ankle amputations are best immobilized postoperatively with well-padded short leg casts. Transtibial and knee disarticulation are managed with rigid plaster dressings. Transfemoral and hip disarticulation are managed with soft compressive dressings.

Continuous epidural anesthesia and postoperative infusional continuous regional anesthesia with an indwelling percutaneous catheter placed at surgery adjacent to the transected nerve enhance postoperative pain control and assist in early ambulation and rehabilitation. These methods are beneficial in the early postoperative period, but are not successful in altering late residual limb pain syndromes. Patients should be mobilized as soon as medically feasible. Weightbearing can be delayed until the residual limb is capable of accepting the load. Tissue breakdown in the early postoperative period is generally related to shearing forces involved when the limb pistons within a cast, rigid dressing, or temporary prosthesis. This can be avoided by changing casts weekly until the residual limb volume stabilizes. Transtibial amputees can bear weight at 5 to 21 days following surgery. Transfemoral amputees can bear weight when their residual limb appears to be capable of accepting load (generally 5 to 21 days). Partial foot amputations and ankle and knee disarticulation can bear weight within the first week, because these levels are end bearing, creating little shearing forces.

Complications

Pain All adults and many posttraumatic pediatric amputees will express phantom limb sensation, ie, the perception that their limb is still attached, following amputation. Phantom limb pain is a condition of severe pain, often described as burning or tearing in the amputated part. When seen in the early postoperative period, anesthetic nerve blocks are beneficial. When seen late, noninvasive therapies include increased prosthetic limb use, intermittent compression, physical therapy modalities, and transcutaneous electrical nerve stimulation.

A more common cause of residual limb pain is a condition similar to reflex sympathetic dystrophy, in which patients describe burning, searing, tearing, or throbbing pain, often severe, in their residual limb. These patients often have undergone amputation following a crushing injury and have symptoms much like a major causalgia. Treatment strategies should be similar to those used in treating patients with reflex sympathetic dystrophy.

Localized residual limb pain is often due to a poorly fitting prosthesis, or a poorly formed residual limb with prominent bone, or a deficient or scar-adherent soft-tissue envelope. The first step in treatment of these problems is prosthetic socket modification. When modification of the prosthetic socket fails, the residual limb can generally be adequately revised by bone shortening combined with resection of the scarred locally adherent tissue. In young patients who would be appreciably functionally impaired by bone shortening, local myocutaneous flaps, free soft-tissue transfer, or tissue expanders can be used. If the soft-tissue envelope is abundant and can tolerate stretching, residual limb bony lengthening can be attempted.

Edema Postoperative residual limb swelling is common. It is uncomfortable and may impede wound healing by increasing tissue and venous pressures. Prevention is the best method of treatment; it is accomplished by a rigid plaster dressing in the transtibial (immediate postoperative prosthesis), knee disarticulation, or foot and ankle amputee. Although such dressings can be used in transfemoral amputation, difficulty in suspension makes their use cumbersome and ineffective. Elastic compressive wraps and shrinker socks are less effective. When compressive stump wrappings are too tight proximally, they may act as a tourniquet, producing appreciable distal swelling or underlying or distal tissue necrosis.

Late residual limb swelling/congestion can be produced by proximal prosthetic socket constriction, venous disease, or cardiac insufficiency. The most severe form, verrucous hyperplasia, is characterized by a wart-like overgrowth of skin combined with darkened pigmentation, fissuring, and serous discharge, which may lead to a secondary cellulitis. This is caused by nonintimate prosthetic socket fit. Creating a more intimate socket fit, often requiring sequential socket modifications, will generally eliminate this problem.

Joint Contracture Hip flexion contracture can be produced during transfemoral amputation by performing the myodesis closure with the hip positioned in a flexed position. Joint contracture can occur between the time of surgery and prosthetic fitting, secondary to positioning. Contractures are best treated by prevention, with early supervised physical therapy and prosthetic limb fitting. When contractures develop, physical therapy or bracing (static or dynamic) is generally not successful. Treatment involves prosthetic limb fitting, weightbearing ambulation, and stretching exercises.

Wound Failure Wound failure occurs in approximately 10% to 15% of patients with diabetes or peripheral vascular disease. Small areas of wound failure can be treated with appropriate debridement and healing by secondary intention. Weightbearing should not be delayed, because the wound will heal much like wounds in total contact cast treatment of diabetic foot ulcers. When the bone is exposed, or an inadequate soft-tissue envelope is available, revision is occasionally necessary. In the young patient, tissue expansion, local tissue transfer, or free tissue transfer can be used to achieve a serviceable residual limb. In the geriatric diabetic dysvascular patient, surgery should entail wedge resection of nonviable tissue, bone shortening, and reconstruction of the soft-tissue envelope.

Dermatologic Problems Most skin problems are related to hygiene. Residual limb skin should be kept clean, dry, and free of residual soap or oils. Acne is common. It is treated with perspiration-absorbing stump socks, meticulous hygiene to prevent buildup of skin oils, and oral tetracycline. Contact dermatitis can also be treated with good hygiene combined with topical steroid creams.

Amputation Levels and Prosthetic Principles

Upper Extremity
The shoulder acts as the center of the functional sphere in which the hand accomplishes prehension. The elbow acts as a caliper to position the hand between the center and periphery of that sphere. Preservation of functional joints and segment length predict ultimate outcomes in the upper extremity amputee. Segment length is valuable for both suspension of the prosthesis and leverage to drive the prosthesis through space. Functional recovery from upper extremity amputation is less satisfactory than from lower extremity amputation, because all insensate upper limb prosthetic function must be under direct visual control.

Prosthetic Principles
Upper limb prostheses should be fitted during the first 30 days after amputation when expected acceptance and use will

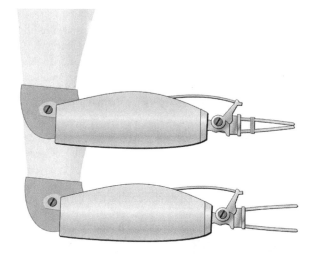

Figure 2

Body-powered upper limb prosthesis is controlled by a cable attached to a shoulder harness. Biscapular abduction lengthens the cable, opening the terminal device. Shoulder relaxation allows the terminal device to be passively closed by the rubber bands at the base of the hook.

approach 85%, as opposed to a 50% usage rate when fitting is delayed. Prosthetic joints can be controlled by body power, electric switch control, or myoelectrically. A body-powered prosthesis has a terminal device, usually a hook, held closed by rubber bands. A figure-of-8 harness is attached by a cable and worn about the shoulders. Biscapular abduction pulls the cable to voluntarily open the terminal device. Relaxing the shoulders allows the terminal device to passively close, because of the action of the rubber bands (Fig. 2). This is opposite of the normal voluntary closing action of the human hand. The myoelectric prosthesis is voluntary opening and phasically "normal", being controlled by electromyographic (EMG) sensors built into the prosthetic socket or suspension harness overlying the motor point of usually a specific agonist muscle for the task to be performed. When the muscle is contracted, the EMG electrode senses the electric signal, activating a battery-powered motor to open or close a terminal device, or flex or extend a prosthetic elbow (Fig. 3). A switch-driven, powered component has a length-activated switch within the harness. Biscapular abduction, or another patient-specific motion, lengthens the sensor to activate the specific component. Regardless of the method of control, each individual prosthetic component, or joint, can only be activated sequentially, as opposed to the simultaneous activity of the normal individual. Therefore, outcomes are improved with the fewest numbers of joints prosthetically replaced. Body-powered systems are lighter and faster than motored systems, but depend on joint excursion and the strength of the individual. Electric systems are limited by the weight of the motors and batteries, which are increased with more powerful, faster motors and longer lasting batteries.

Hand Amputation Complete hand amputations are rare. Whether from trauma or tumors, the most common amputation is one in which only part of the hand or less than the full complement of digits is ablated. Because of the emphasis on function, surgical reconstruction is usually favored over prosthetic fitting for these amputations. Procedures such as ray amputations, pollicizations, and microsurgical options typically yield a functionally superior hand compared to any prosthetic wear. For cosmetic purposes, nonfunctional prostheses have been developed, but are usually worn only during social situations and foregone for conduct of vocational and avocational activities.

Transradial Amputation Wrist disarticulation or maintenance of the pronator quadratus level preserves two thirds of forearm rotation. There are newer body-powered prostheses that accommodate this distal forearm level of amputation. However, the optimal level for transradial amputation if a myoelectric prosthesis is desired is at the junction of the middle and distal thirds of the forearm, allowing an adequate soft-tissue envelope and ease of prosthetic fitting.

Transhumeral Amputation Elbow disarticulation should be avoided, because optimal prosthetic fitting at this level is difficult. Desired length can be obtained with amputation at the diaphyseal-metaphyseal junction. In general, the greater the

humeral length to that point, the better the fit and greater the function.

Shoulder Disarticulation Prostheses at this level provide minimal function. The shoulder is generally passive, with a hybrid combination for elbow and terminal device.

Lower Extremity
The metabolic cost of walking, as well as functional outcomes, are directly related to the length of the residual limb (with an adequate soft-tissue envelope) and the number of usable joints preserved.

Prosthetic Principles
A myriad of dynamic elastic response, or so-called "energy storing" prostheses are presently available. They make use of a carbon-graphite keel that deforms with weightbearing, providing dynamic rebound from active knee extension at push-off. Prosthetic sockets are presently less rigid. They can be composed of rigid outer shells with flexible plastic conformable liners or Silastic gel-type liners. The combination of these materials allows graduated loading to the residual limb, more comfort with weightbearing, and increased performance.

Foot and Ankle Amputation Preservation of the proximal aspect of the great toe proximal phalanx preserves the flexor hallucis brevis and improves walking stability. Ray resection should be limited to a single outer ray for infection, but not gangrene. Transmetatarsal amputation performed through the diaphysis improves the lever arm for propulsion at the risk of developing recurrent plantar ulcers under the residual metatarsal shafts, which can be eliminated with the proximal

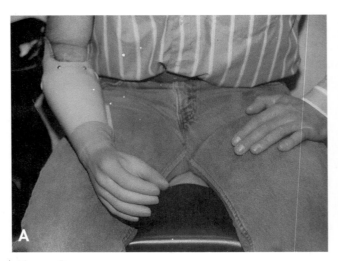 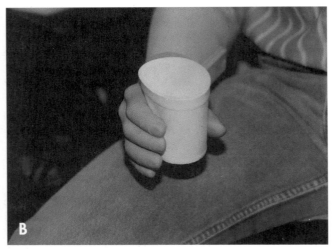

Figure 3
A, Myoelectric transradial prosthesis. B, Close-up view showing the ability to moderate grip strength.

metaphyseal level. Tarsal-metatarsal amputation should be accompanied by percutaneous Achilles tendon lengthening to prevent equinus. Hindfoot amputation should be avoided because of the high risk of severe late ankle equinus. Although this level has been shown to have acceptable outcomes in children, it provides a very short residual limb for push-off, and eliminates the potential use of a dynamic elastic response prosthetic foot. Ankle disarticulation (Syme's) can be safely performed in 1 stage. The articular surface should be preserved to preserve elasticity in weightbearing. The heel pad should be preserved to prevent migration by securing the Achilles tendon or the anterior heel pad to the tibia through drill holes.

Transtibial Amputation Tibial transection at 12 to 15 cm and coverage with a posterior myocutaneous flap is the preferred method. The fibula should be transected just proximal to the tibia. The skew flap technique is constructed with anteromedial and posterolateral skin flaps based on blood flow of the skin.

Knee Disarticulation Knee disarticulation is a muscle-balanced amputation level that is generally reserved for patients who have the biologic capacity to support transtibial amputation wound healing, but will not use a prosthesis. It provides an excellent platform for sitting and a lever arm for transfer. The gastrocnemius muscle should be retained to cover the end of the femur. Skin flaps can be sagittal or posterior myocutaneous. Prosthetically, knee disarticulation provides an excellent residual limb for end bearing. An intrinsically stable 4-bar linkage prosthetic knee joint can be used for secure walking.

Transfemoral Amputation Standard transfemoral amputation disengages the adductors, allowing the femur to be positioned in an abducted position. This leads to an inefficient gait pattern and pain at the lateral/distal residual limb. It has been shown that adductor myodesis positions the femur in a functional position to greatly enhance walking ability. The optimal transfemoral amputation level is 12 to 15 cm above the knee joint, with a medial-based myocutaneous flap (Fig. 4). When the residual limb is thus constructed, modern technology ischial containment sockets can enhance walking ability.

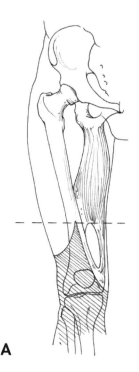

A

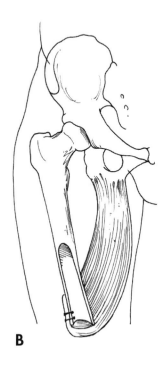

B

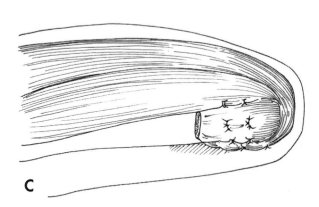

C

Figure 4

A, Diagram depicting the proposed skin flaps and level of bone section. B, Diagram to show attachment of the adductor magnus to the lateral part of femur. C, Diagram depicting attachment of the quadriceps over the adductor magnus. (Reproduced with permission from Gottschalk F: Transfemoral amputation: Surgical procedures, in Bowker JH, Michael JW: American Academy of Orthopaedic Surgeons *Atlas of Limb Prosthetics: Surgical, Prosthetic, and Rehabilitation Principles,* ed 2. St. Louis, MO, Mosby-Year Book, 1992, pp 501–507.)

Annotated Bibliography

Gottschalk F: Transfemoral amputation, in Bowker JH, Michael JW (eds): American Academy of Orthopaedic Surgeons *Atlas of Limb Prosthetics: Surgical, Prosthetic, and Rehabilitation Principles*, ed 2. St. Louis, MO, Mosby-Year Book, 1992, pp 501–507.

This chapter provides the best description on this new technique, which Bowker has called "the most significant surgical advance for the amputee in 20+ years."

Pinzur MS: Amputation surgery in peripheral vascular disease, in Springfield DS (ed): *Instructional Course Lectures 46.* Rosemont, IL, American Academy of Orthopaedic Surgeons, 1997, pp 501–509.

This chapter provides guidelines on amputation level selection for patients undergoing amputation surgery.

Pinzur MS, Garla PG, Pluth T, Vrbos L: Continuous postoperative infusion of a regional anesthetic after an amputation of the lower extremity. *J Bone Joint Surg* 1996;78A:1501–1505.

This article describes a technique for postoperative pain control with a percutaneous catheter placed at the time of surgery.

Classic Bibliography

Bowker JH, Goldberg B, Poonekar PD (eds): Transtibial amputation, in American Academy of Orthopaedic Surgeons *Atlas of Limb Prosthetics: Surgical, Prosthetic, and Rehabilitation Principles*, ed 2. St. Louis, MO, Mosby-Year Book, 1992, pp 429–452.

Dickhaut SC, DeLee JC, Page CP: Nutritional status: Importance in predicting wound-healing after amputation. *J Bone Joint Surg* 1984;66A:71–75.

Kay HW (ed): *The Proposed International Terminology for the Classification of Congenital Limb Deficiencies: The Recommendations of a Working Group of the International Society for Prosthetics and Orthotics.* London, England, Heinemann Medical, 1975.

Pinzur MS, Angelats J, Light TR, Izuierdo R, Pluth T: Functional outcome following traumatic upper limb amputation and prosthetic limb fitting. *J Hand Surg* 1994;19A:836–839.

Pinzur MS, Smith D, Osterman H: Syme ankle disarticulation in peripheral vascular disease and diabetic foot infection: The one-stage versus two-stage procedure. *Foot Ankle Int* 1995;16:124–127.

Wagner FW Jr: Management of the diabetic-neurotrophic foot: Part II. A classification and treatment program for diabetic, neuropathic, and dysvascular foot problems, in Cooper RR (ed): American Academy of Orthopaedic Surgeons *Instructional Course Lectures XXVIII.* St. Louis, MO, CV Mosby, 1979, pp 143–165.

Waters RL, Perry J, Antonelli D, Hislop H: Energy cost of walking of amputees: The influence of level of amputation. *J Bone Joint Surg* 1976;58A:42–46.

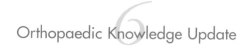
Orthopaedic Knowledge Update 6

Section 2
Systemic Disorders

Chapter 16
Bone Metabolism and
Metabolic Bone Disease

Introduction

Public awareness of bone metabolism and metabolic bone disease has continued to increase because of the impact of osteoporosis on worldwide health. The National Institutes of Health committed a record $105 million to osteoporosis research in 1997. Thus, the diagnosis and treatment of this disease, which is prevalent in the elderly, are sure to continue to change and evolve. Osteoporosis and other disorders of bone metabolism represent an aspect of orthopaedic practice that requires an understanding of both cell biology and endocrinology. This chapter will update current knowledge in the field of bone metabolism and provide a review of current treatments for metabolic bone disease.

Bone metabolism is the study of how bone functions as a part of the body's endocrine system. An abnormality in hormonal control of bone function results in some form of metabolic bone disease or defect in bone remodeling and repair.

Bone metabolism is regulated by 3 types of bone cells that are responsive to a variety of environmental signals. Osteoblasts are generally regarded as bone-forming cells. Because osteoblasts contain the receptors for most factors that regulate bone function, these cells also play a critical role in the overall control of bone metabolism. Osteoclasts are the active cells in bone resorption and are responsible for the remodeling of bone. They produce resorptive cavities, known as Howship's lacunae, on trabecular bone surfaces. Osteocytes are found within mineralized bone matrix, but their function is poorly understood. They may be important in receiving mechanical input signals and transmitting these stimuli to other cells in bone. Osteoblasts and osteocytes arise from the same mesenchymal stem cell precursor (found in bone marrow stroma, periosteum, soft tissues, and possibly peripheral blood vessel endothelium), whereas osteoclasts derive from hematopoietic mononuclear cells.

Mineral Metabolism

Calcium concentration is an important regulator of cellular membrane potentials, blood coagulation, and muscular and cardiovascular functions. Calcium also serves as a messenger for signal transduction in almost every cell in the body. The normal serum level of calcium is 9 to 10 mg/dl; approximately half is bound to plasma protein (primarily albumin), a small fraction is associated with phosphate or citrate, and about 45% exists in the form of free calcium ions. The ionized calcium concentration is maintained within very narrow limits, and bone is used whenever necessary to maintain the ionized calcium level in the physiologic range. At the macroscopic level, calcium homeostasis is maintained by 3 organ systems—the intestines, the skeleton, and the kidneys.

All calcium intake is from the diet. Calcium absorption varies with the perceived requirements of the systems where approximately 20% of dietary calcium is absorbed; the remainder either is not absorbable or is not absorbed and is excreted in the stool. In the intestines, calcium is actively transported across the duodenum in association with a calcium-binding protein. In the jejunum, there is passive diffusion of calcium. Under normal conditions, urinary excretion of calcium balances the amount of calcium absorbed. Absorption of calcium from the gastrointestinal (GI) tract and excretion in the urine averages 150 to 200 mg per day.

Dietary calcium intake requirements vary based on age (Table 1). Substantially more calcium is required during growth, and this requirement continues until achievement of the peak level of bone mass, between the second and third decades of life. Later in life, it is necessary to increase dietary calcium intake to counteract the effect of calcium loss caused by increased bone resorption.

Endocrine Function

The regulation of bone homeostasis depends on the balance between the functions of several organs including the skin, parathyroid glands, liver, kidneys, gonads, adrenals, and thyroid. In addition, in certain pathologic states, pituitary and hypothalamic function also regulate bone physiology. The hormonal balance created by the endocrine system maintains normal serum calcium and phosphate levels.

Table 1
Optimal calcium requirements

Age Group	Optimal Daily Intake of Calcium (mg/day)
Infants	
Birth to 6 months	210
6 months to 1 year	270
Children	
1 to 3 years	500
4 to 8 years	800
9 to 13 years	1,300
Adolescents	
14 to 18 years	1,000
Young Adults	
19 to 30 years	1,000
Adults	
31 to 50 years	1,000
51 to 70 years	1,200
>70 years	1,200
Pregnancy	
≤ to 18 years	1,300
19 to 50 years	1,000
Lactation	
≤ to 18 years	1,300
19 to 50 years	1,000

Recommendations based on National Academy of Sciences guidelines, 1998

Vitamin D

Vitamin D is a fat-soluble, steroid hormone that can modulate calcium homeostasis directly or through its effects on the differentiation and development of the various calcium-regulating cell systems. When skin is exposed to ultraviolet light, vitamin D_3 (cholecalciferol) can be formed endogenously from 7-dehydrocholesterol (Table 2). In light-skinned people, only 15 minutes of daily bright sunlight exposure to the hands and face is required to produce enough vitamin D_3 to be converted physiologically to the minimum requirement (10 mg) of the active metabolite, 1,25-dihydroxyvitamin D_3 (calcitriol, $1,25(OH)_2D_3$). Dark-skinned people may require longer exposure. The other major source of vitamin D is the diet, which provides the 2 isomeric forms of ergocalciferol or vitamin D_2. These 2 forms have the same endogenous function. Both metabolites are stored in several tissues, with the highest concentrations found in adipose tissue and muscle. Because the only significant natural dietary source of vitamin D is cod liver oil and because certain individuals may lack sufficient exposure to sunlight, most milk in the United States is supplemented with vitamin D_2.

Vitamin D metabolism begins with a sequence of steps in which precursor molecules are converted to the active physiologic form. Once ultraviolet light acts to convert 7-dehydrocholesterol to D_3 in the skin, this molecule circulates to the liver where it is hydroxylated at its 25th carbon to produce the major circulating prohormone, 25-hydroxyvitamin D_3 (calcifediol, $25(OH)D_3$). This step is catalyzed by 2 vitamin D 25-hydroxylases, which are located in hepatic microsomes. Once formed, $25(OH)D_3$ becomes the major circulating vitamin D metabolite and is transported bound to an α-globulin. Conditions that affect hepatic function or drugs that induce P-450 microsomal enzymes (for example, phenytoin) will interrupt this conversion pathway leading to inactive polar metabolites of D_3. As discussed later, these conditions can lead to various forms of osteomalacia.

The next step in the metabolism of vitamin D is the 1-α-hydroxylation of $25(OH)D_3$ to form $1,25(OH)_2D_3$, the physiologically active form of the vitamin. Hydroxylation at this first carbon position is the rate-limiting step in the production of the biologically active form. The hydroxylase enzyme for this reaction is located in the mitochondria of renal tubular cells and is activated by parathyroid hormone (PTH). Although PTH is the major molecule that controls 1-α hydroxylase function, serum levels of phosphate, ionized calcium, and $1,25(OH)_2D_3$ itself regulate this activity.

The major target tissues of $1,25(OH)_2D_3$ are kidney, intestine, and bone. In the kidney, it increases proximal tubular

Table 2
Vitamin D and its metabolites

Abbreviation	Vitamin	Drug Name
—	Provitamin D_3	7-dehydrocholesterol
D_2	Vitamin D_2	ergocalciferol
D_3	Vitamin D_3	cholecalciferol
$25(OH)D_3$	25-hydroxyvitamin D_3	calcifediol
$1,25(OH)2D_3$	1,25-dihydroxyvitamin D_3	calcitriol
$24,25(OH)2D_3$	24,25-dihydroxyvitamin D_3	

reabsorption of phosphate. In the intestine, $1,25(OH)_2D_3$ induces the production of the critical calcium-binding protein that is responsible for active calcium transport. When $1,25(OH)_2D_3$ levels increase, or when exogenous $1,25(OH)_2D_3$ is administered, the first effect is increased intestinal calcium absorption, which then leads to increased serum calcium levels.

Bone is the major target tissue for $1,25(OH)_2D_3$; however, here its physiologic role is not as well understood. On the basis of studies with monocytes and macrophages, $1,25(OH)_2D_3$ is thought to promote the differentiation or fusion of osteoclast precursors to osteoclasts, and at pharmacologic doses, it can induce accelerated bone resorption by increasing the activity and number of osteoclasts. Because vitamin D receptors have never been shown to exist in the cytoplasm of osteoclasts, but have been demonstrated in osteoblast-like cells, the mechanism by which $1,25(OH)_2D_3$ modulates bone physiology is probably through an action on the osteoblast (Fig. 1).

Circulating levels of the prohormone $25(OH)D_3$ decrease with age. In addition, aging may lead to reduced activity of 1-α hydroxylase as a consequence of impaired renal function and then result in reduced $1,25(OH)_2D_3$ levels. These alterations in vitamin D metabolism may account for the decreased fractional calcium absorption in the elderly.

Parathyroid Hormone

PTH and vitamin D together form an axis, which is the major metabolic regulator of calcium and phosphate fluxes in the body. The 3 major target organs of PTH are bone, kidney, and intestines. Normally, this peptide hormone is produced in, and secreted exclusively by, the parathyroid gland.

In bone, PTH generally is regarded as a bone resorbing hormone, but PTH receptors are not found on osteoclasts. Instead, these receptors are found on osteoblasts, osteoblast precursors, and very early osteoclast precursors. The effects of PTH on osteoblasts are to: (1) stimulate the release of neutral proteases that degrade surface osteoid and initiate the bone remodeling cycle; (2) stimulate the release of unknown factors from osteoblasts, which then stim-

ulate osteoclasts to resorb bone; and (3) stimulate osteoblasts to synthesize osteoid and form bone. Osteocytes are assumed to have PTH receptors as well, because when PTH stimulates osteocytes, calcium salts in the immediate surrounding lacunar spaces are mobilized.

The rate of PTH synthesis and its release by the cell are related to the extracellular ionized calcium concentration. Intact PTH is relatively short-lived once it enters the circulation. The liver and kidney rapidly cleave the circulating intact molecule into amino-terminal (N-terminal) and carboxy-terminal (C-terminal) fragments. Both the biologically active N-terminal fragment and the intact PTH have a circulating half-life shorter than that of the C-terminal fragment. When kidney function is impaired, clearance of the inactive C-terminal fragment is prolonged. The N-terminal fragment has a

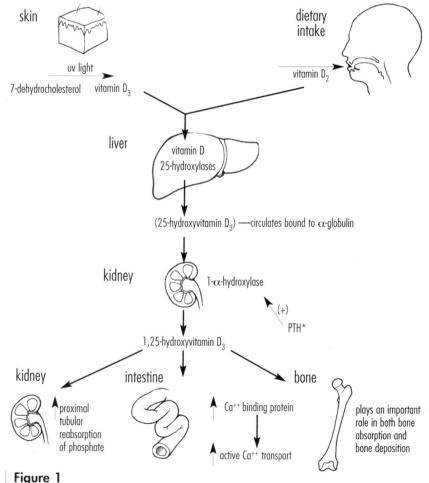

Figure 1

Vitamin D metabolism. *Parathyroid hormone (major regulator), serum phosphate, ionized calcium, and 1,25-dihydroxyvitamin D_3 all influence 1-α-hydroxylase activity.

short half-life and thus provides a more accurate measure of PTH activity in the absence of renal function.

Like calcium homeostasis, secretion of PTH is a very tightly regulated process. The adenylate cyclase and cyclic adenosine monophosphate (cAMP) system in cells of the parathyroid gland regulate its secretion. An increase in serum calcium inhibits cAMP formation and decreases the amount of hormone secreted. In the kidney, PTH activates adenylate cyclases in cells distributed along the length of the renal tubule; in the proximal tubule, PTH decreases phosphorus reabsorption; distally, it increases the reabsorption of calcium.

Increased levels of PTH have been noted in the elderly, possibly as a consequence of reduced fractional calcium absorption in the intestine. These findings support the concept that the PTH and $1,25(OH)_2D_3$ axis may have an aggravating (and possibly pathologic) role in the progressive loss of bone mass during the aging process.

Calcitonin

Calcitonin is an important calcium-regulating hormone whose exact physiologic role remains a matter of controversy. It does not directly regulate the functions of PTH or of vitamin D metabolites, but its ability to modulate serum calcium and phosphate levels is significant. Calcitonin is produced and secreted mainly by the C cells (parafollicular cells) of the thyroid gland; however, small amounts of calcitonin are found in the thymus, pituitary, GI tract, liver, and cerebrospinal fluid.

The major target tissues for calcitonin are bone, kidney, and the GI tract. In bone, its major action is the inhibition of osteoclastic bone resorption. Unlike PTH and $1,25(OH)_2D_3$, osteoclasts do possess specific receptors for this hormone. In the kidney, calcitonin receptors are also known to exist. Calcitonin causes decreased tubular reabsorption of calcium and phosphate. In the GI tract, pharmacologic doses of calcitonin increase the secretion of sodium, potassium, chloride, and water and decrease the secretion of acid.

Estrogens and Corticosteroids

The association among bone loss, fracture risk, and the postmenopausal state (naturally occurring or surgically induced) is a well-known phenomenon. Many studies have shown that accelerated bone loss occurs after menopause when ovarian hormone production ceases. Circulating hormone levels fall to 20% of previous levels; the resulting bone loss can be reversed only by administration of estrogen. Obesity can protect against this bone loss, probably because of higher circulating levels of estrogen metabolites from precursor molecules stored in adipose sites. Although estrogens are known to inhibit bone resorption, the mechanisms responsible for this effect are not fully understood. The effects of estrogen on bone may be mediated by interleukins-1 and/or -6. The presence of estrogen receptors in osteoblasts and osteoclasts has been confirmed.

Both males and females experience age-related bone loss, particularly from trabecular bone. The rate of trabecular bone loss increases in the first few years after menopause and is correlated with decreasing amounts of endogenous estrogens. Estrogen replacement blocks this bone loss in the early postmenopausal years (years 3 to 6), and a decrease in fracture rates in the appendicular skeleton has been documented.

Patients who undergo bilateral oophorectomy before natural menopause also respond to estrogen therapy, and this group is especially at risk for developing osteoporosis because a greater period of time is spent with low estrogen levels. To obtain maximal benefit from estrogen replacement therapy, it should be started as soon as possible after surgical or natural menopause and continued indefinitely. A recent study has confirmed that if estrogen replacement therapy is not started within the first 5 years after menopause, it is of limited benefit in preventing future fractures.

Numerous studies have been undertaken to demonstrate the potential risks of estrogen therapy on the induction of cerebrovascular accident, thrombosis, fluid retention, gallbladder disease, and uterine bleeding. More importantly, studies have demonstrated a potentially higher risk of breast cancer and endometrial cancer in women taking estrogens. Although the information from each of these studies is extremely valuable, some have suffered from certain flaws in methodology. It is accepted that any factor that increases a patient's exposure to estrogen (eg, early menarche, late menopause, estrogen replacement therapy) may predispose that patient to an increased risk of breast or endometrial cancer. Combination cyclic estrogen-progestin (synthetic progesterone) therapy is believed to decrease the occurrence of endometrial but not breast cancer. In patients who have undergone hysterectomy, unopposed estrogen treatment is indicated.

The most important factors to consider in determining whether a patient should or should not take estrogen is the relative risk-benefit ratio. In general, patients who have a strong family history for breast or endometrial cancer may be at increased risk for developing cancers as a result of estrogen treatment. In addition, estrogen therapy is known to exacerbate benign breast diseases and cholecystitis. On the other hand, estrogen is strongly beneficial not only in the prevention of osteoporosis and hip fractures but in the prevention of heart disease in females.

Less information is available on the role of androgens in maintaining skeletal mass in men. In general, it is assumed that the role of androgens is similar to that of estrogens, and androgen receptors have been identified in osteoblasts. Young men with idiopathic hypogonadotropic hypogonadism have reduced cortical and trabecular bone densities, and delayed puberty is associated with osteopenia in men.

Corticosteroids may lead to bone loss by directly inhibiting calcium absorption, increasing renal calcium excretion, and indirectly stimulating secondary hyperparathyroidism. Their principal effects are to decrease production of the intestinal calcium-binding proteins required for absorption. Very high doses of steroids decrease both bone formation and resorption. Even with doses as low as 10 mg of prednisone per day, significant bone loss occurs.

Thyroid Hormones

Thyroid hormones resemble steroid hormones in that they interact with specific cell receptors and eventually bind to nuclear DNA. The thyroid gland produces 2 hormones, thyroxine (T4) and 3,5,3'-triiodothyronine (T3). Both hormones are bound to proteins in the plasma.

Patients with hyperthyroidism or who are undergoing exogenous thyroid treatment show an acceleration in their basal metabolic rates. Bone resorption and bone formation in these patients take place at stimulated rates, but resorption seems to occur at a slightly faster rate than formation. Consequently, chronic hyperthyroidism or thyroid supplementation may contribute to osteoporosis. Recent reports have shown that women who use thyroid hormone have lower bone mass in both the axial and appendicular skeletons and have a higher risk for sustaining hip fractures.

Metabolic Bone Diseases

Metabolic bone diseases result from some failure in the normal processes of bone formation, mineralization, and remodeling. They can be broadly divided into the osteopenic conditions, such as osteoporosis, osteomalacia, and hyperparathyroidism, and the osteosclerotic conditions such as Paget disease and osteopetrosis.

Osteoporosis

Osteoporosis is a bone disorder characterized by decreased bone mass and an increase in fracture risk. One major risk factor for osteoporosis is estrogen withdrawal, whether as a result of a natural or surgically-induced menopause. Additional factors that have been implicated include impaired metabolism, long-term calcium deficiency, secondary hyperparathyroidism, and decreased activity levels. Genetic predisposition (individuals who are fair-skinned and

small, have hypermobile joints, are of Northern European ancestry, or have scoliosis), cigarette smoking, and excessive alcohol intake are other risk factors. Cigarette smokers show significantly increased incidences of bone loss and hip and vertebral fractures that may be due, in part, to the abnormal systemic handling of certain estrogen metabolites. Heavy alcohol users may develop osteoporosis as a result of calcium diuresis or of a direct depressive effect of alcohol on osteoblast function (Outline 1).

Most individuals attain their highest level of bone mass between the ages of 16 and 25 years. The higher this value is, the less chance there is of developing osteoporosis. The reason for this is simply that the possibility of any specific rate of bone loss (from whatever cause) leading to a critically low level depends on the amount of bone present before bone loss begins. In men, bone is normally lost at a rate of 0.3% of total bone mass per year, whereas in women the rate of bone loss is as high as 0.5% per year. The accelerated rate of bone loss, which occurs at a rate of 2% to 3% of total bone mass per year, begins after menopause and may last from 6 to 10 years.

For the purposes of description and understanding of the

Outline 1
Osteoporosis risk factors

Genetic and biologic
 Caucasian race
 Fair skin and hair
 Northern European heredity
 Scoliosis
 Osteogenesis imperfecta
 Early menopause
 Slender body build
Behavioral and environmental
 Cigarette smoking
 Excess alcohol use
 Inactivity
 Malnutrition
 Caffeine use
 Exercise-induced amenorrhea
 High fiber diet
 High phosphate diet
 High protein diet

(Reproduced with permission from Frymoyer JW (ed): *Orthopaedic Knowledge Update 4*. Rosemont, IL, American Academy of Orthopaedic Surgeons, 1993, pp 69–88.)

disease, osteoporosis has been categorized into 2 distinct syndromes. Type I, known as postmenopausal osteoporosis, occurs most commonly in women within 15 to 20 years after menopause. It affects mostly trabecular bone, increasing the patient's susceptibility to vertebral compression fractures, distal radial fractures, and intertrochanteric femoral fractures. Type II osteoporosis, known as senile osteoporosis, occurs in men and women over the age of 70 years with a female-to-male ratio of 2:1. It affects cortical and trabecular bone equally, predisposing patients to multiple wedge vertebral and femoral neck fractures. Thus in type I osteoporosis, estrogen deficiency plays a primary role, while in type II osteoporosis, aging and long-term calcium deficiency are more important.

Clinical Presentation and Diagnosis In general, osteoporosis is a silent and progressive disorder that is often brought to the attention of the patient or the physician only after a fracture. Occasionally, the condition is recognized by asymptomatic thoracic wedge or lumbar compression fractures on a routine lateral chest radiograph. Approximately 30% to 50% of the bone mineral must be lost before bone loss is detectable on radiographs. The differential diagnosis of radiographic osteopenia includes disorders of the cells of the bone marrow, endocrinopathies, primary or secondary osteoporosis, and osteomalacia (Outline 2).

Patient Evaluation The evaluation of a patient with osteopenia is designed to arrive at a diagnosis and to stage the condition for treatment purposes. The medical history is intended to document past and present illnesses, medications, surgery, occupational exposure, nutrition, family history, and social habits, all of which are used to formulate an understanding of the patient's disease risk.

Laboratory Evaluation Serum and urine tests are done routinely to establish the biochemical basis of a patient's condition (Outline 3). A complete blood count and a routine analysis of serum biochemical levels help detect the presence of hematologic disorders, mineral and electrolyte imbalances, and underlying, unrecognized systemic disease. Renal function can be screened by measuring the blood urea nitrogen and serum creatinine levels, whereas hepatic function is assessed using the aspartate amino transferase, alanine amino transferase, alkaline phosphatase, and γ-glutamyl transpeptidase values. If the alkaline phosphatase level is elevated, fractionation of this enzyme is helpful because isoenzymes are secreted by several tissues, including bone, liver, kidney, and intestine. In men, measurement of the serum testosterone is part of the routine workup.

The 24-hour urine collection is used to monitor bone resorption. Pyridinoline and deoxypyridinoline are cross-links of bone and cartilage collagen molecules. They are excreted in the urine during bone resorption, and their measurement is a sensitive indicator of bone turnover. In addition, calcium and phosphate excretion remain important ways for determining the rate of bone loss in patients. If calcium excretion is low, there may be insufficient calcium inges-

---

Outline 2
Differential diagnosis of osteopenia

Primary Osteoporosis
  Type I, postmenopausal
  Type II, senile
Osteomalacia
Endocrine Disorders
  Cushing's disease
  Diabetes mellitus
  Estrogen deficiency
  Hyperparathyroidism
  Hypogonadism
  Iatrogenic glucocorticoid treatment
  Hyperthyroidism or exogenous thyroid medication
Disuse Disorders
  Prolonged immobilization
  Paralysis
Neoplastic Disorders
  Leukemia
  Multiple myeloma
Nutritional Disorders
  Anorexia nervosa
  High protein diet
  High phosphate diet
  Low calcium diet
  Alcoholism
Hematologic Disorders
  Sickle-cell anemia
  Thalassemia
Collagen Disorders
  Homocystinuria
  Osteogenesis imperfecta

(Reproduced with permission from Frymoyer JW (ed): *Orthopaedic Knowledge Update 4.* Rosemont, IL, American Academy of Orthopaedic Surgeons, 1993, pp 69–88.)

Outline 3
Laboratory tests

Routine
Serum
    Complete blood count
    Electrolytes, creatinine, blood urea nitrogen, calcium,
        phosphorus, protein, albumin, alkaline phos-
        phatase, liver enzymes
    Protein electrophoresis
    Thyroid function tests
    Testosterone (men only)
24-hour urine
    Calcium
    Pyridinium cross-links
Special
Serum
    25-hydroxyvitamin D$_3$
    1,25-dihydroxyvitamin D$_3$
    Intact parathyroid hormone
    Osteocalcin (bone Gla protein)
Urine
    Immunoelectrophoresis
    Bence-Jones protein

(Reproduced with permission from Frymoyer JW (ed): *Orthopaedic Knowledge Update 4*. Rosemont, IL, American Academy of Orthopaedic Surgeons, 1993, pp 69–88.)

tion, defective calcium absorption, or vitamin D deficiency. Phosphorus excretion is indicative of the effects of PTH on the kidney and usually is elevated when PTH activity is high.

Patients in whom hypercalcemia has been detected should undergo a workup for primary or secondary hyperparathyroidism. This workup requires the measurement of serum PTH and 1,25-dihydroxyvitamin D$_3$ levels. Although several tests are available for measuring PTH, assay of the intact molecule as opposed to the carboxy or amino terminals is most appropriate. Patients with hypocalcemia, hypophosphatemia, or evidence of renal failure should be checked for vitamin D deficiency by assaying for 25-hydroxyvitamin D.

To complete the biochemical evaluation, a serum protein electrophoresis is performed to rule out multiple myeloma. If there is an elevated globulin region, a serum immunoelectrophoresis can detect a monoclonal immunoglobulin spike. A urine immunoelectrophoresis may demonstrate the presence of a Bence-Jones protein to confirm a diagnosis of multiple myeloma (Outline 3).

Radiologic Assessment Two forms of radiologic assessment are used in the evaluation of patients with metabolic bone disease: radiographs and densitometric scans. Because the vertebral bodies are the most common skeletal elements at risk, the workup of patients suspected of having osteoporosis includes anteroposterior (AP) and lateral radiographs of the thoracic and lumbar spines. Documentation of the fracture status of the vertebrae at the onset of treatment establishes a method for assessing the clinical outcome of any treatment protocol.

Perhaps the greatest contribution to diagnostic efforts in metabolic bone disease has been the development of bone densitometry. At present, the most clinically useful methods are single and dual energy X-ray absorptiometry (SXA and DXA), quantitative computed tomography (QCT), peripheral quantitative computed tomography (pQCT), radiographic absorptiometry (RA), and quantitative ultrasound (QUS). The most important considerations in assessing the utility of each of these methods are the anatomic sites available for study, the radiation dose to the patient, and the precision and accuracy of the test (Table 3).

Quantitative Computed Tomography QCT involves the use of a mineral calibration phantom in conjunction with a computed tomography (CT) scanner. A lateral CT localizes the midplane of 2 to 4 lumbar vertebral bodies and quantitative readings are then obtained from a region of trabecular bone in the anterior portion of the vertebra. The phantom (reference source used to calibrate density measurements in bone) most commonly consists of hydroxyapatite in plastic that is scanned simultaneously with the vertebrae. CT determination of density in the vertebra is then compared to known density readings of solutions in the phantoms. The measurements of the vertebrae are averaged and used to calculate the density of trabecular bone expressed as bone mineral equivalents of $K_2HPO_4 (mg/cm^2)$. QCT is the only method available for assessing both trabecular and cortical areas separately. Also, QCT allows direct measurement of the volume of bone, expressed as density in g/cm^3 versus indirect density measurements expressed as g/cm^2 (bone mineral content in grams divided by the area scanned in cm^2). However, QCT subjects the patient to a higher radiation exposure than other bone densitometry techniques.

pQCT uses the same principle as QCT in measuring bone density. Cortical bone mineral content by pQCT has been shown to be comparable in precision to DXA bone mineral densitometry of the ultradistal radius. Also, the ability of pQCT to differentiate between cortical and trabecular bone density can be used to individually assess the response to the pharmaceutical management of osteoporosis. pQCT can de-

Table 3
Techniques for the measurement of bone mass

Technique	Site	Precision* (%)	Accuracy† (%)	Examination (Time, min)	Dose of Radiation (mrem)
Single-photon absorptiometry	Proximal and distal radius, calcaneus	1–3	5	15	10–20
Dual-energy X-ray absorptiometry	Spine, distal radius, hip, total body	0.5–2.0	3–5	3–7	1–3
Quantitative computed tomography	Spine	2–5	5–20	10–15	100–200

*Precision is the coefficient of variation for repeated measurements over a short period of time in young, healthy persons
†Accuracy is the coefficient of variation for measurements in a specimen the mineral content of which has been determined by other means.

termine the true volumetric density of bone at any skeletal site and delivers a lower radiation dose than conventional QCT.

Single and Dual Energy X-ray Absorptiometry The most widely used methods of bone densitometry technology are SXA and DXA. In these methods, an X-ray tube emits a beam, the attenuation of which is detected by an energy discriminating photon counter. The average scan time for the spine is 5 minutes, and the radiation dose is so low (1 to 3 mrem) that it is essentially unimportant; for comparison, the radiation dose for a chest radiograph is 20 to 50 mrem. Measurement of only 1 site may be adequate to diagnose osteopenia in women over the age of 65, but to assess treatment response, the lumbar spine is usually measured with more precision than the femoral neck.

SXA is most useful in assessing the bone mineral content of the appendicular skeleton because the measurements correlate well with the status of the peripheral long bones but not with the axial skeleton. However, DXA can be used for bone mineral measurements both axially and peripherally. These bone mineral density reports can be affected by articular conditions, such as subchondral bone sclerosis and the presence of osteophytes, so the area scanned must be far enough away from the joint to avoid any such error. The density is given in g/cm², obtained by bone mineral content (the amount of hydroxyapatite) divided by the region scanned. Compared with QCT, DXA has superior precision, lower cost, and lower absorbed doses of radiation. However, one major disadvantage is that the technique does not enable the differentiation between cortical and trabecular bone.

Radiographic Absorptiometry In RA, hand radiographs are taken with an aluminum wedge placed on the films to serve as a density reference. The radiographs are sent to a central facility where they are analyzed using an optical densitometer. The bone mineral density (BMD) is then averaged for the middle phalanges of the second to fourth fingers and reported as a single value. The advantages of this method are low cost and the fact that it can be performed at a standard radiographic facility without the need for special equipment. Because the measurements obtained with RA are sensitive to changes in overlying soft tissues, the technique is limited to the appendicular skeleton.

Ultrasound QUS is emerging as an alternative to photon absorptiometry techniques in the assessment of osteoporosis by using broadband ultrasound attenuation (BUA) and velocity. Ultrasound is a traveling mechanical vibration, and the mechanical properties of the medium progressively alter the shape, intensity (energy per second per unit area), and speed of the propagating wave. Ultrasound is attractive because it is noninvasive, safe, and relatively inexpensive. It is also viewed as having the potential for measuring the mechanical integrity of bone directly, such as strength and stiffness, in contrast to DXA techniques that measure bone mass only. Clinically, the site most often measured is the calcaneus, which lends itself to transmission ultrasound measurements because of its limited amount of overlying soft tissue, relatively parallel medial and lateral bone surfaces, and direct access to both sides of the bone. Ultrasound has been shown to be an effective means for discriminating the prevalence of osteoporotic fractures, having about the same accuracy as absorptiometric techniques. Velocity measured at the calcaneus has been shown to have a sensitivity comparable to femoral neck BMD and a sensitivity better than spine BMD in hip fracture prediction. Also, BUA is still a significant predictor of fracture after adjusting for BMD, and it is better correlated with the type of hip fracture (trochanteric versus cervical) than BMD. Poor precision of calcaneal BUA measurement compared with DXA is one problem that can be resolved by proper transducer positioning and a system that can scan the whole calcaneus.

Bone Biopsy An extremely useful test in certain metabolic bone disease workups is the transilial bone biopsy. Although invasive, it is associated with a minimal degree of pain and inconvenience to the patient, can be performed as an ambulatory procedure, and has a low complication rate. The biopsy can establish a diagnosis in a patient in whom osteomalacia or an occult malignancy is suspected; the tissue obtained can be used to distinguish between osteomalacia and osteitis fibrosa cystica in certain dialysis patients or to elucidate the cause of severe osteopenia in patients whose blood and urine test results are insufficiently informative.

The biopsy is taken from a point 3 cm posterior and 3 cm inferior to the anterior superior iliac spine. Once obtained, the specimen is embedded in methylmethacrylate and cut, processed, and stained using an undecalcified technique. Unstained sections are examined by fluorescence microscopy to determine the dynamic properties of bone. This is made possible by the presence of the tetracycline labels, which are obtained by the preoperative administration of oral tetracycline in 2 doses that are separated in time by a specified number of days (eg, 250 mg of oral tetracycline 3 times a day for 3 days, off for 12 days, repeat for 3 more days, biopsy between 3 and 7 days later). The cellular parameters of bone turnover are assessed by light microscopic examination of hematoxylin and eosin-stained sections. Mineralized osteoid is differentiated from unmineralized osteoid through the use of a salt stain, such as von Kossa, in which calcium and phosphorus salts appear dark, while unmineralized osteoid appears pale. Through the use of a computer-assisted calculating system, an optical drawing tube, and an integrated ocular eyepiece, a number of quantitative parameters of bone statics and dynamics are measured. This technique, known as histomorphometry, enables the clinician to accurately diagnose the disorder and to determine to what extent resorptive or blastic activities are influencing the disease. In patients with renal disease, special stains are used to identify the presence of aluminum in bone as a cause of osteomalacia. This determination is particularly important because dramatic clinical improvements have been reported after removal of the aluminum from the bone.

Osteoporosis Treatment Regimens The goal of any osteoporosis treatment regimen is to prevent further bone loss. Presently, there are no well-accepted treatment protocols that can be shown to safely increase bone mass to normal levels. If there is no history of breast cancer or thromboembolic or endometrial disease, then estrogen replacement therapy is currently thought to be safe. A gynecologic examination is required at the onset of treatment, and an endometrial biopsy is recommended after the first 12 months. If endometrial tissue shows no unusual activity, no further biopsies are required. However, a yearly mammogram is still strongly recommended.

The United States Food and Drug Administration (FDA) recently approved a dosage regimen of alendronate for the treatment of osteoporosis. Alendronate, a bisphosphonate compound, is the first nonhormonal drug approved for the treatment of this disease. It is used in a dose of 5 or 10 mg per day, must be taken orally on an empty stomach, and the patient can only drink water (no other food or beverage) at the time of dosing. Because of the low bioavailability of this compound from the intestinal tract (approximately 0.7%), no food can be taken for at least 30 minutes after dosing. Reports show that alendronate prevents bone loss and is associated with gains in bone mass of up to 10% and almost a 3% decrease in new vertebral fractures with only 3 years of intervention.

Bisphosphonates have a phosphorus-carbon-phosphorus (P-C-P) backbone. They bind to bone mineral through the P-C-P structure and inhibit both the formation and dissolution of calcium phosphate crystals in vitro until the backbone is resorbed. The primary action of the bisphosphonates is to induce prolonged inhibition of bone resorption by decreasing osteoclast activity. They also decrease the number of osteoclasts by decreasing their recruitment and by promoting their apoptosis. Additionally, in vitro studies suggest that osteoblasts secrete an inhibitor of osteoclast production or survival. Thus, there is a marked decrease in bone turnover induced by bisphosphonates.

Calcitonin, a naturally-occurring hormonal compound, has been approved by the FDA for several years in an injectable form. The approved dose of injectable salmon calcitonin is 100 units per day. Recently, the FDA approved a nasal spray formulation of this compound in a dose of 200 units per day.

Raloxifene, a second-generation selective estrogen receptor modulator, is a member of a promising new class of drugs that are agonists for bone and the cardiovascular system, but do not affect the breast or uterus. Raloxifene has demonstrated a 2% increase in bone mineral density over baseline, as compared to a decline with placebo. Also, raloxifene is cardioprotective, reducing overall cholesterol and low density lipoprotein (LDL) cholesterol levels.

If a hypercalciuric component accompanies the active osteoporotic state, 1 to 2 daily doses of thiazide can be given to increase total body calcium retention. Studies have shown that an adequate dietary calcium intake in premenopausal women does not, in itself, protect women against the development of osteoporosis. However, in older postmenopausal women (> 6 years postmenopause), dietary supplementation with calcium can protect against bone loss. Moreover, the role of dietary calcium supplementation in the prevention of osteoporosis appears to be most critical during childhood and adolescent years when peak bone mass is being built. An adequate dietary calcium intake (Table 1) is required at all times, however, to prevent the adverse skeletal effects of secondary hyperparathyroidism. For this reason, all patients under treatment for osteoporosis should take 1.5 g of elemental calcium daily plus 1 or 2 multivitamins, each containing 400 units of vitamin D. Although studies are in progress to determine the best preparation of oral calcium to use in order to enhance intestinal calcium absorption, any calcium is better absorbed when taken with meals. Perhaps the best form of symptomatic relief is achieved through physical therapy and rehabilitation.

Osteomalacia, Renal Bone Disease, and Hyperparathyroidism

Osteomalacia is a metabolic disorder in which there is inadequate mineralization of newly formed osteoid. It can result from vitamin D deficiency, vitamin D resistance, intestinal malabsorption, acquired or hereditary renal disorders, intoxication with heavy metals such as aluminum or iron, and other assorted etiologies (Outline 4). The childhood form of osteomalacia is termed rickets. Rickets of the developing and growing skeleton, which is often caused by the dietary deficiency of vitamin D, has become rare since the widespread supplementation of dairy products with vitamin D (Table 4 and Fig. 2).

Diagnosis The clinical diagnosis of osteomalacia often is difficult because patients usually have nonspecific complaints such as muscle weakness or diffuse aches and pains. Radiographic evidence of osteomalacia often mimics other disorders including osteoporosis. However, the presence of pseudofractures or Looser's transformation zones is good evidence that some degree of osteomalacia is present. Looser's zones are radiolucent areas of bone that result from multiple microstress fractures that heal by the formation of osteomalacic bone, which is not mineralized (Fig. 3).

Outline 4
Causes of osteomalacia

Vitamin D deficiency
  Dietary
      Malabsorption
      Intestinal disease
      Intestinal surgery
  Insufficient sunlight
Impaired vitamin D synthesis
  Liver disease
  Hepatic microsomal enzyme induction
  Anticonvulsant
  Renal failure
Metabolic acidosis
Fanconi's syndrome (renal tubular defect)
Hypophosphatemia
  Malabsorption
  X-linked hypophosphatemic rickets
  Oncogenic
  Oral phosphate-binding antacid excess
Mineralization inhibition
  Bisphosphonate
  Aluminum
  Fluoride
  Iron
  Hypophosphatasia

(Reproduced with permission from Frymoyer JW (ed): *Orthopaedic Knowledge Update 4*. Rosemont, IL, American Academy of Orthopaedic Surgeons, 1993, pp 69–88.)

Although different forms of osteomalacia are biochemically different, the orthopaedist usually can be alerted by elevated alkaline phosphatase, low calcium, or low inorganic phosphorus levels. Serum assays for vitamin D metabolites help clarify the abnormality.

In most patients, transilial bone biopsy is necessary to confirm the diagnosis of osteomalacia. The histologic hallmark of osteomalacia is an increase in the width and extent of osteoid seams, with evidence of decreased rates of mineral apposition as determined by tetracycline labeling. In normally mineralized bone, tetracycline labels show discrete uptake of tetracycline only at times when mineral is being deposited; however, in osteomalacic bone, the slow rate of mineralization leads to an inability of these labels to appear separated in time and results in a smudged appearance.

Table 4
Treatment of rickets in children

Disorder	Calcium (mg)	Vitamin D$_2$ (U)	Phosphorus (mg)	1,25 dihydroxyvitamin D$_3$ (μg)
Nutritional vitamin D deficiency	30/kg/day	1,000 to 2,000/day		
Nutritional calcium deficiency	Standard supplement (ie, 500-mg tablet)			
Vitamin D-dependent rickets, type I*				Up to 3/day initially, then 0.25 to 1.0/day
Vitamin D-dependent rickets, type II†				Up to 35/day (variable success)
Vitamin D malabsorption§		5,000 to 10,000/day		
Nutritional phosphorus deficiency¶	Standard kg-based supplement		20 to 25/kg/day	
X-linked hypophosphatemia			500/day	0.5/day
Anticonvulsant-induced (phenytoin)		400/day		
Renal osteodystrophy**			Restrict dietary intake	Up to 1.5/day

* Defective renal 1-α-hydroxylation of 25-hydroxyvitamin D^3 (pseudovitamin D deficiency rickets)

† Tissue unresponsive to normal levels of 1,25 dihydroxyvitamin D^3 because vitamin D receptor complex fails to bind DNA

§ Can be caused by diseases such as cystic fibrosis, inflammatory bowel disease, celiac disease, and short bowel syndrome

¶ Typically occurs in breast-fed premature infants

** Renal patients with bone aluminum intoxication may require deferoxamine

Etiology of Osteomalacia Osteomalacia is more common in elderly patients, probably because the mild malabsorption in elderly individuals predisposes patients to bone disease. The widespread use of anticonvulsant drugs such as phenytoin also has been shown to cause osteomalacia. The use of these drugs results in the induction of P-450 mixed function oxidases in hepatic cells, and thus the conversion of vitamin D to inactive polar metabolites. This conversion reduces the production of 25-hydroxyvitamin D, which is required for renal conversion to 1,25-dihydroxyvitamin D$_3$. (Note: A milder form of 25-hydroxyvitamin D synthesis impairment by phenytoin may lead to osteoporosis instead of osteomalacia.)

Osteomalacia also is common in chronic renal dialysis patients. The major cause of osteomalacia in these patients is the intoxication of the skeleton with aluminum due to aluminum-containing phosphate-binding antacids, which are used to control phosphate accumulation in patients with renal failure. Phosphate accumulation lowers the serum calcium level, thereby causing the parathyroid gland to become overactive (secondary hyperparathyroidism). This overactivity can lead to a characteristic destruction of trabecular bone known as osteitis fibrosa cystica. Efforts to develop drugs to control serum phosphate levels may lead to a reduction in the occurrence of this complication. However, if aluminum-containing phosphate-binding antacids are absolutely necessary, aluminum levels can be intermittently controlled with the aluminum chelating agent deferoxamine. It is important to note that, in some patients with severe renal secondary hyperparathyroidism, bone pain can be excruciating, serum PTH levels can be difficult to control, and brown tumors can occur (although brown tumors are more common in primary hyperparathyroidism). For severe symptomatic secondary hyperparathyroidism, a parathyroidectomy (partial or total) may be indicated. However, if any aluminum is present in bone, the resultant decrease in bone turnover caused by absence of the parathyroid may increase aluminum accumulation and exacerbate or cause an osteomalacic state. For this reason, bone biopsy with aluminum staining is indicated in

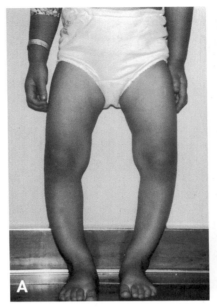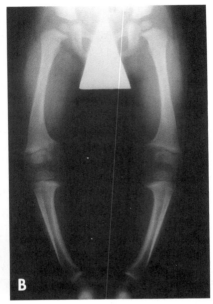

Figure 2

A, Varus deformities of the knee and ankle in a 3-year-old girl with vitamin D-resistant rickets. B, Radiograph shows widening and flaring of femoral and tibial physes.

some hemodialysis patients before a parathyroidectomy is performed.

There are several known hereditary causes of renal rickets in growing children. The most common is X-linked dominant hypophosphatemic rickets. If the disorder is detected early in life, the skeleton may develop normally. Treatment with phosphate and 1,25-dihydroxyvitamin D_3 usually maintains normal growth in these children. Hypophosphatemic rickets is usually due to a renal tubular defect in phosphate reabsorption. In 1948, Albright described a disorder termed "distal renal tubular acidosis," which has a dominant mode of inheritance with variable penetrance. Patients usually show at least 1 of the 3 major features: renal stones, hypophosphatemia, and osteomalacia. High doses of vitamin D and sodium bicarbonate are necessary to treat this condition. In addition, a rare form of osteomalacia associated with the presence of a benign tumor has been reported; the tumor usually is found in the nasopharyngeal cavity or is never identified. The pathophysiology of this type of osteomalacia involves the secretion by the tumor of a phosphaturic substance.

Treatment Treatment depends on the specific etiology of the osteomalacia. However, 1.5 g of elemental calcium per day is prescribed for all patients. For nutritional vitamin D deficiency, patients are given 50,000 U of vitamin D_2 3 to 5 times per week. Patients with malabsorptive states of osteomalacia and anticonvulsant (such as phenytoin)-induced osteomalacia need 50,000 U of vitamin D_2 and 20 to 100 µg of 25-hydroxyvitamin D_3 per day. Patients with renal osteomalacia are given 1 to 2 µg of 1,25-dihydroxyvitamin D_3 a day, and patients who have bone aluminum intoxication also may need deferoxamine. The acid-base disorder of patients in metabolic acidosis is corrected by titrating their blood pH with sodium bicarbonate and giving them 50,000 U of vitamin D_2 and 1 to 2 µg of 1,25-dihydroxyvitamin D_3 a day. For osteomalacia caused by X-linked hypophosphatemia, 2 to 3 µg of 1,25-dihydroxyvitamin D_3 is administered daily until healing, after which the dose is cut to 0.5 to 1.0 µg a day. The hypophosphatemia is treated by administration of 1 to 2 g of phosphorus per day.

Paget Disease of Bone

Etiology Paget disease of bone is the second most common metabolic bone disease after osteoporosis. The prevalence may be as great as 4% of individuals in the Anglo-Saxon population who are older than 55 years of age. Studies have failed to detect a genetic predisposition or an HLA-antigen association type in Paget disease. However, a viral etiology was proposed in 1974 when virus-like inclusion bodies were found in osteoclasts from affected bone. Since then, researchers have focused on a slow virus as the causative agent.

Histologic analyses of specimens of pagetic bone show resorption by large numbers of osteoclasts. This resorption is

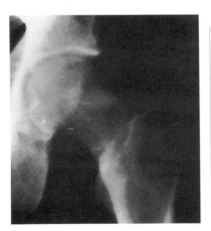

Figure 3

Anteroposterior radiograph of the proximal femur of a patient with osteomalacia. The coarsened appearance of the bone trabeculae suggests abnormal bone quality. In addition, there is a focal area of osteopenia, known as a "Looser zone," on the inferomedial aspect of the femoral neck. This zone, frequently observed in patients with osteomalacia, represents a focal region of unmineralized osteoid.

followed by activation of osteoblasts and the production of new bone. The new bone produced contains widened lamellae and irregular "cement lines," which produce the characteristic "mosaic pattern" appearance of pagetic bone (Fig. 4). This results in the normal fatty or hematopoietic marrow spaces being replaced by loose, highly vascularized fibrous connective tissue. Ultimately, both the osteoclastic and osteoblastic activities decrease, terminating in a burned-out stage with enlarged and deformed bones that are densely sclerotic.

Biochemically, the high rate of bone turnover in Paget disease results in an immediate increase in the excretion of type I collagen breakdown products. The compensatory osteoblastic state is characterized by an increase in alkaline phosphatase activity, and thus, 2 markers, serum alkaline phosphatase and urinary pyridinium cross-links, have been used to follow the course of the disease and its response to treatment.

Paget disease often is discovered as an incidental finding on radiographic examinations because clinical experience has shown that most patients who are afflicted by this condition are asymptomatic. Patients who become symptomatic describe bone and joint pain and, later in the disease, may show deformities. One of the most common manifestations consists of low back pain in patients who, on radiographic examination, show pagetic involvement of the spine. The technetium 99m methylene diphosphonate bone scan is an excellent method for screening areas of pagetic involvement.

Treatment Most patients with Paget disease do not need pharmacologic treatment. Unless there is pain or significant abnormalities in urinary collagen breakdown products or serum alkaline phosphatase, patients can be followed without

the use of drugs. For those patients who do have increased pain and poorly controlled biochemical indices of bone turnover, 3 classes of drugs are available for use: nonsteroidal anti-inflammatory drugs (NSAIDs), calcitonin, and bisphosphonates. For the management of mild symptoms related to Paget disease, indomethacin and other related NSAIDs have been shown to be useful clinically.

Several bisphosphonates are now available for the treatment of Paget disease. One of these, pamidronate, is administered intravenously and is indicated in the treatment of Paget disease that is refractive to other treatments. Alendronate can be given orally or intravenously. Oral alendronate is more effective than pamidronate and does not inhibit the mineralization of bone when used at a 40-mg dose. Furthermore, oral alendronate has similar efficacy to intravenous pamidronate without the associated dose-dependent GI intolerance and severe mucosal erosions of the esophagus and stomach that develop in some patients who have taken oral pamidronate.

Calcitonin has been used extensively in the treatment of Paget disease. This naturally occurring hormone acts through direct inactivation of osteoclasts. The beneficial effects of injectable calcitonin on pain, biochemical indexes of bone turnover, and radiographic abnormalities are well documented. Because approximately 60% of patients develop antibodies, the agent may lose its effectiveness after time. Calcitonin is administered by subcutaneous or intramuscular injection or by nasal spray. Early studies suggest that nasal spray calcitonin leads to fewer side effects and is better tolerated, but its use in Paget disease is limited by a very low bioavailability.

Many patients suffering from Paget disease in the vicinity of joints develop degenerative joint disease, which may result from the biomechanical alteration of subchondral bone. Treatment of degenerative joint disease may involve hip or knee replacement arthroplasty. A 10-year follow-up study of total hip arthroplasty in patients with degenerative coxarthrosis secondary to Paget disease showed the rate of revision was not statistically higher than for patients without Paget disease. Aseptic loosening made revision necessary in approximately 15% of patients.

The polyostotic form of Paget disease typically involves the pelvis and spine. Pelvic lesions are well tolerated unless the acetabulum is involved. Spinal involvement is not as well tolerated. Low back pain is a frequent complaint and is often associated with symptoms of spinal stenosis. The affected spinal segment may become progressively deformed, leading to a narrowing of static canal measurements and resulting in spinal stenosis. These patients often respond well to pharmacologic therapy; however, decompressive laminotomy may be required in patients who do not respond to medical management because radiculopathy or paraplegia may develop.

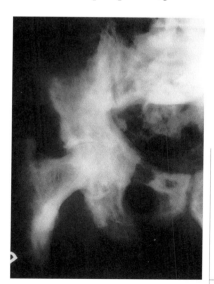

Figure 4

Anteroposterior radiograph of the proximal femur and right hemipelvis of a patient with Paget disease. Note the sclerotic appearance of the bones, coxa vara of the proximal femur, loss of joint space in the hip, and coarsening of the bony trabeculae.

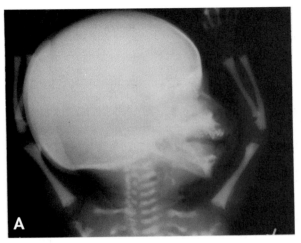
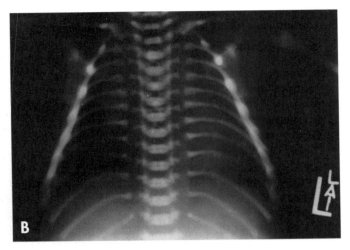

Figure 5

A, Anteroposterior (AP) radiograph of the skull, arms, and forearms of a 6-month-old infant with osteopetrosis. Note extremely dense bones with no radiographic evidence of a patent marrow cavity. B, AP chest radiograph of the same infant.

Sarcomatous degeneration occurs in fewer than 1% of patients with Paget disease. Osteogenic sarcoma is most common but fibrosarcomas, chondrosarcomas, and malignant giant cell tumors also have been reported. A substantial increase in pain in a patient with Paget disease is strongly suggestive of the development of a sarcoma. The prognosis for Paget sarcoma is generally poor.

A benign tumor associated with Paget disease has been described. Intranuclear inclusion bodies similar to those seen in nonneoplastic pagetic tissue were demonstrated in the nuclei of giant cells associated with this tumor. The epidemiologic aspects of this tumor demonstrate that most can be traced to a small town in Italy known as Avellino. This finding further supports an infectious etiology for this condition.

Osteopetrosis

Osteopetrosis (Albers-Schönberg disease or marble bone disease) is a rare metabolic bone disease that is characterized by a diffuse increase in skeletal density and obliteration of marrow spaces (Fig. 5). Histologically, the skeleton shows cores of calcified cartilage that are surrounded by areas of new bone; this new bone formation is normal but there is a deficiency of bone and cartilage resorption. The osteoclasts are abnormal and lack a functional ruffled border.

In humans, osteopetrosis has traditionally been diagnosed as being either the congenital (juvenile, malignant, or infantile) or adult (tarda) form. In the juvenile form, the mode of transmission is autosomal recessive, and this condition is characterized by severe anemia, hepatosplenomegaly, thrombocytopenia, cranial and optic nerve palsy, and a compromised immune system. Death may occur at a young age from anemia and sepsis. The adult or tarda form of osteopetrosis is inherited as an autosomal dominant trait, but some investigators report that autosomal recessive forms of this disease exist as well. Although osteopetrosis tarda is much less severe than the infantile form, a lifelong history of fractures usually characterizes the clinical picture.

Treatment for infantile or juvenile osteopetrosis is bone marrow transplantation at a young age with marrow from an appropriately HLA-matched donor. A successful transplant may resolve the hematologic abnormalities including the defect in the immune system and can result in a gradual restoration of patent marrow cavities. HLA-mismatched transplants are unsuccessful in 30% of patients. A few isolated reports have suggested that high-dose 1,25-dihydroxyvitamin D_3 therapy and a low calcium diet can also treat this condition. Although the mechanism is unclear, it is possible that 1,25-dihydroxyvitamin D_3 either stimulates the development of a normal ruffled border in osteoclasts, or, more likely, increases the fusion of mononuclear osteoclast progenitor cells to multinucleated bone resorbing osteoclasts.

Annotated Bibliography

Endocrine Function

Cauley JA, Seeley DG, Ensrud K, Ettinger B, Black D, Cummings SR: Study of Osteoporotic Fractures Research Group: Estrogen replacement therapy and fractures in older women. *Ann Intern Med* 1995;122:9–16.

The use of estrogen can protect against the risk of hip fracture in older women if it is initiated soon after menopause and continued indefinitely.

Felson DT, Zhang Y, Hannan MT, Kiel DP, Wilson PW, Anderson JJ: The effect of postmenopausal estrogen therapy on bone density in elderly women. *N Engl J Med* 1993;329:1141–1146.

This study shows how estrogen affects bone mass as a function of the time after menopause that treatment is begun and the duration over which it is used.

Bauer DC, Gluer CC, Cauley JA, et al: Study of Osteoporotic Fractures Research Group: Broadband ultrasound attenuation Majeska RJ, Ryaby JT, Einhorn TA: Direct modulation of osteoblastic activity with estrogen. *J Bone Joint Surg* 1994;76A: 713–721.

The authors demonstrate the ability of estrogen to directly affect the osteoblast's capacity to mediate bone formation and resorption.

Schneider DL, Barrett-Connor EL, Morton DJ: Thyroid hormone use and bone mineral density in elderly women: Effects of estrogen. *JAMA* 1994;271:1245–1249.

This is a documentation of the relationship between endogenous or exogenous thyroid hormone and the occurrence of osteoporosis.

Silver JJ, Majeska RJ, Einhorn TA: An update on bone cell biology. *Curr Opin Orthop* 1994;5:50–59.

This is an update of bone cell biology.

Osteoporosis

Bauer DC, Gluer CC, Cauley JA, et al: Study of Osteoporotic Fractures Research Group: Broadband ultrasound attenuation-predicts fractures strongly and independently of densitometry in older women. A prospective study. *Arch Intern Med* 1997;157: 629–634.

This study shows the strength of the association between BUA and fracture is similar to that observed with bone mineral density.

Black DM, Cummings SR, Karpf DB, et al: Fracture Intervention Trial Research Group: Randomised trial of effect of alendronate on risk of fracture in women with existing vertebral fractures. *Lancet* 1996;348:1535–1541.

A prospective study of 5 and 10 mg daily doses of alendronate versus placebo showed that women with low bone mass had reduced incidence of new vertebral fractures with the alendronate group.

Boonen S, Cheng XG, Nijs J, et al: Factors associated with cortical and trabecular bone loss as quantified by peripheral computed tomography (pQCT) at the ultradistal radius in aging women. *Calcif Tissue Int* 1997;60:164–170.

pQCT, as an adjunct to conventional densitometry at the site of the distal radius, is a method of high precision and low radiation.

Bryant HU, Glasebrook AL, Yang NN, et al: A pharmacological review of raloxifene. *J Bone Miner Metab* 1996;14:1–9.

This is an overview of raloxifene, a selective estrogen receptor modulator.

Genant HK, Lang TF, Engelke K, et al: Advances in the noninvasive assessment of bone density, quality, and structure. *Calcif Tissue Int* 1996;59(suppl 1):S10–S15.

The authors compare of the capability of QCT and QUS to determine bone strength and predict fracture risk.

Grampp S, Genant HK, Mathur A, et al: Comparisons of noninvasive bone mineral measurements in assessing age-related loss, fracture discrimination, and diagnostic classification. *J Bone Miner Res* 1997;12:697–711.

This study compares the precision of commonly available methods of noninvasively assessing bone mineral status.

Grodstein F, Stampfer MJ, Colditz GA, et al: Postmenopausal hormone therapy and mortality. *N Engl J Med* 1997;336: 1769–1775.

This prospective study shows that the mortality among women who use postmenopausal hormones, on average, is lower than among nonusers, but the survival benefit diminishes with longer duration of use and is lower for women at low risk for coronary disease.

Kaufman JJ, Einhorn TA: Ultrasound assessment of bone. *J Bone Miner Res* 1993;8:517–525.

The authors review the fundamentals of US as it may be applied to the noninvasive assessment of bone.

Liberman UA, Weiss SR, Bröll J, et al: The Alendronate Phase III Osteoporosis Treatment Study Group: Effect of oral alendronate on bone mineral density and the incidence of fractures in postmenopausal osteoporosis. *N Engl J Med* 1995;333:1437–1443.

This double-blinded, randomized multicenter study established the efficacy of alendronate as a treatment for postmenopausal osteoporosis.

Lloyd T, Andon MB, Rollings N, et al: Calcium supplementation and bone mineral density in adolescent girls. *JAMA* 1993;270: 841–844.

This is a report of the role of calcium in the acquisition of peak bone mass by teenage girls.

Mirsky EC, Einhorn TA: Bone densitometry in orthopaedic practice. *J Bone Joint Surg* 1998;80A:1687-1698.

The tools currently used for determination of bone density, clinical indications for their use, and interpretation of results are discussed.

Morton DJ, Barrett-Connor EL, Edelstein SL: Thiazides and bone mineral density in elderly men and women. *Am J Epidemiol* 1994;139:1107–1115.

This is an update of the use of thiazide diuretics in the maintenance of total body calcium.

Njeh CF, Boivin CM, Langton CM: The role of ultrasound in the assessment of osteoporosis: A review. *Osteoporosis Int* 1997;7:7–22.

Quantitative ultrasound (US) and BUA and velocity are discussed as alternative to photon absorptiometry techniques in the assessment of osteoporosis.

Pak CY, Sakhaee K, Adams-Huet B, Piziak V, Peterson RD, Poindexter JR: Treatment of postmenopausal osteoporosis with slow-release sodium fluoride: Final report of a randomized controlled trial. *Ann Intern Med* 1995;123:401–408.

This randomized, placebo-controlled trial showed that slow-release sodium fluoride and calcium citrate, administered for 4 years, inhibited new vertebral fractures and augmented spinal and femoral neck bone mass.

Rodan GA: Bone mass homeostasis and bisphosphonate action. *Bone* 1997;20:1–4.

Bone resorption inhibitors, such as alendronate, can play a role in the feedback regulation in the coupling of bone formation and bone resorption through the alteration of bone mass.

Osteomalacia, Renal Bone Disease, and Hyperparathyroidism

Mankin HJ: Metabolic bone disease, in Jackson DW (ed): *Instructional Course Lectures 44.* Rosemont, IL, American Academy of Orthopaedic Surgeons, 1995, pp 3–29.

This is an excellent comprehensive overview of metabolic bone disease including the various types of osteomalacia.

Paget Disease

Case Records of the Massachusetts General Hospital: Weekly clinicopathological exercises. Case 1-1986: A 67-year-old man with Paget's disease and progressive leg weakness. *N Engl J Med* 1986;314:105–113.

This is a review of the case records of an unusual presentation of giant cell tumor in Paget disease, which suggests a familial form of inheritance traced to the town of Avellino, Italy.

Delmas PD, Meunier PJ: The management of Paget's disease of bone. *N Engl J Med* 1997;336:558–566.

The authors discuss current aspects and pharmaceutical modalities of the treatment of Paget disease.

Osteopetrosis

Shapiro F: Osteopetrosis: Current clinical considerations. *Clin Orthop* 1993;294:34–44.

This review of the classification of osteopetrosis includes a description of the physical, biochemical, and radiographic findings.

Classic Bibliography

Cai Q, Hodgson SF, Kao PC, et al: Brief report: Inhibition of renal phosphate transport by a tumor product in a patient with oncogenic osteomalacia. *N Engl J Med* 1994;330:1645–1649.

Colditz GA, Stampfer MJ, Willett WC, Hennekens CH, Rosner B, Speizer FE: Prospective study of estrogen replacement therapy and risk of breast cancer in postmenopausal women. *JAMA* 1990;264:2648–2653.

Dawson-Hughes B, Dallal GE, Krall EA, Sadowski L, Sahyoun N, Tannenbaum S: A controlled trial of the effect of calcium supplementation on bone density in postmenopausal women. *N Engl J Med* 1990;323:878–883.

Felsenfeld AJ, Harrelson JM, Gutman RA, Wells SA Jr, Drezner MK: Osteomalacia after parathyroidectomy in patients with uremia. *Ann Intern Med* 1982;96:34–39.

Finkelstein JS, Neer RM, Biller BM, Crawford JD, Klibanski A: Osteopenia in men with a history of delayed puberty. *N Engl J Med* 1992;326:600–604.

Gabel GT, Rand JA, Sim FH: Total knee arthroplasty for osteoarthrosis in patients who have Paget disease of bone at the knee. *J Bone Joint Surg* 1991;73A:739–744.

Hadjipavlou A, Lander P: Paget disease of the spine. *J Bone Joint Surg* 1991;73A:1376–1381.

Jilka RL, Hangoc G, Girasole G, et al: Increased osteoclast development after estrogen loss: Mediation by interleukin-6. *Science* 1992;257:88–91.

Johnston CC Jr, Slemenda CW, Melton LJ III: Clinical use of bone densitometry. *N Engl J Med* 1991;324:1105–1109.

Kaplan FS, August CS, Fallon MD, Dalinka M, Axel L, Haddad JG: Successful treatment of infantile malignant osteopetrosis by bone-marrow transplantation: A case report. *J Bone Joint Surg* 1988;70A:617–623.

Kiel DP, Felson DT, Anderson JJ, Wilson PW, Moskowitz MA: Hip fracture and the use of estrogens in postmenopausal women: The Framingham Study. *N Engl J Med* 1987;317:1169–1174.

Lindsay R, Hart DM, Aitken JM, MacDonald EB, Anderson JB, Clarke AC: Long-term prevention of postmenopausal osteoporosis by oestrogen: Evidence for an increased bone mass after delayed onset of oestrogen treatment. *Lancet* 1976;1:1038–1041.

Malluche HH, Smith AJ, Abreo K, Faugere MC: The use of deferoxamine in the management of aluminum accumulation in bone in patients with renal failure. *N Engl J Med* 1984;311:140–144.

Marcus R, Cann C, Madvig P, et al: Menstrual function and bone mass in elite women distance runners: Endocrine and metabolic features. *Ann Intern Med* 1985;102:158–163.

Mills BG, Singer FR: Nuclear inclusions in Paget's disease of bone. *Science* 1976;194:201–202.

Mills BG, Yabe H, Singer FR: Osteoclasts in human osteopetrosis contain viral-nucleocapsid-like nuclear inclusions. *J Bone Miner Res* 1988;3:101–106.

Prince RL, Smith M, Dick IM, et al: Prevention of postmenopausal osteoporosis: A comparative study of exercise, calcium supplementation, and hormone-replacement therapy. *N Engl J Med* 1991;325:1189–1195.

Prior JC, Vigna YM, Schechter MT, Burgess AE: Spinal bone loss and ovulatory disturbances. *N Engl J Med* 1990;323:1221–1227.

Riggs BL, Melton LJ III: The prevention and treatment of osteoporosis. *N Engl J Med* 1992;327:620–627.

Riggs BL, Melton LJ III: Evidence for two distinct syndromes of involutional osteoporosis. *Am J Med* 1983;75:899–901.

Riis B, Thomsen K, Christiansen C: Does calcium supplementation prevent postmenopausal bone loss? A double-blind, controlled clinical study. *N Engl J Med* 1987;316:173–177.

Schajowicz F, Santini Araujo E, Berenstein M: Sarcoma complicating Paget's disease of bone: A clinicopathological study of 62 cases. *J Bone Joint Surg* 1983;65B:299–307.

Silverberg SJ, Shane E, de la Cruz L, Segre CV, Clements TL, Bilezikian JP: Abnormalities in parathyroid hormone secretion and 1,25-dihydroxyvitamin D3 formation in women with osteoporosis. *N Engl J Med* 1989;320:277–281.

Sinaki M, Mikkelsen BA: Postmenopausal spinal osteoporosis: Flexion versus extension exercises. *Arch Phys Med Rehabil* 1984;65:593–596.

Siris ES, Clemens TL, Dempster DW, et al: Tumor-induced osteomalacia: Kinetics of calcium, phosphorus, and vitamin D metabolism and characteristics of bone histomorphometry. *Am J Med* 1987;82:307–312.

Steinberg KK, Thacker SB, Smith SJ, et al: A meta-analysis of the effect of estrogen replacement therapy on the risk of breast cancer. *JAMA* 1991;265:1985–1990.

Uebelhart D, Gineyts E, Chapuy MC, Delmas PD: Urinary excretion of pyridinium crosslinks: A new marker of bone resorption in metabolic bone disease. *Bone Miner* 1990;8:87–96.

Chapter 17
Musculoskeletal Oncology

Evaluation

The initial evaluation of a patient with a suspected bone or soft-tissue lesion is no different than for any other patient: a complete history and physical examination. Good quality radiographs are invaluable for forming an initial differential diagnosis and should be obtained on all patients before surgical intervention and before ordering magnetic resonance imaging (MRI). Plain radiographs usually are adequate for forming a differential diagnosis for bone lesions and an initial educated guess as to whether a lesion is benign or malignant. Radiographs of soft-tissue lesions can show if there are calcifications present and if there is erosion into bone, which is uncommon.

MRI is an invaluable tool for gaining additional diagnostic clues and determining anatomic extent. When ordering an MRI for a suspected aggressive or malignant bone lesion, it is important to image the entire bone because skip metastases are known to occur with both osteosarcoma and Ewing's sarcoma. An MRI of the knee rarely shows the complete extent of a distal femoral lesion. Gadolinium contrast should be ordered selectively. Gadolinium is useful for delineating intra-articular and periarticular tumor extension and for distinguishing between edema and tumor infiltration around soft-tissue sarcoma. Gadolinium enhanced MRI scans before and after chemotherapy can also predict the histologic response to chemotherapy. This information can be used by the medical oncologist to alter chemotherapy agents. Knowing the response to chemotherapy preoperatively can help the surgeon with surgical planning. If the apparent response is poor, margins (Fig. 1 and Table 1) may need to be wider. If a tumor is barely resectable and the response is poor, amputation may be selected rather than limb salvage. Thallium scans also have been used successfully to evaluate the response to chemotherapy, but because a preoperative MRI is done to plan the extent of anatomic resection and has better spatial resolution than thallium scintigraphy, the latter probably has limited usefulness.

Some lesions are notorious for being diagnostic dilemmas on imaging studies. Examples include distinguishing between Ewing's sarcoma and eosinophilic granuloma, and distinguishing enchondroma from chondrosarcoma. Although not 100% sensitive or specific, MRI is helpful in distinguishing between these benign and malignant lesions.

MRI for soft-tissue lesions should be performed before biopsy or excision for all but small subcutaneous masses for which the entire tumor bed can be resected if the lesion is found to be a subcutaneous sarcoma. If this will not be possible because of location, imaging and incisional biopsy should

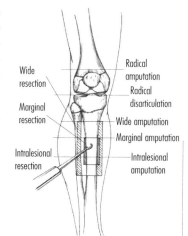

Figure 1

Enneking description of surgical margins. (Reproduced with permission from Springfield D: Musculoskeletal tumors, in Canale ST, Beaty JH (eds): *Operative Pediatric Orthopaedics*, ed 2, St. Louis, MO, Mosby-Year Book, 1995, p 1155.)

Table 1
Surgical margins

Margin	Local	Amputation
Intracapsular	Curettage or debulking	Debulking amputation
Marginal	Marginal excision	Marginal amputation
Wide	Wide local excision	Wide through-bone amputation
Radical	Radical local resection	Radical disarticulation

(Reproduced with permission from Enneking WF: *Musculoskeletal Tumor Surgery*. New York, NY, Churchill Livingstone, 1983, p 91.)

be performed before resection. MRI accurately determines anatomic extent and can help distinguish some benign from malignant vascular and lipomatous tumors. Computed tomography (CT) is useful for cortical lesions such as osteoid osteomas and surface lesions such as osteomas and surface osteosarcoma.

Distant disease is detected with a chest radiograph and chest CT. A bone scan is performed in patients with bone lesions, but not ordinarily in patients with soft-tissue tumors because soft-tissue sarcomas rarely metastasize to bone. Occasionally a bone scan can be helpful in conjunction with CT for judging cortical invasion. Bone scans are useful for identifying abnormalities in children who have unexplained or poorly localized pain. Bone scans are also useful in adults with unexplained pain that does not respond to conservative measures or if there is a history or suspicion of malignancy. Evaluation for distant disease can wait until after a biopsy; this will save some patients unnecessary testing because all lesions biopsied do not prove to be malignant.

The following laboratory studies are also useful: complete blood cell count (CBC) and sedimentation rate, serum calcium, lactic dehydrogenase (LDH), and alkaline phosphatase. The sedimentation rate can be elevated in patients with both osteomyelitis and Ewing's sarcoma. The levels of elevation of the LDH and alkaline phosphatase have been shown to correlate with survival in Ewing's sarcoma and osteosarcoma, respectively. Patients with presumed giant cell tumors may actually have brown tumors, and these 2 entities may be difficult to distinguish histologically. If serum calcium is elevated or serum phosphate depressed, parathyroid hormone level should be checked.

Evaluation of patients for possible metastatic disease with no known primary tumor consists of history and physical examination, routine laboratory analysis including serum protein electrophoresis, plain radiography of the involved bone and the chest, whole-body technetium-99m-phosphonate bone scintigraphy, and CT of the chest, abdomen, and pelvis. After this evaluation, a biopsy of the most accessible osseous lesion is done. This diagnostic strategy is successful in identifying 85% of the primary tumors. If the biopsy is not diagnostic of the tissue type and the previous tests do not identify the primary tumor, further testing has not been found to be useful, and these tumors usually fall into the category of adenocarcinoma of unknown primary.

Biopsy

A biopsy is a serious undertaking that if not performed properly can adversely affect the patient. The biopsy incision should be placed longitudinally and in a place where it can be excised en bloc with the tumor at the time of resection. There should be no dissection of structures; the biopsy should be through muscle, which can be resected with the specimen and will contain any tumor spillage from the biopsy, rather than between muscles, which can result in extensive contamination. The tumor should be biopsied through the compartment in which it has arisen so as not to contaminate additional structures. It is important to not contaminate major vessels and nerves because contamination may preclude a limb salvage procedure. If a soft-tissue mass is present, there is no need to biopsy the bone. If the cortex and intramedullary contents must be sampled, the biopsy defect should be round or oval, the path to the bone should be through a structure that can be resected, and care should be taken to biopsy a representative portion of the tumor. The interface between the host bone and the lesion can be the most informative, whereas the central part of the lesion may be necrotic and the tissue nondiagnostic. Intraoperative frozen pathology should be obtained to ensure that diagnostic tissue has been obtained. Preoperative discussion with the pathologist is useful to ensure that tissue is processed for the appropriate studies, which may include electron microscopy, immunohistochemistry, and cytogenetics. Cytogenetics requires fresh tissue and cannot be done after tissue has been fixed in formalin. Tissue should also be sent for aerobic, anaerobic, fungal, and tuberculous cultures, because some lesions that appear to be neoplasms may prove to be infectious, and in rare instances, tumor and infection may coexist. Although in most instances it is clear preoperatively whether infection is a possibility, it is reasonable to culture all biopsies and submit tissue for pathologic examination on all cultures. Careful hemostasis should be obtained before wound closure to minimize contamination. Sometimes the bone defect must be filled with bone cement or thrombin soaked gel foam to control bleeding. If a drain is used, it should be placed in line with and close to the biopsy incision, and the drain site should be excised along with the biopsy tract at the time of resection. After biopsy, the limb may need to be protected in a cast to prevent fracture or protected by using crutches and limited weightbearing.

Several major centers have reported that both fine needle aspiration and core needle biopsy are successful for the diagnosis of bone and soft-tissue neoplasms and that even cytogenetic analysis can be performed on fine needle aspirations from Ewing's sarcoma. Successful use of this technique requires cooperation among the surgeon, pathologist, and radiologist. If the histopathology is not consistent with the radiograph, or if the biopsy is nondiagnostic, an open biopsy should be performed. Needle track recurrences are uncommon, but do occur; therefore, needle and incisional biopsy tracks should be excised in continuity with the underlying tumor at the definitive resection.

In 1992 the Musculoskeletal Tumor Society (MSTS) repeated a study it had performed in 1982 to determine if biopsy-related rates of complications, errors, and deleterious effects had changed. In the original study, complications were 2 to 12 times more frequent in biopsies performed at the referring institutions compared to those done at the treatment centers, and unfortunately, no progress had been made between 1982 and 1992 in decreasing the complication rates at referring institutions or in increasing the referral of patients to treatment centers before the biopsy is performed. Ideally, the biopsy should be done by the surgeon who will perform the definitive treatment.

Bone Tumor Staging

There are two staging systems in use for bone sarcomas: the American Joint Committee on Cancer (AJCC) system and Musculoskeletal Tumor Society (MSTS) system (Table 2). The AJCC system uses the same variables as the MSTS system for malignant tumors, but weights them differently. The MSTS system also stages benign bone tumors.

Benign tumors are classified into stages 1, 2, and 3. The system attempts to integrate clinical, histologic, and imaging characteristics to rank the tumors into increasing stages of aggressiveness. Usually a differential diagnosis can be developed based on the plain radiographs and the patient's age. Benign appearing lesions that are asymptomatic, stage 1, are called latent and can be observed. Examples include nonossifying fibroma, enchondroma, and some unicameral bone cysts. Benign, active or aggressive lesions, stages 2 and 3, often need to be imaged with CT or MRI to obtain additional data that may be of help in ruling out a malignancy and to aid in preoperative planning. For example, a giant cell tumor that has completely eroded the cortex may have a large extraosseous mass that will be detected with MRI.

Malignant tumors are divided into low (stage I) and high (stage II) grade tumors based on histologic criteria. Tumors are further classified into intracompartmental (A) and extracompartmental (B) based on local anatomic extent. Stage III patients are

those with metastatic disease. The purpose of staging is to give a prognosis and to guide treatment. Chemotherapy generally is used for high grade osteosarcoma, malignant fibrous histiocytoma (MFH) of bone, and Ewing's sarcoma, but not for low grade lesions or any grade chondrosarcoma. Anatomic extent helps to plan the resection and reconstruction.

Although additional variables have been shown to have prognostic significance, they have not yet been incorporated into any of the staging systems. For osteosarcoma, these variables include tumor size, skip metastases, response to chemotherapy, and expression of the multidrug resistance (MDR) gene.

The MSTS system does not apply to Ewing's sarcoma, which has its own list of prognostic variables, including extremity versus central site, tumor volume, response to chemotherapy, and presence or absence of metastases. It is not clear how the MSTS system applies to grade II chondrosarcoma. Because of their metastatic potential, these tumors generally are considered to be stage II in the MSTS system. However, the treatment for grade II and III, and in some authors' opinions grade I, chondrosarcoma is surgical resection. In general, compartment status does not change treatment but in part guides the surgical planning. Whether intra- or extracompartmental, the surgical goal is resection with a wide margin. Radical margins, ie, resection of all involved compartments, are rarely used, because equivalent results are obtained with wide margins and the use of adjuvants: chemotherapy for

Table 2
Staging of bone sarcomas

AJCC*					MSTS (Enneking)†			
Stage	Grade	T	N	M	Stage	Grade	Site	M
IA	G1-G2	T1	0	0	IA	G1	T1	0
IB	G1-G2	T2	0	0	IB	G1	T2	0
IIA	G3-G4	T1	0	0	IIA	G2	T1	0
IIB	G3-G4	T2	0	0	IIB	G2	T2	0
III	NA							
IVA	Any	Any	1	0	IIIA	G1-G2	T1	1
IVB	Any	Any	Any	1	IIIB	G1-G2	T2	1

* AJCC: G1, well differentiated; G2, moderately differentiated; G3 to G4, poorly differentiated, undifferentiated; T1, tumor confined within cortex; T2, tumor invades beyond the cortex; N0, no regional lymph node metastases; N1, regional lymph node metastases; M0, no distant metastasis; and M1, distant metastasis; NA, not applicable

† Musculoskeletal Tumor Society: G1, low grade; G2, high grade; T1, intracompartmental; T2, extracompartmental; M0, no distant metastasis; and M1, regional or distant metastasis

(Adapted with permission from Fleming J, Cooper J, Henson DE, et al (eds): *Manual for Staging of Cancer*, ed 5, Philadelphia, PA, JB Lippincott, 1997, p 143.)

osteosarcoma, Ewing's sarcoma, and MFH of bone, and sometimes radiotherapy for Ewing's sarcoma.

Soft-Tissue Sarcoma Staging

Three staging systems are currently in use for soft-tissue sarcomas: the AJCC, Memorial Sloan-Kettering Cancer Center, and MSTS staging systems (Table 3). The AJCC system was modified in 1997 and is based on histologic grade (G1, G2, G3, G4), size (more or less than 5 cm), superficial or deep to the investing fascia, regional lymph node involvement, and distant metastasis. The Memorial Sloan-Kettering Cancer Center system is based on histologic grade (high or low), size (more or less than 5 cm), depth relative to the investing fascia (superficial or deep), and presence or absence of metastasis. The MSTS system is based on grade (high or low), anatomic extent (intracompartmental or extracompartmental), and presence or absence of distant metastasis. Other pathologic variables and molecular markers have been identified as having prognostic significance but have not been incorporated into the staging systems. A recent study concluded that the MSTS system is better for surgical planning and that systems that take into account grade and size are better for staging and prognosis. The goal is to identify the subgroups of patients at high risk of developing distant metastases so that they can be included in trials of adjuvant therapy, which is necessary to improve survival for this disease. The most important variables at this point are size and histologic grade.

None of the above staging systems applies to rhabdomyosarcoma, the most common soft-tissue sarcoma in children. A clinical staging system is used for rhabdomyosarcoma; it takes into account histologic subtype, location (extremity is one location), confinement to anatomic site of origin (similar to intra and extracompartmental), size, regional lymph node metastases (which occur frequently), distant metastases, and completeness of resection. Unlike other musculoskeletal neoplasms, regional nodal sampling is a required step in staging because nodal involvement is so common in extremity rhabdomyosarcoma. A staging system that is partly based on the completeness of surgical resection might lead to the conclusion that less than a wide margin is acceptable. This is not the case, because incomplete resection has a negative impact on survival. Unlike other sites, such as the head and neck or abdomen, wide margins should be obtainable in the extremity.

Molecular Biology of Sarcomas

The current staging of sarcomas is based on gross histopathologic assessment. Although there is some prognostic value to the current staging system, further study is required to refine the current system for defining tumor biology. In addition, it is hoped that the understanding of genetic abnormalities of sarcoma will lead to more effective treatments for targeted high risk patients.

Abnormalities in gene expression presumably underlie all pathologic states of malignancy. At the simplest level, genes that control growth and differentiation can be divided into 2 types: tumor suppressor genes and oncogenes. Suppressor genes ordinarily restrain the cell from undergoing uncontrolled division. A mutation in a suppressor gene may abolish the growth regulatory mechanism. However, an oncogene stimulates cell growth and division. In reality, the molecular defects and inter-

Table 3
Staging of soft-tissue sarcoma

	AJCC*					MSTS (Enneking)†		
Stage	Grade	T	N	M	Stage	Grade	Site	M
IA	1-2	1a-1b	0	0	IA	1	T1	0
IB	1-2	2a	0	0	IB	1	T2	0
IIA	1-2	2b	0	0	IIA	2	T1	0
IIB	3-4	1a-1b	0	0	IIB	2	T2	0
IIC	3-4	2a	0	0	IIIA	1-2	T1-T2	1
III	3-4	2b	1	0	IIIB	1-2	T1-T2	1
IV	Any	Any	N1	0				
			N0	M1				

(Adapted with permission from Fleming J, Cooper J, Henson DE, et al (eds): *Manual for Staging of Cancer*, ed 5, Philadelphia, PA, JB Lippincott, 1997, p 149.)

* AJCC: G1, well differentiated; G2, moderately well differentiated; G3 to G4, poorly differentiated; T1 ≤ 5 cm, T1a superficial, T1b deep; T2 > 5 cm, T2a superficial, T2b deep; N0, no lymph node metastasis; N1, regional lymph node metastasis; M0, no distant metastasis; and M1, distant metastasis

† Musculoskeletal Tumor Society: G1, low grade; G2, high grade; T1, intracompartmental; T2, extracompartmental; M0, no regional or distant metastasis; and M1, regional or distant metastasis

Table 4
Characteristic cytogenetic aberrations in malignant bone and soft-tissue tumors

Histology	Characteristic Cytogenetic Events	Frequency (%)	
Ewing's sarcoma	t(11;22)(g24;q11.2-12)	95	Fusion protein EWS/Fli-1, which is a transcription factor
Alveolar rhabdomyosarcoma	t(2;13)	80	Fusion of PAX3 with ALV, a DNA transcription factor
Embryonal rhabdomyosarcoma	+2q, +20	80	
Synovial sarcoma	t(X;18)	95	Fusion of SSX with SYT
Malignant fibrous histiocytoma	Complex	90	
Malignant peripheral nerve sheath tumor	Complex	90	
Leiomyosarcoma	1p-	75	
Infantile fibrosarcoma	+11, +17, +20	90	
Dermatofibrosarcoma protuberans	Ring chromosome 17	90	
Myxoid liposarcoma	t(12;16)	75	Fusion of CHOP with TLS which results in a DNA transcription factor
Pleomorphic liposarcoma	Complex	90	
Well-differentiated liposarcoma	Ring chromosome 12	80	
Clear cell sarcoma	t(12;22)	90	Fusion EWS and AFT 1, a DNA transcription factor
Endometrial stromal sarcoma	t(7;17)	50	
Intra-abdominal desmoplastic small round cell tumor	t(11;22)(p13;q12)	> 50	Fusion of EWS and WT1, a DNA transcription factor
Mesothelioma	1p-, 3p-, -22	90	
Myxoid chondrosarcoma	t(9;22)	50	
Multiple hereditary exostosis	8q24.1, 11p13, 19q		Mutations in EXT1, 2, or 3

(Adapted with permission from Fletcher JA: Cytogenetics and experimental models of sarcomas. *Curr Opin Oncol* 1994;6:367–371.)

actions are much more complicated than described. There are multiple layers of gene interaction and regulation and numerous possibilities for abnormal gene expression. These mechanisms include gene mutations, deletions, and rearrangements. Mutations that regulate the activity of both suppressor genes and oncogenes can give similar results to mutations affecting the suppressor genes or oncogenes themselves. One difficulty is that tumors usually have multiple genetic abnormalities. Whereas for some tumors, such as colon cancer, it is possible to trace out the progression of genetic abnormalities between a premalignant polyp and an invasive cancer, this is not yet possible for sarcoma. In addi-

tion, there are multiple genetic abnormalities in a high grade tumor. It is not always clear which genetic mutations are the primary defects and which are the secondary defects.

Chromosomal Translocations
Radiation injury has been implicated in the formation of sarcomas. Radiation is known to cause DNA breaks that can result in chromosomal translocations and possible malignant transformation. Table 4 outlines chromosomal translocations that have been documented in a large number of sarcomas. As can be seen, chromosomal translocations are frequent events, occurring in up to 95% of some sarcomas. These

chromosomal translocations allow for some genes, particularly oncogenes, to be brought in to the proximity of a different gene promoter. The fusion of a gene that normally is expressed with an oncogene, which normally is not expressed, results in inappropriate expression of the oncogene, because it is now activated, under control of the promoter of the normal gene. The activation of oncogenes results in increased cell growth and malignant transformation. Such is the case with *bcr/abl* in chronic myelogenous leukemia and *bcl-2* in non-Hodgkin's B-cell lymphoma.

Alveolar rhabdomyosarcoma has a characteristic chromosomal translocation between the long arm of chromosome 2 and the long arm of chromosome 13 referred to as t(2;13)(q35;q14). This translocation places the *PAX3* gene (which is involved in transcriptional regulation of neuromuscular development) in proximity to the *ALV* gene (a member of the forkhead family of transcriptional factors). When a consistent translocation is found in a type of tumor, it is presumed that the genes affected by the translocation are involved in the pathobiology of the tumor. This is usually borne out by functional analysis of the affected genes, which are either inactivated by the translocation, in which case the gene is a tumor suppressor gene, or activated by the mutation as above.

Ewing's sarcoma has a translocation between chromosomes 11 and 22 in 95% of cases that affects the same break point. It has long been postulated that a gene at this location is responsible for development of Ewing's sarcoma. The translocation produces a fusion protein between the *EWS* and *Fli-1* genes. The latter is a member of the ets transcription factor family. The discovery of *EWS/Fli-1* has helped add some order to the general class of small round cell tumors, which includes PNET (peripheral primitive neuroectodermal tumor), Ewing's sarcoma, and Askin tumor, because many share the common feature of fusion of *EWS* with a transcription factor.

Tumor Suppressor Genes

The 2 most well studied tumor suppressor genes are the retinoblastoma (Rb) and p53 genes. The Rb gene was the first of such genes to be discovered. The tumor suppressor effect was initially hypothesized based on the differences in epidemiology between hereditary and spontaneous retinoblastoma. Mutations in the Rb gene are the basis for virtually all retinoblastomas. Patients with hereditary retinoblastoma are at risk for other neoplasms, with approximately 15% of these patients developing additional tumors, half of which will be osteosarcomas. Analysis of a series of patients with osteosarcoma without known retinoblastoma revealed 35% had Rb mutations.

The Rb gene has been cloned and its function defined as a regulator of cell proliferation. When in its hypophosphorylated state, Rb binds to DNA and prevents cell replication. When it becomes phosphorylated, it does not bind DNA and the cell divides. Many growth factors and cytokines affect the phosphorylation state of Rb. Mutations in the Rb gene inactivate it and in some settings allow ungoverned cell proliferation and tumor development. Rb is a recessive suppressor gene because both copies of the gene must be mutated to lose its suppressor activity. Thus, as long as 1 copy of the gene is normal, there will be enough activity in the normal protein to effectively regulate the cell because there is no interaction between the wild type and mutant Rb protein.

The most commonly mutated tumor suppressor gene in human cancer is the p53 gene, which is mutated in approximately 50% of all tumors. The Li-Fraumeni syndrome is an inherited defect in this tumor suppressor gene. One postulated role for p53 is to arrest the cell cycle when there is DNA damage so that the cell can repair itself before dividing. Cells lacking normal p53 function continue to divide before the DNA damage can be repaired and pass along potentially tumorigenic mutations. The p53 gene can also suppress transcription of other growth related genes, such as c-*fos* and c-*jun*. It is called a dominant suppressor gene because a mutation in just one copy of the gene is capable of inactivating the normal wild type protein. The mutated protein binds to the wild type protein and the complex becomes inactive. It was found that 28% to 65% of osteosarcomas have p53 mutations. Only a few patients with osteosarcoma have a new germ-line p53 mutation (a mutation affecting all of the cells in the individual). Half of the somatic mutations (mutations in the tumor cells only) are point mutations and others are gross rearrangements or deletions.

The murine double minute-2 (MDM2) gene inhibits p53 by binding to p53, thereby preventing the p53 from binding to DNA. When the MDM2 is overexpressed, p53 is inactivated. The overexpression of MDM2 by gene amplification has been found to occur in 37% of soft-tissue sarcomas, 10% of osteosarcomas, and 13% of Ewing's sarcomas, but not in chondrosarcoma.

Undoubtedly, there are yet to be discovered tumor suppressor gene mutations that account for the tumors in which Rb, p53, and MDM2 expression is normal. Although the suppressor gene mutations occur in sarcomas, this knowledge has not been translated into therapeutic use. In cell culture, the normal gene can be inserted into a cell and normal Rb or p53 function restored. With advances in gene therapy, hope for future treatment is to be able to restore the normal growth regulatory mechanism in patients.

Oncogenes

Oncogenes are normal genes that are similar to viral oncogenes. Many of these genes are normally expressed during growth and development. However, when they are abnormally expressed because of an activating mutation or fusion with a normal gene they have the ability to induce uncontrolled growth. The first identified transforming oncogene was c-*src*, the cellular homologue of v-*src*, the Rous sarcoma virus oncogene that is capable of inducing sarcomas in animals. The protein product pp60^{c-src} is a tyrosine kinase. Functions of oncogenes can be grouped into growth factors, growth factor receptors, which usually have tyrosine kinase activity, guanine binding proteins, which are part of the signal transduction pathway for growth factor receptors, cytoplasmic oncoproteins with serine/threonine protein kinase activity, nuclear transcription factors, and those that are unclassified.

Well over 50 oncogenes have been described. Some of these have been evaluated in sarcoma. In a series of 26 sarcomas, analyzed with Southern blot for amplification of a number of oncogenes, only 3 tumors had amplifications or rearrangements. *Erb-2 (HER-2/neu)* is a truncated version of the epidermal growth factor receptor that has high intrinsic autophosphorylating protein kinase activity. Amplification of *erb-2* has been suggested to carry a poor prognosis in some subsets of breast cancer patients. The functional role of *erb-2* in soft-tissue sarcoma has not been clearly defined. Immunostain study of *erb-B-2* expression in sarcoma did not find overexpression in 87 soft-tissue sarcomas or 45 bone sarcomas. In another study, 2 of 6 benign soft-tissue tumors and 6 of 105 sarcomas had amplification of c-*erb*-B-2 and a 37% increase of messenger ribonucleic acid (mRNA). There was no correlation between *erb*-B-2 gene amplification or mRNA level with protein expression or histologic grade. This indicates that a complete analysis of each oncogene must include Southern blot for gene amplification and rearrangements, Northern blot for increased mRNA expression, which can occur in the absence of gene amplification, and Western blot to assess protein expression resulting from translational changes without alteration in DNA or RNA.

The focal adhesion kinase (FAK) gene codes for p125^{FAK} tyrosine kinase and is involved in cell adhesion, motility, and anchorage independent growth. Increased amounts of p125^{FAK} have been found by Western blot in all of 13 sarcomas when compared to normal tissue or hyperplastic lesions, suggesting that p125^{FAK} may be related to invasion and metastasis.

Malignant transformation usually is an end result of interplay of tumor suppressor gene(s) and oncogene(s). Given the sheer number of genes that seem to be related to tumorigen-esis, and the labor intensive nature of testing tumors for each gene abnormality, the relative contribution of each of these genes to tumor development is currently unclear. Newer methods for quantitatively and simultaneously assessing expression of a large number of genes in a tissue may allow for a more complete analysis of abnormalities in gene expression in tumors.

Benign Bone Tumors

Unicameral Bone Cyst

The unicameral bone cyst is a tumor that develops in metaphyseal bone adjacent to the physis and most commonly involves the proximal humerus and the proximal femur. Radiographic features include a geographic pattern of bone destruction with cortical thinning and expansion (Fig. 2). Unlike aneurysmal bone cysts, which are typically eccentric, unicameral cysts have a central location in the bone. Periosteal reaction occasionally occurs in the setting of a pathologic fracture. These tumors are typically asymptomatic until pathologic fracture occurs.

The etiology of unicameral bone cysts remains unknown. The cyst lining is composed of a thin fibrous membrane containing hemosiderin, chronic inflammatory cells, and multinucleated giant cells. Analysis of fluid from unicameral cysts has revealed high levels of cytokines and prostaglandins, which stimulate osteoclast activity, as well as osteoclast associated enzymes, including lysozomal enzymes and acid phosphatase. Increased hydrostatic pressure has been documented in the cysts and has been postulated to be responsible for resorptive erosion.

Pathologic fracture occurs in a large number of unicameral cysts, and fracture was found to be most highly associated with lesions that occupy more than 85% of the involved bone in the transverse plane on both the anteroposterior (AP) and lateral radiographs. In the setting of pathologic fracture, the fracture should be permitted to heal. Although fracture occasionally stimulates cyst healing, in most cases the cyst remains unchanged.

Treatment for unicameral cysts has primarily consisted of either aspiration and injection of methylprednisolone acetate or intralesional curettage and bone grafting. Aspiration and injection typically requires multiple injections at 6- to 8-week intervals, but results in healing in up to 75% of cases, a rate similar to that observed with open bone grafting. Rates of healing are lower in multiloculated cysts adjacent to the physis that are more biologically active. Curettage and bone graft have been advocated in lesions recalcitrant to steroid injection or in weightbearing bones, including the calcaneus

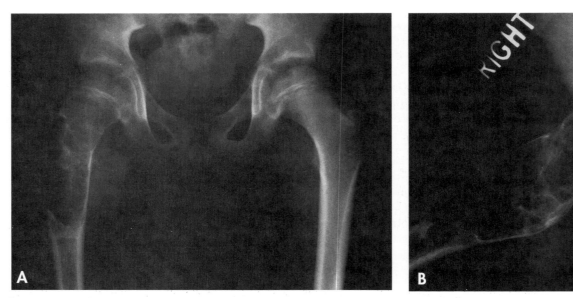

Figure 2

Anteroposterior (A) and lateral (B) radiographs of the hip in an 8-year-old with a unicameral bone cyst. The cyst is expansile, centrally located, and involves both the metaphysis and the diaphysis. The cortex is thinned, but has well-defined borders consistent with a slow rate of growth and a geographic pattern of bone destruction. The cyst has a characteristic septated appearance.

and proximal femur. However, curettage is risky in active lesions adjacent to the physis in young children. The natural history of unicameral bone cysts involves penetration of the physis with epiphyseal involvement in 2% of patients. Recently, aspiration and injection of autologous bone marrow have been reported in 10 patients, with a single injection resulting in healing of all 10 bone cysts within 4 months. Although these results are promising, they have yet to be reproduced by other investigators. Unicameral cysts typically resolve by adulthood, but they require close follow-up and often repeated treatment because of their propensity for recurrence. Small cysts can be treated with observation.

Giant Cell Tumor

Giant cell tumor of bone is an aggressive benign neoplasm involving the metaphysis and epiphysis of the long bones; it usually occurs in young adults between the ages of 20 and 40 years. The tumor is purely lytic and usually is associated with cortical disruption (Fig. 3). The tumor is composed of abundant osteoclast-like giant cells within a fibrous stroma. The stromal cells express a combination of histiocytic, myofibroblastic, and osteoblastic features and are the proliferating, neoplastic component of the tumor. In contrast, the giant cells are reactive, nonproliferating cells that express osteoclast characteristics and are responsible for the bone resorption observed in these tumors. Several investigations have demonstrated the ability of isolated stromal cells to induce mono-

cyte fusion and osteoclast formation in vitro. The giant cell component of the tumors may also have a role in the perpetuation of these tumors through expression of high levels of interleukin-1 and -6, and tumor necrosis factor-alpha. These cytokines stimulate osteoclast progenitor cells and mature osteoclasts and can enhance bone resorption in an autocrine fashion.

Giant cell tumor has a high propensity for local recurrence, in spite of the use of adjuvant treatments. In 2 recent series, recurrence developed in 3 of 38 patients (8%) and in 15 of 60 patients (25%) after curettage and methylmethacrylate cementation. In the latter series, the recurrence rate was reduced to 7 of 41 (17%) in those receiving additional treatment of the bone cavity with phenol or a high speed burr before cementation. Cryosurgery with liquid nitrogen is another accepted adjuvant therapy for giant cell tumor and is associated with similar rates of recurrence. Nearly all recurrences occur within 2 years, although late recurrences, up to 18 years, have been reported.

Pulmonary metastases develop in approximately 2% of patients with giant cell tumors. Flow cytometry demonstrates a normal or diploid pattern in both primary and metastatic tumors, and is thus not predictive of the risk of metastasis. Likewise, a similar rate of proliferation has been observed in both primary and metastatic lesions. Recently, it has been shown that giant cell tumors constitutively express both 72 kd and 92 kd gelatinases (MMP2 and MMP9), proteins

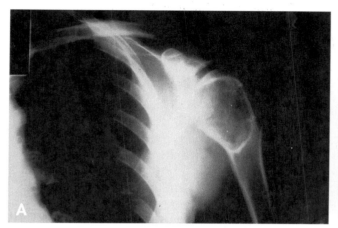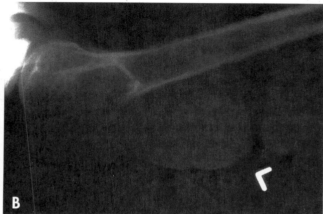

Figure 3

Anteroposterior (A) and lateral (B) radiographs of the shoulder in a 28-year-old with a giant cell tumor of bone. The lesion has a septated, lytic appearance with well-defined sclerotic borders and is located in the epiphysis and metaphysis. The tumor has thinned the cortex and extends to the subchondral bone.

implicated in both local aggressiveness and metastasis. Inhibitors of the matrix metalloproteinases are being developed and may have a therapeutic role in the future.

Approximately 7% of giant cell tumors occur in the spine, with neurologic deficits on presentation in 50% of patients with spine and nearly 90% of patients with sacral tumors. The reported recurrence rates of spine tumors at 2 institutions were 10 of 24 (42%) and 7 of 21 (33%). Limited surgery combined with radiation therapy, including proton beam therapy, has led to control rates similar to those observed in other locations. However, radiation is associated with the malignant transformation of giant cell tumors and should be reserved for inoperable tumors.

Osteoid Osteoma

Osteoid osteoma occurs in young adults and is a benign neoplastic proliferation of immature osteoblasts that is typically surrounded by dense reactive lamellar bone. This results in a characteristic radiographic appearance of a small lytic "nidus" surrounded by dense reactive bone (Fig. 4). The neoplastic cells produce immature or woven bone with characteristic osteoblastic rimming of the osteoid surfaces. The lesions are less than 1 cm in size. Patients usually present with aching pain that is often severe, typically worse at night, and that often is relieved with nonsteroidal anti-inflammatory agents (NSAIDs).

Osteoid osteomas may spontaneously resolve after 5 to 7 years. Conservative management with close follow-up is advocated for patients with excellent pain relief with NSAIDs, provided that the lesions have characteristic radiographic and clinical features. In patients with poor pain relief, surgical excision of the nidus is the traditional treatment. However, the nidus often is difficult to identify during surgery, and excision frequently is performed with excessive removal of bone. Preoperative labeling of the lesion with technetium 99 can assist in identification of the lesion by using an intraoperative probe.

Recently, radiologic procedures have been described for treatment of osteoid osteoma that may lessen the morbidity of surgical intervention. Sixteen of 18 patients were successfully treated by thermal necrosis using a small radiofrequency electrode inserted into the lesion by CT guidance. Fourteen of 16 patients were treated with a CT guided excision of the nidus in another study.

Benign Cartilage Tumors

Benign cartilage tumors arise from rests of physeal cartilage and are the most common neoplasms involving bone, although the exact incidences of some of the tumors are uncertain because they remain clinically inapparent. The various tumors have distinct clinical and radiographic features and are listed in Table 5. Because some of the tumors have malignant potential, a major challenge in their management is recognizing sarcomatous transformation. In general, benign cartilage lesions are inactive in adults. Serial radiographs demonstrating activity of a lesion with progressive cortical erosion or intramedullary extension is highly associated with malignant degeneration. Chondrosarcomas typically are associated with aching discomfort and occur in a more elderly population.

Enchondromas and osteochondromas are the 2 benign cartilaginous neoplasms that most frequently undergo sarcoma-

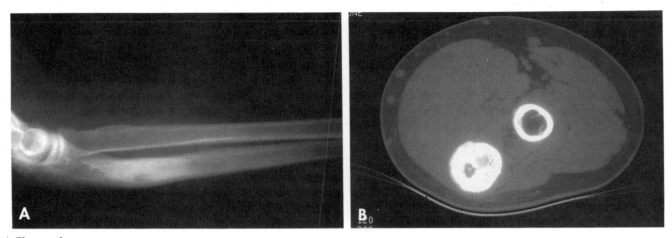

Figure 4

A lateral radiograph (A) and a computed tomogram (B) of an osteoid osteoma in a 24-year-old. Abundant reactive bone formation surrounds a well-defined lytic area in the proximal ulna. The lesion is located in the cortex, and the medullary space is replaced by reactive bone formation.

Table 5
Benign cartilage tumors

Tumor	Age of Presentation	Location	Radiographic Findings	Treatment Potential	Malignant Potential
Enchondroma	Adolescence through adulthood	Intramedullary, tubular bones, hand common	Speckled calcification in pattern of rings and arcs	Observation	Small
Chondroblastoma	Adolescence	Epiphysis, proximal humerus and knee most common	Lytic lesion in epiphysis	Curettage and bone graft; adjuvant phenol or cryotherapy	None
Osteocartilaginous exostosis	Adolescence/ adulthood	Metaphysis, proximal humerus and knee, can involve axial skeleton	Peduculated or sessile exostosis, cartilaginous cap, trabecular bone extend into lesion	Observation unless mechanical symptoms on surrounding structures	Small
Chondromyxoid fibroma	Adolescence/ young adult	Metaphysis, proximal tibia most common	Lytic, "soap bubble" appearance with sclerotic margins, eccentric	Curettage and bone graft	None
Parosteal chondroma	Adolescence/ young adult	Metaphysis, hands and feet most common, also long bones; rare in axial skeleton	Extracortical scalloping, occasional speckled calcification	Curettage and bone graft	Rarely

tous degeneration, although this process occurs in fewer than 1% of these tumors. In the absence of evidence of malignancy, these tumors should be followed up clinically as well as radiographically, depending on the size, location, and clinical symptoms. Secondary chondrosarcomas most frequently arise in large lesions located in the axial skeleton or proximal appendicular skeleton. Most of these tumors are low grade malignancies.

Malignant degeneration of osteocartilaginous exostoses is marked by an increase in the thickness of the cartilaginous cap, which is typically only a few millimeters in adults, to a thickness of more than 2 cm. The potential for malignant degeneration is much greater in individuals with hereditary multiple exostoses; the tumors in these patients are more likely to be high grade, and they typically occur at an earlier age in this population. Three-dimensional imaging studies, including CT and MRI scan, are extremely helpful in evaluating the thickness of the cartilaginous cap. Benign osteocartilaginous exostoses occasionally require marginal excision because of mechanical symptoms on surrounding soft tissues or nerves. In children in whom the cap is active and the lesion is growing, the potential for recurrence is approximately 5%. Because these lesions also tend to be close to the physis, delaying surgery until adolescence is optimal, when possible.

Chondroblastomas are aggressive lesions involving the epiphysis that almost exclusively affect adolescents. These lesions are more common in boys, occur near the end of growth, and frequently cross the physis to involve the metaphysis. The lesions are lytic and can cause joint destruction. Management involves aggressive curettage and bone graft. Because these lesions have a tendency to recur, local adjuvant therapy, such as phenol or cryotherapy, has been recommended. In 1 series, the use of phenol decreased the rate of recurrence in benign aggressive bone lesions from 41% to 7%. A recent study found a 5% concentration of phenol to be optimal for the treatment of benign tumors.

rent neoadjuvant (preoperative and postoperative) chemotherapeutic regimens, the long-term survival is now approaching 70%. The importance of the chemotherapeutic responsiveness of the primary tumor for long-term survival has been demonstrated in numerous studies. The Children's Cancer Group recently reported a multi-institutional 8-year survival rate of 87% in good responders (< 5% viable tumor cells in resected specimen), compared to a survival rate of 52% in all others. Chemotherapeutic responsiveness also is associated with a decreased risk of local recurrence in limb salvage surgery. It has been shown that the amount of chemotherapy induced tumor necrosis is the most important prognostic variable for survival and local recurrence.

Local recurrence carries a particularly poor prognosis in osteosarcoma, with recently reported recurrence rates of 8% for wide amputation, 10% for limb salvage, and 0% for radical amputation. Only 3 of 29 patients (11%) with local recurrence survived long-term. One of the most important negative factors for long-term survival is the expression of the multidrug resistance (MDR) gene. MDR-1 codes for p-glycoprotein, a calcium-dependent adenosine triphosphatase located on the cell membrane that has the capacity to pump chemotherapeutic agents, particularly adriamycin, outside the cell. p-Glycoprotein expression was recently found to increase the risk of an adverse outcome in osteosarcoma

Malignant Bone Tumors

Osteosarcoma

Osteosarcoma is the most common primary bone sarcoma and typically involves adolescents and young adults, although a second peak of incidence occurs in the elderly in association with Paget disease. The most common form is the high grade intramedullary variant that typically occurs in the metaphysis of the long bones and that accounts for more than 85% of osteosarcomas (Fig. 5). Metastases most commonly involve the lungs (90%), but frequently occur in bone (20%). In advanced disease, widespread metastases are common.

Before the use of chemotherapy for the treatment of osteosarcoma in the early 1970s, the long-term survival ranged between 10% and 20%, despite aggressive local management of this tumor. With cur-

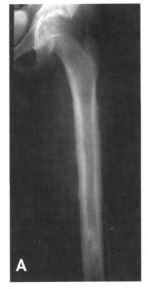
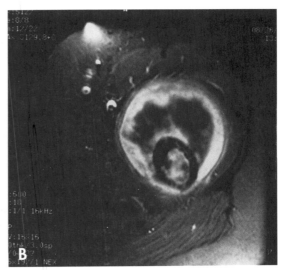

Figure 5

An anteroposterior radiograph (A) and contrast-enhanced T1-weighted axial magnetic resonance image (B) of the femur in a 12-year-old with an osteosarcoma presenting as a mixed lytic and blastic lesion. There is a permeative pattern of bone destruction with periosteal reaction and a large soft-tissue mass that enhances with contrast. The bone marrow is replaced by tumor.

Table 6
Local recurrence in Ewing's sarcoma treated with radiation and surgery

Year of Study	Patients (No.)	Location	Radiation (%)	Surgery (%)	Radiation + Surgery (%)
1995	39	Pelvis	15	–	16
1995	177	All sites	14	0	05
1996	242	All sites	31	4	07
1997	69	Femur	80	3.5	3.3

patients by 3.37-fold. In a series of 105 tumors, p-glycoprotein was detected in 23% of primary and 50% of metastatic tumors. Expression of the MDR gene has been shown to correlate with tumor necrosis in 1 study and survival in another. By assessing tumors for MDR expression at the time of biopsy, it may be possible to give agents that counteract the effect of MDR along with chemotherapy to increase the effectiveness of the chemotherapy or to use dose-intensified chemotherapy with bone marrow transplantation for high risk patients. Although MDR reversing agents work in cell culture, clinical trials have not been able to demonstrate efficacy. There is continued debate regarding induction of p-glycoprotein by chemotherapy, but most evidence suggests an absence of induction. Current research is focused on the design of pharmacologic agents to block p-glycoprotein activity.

Metastatic disease at the time of presentation is associated with a poor outcome. However, aggressive, simultaneous surgical management of both the primary site and pulmonary metastases results in disease-free survival in 55% of patients at 30 months. Two recent studies examined the controversial role of limb salvage surgery in osteosarcoma patients with pathologic fracture. Recurrence rates with limb salvage were 19% and 30% compared with no recurrences in either study when fracture patients were treated with amputation. Despite the high recurrence rate, there was no survival advantage in the populations undergoing amputation, although these results must be carefully interpreted because of the small size of the populations.

In contrast to high grade osteosarcomas, low grade tumors, including parosteal osteosarcomas, which make up fewer than 5% of osteosarcomas, do not typically require chemotherapy and rarely metastasize. However, a recent series described high grade, dedifferentiated areas in up to 16% of parosteal osteosarcoma. Although medullary invasion by these tumors has previously been considered a poor prognostic sign, this was not associated with a negative outcome.

Ewing's Sarcoma/Primitive Neuroectodermal Tumor

Ewing's sarcoma and primitive neuroectodermal tumor (PNET) are closely related small round cell tumors that most likely are derived from cells of neural crest origin. The tumors behave in an identical fashion, but are distinguishable by relatively more neural crest differentiation in PNET. These tumors are the second most common bone malignancies, and like osteosarcoma, most commonly occur in individuals between 10 and 30 years of age. They share a classic chromosomal translocation between chromosome 11 and chromosome 22 t(11;22), with the production of a chimeric protein that appears to act as a transcriptional activator. These translocations are found in 95% of Ewing's sarcomas and PNETs.

These tumors are extremely aggressive locally and have a high propensity for metastasis, most commonly to the lungs. The tumors typically occur in the metaphysis of the long bones and generally are associated with a large soft-tissue mass. Diaphyseal involvement is common and approximately 25% of the tumors involve the pelvis, where the prognosis is particularly grim, with survival rates of approximately 40%. Similar to chondrosarcoma, the prognosis is improved with a more distal lesion, although the improved prognosis may be related to tumor size, because smaller tumors have less propensity for metastasis.

Neoadjuvant chemotherapy has led to dramatic improvements in survival, with current long-term survival rates approaching 60% to 70%. A recent study of 118 Ewing's sarcoma patients treated with preoperative chemotherapy identified 5-year disease-free survival rates of 95% in patients with no histologically viable tumor, 68% in patients with microscopically viable tumor, and 34% in patients with macroscopically viable tumor. Although chemotherapy is effective in the management of micrometastatic disease, presentation with identifiable metastasis is associated with an extremely poor prognosis. In 1 study, the survival rate at 6.8 years was only 13% in patients presenting with evidence of metastases compared to 64% in patients without metastasis.

In recent years, emphasis on surgical resection in the treatment of Ewing's sarcoma has increased; studies have demonstrated reduced rates of local recurrence in surgically treated compared to radiation treated tumors (Table 6). However, radiation continues to have a role, particularly in tumors where adequate surgical margins cannot be obtained. Data from the Cooperative Ewing's Sarcoma study demonstrate the lowest rate of local recurrence with radical or wide margins with or without radiation therapy (5%), but similar rates of recurrence were found in marginal resections with or without radiation (12%) and intralesional surgeries with radiation (14%). In addition to reducing the incidence of local recurrence, surgery appears to have an advantage over radiation therapy in terms of long-term disease-free survival, although a few studies have not shown a survival advantage in surgically treated patients. Definitive information regarding the role of surgery versus radiation is uncertain in the absence of carefully designed prospective studies.

Chondrosarcoma

Chondrosarcoma is a malignancy of cartilage cells and most commonly arises secondarily from benign cartilaginous neoplasms, such as enchondromas and osteochondromas. Chondrosarcomas typically occur in an older age group than the other primary bone sarcomas and have a peak incidence in the fifth through seventh decades. Fewer than 5% of chondrosarcomas occur in individuals younger than 20 years.

Unlike other bone sarcomas, most chondrosarcomas are low grade, and there is a large degree of histologic overlap between benign and low grade malignant lesions. For this reason, these tumors in particular require a comprehensive approach with careful consideration of patient symptoms and radiographic and histologic findings. Malignant cartilage tumors typically have an unstable radiographic appearance over time with evidence of endosteal erosion (Fig. 6), cause aching and nonactivity related pain, and occur in older individuals. Evaluation of a biopsy specimen requires close collaboration between an experienced musculoskeletal pathologist and oncologist for accurate diagnosis, because tumors that otherwise appear identical behave much more aggressively when located in a more central location in the body.

Consideration of location of the tumor is a particularly important feature in the evaluation of cartilage neoplasms. Cartilaginous neoplasms that occur in the axial or proximal appendicular skeleton have a much more aggressive course than those arising in the distal skeleton. A neoplasm in the hand or foot with more aggressive histologic and radiographic characteristics than a pelvic tumor may be considered benign while the pelvic neoplasm is considered malignant. Approximately 25% of chondrosarcomas occur in

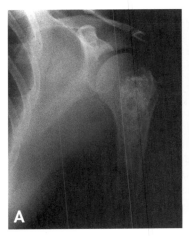
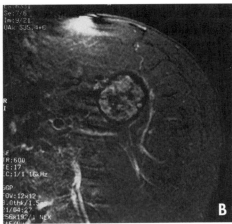

Figure 6

An anteroposterior radiograph (A) and contrast-enhanced T1-weighted axial magnetic resonance image (B) of the proximal humerus in a 55-year-old with a grade 1 chondrosarcoma. Stippled calcification in the proximal metaphysis and diaphysis is associated with endosteal erosion of the cortex. Enchondromas usually are not associated with erosive changes in the bones except when in the hands and feet.

the pelvis but they are rare in the hand, the most common location for benign cartilaginous tumors. The features of malignant cartilaginous neoplasms of the hands and feet were recently reviewed in 163 patients. The tumors were considered low grade in 116 patients, intermediate grade in 44 patients, and high grade in only 3 patients. Despite highly aggressive characteristics in these tumors, including cortical destruction in 92% and a soft-tissue mass in 80%, only 12 patients developed metastases, with 7 patients dying of disease. In contrast, 2 recent reviews of pelvic chondrosarcomas demonstrated high grade neoplasms in 45% and 48% of patients and long-term survival in approximately 50%.

The histologic grade of the tumor correlates with metastasis and is the most important determinant of long-term survival. In a study of 67 pelvic chondrosarcomas, metastasis occurred in 0 of grade I, 20% of grade II, 60% of grade III, and 75% of dedifferentiated tumors. Because chondrosarcomas are essentially resistant to radiation therapy and chemotherapy, metastatic disease is catastrophic and difficult to treat. A recent study of 74 dedifferentiated chondrosarcomas identified a 5-year survival rate of 13%. Constitutive expression of the MDR gene, p-glycoprotein, has recently been identified in normal and neoplastic cartilage and may account for the resistance of these tumors to chemotherapy. As agents designed to block p-glycoprotein become available, chemotherapy may become effective in these tumors, with improvement in the survival of patients with high grade tumors.

Because of the low propensity of low grade chondrosarcomas to metastasize, intralesional management of these tumors, with the addition of adjuvant therapies including cementation with polymethylmethacrylate, has been advocated. However, this approach remains controversial. In 1 study of 23 patients with low grade chondrosarcoma treated with intralesional curettage, the 10-year local recurrence rate was 9%. However, a more recent study of 26 patients, including 14 grade I, 8 grade II, and 4 grade III tumors, demonstrated a 20-year relapse-free survival of only 7% compared with a 64% relapse-free rate in 38 patients with wide or marginal surgery. Another recent study suggested that acceptably low recurrence risk can be achieved when local adjuvants such as cementation are used. Because of the ineffectiveness of current adjuvant therapies, adequate surgical excision of chondrosarcoma is necessary for cure, and the role of less aggressive intralesional surgery is yet to be determined.

Recently, genes associated with the development of multiple osteochondromas, a autosomal dominant familial disorder associated with the development of multiple exostoses, derangements of epiphyseal cartilage, and a propensity for malignant degeneration, have been identified. Exostosis or EXT genes have been identified at 3 chromosomal loci, including EXT 1 on chromosome 8 (8q24), EXT 2 on chromosome 11 (11p13), and EXT 3 on chromosome 19 (19q). A tumor suppresser function has been proposed for these genes, although their mechanism of action is unknown. It appears that abnormality or loss of heterozygosity at the EXT genes in addition to other genetic events is necessary for the development of chondrosarcomas in multiple hereditary exostosis. However, these genes appear to have a role in the development of other chondrosarcomas as well. Loss of heterozygosity was observed for markers linked to EXT 1 and EXT 2 in 44% of 18 sporadic chondrosarcomas. Similarly, the development of extraskeletal myxoid chondrosarcoma has been linked to a specific genetic event, consisting of a chromosomal translocation from chromosome 9 to 22. This results in the rearrangement of a gene with DNA binding characteristics. As the genetic determinants of chondrosarcoma become elucidated, potential new adjuvant therapies, which are critically needed for this tumor, will emerge.

Chemotherapy

Since its introduction in the early 1970s, chemotherapy has had a remarkable impact on major childhood bone and soft-tissue sarcomas, osteosarcoma, Ewing's sarcoma, and rhabdomyosarcoma. While chemotherapy has assisted in improving local control and has facilitated modern techniques in limb salvage surgery, the major role of this adjuvant is to eradicate micrometastatic disease. It is estimated that micrometastases, most commonly to the lungs, are present in 80% to 90% of osteosarcoma and Ewing's sarcoma patients at presentation.

Chemotherapy is extremely effective for the treatment of rhabdomyosarcoma, with a 70% overall long-term survival and with cure rates of 20% in children who present with metastasis. Local disease is treated with surgical resection, with addition of radiation when excision is incomplete. Osteosarcoma and Ewing's sarcoma are treated with neoadjuvant chemotherapeutic regimens, consisting of several courses of chemotherapy before surgical resection, followed by the completion of chemotherapy. The extent of tumor necrosis as a measure of tumor responsiveness to chemotherapy is an important prognostic factor in children with osteosarcoma and Ewing's sarcoma. Chemotherapy protocols take nearly a year to complete and are associated with intense emotional, psychological, and physical hardships. However, recent study of 39 long-term survivors of osteosarcoma did not identify any persistent psychosocial disability.

Current chemotherapeutic regimens use simultaneous administration of multiple drugs to permit synergistic activity of complementary chemotherapeutic agents. That is, regimens typically use complex combinations of agents with different activities. Table 7 lists the common agents, their drug classification, and mechanisms of action. There is substantial overlap among the drugs used for the treatment of the pediatric sarcomas; drugs such as adriamycin, cyclophosphamide, and actinomycin D are important components of each of these regimens. However, high dose methotrexate and cisplatin are uniquely important in the treatment of osteosarcoma. A recent analysis of 30 studies involving 1,909 osteosarcoma patients found the dose intensity of methotrexate to be the most important factor in disease-free survival. Prevention of methotrexate toxicity, including myelosuppression, gastrointestinal mucositis, nephrotoxicity, and liver toxicity, requires hydration, alkalinization of the urine, monitoring of serum drug levels, and administration of a leucovorin (a folate analog) rescue dose. The major toxic effects of methotrexate occur between 5 and 14 days after dosing.

Carefully controlled prospective multicenter clinical trials are essential for the evaluation of chemotherapeutic efficacy. These trials permit enrollment of enough patients so that statistically meaningful assumptions regarding the treatment of these rare tumors can be made in a relatively brief period of time. Most patients with pediatric sarcomas are enrolled in these studies, typically under the auspices of groups such as the Pediatric Oncology Group and the Eastern Collective Oncology Group.

The agents most commonly used in the treatment of osteosarcoma include adriamycin, high dose methotrexate, and cisplatin. Cyclophosphamide, actinomycin D, and bleomycin also are frequently used. Ifosfamide and etoposide

Table 7
Chemotherapuetic agents commonly used to treat bone sarcomas

Drug	Drug Class	Mechanism of Action	Complication/Side Effects*
Cyclophosphamide Ifosfamide	Alkylating agents	Reactive intermediates cause DNA cross-links	Myelosuppression, hemorrhagic cystitis/infertility (Co-administration of Mesna reduces cystitis)
Cisplatin	Alkylating agent activity		Nephrotoxicity/ototoxicity/ myelosuppression
Adriamycin	Antitumor antibiotics (Produced by Streptomyces species)	DNA intercalation impairs DNA/RNA synthesis, leads to strand breaks	Myelosuppression/**cumulative cardiac toxicity**
Actinomycin D Bleomycin			**Pneumonitis/pulmonary fibrosis**
Vincristine	Plant alkyloids (Extracts from Vinca rosea)	Bind tubulin, inhibit microtubules with metaphase arrest	**Neurotoxicity**
Etoposide	(Etoposide is synthetic derivative)		**Myelosuppression, transient hypotension**
Methotrexate	Antimetabolites	Dihydrofolate reductase inhibitor, interferes with purine synthesis and prevents DNA synthesis; affects S phase cells	Myelosuppression

*All of the agents are associated with nausea and vomiting. For each drug class, side effects specific for a certain drug are listed in bold faced type

have more recently been included in chemotherapeutic trials. Agents effective in the treatment of Ewing's sarcoma include vincristine, actinomycin D, cyclophosphamide, adriamycin, ifosfamide, and etoposide. Rhabdomyosarcoma is effectively treated with a combination of vincristine, actinomycin D, cyclophosphamide, and adriamycin. Current investigations are examining the efficacy of ifosfamide and etoposide in the treatment of rhabdomyosarcoma.

The side effects of chemotherapy are severe and often life-threatening. The plant alkyloid adriamycin, which is highly effective for treatment for all of the pediatric sarcomas, is associated with both acute and chronic cardiac toxicity. The chronic cardiac toxicity consists of a dilated cardiomyopathy and is cumulative, limiting the total dose of adriamycin to approximately 450 mg/m^2 (body surface area). Fever and neutropenia are 2 of the most common side effects of chemotherapy and are associated with the effectiveness of chemotherapeutic agents in targeting dividing cells. A recent study of 54 Ewing's sarcoma patients treated with 7 cycles of vincristine, adriamycin, and cyclophosphamide and 11 cycles of ifosfamide and etoposide demonstrated an incidence of febrile neutropenia after 49% of cycles. Subclinical cardiac dysfunction occurred in 40%, while 7% had clinically apparent cardiac dysfunction.

Chemotherapeutic adjuvants have markedly reduced the complications associated with chemotherapy and have permitted the institution of more aggressive and beneficial therapeutic protocols. Administration of recombinant human granulocyte colony stimulating factor has been found to significantly reduce the duration of severe leukopenia (absolute neutrophil count < 100) and decrease the rate of hospital admission for cytopenic fever. In addition, it also theoretically permits more aggressive dosing and scheduling of chemotherapy. Ondansetron is an effective antiemetic with minimal side effects in children receiving chemotherapy. The alkylating agents, cyclophosphamide and ifosfamide, produce an acrolein metabolite that causes an acute sterile hemorrhagic cystitis in approximately 10% of patients. This compound is neutralized by MESNA (2-mercaptoethanesulfonate) and prevents the cystitis. Leucovorin is an important adjuvant in the use of high dose methotrexate. Methotrexate is a dihydrofolate reductase inhibitor that blocks DNA synthesis by reducing the levels of reduced folates necessary for purine metabolism. Following methotrexate delivery at a toxic concentration several orders of magnitude higher than conventional therapy, leucovorin is administered as a rescue dose. Because leucovorin is a folic acid analog that does not require reduction by the enzyme dihydrofolate reductase for activity, it bypasses the effects of methotrexate. The high dosing regimen of methotrexate facilitated by leucovorin is extremely beneficial in the treatment of osteosarcoma. Intense research is currently underway to develop chemotherapeutic adjuvants capable of reversing the effects of the cellular drug resistance mechanisms, including p-glycoprotein, and will result in a major breakthrough in childhood cancer therapy.

Limb Salvage Surgery

Most patients with extremity sarcomas currently undergo limb salvage surgery, with primary amputations performed in only 10% to 15% of patients. During limb salvage, the surgeon must strictly adhere to the principles of oncologic surgery, and tissue planes free of tumor involvement must be developed. Three-dimensional imaging is critical for surgical planning and identifies the location of important neurovascular structures that must be spared for adequate limb function and whether an intra- or extra-articular resection must be done.

The rate of local recurrence in patients with high grade bone sarcomas treated with limb salvage is approximately 10%. Although this rate is perhaps slightly higher than that observed with amputation, long-term survival rates are not improved by amputation. Similarly, although limb disarticulation is associated with local recurrence rates approaching 0%, this mutilating procedure also does not improve overall survival. The use of adjuvant treatments, including chemotherapy and radiation therapy, has largely been responsible for the low recurrence rates in limb salvage surgeries. A recent study examining local recurrence rates in osteosarcoma patients found the adequacy of surgical margins and the response to chemotherapy to be important predictors of local recurrence. Radiation therapy is an equally important component of local control in patients with soft-tissue sarcomas.

Numerous methods have been devised for the reconstruction of bone defects after tumor resections, all of which have high complication and failure rates. The results of 1,001 custom-made cemented endoprostheses implanted at a single institution were recently reviewed, and results varied according to the anatomic location of the implant. The probability of implant survival at 10 years was 93.8% for a proximal femoral replacement, 67.4% for a distal femoral prosthesis, and 58% for a proximal tibial prosthesis. Prosthetic survival in 82 patients treated at another institution was similar, with overall survival rates of 83% at 5 years and 67% at 10 years; the failure of proximal tibial prostheses were the highest and approached 50%.

Allografts are used at many tumor centers to avoid the possibility of aseptic loosening. Large structural allografts are sterilely procured from carefully tested donors and are typically stored fresh-frozen in licensed tissue banks. Articular cartilage is preserved during freezing with a solution of 10% dimethylsulfoxide and up to 50% viability of the cells has been observed. Tissue typing is not performed, and allografts are selected for implantation on the basis of size. Allografts can be inserted as osteoarticular implants after intra-articular resection, with preservation of the allograft cartilage, or as allograft-prosthetic composites. Osteoarthritis frequently develops in osteoarticular allografts by 6 years.

Allografts also are associated with a high complication rate. The rate of infection is approximately 10% in the first year. Allograft fractures typically occur between 2 and 3 years, with rates ranging from 19% to 54% recently described. Although allograft fractures are through necrotic bone and are thus catastrophic, healing rates of more than 50% have been reported with autologous bone grafting. Nonunion of the allograft-host junction occurs in 17% to 33% of patients and is more frequent in those receiving chemotherapy and radiation therapy. Most nonunions can be salvaged with bone grafts. Despite the high complication rate, satisfactory results have been reported in 75% of patients after more than 20 years. Few studies have directly compared the results of allograft with endoprosthetic replacement, but the studies performed suggest a similar degree of success.

Reconstructive procedures in young children present a unique challenge because of remaining growth. Expandable prostheses permit limb lengthening during development but require multiple procedures. In one recent series, an average of more than 8 procedures were required to gain a mean lengthening of 13.2 cm. Allografts have also been used in children and adolescents, but limb length discrepancies of more than 2 cm have been described in one third of patients.

Studies on the outcome of limb salvage surgery have indicated that functional results are similar to or slightly better than those with amputation. Although amputations are typically more durable and require less surgical intervention, most patients clearly prefer limb salvage and have improved self images with this procedure. The cost-effectiveness of limb salvage was compared with that of amputation in a recent study; historic data were used to determine the likelihood of further surgery or revision. Although the initial cost of limb salvage is higher, the accumulated costs associated with amputation and prostheses exceeded those of limb salvage by approximately $114,000 over a 20-year period.

Bone Metastasis

The skeleton is 1 of the 3 most common sites of metastases and accounts for a significant degree of morbidity in patients with systemic cancer. Although bone metastases have been reported with nearly all cancers, carcinomas of the breast, prostate, lung, kidney, and thyroid have a particularly high predilection for bone involvement. It has been estimated that up to three fourths of the patients that succumb to cancer have bone metastases at the time of death.

Tumor cells most commonly involve bone in the axial and proximal portion of the appendicular skeleton where there is abundant blood supply and marrow content. Bone metastasis most commonly results in destruction of host bone with the development of a lytic lesion. However, sclerotic lesions also can occur and are the most common lesions found in prostate carcinoma. Other tumors, such as lymphoma, frequently result in a mixed lytic and blastic lesion, a pattern that sometimes occurs in breast and other carcinomas.

Tumor cells contribute minimally to direct bone resorption, but instead secrete factors that stimulate osteoclast recruitment and activation. Thus, large numbers of host osteoclasts are typically observed adjacent to tumor deposits. Factors implicated in tumor mediated bone resorption include parathyroid related protein (PTHrP), interleukins 1 and 6, and tumor necrosis factor-alpha. PTHrP expression in breast carcinoma has been found to be highly associated with the development of bone metastases. Unlike normal bone remodeling, bone resorption in metastatic disease is not associated with compensatory bone formation.

The development, progression, and expansion of bone metastases depend on osteoclast bone resorption. Bisphosphonates, inhibitors of osteoclast activity, markedly reduce skeletal metastases and overall tumor burden while prolonging life span in animal models. Similarly, in a randomized trial of 380 breast cancer patients with bone metastases, intravenous pamidronate (90 mg monthly for 12 months) decreased the rate of skeletal complications and delayed the median time for the first occurrence of a skeletal complication from 7.0 to 13.1 months. The patients treated with pamidronate had decreased pain and improved function. Thus, intravenous pamidronate has become a standard treatment for patients with bone metastases. Oral bisphosphonates are also efficacious.

Progression of bone metastases leads to skeletal compromise and frequently is associated with pain, fracture, hypercalcemia, and potential neurologic compromise in tumors involving the spine. Criteria for impending fracture have been developed and include weightbearing pain, size larger than 3 cm, and involvement of more than 50% of the cortex.

Aggressive surgical management of impending and pathologic fractures results in improvements in both life span and quality of life. Postoperative radiation therapy has been shown to be an important adjunct and improves the results of surgical stabilization.

Soft-Tissue Tumors

Patients presenting with soft-tissue tumors require a careful evaluation because there is substantial overlap between benign and malignant soft-tissue tumors. However, patients with malignant lesions typically present with relatively large tumors that frequently are associated with aching discomfort and are most commonly located in the deep, subfascial tissues. Because many soft-tissue sarcomas, including synovial sarcoma, often have an insidious course, the presence of a slowly enlarging, painless mass often results in a false sense of security. MRI scans are extremely helpful in the evaluation of soft-tissue masses because nearly all sarcomas enhance with gadolinium and have a heterogeneous signal of high intensity on T-2 images, indicating the presence of a highly cellular tumor with a rich blood supply. Nearly all major tumor centers routinely diagnose soft-tissue sarcomas on the basis of aspiration and needle biopsy specimens, which are typically obtained in an outpatient clinic setting with minimal morbidity. Poorly planned excisions of soft-tissue masses without prior biopsy or imaging studies frequently result in contamination of normal surrounding tissues with disastrous consequences.

Benign Soft-Tissue Tumors

Benign soft-tissue tumors are a clinically diverse group of tumors ranging from dormant lesions, such as subcutaneous lipomas, to highly invasive and aggressive tumors, such as desmoids (aggressive fibromatosis) that can be limb and life threatening. Lipomas are the most common benign soft-tissue neoplasm. They typically occur in adults, are most commonly present in the subcutaneous tissues, and have minimal malignant potential. Intramuscular lipomas are deep tumors, which are often more clinically aggressive. These tumors frequently increase in size, often have atypical histologic characteristics, and are more likely to recur after excision. On MRI imaging, lipomas have a characteristic fat signal that clearly distinguishes them from high grade liposarcomas, but they can be difficult to distinguish from a well differentiated liposarcoma.

Hemangiomas also frequently occur intramuscularly. These tumors have a variable clinical course ranging from dormant to highly aggressive with continued invasion and replacement of normal tissue. Hemangiomas frequently are painful and are associated with limb swelling in the dependent posi-

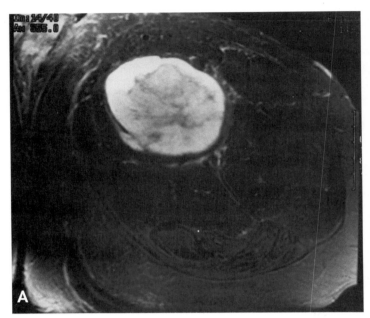
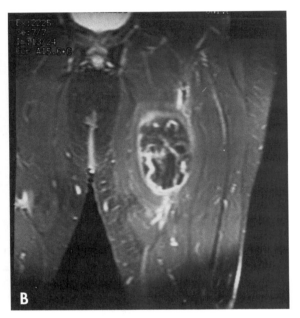

Figure 7

Axial T2-weighted (A) and coronal contrast-enhanced T1-weighted (B) magnetic resonance images of the proximal thigh in a 64-year-old with a high grade malignant fibrous histiocytoma. The mass is in the adductor compartment of the thigh, is adjacent to the neurovascular bundle, and has a characteristic heterogeneous high signal intensity on the T2-weighted image. The signal intensity is low on T1-weighted images but enhances with contrast. Areas with poor enhancement represent regions of tumor necrosis.

tion. Excision is appropriate for symptomatic or progressive small localized tumors. However, because these tumors have a very high rate of recurrence, diffuse tumors frequently are managed with compression stockings with improvement in symptoms. Aggressive fibromatosis is the most aggressive benign soft-tissue neoplasm. These tumors are poorly encapsulated and invade surrounding normal muscle planes. They are typically treated with wide resection and recurrence rates are similar to those observed with high grade malignancies. Radiation therapy reduces the incidence of recurrent disease. Low dose chemotherapy, using adriamycin and decarbazine, has been effective in controlling unresectable tumors. Successful therapy with a less toxic regimen, consisting of tamoxifen and diclofenac, has recently been described, and as the biology of these tumors is better defined, it is likely that additional therapies will emerge. Although hemangioma and aggressive fibromatosis affect adults, they are the most common benign soft-tissue tumors in the pediatric population.

Soft-Tissue Sarcoma

Soft-tissue sarcomas are a heterogeneous group of tumors derived from mesenchymal stem cells. The tumors are more frequent than bone sarcomas, but are still quite rare, with approximately 6,000 new cases each year in the United States.

Although the tumors are classified into various histologic subtypes based on patterns of tissue-specific differentiation, adult soft-tissue sarcomas frequently are lumped together and considered as a group because of the similarity of their clinical behavior (Fig. 7). The various histologic subtypes have predilections for certain age groups and, in some cases, for anatomic sites (Table 8).

Rhabdomyosarcoma is the most common pediatric soft-tissue sarcoma and has a peak incidence in children younger than 10 years of age. Unlike the soft-tissue sarcomas in adults, which are relatively chemoresistant, rhabdomyosarcomas are highly responsive to chemotherapeutic intervention, and long-term survival has improved dramatically with the advent of multiagent chemotherapy. Current long-term survival rates are between 60% and 70%. The prognosis of rhabdomyosarcoma depends on the histologic subtype; the more malignant variety, alveolar rhabdomyosarcoma is more common in the trunk and extremities. Local treatment of rhabdomyosarcoma consists of wide excision, with the addition of radiation therapy for inadequate excision. Approximately 25% percent of synovial sarcomas occur in an adolescent population and are the most common nonrhabdomyosarcoma soft-tissue tumors in this age group. Synovial sarcomas in this age group behave similarly to other soft-tissue sarcomas in adults.

Table 8
Incidence and clinical features of selected soft-tissue sarcomas

Histology	Relative Incidence (%)	Peak Age Range	Clinical/Histologic Features
Malignant fibrous histiocytoma (MFH)	25-30	50-80	Fibroblasts and histocytes arranged in a whirling, storiform pattern; 5 subtypes: storiform-pleomorphic, myxoid, giant cell, inflammatory, and angiomatoid
Liposarcoma	20-25	40-60	4 histologic types; myxoid most common (50%); well differentiated with best prognosis, pleomorphic with the worst
Synovial sarcoma	10-15	20-40	Most common soft-tissue sarcoma of the foot and ankle; histologically cytokeratin (+); biphasic tumors (epithelial and fibrous areas) with better prognosis than monophasic tumors (fibroblastic); calcification common, improves prognosis; lymph node metastases
Fibrosarcoma	8-12	30-50	Previously most common soft-tissue sarcoma prior to reclassification of many tumors as MFH; historically presents with herringbone pattern; low grade tumors need to be distinguished from desmoid tumor
Leiomyosarcoma	5-10	50-70	Occur most commonly in retroperitoneum or intra-abdominal area; more common in women
Peripheal nerve sheath tumor	5-10	20-50	Most cases associated with neurofibromatosis or prior radiation; most commonly develop in association with major nerves
Epithelioid sarcoma	< 5	20-40	The majority occur in the forearm and hand, making it among the most common sarcomas in this location; epithelial markers are positive on histologic stains; metastases to lymph nodes
Clear cell sarcoma	< 5	20-40	Arises from tenosynovial structures and common in the distal lower extremity and foot; probable neuroectodermal origin and histologically similar to melanoma and renal cell carcinoma
Angiosarcoma	< 1	Adult	Majority of tumors associated with chronic lymphedema; unlike other sarcomas, typically cutaneous, presents with multiple blue-purple spots

Although the overall survival of adults with soft-tissue sarcomas in the United States is approximately 50%, survival is highly dependent on the grade and size of the tumor. The 5-year rate of distant recurrence in 1,041 patients presenting with localized extremity soft-tissue sarcomas was found to be 7% for low grade tumors and 37% for high grade tumors. A recent study of 471 sarcoma patients identified 20%, 41%, and 53% rates of metastasis in tumors from 1 to 5, 6 to 10, and 11 to 15 cm, respectively. Although tumors located in the subcutaneous tissues have a lower propensity for metastasis, data from a recent study indicated that differences in metastasis in superficial and deep sarcomas are due primarily to differences in size.

Local recurrence is a risk factor for metastasis, with data from the Swedish National Tumor Registry demonstrating a 29% incidence of metastasis in all primary soft-tissue sarcomas compared to a 53% incidence in recurrent tumors.

Metastases are primarily to the lungs and rarely to regional lymph nodes, except for synovial sarcoma, rhabdomyosarcoma, and epithelioid sarcoma, all of which have a rate of regional nodal metastases of between 20% and 30%. Bone metastases from soft-tissue sarcoma were recently documented in 10.1% of 277 soft-tissue sarcoma patients, with a pathologic fracture apparent in 21 of 44 lesions. Although pulmonary metastases are typically evident within 1 year, the mean time to onset of bone metastases was 18 months.

The reported incidence of local recurrence in soft-tissue sarcoma has varied in recent large series from rates of 6% to 21%. Risk factors include a prior local recurrence, inadequate surgical margins, and tumor grade; radiation therapy is a negative risk factor. Certain histologic subtypes, including fibrosarcoma and malignant peripheral nerve tumor, are associated with increased local recurrence. The presence of positive margins is highly associated with the development of recurrent tumor. In a study of 271 patients with malignant fibrous histiocytoma, positive surgical margins were associated with a 39% local recurrence rate compared to a recurrence rate of 17% in patients with negative margins. Two recent studies examined the findings in 95 and 67 patients with inadequate resections. Residual tumor was found in 56 of the 95 and 30 of the 67 patients, respectively, on reexcision. Because metastases are more likely to occur after local recurrence, primary reexcision is recommended for incompletely excised soft-tissue sarcomas. Local recurrence has been associated with decreased long-term survival.

Management of Soft-Tissue Sarcoma in Adults

The local control of soft-tissue sarcoma generally requires a combination of surgical and adjuvant radiation therapy. Adequate surgical resection involves complete tumor removal with surgical margins free of tumor involvement. Marginal resections, which are through the reactive tissue surrounding the tumor, are inadequate because this region is typically penetrated by tumor cells. While radical, or extracompartmental, surgery is associated with local recurrence rates approaching zero, the functional deficits associated with these surgeries are not generally compatible with limb salvage. For this reason, most surgical resections are done with wide margins, and the adequacy of the resection is very dependent on the tissues present at the margins. Fascial tissues are excellent barriers to tumor spread and 1-mm fascial margins are typically acceptable. However, muscle and fat are poor barriers to tumor spread and at least 2 or 3 cm of normal tissue is optimal.

Adjuvant radiation therapy, which is highly effective at controlling microscopic residual tumor, is a critical component of limb salvage surgery. Radiation therapy decreases the rate of local recurrence by more than 50%. Radiation therapy for soft-tissue sarcomas is generally at doses in excess of 50 Gy, approaching the toxic dose for many tissues, and thus must be carefully planned. Rates of tumor control are similar regardless of whether radiation therapy is given preoperatively or postoperatively, although wound healing complications are more common in patients receiving preoperative radiation therapy. To decrease wound healing complications, doses of preoperative radiation therapy are typically limited to 50 Gy, with additional radiation given postoperatively. Free tissue transfer has become an essential component for limb salvage surgery in the setting of wound complications. Because of the risk of wound healing, as well as a long-term risk of a secondary radiation-induced sarcoma, it is probably reasonable to avoid radiation therapy in selected low grade sarcomas in which adequate resections have been performed. Delivery of radiation through the use of indwelling brachytherapy catheters, which are implanted at the time of surgical resection, is another acceptable method of adjuvant radiation therapy to the surgical bed.

Chemotherapy has been controversial in the treatment of soft-tissue sarcomas and continues to be given on an experimental basis. However, soft-tissue sarcomas have been shown to respond to some chemotherapeutic agents, including adriamycin and ifosfamide. In combination, response rates of between 18% and 45% have been reported with these agents in patients with metastatic disease. Synovial sarcoma appears to be particularly responsive to ifosfamide. A recent study demonstrated 9 partial responses and 4 complete responses in 13 patients with metastatic synovial sarcoma. However, a clear survival benefit has not been demonstrated with chemotherapeutic agents, and controlled, randomized trials are ongoing. Ifosfamide and adriamycin are typically used in current trials. A protocol using MAID chemotherapy, (ifosfamide, adriamycin, decarbazine, and the bladder protective agent, MESNA), is being used at several tumor centers in the United States Because of the toxicity of these agents, chemotherapy trials typically include only patients with large, high grade tumors, which are at significant risk for metastasis.

Thoracotomy for the treatment of lung metastasis is another useful adjuvant in the management of soft-tissue sarcomas. Aggressive management of pulmonary metastases in patients with soft-tissue sarcoma results in 5-year disease free survival rates as high as 40% and frequently requires multiple thoracotomies.

Annotated Bibliography

Evaluation and Staging

Ayala AG, Ro JY, Fanning CV, Flores JP, Yasko AW: Core needle biopsy and fine-needle aspiration in the diagnosis of bone and soft-tissue lesions. *Hematol Oncol Clin North Am* 1995;9: 633–651.

This review of a 16-year experience with over 800 percutaneous biopsies of bone and soft-tissue lesions indicates that in most instances needle biopsy will be diagnostic and that it has many advantages over open biopsy.

Brien EW, Terek RM, Geer RJ, Caldwell G, Brennan MF, Healey JH: Treatment of soft-tissue sarcomas of the hand. *J Bone Joint Surg* 1995;77A:564–571.

This study documents the aggressive nature, difficulty in obtaining negative margins, and poor survival of seemingly innocuous small soft-tissue sarcomas occurring in the hand.

Fleming J, Cooper J, Henson DE, et al (eds): *Manual for Staging of Cancer*, ed 5. Philadelphia, PA, JB Lippincott, 1997.

This is the standard reference for staging of cancer used by medical and surgical oncologists.

Mankin HJ, Mankin CJ, Simon MA: The hazards of the biopsy, revisited: For the members of the Musculoskeletal Tumor Society. *J Bone Joint Surg* 1996;78:656–663.

Errors in diagnosis, complications of the biopsy, and changes in the course of treatment were 2 to 12 times greater if the biopsy was done in a referring institution rather than a treatment center; 27% of biopsies done at referring institutions had an error in diagnosis.

O'Reilly R, Link M, Fletcher B, et al: NCCN pediatric osteosarcoma practice guidelines. The National Comprehensive Cancer Network. *Oncology* 1996;10:1799–1812.

These are current treatment recommendations for pediatric osteosarcoma.

Pisters PWT, Leung DHY, Woodruff J, Shi W, Brennan MF: Analysis of prognostic factors in 1041 patients with localized soft tissue sarcomas of the extremities. *J Clin Oncol* 1996;14: 1679–1689.

In the largest series of prospectively studied patients with extremity soft-tissue sarcoma, the significant variables differ depending on the end point. Prognostic factors for disease-specific survival are size > 10 cm, high grade, deep location, recurrent disease at presentation, leiomyosarcoma and malignant peripheral-nerve tumor, microscopically positive surgical margins, and lower extremity site.

Skrzynski MC, Biermann JS, Montag A, Simon MA: Diagnostic accuracy and charge-savings of outpatient core needle biopsy compared with open biopsy of musculoskeletal tumors. *J Bone Joint Surg* 1996;78:644–649.

The diagnostic accuracy of core needle biopsy in 62 patients was 84%, and hospital charges were considerably less than for open biopsy. Clinical acumen is critical for the successful use of this technique.

Soft-tissue sarcoma surgical practice guidelines. *Oncology* 1997;11:1327–1332.

These are the current staging and treatment practice guidelines by the Society of Surgical Oncology for soft-tissue sarcoma.

Imaging

Davies AM, Pikoulas C, Griffith J: MRI of eosinophilic granuloma. *Eur. J Radiol* 1994;18:205–209.

This study showed that eosinophilic granuloma had less peritumoral edema than osteomyelitis or Ewing's sarcoma and that it had a low signal intensity rim on short tau inversion recovery (STIR) sequence.

De Beuckeleer LH, De Schepper AM, Ramon F, Somville J: Magnetic resonance imaging of cartilaginous tumors: A retrospective study of 79 patients. *Eur J Radiol* 1995;21:34–40.

In this series, the combination of low signal intensity on T2-weighted images and ring and arc enhancement after gadolineum administration had a specificity of 92.3% and sensitivity of 76.5% in distinguishing low-grade chondrosarcoma from enchondroma.

De Beuckeleer LH, De Schepper AM, Ramon F: Magnetic resonance imaging of cartilaginous tumors: Is it useful or necessary? *Skeletal Radiol* 1996;25:137–141.

MRI improves accuracy in diagnosing low-grade chondrosarcomas. Because osteochondromas have a characteristic appearance on plain films, MRI contributes only in the diagnostic workup of cases in which malignant transformation is suspected.

Fletcher BD, Hanna SL: Pediatric musculoskeletal lesions simulating neoplasms. *Magn Reson Imaging Clin N Am* 1996;4: 721–747.

This article describes the common developmental, infectious, traumatic, and iatrogenic lesions in which the initial presentation is that of a malignant, musculoskeletal neoplasm.

Gelineck J, Keller J, Myhre Jensen O, Nielsen OS, Christensen T: Evaluation of lipomatous soft tissue tumors by MR imaging. *Acta Radiol* 1994;35:367–370.

The MRI findings in 43 patients with lipomatous tumors ≥5 cm in diameter were correlated to histologic features and diagnosis. Twenty-six tumors were classic lipomas on MRI and at microscopy; 8 lipomas raised suspicion of malignancy at MRI but all were histologically benign; and 9 tumors considered malignant at MRI proved to be malignant by microscopy

Holscher HC, Bloem JL, Van Der Woude HJ, et al: Can MRI predict the histopathological response in patients with osteosarcoma after the first cycle of chemotherapy? *Clin Radiol* 1995;50: 384–390.

Increase in tumor volume and of the T2 signal intensity of an extraosseous tumor can predict a poor response after 1 cycle of chemotherapy.

Janzen L, Logan PM, O'Connell JX, Connell DG, Munk PL: Intramedullary chondroid tumors of bone: Correlation of abnormal peritumoral marrow and soft-tissue MRI signal with tumor type. *Skeletal Radiol* 1997;26:100–106.

Abnormal marrow or soft-tissue signal around a chondroid tumor is suggestive of chondrosarcoma, even in the absence of bone destruction. STIR images are necessary for adequate detection of peritumoral signal abnormalities.

Kawai A, Sugihara S, Kunisada T, Uchida Y, Inoue H: Imaging assessment of the response of bone tumors to preoperative chemotherapy. *Clin Orthop* 1997;216–225.

This study compares the ability to predict response to chemotherapy of digital subtraction angiography, thallium scintigraphy, and dynamic MRI. Dynamic MRI had a 100% sensitivity, 85.7% specificity, and 90.9% accuracy.

Munk PL, Lee MJ, Janzen DL, et al: Lipoma and liposarcoma: Evaluation using CT and MR imaging. *Am J Roentgenol* 1997;169:589–594.

This article describes CT and MRI characteristics of benign and malignant fatty tumors.

Sundaram M: The use of gadolinium in the MR imaging of bone tumors. *Semin Ultrasound CT MR* 1997;18:307–311.

The author suggests that gadolinium is not necessary for routine evaluation of solitary bone lesions, but may be useful for evaluating intra-articular extention of osteosarcoma and response of osteosarcoma to chemotherapy.

Molecular Biology of Sarcoma

Ahn J, Ludecke H-J, Lindow S, et al: Cloning of the putative tumor suppressor gene for hereditary multiple extoses (EXT1). *Nat Genet* 1995;11:137–143.

Baldini N, Scotlandi K, Barbanti-Brodano G, et al: Expression of p-glycoprotein in high-grade osteosarcomas in relation to clinical outcome. *N Engl J Med* 1995;333:1380–1385.

Increased levels of p-glycoprotein in osteosarcoma were associated with a decreased probability of event-free survival but did not correlate with tumor necrosis.

Gebhardt MC: Molecular biology of sarcomas. *Orthop Clin North Am* 1996;27:421–429.

This is an excellent review of molecular genetics for the orthopaedist.

Kawai A, Woodruff J, Healey JH, Brennan MF, Antonescu CR, Ladanyi M: SYT-SSX gene fusion as a determinant of morphology and prognosis in synovial sarcoma. *N Eng J Med* 1998; 338:153–160.

The type of SYT-SSX fusion has prognostic and diagnostic significance. Tumors with a SYT-SSX1 fusion have a worse prognosis and may be monophasic or biphasic, whereas those with a SYT-SSX2 fusion were all monophasic and had a better prognosis.

Bone Tumors

Abudu A, Sferopoulos NK, Tillman RM, Carter SR, Grimer RJ: The surgical treatment and outcome of pathological fractures in localised osteosarcoma. *J Bone Joint Surg* 1996;78B:694–698.

Limb salvage surgery was performed in 27 of 40 patients and amputation in the other 13. Recurrence rates were 19% for limb salvage and zero for amputation. The 5-year survival rate was 64% with limb salvage and 47% with amputation.

Grimer RJ, Carter SR, Pynsent PB: The cost-effectiveness of limb salvage for bone tumours. *J Bone Joint Surg* 1997;79B: 558–561.

The authors developed a formula for calculating the ongoing costs of limb salvage with an endoprosthesis compared to amputation, using historic data to show the likelihood of further surgery and revision.

Lokiec F, Ezra E, Khermosh O, Wientroub S: Simple bone cysts treated by percutaneous autologous marrow grafting: A preliminary report. *J Bone Joint Surg* 1996;78B:934–937.

The authors describe 10 consecutive cases in which unicameral cysts were treated with percutaneous biopsy, aspiration, and injection of autogenous bone marrow aspirated from the iliac crest. Pain was relieved in all patients by 2 weeks with return to full activities within 6 weeks. Complete healing and remodeling occurred by 4 months.

O'Donnell RJ, Springfield DS, Motwani HK, Ready JE, Gebhardt MC, Mankin HJ: Recurrence of giant-cell tumors of the long bones after curettage and packing with cement. *J Bone Joint Surg* 1994;76A:1827–1833.

The authors report local recurrence in 15 of 60 patients with a giant cell tumor of the long bone treated with curettage and polymethyl-methacrylate cementation. The recurrence rate was reduced to 17% (7 of 41) in patients in which the tumor cavity was treated with phenol or a high speed burr prior to cementation.

Ozaki T, Hillmann A, Hoffmann C, et al: Significance of surgical margin on the prognosis of patients with Ewing's sarcoma: A report from the Cooperative Ewing's Sarcoma Study. *Cancer* 1996;78:892–900.

Surgical management of 242 patients with or without radiation treatment resulted in a 7% recurrence rate compared to a recurrence rate of 31% with radiation alone. The 10-year overall survival was similar in the surgically treated cases.

Rosenthal DI, Springfield DS, Gebhardt MC, Rosenberg AE, Mankin HJ: Osteoid osteoma: Percutaneous radio-frequency ablation. *Radiology* 1995;197:451–454.

The authors present their results in 18 patients with osteoid osteoma treated by thermal necrosis using a small radiofrequency electrode that creates a 1-cm area of thermal necrosis. Symptoms were relieved in 16 of 18 patients; one patient had a second procedure. There were no recurrences or complications.

Velez-Yanguas MC, Warrier RP: The evolution of chemotherapeutic agents for the treatment of pediatric musculoskeletal malignancies. *Orthop Clin North Am* 1996;27:545–549.

The authors review the principles of chemotherapeutic treatment of osteosarcoma, Ewing's sarcoma, and rhabdomyosarcoma, including potential complications of treatment.

Chondrosarcoma

Ozaki T, Lindner N, Hillmann A, Rodl R, Blasius S, Winkelmann W: Influence of intralesional surgery on treatment outcome of chondrosarcoma. *Cancer* 1996;77:1292–1297.

The authors reviewed the results in 26 chondrosarcoma patients treated with intralesional surgery, including 18 in the axial skeleton, and 8 in an extremity. The 20-year overall survival rate was 68% for intralesional surgery and 66% for wide or marginal. Survival was 85% in grade 1 or 2 tumors, and only 44% in grade 3 tumors. Central tumors had a 57% survival compared with 87% in extremity tumors.

Raskind WH, Conrad EU, Chansky H, Matsushita M: Loss of heterozygosity in chondrosarcomas for markers linked to hereditary multiple exostoses loci on chromosomes 8 and 11. *Am J Hum Genet* 1995;56:1132–1139.

The authors evaluated 18 sporadic chondrosarcomas for loss of constitutional heterozygosity (LOH) at polymorphic loci. Four of 17 sporadic chondrosarcomas had LOH for markers linked to EXT 1, and 7 showed LOH for markers linked to EXT 2. The findings support a possible tumor suppresser function for these genes in cartilage.

Metastases

Hicks DG, Gokan T, O'Keefe RJ, et al: Primary lymphoma of bone: Correlation of magnetic resonance imaging features with cytokine production by tumor cells. *Cancer* 1995;75:973–980.

The authors identified channels of tumor permeation through the cortex in 4 patients with primary lymphoma of bone on both MRI scans and histology sections. These channels were produced and lined by host osteoclasts that were actively resorbing bone. The tumor cells produced large amounts of interleukin-1, interleukin-6, and tumor necrosis factor-alpha.

Hortobagyi GN, Theriault RL, Porter L, et al: Efficacy of pamidronate in reducing skeletal complications in patients with breast cancer and lytic bone metastases: Protocol 19 Aredia Breast Cancer Study Group. *N Engl J Med* 1996; 335: 1785–1791.

In this study, 380 women receiving chemotherapy for stage IV breast cancer and at least one lytic bone lesion were randomized to receive placebo or intravenous pamidronate. Mean time to first skeletal complication was longer in the pamidronate group (13.1 versus 7.0 months), and the proportion of patients in whom a skeletal complication occurred was smaller (43% versus 56%).

Soft-Tissue Sarcoma

Choong PF, Pritchard DJ, Rock MG, Sim FH, Frassica FJ: Survival after pulmonary metastasectomy in soft tissue sarcoma: Prognostic factors in 214 patients. *Acta Orthop Scand* 1995;66:561–568.

The authors describe the outcome in 214 patients with metastatic soft-tissue sarcoma who underwent pulmonary metastasectomy. The tumors were high grade in 88%, and adjuvant chemotherapy was given to 163 patients. The 5-year overall survival was 40%. Prognostic factors included the size and number of metastases; a metastasis-free interval of less than 18 months was an unfavorable factor.

Goodlad JR, Fletcher CD, Smith MA: Surgical resection of primary soft-tissue sarcoma: Incidence of residual tumour in 95 patients needing re-excision after local resection. *J Bone Joint Surg* 1996;78B:658–661.

The authors performed a reexcision in 95 patients with soft-tissue sarcomas initially excised at other institutions with inadequate margins. Tumor tissue was found in 29 of 55 lower limb, 16 of 25 upper limb, 7 of 10 trunk, and 4 of 5 head and neck tumor specimens. The tumor was macroscopically detectable in 31 specimens.

Classic Bibliography

Enneking WF: A system of staging musculoskeletal neoplasms. *Clin Orthop* 1986;204:9–24.

Finn HA, Simon MA: Staging systems for musculoskeletal neoplasms. *Orthopedics* 1989;12:1365–1371.

Nelson TE, Enneking WF: Staging of bone and soft tissue sarcomas revisited, in Stauffer RN (ed): *Advances in Operative Orthopedics*. St Louis, MO, Mosby Year-Book, 1994, vol 2, pp 379–291.

Schima W, Amann G, Stiglbauer R, et al: Preoperative staging of osteosarcoma: Efficacy of MR imaging in detecting joint involvement. *Am J Roentgenol* 1994;163:1171–1175.

Simon MA, Biermann JS: Biopsy of bone and soft-tissue lesions, in Schafer M (ed): *Instructional Course Lectures 43*. Rosemont, IL, American Academy of Orthopaedic Surgeons, 1994, pp 521–526.

Simon MA, Finn HA: Diagnostic strategy for bone and soft-tissue tumors, in Schafer M (ed): *Instructional Course Lectures 43*. Rosemont, IL, American Academy of Orthopaedic Surgeons, 1994, pp 527–536.

Springfield DS: Staging systems for musculoskeletal neoplasia, in Schafer M (ed): *Instructional Course Lectures 43*. Rosemont, IL, American Academy of Orthopaedic Surgeons, 1994, pp 537–542.

Chapter 18
Infection

Introduction

Despite recent advances in diagnosis, antibiotic development, and refined surgical techniques, the management of orthopaedic infections remains a challenging clinical problem. Even as new antimicrobials are introduced, microorganisms are developing resistance to related antibiotics. Preventing iatrogenic infection, limiting nosocomial transmission, and combating multiple-drug resistant organisms have developed into important issues. Hospital restrictions on antibiotic use have complicated drug selection and made infectious disease consultation mandatory in many instances. The economic impact of infection has become increasingly obvious. Under the influence of managed care, the cost and effectiveness of various treatment alternatives have been questioned and efforts have been made to decrease hospitalization and limit parenteral antibiotics. A high index of suspicion, early intervention, and aggressive treatment are important, as bacteria become less responsive to medical management. Several unusual inflammatory conditions have been described that mimic pyogenic orthopaedic infections, and for pediatric cases, these conditions must often be considered in the differential diagnosis.

Bacterial Virulence

Infection reflects a complex interaction between the host, a pathogen, and the response of each to the other. Virulence factors are the mechanisms pathogens use to circumvent the normal host defenses and are critical in the pathogenesis of any infection. *Escherichia coli* produces a cytotoxic necrotizing factor, a hemolysin, and a toxic extracellular superoxide. *Pseudomonas aeruginosa* produces an extracellular fibrinogen binding protein, and at least 2 exoproteases that cleave and inactivate immunoglobulins. *Staphylococcus aureus* virulence factors include alpha hemolysin, protein A, fibronectin binding proteins, and a neutrophil toxin, leukocidin. A capsular polysaccharide on *S aureus* acts as a type II collagen receptor mediating adhesion to cartilage, and has been implicated in the development of septic arthritis. Streptococcal virulence factors include pyrogenic exotoxins A, B, and C; streptoki-

nase; streptolysin O and S; and M protein. M protein is a surface molecule that binds serum kininogens, the precursors to vasoactive kinins.

Streptococcal strains responsible for toxic shock-like syndrome produce pyrogenic exotoxin A. This syndrome, first identified in 1983, has a mortality rate of nearly 30%. The usual infectious focus is skin or soft tissues, and the salient features on presentation include hypotension, fever, rash, desquamation, and multiorgan failure. This disease is difficult to manage medically because of the invasive nature and extensive associated tissue necrosis. Early diagnosis and prompt surgical debridement are mandatory to prevent mortality in severe infections. As an adjunct to surgery, antibiotic coverage with cephalosporins, clindamycin, or vancomycin is most appropriate for an aggressive streptococcal infection.

Expression of the exopolysaccharide glycocalyx secludes bacteria from host defenses and antibiotics, accounting for their resistance to treatment. Bacteria enveloped in this extracellular coating, often considered a form of slime, are readily demonstrated on tissues and biomaterials retrieved from infections related to prostheses and internal fixation devices. Glycocalyx is composed of protein and carbohydrate, and is an important factor facilitating bacterial adherence to orthopaedic implants. Other factors affecting adherence to biomaterials include surface charges and alterations in the host immune response.

Antibiotic Resistance

Microorganisms resistant to standard antibiotic regimens are becoming more common and pose a major health threat at the close of this century. Resistance to available antimicrobial agents is increasing, including resistance to both penicillinase-resistant penicillins (oxacillin and methicillin) and fluoroquinolones by staphylococci, resistance to the glycopeptides (vancomycin and teicoplanin) by enterococci, and resistance to imipenem by pseudomonads. New compounds for effective therapy against antimicrobial-resistant gram-positive species are needed. Development of resistance is facilitated by inadequate dosing regimens, empiric prescription of broad-spectrum antibiotics, and failure to adhere to

Table 1
Adverse reactions to antibiotics

Reaction	Frequent	Occasional	Rare
Dermatologic			
rash	ampicillin	cephalosporins	metronidazole
	co-trimoxazole	clindamycin	erythromycin
	penicillins		
	vancomycin		
Gastrointestinal			
abdominal pain/cramping	erythromycin	metronidazole	
diarrhea	clindamycin	all antibiotics	
	ampicillin		
nausea/vomiting	erythromycin (IV and PO)	imipenem (with rapid infusion)	
	co-trimoxazole		
pseudomembranous colitis	clindamycin	beta-lactams	
	ampicillin		
Hematologic			
anemia	amphotericin B	penicillins (hemolytic)	
	(normochromic, normocytic)	co-trimoxazole (megaloblastic)	
hypoprothrombinemia	moxalactam	cefoperazone	
		cefamandole	
		cefotetan	
		cefamandole	
neutropenia		co-trimoxazole	
		vancomycin	
		penicillins	
		cephalosporins	
platelet dysfunction	moxalactam		
	carbenicillin		
	ticarcillin		
Hepatobiliary			
biliary sludging			erythromycin
cholestatic hepatitis			co-trimoxazole
transaminase enzyme elevations		nafcillin	
		ticarcillin	
		aztreonam	
		imipenem	
		co-trimoxazole	
		ceftriaxone	
Neurologic			
neuropathy		metronidazole	
ototoxicity		aminoglycosides	vancomycin
			erythromycin
seizures		imipenem	penicillins
		ciprofloxacin	
Phlebitis	erythromycin	cephalosporins	penicillins
	vancomycin	metronidazole	clindamycin
	amphotericin B		
	nafcillin		
Renal			
acute tubular necrosis		aminoglycosides	beta-lactams
		amphotericin B	
dose-dependent renal insufficiency	aminoglycosides		
	amphotericin B		
hypokalemia	amphotericin B	carbenicillin	aminoglycosides
		ticarcillin	
interstitial nephritis		methicillin	rifampin

(Reproduced with permission from Kasser JR (ed): *Orthopaedic Knowledge Update 5*. Rosemont, IL, American Academy of Orthopaedic Surgeons, 1996, pp 149–161.)

standard principles of management of infectious diseases. Proper antibiotic selection is based on cultures and sensitivities, and narrow-spectrum antibiotics diminish the risk of developing resistance. Resistance develops by either direct genetic exchange or spontaneous mutation. Direct genetic exchange often involves transfer of plasmids, small independently reproducing strands of DNA. Bacteria are able to survive in the presence of antibiotic if transferred genetic material confers resistance by encoding proteins that alter surface receptors, change cell wall permeability, or enhance metabolism of the drug itself. Spontaneous mutations may affect the specific target of the antibiotic, subtly altering the interaction at the molecular level.

Enterococci are second only to staphylococci in causing hospital-acquired infections, and drug resistance among these organisms is a growing problem. Vancomycin-resistant enterococci (VRE) now account for 7.9% of nosocomial enterococcal infections, and many hospitals have found it necessary to enforce strict isolation precautions to limit further spread. Use of gloves, gowns, and hand washing by physicians and nurses are the most important means of controlling nosocomial transmission. Treatment regimens for these pathogens have been developed, but efficacy is not yet clearly established. Multiple antibiotic resistant organisms are an even greater threat and to date no effective treatment regimen is available.

Antimicrobial Treatment of Osteomyelitis

Appropriate antibiotic coverage based on cultures and sensitivities of adequate specimens is still the mainstay of medical management. The duration of treatment is empiric and partially based on the clinical response and on any adverse reactions to the antibiotic (Table 1). The often recommended standard length of antibiotic administration has been 4 to 6 weeks, but there is no evidence this regimen is superior to treatment for shorter periods. Successful treatment correlates best with serum levels of antibiotic and not the route of administration. Although parenteral antibiotics at home have led to a decrease in the total cost of therapy, patients may often be transferred to an oral antibiotic without a significant decrease in efficacy. Patient compliance is more difficult to monitor with oral administration, and parenteral routes may be preferred in some patients. Oral antibiotic coverage is appropriate for responsible patients but must still be based on the results of microbiology studies, and its use should be monitored by serum bactericidal levels at intervals during treatment.

New Antibiotics

The prevalence of multidrug resistant strains of common gram-positive organisms has grown rapidly. Increasingly, methicillin resistant *S aureus* (MRSA), methicillin resistant *S epidermidis* (MRSE), and VRE are identified as pathogens in serious infections. This increase in resistance highlights the need for new antimicrobials to expand our therapeutic options.

Quinupristin/dalfopristin is the first of a unique class of antibiotics called streptogramins. Streptogramin antibiotics are each composed of 2 chemically distinct compounds, and when administered together act synergistically to inhibit bacterial protein synthesis. The combination of these 2 components results in a drug less susceptible to the development of resistance. Streptogramins are characterized by their unique mechanism of action, intracellular activity, synergistic components, and broad spectrum of activity against gram-positive cocci. Clinical evidence suggests they may be effective against multidrug resistant organisms including both MRSA and VRE. Novobiocin is one of the coumarin group of antibacterials, classical inhibitors of DNA gyrase, and several studies suggest it may be useful for treating VRE. It also inhibits adenosine triphosphatase (ATPase) activity and hydrolysis and acts as an antiviral agent by interfering with viral assembly.

Teicoplanin, a new semisynthetic glycopeptide antibiotic similar to vancomycin, has proved effective in the treatment of various gram-positive infections. Glycopeptides act by binding the peptidoglycan precursor terminus, the target of transglycosylase and transpeptidase enzymes. Teicoplanin exhibits in vitro activity against gram-positive pathogens equal to or greater than that of vancomycin. The pharmacokinetics of teicoplanin allow for once-daily dosing, either intravenous or intramuscular with reliable absorption for patients with limited venous access. Teicoplanin is potentially safer than vancomycin and associated with less nephrotoxicity or ototoxicity.

There continues to be tremendous interest in the development of alternative fluoroquinolones, although there are concerns regarding the toxic effect of fluoroquinolones on both adult and pediatric cartilage. The quinolones are related to nalidixic acid, and fluorinated quinolones have been the most effective clinically. Fluoroquinolones are bactericidal by interfering with bacterial DNA synthesis, inhibiting the A subunit of bacterial topoisomerase resulting in uncontrolled messenger RNA and protein synthesis. Tissue bioavailability is excellent, and oral administration is virtually equivalent to parenteral routes. Fluoroquinolones are active against a broad spectrum including gram-negative and gram-positive aerobic and facultative anaerobic bacteria. Ciprofloxacin is a potent oral anti-Pseudomonal drug, but less active against common Staphylococcal clinical isolates than cephalosporins and other less expensive oral alternatives. Ofloxacin contains an even mix of its own levo- and dextrorotatory isomers, but the levorotatory isomer is far more potent. Levofloxacin has been developed as the more active isomer of ofloxacin.

Local Antibiotic Depots

Use of antibiotic-laden polymethylmethacrylate (PMMA) beads and spacers has become a very popular means of local antibiotic delivery and dead space management. This technique can be used to deliver tremendously high local concentrations of antibiotic with very little concomitant systemic administration. Powdered antibiotics such as vancomycin and tobramycin can be used, although only gentamicin-laden beads are available commercially. PMMA beads can be used acutely for open fracture management, and the bead pouch technique is useful as a temporizing measure for difficult wounds until formal coverage can be arranged. Antibiotic impregnated beads facilitate staged management of chronic musculoskeletal infections, obliterating the debridement defect and simultaneously delivering high local concentrations of antibiotic. Although concentrations may be so high locally they are potentially toxic to osteoblasts, very little of this antibiotic is distributed systemically. Use of antibiotic-laden PMMA beads often requires a second surgical procedure, although removal and exchange for bone graft is not mandatory in all cases.

Use of a biodegradable carrier for local antibiotic delivery and dead space obliteration offers the advantages of PMMA beads, with the additional distinct benefit of gradual spontaneous degradation. Several materials are currently under investigation as potential carriers of antibiotic, including polylactic acid and poly(DL-lactide)-coglycolide. Bio-degradable antibiotic depots may take the form of beads, microspheres, or can be applied as a thin coating on orthopaedic implants.

Osteomyelitis in Adults

Indium-labeled leukocyte scintigraphy and magnetic resonance imaging (MRI) have made it possible to diagnose subclinical osteomyelitis and its extent within the medullary canal. Sequential technetium-gallium imaging is preferred if the focus involves the vertebral column, because the hematopoietic nature of the vertebral marrow makes interpretation of indium-labeled leukocyte scintigraphy images difficult.

MRI is superior to indium-labeled leukocyte scintigraphy in defining the extent of infection. The extent of intra- and extramedullary disease seen on MRI correlates directly with

that seen on serial sectioning of amputated specimens. MRI cannot differentiate between edema and bacteria-induced cellulitis; and it differentiates poorly between areas of abnormal marrow resulting from chronic inactive osteomyelitis and areas previously disrupted by trauma or surgery. MRI is unable to define the presence of a cortical osteomyelitis if there is no cortical disruption or medullary involvement.

Lack of a standardized classification and clinical staging system hampers evaluation of different treatment regimens. Considerations include the bone involved, the duration of infection (acute versus chronic), the mechanism of infection (hematogenous versus exogenous), the site of infection (medullary versus cortical, periarticular versus diaphyseal, localized versus diffuse), and the local and systemic quality of the host.

Surgical treatment of osteomyelitis consists of the excision of all necrotic and infected tissue. Aggressive debridement, appropriate antibiotics, and adequate dead space management can eradicate the infection in nearly all patients. Management may include antibiotic-impregnated methylmethacrylate beads, local or vascularized soft-tissue flaps, autogenous bone grafting (Fig. 1), distraction osteogenesis, or the use of vascularized bone grafts. Staging of reconstruction is important. Bone grafting is not effective if the donor material is placed into an inadequately prepared, inflammatory soft-tissue bed.

A complication of persistent, chronic osteomyelitis is the development of squamous cell carcinoma, which occurs in 0.2% to 1.7% of patients. Difficult cases may require amputation.

Septic Arthritis in Adults

Nongonococcal Bacterial Arthritis

Bacteria can reach a joint by direct inoculation or by contiguous spread from adjacent osteomyelitis, cellulitis, or septic bursitis. Bacterial phagocytosis, synovial proliferation, granulation tissue formation, and bone and cartilage destruction then begin. This destruction is mediated by the direct toxic effects of the bacteria and by the increased intracavitary pressure. Host cell phagocytosis and the release of proteolytic enzymes contribute to the tissue destruction. Lysosomal enzyme release within 24 hours of infection in animal models has been demonstrated. Glycosaminoglycan depletion occurs by day 5. Sterile inflammatory synovial fluids have been shown to contain proteinase capable of destroying articular cartilage.

Most patients with nongonococcal bacterial arthritis present with arthritis in only 1 joint, monoarticular septic arthritis (MASA). The knee is most affected. Although sys-

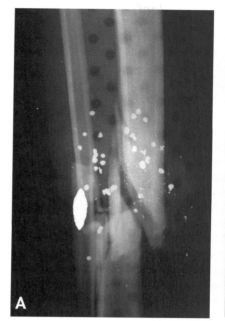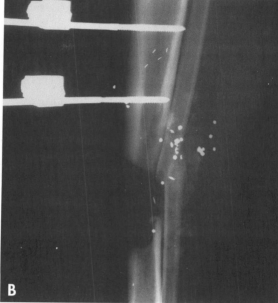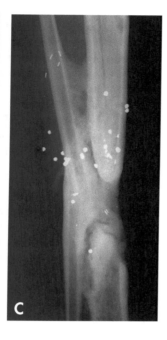

Figure 1

A, Emergency room radiograph of right tibia and fibula of 31-year-old male who had just sustained a close-range shotgun injury. B, Lateral radiograph of right tibia after debridement of all necrotic bone and soft tissue, external fixator stabilization, microvascular soft-tissue reconstruction at 5 days, and placement of autogenous cancellous iliac crest bone graft through Harmon posterolateral approach at 7 weeks. C, Anteroposterior radiograph view at 24 months, showing consolidation of bone graft with reconstitution of infection-free, weightbearing extremity. (Reproduced with permission from Kasser JR (ed): *Orthopaedic Knowledge Update 5*. Rosemont, IL, American Academy of Orthopaedic Surgeons, 1996, pp 149–161.)

temic symptoms of fever and chills are common, the local sign of infection is incapacitating joint pain.

Approximately one fourth of all septic arthritis patients may have more than 1 joint involved. In polyarticular septic arthritis (PASA), 3 or 4 joints are usually infected, and 40% of patients have extra-articular septic foci, such as pulmonary infections, endocarditis, and subcutaneous abscesses. Over 50% of patients with PASA have some form of rheumatologic disorder, which is usually in its more severe form at the time that the infection develops. The most common disease is rheumatoid arthritis (RA). Although RA affects more women than men, more men than women develop PASA. Patients with RA have a higher incidence of fatality. Delayed diagnosis of these infections because of the difficulty in distinguishing a rheumatoid flare from an acute infection contributes to the poor outcome in RA patients.

An important risk factor for the development of a joint infection is the presence of a prosthesis. Approximately 1% to 2% of all hip and knee arthroplasties are complicated by infection. Human immunodeficiency virus (HIV) infection also increases the risk of joint infection, although studies have shown no significant difference in the causative organisms, clinical presentation, treatment, or outcome in this group. However, the variety of infectious agents increases with the onset of clinical AIDS, while the chance of a successful outcome decreases. RA, diabetes mellitus, hemophilia, and sickle-cell anemia also predispose to infectious arthritis. In sickle-cell anemia, salmonella causes more than 50% of the infections.

The diagnosis of bacterial arthritis is based on the physical examination and on the analysis of synovial fluid. Although the white blood cell (WBC) count in the synovial fluid can vary, counts above 50,000 to 100,000 cells/ml in the immune competent host strongly suggest the presence of infection.

Patients with acute arthritis should be screened for both infectious and crystal-induced causes. The coexistence of these diseases can be missed by the failure to examine synovial fluid for bacteria or crystals if one or the other is found. Crystal-induced arthritis and septic arthritis may occur simultaneously because the decreased joint pH associated with infection decreases the solubility of urate.

Parenteral antibiotics should be initiated as soon as material for culture has been obtained. The goals of treatment include sterilization of the joint; decompression and removal of all inflammatory cells, enzymes, debris, or foreign bodies; elimination of the destructive pannus; and return to full function.

The best methods for drainage, decompression, and cleansing of the joint are debated. The physician must weigh the benefit of repeated aspiration versus arthroscopy or arthrotomy. Surgical drainage is indicated for all joints that do not respond to antibiotic therapy and aspiration within 72 hours, for those in which the synovial fluid appears to be loculated, and for infections involving the hip. Arthroscopy of the knee, when technically feasible, seems to be the best treatment to accompany antibiotic therapy in early septic arthritis.

Gonococcal Bacterial Arthritis

Neisseria gonorrhoeae is the most common cause of septic arthritis among young adults. The disease is 4 times more common in women than in men. Recent menstruation and the immediate postpartum period increase the risk of gonococcal dissemination. The disease most commonly presents with acute onset of migratory polyarthralgia, low-grade fever, and chills. Tenosynovitis and skin involvement are seen in two thirds of patients. Fewer than 50% of patients develop a true arthritis. The disease is frequently divided into the bacteremic form, characterized by dermatitis, tenosynovitis, fever, and chills, and the less frequent suppurative form in which arthritis is the primary manifestation. In these latter patients, there can be large purulent effusions. In all types of disseminated gonococcal infection, blood cultures are frequently negative, and only 50% of joint effusions are culture positive. Frequently, the patient will present without symptoms at the primary site of infection, whereas other patients will complain of vaginal or urethral discharge, urethritis, or dysuria.

Synovial fluid aspiration usually yields a WBC count between 30,000 and 100,000, primarily polymorphonuclear neutrophils. Gram stains are frequently negative, although concentrating the synovial fluid prior to staining can increase the sensitivity of this test. Gram stains and culture of skin lesions are rarely positive; blood cultures are positive in only 30% of patients. The best yield for positive cultures is the genitourinary tract. Cultures of the cervix or urethra are positive in 80% to 90% of women and 50% to 75% of men.

Patients, especially those with purulent effusions, should be hospitalized. Most infections are caused by penicillin-resistant strains of *N gonorrhoeae*, and a beta-lactamase-resistant cephalosporin, such as ceftriaxone, is usually the first line of therapy. After local signs of infection have subsided, oral antibiotics, such as amoxicillin with clavulanic acid, may be substituted. Antibiotic therapy should continue for at least 7 days. Large, purulent synovial effusions may require longer-term antibiotics with repeated aspiration. Open drainage is rarely necessary except with hip involvement. Patient educa-

tion and the treatment of sexual partners are crucially important in the prevention of recurrence.

Lyme Disease

Lyme disease, the most common vector-borne illness in the United States, is carried by the tick *Ixodes dammini* in the eastern and central United States and by *I pacificus* in the Pacific northwest. These ticks carry the causative gram-negative agent, *Borrelia burgdorferi*, between humans and their animal reservoirs: deer and rodents. The disease is seen throughout the United States. It is divided into the clinical stages of early localized infection (stage 1), early disseminated infection (stage 2), and persistent infection (stage 3). In stage 1, erythema migrans, the characteristic skin lesion, occurs within 3 to 32 days after the tick bite. Stage 2 is the first to have musculoskeletal involvement, usually migratory pain without swelling of both articular and periarticular structures.

Arthritis, the dominant feature of late Lyme disease, typically becomes symptomatic 6 months after infection, with intermittent inflammatory mono- or oligoarthritis of large joints, most frequently the knee. Initial attacks present with large effusions but are usually brief in duration. Episodes occurring in the second or third year usually last months. Of untreated patients, 19% progress to chronic Lyme arthritis (an episode of continual joint involvement lasting at least 1 year). Local factors may affect clinical presentation. Patients with high concentrations of interleukin-1 receptor antagonist and low levels of interleukin-1β had more rapid resolution of arthritis attacks than those with the opposite cytokine profile.

Diagnosis is complicated by the absence of a readily available, highly sensitive test. Enzyme-linked immunosorbent assay (ELISA) is 90% sensitive and specific in late disease, but in the early stages as few as 26% of patients have an immunoglobulin G (IgG) response. There is also very little standardization between, or even within, laboratories, and false positives and negatives occur. Immunoblotting may be as high as 95% specific, but again there is little standardization. Other possible modalities for diagnostic testing under development include polymerase chain reaction (PCR) and recombinant protein ELISA.

Treatment of Lyme disease is based on the stage of the infection. In early disease, oral treatment with amoxicillin for 10 to 30 days, depending on disease severity and clinical response, is adequate. Lyme arthritis initially should be treated with a course of doxycycline or amoxicillin for 30 days, with parenteral ceftriaxone reserved for nonresponders. In persistent arthritis, other therapies include intra-articular steroid injections or synovectomy.

Reactive Arthritis

Reactive arthritis (ReA), although not a true infection, is believed to have an infectious component. It is defined as an arthritis preceded by an immunologic sensitization. The pathogenesis of the disease is not clearly defined, but it is believed that spondyloarthropathies result from an inherited susceptibility, the HLA-B27 haplotype, combined with an infectious agent that serves as the inciting factor. It was previously thought that the infectious trigger only started the disease process. More recently, detection of DNA from various inciting agents at all stages of the disease indicates some continued role for the trigger. The Yersinia urease B subunit is an antigen that has been identified as one protein responsible for the disease process. It is believed that an interaction between the responsible infectious agents and the HLA-B27 haplotype leads to the progression of the disease via stimulation of CD8$^+$ cytotoxic T cells.

ReA is divided into urogenic, enterogenic, respiratory tract-associated, and idiopathic arthritis. *Clostridia, Salmonella, Shigella, Staphylococcal, Streptococcal, Neisseria* and *Mycobacteria* species all cause ReA. Idiopathic causes are decreasing as other causes are discovered. Some newly discovered triggers include hepatitis B vaccine, *Chlamydia pneumoniae,* and *Vibrio parahaemolyticus.* It is often difficult to separate ReA from bacterial arthritis, given their similar presentations and causative agents. In patients in whom an organism cannot be identified despite a preceding infection, the diagnosis of ReA should be considered.

The treatment of ReA has long relied on nonsteroidal anti-inflammatory agents (NSAIDs). Intra-articular steroids have also proven useful, as have systemic steroids in severe cases. The use of antibiotics has recently been investigated. In some studies, long-term (3 months) tetracycline therapy shortened the duration of arthritis in patients with *Chlamydia trachomatis*-induced ReA, but tetracycline efficacy may be due to its ability to resist collagen lysis rather than its antimicrobial properties. An investigation of the effectiveness of the quinolone treatment of enterogenic ReA showed some improvement in certain categories, but did not conclusively demonstrate the antibiotic's efficacy. Sulfasalazine has reduced the occurrence of peripheral joint symptoms in spondyloarthropathy patients, and it may be of some use in ReA.

Human Immune Deficiency Arthropathy

Infection with HIV can lead to a variety of musculoskeletal manifestations. The most common of these is a sterile polyarthritis that is believed to involve a mechanism similar to ReA. HIV itself is believed to be the causative agent in most of these patients, rather than the disease being a result of bacterial infection secondary to decreased immune response.

The HIV type of ReA is frequently refractory to treatment. Although NSAIDs are usually administered, they seem to be less effective than in other cases of ReA. Sulfasalazine appears to be beneficial in some patients. Immunosuppressive drugs, such as methotrexate and azathioprine (AZT), should be avoided given the increased incidence of opportunistic infections and Kaposi's sarcoma. Also common in HIV patients is psoriatic arthritis. The disease is almost identical to classic psoriatic arthritis, except that the skin lesions may be found in unusual locations and may be particularly aggressive. Treatment involves the use of NSAIDs, and some patients respond to AZT and etidronate. Other noninfectious bone and joint diseases seen in patients with HIV include non-Hodgkin's lymphoma and Kaposi's sarcoma.

These aseptic articular manifestations are much more common than true musculoskeletal infections. Even with HIV's increased incidence of bacterial and fungal infections, the number of infections with bone and joint involvement are few. One study found 0.3% of HIV patients with an infection of the musculoskeletal system; the most common infections were septic arthritis and osteomyelitis. Other infections include bursitis, bacterial myositis, and polymyositis. These infections are caused by both common bacteria such as *S aureus* and by opportunistic infections such as *Cryptococcus neoformans, Nocardia asteroides, Mycobacterium kansasii,* and *Histoplasma capsulatum.*

The diagnosis of musculoskeletal infections in patients with HIV is especially challenging. These manifestations are rare and, as such, are frequently not considered. This omission is especially true in the patients who are beginning to have multiple systemic problems. Because many patients are receiving antibiotics at the time of first presentation with a bone or joint symptom, organism isolation and identification is even more difficult. The clinical manifestations are also altered by the HIV infection. A low WBC count, for example, cannot be used to rule out an infection in this population. One study contained 2 patients in whom multiple organisms could be visualized in the synovial fluid, but the fluid itself was clear, with less than 10,000 WBC. Finally, the incidence of a concomitant infection in the HIV-positive patient is high, so systemic symptoms are frequently attributed to the other source.

Early diagnosis and aggressive treatment can lead to cure rates approaching 80%. Treatment for these individuals is similar to that for other patients, except that the antibiotic choices will differ, as will the length of antibiotic administration. Prior to identification of the organism and its sensitivities, several antibiotics are given to cover a variety of bacteria that may include the causative agent. Identification of an organism in the blood does not mean the causative agent of the joint infection has been identified. In several cases, bone and joint infections caused by an opportunistic infection of one type have coincided with bacteremia of a different species. Long-term parenteral antibiotics are required to treat these infections, and no data currently exist to support a switch to oral antibiotics.

Pediatric Infection

Pathogenesis, location, causative organisms, and presenting signs and symptoms of pediatric orthopaedic infections make their management unique. Diseases such as congenital syphilis are unique to the pediatric population.

Acute Hematogenous Osteomyelitis

Hematogenous osteomyelitis occurs more frequently in children than in adults because of the vascular anatomy of growing bones, the more frequent bacteremia, and repeated trauma in the pediatric population.

Microbiology S aureus, the most common causative agent, accounts for 80% of all osteomyelitis; unfortunately, many strains are resistant to penicillin and methicillin. In children younger than 3 years of age, *Haemophilus influenzae* type B (HIB) may be responsible for septic joints and, rarely, osteomyelitis. Vaccination against *H influenzae* has largely eliminated it as a musculoskeletal pathogen. *Pseudomonas aeruginosa* is more commonly found in the peripubertal (9 to 12 years old) age group. These infections are often related to a penetrating foot injury. The patients may have a normal WBC count and an elevated erythrocyte sedimentation rate (ESR).

Clinical Presentation A history of prior infection, unexplained bone pain, fever, and local inflammation all suggest this diagnosis. Other symptoms include irritability, anorexia, lethargy, and vomiting. It is important to obtain material for culture before administering antibiotics.

Diagnosis Several laboratory values are helpful in the diagnosis and management of acute hematogenous osteomyelitis. The WBC count is frequently elevated. An elevated ESR is found in most patients; however it takes 3 to 5 days for the ESR to rise to its peak level, and it does not fall with improvement of the clinical condition. Measurement of C-reactive protein (CRP), appears to be a better means of monitoring the course of the infection. CRP levels, usually elevated (>19 mg/l) at the time of admission, peak by day 2, and drop rapidly with treatment, returning to normal within a week. CRP levels are higher and take longer to return to normal in patients with concomitant osteomyelitis and septic arthritis.

Blood cultures and bone aspiration should be done in all cases of acute hematogenous osteomyelitis. Aspiration, the single most valuable test, should be postponed only if a malignant process is suspected; it should not be delayed for a bone scan. Radiographs frequently offer little early diagnostic help. Soft-tissue swelling may be evident by day 3; more commonly, no radiographic changes are seen for up to 2 weeks after symptoms begin. Technetium 99m diphosphonate bone scanning can detect changes within 24 hours of infection. Unfortunately, when performed this early, the test has low sensitivity (missing up to 20% of infections) and low specificity (increased uptake may also indicate either trauma or tumor). MRI has been described as having 100% sensitivity with a much greater specificity. MRI may distinguish cellulitis from acute hematogenous osteomyelitis; can locate abscesses, sequestra, and sinus tracts; and may be useful to differentiate between acute and chronic osteomyelitis.

Treatment After completion of the required cultures, empiric antibiotic therapy should begin. The choice of first line antibiotics should be based on organism prevalence. In children, it is crucial to cover S aureus with an antibiotic such as oxacillin. In neonates, additional coverage of HIB with gentamicin is required. In patients with sickle-cell anemia, both cefotaxime and oxacillin should be used to cover salmonella and S aureus. Infection caused by deep penetrating wounds should be treated by an antibiotic that covers pseudomonads, and tetanus prophylaxis is required. When culture results are available, antibiotic therapy is tailored to the specific organisms found.

Choosing the proper antibiotic dose for neonates, infants, and children is important. Close monitoring of peak and trough serum levels assures that the minimal inhibitory concentration is reached. All children are started on parenteral antibiotics. Although 6 weeks of intravenous antibiotics is frequently recommended, the current trend is to switch to oral antibiotics after 2 weeks when clinically appropriate. Criteria used to help decide if oral antibiotics will be effective include clinical response as noted by changes in the physical examination, by defervescence, and by evaluation of laboratory values such as CRP and ESR. Other criteria include isolation of a bacterial pathogen sensitive to an oral antibiotic, the ability of this antibiotic to reach appropriate serum levels without excessive toxicity, the patient's ability to tolerate the medication by oral route, and the assurance of proper patient and parental compliance.

If necrotic bone and exudate have formed an abscess, antibiotics alone will not be effective. Aspiration of exudate is an indication for surgery. Patients with clinically diagnosed

Menschik M, Neumuller J, Steiner CW, et al: Effects of ciprofloxacin and ofloxacin on adult human cartilage in vitro. *Antimicrob Agents Chemother* 1997;41:2562–2565.

Chondrocyte toxicity and necrosis was demonstrated by electron microscopy after incubation of adult cartilage biopsy specimens in media containing ciprofloxacin or ofloxacin. The clinical significance is uncertain, but the possibility of cartilage damage related to fluoroquinolone treatment cannot be excluded.

Shea KW, Cunha BA: Teicoplanin. *Med Clin North Am* 1995;79: 833–844.

This review article discusses the potential advantages of teicoplanin, a new glycopeptide antibiotic related to vancomycin. Teicoplanin may be delivered intramuscularly in those patients with limited venous access, and maintenance therapy can be administered on a daily basis.

PMMA Local Antibiotic Depots

Edin ML, Miclau T, Lester GE, Lindsey RW, Dahners LE: Effect of cefazolin and vancomycin on osteoblasts in vitro. *Clin Orthop* 1996;333:245–251.

Osteoblast-like cell cultures were exposed to various concentrations of 2 antibiotics. In this model, vancomycin was less toxic than cefazolin at high concentrations and may be a better choice for local antibiotic depot administration.

Henry SL, Galloway KP: Local antibacterial therapy for the management of orthopaedic infections: Pharmacokinetic considerations. *Clin Pharmacokinet* 1995;29:36–45.

This is a complete review of the important pharmacokinetic considerations for the optimal use of antibacterial agents in the treatment of osteomyelitis. The indications for the use of local antibiotic therapy are thoroughly discussed, and the advantages and disadvantages are compared to systemic antibiotic administration.

Ostermann PA, Seligson D, Henry SL: Local antibiotic therapy for severe open fractures: A review of 1085 consecutive cases. *J Bone Joint Surg* 1995;77B:93–97.

This retrospective study compares a group receiving systemic antibiotics alone to a group receiving supplemental local aminoglycoside delivered via PMMA beads. The infection rate was reduced overall from 12% to 3.7% in the group managed with antibiotic beads. These results suggest the adjuvant use of local antibiotic may reduce the incidence of infection after severe open fractures.

Biodegradable Local Antibiotic Depots

Jacob E, Cierny G III, Zorn K, McNeill JF, Fallon MT: Delayed local treatment of rabbit tibial fractures with biodegradable cefazolin microspheres. *Clin Orthop* 1997;336:278–285.

Biodegradable microspheres containing cefazolin were constructed using poly(DL-lactide)-coglycolide, and used for delayed treatment of simulated open fractures in a rabbit model. The results suggest local antibiotic therapy with biodegradable cefazolin microspheres may be beneficial in the treatment of open fractures even if treatment is delayed several hours.

Mader JT, Calhoun J, Cobos J: In vitro evaluation of antibiotic diffusion from antibiotic-impregnated biodegradable beads and polymethylmethacrylate beads. *Antimicrob Agents Chemother* 1997;41:415–418.

Comparison of antibiotic elution from beads made of PMMA, polylactic acid (PLA), and poly(DL-lactide)-coglycolide (PL:CG). Antibiotic beads composed of PLA and PL:CG have superior elution characteristics compared to the PMMA beads currently used; they are also biodegradable and do not require additional surgery for removal.

Price JS, Tencer AF, Arm DM, Bohach GA: Controlled release of antibiotics from coated orthopedic implants. *J Biomed Mater Res* 1996;30:281–286.

Polylactic-co-glycolic acid copolymer (PLGA) was applied to implants and used as a biodegradable carrier of gentamycin in an in vitro model. Local concentrations very near the implants were found to have bactericidal antibiotic levels, demonstrating the possible use of a thin biodegradable antibiotic coating for orthopaedic implants.

Osteomyelitis

Boutin RD, Brossmann J, Sartoris DJ, Reilly D, Resnick D: Update on imaging of orthopedic infections. *Orthop Clin North Am* 1998;29:41–66.

The imaging appearance of musculoskeletal infections is described and the advantages and disadvantages are discussed for 5 imaging methods: radiography, sonography, CT, scintigraphy, and MR imaging. Chronic recurrent multifocal osteomyelitis, musculoskeletal infections in AIDS patients, and pedal infections in diabetic infections are emphasized.

Cho SH, Song HR, Koo KH, Jeong ST, Park YJ: Antibiotic-impregnated cement beads in the treatment of chronic osteomyelitis. *Bull Hosp Jt Dis* 1997;56:140–144.

Thirty-one patients with chronic osteomyelitis of long bones were treated with primary saucerization and implantation of antibiotic-impregnated PMMA beads, followed by secondary bone grafts. At an average follow-up of 4 years, 17 (55%) were completely free of infection; 10 (32%) required repeated procedures, and 4 required amputations.

Cottias P, Tomeno B, Anract P, Vinh TS, Forest M: Subacute osteomyelitis presenting as a bone tumour: A review of 21 cases. *Int Orthop* 1997;21:243–248.

Twenty-one patients with subacute osteomyelitis were initially considered to have bone tumors. Clinical symptoms were not specific and laboratory investigations were normal. Definitive diagnosis was made by surgical biopsy, histology, and cultures, which grew Staphylococcus in 9 patients. There was no recurrence of infection after currettage and excision of the infected tissues.

Hadjipavlou AG, Cesani-Vazuqez F, Villaneuva-Meyer J, et al: The effectiveness of gallium citrate Ga 67 radionuclide imaging in vertebral osteomyelitis revisited. *Am J Orthop* 1998;27: 179–183.

Gallium scanning proved to be 100% sensitive, specific, and accurate. Complementary bone and gallium scans are recommended for patients suspected of having spinal infections. If the scans are positive, a biopsy should be done; if the scans are negative, no further investigation is needed.

Kawanabe K, Okada Y, Satsusue Y, Iida H, Nakamura T: Treatment of osteomyelitis with antibiotic-soaked porous glass ceramic. *J Bone Joint Surg* 1998;80-B:527–530.

A new drug delivery system using porous apatite-wollastonite glass ceramic was successful in eliminating infection in 4 patients with infected total hip arthroplasties and 1 with osteomyelitis of the tibia.

Maynor ML, Moon RE, Camporesi EM, et al: Chronic osteomyelitis of the tibia: Treatment with hyperbaric oxygen and autogenous microsurgical muscle transplantation. *J South Orthop Assoc* 1998;7:43–57.

Thirty-four patients with chronic osteomyelitis were treated with antibiotics, surgery (average of 8.3 procedures), and hyperbaric oxygen (average, 35 treatments). Twenty patients (59%) also had free vascularized muscle flaps. Of 26 patients with 24 months of follow-up, 21 (81%) were drainage-free. At long-term follow-up (84 months), patients who had muscle flaps were more likely to be drainage-free than patients who had only debridement.

Panda M, Ntungila N, Kalunda M, Hisenkamp M: Treatment of chronic osteomyelitis using the Papineau technique. *Int Orthop* 1998;22:37–40.

Forty-one patients with chronic osteomyelitis were treated with a modified Papineau technique. Wound healing was complete at an average of 3 months with spontaneous healing and at 4.5 months after skin grafting. Control of infection and bone healing were obtained in 89% after 3 to 7 months.

Septic Arthritis

Berbari EF, Hanssen AD, Duffy MC, Steckelberg JM, Osmon DR: Prosthetic joint infection due to Mycobacterium tuberculosis: A case series and review of the literature. *Am J Orthop* 1998; 27:219–227.

To decrease the risk of reactivation after prosthesis implantation in patients with quiescent tuberculous septic arthritis who have not received prior antituberculous therapy, consideration should be given to preoperative or perioperative antituberculous prophylaxis.

Donatto KC: Orthopedic management of septic arthritis. *Rheum Dis Clin North Am* 1998;24:275–286.

The goals of treatment of septic arthritis are joint decompression, joint sterilization, and preservation of joint function. Arthrotomy has several advantages over serial aspirations: a more complete decompression, a lower intra-articular bacterial count after lavage, the possibility of synovectomy, and no delay in infections that may be unresponsive to simple aspiration and antibiotics.

Marsh JL, Watson PA, Crouch CA: Septic arthritis caused by chronic osteomyelitis. *Iowa Orthop J* 1997;17:90–95.

Four patients with previously quiescent osteomyelitis developed septic arthritis in an adjacent joint. The osteomyelitis focus was in the bone proximal (up to 10 cm) to the involved joints. Aggressive surgical debridement of both bone and joint, followed by a prolonged course of antibiotics, led to resolution in all patients.

Williams RJ III, Laurencin CT, Warren RF, et al: Septic arthritis after arthroscopic anterior cruciate ligament reconstruction: Diagnosis and management. *Am J Sports Med* 1997;25: 261–267.

Of 2,500 patients with arthroscopic ACL reconstruction, 7 (0.3%) had postoperative deep infections of the knee. Six had concomitant open procedures. All patients had immediate arthroscopic debridement and irrigation, intravenous antibiotics for 4 to 6 weeks, protected weight-bearing, and physical therapy. Six of the 7 patients had minimal or no pain and were satisfied with their functional results.

Atypical Osteomyelitides

Demharter J, Bohndorf K, Michl W, Vogt H: Chronic recurrent multifocal osteomyelitis: A radiological and clinical investigation of 5 cases. *Skeletal Radiol* 1997;26:579–588.

The authors describe in detail the radiographic, scintigraphic, and clinical findings in 5 cases of CRMO. Only careful correlation between these features allows an accurate assessment of disease activity in this syndrome. Radiographs of bone lesions found soon after symptoms begin resemble those of acute osteomyelitis.

Stahlman GC, DeBoer DK, Green NE: Fusobacterium osteomyelitis and pyarthrosis: A classic case of Lemierre's syndrome. *J Pediatr Orthop* 1996;16:529–532.

The authors report a case of anaerobic septic arthritis and multifocal acute hematogenous osteomyelitis as part of a classic presentation of Lemierre's syndrome.

Classic Bibliography

Calhoun JH, Henry SL, Anger DM, et al: The treatment of infected nonunions with gentamicin-polymethylmethacrylate antibiotic beads. *Clin Orthop* 1993;295:23–27.

Cushing AH: Diskitis in children. *Clin Infect Dis* 1993;17:1–6.

Dagan R: Management of acute hematogenous osteomyelitis and septic arthritis in the pediatric patient. *Pediatr Infect Dis J* 1993;12:88–92.

Evans RP, Nelson CL, Harrison BH: The effect of wound environment on the incidence of acute osteomyelitis. *Clin Orthop* 1993;286:289–297.

Frederiksen B, Chritiansen P, Knudsen FU: Acute osteomyelitis and septic arthritis in the neonate, risk factors and outcome. *Eur J Pediatr* 1993;152:577–580.

Henry SL, Osterman PA, Seligson D: The antibiotic bead pouch technique: The management of severe compound fractures. *Clin Orthop* 1993;295:54–62.

Kalish R: Lyme disease. *Rheum Dis Clin North Am* 1993;19: 399–426.

Laurencin CT, Gerhart T, Witschger P, et al: Bioerodible polyanhydrides for antibiotic drug delivery: In vivo osteomyelitis treatment in a rat model system. *J Orthop Res* 1993;11:256–262.

Lerner RK, Esterhai JL Jr, Polomano RC, et al: Quality of life assessment of patients with posttraumatic fracture nonunion, chronic refractory osteomyelitis, and lower-extremity amputation. *Clin Orthop* 1993;295:28–36.

Levine SE, Esterhai JL Jr, Heppenstall RB, et al: Diagnoses and staging: Osteomyelitis and prosthetic joint infections. *Clin Orthop* 1993;295:77–86.

Mader JT, Landon GC, Calhoun J: Antimicrobial treatment of osteomyelitis. *Clin Orthop* 1993;295:87–95.

Malin JK, Patel NJ: Arthropathy and HIV infection: A muddle of mimicry. *Postgrad Med* 1993;93:143-146,149–150.

Nocton JJ, Dressler F, Rutledge BJ, et al: Detection of Borrelia burgdorferi DNA by polymerase chain reaction in synovial fluid from patients with Lyme arthritis. *N Engl J Med* 1994;330: 229–234.

Schauwecker DS: The scintigraphic diagnosis of osteomyelitis. *Am J Roentgenol* 1992;158:9–18.

Scopelitis E, Martinez-Osuna P: Gonococcal arthritis. *Rheum Dis Clin North Am* 1993;19:363–377.

Tehranzadeh J, Wang F, Mesgarzadeh M: Magnetic resonance imaging of osteomyelitis. *Crit Rev Diagn Imaging* 1992;33: 495–534.

Unkila-Kallio L, Kallio MJ, Eskola J, et al: Serum C-reactive protein, erythrocyte sedimentation rate, and white blood cell count in acute hematogenous osteomyelitis of children. *Pediatrics* 1994;93:59–62.

Chapter 19
Arthritis

Arthritis and related disorders are leading causes of activity limitation and disability in the adult population of the United States, where the economic costs of musculoskeletal illness have been conservatively estimated to be approximately 1% of our gross national product. A significant portion of these costs is attributable to arthritis. As the population ages, the impact of arthritis in terms of disability and associated economic cost is expected to increase. Research efforts continue to advance understanding of the pathogenesis and treatment of rheumatic diseases.

Normal Joint Physiology

The function of the normal synovial joint is dependent on the important relationships between synovium, articular cartilage, and the underlying subchondral bone. Articular cartilage, being avascular, receives its nutrition solely via diffusion of nutrients from the synovial fluid, through the extracellular matrix. Alterations in the normal properties of the synovium, the subchondral bone, or the synovial tissue itself have been demonstrated to have significant effects on the integrity of articular cartilage. Unfortunately, the ability of articular cartilage to heal or repair itself in vivo after significant damage is extremely limited.

Relatively large joint reaction forces typically occur in weightbearing joints. Because of the effects of muscular forces exerted across these joints, joint reaction forces are usually several times those forces resulting from body weight alone. The effects of these large joint reaction forces on the cartilage matrix and subchondral bone may be responsible for degeneration of articular cartilage seen in certain types of osteoarthritis. The lubricating properties of the synovial fluid and the cartilage matrix minimize the shear stresses generated by these large joint reaction forces occurring during joint movement. Both boundary and fluid film lubrication mechanisms contribute to reduction of shear stresses.

Structure of Articular Cartilage

The Matrix
The extracellular matrix is the most distinctive component of articular cartilage and is responsible for its physiologic and mechanical properties. Articular cartilage is approximately 80% water and 20% organic solid. Approximately 50% of the dry weight of cartilage can be attributed to collagen. Although type II collagen is the predominate form found in articular cartilage, other cartilage-specific collagens include types IX, X, and XI. The specific arrangement of collagen fibers within the different zones of the matrix contribute to the ability of articular cartilage to resist various mechanical forces occurring under loading and provide anchorage to the underlying subchondral bone at the tidemark.

The remainder of the organic portion of the cartilage matrix is composed of the matrix proteoglycans. Aggrecan is the principle proteoglycan, in terms of size and abundance, within the articular cartilage matrix. Individual aggrecan molecules are complex anionic glycoproteins consisting of a linear protein core with attached long-chain glycosaminoglycans (GAGs). Chondroitin 4-sulfate, chondroitin-6 sulfate, and keratan sulfate are the GAGs found in human articular cartilage. Proteoglycan macromolecules form when a single long filament of hyaluronic acid interacts, via link protein, with several of these aggrecan molecules. The resultant aggregates are held together by electrostatic forces and link proteins. These macromolecules interact with matrix water and other organic components of the matrix (collagen) to provide for the unique mechanical properties of articular cartilage and lubrication of the joint.

Chondrocytes
Chondrocytes, the cellular elements of articular cartilage, are metabolically active cells that synthesize the collagenous and proteoglycan constitutents of the matrix, as well as the enzymes and protease inhibitors responsible for both the maintenance and degradation of cartilage. Under normal circumstances, mature chondrocytes are terminally differentiated cells incapable of mitosis. Chondrocyte functions are influenced by a number of different growth factors, cytokines, medications, and alterations in mechanical loading. These extracellular stimuli are responsible for the initiation of a cascade of intracellular events (via second messenger signals), ultimately resulting in activation of specific DNA binding proteins and induction of target genes within the articular chondrocyte.

Maintenance of homeostasis within the cartilage matrix is regulated by the complex and incompletely understood interactions between chondrocytes, matrix components, and a number of different growth factors, cytokines, and mechanical stimuli from the environment. In general, cartilage growth factors, such as insulin-like growth factor-I (IGF-I), basic fibroblast growth factor (bFGF), and transforming growth factor-beta (TGF-β) are typically associated with stimulation of cartilage matrix production. Recent evidence suggests that these polypeptide growth factors play an important role, both in maintaining within the matrix the precise balance between anabolic and catabolic activities necessary for the preservation of normal articular cartilage, and in potentially limiting the reparative response of articular cartilage to joint disease and injury. IGF-I has been shown to stimulate mitotic activity and matrix synthesis by articular chondrocytes. Observed age-related decreases in human serum IGF-I levels and reduction in responsiveness of chondrocytes to IGF-I may render articular cartilage less capable of maintaining its integrity with aging.

TGF-β has been shown to stimulate matrix proteoglycan and collagen production, and inhibit its matrix degradation, thus antagonizing the catabolic effects of interleukin-1 (IL-1). TGF-β also increases the expression of tissue inhibitors of metalloproteinases (TIMPs) in chondrocytes. bFGF has a mitogenic effect on chondrocytes and appears to be capable of initiating repair of superficial articular cartilage defects in vivo. Because of their complex interactions with other growth factors, cytokines, and matrix metalloproteinases (MMPs), the net anabolic or catabolic effects of TGF-β and bFGF likely differ depending on the state of the target cells.

MMPs are a group of enzymes capable of degrading many matrix macromolecules found in articular cartilage and other connective tissues. Collagenase, stromolysin, and gelatinase are currently thought to be the important MMPs responsible for cartilage matrix degradation occurring in various arthritic disorders. In response to a variety of mediators of inflammation, these MMPs can be synthesized by chondrocytes, synovium, and infiltrating leukocytes. The activity of these metalloproteinases can be inhibited in vivo by TIMPs. TIMP-1 and TIMP-2 have been demonstrated to have broad inhibitory activity against a variety of MMPs.

Cytokines, such as IL-1, tumor necrosis factor alpha (TNF-α), and tumor necrosis factor beta (TNF-β), have been shown to stimulate net matrix degradation through several mechanisms. IL-1 has been demonstrated to stimulate expression of the MMPs collagenase and stromolysin, and to inhibit type II collagen and proteoglycan synthesis in chondrocytes. IL-1 also inhibits the growth stimulatory effect of TGF-β on articular chondrocytes, and it is a potent stimula-

tor of prostaglandin E_2 (PGE$_2$). TNF-α and TNF-β have also been shown to induce collagenase and PGE$_2$ production by synovial cells. IGF-I has been shown to partially reverse the catabolic effects of IL-1.

Another member of the interleukin family, IL-4, appears to be a chondroprotective factor that inhibits cartilage matrix degradation by suppressing TNF-α, IL-1, and PGE$_2$ production. Certain members of the IL-6 cytokine family (IL-6, IL-11, and leukemia inhibitor factor) may also have a chondroprotective effect by stimulation of TIMP expression in chondrocytes.

In the past, the articular cartilage has been regarded as the target of, rather than an active contributor to, inflammation within a synovial joint. Recently, however, articular chondrocytes have been shown to be capable of producing a number of proinflammatory mediators, which result in leukocyte migration into the synovial joint. Thus, even chondrocytes have the potential to initiate and maintain an inflammatory process within the synovial joint.

Recent evidence suggests that nitric oxide is an important mediator of inflammation in both rheumatoid arthritis and osteoarthritis. Both synovial fibroblasts and macrophages appear to be the major sources of synovial nitric oxide, which may be produced as a nonspecific synovial response to injury or inflammation. The tissue effects of nitric oxide are complex, and it appears to have both inflammatory and anti-inflammatory properties. Synovial cells have been shown to be activated by nitric oxide to produce TNF-α, and possibly other proinflammatory cytokines. Nitric oxide also has been shown to regulate MMP production and may also inhibit matrix proteoglycan synthesis via IL-1β. Nitric oxide production within the chondrocyte is stimulated by the induction of nitric oxide synthase by IL-1 and TNF-α. Current evidence supports the association of nitric oxide with net catabolic activity in human articular cartilage.

Subchondral Bone

Important relationships exist between the subchondral bone and articular cartilage that are essential for maintenance of integrity and health of the synovial joint. Under the relatively narrow range of normal joint forces, the subchondral bone supporting the articular cartilage is cushioned from excessive loads by the ability of articular cartilage to effectively absorb compressive loads. Damage to the articular cartilage may result in alteration of the microarchitecture and mechanical properties of the subchondral bone. Similarly, alteration of the integrity or mechanical properties of the subchondral bone can result in damage to the overlying articular cartilage (Fig. 1). Conditions associated with decreased strength of the subchondral bone, as is seen in osteonecrosis, result in loss of structural support of the articular cartilage and collapse. Conditions associated with increased stiffness of the supporting subchondral bone result in increased compressive stresses in the articular cartilage and damage to the articular surface. There is some evidence that similar biomechanical changes in the subchondral bone may precede the appearance of degenerative changes in the articular cartilage in osteoarthritis, suggesting that this process is initiated by an abnormality of the subchondral bone, rather than an abnormality of the cartilage itself.

Osteoarthritis

Osteoarthritis (OA) is a common joint disorder of multifactorial etiology, the prevalence of which increases progressively with age. Despite the inflammatory connotations of the "itis" suffix, the initiating events in OA appear to be mechanical, rather than inflammatory, in nature. Inflammation does, however, appear to play a lesser role in the progression of disease in OA. Osteoarthrosis is, however, probably a more accurate description of the clinical syndrome commonly and synonymously referred to as OA.

Two philosophically differing paradigms have been suggested to explain the pathogenesis of OA. The most widely accepted considers OA as a disease process (or group of processes) with common pathologic features that ultimately lead to joint failure. Another less widely held theory suggests that OA is the end result of two features of human evolution—the change in posture (from quadruped to upright biped gait) and the development of a long "postreproductive life span" relative to ancestral predecessors. This later paradigm views OA as a consequence of evolution, as the articular damage in joints that are "underdesigned" for upright posture accumulates with age and is less adequately repaired in individuals of advancing age.

Primary and Secondary Osteoarthritis

OA can be classified into primary (idiopathic) or secondary types. In most patients with OA, a definite underlying etiology cannot be established, and these are considered idiopathic. Occasionally, cases of apparent primary OA present at a relatively early age, with more generalized clinical findings and distribution of disease, and a strong family history or pattern of inheritance. Subtle genetic aberrations, and resultant alterations in the structural macromolecules responsible for the normal integrity of articular cartilage, have been identified in a small number of these patients. Mutations in the

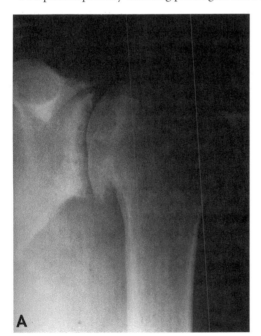 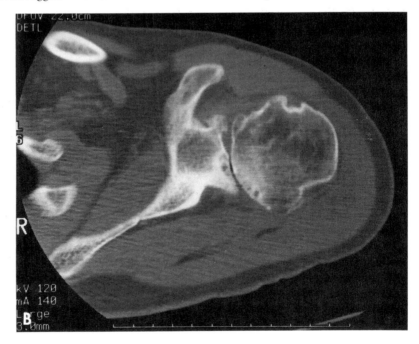

Figure 1

A, Typical anteroposterior radiograph of glenohumeral osteoarthritis. Note the inferior spurring of the humerus, and subchondral sclerosis and cysts in the glenoid. B, Computed tomographic scan of the same shoulder demonstrates the degree of posterior glenoid wear and posterior humeral head subluxation (arrow). (Reproduced with permission from Green A: Current concepts of shoulder arthroplasty, in Cannon WD Jr (ed): *Instructional Course Lectures 47.* Rosemont, IL, American Academy of Orthopaedic Surgeons, 1998, pp 127–133.)

type II collagen gene have been identified in several kindreds of familial OA. An ultimate genetic etiology for additional clinical presentations of primary OA may be likely, as point mutations in critical genes responsible for normal structure and function of articular cartilage are identified. It is likely that such minor genetic variations are somehow responsible for an increased susceptibility to age-related, accumulated articular damage in these patients. In these cases, initiation and progression of disease would be expected to occur as a consequence of normal loading of articular cartilage that has subtle structural abnormalities.

Secondary OA can be the result of various causes, which adversely affect the structural integrity and resultant biomechanical properties of cartilage, or the mechanical forces transmitted to the articular cartilage. These are typically associated with a recognized systemic or metabolic disorder, or articular trauma of a singular or repetitive nature. In many instances, the underlying etiology responsible for secondary OA will be obvious (eg, developmental dysplasia of the hip, osteonecrosis, Legg-Calvé-Perthes disease, or intra-articular fracture). Secondary OA develops in direct response to abnormal mechanical loading in these patients with articular cartilage that is, at least initially, structurally normal. Obesity is an example of a common, potentially modifiable risk factor for secondary OA of the knee, which appears to develop as a direct result of repetitive mechanical overloading of structurally normal articular cartilage.

A growing body of evidence suggests that OA may be the indirect result of structural and biomechanical alterations in the subchondral bone, rather than simply the direct result of mechanical overloading of the articular cartilage itself. Microstructural and biomechanical changes within the subchondral bone have been demonstrated to precede the characteristic biochemical and histologic changes typically associated with OA. Alterations in the mechanical properties of the subchondral bone have significant effects on the mechanical stresses experienced by the overlying articular cartilage. OA should perhaps more appropriately be considered to be a disorder of disturbed balance between the degradation and repair of the articular cartilage and subchondral bone (Figs. 2 and 3). In many cases of either primary or secondary OA, initiation of damage to the articular cartilage is probably a result of the complex, and yet unknown, interactions between multiple genetic and environmental factors.

Molecular Markers of Arthritic Disease

Articular cartilage and subchondral bone are dynamic tissues with continuous matrix turnover. Maintenance of health within the synovial joint requires maintenance of matrix homeostasis and structural integrity within both of these tissues. Pathologic conditions, such as OA, rheumatoid arthritis (RA), or trauma, disrupt the delicate balance between anabolic and catabolic processes within the matrix of these tissues, ultimately resulting in loss of articular cartilage. Structural macromolecules, or their fragments, are constantly released from the cartilage matrix by these metabolic

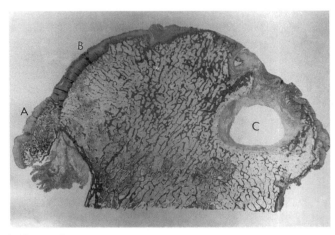

Figure 2

A low-power photomicrograph of a femoral head with osteoarthritis. A is an osteophyte covered by a mixture of hyaline and fibrocartilage. B is remaining true articular hyaline cartilage. C is a subchondral bone cyst. (Reproduced with permission from Schiller AL: Pathology of osteoarthritis, in Kuettner KE, Goldberg VM (eds): *Osteoarthritic Disorders*. Rosemont, IL, American Academy of Orthopaedic Surgeons, 1995, pp 95–101.)

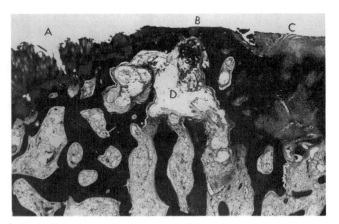

Figure 3

The surface of a femoral head with osteoarthritis. A, remaining true hyaline articular cartilage; B, articular cartilage totally gone, exposing thickened eburnated subchondral bone plate; C, surface plug of fibrocartilage bordered by reactive woven bone; and D, early subchondral bone cyst. (Reproduced with permission from Schiller AL: Pathology of osteoarthritis, in Kuettner KE, Goldberg VM (eds): *Osteoarthritic Disorders*. Rosemont, IL, American Academy of Orthopaedic Surgeons, 1995, pp 95–101.)

processes. Quantification of these "molecular markers" of joint disease is of considerable scientific and clinical interest, because they are potentially reflective of the relative state of matrix homeostasis within articular cartilage. Analysis of these markers of disease may help in elucidating the specific molecular events occurring in damaged or arthritic cartilage, and identify potential sites of therapeutic intervention.

As a result of the distinct zonal organization of articular cartilage, these molecular markers may allow for characterization of the anabolic and catabolic processes occurring in different zones (superficial, middle, or deep), or different regions of proximity to the chondrocytes (pericellular, territorial, or interterritorial). Because the recognized structural zones of articular cartilage each appear to be organized to serve a specific function, the consequences of damage in one zone may differ from that in another zone. Due to the relative location with respect to chondrocyte proximity, matrix damage in the interterritorial region would not be expected to be as effectively repaired as damage in the pericellular region. Experimental evidence also suggests that while loss of proteoglycan from the matrix may be reparable and potentially reversible, damage to matrix collagen may be considerably more difficult to repair. Identification of clinically relevant molecular markers of disease may thus be of diagnostic value, by establishing the presence of subclinical disease or the extent of disease within a joint. Molecular markers may also be useful in monitoring response to treatment or activity of disease.

Several potentially relevant molecular markers have been identified in RA and OA. A catabolic product of aggrecan degradation, hyaluronan binding region, has been shown to be associated with advanced, and probably irreversible RA. Another cartilage matrix protein, cartilage oligomeric protein (COMP) appears to be a potentially useful serum marker for OA and possibly RA. COMP levels appear to increase with advancing OA and remain constant in patients with nonprogressive OA. Bone sialoprotein is a bone specific protein that appears to be increased in advanced, irreversible RA. Antibodies have also been generated that recognize epitopes of matrix macromolecules, including type II collagen and proteoglycans that are exposed during proteolytic cleavages associated with degradation. These epitopes are not recognized in normal cartilage but can be detected in the serum or joint fluid, and thus show promise as additional markers for arthritis.

Therapeutic Options for Treatment of OA
Activity modification, analgesics, nonsteroidal anti-inflammatory drugs (NSAIDs), and appropriate physical therapy have been the mainstay of treatment for OA. Obesity is a potentially modifiable risk factor for development of OA, and weight loss has been shown to slow progression of disease and to relieve symptoms in obese patients with OA of the knee. Although low impact exercise has not been shown to be a risk factor, several studies have documented the adverse effects of high impact and high intensity activity on the eventual development of OA. Patients with abnormal joints as a result of previous ligament, meniscal, or articular cartilage injuries will subject their joints to relatively increased mechanical loads, potentially accelerating the development of OA. Secondary OA developing as a result of a developmental or acquired skeletal deformity may potentially be reversed by a realignment osteotomy that normalizes the biomechanical loads on the involved joint. Unfortunately, these patients frequently present with degenerative changes that are too far advanced for an osteotomy to provide a reliable and satisfactory clinical result. Newer NSAIDs, with potentially reduced side effects and increased efficacy, become available yearly. However, the potential side effects of these medications are considerable in the older patient population typically afflicted with OA. In general, the treatment of OA in the past has been based primarily on alleviation of symptoms, rather than altering the normal progression of disease. Several recently available therapies and experimental therapies under development offer alternatives to previous treatment modalities, and may represent an opportunity to significantly alter the clinical course of OA.

Autogenous Chondrocyte Transplantation New therapeutic approaches incorporating cell-based technologies have been the subject of considerable interest in both the scientific and lay press. In general, these different techniques have been directed toward the repair of isolated, limited sized (2 to 7 cm²) chondral defects of the knee. Although these lesions are likely prearthritic in nature, it is unknown if these techniques will be applicable for the treatment of more extensive disorders of articular cartilage, such as established OA.

The most popular of these procedures initially involves the arthroscopic harvesting of healthy autogenous articular chondrocytes from an uninvolved and nonloadbearing area of the knee. The isolated chondrocytes are then cultured for 2 to 3 weeks to increase the number of cells, and subsequently surgically reimplanted into the chondral defects to be treated. These autogenous transplants are held in place by a periosteal flap sutured over the defect. The early (2 to 3 year) reported clinical results with this technique are favorable, with 60% to 70% of patients experiencing a reduction in mechanical symptoms and improved function. Early clinical results with the treatment of chondral defects of the patella do not appear to be as favorable as the results of treatment of tibiofemoral defects.

Critics of this technique argue that it has not been subjected to the necessary scientific scrutiny obtainable only by a randomized clinical trial, or by comparing outcomes with untreated patients. It is not yet evident whether the same results may be obtainable with the use of a periosteal flap alone, considering the favorable reported results with the use of periosteal and perichondrial interpositional grafts for treatment of similar defects. In fact, results of a recent study using a canine model suggested no difference between periosteal flaps with and without transplanted autologous chondrocytes. The durability of the repair or regenerated tissue has not been established because of the short-term follow-up and the few clinical reports of this technique. Experimental evidence also suggests that cartilage regeneration following transplantation of mesenchymal stem cells may be superior to results obtained using autogenous chondrocytes. Autogenous chondrocyte transplantation (including the 2 associated surgical procedures) is expensive, and further documentation of the efficacy and cost-effectiveness of this procedure is warranted in this era of dwindling health care resources.

Focal chondral or osteochondral defects can also be managed by transplantation of osteochondral autografts. A technique, commonly referred to as "mosaicplasty," of transplantation of multiple osteocartilagenous plugs or pegs from a nonweightbearing or peripheral area of the joint into small defects has become more widely used. Autografts of up to 10 mm in diameter can be transferred into prepared defects in the femoral condyles. Reported clinical results with this technique are limited, however.

Other Therapies Intra-articular administration of hyaluronic acid has become widely used for the treatment of OA in Europe and Japan, and recently became available in the United States. Although its mechanism of action is incompletely understood, exogenous synovial fluid hyaluronic acid acts as a lubricant in joints and has a pharmacologic effect that results in stimulation of de novo synthesis of hyaluronic acid, inhibition of arachidonic acid release, and inhibition of IL-1α induced PGE_2 synthesis by synoviocytes. Hyaluronic acid also influences leukocyte adherence, proliferation, migration, and phagocytosis, and it protects against cellular damage caused by reactive oxygen species. Intra-articular injection of hyaluronic acid seems to be as effective as commonly used NSAIDs in relieving pain and improving function in patients with OA of the knee, with a reduced incidence of side effects. Intra-articular hyaluronic acid may be especially useful for the symptomatic treatment of OA of the knee in elderly patients with a prior history of NSAID intolerance or unresponsiveness, or in patients with contraindications to the use of NSAIDs. Typically, a series of 3 to 5 hyaluronic acid injections, administered weekly, is recommended. Although the positive therapeutic effects of intra-articular hyaluronic acid have been documented to last for at least 6 months, long-term efficacy and the need for repeated series of injections are uncertain.

Glucosamine sulfate, administered orally, has been demonstrated to stimulate proteoglycan synthesis by chondrocytes and has mild anti-inflammatory properties. Several clinical trials in patients with OA have demonstrated superior results with glucosamine sulfate compared to placebo. Efficacy of glucosamine sulfate appears to be comparable to that obtained with commonly used NSAIDs. Unlike NSAIDs, which exert their anti-inflammatory effects by inhibition of the cyclooxygenase system and prostaglandin synthesis, glucosamine sulfate appears to exert its therapeutic effects through a prostaglandin independent mechanism. The reduced incidence of adverse events (principally gastrointestinal) with glucosamine sulfate, compared to NSAIDs, has been suggested to result from their differential effects on prostaglandin synthesis.

Future Directions Although not yet clinically feasible, manipulation of the biologic and environmental regulators of the chondrocyte would be logical targets of investigation into new therapies for the treatment of OA and RA. The ability to stimulate the intrinsic self-reparative properties of damaged cartilage by growth factors, such as IGF-I and TGF-β, and to simultaneously inhibit the catabolic effects of cytokines, such as IL-1 and TNF, or matrix metalloproteinases, would likely have a profound effect on the treatment of these disorders. Further understanding of the specific events associated with the initiation and progression of cartilage degeneration and arthritis will likely result in the development of more effective therapies for these disorders.

Rheumatoid Arthritis

RA is a relatively uncommon, immunologically mediated, inflammatory disorder of synovial joints. Although the pathogenesis of RA is incompletely understood, the initial target of this inflammatory process appears to be the synovium. Although it may present in several variant forms, multiple joint involvement, initially with synovitis and later with arthritis, is the rule (Fig. 4). In certain patients, who typically have a more aggressive form of the disease, systemic manifestations can occur. The result of this process, if unsuccessfully treated, all too frequently progresses to a chronic, progressive, disabling polyarticular form of arthritis. Life expectancy is shortened significantly in patients with RA as a result of complications associated with immobility and the extra-articular, systemic manifestations of the disease.

Etiology

RA is thought to develop in individuals with a genetically determined, immunologic predisposition for the disease. Several human leukocyte antigen (HLA) types have been associated with the development of RA, the most prevalent being type HLA-DR4. Although the exact "trigger" postulated to be responsible for the initiation of RA is unknown, the subsequent sequence of immunologic events leading to the development of the rheumatoid synovitis is generally accepted (Fig. 5). The factor responsible for initiating this complex process has been postulated to be an environmental antigen, possibly of infectious origin. The etiologic role of infection has been firmly established in 2 related inflammatory arthropathies, Lyme disease and reactive arthritis, and has been suggested as the etiologic agent in several other immunologic or autoimmune diseases, including sarcoidosis, Crohn's disease, ulcerative colitis, psoriasis, and giant cell arteritis. Recent studies in humans suggest that retroviruses or the Epstein-Barr virus may be the most likely etiologic agent responsible for RA.

Presentation of the responsible environmental antigen from the antigen presenting cell (APC) macrophage to the T cell initiates the pathophysiologic cascade of cytokine production, B cell proliferation, and antibody production seen in RA. T cells of the CD4 phenotype are the most populous member of this cellular lineage in pannus, and CD4 lymphocytes have been thought to play a critical role in magnifying the immune response. Cytokines produced by T cells exert their catabolic effects on the cartilaginous matrix, and are responsible for activation of B cells and

their differentiation into antibody producing plasma cells, which then produce immunoglobins IgG and IgM.

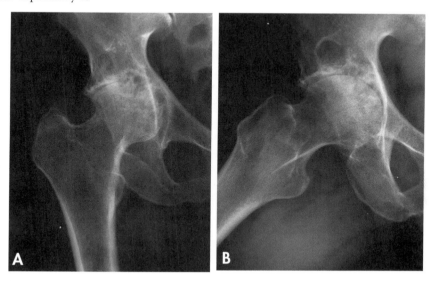

Figure 4

Anteroposterior (A) and lateral (B) radiographs of the hip of a 56-year-old-man with rheumatoid arthritis involving both wrists, both feet, and the right hip show moderate periarticular osteopenia, loss of joint space, and extensive acetabular cyst formation. (Reproduced with permission from Lachiewicz PF: Rheumatoid arthritis of the hip. *J Am Acad Orthop Surg* 1997;5:332–338.)

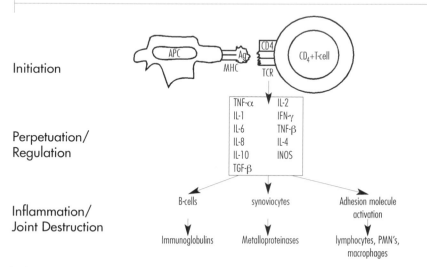

Figure 5

Major cells and cellular products implicated in the immune-mediated inflammatory process of rheumatoid arthritis. APC, antigen-presenting cell; Ag, antigen; MHC, major histocompatibility complex; TCR, T cell receptor; TNF-α, tumor necrosis factor α; IL-1, interleukin-1; TGF-β, transforming growth factor-β; IFN-γ, interferon-γ; TNF-β, tumor necrosis factor β; iNOS, inducible nitric oxide synthase; PMNs, polymorphonuclear cells. (Reproduced with permission from Moreland LW, Heck LW Jr, Koopman WJ: Biologic agents for treating rheumatoid arthritis: Concepts and progress. *Arthritis Rheum* 1997;40:397–400.)

Cellular Response

Synovial angiogenesis, which is essential for synovial proliferation and development of the characteristic rheumatoid pannus, occurs in response to cytokines such as IL-1 and TNF-α. Recent experimental evidence suggests that hepatocyte growth factor (HGF) is produced by rheumatoid synovial fibroblasts in response to IL-1, and that this may be an important factor resulting in synovial angiogenesis. Fibroblast-like cells in the pannus and synovium produce MMPs (collagenase and stromolysin), resulting in degradation of the cartilaginous matrix and erosion of bone. Antibodies to type II collagen, and other minor collagen types present in articular cartilage, may result in immune complexes that form deposits within the cartilage or are released into the synovial fluid, further augmenting the inflammatory process. This altered immune reactivity or autoantibody response appears to play a significant role in the progression of RA, but not in the initiation of the disease. Neutrophils attracted into the synovial fluid become activated by the phagocytosis of cellular debris and immune complexes, resulting in further release of MMPs, prostaglandins, and production of superoxide species. Despite the presence of multiple factors that tend to inhibit these catabolic processes, irreversible articular damage typically occurs because the anabolic activities are overwhelmed by the inflammatory processes outlined above.

This widely accepted T cell paradigm for the pathogenesis of RA has been recently challenged for a variety of reasons. In spite of an exhaustive search for the environmental antigen responsible for initiation of rheumatoid synovitis, none has been definitively identified to date. Alternative theories regarding the pathogenesis of RA have been proposed, which appear to downplay the importance of the T cell in the initiation of RA. One of these hypothesizes that the initiating event in RA may be the production of cytokines in the synovium, in response to nonspecific stimuli (minor trauma, infections, allergic reactions, or immunologic materials), with resultant stimulation of synovial macrophages and fibroblasts (Fig. 6). With repeated nonspecific stimulation, local conditions develop that promote differentiation of dendritic cells in the rheumatoid synovium, which then become capable of presenting autoantigen or self peptide to an autoreactive T cell. These dendritic cells, rather than the APC macrophage, are responsible for presentation of autologous antigen, rather than exogenous antigen, to the T cells. This scheme does not require the presence of the T cell or exogenous antigen for initiation of the disease process. Progression of disease continues as memory T cells perpetuate the autoimmune response, resulting in recruitment of other effector cells. Whether any of these new explanations for the patho-

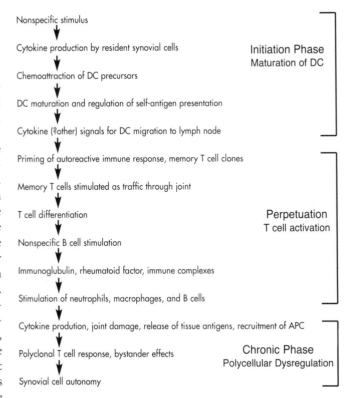

Figure 6

A model for the initiation and perpetuation of rheumatoid arthritis (RA). The model proposes that there are 3 phases of RA: initiation, characterized by cytokine production, dendritic cell (DC) infiltration, and differentiation; perpetuation, associated with T cell proliferation in response to antigen presented by DC; and the chronic phase, characterized by polycellular dysregulation. (Reproduced with permission from Thomas R, Lipsky PE: Presentation of self peptides by dendritic cells: Possible implications for the pathogenesis of rheumatoid arthritis. *Arthritis Rheum* 1996;39:183–189.)

genesis of RA replace the widely accepted T cell paradigm previously considered as dogma is uncertain.

Treatment of Rheumatoid Arthritis

Drugs used for the treatment of RA have been classified into "first-line" and "second-line" drugs. The rationale for this classification was based primarily on the observed toxicity and risks of the various medications, rather their efficacy in halting the progress of the disease. In the past, use of second-line drugs was typically postponed until later in the course of the disease because of concerns about the potential side-effects of some of these medications. The adverse effects of these drugs are almost always reversible; however, articular damage due to inadequately controlled RA is virtually never reversible. The clinical course of RA is self-limited in fewer than 10% of patients, with the remainder of patients eventually progressing to chronic polyarticular RA. Recently, the necessity of early diagnosis and aggressive initial medical management in preventing irreversible articular damage in patients with RA has become more widely accepted. Unlike first-line drugs, several second-line drugs have been demonstrated to decrease the number of painful and swollen joints, suppress the acute phase response, decrease the titer of rheumatoid factor, and retard the radiographic progression of RA. In view of the above, a more useful classification of drugs used to treat RA has been proposed, based on their effects and their ability to control the disease process. This classification categorizes therapeutic agents into symptom-modifying antirheumatic drugs (SMARDs) or disease modifying antirheumatic drugs (DMARDs). NSAIDs traditionally are considered to be first-line drugs, and corticosteroids belong to the SMARD group.

Methotrexate and sulfasalazine are 2 of the most effective and widely used members of the DMARD group. Unlike many of the traditional second-line drugs, such as gold or hydroxychloroquine, which have a slow onset of action of 3 to 6 months, evidence of a positive clinical response may be seen after 3 to 6 weeks with methotrexate and sulfasalazine. Considering that irreversible joint destruction can occur rapidly after onset of rheumatoid synovitis, this is a significant advantage that allows for prompt modification of dosage or institution of other changes in the therapeutic regimen as necessary. Results of combined pharmacologic therapy with both methotrexate and sulfasalazine may be superior to results obtained with either drug alone. Cyclosporine, a known inhibitor of T lymphocyte function, in combination with methotrexate, has recently been shown to be effective in the treatment of severe RA.

Serum markers of disease may be helpful in predicting severity of disease and response to treatment, and may be useful in monitoring disease activity during treatment. Experimental evidence suggests that COMP levels in the first year following diagnosis are elevated in patients who have rapid progression of disease. Genetic typing and analysis of HLA type in patients with RA show promise as potentially useful prognostic tools.

Biologic Agents for Treatment of RA

Recent technologic advancements have made it possible to identify cellular subtypes, cell surface markers, and cell products important in the immunopathogenesis of RA. This evolving understanding of RA provides the opportunity for development of new therapies specifically targeted at many potential points along the disease pathway. Clinical use of these biologic agents has been preliminary and, in general, limited to patients with refractory or longstanding disease.

Some of these therapies, which may be relatively ineffective in the later stages of RA, may be effective in the early stages of the disease. In addition, successful treatment of RA may require combination therapy directed toward several targets involved in the disease process. Potential biologic therapeutic agents for RA include monoclonal antibodies directed against cell surface markers (eg, anti CD4 antibodies, anticytokine antibodies), recombinant forms of natural inhibitor molecules (eg, rIL-1Ra), or MMP inhibitors.

T-cell Receptor Response The central role of the T cell in the most widely accepted paradigm for the pathogenesis of RA has made it the target of many of these immunologic therapies. Monoclonal antibodies directed at various T cell surface markers (including CD4, CD7, CD5 and CD52) and at IL-2 receptors of activated T cells have been used in limited clinical trials. In general, the results of these attempts have been disappointing, prompting some to question the importance of the T cell in the perpetuation of RA.

T-cell receptor (TCR) peptides and attenuated autologous T lymphocytes have been used as vaccines in several controlled clinical trials in patients with RA. TCR vaccination may induce tolerance, depletion, suppression, or inactivation of receptors on T cells that are specific for an inciting autoantigen. The lack of identification of a specific disease-inducing antigen in RA is the major potential limitation to this therapeutic approach.

APC activation of T cells can potentially be prevented by agents that block T cell recognition by the APC. In RA, the obvious targets for this therapeutic approach are the class II major histocompatability complex (MHC) alleles associated with the disease (eg, HLA-DR1 and HLA-DR4). Encouraging clinical responses have been noted in the few studies investigating the use of MHC antagonists.

Cytokine Inhibition The principal proinflammatory cytokines implicated in the pathogenesis of RA have been the target of many biologic agents. Binding of IL-1 to its specific receptor (IL-1R) is the key event in the activation of target cells by this cytokine. Tenidap, a new antirheumatic drug, appears to reduce the number of IL-1 receptors and level of collagenase expression in human synovial fibroblasts in OA and RA. Tenidap is also a potent inhibitor of cyclooxygenase, resulting in additional anti-inflammatory effects due to suppression of prostanglandin synthesis.

Several naturally occurring inhibitors of the cytokines IL-1 and TNF-α have been isolated, including IL-1 receptor antagonist (IL-1Ra), soluble IL-1 receptors I and II (sIL-1R), and soluble TNF-α receptors I and II (sTNFR). Although levels of these inhibitors in serum and in the tissues (at sites of inflammation) are increased in RA, a relative excess of these cytokines in RA favors the proinflammatory effects of IL-1 and TNF-α.

IL-1Ra is a specific inhibitor of IL-1 activity that blocks the binding of IL-1 to cell surface receptors. The proinflammatory effects of IL-1 are overwhelmingly favored because all IL-1 receptors on the cell surface must be blocked by IL-1Ra for complete inhibition of IL-1 induced functions. IL-1Ra concentrations over 100 times those of IL-1 are required to inhibit the activities of IL-1 in vitro. Clinical trials with recombinant human IL-1Ra have demonstrated promising short-term results in treatment of RA.

TNF Inhibition Another potentially useful therapeutic approach to the treatment of RA is inhibition of TNF. The biologic effects of TNF-α and TNF-β are mediated through 2 cell surface receptors designated type I and type II. sTNFR are the shed extracellular portions of these 2 cell surface receptors. As is the case for IL-1Ra, there appears to be an excess of TNF compared with its natural inhibitor, sTNFR. To improve the pharmacokinetics of sTNFR, a recombinant sTNFR has been fused to the Fc portion of an IgG1 immunoglobulin forming a recombinant sTNFR fusion protein (rTNFR:Fc). Soluble TNFRs, including rTNFR:Fc, function like antibodies by binding TNF and preventing its binding with the surface receptors on target cells and cell activation. Initial clinical trials with rTNFR:Fc have been encouraging.

IL-10 and IL-4 are regulatory cytokines that inhibit the release of and interfere with the activity of IL-1, TNF-α and other proinflammatory cytokines (IL-6 and IL-8), and increase synthesis of natural cytokine inhibitors including IL-1Ra and sTNFR. IL-10 and IL-4 also inhibit production of matrix metalloproteinases (MMPs) and thus may be clinically useful inhibitors of proinflammatory cytokines involved in RA.

Collagen degradation products have been suggested as potential antigenic stimuli for the initiation and/or perpetuation of synovitis in RA. Oral tolerance is a reduction in the systemic immune response to an antigen that occurs in response to feeding of the oral antigen. The exact mechanism underlying the development of oral tolerance is unknown. Several small studies of oral administration of type II collagen in RA have shown some decrease in disease activity.

Adhesion molecules expressed on the surface of endothelial cells and complementary sites on the surfaces of immune cells are important in recruitment and transvascular migration of a variety of cells (including neutrophils and macrophages) participating in the inflammatory synovitis of RA. Use of antiadhesion molecules that block the above process may be a potential site of intervention into the pathogenesis of RA. Monoclonal antibodies to intracellular adhesion molecule 1 (ICAM-1) have been used in several clinical studies with promising results.

Therapeutic approaches directed towards modulation of MMPs are logical in the treatment of RA. Administration of exogenous TIMP, agents such as retinoids that can increase local production of TIMP, and synthetic inhibitors of MMPs have been used experimentally and may be clinically useful. Tetracycline and related antibiotics are inhibitors of MMPs and have been the subject of limited clinical trials in patients with RA.

The encouraging short-term clinical results with several of these biologic therapies for RA require further investigation to establish if these agents can truly modify the course of this disease and can be administered safely over long periods of time. Potential long-term toxicities of these biologic agents include development of antibodies, opportunistic infections, and lymphomas, which might potentially seriously limit their clinical usefulness. Combinations of biologic agents or the use of these agents in combination with traditional DMARDs may significantly enhance their clinical utility. As understanding of the pathogenesis of RA is refined by these investigations, more effective biologic therapies that inhibit the critical events in the disease process will emerge.

Annotated Bibliography

American College of Rheumatology Ad Hoc Committee on Clinical Guidelines: Guidelines for the management of rheumatoid arthritis. *Arthritis Rheum* 1996;39:713–722.

This article thoroughly outlines the clinical evaluation and current treatment recommendations for patients with RA. The rationale for early diagnosis and timely initiation of DMARDs to prevent irreversible joint damage is emphasized and presented in an algorithmic form. A succinct review of drug treatment of RA is presented.

American College of Rheumatology Ad Hoc Committee on Clinical Guidelines: Guidelines for monitoring drug therapy in rheumatoid arthritis. *Arthritis Rheum* 1996;39:723–731.

This companion article to the previous reference thoroughly reviews the American College of Rheumatology recommendations regarding clinical monitoring of drug therapies used in the treatment of RA. Drug toxicities and side effects, and their associated risk factors are reviewed in detail. These guidelines developed for the nonrheumatologist are presented in a practical and clinically useful manner.

Arend WP: Editorial: The pathophysiology and treatment of rheumatoid arthritis. *Arthritis Rheum* 1997;40:595–597.

This provocative editorial succinctly presents the evidence for and against the T cell paradigm for the immunopathogenesis of RA and provides direction for basic and clinical research efforts in RA.

Blackburn WD: Management of osteoarthritis and rheumatoid arthritis: Prospects and possibilities. *Am J Med* 1996;100: 24S–30S.

This article reviews the pharmacologic management of RA and OA, and discusses several promising new therapeutic prospects for these disorders. The traditional therapeutic pyramid for treatment of RA and the rationale for reconfiguring the pyramid by earlier use of DMARDs to prevent irreversible joint destruction is presented.

Buckwalter JA, Mankin HJ: Articular Cartilage: Part I. Tissue design and chondrocyte-matrix interactions, in Cannon WD (ed): *Instructional Course Lectures 47.* Rosemont, IL, American Academy of Orthopaedic Surgeons, 1998, pp 477–486.

Buckwalter JA, Mankin HJ: Articular Cartilage: Part II. Degeneration and osteoarthrosis, repair, regeneration, and transplantation, in Cannon WD (ed): *Instructional Course Lectures 47.* Rosemont, IL, American Academy of Orthopaedic Surgeons, 1998, pp 487–504.

The authors present a comprehensive review of the composition, structure, and function of articular cartilage in Part I. A comprehensive review of our current understanding of the processes involved in the degeneration of articular cartilage, osteoarthrosis, and therapeutic approaches to repair or regenerate articular cartilage is presented in Part II.

Di Cesare PE, Carlson CS, Stolerman ES, Hauser N, Tulli H, Paulsson M: Increased degradation and altered tissue distribution of cartilage oligomeric matrix protein in human rheumatoid and osteoarthritic cartilage. *J Orthop Res* 1996;14:946–955.

Degradation and tissue distribution of COMP in normal, OA, and RA articular cartilage was investigated. Degradation fragments released from the matrix into synovial fluid reflect the pathologic processes occurring within the matrix. Distribution of COMP in articular cartilage varied with the underlying disease.

Dieppe P: Osteoarthritis and molecular markers: A rheumatologist's perspective. *Acta Orthop Scand* 1995;266(suppl):1–5.

General hypotheses regarding the etiology and pathogenesis of OA are reviewed. The potential role of molecular markers in diagnosis and treatment of OA are discussed.

Fox DA: The role of T cells in the immunopathogenesis of rheumatoid arthritis: New perspectives. *Arthritis Rheum* 1997; 40:598–609.

This article reviews the T-cell paradigm for the immunopathogenesis of RA and focuses on recent experimental evidence in conflict with this widely accepted explanation for RA. The author suggests that a new model for the pathogenesis of RA, which downplays the role of the T cell, is necessary.

Fries JF, Williams CA, Morfeld D, Singh G, Sibley J: Reduction in long-term disability in patients with rheumatoid arthritis by disease-modifying antirheumatic drug-based treatment strategies. *Arthritis Rheum* 1996;39:616–622.

This large prospective, multicenter study investigated the effects of treatment on long-term functional outcome in patients with RA. Increased DMARD use was associated with significantly better long-term Disability Index values.

Hochberg MC, Altman RD, Brandt KD, et al: Guidelines for the medical management of osteoarthritis: Part I. Osteoarthritis of the hip: American College of Rheumatology. *Arthritis Rheum* 1995;38:1535–1540.

Hochberg MC, Altman RD, Brandt KD, et al: Guidelines for the medical management of osteoarthritis: Part II. Osteoarthritis of the knee: American College of Rheumatology. *Arthritis Rheum* 1995;38:1541–1546.

This two part article outlines the current recommendations of the ACR regarding nonsurgical treatment of OA of the hip and knee. Both pharmacologic and nonpharmacologic modalities, including patient education and physical and occupational therapy are reviewed.

Martel-Pelletier J, Mineau F, Tardif G, et al: Tenidap reduces the level of interleukin 1 receptors and collagenase expression in human arthritic synovial fibroblasts. *J Rheumatol* 1996;23: 24–31.

Synovial fibroblasts from patients with RA and OA demonstrate a dose-dependant decrease in the number of IL-1 binding sites/cell and collagenase expression in response to tenidap in vitro. The biologic activity of this new antiarthritic drug is reviewed.

Messner K, Gillquist J: Cartilage repair: A critical review. *Acta Orthop Scand* 1996;67:523–529.

The authors present a critical review of published reports regarding various techniques to promote cartilage repair, including autologous chondrocyte transplantation, perichondrium or periosteum grafting, subchondral drilling, and abrasion chondroplasty.

Moreland LW, Heck LW Jr, Koopman WJ: Biologic agents for treating rheumatoid arthritis: Concepts and progress. *Arthritis Rheum* 1997;40:397–409.

This article presents a thorough review of the concepts and rationale for the use of biologic agents as potential therapies for RA and provides a summary of the published results of related clinical trials. Biologic agents, including antibodies to cell surface markers, TCR and MHC vaccines, recombinant cytokine inhibitors, anti-TNF and adhesion molecule antibodies, and MMP inhibitors, are discussed.

Müller-Fassbender H, Bach GL, Haase W, Rovati LC, Setnikar I: Glucosamine sulfate compared to ibuprofen in osteoarthritis of the knee. *Osteoarthritis Cartilage* 1994;2:61–69.

In this prospective, randomized, double-blind study of glucosamine sulfate versus ibuprofen for OA of the knee, efficacy was comparable between orally administered glucosamine and ibuprofen, but side effects were considerably less with glucosamine sulfate. The pharmacologic activities of this therapeutic agent, which has received considerable attention in the lay press, are reviewed.

Murphy G: Matrix metalloproteinases and their inhibitors. *Acta Orthop Scand* 1995;266(suppl):55–60.

The author presents an in depth review of MMPs and their inhibitors with specific emphasis on their role in the development of arthritis.

Saxne T: Differential release of molecular markers in joint disease. *Acta Orthop Scand* 1995;266(suppl):80–83.

The author reviews the theoretical and experimental rationale and potential clinical usefulness of molecular markers in RA and OA.

Thomas R, Lipsky PE: Presentation of self peptides by dendritic cells: Possible implications for the pathogenesis of rheumatoid arthritis. *Arthritis Rheum* 1996;39:183–190.

This article reviews the role of the dendritic cell in the pathogenesis of RA and proposes an alternative hypothesis for the initiation and perpetuation of RA in which endogenous antigens are presented to the T cell by the dendritic cell.

Trippel SB: Growth factor actions on articular cartilage. *J Rheumatol* 1995;43(suppl):129–132.

This is a concise review of the actions of relevant polypeptide growth factors in the regulation of cell behavior of articular chondrocytes. The potential to stimulate the intrinsic self-reparative properties of damaged cartilage by growth factors, such as IGF-1 and TGF-β, are discussed.

Classic Bibliography

Brittberg M, Lindahl A, Nilsson A, Ohlsson C, Isaksson O, Peterson L: Treatment of deep cartilage defects in the knee with autologous chondrocyte transplantation. *N Engl J Med* 1994; 331:889–895.

Felson DT: The epidemiology of knee osteoarthritis: Results from the Framingham Osteoarthritis Study. *Semin Arthritis Rheum* 1990;20(3 suppl 1):42–50.

Jimenez SA, Dharmavaram RM: Genetic aspects of familial osteoarthritis. *Ann Rheum Dis* 1994;53:789–797.

Shapiro F, Koide S, Glimcher MJ: Cell origin and differentiation in the repair of full-thickness defects of articular cartilage. *J Bone Joint Surg* 1993;75A:532–553.

Wakitani S, Goto T, Pineda SJ, et al: Mesenchymal cell-based repair of large, full-thickness defects of articular cartilage. *J Bone Joint Surg* 1994;76A:579–592.

Chapter 20
Connective Tissue Disorders

Joint hypermobility is a common characteristic of connective tissue disorders (Ehlers-Danlos syndrome, osteogenesis imperfecta, Marfan syndrome, and some chondrodysplasias). It is attributed to laxity of the supporting ligaments as a result of mechanical failure of their structural components, particularly collagen. It is diagnosed using the Carter-Wilkinson criteria (Beighton modifications) and requires at least 3 of the following: passive opposition of the thumb to the flexor aspect of the forearm; passive hyperextension of the fingers until parallel with the extensor aspect of the forearm; hyperextension of the elbows beyond 10°; hyperextension of the knees beyond 10°; and forward trunk flexion with straight knees and the palms of the hands on the floor.

Marfan Syndrome

This autosomal dominant syndrome is characterized by musculoskeletal, ocular, and cardiovascular problems. The genetic defect is an abnormal FBN1 gene on the long arm of chromosome 15, which encodes the glycoprotein fibrillin, a component of elastic microfibrils in the extracellular matrix. The incidence has been estimated as high as 1 in 10,000 in the general population. The actual incidence is difficult to assess because the variable penetrance of the disorder results in a group of mildly affected individuals, many of whom are never diagnosed. Spontaneous mutation may account for up to 25% of new cases.

New, more stringent criteria for establishing the diagnosis of Marfan syndrome have been presented (Table 1). To diagnose an index case in an individual whose family history is not contributory, major criteria in at least 2 organ systems and involvement of a third organ system are required. DNA testing is not yet clinically available.

Musculoskeletal manifestations of Marfan syndrome include dolichostenomelia (an arm-span-to-height ratio greater than 1.05) and a disproportionate upper to lower body length (a ratio of less than 0.85 in whites and 0.78 in blacks). Additional orthopaedic findings include the wrist sign (positive when the thumb overlaps the fifth finger as these two digits encircle the contralateral wrist) and the Steinberg sign (positive when the thumb, held in the clasped fist, protrudes beyond the ulnar border of the hand), chest wall deformity (pectus excavatum or pectus carinatum), reduced elbow extension, protrusio acetabuli, and pes

planovalgus. Height throughout childhood is just above the 97th percentile.

Scoliosis occurs in 50% of those with Marfan syndrome. The type and frequency of scoliosis is similar to that in idiopathic scoliosis. Generally, the technique for instrumentation is the same as that for idiopathic scoliosis. The mean kyphosis is mildly greater than in the general population. However, the sagittal profile can be quite variable depending on whether the transition between kyphosis and lordosis occurs at or caudad to the normal levels. Pulmonary function may be restricted by thoracic lordoscoliosis (Fig. 1). Adults frequently have pain attributed to degenerative arthritis of the spine.

In the past, 90% of affected individuals succumbed to cardiovascular complications. However, beta-blocker therapy to slow aortic root dilatation and elective surgery for documented aortic root dilatation have increased life expectancy. Aortic root dilatation and rupture and mitral valve prolapse may be diagnosed by ultrasonography. Most patients are myopic, and premature cataracts are common. Bilateral superior lens dislocation occurs in 60% of affected individuals. Regular cardiovascular and ophthalmologic evaluations are essential.

Many clinical features of Marfan syndrome are shared by other connective tissue disorders. Therefore, Marfan syndrome may be confused with other connective tissue disorders, particularly congenital contractural arachnodactyly (CCA or Beals syndrome) and homocystinuria. Individuals with CCA have skeletal features, such as arachnodactyly, dolichostenomelia, and scoliosis, but have joint contractures instead of joint hyperlaxity. They also have ear deformities. Cardiac and ophthalmologic anomalies are absent. Patients with homocystinuria display a body habitus similar to that of Marfan syndrome. Hypermobility syndrome and Stickler syndrome also must be considered in the differential diagnosis.

Ehlers-Danlos Syndrome

Ehlers-Danlos syndrome (EDS) is a heterogeneous group of inherited connective tissue disorders characterized by joint hypermobility; fragile, hyperextensible, doughy skin; atrophic scars; connective tissue fragility; and easy bruising. Traditionally, there were 11 genetically distinct disorders; more recently, this number has been reduced to 9. Symptoms, natural history, and mode of inheritance vary substantially

Table 1
Diagnostic criteria for Marfan syndrome

System	Major Criteria	Minor Criteria
Musculoskeletal*	Pectus carinatum; pectus excavatum requiring surgery; dolichostenomelia; wrist and thumb signs; scoliosis > 20° or spondylolisthesis; reduced elbow extension; pes planus; protrusio acetabulae	Moderately severe pes excavatum; joint hypermobility; highly arched palate with crowding of teeth; facies (dolichocephaly, malar hypoplasia, enophthalmos, retognathia, down-slanting palebral fissures)
Ocular†	Ectopia lentis	Abnormally flat cornea; increased axial length of globe; hypoplastic iris or hypoplastic ciliary muscle causing decreased miosis
Cardiovascular§	Dilatation of ascending aorta ± aortic regurgitation, involving sinuses of Valsalva; or dissection of ascending aorta	Mitral valve prolapse ± regurgitation; dilatation of main pulmonary artery without valvular or peripheral pulmonic stenosis or obvious cause below 40 years; calcification of mitral anulus below 40 years; or dilatation or dissection of descending aorta below 50 years
Family/ genetic history¶	Parent, child, or sibling meets diagnostic criteria; mutation in *FBN1* known to cause Marfan syndrome; or inherited haplotype around *FBN1* associated with Marfan syndrome in family	None
Skin and integument**	None	Stretch marks not associated with pregnancy, weight gain, or repetitive stress; or recurrent or incisional hernias
Dura¶	Lumbosacral dural ecstasia	None
Pulmonary**	None	Spontaneous pneumothorax or apical blebs

* Two or more major or 1 major + 2 minor criteria required for involvement
† At least 2 minor criteria required for involvement
§ One major or minor criterion required for involvement
¶ One major criterion required for involvement
** One minor criterion required for involvement
(Data taken from Paepe A, Devereux RB, Dietz HC, Hennekam RCM, Pyeritz RE: Revised diagnostic criteria for the Marfan Syndrome. Am J Med Gen 1996;62:417–426.)

(Table 2). Types I, II, and III are most common. The molecular mechanisms of many EDS subtypes are now known. Most disrupt collagen fibril assembly, leading to abnormalities in the skin, vasculature, pleuroperitoneum, intestinal walls, ligaments, tendons, cartilage, and eyes. Diagnosis of most types can be made on the basis of family history and physical examination.

Orthopaedic problems in EDS arise from joint hypermobility. Dislocations (patellar subluxation/dislocation, multidirectional shoulder instability) are particularly common in type III EDS. Ambulation may be delayed because of instability and hypermobility. Pes planus is common. Developmental hip dislocation may be seen in types I, IV, and VII. Scoliosis occurs in up to 50% of type III EDS patients, and kyphoscoliosis is a hallmark of type VI EDS. The scoliosis should be treated like idiopathic scoliosis. Because increased flexibility leads to a higher risk of progression, however, early spinal fusion may be indicated.

Joint pain is a significant problem and worsens over time, while joint instability decreases over time. Pain is usually refractory to pharmacologic and physical interventions and chronic pain is common. Treatment is generally nonsurgical and includes physical therapy and orthoses when appropriate. Contact sports and other activities that place the joints at risk should be avoided. Efforts to stabilize the soft tissues eventually fail because of the patient's collagen abnormalities, thus arthrodesis is preferred to arthroplasty. Surgical wounds heal slowly and may dehisce.

Type IV EDS is rare and unique. Joint hypermobility is usually minimal, except in the small joints of the hands and feet. The skin is thin and translucent but not hyperelastic. The venous pattern over the trunk, abdomen, and extremities is visible. A history of easy bruising is common. Of great concern is the high incidence of spontaneous rupture of arteries, the colon, and the gravid uterus. Orthopaedically, these individuals may have clubfeet, developmental hip dislocation, and tendon contractures, particularly of the Achilles tendon or foot extensors.

Homocystinuria

Homocystinuria (HCU) is caused by a deficiency in the enzyme cystathionine beta synthase; it is transmitted as auto-

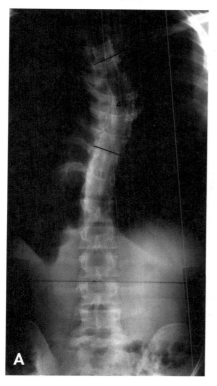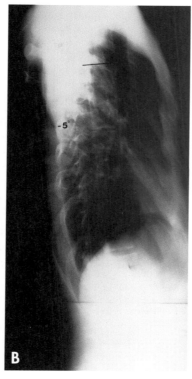

Figure 1

A and B, Thoracic lordosis in a patient with Marfan syndrome. (Reproduced with permission from Freeman BW III, Betz RR: The pediatric spine, in Canale ST, Beaty JH (eds): *Operative Pediatric Orthopaedics,* ed 2. St. Louis, MO, Mosby-Year Book, 1995, p 622.)

ness, gait abnormality, and osteoporosis. Pes cavus is very common and differs from the long, narrow, flatfoot of Marfan syndrome.

A long, thin foot with a disproportionately long great toe and lax ankle support in patients with Marfan syndrome makes shoe-fitting difficult. Pes planovalgus is the most common finding; however, cavus and cavovarus deformities have been reported. The majority of children can be managed with regular shoes, with or without orthoses; few require triple arthrodesis.

Other manifestations include fine or brittle hair, thin skin, malar rash, high arched palate with crowded and protruding teeth, fatty changes in the liver, myopia, cataracts, glaucoma, inguinal hernia, and myopathy. Mental retardation and spasticity are common central nervous system manifestations. Surgery should be avoided whenever possible because of increased risk for thrombosis (both arterial and venous). Life expectancy is decreased.

Osteogenesis Imperfecta

Osteogenesis imperfecta (OI) is a group of hereditary disorders of type I collagen that result in bone fragility. Clinical expression ranges from mild osteoporosis to intrauterine fractures and perinatal death. Males and females are equally affected. The incidence of OI is approximately 1 in 20,000 births. The Sillence classification (Table 3) is based on genetic and extraskeletal features as well as skeletal fragility. The long-term prognosis is strongly related to the Sillence type.

OI is genetically homogeneous within families; however, the phenotype among affected members of the same family may be variable, and unrelated patients with the same phenotypes may have different molecular defects. Germ line mosaicism (ie, the existence of normal and mutant cell populations in a single individual) has been implicated as a cause of OI in families in whom phenotypically normal parents have 1 or more children with OI.

The diagnosis is usually based on clinical examination, growth rate, fracture rate, and radiographic appearance of the bone. It is confirmed by collagen assay using fibroblast cultures from skin biopsy. Clinical features include bone fragility with numerous fractures and bowing, scoliosis, wormian cranial bones, triangular facies, and trefoil-shaped pelvis. Orthopaedic treatment is directed toward prevention and treatment of long bone fractures.

somal recessive with heterozygote and homozygote forms. Approximately 40% of patients respond to high doses of vitamin B6 (pyridoxine); these patients usually have milder clinical manifestations, later onset of disease, and fewer complications than those who do not respond to vitamin B6. Urine analyses for homocysteine and methionine are effective screening measures.

Clinical features are inferior optic lens dislocation (in contrast to Marfan syndrome, which is superior), mental retardation, skeletal abnormalities, and thrombotic events. Patients with this disorder have a marfanoid habitus with arachnodactyly, dolichostenomelia, scoliosis, and pectus excavatum. Distinguishing between two conditions is essential. Scoliosis occurs in up to one third of patients, but it is generally less severe than in Marfan syndrome. Progressive kyphosis is the more frequent spinal deformity. Most importantly, individuals with HCU have joint tightness, whereas joints in Marfan syndrome are lax. Other orthopaedic findings include flaring of the distal femur, bowing of the tibia, enlargement of the carpal bones, genu valgum, muscle weak-

Table 2
Ehlers-Danlos syndrome (cutis hyperelastica)

Type	Acronym	Transmission*	Clinical Findings	Miscellaneous	Basic Defect
I	Gravis type	AD	Hyperextensible skin, poor wound healing, scoliosis, pes planus; hypermobility of small and large joints; osteoarthritis, clubfoot and hip dislocation in the newborn	Easy bruising, "cigarette paper" scars, varicose veins, miscarriages, prematurity, mitral valve prolapse	COL5A1 mutations
II	Mitis type	AD	Similar to EDS I; joint laxity less severe but remarkable in small joints	Less severe than EDS I, no prematurity	COL5A1 mutations, COL1A2 null alleles
III	Hypermobile type	AD	Early onset osteoarthritis, joint dislocations, marked large and small joint hypermobility	Soft skin, no scarring	Unknown
IV	Vascular type	AR (rare)	Hands and feet appear prematurely aged, thin skin without hyperextensibility, minimal joint hypermobility	Severe vascular fragility; uterine and bowel ruptures; stroke; abnormal facies with large eyes, thin nose, thin lips; short life expectancy	COL3A1 mutations; numerous point mutations and exon skips, rarely deletions
	IVA acrogeric IVB acrogeric IVC ecchymotic	AD AR AD			
V	X linked type	XR	Joint laxity	Very rare; similar to EDS I, II, III	Unknown
VI	Ocular scoliotic VIA decreased lysyl hydroxylase levels, VIB normal levels	AR	Kyphoscoliosis (occasionally intractable), muscle hypotonia, moderate joint laxity, skin hyperextensibility	Easy bruising, arterial rupture, ocular fragility	Lysyl hydroxylase point mutations or exon skips (homozygosity and double heterozygosity)
VII	A and B arthrochalasis multiplex congenita	AD	Multiple joint dislocations, bilateral hip dislocation at birth, increased skin elasticity without fragility; diffuse hypotonia, increased bone fragility	Easy bruising, short stature	A: COL1A1 exon 6 skipping mutations; B: COL1A2 exon B skipping mutations
	C	AR	Soft fragile, bruisable skin; marked joint hypermobility	Blue sclera	C: procollagen peptidase deficiency
VIII	Periodontis type	AD	Joint laxity, increased skin elasticity with fragility	Periodontal disease with early tooth loss, easy bruising	Some are COL3A1, others not
IX†	Vacant				
X	Fibronectin abnormality	AR	Mild, similar to EDS II or EDS III without dislocations	Platelet aggregation dysfunction resulting in poor clotting	Defect in fiber section
XI§	Vacant				

*AD, autosomal dominant; AR, autosomal recessive; XR, x-linked recessive
†EDS type IX is no longer part of EDS; it has been reclassified as a disease of copper metabolism
§EDS type XI is now reclassified as a disorder of joint instability

Table 3
Osteogenesis Imperfecta

Type		Transmission*	Biochemistry	Orthopaedic	Miscellaneous
I	A	AD	Half normal amount of type I collagen	Mild to moderate bone fragility, osteoporosis	Blue sclerae, hearing loss, easy bruising, dentinogenesis imperfecta absent
	B	AD		Short stature	More severe than IA with dentinogenesis imperfecta
II		AD, AR and mosaic	Unstable triple helix	Multiple intrauterine fractures, extreme bone fragility	Usually lethal in perinatal period, delayed ossification of skull, interuterine growth retardation
	A		Long bones broad, crumpled; ribs broad with continuous beading		
	B		Long bones broad, crumpled; ribs discontinuous or no beading		
	C		Long bones thin, fractured; ribs thin, beaded		
	D		Severely osteopenic with generally well-formed skeleton; normally shaped vertebrae and pelvis		
III		AD (new mutation) and AR (rare)	Abnormal type I collagen	Progressive deforming phenotype, severe bone fragility with fractures at birth, scoliosis, severe osteoporosis, extreme short stature	Hearing loss, short stature, blue sclerae becoming less blue with age, shortened life expectancy, dentinogenesis imperfecta, relative macrocephaly with triangular faces
IV	A	AD	Shortened pro alpha, (I) chains	Mild to moderate bone fragility, osteoporosis, bowing of long bones, scoliosis	Light sclerae, normal hearing, normal dentition, dentinogenesis imperfecta absent
	B	AD			Dentinogenesis imperfecta present

*AR, autosomal recessive; AD, autosomal dominant

In the young child, lightweight bracing is helpful. If 2 or more fractures of the femur or tibia have occurred in less than 12 months, the use of expandable Bailey-DuBow rods or Rush nails is reasonable. The rods will assist in fracture management and maintain reasonable lower limb alignment as the child grows.

Progressive scoliosis may be difficult to control, despite internal fixation. Bracing is not recommended because it may produce chest deformity as a result of the patients' bone plasticity. Early stabilization with segmental fixation and spinal fusion may be required.

Basilar impression (BI) has been reported in 25% of individuals with OI. It occurs most frequently in patients with Sillence type IVB (71%), and 50% of these patients have neurologic signs of posterior fossa compression. Signs of BI include nystagmus, facial spasm, nerve paresis, pyramidal tract signs, proprioceptive defects, and papilledema. They may be apparent before the patient experiences symptoms (eg, headache, trigeminal neuralgia, imbalance weakness in the arms or legs, and bladder disorders). More severe consequences of BI include brain stem compression, tetraplegia, respiratory arrest, and sudden death.

Unexplained fractures are characteristic of both OI and child abuse. It is difficult to distinguish children with OI from those who are abused. Skin biopsy is not a definitive test for OI, and mutation analysis is currently available only on a research basis. Routine biochemical studies for children suspected to have been abused are unwarranted; therefore, clinical and radiologic evaluation are key. Signs of child abuse not typical of OI include retinal hemorrhage, intracranial injury, lacerations, burns, and sexual abuse. OI can occur without a family history, blue sclera, or metaphyseal fracture.

If any doubt remains after the initial evaluation, the physician should assume the child was abused and act accordingly.

Annotated Bibliography

Cole WG: The molecular pathology of osteogenesis imperfecta. Clin Orthop 1997;343:235–248.

This article reviews the molecular pathology of 200 cases of OI and correlates the finding with clinical, radiologic, and pathologic features of the disorder. As a result of this work, the clinical classification of OI was expanded, and a new biochemical classification was developed.

De Paepe A, Devereux RB, Dietz HC, Hennekam RC, Pyeritz RE: Revised diagnostic criteria for the Marfan syndrome. Am J Med Genet 1996;62:417–426.

This article reviews the new, more stringent requirements for the diagnosis of Marfan syndrome. It delineates initial criteria for diagnosis of other inheritable conditions with partially overlapping phenotypes.

Gray JR, Davies SJ: Marfan syndrome. J Med Genet 1996;33: 403–408.

This is a thorough review of the clinical presentation, genetics, and molecular abnormalities of Marfan syndrome.

Hobbs WR, Sponseller PD, Weiss AP, Pyeritz RE: The cervical spine in Marfan syndrome. Spine 1997;22:983–989.

This review of 104 patients with Marfan syndrome found a large number of individuals with increased atlanto-axial translation and basilar impression. Based on the increased prevalence of severe cervical and ligamentous abnormalities, the authors recommend that patients with Marfan syndrome avoid sports with risks of high impact loading on the cervical spine. Because neurologic injuries in Marfan syndrome are rare, the authors do not recommend radiographs for patients undergoing general anesthesia.

Lipscomb KJ, Clayton-Smith J, Harris R: Evolving phenotype of Marfan's syndrome. Arch Dis Child 1997;76:41–46.

The musculoskeletal features of Marfan syndrome generally predominate and evolve throughout childhood. Awareness of the musculoskeletal presentation of Marfan syndrome aids diagnosis.

Luhmann SJ, Sheridan JJ, Capelli AM, Schoenecker PL: Management of lower-extremity deformities in osteogenesis imperfecta with extensible intramedullary rod technique: A 20-year experience. J Pediatr Orthop 1998;18:88–94.

This is a thorough review of the technique and rationale for the use of extensible rods in OI.

Marini JC, Gerber NL: Osteogenesis imperfecta: Rehabilitation and prospects for gene therapy. JAMA 1997;277:746–750.

This is an excellent review of the genetics and biochemistry of OI, rehabilitation goals and issues, growth hormone treatment, and current knowledge on the possible role for gene therapy.

Pope FM, Burrows NP: Ehlers-Danlos syndrome has varied molecular mechanisms. J Med Genet 1997;34:400–410.

This is a thorough review of the clinical presentation, genetics, and molecular abnormalities found in the various types of Ehlers-Danlos syndrome.

Raff ML, Byers PH: Joint hypermobility syndromes. Curr Opin Rheumatol 1996;8:459–466.

The authors describe how to recognize joint hypermobility and review common joint hypermobility syndromes. They emphasize the strong association between hypermobility and musculoskeletal complaints.

Sillence DO: Craniocervical abnormalities in osteogenesis imperfecta: Genetic and molecular correlation. Pediatr Radiol 1994;24:427–430.

This comprehensive review of clinical science and symptoms of basilar impression in OI patients includes a thoughtful discussion of prevention strategies.

Sotos JF: Overgrowth: Section V. Syndromes and other disorders associated with overgrowth. Clin Pediatr (Phila) 1997;36: 89–103.

This is an excellent overview of 4 disorders commonly associated with overgrowth: Marfan syndrome, congenital contractual arachnodactyly (Beals syndrome), homocystinuria, and Sotos syndrome.

Sponseller PD, Hobbs W, Riley LH III, Pyeritz RE: The thoracolumbar spine in Marfan syndrome. J Bone Joint Surg 1995;77A:867–876.

In a review of 113 patients with Marfan syndrome, 82 of whom were skeletally immature, scoliosis was present in about 63% of the adults of both sexes. Curve progression was likely for curves of more than 20° during growth and for those of 30° to 40° during adulthood. The mean kyphosis was increased. Back pain and impairment were more common than in the general population.

Sponseller PD, Sethi N, Cameron DE, Pyeritz RE: Infantile scoliosis in Marfan syndrome. Spine 1997;22:509–516.

Infantile Marfan syndrome is the most severe form. Bracing has a limited role in infantile scoliosis and is appropriate only if the curve is less than 40°. Surgery should not be performed on patients younger than 4 years of age, because many patients with large curves succumb spontaneously to cardiac complications.

Steiner RD, Pepin M, Byers PH: Studies of collagen synthesis and structure in the differentiation of child abuse from osteogenesis imperfecta. J Pediatr 1996;128:542–547.

The authors note that although OI can be diagnosed by biochemical studies, clinical evaluation by experienced physicians is usually sufficient to differentiate OI and child abuse. Routine biopsy is unwarranted.

Classic Bibliography

Ainsworth SR, Aulicino PL: A survey of patients with Ehlers-Danlos syndrome. *Clin Orthop* 1993;286:250–256.

Beighton P, Solomon L, Soskolne CL: Articular mobility in an African population. *Ann Rheum Dis* 1973;32:413–418.

Boers GH, Polder TW, Cruysberg JR, et al: Homocystinuria versus Marfan's syndrome: The therapeutic relevance of the differential diagnosis. *Neth J Med* 1984;27:206–212.

Carter C, Wilkinson J: Persistent joint laxity and congenital dislocation of the hip. *J Bone Joint Surg* 1964;46B:40–45.

Dietz FR, Mathews KD: Update on the genetic bases of disorders with orthopaedic manifestations. *J Bone Joint Surg* 1996;78A:1583–1598.

Gamble JG, Rinsky LA, Strudwick J, Bleck EE: Non-union of fractures in children who have osteogenesis imperfecta. *J Bone Joint Surg* 1988;70A:439–443.

Hanscom DA, Winter RB, Lutter L, Lonstein JE, Bloom BA, Bradford DS: Osteogenesis imperfecta: Radiographic classification, natural history, and treatment of spinal deformities. *J Bone Joint Surg* 1992;74A:598–616.

Joseph KN, Kane HA, Milner RS, Steg NL, Williamson MB Jr, Bowen JR: Orthopaedic aspects of the Marfan phenotype. *Clin Orthop* 1992;277:251–261.

Marini JC: Osteogenesis imperfecta: Comprehensive management. *Adv Pediatr* 1988;35:391–426.

Mudd SH, Skovby F, Levy HL, et al: The natural history of homocystinuria due to cystathionine beta-synthase deficiency. *Am J Hum Genet* 1985;37:1–31.

Nicholas RW, James P: Telescoping intramedullary stabilization of the lower extremities for severe osteogenesis imperfecta. *J Pediatr Orthop* 1990;10:219–223.

Sillence DO, Senn A, Danks DM: Genetic heterogeneity in osteogenesis imperfecta. *J Med Genet* 1979;16:101–116.

Chapter 21
Genetic Disorders and Skeletal Dysplasias

Genetic Disorders

Overview

Many of the diseases treated by orthopaedic surgeons have a genetic basis, and an understanding of genetics is becoming important in these conditions. The human genome contains about 3 billion nucleotides making up 100,000 genes located on 23 pairs of chromosomes. The Human Genome Organization aims to sequence the entire genome in the next 10 to 15 years. Up-to-date information about specific disorders, mapping information, and references is available through Online Mendelian Inheritance in Man (OMIM) on the worldwide web at http://www3.ncbi.nim.nih.gov/omim/.

Chromosomal disorders occur more frequently than single gene disorders, affecting 0.7% of live births, and are found in half of all spontaneous abortions. They may be detected by cytogenetic techniques because of their major effect on the number or structure of chromosomes. The most common autosomal trisomies involve chromosome 21 (Down syndrome), 18 (microcephaly, overlapping third and fifth fingers, cardiac defects), or 13 (polydactyly with encephalocele, thin ribs). Trisomy of the sex chromosomes may be seen, such as in Klinefelter's syndrome (47, XXY), which results in tall individuals with developmental delay and valgus knees, or there may be monosomy as in Turner's syndrome (45, X), which causes gonadal dysgenesis and webbing of the neck. An example of partial deletion of a chromosome is the Langer-Geidion syndrome, with deletion of the region of q 24.11 to 24.23 on chromosome 8, resulting in mental retardation and osteochondromas.

Trisomy 21: Down Syndrome

Clinical Presentation and Natural History Down syndrome occurs once in every 700 to 800 live births. Growth and development are retarded, and affected children are of short stature. The intelligence range is wide but generally lower than normal. Factors influencing intellectual achievement include family background, early institutionalization, early intervention programs, presence of congenital heart disease, and phys-ical abnormalities. Because 50% of children have some hearing loss that can affect intellectual development, audiology examinations are necessary. Ambulation is delayed (2 to 3 years of age); the gait is broad-based and waddling. Congenital heart defects occur in 30% to 50% of affected individuals, and gastrointestinal malformations are present in 5% to 7%. The mortality is increased during the first 10 years, even when deaths from congenital heart defects are excluded. This is the result of an increased susceptibility to infections, caused either by abnormal function of the T lymphocytes or an anatomic abnormality of the respiratory system (eg, gastroesophageal reflux, primary pulmonary hypertension, and obstructive sleep apnea). Ninety percent of children without significant congenital defects live to adulthood.

Individuals with Down syndrome are at increased risk for other medical problems, including cataracts, juvenile onset diabetes mellitus, thyroid conditions, and seizures. Leukemia is present in 1% of patients. A progressive dementia similar to Alzheimer's disease may develop by the fourth decade.

Orthopaedic Problems and Treatment Orthopaedic problems are predominantly related to ligamentous laxity (Fig. 1). Recurrent patellar subluxation occurs in one third of the individuals; 10% have frank dislocations. Physical therapy is difficult in these children, and surgical results are compromised by recurrence caused by ligamentous laxity. One out of 20 children develops hip instability during the first decade (acute dislocation, habitual dislocation, subluxation, progressive instability, and acetabular dysplasia). Treatment must be tailored to each anatomic problem; soft-tissue procedures must be supplemented by correction of bony deformities with femoral and/or pelvic osteotomy to obtain stability. Slipped capital femoral epiphysis also occurs, and hypothyroidism should be investigated. Pes planus is common and needs only symptomatic treatment. Hallux valgus is also common and is associated with predisposing factors, such as external tibial torsion, hindfoot valgus, and/or pronation. Persistent pain and difficulties with shoeing that cannot be managed with orthoses may necessitate surgical correction.

The most significant problem is atlantoaxial instability, with

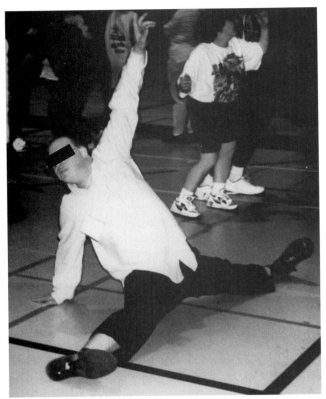

Figure 1

Ligamentous laxity as this patient is demonstrating is central to most of the musculoskeletal problems of Down syndrome.

or without atlanto-occipital instability. The reliability and utility of plain radiographic measurements of both occiput-C1 and C1-C2 have been questioned. Recent reviews have demonstrated a significant complication rate with cervical fusions. Fusion should be reserved for myelopathy or severe instability with marginal space available for the spinal cord and an atlanto-dens interval > 10 mm. Newer techniques, such as a Luque loop rod or large autogenous iliac crest grafts with occiput to C2 fusion are reported to have fewer complications than standard C1-C2 fusion. The American Academy of Pediatrics' Committee on Sports Medicine and Fitness has questioned the practice of obtaining flexion-extension lateral radiographs of the cervical spine to determine participation in Special Olympics. They observed, after a careful review of the existing literature, that "identification of those patients who already have or who later have complaints or physical findings consistent with symptomatic spinal cord injury is a greater priority than obtaining radiographs. Recognition of these symptomatic patients is challenging and requires frequent interval histories and physical examinations...."

Neurofibromatosis

Incidence and Genetics Neurofibromatosis, the most common single gene disorder in humans, occurs in 2 forms, NF-1, with an incidence of 1 in 3,500 live births, and NF-2, with an incidence of 1 in 50,000 births. It is autosomal dominant, with nearly complete penetrance. Half the reported cases are new mutations.

The NF-1 gene is located on chromosome 17. This gene codes for the protein named neurofibromin, believed to be a tumor-suppressor gene that normally functions to control cell growth and differentiation. Neurofibromas occur if the unaffected allele coding for neurofibromin (that is, the allele not carrying the mutation causing NF-1) undergoes a somatic mutation. This "two hit" hypothesis of neurofibroma causation is supported by mutation analysis of neurofibromas from a large number of individuals in different families.

The NF-2 gene is located on chromosome 22. The mutant gene codes for merlin or schwannomin, which is a protein that links the cytoskeleton to the plasma membrane. This gene also appears to be a tumor-suppressor gene, and the severity of the disorder correlates with how severe a truncation of the protein is caused by the specific mutation. In NF-2 there are fewer peripheral lesions, but more significant intracranial ones, including bilateral acoustic neuromas and other tumors of the meninges and Schwann cells (Outline 1). Affected individuals tend to be short with large heads and frequently experience precocious puberty. Seizures and varying degrees of intellectual deficiency are present in 50%.

Clinical Presentation The clinical presentation of the disease varies widely, and many affected individuals appear normal at birth. Numerous organ systems are affected. In the more common NF-1, characteristic features are café-au-lait spots, axillary freckles, hyperpigmented nevi, and neurofibromas of the peripheral and central nervous systems. The café-au-lait spots are usually present at birth but may take up to a year or more to appear. Their number and size increase after their initial presentation, rendering an inaccurate diagnosis based on numbers and size during the first decade of life. The hyperpigmented nevus is often associated with a deep plexiform neurofibroma.

The typical neurofibromas begin to appear by age 10 years. They increase in size and number during puberty. Lesions are composed of benign Schwann cells and fibrous connective tissue. They are either sessile or peduncular and may develop along the path of a peripheral nerve or motor root. They rarely cause neurologic deficit. Plexiform neurofibromas are more serious. Usually present at birth, they are characterized by a deep brown skin pigmentation with pendulous skin

Outline 1
Criteria for Neurofibromatosis-1 and Neurofibromatosis-2

Criteria for NF-1 (2 or more of the following):

1. Six or more café-au-lait macules whose greatest diameter is 5 mm in perpubertal patientsand 15 mm in postpubertal patients

2. Two or more neurofibromas of any type or one plexiform neurofibroma

3. Freckling in the axillary or inguinal regions

4. Optic glioma

5. Two or more Lisch nodules (iris hamartomas)

6. A distinctive osseous lesion, such as sphenoid dysplasia or thinning of long bone cortex, with or without pseudarthrosis

7. A first-degree relative (parent, sibling, or child) with NF-1 by the above criteria

Criteria for NF-2 (1 of the following):

1. Bilateral eighth nerve masses seen with appropriate imaging techniques (eg, computed tomography or magnetic resonance imaging)

2. NF-2 in a first degree relative, and either a unilateral eighth nerve mass or 2 of the following: neurofibroma, meningioma, glioma, schwannoma, or juvenile posterior subcapsular lenticular opacity.

(Reproduced with permission from Aoki S, Barkovich AJ, Nishimura K, et al: Neurofibromatosis types 1 and 2: Cranial MR findings. *Radiology* 1989;172:527-534.)

folds. Although histologically benign, they cause significant limb overgrowth and gigantism, infiltration of the neuraxis, and grotesque facial disfigurement. Their highly vascular nature renders surgical removal impractical. Skeletal overgrowth is asymmetric, and variable skeletal components are involved. Erosion and cystic changes may occur within bones and mimic other diseases.

Malignancies can occur in 5% to 15% of affected individuals. Neurofibromas in adolescence and adulthood may undergo malignant degeneration, or malignant neurofibrosarcomas may appear de novo. Rapid increase in size

necessitates excisional biopsy. Other concomitant malignancies, including Wilm's tumor, leukemia, and rhabdomyosarcoma, are also more likely to occur.

Radiographic Findings Magnetic resonance imaging (MRI) studies have a demonstrated high sensitivity and allow the detection of intracranial lesions and the differentiation of type I from type II neurofibromatosis. Such studies of the spine are mandatory before surgery to detect the intraspinal lesions of neurofibroma, dural ectasias, and meningocele. MRI may also detect large neurofibromas in the spine, pelvis, or neck that should undergo excisional biopsy.

Orthopaedic Problems A major orthopaedic problem is present in at least 40% of these individuals. Neurofibromatosis must be considered when evaluating a patient with pseudarthrosis of a long bone, hypertrophy of a part, an unusual radiographic lesion, or a significant scoliosis or spinal deformity. For a discussion of the spinal abnormalities and their treatment, see chapter 47.

Pseudarthrosis usually involves the tibia and appears in infancy with the classic anterolateral bow. The ulna, femur, clavicle, radius, and humerus may also be involved. The relationship of pseudarthrosis to neurofibromatosis is well established, but the mechanism remains unknown. The Boyd classification for pseudarthrosis of the tibia generally is used. The common types are I, pseudarthrosis at birth; II, anterolaterally bowed tibia; III, cyst in the medullary canal; and IV, stress fractures. Initial bracing for the anterolaterally bowed tibia is recommended. Once fracture or pseudarthrosis occurs, surgical treatment is indicated. The prognosis for establishing a solid union remains guarded. Recent reports suggest a good union rate with intramedullary rodding and bone grafting; vascularized fibula transfer and the Ilizarov technique are reserved for failure of rodding and grafting.

Turner's Syndrome

This relatively common disorder, with an incidence of 1 in 2,500 live births, is caused by presence of a single sex chromosome (X). At birth, a webbed neck, persistent edema of the dorsum of the hands and feet, and widely-spaced nipples are present. Stature remains low, and sexual maturation never happens unless estrogen supplementation is given. Growth hormone produces a mild increase in height. Patients are vulnerable to X-linked recessive disorders normally affecting only males, such as Duchenne muscular dystrophy. Social acceptance is high, and with hormone supplementation and ovum transport, affected individuals may become pregnant. Orthopaedic problems include scoliosis, osteoporosis, and asymptomatic valgus of the elbows and knees.

Stickler Syndrome

The inheritance in this condition, also termed hereditary arthro-ophthalmopathy, is autosomal dominant, and the defect appears to be in type II collagen. Stickler syndrome resembles Marfan syndrome in that affected individuals are tall and slender. They are different, however, in having irregular epiphyses, with subsequent osteochondritis dissecans and arthritis. Morning stiffness is a common complaint. Coxa valga and protrusio acetabulae may develop. Aortic enlargement is not common, but retinal detachment may occur.

Skeletal Dysplasias

The skeletal dysplasias are a group of genetic disorders that have generalized disorder of growth and development of bone and cartilage. Their heterogeneity has multiple different causes. The clinical problems in patients with skeletal dysplasia fall into certain predictable categories: lower extremity length or angular disturbances, joint stiffness or degenerative change, short stature (height < 2 standard deviations below the mean of the population), cervical instability, thoracolumbar kyphosis or scoliosis, and spinal stenosis. Patients with each dysplasia have some of these problems, but not all of them. Table 1 lists the spinal abnormalities seen in various skeletal dysplasias. Dysplasias that are relatively common include achondroplasia, spondyloepiphyseal dysplasia, metaphyseal dysplasia, and multiple exostoses.

Achondroplasia

Achondroplasia is the most common of the skeletal dysplasias. It is transmitted in an autosomal dominant fashion, although two thirds of cases arise through new mutations, with advanced paternal age as a risk factor. It has been recently shown to arise from a mutation in the gene for fibroblast growth factor receptor protein. Patients are recognizable from birth, because of the frontal bossing, midface hypoplasia, and extreme shortening of the proximal segments of the limbs, especially of the humerus and the femur, a pattern termed rhizomelic shortening. The ilia are squared, with hor-

Table 1					
Characteristic spinal problems in skeletal dysplasias					
Condition	**Deformity**	**Anomaly**	**Instability**	**Stenosis**	**Special Features**
Achondroplasia	T-1 kyphosis ages 0-2	0		Foramen magnum; entire spine	Adult weakness due to stenosis
Diastrophic dysplasia	Cervical kyphosis; T-1 scoliosis	Cervical spina bifida occulta			Cervical kyphosis may resolve; scoliosis usually rigid
SED congenita	Scoliosis	Odontoid hypoplasia	C1-C2		
Morquio syndrome	T-1 scoliosis	Odontoid hypoplasia	C1-C2		
Hurler's syndrome	T-1 kyphosis; scoliosis		C1-C2		Most live 1-2 decades
Osteogenesis imperfecta	Kyphosis; scoliosis				Scoliosis related to overall severity
Larsen syndrome	Cervical kyphosis	Cervical spondylolisthesis; cervical spina bifida	Midcervical		Kyphosis should be fused posteriorly

izontal acetabulae and sharp sciatic notches. Although the cranium is large and the ventricles may be enlarged, true hydrocephalus is rare. Patients are often hypotonic and slow in meeting motor milestones, although they usually have normal coordination in later childhood. Mild foramen magnum stenosis is common but there is a subgroup of patients who have clinically significant stenosis that requires foramen magnum decompression. Some advocate evaluating all infants with achondroplasia for this stenosis.

Ligaments are surprisingly lax in achondroplasia, leading to recurvatum in infancy, which commonly resolves. Genu varum occurs in a number of patients, possibly as a result of overgrowth of the fibula relative to the tibia. In most patients it is mild and asymptomatic. However, if it becomes severe or painful, valgus osteotomy may be performed for symptoms or appearance; the long-term effect of the deformity on degenerative joint disease is not known. Elbow flexion contractures or radial head subluxation may occur but are asymptomatic, and degenerative disease of any joint is rare.

Some means are available to increase stature. Growth hormone has been shown to have a mild stimulatory effect on the patients with the lowest growth velocities, but it is not widely used. Surgical limb lengthening may produce dramatic gains because the bone, muscles, and nerves tolerate major elongation compared to congenital limb deficiencies. The lengthening rarely brings patients into the normal range of stature, however. For this reason, and because treatment is so prolonged, most patients do not elect to have this done. Life expectancy and intelligence are typically normal.

Thoracolumbar kyphosis, extremely common in the first years of life (Fig. 2), results from a developmental overload at the thoracolumbar junction from unsupported body weight. It usually resolves as trunk muscle strength is gained. When the kyphosis persists past the age of 2 years, hyperextension bracing often promotes resolution. When kyphosis persists into later childhood, fusion may be indicated, but this is rare. Scoliosis does not typically occur in achondroplasia. Instability of the cervical spine is uncommon, in contrast to many other forms of dysplasia, but cervical stenosis may occur, as in the lumbar spine. Spinal stenosis results from undergrowth of the pedicles and close spacing, which become more pronounced in the descending regions of the spine. Radiographs of the lumbar spine demonstrate narrow interpedicular distance. The patient often becomes symptomatic when degenerative changes are superimposed on the already tight canal. Neurogenic claudication is relieved by hunching over, resting the hands on the thighs to decrease the lumbar lordosis and open up the canal. Cauda equina syndrome may occur in the lower spine, or myelopathy may ensue if the stenosis includes the cervical or thoracic spine.

Decompression should include all stenotic areas of the spine, usually proceeding distally to the sacrum. Any serious preexisting thoracolumbar kyphosis should be fused at the time.

Pseudoachondroplasia

Pseudoachondroplasia is transmitted as autosomal dominant in many cases. In those where the pattern of transmission is less typical, it is believed to result from germ line mosaicism. A gene for this disorder has recently been localized to chromosome 19, and appears to code for cartilage oligomeric matrix protein (COMP). This protein is normally present at high levels in cartilage matrix, and it is possible that failure of

proteoglycan binding by COMP results in accumulation of proteoglycan in the chondrocytes.

This disorder resembles achondroplasia because of its rhizomelia but otherwise has little in common with it. It is rarely distinguishable at birth, but becomes more distinct with age, leading to diagnosis by 4 years when relative shortening of the trunk, limbs, and ligamentous laxity develop. Craniofacial features are normal. Life expectancy is unaffected.

The long bones develop changes in the epiphyses as well as the metaphyses. The epiphyses have delayed and fragmented ossification; in the proximal femur this may be mistaken for bilateral Legg-Calvé-Perthes disease. The epiphyseal irregularity may lead to restricted range of motion and, eventually, to degenerative joint disease. Epiphyseal extrusion may develop progressively, especially if there is adduction of the femur or genu valgum. Whether surgical intervention affects the long-term fate of the hip is not known. The knees often develop varus, valgus, or "windswept" malalignment. Surgery is appropriate when the angulation is severe. An arthrogram or MRI may be necessary to see the true surface of the joint, because of the delay in ossification. Recurrence is common, and repeat surgery may be needed. The spine is less frequently involved, although the vertebrae may show anterior indentations on the margins, similar to Morquio syndrome. Upper cervical instability and scoliosis occur in a few patients.

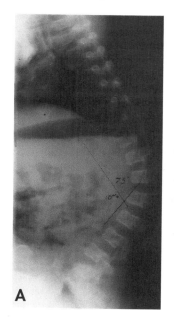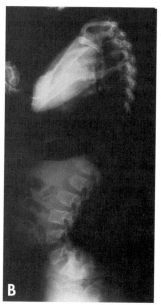

Figure 2

Thoracolumbar kyphosis is very common in infants with achondroplasia (A). The kyphosis in this patient persisted past the age of 2 ½ years, so bracing was initiated. The curve improved so that the patient had only a negligible kyphosis (B) by age 5 years.

Spondyloepiphyseal Dysplasia (SED)

This group of disorders are all due to a defect in the gene for type II collagen. The more common SED congenita is usually autosomal dominant, while SED tarda is X-linked recessive. Vertebral flattening and scoliosis lead to shortening of the trunk, even greater than that of the rhizomelic shortened extremities. The midface is flat and the chest barrel-shaped. The hands and feet are usually normal, but talipes equinovarus may be seen. There is usually increased lumbar lordosis, either primarily or due to hip flexion contractures.

Radiographic Findings The ilia are square, and the epiphyses are delayed in ossification and are fragmented. In the hip, this may be mistaken for bilateral Legg-Calvé-Perthes disease, but the synchronous nature of the changes, as well as presence of changes in other epiphyses, should be a clue to diagnosis. Coxa vara may also occur. The metaphyses of long bones may show mild irregularity. The vertebral bodies are initially biconvex, but become progressively flattened with age, and the end plates become irregular. The odontoid may be hypoplastic or absent, leading to instability that may cause neurologic compromise, even in early childhood.

Orthopaedic Problems Motor milestones are usually met on time; therefore, a delay should prompt a search for atlantoaxial instability. A positive Trendelenburg gait may be manifest because of the hip disorder. Presenting problems may include short stature, scoliosis, hip pain, or increasing spasticity. Retinal detachment may occur, so periodic ophthalmologic surveillance is indicated. These patients are not particularly good candidates for limb lengthening because of the epiphyseal involvement. Degenerative arthritis of the hips or the knees may be treated with arthroplasty.

Osteotomy of the proximal femur may be indicated to correct coxa vara or to provide containment, although proof of increased longevity of the joint following the procedures is lacking. Osteotomy about the knee for severe angular disturbances is usually successful. Upper cervical instability should be treated with posterior fusion if significant; decompression should be added if there is stenosis. Scoliosis may be treated in the standard fashion, with addition of anterior fusion for large or rigid curves, or those at risk of continued postoperative deterioration (usually under age 11 years).

Multiple Epiphyseal Dysplasia

This relatively common skeletal dysplasia is characterized by abnormal epiphyses in multiple joints and often presents late. Inheritance is autosomal dominant. Stature is in the lower range of normal. The hips and knees are most commonly affected. Joint pain, stiffness, and genu valgus may be initial complaints. Patients may present with the diagnosis of bilateral Legg-Calvé-Perthes disease. This should be an indication for a skeletal survey. Redirectional osteotomies are often inappropriate because of the nonspherical femoral head. Proximal tibial osteotomy is indicated for bothersome genu valgum. Premature osteoarthritis may develop in middle age.

Metaphyseal Chondrodysplasia

The metaphyseal chondrodysplasias are characterized by metaphyseal deformity and irregularity adjacent to the physes, with little or no epiphyseal involvement. They must be differentiated from the various forms of rickets.

The Schmid type, diagnosed at 2 to 3 years, is an autosomal dominant condition with a mutation in the gene for type X collagen. Patients may show genu varum, increased lumbar lordosis, and a Trendelenburg gait. The physis is wide in comparison to other types, and the metaphyses are cupped and flared. Proximal femoral osteotomy for coxa vara, or tibial osteotomy for genu varum, may be helpful if the deformities are severe.

The Jansen type is autosomal dominant and recently has been associated with a mutation of the receptor for parathyroid hormone-parathyroid hormone-related peptide. There is severe shortening of the limbs at birth, frontal bossing, and micrognathia. Bowing of the diaphyses occurs with growth as a result of the elongation of the abnormal metaphyses. Flexion contractures develop in the major joints.

McKusick type (cartilage-hair hypoplasia), usually diagnosed at age 2 or 3 years, was first described by McKusick in the Amish population and is autosomal recessive. Progressive dwarfing results in markedly short adult stature. The fingers are broad and the ligaments are lax. The hair is fine and light. There is metaphyseal cupping in the distal femur but no significant coxa vara. Significant systemic problems have been reported, including lymphopenia, neutropenia, immune deficiency, Hirschsprung's disease, and malabsorption.

Multiple Cartilaginous Exostoses (Diaphyseal Aclasia)

This condition, also known as multiple osteochondromatosis, is one of the more common osteochondrodysplasias seen by orthopaedic surgeons. It is usually transmitted in an autosomal dominant fashion. The disorder is genetically heterogeneous, with abnormalities found in different individuals on chromosomes 8, 11, and 19, designated EXT1, EXT2, and EXT3. This may account for some of the phenotypic heterogeneity. Some of these genes are tumor-suppressor genes. The exostoses usually appear after age 3 to 4 years. There is a generalized disturbance in physeal regulation; nests of growth cartilage "escape" from the confines of the ring of Lacroix and grow perpendicular to the bone in a sessile or pedunculated fashion. The cortex of the exostosis is contiguous with that of the bone itself. The smaller the diameter of the affected bone, the more affected its growth will be. The metaphyses of most long bones display a broadening caused by failure of remodeling in the cut-back zone.

Problems from this condition may be divided into four categories: (1) local prominence and impingement by the osteochondromas; (2) asymmetric growth of 2-bone segments, such as the forearm and the leg; (3) limb-length inequality; and (4) late degeneration into chondrosarcoma. Local prominence may cause pressure on muscles, nerves, or adjacent bones. These tend to become symptomatic in the prepubertal period. Examples include peroneal palsy from a proximal fibular lesion; tendonitis of the pes anserinus or vastus lateralis and medialis; and restriction of forearm rotation or snapping shoulder from a lesion under the scapula. Asymmetric growth often results in genu valgum, ankle valgus, ulnar subluxation of the carpus, and radial head subluxation. Limb-length inequality is usually inconsequential but has been reported to be as much as 4 cm. Malignant degeneration is difficult to monitor because it may occur at any time. Some authors recommend a bone scan every 2 years, but periodic careful examination or self-examination with reporting of any growth of the mass or increase in pain is the most practical solution.

Locally prominent lesions should be excised with their cartilage cap if bothersome. Parents should be advised that some bony prominence may recur if the child is young. Unfortunately, removing osteochondromas does not restore the growth potential to an affected bone, nor does it restore much rotation to a severely restricted forearm. Angular disturbances are treated by hemiepiphyseodesis when young, or osteotomy when older. Ulnar tethering may be treated by osteotomy, ulnar lengthening, and radial hemiepiphyseodesis or shortening if indicated. Painful radial head dislocations may be excised at skeletal maturity. Recent studies have shown that most forearm deformities in this condition are relatively well tolerated.

Leg-length inequality arises with differentiated involvement by osteochondromas; epiphyseodesis is the most appropriate treatment.

Enchondromatosis (Ollier Disease)

This uncommon condition is characterized by asymmetric, intraosseous cartilage masses. Radiographically, there are streak-like geographic lucencies, greatest in the metaphyses. Shortening and angulation occur in the bones with greatest involvement. The lesions expand with growth, ceasing at puberty. In some patients, hemangiomas also occur

(Maffucci syndrome). Treatment depends on the magnitude of the angulation and limb-length inequality and may include epiphyseodesis, osteotomy, and/or lengthening. Transformation to a low-grade chondrosarcoma may occur in adults.

Diastrophic Dysplasia

This cartilaginous disorder affects trachea, ear, and the ligaments. It is due to a defect in a cellular sulfate transport protein, resulting in undersulfation of proteoglycans, critical components of cartilage, thereby impairing the hydraulic properties of cartilage.

Affected persons have rhizomelic short stature from birth, which becomes progressively more noticeable. The pinnae of the ears develop a characteristic idiopathic swelling at about 6 to 8 weeks, followed by the development of the classic "cauliflower ear." A small proportion of neonates develop severe tracheomalacia, which may be fatal. A widely abducted or "hitchhiker" thumb is a characteristic feature, caused by a short, proximally placed, triangular first metacarpal. The proximal interphalangeal joints of the digits are often fused. The neonatal hip flexion contracture fails to improve, and the proximal femoral epiphyses progressively deform. The knees have flexion contractures, epiphyseal deformation, valgus angulation, and, often, patellar subluxation. The feet usually demonstrate a rigid equinovarus deformity (Fig. 3). Surgery is usually required with poorer results than idiopathic clubfeet. Bony procedures or talectomy may be necessary.

Premature degenerative joint disease is common, especially in the hip; the mean age of patients at arthroplasty in 1 series was 37 years. Special custom components are necessary. The 5-year survival of the implant is at least 90%.

The midcervical spine is often bifid posteriorly; a kyphosis may develop, which may or may not resolve. Surgical intervention may be necessary to prevent neurologic impairment in severe kyphoses. Cervical instability is common. Kyphoscoliosis is present in one half to one third of patients. Response to bracing is not uniform; surgery may be necessary, but results in modest correction.

Mucopolysaccharidoses

The mucopolysaccharidoses are a group of inherited metabolic disorders caused by a deficiency of specific lysosomal enzymes, which results in intracellular accumulation of partially degraded glycosaminoglycans. There is phenotypic variability within a given diagnosis. Common features include corneal clouding, organomegaly, epiphyseal deformation with limitation of joint motion, deafness, and cardiac disease. Diagnosis is made using urine analysis for glyscosaminoglycan, tissue samples, and leukocyte enzyme analysis. Anesthesia is often difficult because of size, cervical instability, and the need for fiber optic intubation. Hurler syndrome (Fig. 4) is one of the most common and is due to a deficiency of L-iduronidase. It is usually diagnosed by age 2 years and fatal by age 10 years. Bone marrow transplant may be successful in arresting, but not reversing, disease progression; thus, the youngest siblings are benefited the most by marrow transplant. Thoracolumbar kyphosis or cervical instability may require surgery. Hunter syndrome is milder than Hurler syndrome, with a normal life expectancy. Morquio syndrome includes pectus carinatum, normal intelligence, and flame-shaped projections from the anterior vertebral bodies. Atlantoaxial instability may require cervical fusion.

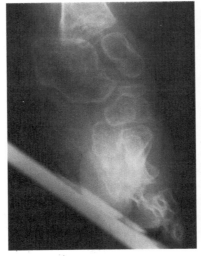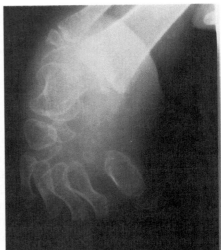

Figure 3

The most common foot deformity in diastrophic dysplasia is a rigid equinovarus.

Cleidocranial Dysostosis

Although its name highlights the 2 most prominent features of this disorder, this autosomal dominant dysplasia involves multiple skeletal abnormalities, especially in bones of intramembranous origin. The abnormal gene *CBFA* appears important for normal osteogenesis. The clavicles are deficient distally or totally. There may be coxa vara, which should be treated according to standard indications. The symphysis pubis is delayed in its midline ossification. The skull displays frontal bossing with a midfrontal groove, as well as widened sutures and persistent fontanelles. Patients (especially females) may present initially with short stature; males eventually reach a stature of the fifth to fiftieth percentile, while women are usually below the fifth percentile. There may be underdevelopment of the distal phalanges. Scoliosis occurs in a minority of cases, although it has been reported in association with syringomyelia in several.

Larsen Syndrome

Autosomal dominant as well as recessive forms of this syndrome have been observed. The genetic locus is in the short arm of chromosome 3 near the collagen VII locus but the biochemical defect is unknown. It is characterized by multiple dislocations of large joints (hips, knees, elbows), a broad face with hypertelorism, and ligamentous laxity. Clubfeet are also common. Tracheomalacia, cleft palate, and cardiac valvular defects occur with increased frequency and may limit management in infancy. Differential diagnosis includes

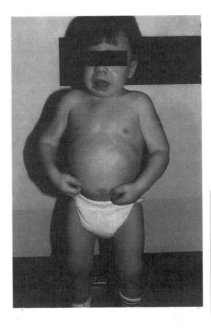

Figure 4

Patient with severe mucopolysaccharidosis type I (Hurler syndrome) has the typical appearance of a storage disorder, with organomegaly, characteristic facial appearance, corneal clouding and developmental delay.

Ehlers-Danlos syndrome and arthrogryposis.

Open reduction is usually needed for knee dislocation. Following this, the hips and feet may be treated surgically. Before general anesthesia, cervical kyphosis or instability should be assessed; when present, fusion is appropriate to prevent myelopathy.

Annotated Bibliography

Down Syndrome

American Academy of Pediatrics Committee on Sports Medicine and Fitness: Atlantoaxial instability in Down syndrome: Subject review. *Pediatrics* 1995;96:151–154.

This is a careful review of the literature to date. The authors concluded that routine lateral radiographs are of unproved value and that identification of prodromal symptoms and signs of spinal cord compression is of paramount importance.

Karol LA, Sheffield EG, Crawford K, Moody MK, Browne RH: Reproducibility in the measurement of atlanto-occipital instability in children with Down syndrome. *Spine* 1996;21:2463–2467.

Another report of an unreproducible clinical measurement of plain radiographs. The authors recommend MRI if there is suspicion of instability.

Rizzolo S, Lemos MJ, Mason DE: Posterior spinal arthrodesis for atlantoaxial instability in Down syndrome. *J Pediatr Orthop* 1995;15:543–548.

Nine patients were treated; 3 developed a fibrous union but all became stable.

Neurofibromatosis

Ruttledge MH, Andermann AA, Phelan CM, et al: Type of mutation in the neurofibromatosis type 2 gene (NF2) frequently determines severity of disease. *Am J Hum Genet* 1996;59:331–342.

The more severe the truncation in the protein merlin (schwannomin) a mutation causes, the more severe the disorder. Patients with single amino acid mutations have a mild phenotype.

Serra E, Puig S, Otero D, et al: Confirmation of a double-hit model for the NF1 gene in benign neurofibromas. *Am J Hum Genet* 1997;61:512–519.

Data are presented showing that neurofibromas occur when the normal allele of the gene coding for neurofibromin in patients inheriting a mutated allele undergoes somatic mutation.

Skeletal Dysplasias

Dietz FR, Mathews KD: Update on the genetic bases of disorders with orthopaedic manifestations. *J Bone Joint Surg* 1996;78A: 1583–1598.

This review of genetics and research techniques includes a table of orthopaedically important disorders and overview of clinicopathologic basis of selected conditions.

McKusick VA (ed): *Mendelian Inheritance in Man: A Catalog of Human Genes and Genetic Disorders*, ed 11. Baltimore, MD, Johns Hopkins University Press, 1994.

This is the "bible" for information on rare genetic disorders, edited by the founder of the specialty of medical genetics.

Achondroplasia

Ganel A, Horoszowski H: Limb lengthening in children with achondroplasia: Differences based on gender. *Clin Orthop* 1996;332:179–183.

In this series of 12 patients, the authors recommend delaying lengthening in females until skeletal maturity.

Horton WA, Hecht JT, Hood OJ, Marshall RN, Moore WV, Hollowell JG: Growth hormone therapy in achondroplasia. *Am J Med Genet* 1992;42:667ñ670.

This pilot study of 6 children treated for 6 months and followed up for 6 months afterward showed a modest effect only in the children with the lowest growth velocities; no untoward effects were noted.

Pauli RM, Breed A, Horton VK, Glinski LP, Reiser CA: Prevention of fixed, angular kyphosis in achondroplasia. *J Pediatr Orthop* 1997;17:726–733.

The authors outline a program of parental counseling and bracing when needed that they feel was able to alter the risk of kyphosis in 66 patients.

Pauli RM, Horton VK, Glinski LP, Reiser CA: Prospective assessment of risks for cervicomedullary-junction compression in infants with achondroplasia. *Am J Hum Genet* 1995;56: 732–744.

Infants with achondroplasia are at risk for potentially lethal sequelae of craniocervical junction abnormalities; the authors recommend evaluation of all achondroplastic children for this in infancy.

Shiang R, Thompson LM, Zhu YZ, et al: Mutations in the transmembrane domain of FGFR3 cause the most common genetic form of dwarfism, achondroplasia. *Cell* 1994;78:335–342.

This is the first report of the defect causing achondroplasia, which is located on chromosome 4.

Uematsu S, Wang H, Kopits SE, Hurko O: Total craniospinal decompression in achondroplastic stenosis. *Neurosurgery* 1994;35:250–257.

Seven patients are reported who underwent posterior decompression of the spine over the entire neuraxis in 1 or several stages. In addition to multiple areas of stenosis, some patients had Arnold-Chiari syndrome, syringomyelia, or basilar impression.

Pseudoachondroplasia

Breur GJ, Farnum CE, Padgett GA, Wilsman NJ: Cellular basis of decreased rate of longitudinal growth of bone in pseudoachondroplastic dogs. *J Bone Joint Surg* 1992;74A:516–528.

The alteration in the matrix causes a change in the shape and size of the hypertrophic cells, resulting in decreased longitudinal growth.

Metaphyseal Chondrodysplasia

Schipani E, Langman CB, Parfitt AM, et al: Constitutively activated receptors for parathyroid hormone and parathyroid hormone-related peptide in Jansen's metaphyseal chondrodysplasia. N Engl J Med 1996;335:708–714.

A defect in these proteins may explain the protean manifestations of this disease.

Multiple Cartilaginous Exostoses

Stanton RP, Hansen MO: Function of the upper extremities in hereditary multiple exostoses. J Bone Joint Surg 1996;78A: 568–573.

Standardized testing of 28 patients revealed little objective loss of function.

Wells DE, Hill A, Lin X, Ahn J, Brown N, Wagner MJ: Identification of novel mutations in the human EXT1 tumor suppressor gene. Hum Genet 1997;99:612–615.

Six mutations in the human EXT1 gene on chromosome 8 were identified in 6 different families.

Diastrophic Dysplasia

Hastbacka J, de la Chapelle A, Mahtani MM, et al: The diastrophic dysplasia gene encodes a novel sulfate transporter: Positional cloning by fine-structure linkage disequilibrium mapping. Cell 1994;78:1073–1087.

This study demonstrated the disorder of a sulfate transport enzyme by positional cloning and fine-structure linkage in a Finnish population.

Peltonen JI, Hoikka V, Poussa M, Paavilainen T, Kaitila I: Cementless hip arthroplasty in diastrophic dysplasia. J Arthroplasty 1992;7(suppl):369–376.

Results were generally good in this series of 15 hips. Complications included 2 intraoperative fractures and 2 femoral palsies. Two components were loose at 5 years.

Ryoppy S, Poussa M, Merikanto J, Marttinen E, Kaitila I: Foot deformities in diastrophic dysplasia: An analysis of 102 patients. J Bone Joint Surg 1992;74B:441–444.

In this Finnish study the most common finding was adduction and hindfoot valgus (seen in 43%), followed by equinovarus (37%) and pure equinus. There was often additional varus of the great toe, which was analogous to the hitchhiker deformity seen in the thumb. The deformities were stiff and involved bony malformation as well as malalignment.

Mucopolysaccharidoses

Wraith JE: The mucopolysaccharidoses: A clinical review and guide to management. Arch Dis Child 1995;72:263–267.

This is an excellent review and clinical discussion of these rare disorders.

Cleidocranial Dysostosis

Ramesar RS, Greenberg J, Martin R, et al: Mapping of the gene for cleidocranial dysplasia in the historical Cape Town (Arnold) kindred and evidence for locus homogeneity. J Med Genet 1996;33:511–514.

A gene for this condition maps to the short arm of chromosome 6.

Larsen Syndrome

Johnston CE II, Birch JG, Daniels JL: Cervical kyphosis in patients who have Larsen syndrome. J Bone Joint Surg 1996;78A: 538–545.

Cervical kyphosis should be sought in the initial evaluation of these infants. Early posterior fusion may prevent myelopathy and may allow curves to correct.

Vujic M, Hallstensson K, Wahlstrom J, Lundberg A, Langmaack C, Martinson T: Localization of a gene for autosomal dominant Larsen syndrome to chromosome region 3p21.1-14.1 in the proximity of, but distinct from, the COL7A1 locus. Am J Hum Genet 1995;57:1104–1113.

The location of a gene for Larsen syndrome has been approximated using a large Swedish kindred.

Classic Bibliography

Bennett JT, McMurray SW: Stickler syndrome. J Pediatr Orthop 1990;10:760–763.

Jarvis JL, Keats TE: Cleidocranial dysostosis: A review of 40 new cases. Am J Roentgenol Radium Ther Nucl Med 1974;121:5–16.

Narod SA, Parry DM; Parboosingh J, et al: Neurofibromatosis type 2 appears to be a genetically homogeneous disease. Am J Hum Genet 1992;51:486–496.

Richie MF, Johnston CE II: Management of developmental coxa vara in cleidocranial dysostosis. Orthopedics 1989;12: 1001–1004.

Segal LS, Drummond DS, Zanotti RM, Ecker ML, Mubarak SJ: Complications of posterior arthrodesis of the cervical spine in patients who have Down syndrome. J Bone Joint Surg 1991;73A:1547–1554.

Shapiro F, Simon S, Glimcher MJ: Hereditary multiple exostoses: Anthropometric, roentgenographic, and clinical aspects. J Bone Joint Surg 1979;61A:815–824.

Shaw ED, Beals RK: The hip joint in Down's syndrome: A study of its structure and associated disease. Clin Orthop 1992; 278:101–107.

Tredwell SJ, Newman DE, Lockitch G: Instability of the upper cervical spine in Down syndrome. J Pediatr Orthop 1990;10: 602-606.

Chapter 22
Neuromuscular Disorders in Children

Cerebral Palsy

Cerebral palsy (CP) is a nonprogressive encephalopathy with varying degrees of severity and patterns of involvement. Patients are classified based on the number of limbs affected, usually hemiplegia or quadriplegia, and the type of abnormal muscle tone, usually spasticity. CP leads to deficits of the musculoskeletal system including motor control, muscle strength and tone, balance, and coordination. Specific treatments are directed to correct or compensate for these deficiencies (Fig. 1).

Deformities develop as a result of muscle imbalance. Dynamic deformities lead to abnormal gait; static deformities, such as joint contractures and abnormal bony alignment, may develop over time secondary to the long-term effects on a growing skeleton. Treatment is directed toward rebalancing the dynamic forces and correcting the static deformity. The keys to treatment are identifying the primary deformities, understanding the interactions of all joints in all planes, and not treating specific areas in isolation. Gait analysis documents gait deformities and assists in formulation of a treatment plan.

This section is organized into treatment of specific joint deformities, options in the treatment of abnormal muscle tone, and outcomes of treatment.

Joint-Specific Treatment

The foot-ankle complex may develop 3 specific deformities. The equinus deformity is the most recognizable deformity. The gastrocnemius-soleus complex generates 36% of the power needed for gait. The focus has been to maintain this power through selective lengthening of the gastrocnemius by a musculotendinous recession at the midcalf level while preserving soleus strength. The surgeon must be sure the equinus seen is not due to flexion at the knee (crouch) or forward lean at the hip. Inappropriate lengthening of the Achilles tendon only exacerbates those deformities and produces further "crouching." Experienced observational skills and gait analysis assist in identifying this subgroup of patients.

Equinovarus of the foot is commonly seen in patients with hemiplegic involvement. Treatment options include a split anterior or split posterior tibialis tendon transfer. Treatment of patients with strong anterior tibialis muscle should be a

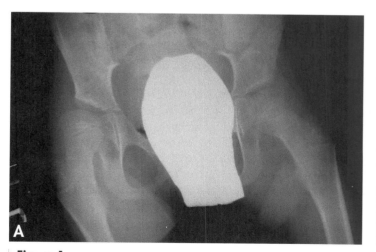
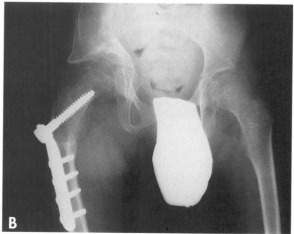

Figure 1

A, Subluxation of the right hip in an 8-year old child with cerebral palsy. B, After femoral varus derotation and pelvic osteotomies. (Reproduced with permission from Kasser JR (ed): *Orthopaedic Knowledge Update 5.* Rosemont, IL, American Academy of Orthopaedic Surgeons, 1996, pp 195–202.)

posterior tibialis tendon lengthening with split anterior tibial tendon transfer to the lateral aspect of the foot. If the anterior tibial muscle is weak, then a split posterior tibial transfer to the peroneus brevis will equalize the pull across the subtalar joint and correct the inversion deformity.

The equinovalgus foot with a prominent medial talar head may cause pain and difficulty with orthoses. A reliable and predictable treatment in the stiff foot is an extra-articular subtalar arthrodesis with internal fixation and autogenous cancellous graft. Interest has been renewed in lengthening of the lateral column by calcaneal osteotomy, a procedure that has the theoretical advantage of maintaining subtalar motion. Long-term results will compare osteotomy with arthrodesis.

Knee deformities may be secondary to ankle calcaneus deformity or hip flexion contracture, which must be assessed before implicating "tight" hamstrings as the cause. Crouch gait is commonly associated with a stiff knee (the lack of adequate knee flexion in swing phase and decrease in the total arc of motion). In addition to hamstring lengthening, rectus femoris transfer medially may correct both kinematic deformities. Other factors (speed of gait, ankle power, limb acceleration) may preclude the effectiveness of the rectus transfer.

Hip deformities include dynamic deformities of flexion and adduction. The release of the iliopsoas over the brim (intramuscular lengthening) has become a popular method to treat the flexion deformity with traditional adductor releases used for scissoring gait. Adductor transfers have fallen out of favor because they may create asymmetric gait.

Transverse plane deformities are now treated more frequently. Realigning the knee and foot in the sagittal plane and the line of progression is a way to improve gait efficiency. Internal femoral rotation can be treated with either proximal or distal rotational osteotomy, aiming for slightly more external than internal rotation. In theory, proximal osteotomy may affect the iliopsoas, resulting in functional lengthening. Correction of foot and tibial rotation is needed to maintain the role of the foot as a lever in the plantarflexion-knee extension couple.

Spasticity Management

Methods are available for reducing spasticity, which is only one component of the motor deficit in CP. Abnormalities of balance, strength, and motor control also influence ambulation. Despite this, parents observe the spasticity and often believe that its reduction can normalize their child. It is imperative that the parents be counseled regarding what effect spasticity reduction can have on their child's function.

Selective dorsal rhizotomy has been popularized by Peacock. Rhizotomy produces "permanent" loss of spasticity

with minimal recurrence of velocity dependent tone. Spasticity is reduced by the sectioning of dorsal rootlets, which are intraoperatively selected using electrical stimulation and the subsequent electromyography pattern. As experience with the procedure increases, fewer rootlets are sectioned (30% to 50%). Functional gains are related to patient selection and the extent of underlying deficits. The ambulatory patient without assistive devices, joint contractures, or ataxia is the ideal patient. Broadening patient selection criteria compromises the results. Previous reports of progressive hip subluxation and scoliosis have not been borne out in this walking population.

Botulinum toxin A recently has been used for spasticity management. It is the purified toxin from a species of Clostridia with proven clinical effectiveness in the treatment of blepharospasm. This paralyzing agent works at the myoneural junction by blocking acetylcholine release. It is injected into the offending muscle groups to reduce spasticity and improve joint position and function. Administered in the outpatient setting with some form of conscious sedation, its duration of action is 6 weeks to 3 months. This reversibility has both advantages and disadvantages. Its short-term effect allows the toxin to be used in a diagnostic manner to determine which muscles are contributing to deformity or if the weakness created could worsen the patient. It may allow more aggressive stretching and subsequent bracing with functional improvement obviating the need for surgery in patients with mild deformity. A disadvantage of the short duration of action is the need for repeated injections to continue the toxin's effect. Due to the limited total body dose at a single setting, not all muscles can be treated, and ultimately the rate of surgical intervention is not changed by this treatment.

Oral baclofen has been widely used for muscle relaxation. The side effect of sedation and the variable response to oral baclofen has limited its use in CP. The efficacy of intrathecal baclofen has now been explored. Direct delivery of the drug to the spinal cord achieves the desired effect with a smaller dose and decreased side effects. The dose can be titrated to achieve the desired amount of spasticity reduction. The advantages of intrathecal baclofen are its reversibility and its titratability; its disadvantages are the problems associated with any internalized pump device (mechanical, infectious, invasiveness). The nonambulatory spastic quadriplegic patient whose spasticity interferes with positioning and posturing may be the ideal candidate for intrathecal baclofen. Recent clinical trials have shown it may also be efficacious in ambulatory patients. There have been some recent positive results in patients with dystonia, an area with few treatment options.

Muscle Management

Muscle strength, a common deficit in patients with CP, can be improved with a physical therapy program. Quadriceps strength can be quantitatively increased and translates into positive gains of knee extension in gait. Ankle dysfunction caused by muscle weakness can be managed with appropriate bracing. Plastic ankle-foot orthoses (AFOs) are frequently prescribed. Varying designs exist with differing theoretical biomechanical characteristics. A common choice is a posterior leaf spring orthosis that provides support, maintains functional skills, and is well tolerated.

Outcome Measures

The most widely used questionnaire for the CP population is the GMFM (gross motor function measure). This validated, standardized assessment tool evaluates various aspects of sitting, standing, walking, running, and jumping. Its sensitivity may be limited in the less involved child with CP as the more functional patient maximizes the score in many of the simpler tasks. However, studies are now correlating score changes before and after orthopaedic intervention. In adult patients with CP the most important quality of life factor is educational level and cognitive ability, with mobility lower on the list. This must not be forgotten while treating the child and related parental desires. Preservation of function and the prevention of pain must be guiding principles in treatment, not necessarily the normalization of gait graphs.

CP treatment continues to improve with a multidisciplinary approach. The integration of physical therapy, spasticity reduction, orthoses, and surgery has been proven effective as evidenced by objective measurement changes in gait and functional outcome assessment tools.

Myelomeningocele (Myelodysplasia, Spina Bifida, Neural Tube Defects)

Myelomeningocele is a major birth defect involving the spine and spinal cord with motor paralysis ranging from minimal to high thoracic levels (Table 1). It has an incidence of 1 in 1,000 live births in the United States. The etiology in 50% of patients is a dietary folate deficiency that is preventable with the periconceptual administration of folate. The other 50% are sporadic or caused by unknown factors, including teratogen exposure in the first 8 weeks of fetal life; inherited and genetic causes are rare. Survival is related to the degree of brain stem involvement.

During the first year of life, treatment is primarily neurosurgical and developmental. Chiari II abnormalities are common and treatment of hydrocephalus in the neonatal period

is necessary in 90% of patients. Urologic abnormalities are also common. Physical therapy assesses and intervenes for developmental delay and prepares the child for the upright position after 1 year of age. Clubfeet and other congenital foot deformities are typically corrected between 12 and 18 months of age. Although most children obtain an acceptable result from clubfoot surgery, the highest rates of unacceptable results occur in those with thoracic or high lumbar motor levels. The goal in correcting any foot deformity is a flexible, braceable foot. The goal of standing and/or ambulation is sought after 15 to 18 months of age depending on the motor level and central nervous system involvement (ie, problems with independent sitting or standing balance). Progressive deterioration of function as a result of motor loss, contractures, or progressive scoliosis may be caused by a tethered cord and need not be accepted as the natural history of spina bifida.

Acquired deformities during childhood include hip subluxation and dislocation and contractures about the hip, knee, or foot and ankle. Treatment of the hip should be focused on motion and symmetry, with less emphasis on reduction of the subluxation or dislocation. Exceptions to this rule are highly functioning community ambulators who have L4/L5 or sacral motor level, unilateral dislocations, or severe asymmetry in range of motion or gait that may require muscle balancing and osteotomies.

Ambulation correlates primarily with motor level and sitting balance. Predicted adolescent and adult walkers are children with low lumbar or sacral motor levels (Fig. 2) and normal sitting balance. In ambulatory children, posterior surgical release with capsulotomy or occasional supracondylar femoral osteotomy for knee flexion contractures will improve the gait. Recurrence of knee flexion contractures is most common in nonambulatory thoracic level children without independent walking skills. As many as 15% of children with myelomeningocele report a history of latex sensitivity or allergy, with the potential risks of anaphylaxis and death. These children must be maintained in a latex-free environment, particularly during their medical care and any surgical intervention. Scoliosis and myelomeningocele are discussed in chapter 47.

The Progressive Neuromuscular Diseases

A group of conditions that affect either the central nervous system, peripheral nerves, or muscles share the characteristics of being inherited and associated with progressive loss of function as a result of increasing weakness with the passage

Table 1
Function, clinical problems, and common brace alternatives for different motor levels in myelomeningocele

Myelomeningocele Level*	Probable Adolescent/ Adult Function†	Clinical Problems	Common Brace Alternatives†
Thoracic	Sitter	Spinal deformity Hip subluxation/dislocation (acquired) Congenital clubfoot Congenital vertical talus	Parapodium or swivel walker Seating devices Mobility devices
L1-L2	Independent sitter, hands free; possible household ambulation with RGO braces	Spinal deformity Hip flexion deformity Hip subluxation/dislocation (acquired) Congenital clubfoot Congenital vertical talus	RGO seating devices Mobility devices
L3	Household, community ambulator with KAFO or AFO braces (presence of strong quadriceps makes possible)	Hip flexion, adduction deformity Higher incidence of hip subluxation or dislocation Hip subluxation/dislocation (acquired) Congenital clubfoot Congenital vertical talus	KAFO, occasionally AFO
L4-L5	Community ambulator with AFO braces	Acquired calcaneus foot deformities Foot ulcerations (insensitivity and high level of activity) Hip subluxation/dislocation (acquired) Congenital clubfoot Congenital vertical talus	KAFO initially, then AFO
Sacral	Community ambulator or normal with or without AFOs	Acquired cavus feet, claw toes, ulcers Hip subluxation/dislocation (acquired) Congenital clubfoot Congenital vertical talus Major urologic problems common	AFO or UCBL or none

* Functional level is defined as distal level with grade III-V strength. Changes in function, such as disabling spasticity, loss of function or strength, or scoliosis may be a result of associated hydrocephalus, Chiari II malformation, or tethered cord syndrome. Factors affecting ambulation as adolescent or adult include motor level, central nervous system deficits, obesity, scoliosis, lower extremity contractures, motivation, and intelligence

† RGO, reciprocating gait orthosis; KAFO, knee-ankle-foot orthosis; AFO, ankle-foot orthosis; UCBL, University of California Berkeley Lab orthosis

of time. In the past few years there has been an explosion of knowledge regarding the basic genetic defects underlying these diseases. A variety of different genetic abnormalities responsible for these conditions include point mutations, deletions (Duchenne's muscular dystrophy), duplications (Charcot-Marie-Tooth disease), and amplification of repeating base pair triplets (myotonic dystrophy). Absolute diagnosis can be obtained, in many cases, by genetic techniques, and the future holds promise for treatment and cure by gene replacement therapy.

Presently there is no specific medical treatment for any of these conditions; however, a variety of intervention strategies can be used to either prolong functional skills or adapt to functional losses to allow for a more independent life-style. Because these conditions are associated with progressive loss of strength, which is not homogeneous, certain muscle groups overpower their antagonists, and the imbalance limits motion and leads to the development of secondary contractures. Patients typically develop hip and knee flexion contractures and equinovarus and cavus deformities of the foot and ankle. Scoliosis also is common. Although the specific approach to treatment varies with the individual disease, some general principles can be universally applied.

Duchenne's Muscular Dystrophy

Natural History and Pathophysiology
Patients with Duchenne's muscular dystrophy (DMD) demonstrate progressive weakness with characteristic histologic changes of muscle necrosis and fibrofatty muscle infiltration. Affected boys walk late (usually > 18 months), generally lose ambulatory ability by age 12, and often die from pulmonary insufficiency by age 20. However, positive pressure ventilation may increase their life span.

This condition results from a complete absence of the cell membrane associated protein dystrophin. The dystrophin gene resides on the X chromosome, making its absence an X-linked recessive trait. In DMD all of the deletions are "in-frame" (the deletions begin and end within a triplet base pair that codes for a specific amino acid). As a result, when the gene is respliced, all of the downstream triplets are shifted by 1 or 2 base pairs so that the DNA downstream from this deletion codes for a nonsense protein, and, therefore, no dystrophin is produced. In Becker muscular dystrophy, there also is a deletion within the dystrophin gene, but it is between triplets (out of frame) and, therefore, does not disrupt the reading frame of the base pair triplets. This deletion results in synthesis of a reduced quantity of a smaller dystrophin molecule and causes a disease relatively similar to DMD, but with a later age of onset, slower clinical progression, and longer life span.

This genetic information has led to marked improvement and simplification of the diagnosis of DMD. In the 65% of patients with DMD who have a large segment deleted from the dystrophin gene, DNA testing from peripheral blood can provide a precise diagnosis. The remaining one third of patients have only a small deletion or substitution, which is not detectable on clinical testing, thus a standard diagnostic evaluation will have to proceed when the diagnosis is suspected in this group. This evaluation should include clinical examination and serum creatine kinase (CK), which is often 50 to 100 times normal (5,000 to 15,000 units). The only other condition with CK values this high is dermatomyositis. An absolute diagnosis requires a muscle biopsy. The muscle should not be fixed in formalin but frozen for histochemical evaluation, as well as immunohistochemical staining for dystrophin (complete absence in DMD). Western blot analysis confirms a total absence of dystrophin and an absolute diagnosis of DMD. For mothers who are known carriers and show a large deletion, amniocentesis or chorionic villus sampling (CVS) is appropriate.

Medical Treatment
There is renewed interest in the use of steroids, particularly prednisone, which may prevent, at least on a short-term basis, the loss of muscle strength in DMD

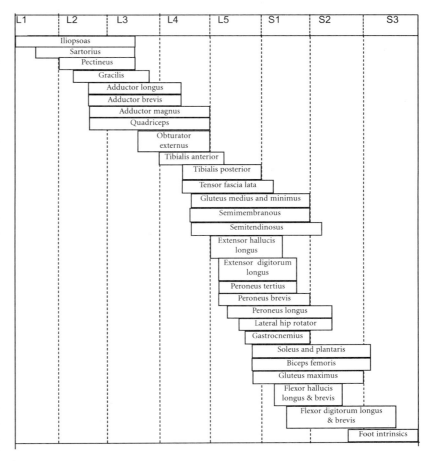

Figure 2

Neurosegmental innervation of lower limb muscles. (Reproduced with permission from Sharrard WJW: Posterior iliopsoas transplantation in the treatment of paralytic dislocation of the hip. *J Bone Joint Surg* 1964;46B:427.)

patients. However, it is not clear if the secondary cost of chronic steroid treatment outweighs the measurable benefits. Longer-term studies are needed; many clinicians remain skeptical that the ultimate effect on outcome outweighs the side effects. The ultimate treatment for DMD will involve introduction of the normal dystrophin gene into the muscle of boys with DMD. This has been successful in experimental systems at the zygote stage, but several technical hurdles remain before human use and proven benefit.

Orthopaedic Treatment Patients with DMD as well as other muscle diseases are at risk for malignant hyperthermia, so proper precautions should be taken if surgery, including biopsy, is done. Hamstring lengthening may prolong walking in those patients with premature contractures and adequate muscle strength. Night use of AFOs may delay progression of the inevitable equinus contracture, but AFOs should not be used for ambulation, because they adversely affect walking stability. Tenotomy of the Achilles and posterior tibialis tendons will correct equinovarus deformity, but it is likely to recur unless the posterior tibialis is transferred to the mid dorsum of the foot. Once the Achilles tendon is lengthened or released, floor reaction force is significantly diminished. Patients and families should be told preoperatively that the patient may require knee-ankle-foot orthoses after this surgery and that patients should resume standing on the first postoperative day after soft-tissue surgery to prevent progressive loss of strength.

The most critical surgical procedure for these patients is spinal fusion. Spinal stabilization has been shown to maintain pulmonary function and prolong life. There is an almost universal consensus that spinal fusion should be done before scoliosis becomes severe, because once curves become apparent, they will always progress, and these severe curves limit the independence and comfort of the adolescent with DMD. Orthoses, which only slow curve progression, are contraindicated because of loss of pulmonary function in the early teen years. Spinal fusion usually should be performed between the ages of 11 and 13 years while the vital capacity is still greater than 50% of expected to significantly reduce the risk of postoperative pulmonary complications. Segmental stabilization techniques are recommended; fusion to the pelvis and sacrum is controversial. When undertaken before the curvature becomes severe and before the onset of pelvic obliquity, fusion from the upper thoracic spine to L5 is sufficient and inclusion of the pelvis is unnecessary. Patients should be mobilized rapidly after surgery and usually can return to school within 2 weeks. Once the spine is stabilized, no further orthopaedic surgical intervention will be necessary, but patients require appropriate adaptive equipment including a

power chair. With the onset of pulmonary failure, between 17 and 20 years of age, ventilatory support can be considered, beginning with nighttime nasal ventilation and progressing to tracheostomy with full-time ventilation, which may increase life span by several decades.

Spinal Muscular Atrophy

Natural History and Pathophysiology Spinal muscular atrophy (SMA) is characterized by progressive muscular weakness caused by a progressive loss of anterior horn cells of the spinal cord. This condition is now classified as follows.

Type I (also known as Werdnig-Hoffmann disease) is characterized by severe weakness in the neonatal or infant period, inability to achieve independent sitting, and death from respiratory failure, usually by age 2 years. A few patients in this group may survive until age 10 years.

Type II patients frequently have a history of normal development for the first 4 to 6 months, achieve independent sitting balance, but never stand or walk. Scoliosis is universal and may appear by age 4 years. Most will experience a dislocation of 1 or both hips by age 10 years.

Type III: Patients with type IIIa involvement are able to stand and independently walk and have onset of disease before 3 years of age. They usually lose the ability to walk by age 15 years, but at least one third of these patients will walk up to age 40 years. Life expectancy may be normal in many cases.

Patients with type IIIb involvement (Kugelberg-Wellander disease) have an onset of disease at age 3 years or older. Weakness may cause foot drop and limit endurance, but these patients remain adult ambulators with a normal life span.

Approximately 95% of patients with SMA I, II, and IIIa have a deletion on chromosome 5 in the region that contains the *SMN* (survival motor neuron) gene. This gene is normally inactive during fetal development and allows normal programmed cell death in the developing fetus. In normal situations, this gene becomes active in the mature fetus to stabilize the neuronal population, but in its absence neuronal cell death (apoptosis) persists. A heterozygous deletion leads to the asymptomatic carrier state, so that SMA is inherited in an autosomal recessive fashion.

Medical Treatment There is some interest in medical treatment for these patients using inhibitors of gamma aminobutyric acid synthesis, with promising early trials.

Orthopaedic Treatment Most patients with type II SMA will develop hip dislocations, which are temporarily symptomatic and do not influence function in these nonambulatory patients. Surgical reconstruction may be successful, but continued dislocation may occur even after a surgical attempt at hip stabilization. Therefore, hip surgery is not indicated in most patients. Contracture release is rarely indicated in types II and IIIa, because loss of function primarily results from weakness rather than contracture. Tendon transfers occasionally may be indicated in type IIIb patients to correct specific functional defects of the foot and ankle.

All patients with type II and most with type IIIa SMA will develop scoliosis. These are usually long "C" shaped curves that progress to severe, incapacitating deformities if untreated. To provide for proper and comfortable sitting, thoracolumbosacral orthoses (TLSOs) may be used in younger children with flexible curves until they are old enough for surgery. Young patients whose curves cannot be controlled with a TLSO or those older than 10 years need definitive surgery, consisting of a long posterior spinal fusion with segmental instrumentation to the pelvis if pelvic obliquity is present. Concomitant anterior spinal fusion, if the child can tolerate it, may be required as well to prevent the crankshaft phenomenon. However, for many patients, even with severe curves, posterior fusion alone is sufficient. Patients with type III disease who are ambulatory should probably undergo spinal fusion that excludes the pelvis.

Charcot-Marie-Tooth Disease

Charcot-Marie-Tooth disease is a heterogeneous family of disorders now referred to as hereditary motor and sensory neuropathies (HMSN) types I-VII. HMSN I is the common peripheral neuropathy characterized by weakness in the distal extremities associated with diminished sensation and delayed nerve conduction caused by demyelination.

Children and adolescents may develop progressive cavus or cavovarus foot deformities (Fig. 3). Peroneal nerve atrophy results in weakness of the anterior and lateral compartment muscles. Considerable variability exists with the patterns of leg atrophy; magnetic resonance imaging axial T1 images show asymmetry from side to side. Consideration of this asymmetric involvement is important when planning treatment. Children and adolescents with Charcot-Marie-Tooth disease should be evaluated for acquired hip dysplasia and subluxation. Severe cases may require acetabuloplasty.

Pathophysiology and Natural History The most common type is Charcot Marie Tooth IA (HMSN type 1A), which is caused by peripheral nerve myelin sheath loss with delay in nerve conduction velocity as defined by electrodiagnostic studies. Type IA is caused by the complete duplication of the peripheral myelin protein gene located on chromosome 17. This autosomal dominant condition can now be easily

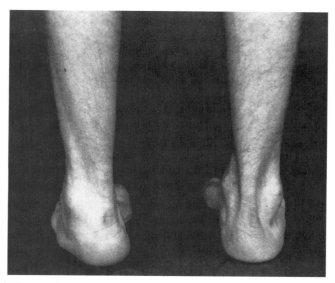

Figure 3

Foot deformity in a 17-year-old patient with Charcot-Marie-Tooth disease. (Reproduced with permission from Kasser JR (ed): *Orthopaedic Knowledge Update 5*. Rosemont, IL, American Academy of Orthopaedic Surgeons, 1996, pp 195–202.)

(although not inexpensively) diagnosed by DNA blood studies, and patients can avoid the discomfort of nerve conduction studies if type IA is suspected.

The primary clinical problem for these patients is progressive foot weakness and deformity. This usually becomes apparent between 10 and 14 years of age. Progressive claw toes and cavovarus deformities develop as a result of weakness of the anterior tibialis and peroneals, and contracture and weakness of the plantar intrinsic musculature. Hand involvement also occurs in adulthood, primarily because of the intrinsic muscles leading to an intrinsic minus deformity.

Orthopaedic Treatment Tendon transfers are performed when the foot is flexible but beginning to assume a cavovarus posture. The most frequent combination is the Jones/Hibbs transfer, plantar release, and posterior tibialis transfer to the mid dorsum of the foot. Achilles tendon lengthening should be avoided when the apparent "equinus" is caused by cavus and not hindfoot deformity. Triple arthrodesis should be avoided if possible because the long-term outcomes of this procedure have been shown to be poor. Osteotomy of the first metatarsal and the calcaneus may be necessary to support soft-tissue procedures if the cavus has become relatively rigid.

Myotonic Dystrophy

Myotonic dystrophy (Fig. 4) is an autosomal dominant condition that varies from mild and subclinical to very severe.

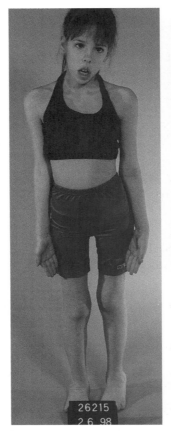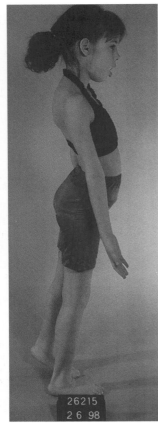

26215
2 6 98

26215
2 6 98

Figure 4

Child with myotonic dystrophy.

number tends to amplify with successive generations, more in the ovum than the sperm. This amplification process is known as anticipation, and it explains the appearance of congenital myotonic dystrophy wherein affected infants of affected mothers are very severely affected and may be profoundly hypotonic at birth, requiring ventilatory support. This problem was previously attributed to some maternal serum factor, but actually is caused to a greater degree by amplification of this triplet within the ovum of the affected mother.

Orthopaedic Treatment Severely involved patients may not walk until 2 to 4 years of age. Achilles tendon contractures may require lengthening. Kyphosis and/or scoliosis should be treated by orthoses when progressive and may ultimately require surgery.

Arthrogryposis

The term arthrogryposis is a descriptive one indicating contractures in 2 or more different joints. There are an estimated 150 different conditions—sporadic, genetic, neurologic—that feature multiple joint contractures. The evaluation and specific diagnosis of these children often requires evaluation by a medical geneticist. The most common and classic form of arthrogryposis is amyoplasia. Functional outcomes indicate that at age 5 years, 85% of children with amyoplasia are ambulatory, most are independent in their activities of daily living, and most are in regular classrooms at the appropriate grade level.

The initial approach to management of the multiple joint contractures is an intensified program of passive range of motion of all involved joints by a physical therapist, which is carried out further by the family at home on a daily basis. Passive range of motion therapy is most successful when begun in a child younger than 1 year of age.

Although the treatment of bilateral hip dislocations remains controversial for patients with amyoplasia, reduction by a medial open approach has been shown to result in stable reductions without stiffness or asymmetry. Unilateral dislocations are less controversial and should be surgically reduced. Prolonged immobilization should be avoided.

Severe knee flexion contractures may be treated by posterior release with joint capsulotomy with or without femoral supracondylar osteotomy. Distal femoral extension osteotomy allows for significant correction but is associated with recurrence in all children because of remodeling at a rate of approximately 1.0° per month necessitating repeat procedures.

Adult patients exhibit myotonia with an inability to relax a muscle after contraction. Myotonia may not occur until the second decade, and children usually present with hypotonia. Patients show varying degrees of mental retardation, cataracts, and progressive distal weakness; typical facies may occur and are more apparent with more severe degrees of involvement. Scoliosis or more characteristically kyphosis may develop, be progressive, and require surgical treatment, even before age 10 years. Cardiac conduction abnormalities may occur and be life threatening, with sudden death in the third or fourth decade.

This condition is caused by amplification of a noncoding CTG triplet in an untranslated region on chromosome 19. Normal individuals have 5 to 27 copies of this repeating triplet in this gene. Affected individuals may have 50 to 1,000 or more of these repeating units, and clinical severity is directly related to the number of CTG triplets present. The

Friedreich's Ataxia

Friedreich's ataxia, the most common inherited ataxia, is autosomal recessive and caused by a mutation on chromosome 9 (frataxin gene). The clinical spectrum is broad, and a direct molecular test on chromosome 9 is useful for diagnosis and genetic counseling. In general, patients become non-ambulatory at a mean age of 20 years when lower limb strength has declined to 56% of normal. Ataxia, rather than weakness, is the primary cause for loss of ambulation. Hip extensor weakness occurs first; upper limb and trunk muscles are spared until late in the disease. Scoliosis may occur and should be treated as adolescent idiopathic scoliosis.

Annotated Bibliography

Cerebral Palsy

Renshaw TS, Green NE, Griffin PP, Root L: Cerebral palsy: Orthopaedic management. *J Bone Joint Surg* 1995;77A: 1590–1606.

This is a thorough review of the orthopaedic principles for treatment of the patient with cerebral palsy. Aspects of management of the lower extremity and spine are discussed. Specific deformities are discussed and treatment alternatives are presented based on the authors' vast experience.

Gage JR, DeLuca PA, Renshaw TS: Gait analysis: Principles and applications. Emphasis on its use in cerebral palsy. *J Bone Joint Surg* 1995;77A:1607–1623.

This review article by experienced authors in the field of gait analysis provides the reader with an overview of the principles of gait and the use of 3-dimensional joint centered kinematics and kinetics with the electromyography data to analyze the deviations in gait seen in patients with CP. Specific examples illustrate the usefulness of gait analysis both diagnostically and as an outcome measure.

Myelomeningocoele

Brinker MR, Rosenfeld SR, Feiwell E, Granger SP, Mitchell DC, Rice JC: Myelomeningocele at the sacral level: Long-term outcome in adults. *J Bone Joint Surg* 1994;76A:1293–1300.

This long-term outcome study of patients with sacral level spina bifida documented a decline in ambulatory status as they reached adulthood. A change in motor level occurred in 22%.

de Carvalho Neto J, Dias LS, Gabrieli AP: Congenital talipes equinovarus in spina bifida: Treatment and results. *J Pediatr Orthop* 1996;16:782–785.

A radical posteromedial and lateral release can produce an overall acceptable result in 77% of the cases. The poor results seen in the thoracic-high lumbar patients are likely to be related to the lack of weight-bearing in view of their motor paralysis.

Mannor DA, Weinstein SL, Dietz FR: Long-term follow-up of Chiari pelvic osteotomy in myelomeningocele. *J Pediatr Orthop* 1996;16:769–773.

The management of hip instability in myelomeningocele patients is controversial. The Chiari osteotomy alone did not achieve long-term hip stability in the majority of patients.

Marshall PD, Broughton NS, Menelaus MB, Graham HK: Surgical release of knee flexion contractures in myelomeningocele. *J Bone Joint Surg* 1996;78B:912–916.

Surgical release of knee flexion contractures in myelomeningocele improves gait in all children who walk, particularly those with low lumbar lesions. Recurrence of knee flexion contractures after surgical release is most common in those with thoracic lesions who do not achieve independent walking.

Oakley GP, Erickson JD, James LM, Mulinare J, Cordero JF: Prevention of folic acid-preventable spina bifida and anencephaly: Neural tube defects, in Bolk G, Marsh JH (eds): *CIBA Foundation Symposium 181.* New York, NY, John Wiley & Sons, 1994, pp 212–231.

This review emphasizes the preventable cases of spina bifida and anencephaly resulting from nutritional deficiency of folate.

Swank M, Dias LS: Walking ability in spina bifida patients: A model for predicting future ambulatory status based on sitting balance and motor level. *J Pediatr Orthop* 1994;14:715–718.

The 2 variables that were significantly predictive (89%) of a patient's independent ambulatory ability were motor level and sitting balance. The 3 groups likely to be independent ambulators were lumbar and sacral level patients with no sitting balance deficit. Thoracic level patients are not community ambulators in and after adolescence. Sitting balance is an easily applicable screening tool during childhood.

Tosi LL, Buck BD, Nason SS, McKay DW: Dislocation of hip in myelomeningocele: The McKay hip stabilization. *J Bone Joint Surg* 1996;78A:664–673.

Recent data have shown that not all hips in these children are at risk. The operation is performed if there is documented instability of the hip in select patients.

Worley G, Schuster JM, Oakes WJ: Survival at 5 years of a cohort of newborn infants with myelomeningocele. *Dev Med Child Neurol* 1996;38:816–822.

Brain stem dysfunction was associated with a significantly greater mortality, despite aggressive neurosurgical management. Survival is related to brain stem dysfunction.

Neuromuscular Diseases, General

OMIM-*Online Mendelian Inheritance in Man, OMIM* ™. Center for Medical Genetics, Johns Hopkins University (Baltimore, MD) and National Center for Biotechnology Information, National Library of Medicine (Bethesda, MD), 1996.

This is the catalog of human genes and genetic disorders, authored and edited by Dr. Victor A. McKusick and his colleagues at Johns Hopkins and elsewhere. It is now available, totally free, on the Internet at http://www3.ncbi.nlm.hig.gov/omim/. It will provide a clinical summary, historical perspective, and most recent research along with an extensive reference list of all known genetic diseases of humans. Clicking on "Mini-mim" will provide a capsule look at any of the heritable diseases. In addition, a variety of hyperlinks throughout the text are linked with the National Library of Medicine so that abstracts are immediately available with the click of a mouse. This useful resource, not only for neurologic diseases, but any heritable diseases, is now available to everyone with Internet access.

Dubowitz V (ed): *Muscle Disorders in Childhood*, ed 2. Philadelphia, PA, WB Saunders, 1995.

Photos and concise clinical description are provided of all of the common and many of the uncommon neuromuscular diseases. Clinical patient photos are excellent and descriptions are concise, accurate, and to the point.

Duchenne's Muscular Dystrophy

Galasko CS, Delaney C, Morris P: Spinal stabilisation in Duchenne muscular dystrophy. *J Bone Joint Surg* 1992;74B: 210–214.

This review of a group of patients, some of whom had spinal stabilization and some of whom did not, compares their long-term outcomes. The authors showed that there was improvement in pulmonary function and survival in the patients who underwent spinal stabilization.

Mendell JR, Moxley RT, Griggs RC, et al: Randomized, double-blind six-month trial of prednisone in Duchenne's muscular dystrophy. *N Engl J Med* 1998;320:1592–1597.

This study demonstrated improvement in strength and function in patients with DMD on a daily dose of prednisone. The authors felt that the benefits outweighed the risks and subsequent studies by the same multicenter group have demonstrated even longer-term effects.

Miller RG, Hoffman EP: Molecular diagnosis and modern management of Duchenne muscular dystrophy. *Neurol Clin* 1994;12:699–725.

This is a comprehensive discussion of the genetics/molecular pathophysiology of DMD and strategies for disease correction.

Rideau Y, Duport G, Delaubier A, Guillou C, Renardel-Irani A, Bach JR: Early treatment to preserve quality of locomotion for children with Duchenne muscular dystrophy. *Semin Neurol* 1995;15:9–17.

The authors discuss the role of early muscle release in maintenance of ambulation in patients with DMD. This approach has been very popular in Europe.

Rideau Y, Delaubier A, Guillou C, Renardel-Irani A: Treatment of respiratory insufficiency in Duchenne's muscular dystrophy: Nasal ventilation in the initial stages. *Monaldi Arch Chest Dis* 1995;50:235–238.

Current techniques for ventilatory support for patients with DMD are presented.

Shapiro F, Specht L: The diagnosis and orthopaedic treatment of inherited muscular diseases of childhood. *J Bone Joint Surg* 1993;75A:439–454.

The authors review orthopaedic management of DMD as well as other muscle diseases.

Sussman MD: Advantage of early spinal stabilization and fusion in patients with Duchenne muscular dystrophy. *J Pediatr Orthop* 1984;4:532–537.

This is a concise explanation of the rationale for early surgical stabilization of spinal deformity for patients with DMD.

Vignos PJ, Wagner MB, Karlinchak B, Katirji B: Evaluation of a program for long-term treatment of Duchenne muscular dystrophy: Experience at the University Hospitals of Cleveland. *J Bone Joint Surg* 1996;78A:1844–1852.

In this review of 144 patients over a 40-year period, managed at 1 institution, the focus is on the role of bracing and contracture release. The senior author has been responsible for the treatment of these patients over this significant period of time.

Spinal Muscular Atrophy

Merlini L, Granata C, Bonfiglioli S, Marini ML, Cervellati S, Savini R: Scoliosis in spinal muscular atrophy: Natural history and management. *Dev Med Child Neurol* 1989;31:501–508.

This is a review of the literature on scoliosis in SMA as well as a report on the natural history of 109 patients over a 12-year period.

Phillips DP, Roye DP Jr, Farcy JP, Leet A, Shelton YA: Surgical treatment of scoliosis in a spinal muscular atrophy population. *Spine* 1990;15:942–945.

This is a retrospective analysis of 31 patients with all 3 clinical forms of SMA treated over a 20-year period, with an average follow-up of 11.3 years.

Shapiro F, Specht L: The diagnosis and orthopaedic treatment of childhood spinal muscular atrophy, peripheral neuropathy, Friedreich ataxia, and arthrogryposis. *J Bone Joint Surg* 1993;75A:1699–1714.

This article reviews SMA, hereditary motor and sensory neuropathies, Friedreich's ataxia, and arthrogryposis. Clinical features, natural history, and orthopaedic treatment are summarized.

Thompson CE, Larsen LJ: Recurrent hip dislocation in intermediate spinal atrophy. *J Pediatr Orthop* 1990;10:638–641.

The authors report 4 patients treated for unilateral hip dislocation using a variety of methods.

Zerres K, Rudnik-Schoneborn S, Forrest E, Lusakowska A, Borkowska J, Hausmanowa-Petrusewicz I: A collaborative study on the natural history of childhood and juvenile onset proximal spinal muscular atrophy (type II and III SMA): 569 patients. *J Neurol Sci* 1997;146:67–72.

In this clinical data analysis of 569 patients with type II and III SMA, the authors found the survival of the type II patients to be 98.5% at 5 years and 68.5% at 25 years. They found the likelihood of type IIIa patients being able to walk at 10 years was 70.3% and at 40 years was 22%, while that for type IIIb patients was 96.7% at 10 years and 58.7% at 40 years.

Charcot-Marie-Tooth Disease

Stilwell G, Kilcoyne RF, Sherman JL: Patterns of muscle atrophy in the lower limbs in patients with Charcot-Marie-Tooth disease as measured by magnetic resonance imaging. *J Foot Ankle Surg* 1995;34:583–586.

The worst areas of involvement, on a scale of 1 to 4, with 4 being worst, were in the lateral compartment in the mid calf and in the anterior, posterior, and lateral compartments of the distal calf. Considerable variation in the pattern of involvement from patient to patient was seen; all 4 calf muscle compartments may be asymmetrically involved to varying degrees.

Wise CA, Garcia CA, Davis SN, et al: Molecular analyses of unrelated Charcot-Marie-Tooth (CMT) disease patients suggest a high frequency of the CMTIA duplication. *Am J Hum Genet* 1993;53:853–863.

This article describes the finding of a gene duplication which is associated with Charcot-Marie-Tooth IA, the most common type of CMT, associated with delayed nerve conductions and autosomal dominant inheritance.

Arthrogryposis

DelBello DA, Watts HG: Distal femoral extension osteotomy for knee flexion contracture in patients with arthrogryposis. *J Pediatr Orthop* 1996;16:122–126.

Distal femoral extension osteotomy is effective and safe for the correction of knee flexion contracture. A significant problem with the procedure is that recurrence occurs in all growing children at a rate of 1.0°/month.

Sarwark JF, MacEwen GD, Scott CI Jr: Amyoplasia (a common form of arthrogryposis). *J Bone Joint Surg* 1990;72A:465–469.

This article reviews the etiologies of multiple joint contractures and discusses the current thinking on orthopaedic evaluation and treatment of the manifestations of the most common and familiar form of arthrogryposis-amyoplasia (formerly known as arthrogryposis multiplex congenita).

Sells JM, Jaffe KM, Hall JG: Amyoplasia, the most common type of arthrogryposis: The potential for good outcome. *Pediatrics* 1996;97:225–231.

Although children with amyoplasia have pronounced isolated musculoskeletal involvement at birth, which requires orthopaedic and rehabilitative interventions during their childhood, their functional outcome in both physical and educational areas is excellent.

Szoke G, Staheli LT, Jaffe K, Hall JG: Medial-approach open reduction of hip dislocation in amyoplasia-type arthrogryposis. *J Pediatr Orthop* 1996;16:127–130.

Hip dislocations in infants with amyoplasia may be successfully reduced by medial-approach open reduction. Bilateral reduction and concurrent correction of other lower limb contractures may be done during the same surgical session.

Friedreich's Ataxia

Beauchamp M, Labelle H, Duhaime M, Joncas J: Natural history of muscle weakness in Friedreich's ataxia and its relation to loss of ambulation. *Clin Orthop* 1995;311:270–275.

Patients became totally unable to walk at a mean of age 20.5 years, with a further decline in lower limb strength to 56% of normal. Weakness does not appear to be the primary cause for loss of ambulation in patients with Friedreich's ataxia.

Durr A, Cossee M, Agid Y, et al: Clinical and genetic abnormalities in patients with Friedreich's ataxia. *N Engl J Med* 1996; 335:1169–1175.

The clinical spectrum of Friedreich's ataxia is broader than previously recognized, and the direct molecular test on chromosome 9 is useful for diagnosis, determination of prognosis, and genetic counseling.

Classic Bibliography

Birmingham KP, Dsida RM, Grayhack JJ, et al: Do latex precautions in children with myelodysplasia reduce intraoperative allergic reactions? *J Pediatr Orthop* 1996;16:799–802.

Kumar SJ, Marks HG, Bowen JR, MacEwen GD: Hip dysplasia associated with Charcot-Marie-Tooth disease in the older child and adolescent. *J Pediatr Orthop* 1985;5:511–514.

Peacock WJ, Staudt LA: Functional outcomes following selective posterior rhizotomy in children with cerebral palsy. *J Neurosurg* 1991:74:83.

Sarwark JF, Weber DT, Gabrieli AP, McLone DG, Dias L: Tethered cord syndrome in low motor level children with myelomeningocele. *Pediatr Neurosurg* 1996;25:295–301.

Walker JL, Nelson KR, Heavilon JA, et al: Hip abnormalities in children with Charcot-Marie-Tooth disease. *J Pediatr Orthop* 1994;14:54–59.

Chapter 23
Pediatric Hematologic
and Related Conditions

Hemophilia

Classic hemophilia or hemophilia A (factor VIII deficiency) is
an inherited sex-linked recessive disorder. The incidence in
the United States is 1 per 10,000 live male births. Christmas
disease, or hemophilia B, is a sex-linked recessive factor IX
deficiency and occurs in 1 per 40,000 live births.
Musculoskeletal complications encountered in these children
are acute hemarthroses (knee, elbow, and ankle in decreasing
order of frequency), soft-tissue and muscle bleeds, acute
compartment syndrome, carpal tunnel syndrome, and
femoral neurapraxia. Patients are classified as severe when
clotting activity is < 1%, moderate when 1% to 5%, and mild
when > 5%. Early diagnosis and aggressive management are
key to lessening complications.

Several different treatment plans exist. "On demand therapy" is the traditional method of hemophilia management;
factor replacement is given at the first sign of a bleeding
episode. "Primary prophylaxis" involves initiation of regular
factor replacement therapy soon after the diagnosis of severe
hemophilia (usually 1 to 2 years of age) with the intention of
preventing joint bleeds. "Secondary prophylaxis" is used after
a child has established a pattern of frequent bleeding but
before frequent joint bleeds occur.

A target joint is defined as one with 4 bleeding episodes in
a 6-month period. Treatment involves regular replacement
therapy with either recombinant or plasma derived factor for
at least 6 to 12 weeks to interrupt bleeding cycles. Most
patients use recombinant factor. In general, 1 unit of factor
VIII concentrate per kg of body weight provides a 2%
increase in the factor VIII plasma activity. Acute joint bleeds
are presently treated with a more intensive therapy than in
the past. The deficient coagulation factor level is raised to
100% for most surgical procedures.

The chronic phase of articular involvement with recurrent
bleeds and effusions can lead to articular cartilage degeneration. Initially, synovial hypertrophy and chronic hyperemia
occur, followed by epiphyseal overgrowth. Articular involvement may be graded as follows: grade 1, transitory synovitis,
no bleeding sequelae, and no more than 3 episodes in 3
months; grade 2, permanent synovitis with increased joint

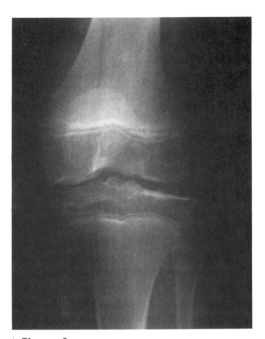

Figure 1

This patient's hemophilic knee arthropathy was treated with arthroscopic synovectomy, and
there was a satisfactory result at 2-year follow-up. (Reproduced with permission from Kasser
JR (ed): *Orthopaedic Knowledge Update 5.* Rosemont, IL, American Academy of
Orthopaedic Surgeons, 1996, pp 203–207.)

size, synovial thickening, and limitation of movement; grade
3, chronic arthropathy with axial deformity and muscular
atrophy; and grade 4, ankylosis.

Management of the patient with chronic articular involvement is aimed at preventing further deterioration with a prophylactic factor replacement regimen. Persistent, painful, or
progressive synovitis can be managed with open or arthroscopic synovectomy for breakthrough bleeds (especially the
knee and elbow) (Fig. 1). There is waning enthusiasm for
chemical (rifampicin) and radioactive (gold 198) synovectomy. Intra-articular dexamethasone, a nonsteroidal anti-
inflammatory drug (NSAID), may provide temporary relief.
Total joint arthroplasty may be helpful in selected adult candidates.

Factor inhibitors develop in 15% to 25% of patients with severe factor VIII deficiency (up to 50% if one includes transient or insignificant inhibitors). Many children with high titer factor VIII inhibitors are treated with daily high doses of factor VIII (immune tolerance) to reduce or eliminate the inhibitor. A substantial percentage of the adult hemophiliac population treated with concentrated plasma derived factor before 1985 became human immunodeficiency virus (HIV) positive. All hemophilia patients are monitored for development of treatment-related viral infection; the incidence of infection today is extremely low. Serial examinations of T4 lymphocyte counts are performed for patients at risk. Medical therapies are still evolving for the AIDS (acquired immune deficiency syndrome) patient with hemophilia. Current gene therapy efforts for hemophilia are focused on developing a vector that is safe and gives long-term expression of the missing factor at levels that will significantly change the phenotype.

Sickle Cell Disease

Sickle cell trait affects 8% to 10% of the African American population and other groups less frequently. Clinical manifestations are usually not apparent. Those patients with sickle cell trait have inherited a beta-S globin gene and a beta-A globin gene. Sickle cell disease (SCD) affects approximately 1 in 400 African Americans. The most common type of SCD, termed SS, is a homozygous condition in which individuals inherit the beta-S globin gene from each parent. In addition to musculoskeletal complications, SCD has systemic effects, particularly on splenic function and on central nervous, renal, and hepatic function.

Musculoskeletal involvement includes bone infarction, osteonecrosis, and osteomyelitis. Bone infarction is caused by blockage of marrow vascular channels by sickled erythrocytes. It is seen as early as 6 to 12 months of age and ultimately occurs in up to 74% of patients. Sickle cell dactylitis may resemble infection with pain and swelling and may last for 1 to 2 weeks. Vaso-occlusive episodes are managed with NSAIDs, oxygen, and hydration. Osteonecrosis of the femoral head is an especially difficult problem. Treatment options include conservative measures and core decompression (multicenter trial underway). Total joint replacement is rarely indicated in young adults. Osteomyelitis occurs in less than 1% of affected patients. Patients present with a warm, swollen, painful extremity. Routine evaluation should include blood cultures and needle aspiration of the affected area. Differentiation from infarction is aided by aspiration and by comparing the results of a technetium 99 scan to

those of a bone marrow scan. Causative organisms include *Staphylococcus aureus, Salmonella, and Streptococcus pneumoniae*. Septic arthritis is rare in patients with SCD; surgical drainage of septic joints, osteomyelitis, and subperiosteal abscesses is indicated. Patients with SCD require preoperative evaluation and treatment. Simple transfusion to raise hemoglobin levels to 10 g/dl is as effective as exchange transfusion (to reduce HgS to less than 30%) in reducing complications. Pneumococcal sepsis is the leading cause of death in young children with SCD.

Thalassemia

The thalassemia syndromes are a diverse group of inherited microcytic hemolytic anemias resulting in absence or decreased production of the normal globin chains. Thalassemia major (Cooley's anemia), the homozygous form of beta thalassemia, is a disorder featuring severe chronic hypochromic, microcytic hemolytic anemia. Children with this disorder usually develop jaundice and hepatosplenomegaly by 1 year of age. The resulting hyperplastic marrow contributes to the radiographic findings of long-bone thinning, metaphyseal expansion, a "hair-on-end" appearance of the skull, pathologic fractures, and premature physeal closure (especially of the proximal humerus and distal femur). The altered skeleton may predispose to degenerative osteoarthritis, usually in the second and third decades. Paraparesis resulting from spinal cord compression from extramedullary hematopoiesis may occur. Current therapies include transfusion, splenectomy, parenteral chelation of transfusional iron overload, bone marrow transplantation, and ancillary medical management.

Thalassemia intermedia patients are not usually transfusion dependent but may have organomegaly and musculoskeletal manifestations similar to those of thalassemia major patients. Thalassemia minor is the heterozygous form with mild microcytic anemia, normal longevity, and few symptoms. Prenatal detection of beta thalassemia is now available.

Leukemias

Leukemia accounts for over 30% of all childhood cancers. Acute lymphocytic leukemia (ALL) accounts for 80% of pediatric leukemias. There is an increased occurrence of lymphoid leukemias in patients with Down syndrome, immunodeficiencies, and ataxia telangiectasia. The peak incidence is at 4 years of age. Patients present with fatigue, pallor, purpura, fever, hepatosplenomegaly, or bone and joint pain, and are

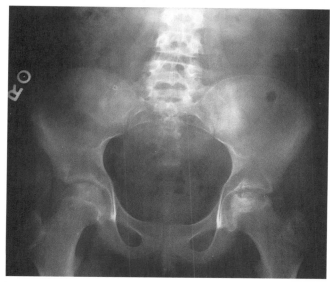

Figure 2

Osteonecrosis of both femoral heads in a patient on a chemotherapeutic protocol for acute lymphocytic leukemia.

diagnosed by the identification of abnormal cells in the peripheral smear or bone marrow. In the early phase of the disease, anemia, neutropenia, and thrombocytopenia occur in 80% of patients; 10% of children have normal peripheral blood counts. Twenty percent to 60% of patients present with musculoskeletal signs or symptoms. Skeletal involvement occurs in approximately 50% of cases with diffuse osteopenia the most frequent manifestation. Lucencies and periostitis may mimic osteomyelitis. Nonspecific juxtaepiphyseal lucent lines, a result of generalized metabolic dysfunction, are also seen. Sclerotic bands of bone trabeculae are more typical in older children. Fractures, including vertebral compression fractures, may also be seen. Bone scan may aid in identifying clinically silent areas but may not correlate with areas of obvious destruction on radiographs.

Chemotherapy usually includes vincristine, prednisone, and asparaginase or methotrexate, vincristine, L asparaginase, and dexamethasone. Remission rates up to 98% are now seen, with cure rates approaching 80%. The complication most frequently seen by orthopaedic surgeons is osteonecrosis (ON), most commonly of the femoral head (Fig. 2). This may be seen after chemotherapy, after chemotherapy and allogenic bone marrow transplantation (BMT), or after graft versus host disease related to BMT. Although most ON is attributed to corticosteroid therapy, L asparaginase can contribute to thrombophilia and has been implicated in the production of ON. The risk of ON is especially high in males

older than 16 years who are treated for graft versus host reaction with steroids or irradiation. Magnetic resonance imaging (MRI) is best for the early detection of ON. Treatment may include protected weightbearing, symptomatic treatment, core decompression, and total hip replacement. Complications of radiation include slipped capital femoral epiphysis, ON, mild scoliosis, osteochondromas, and sarcomas.

Gaucher's Disease

Gaucher's disease is the most common sphingolipidosis caused by a deficiency of lysosomal enzyme glucocerebrosidase; abnormal accumulation of glucocerebroside (glucosylceramide) occurs in the reticuloendothelial system macrophages. It is inherited as an autosomal recessive trait. Type I is a chronic nonneuropathic form with visceral (spleen and liver) and osseous involvement. This is the most common form (> 90%) and has a high incidence in Ashkenazi Jews. Type II is an acute, neuropathic form with central nervous system (CNS) involvement and early infantile death; type III is a subacute nonneuropathic type with chronic CNS involvement. Anemia, leukopenia, and thrombocytopenia result from both hypersplenism and marrow replacement. Osseous lesions result from marrow accumulation and include Erlenmeyer flask appearance of the femur, ON (particularly of the femoral head) (Fig. 3), and pathologic fractures, especially of the spine and femoral neck. MRI is more sensitive than radiographs or computed tomography in demonstrating marrow involvement. Femoral head ON is first managed symptomatically, with osteotomy or joint replacement later

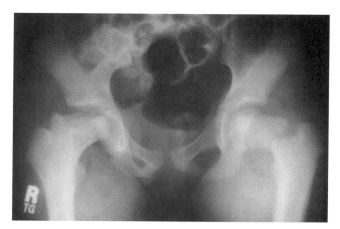

Figure 3

Gaucher's disease in a 12-year-old girl; note osteonecrosis of right hip femoral head and pathologic fracture of the left femoral neck.

when necessary. Pathologic fractures (especially of the femoral neck or shaft after biopsy and spine compression fractures) may be managed conservatively, but surgery can be performed with a known increased risk of infection.

Bone crisis and osteomyelitis in patients with Gaucher's disease demonstrate similar symptoms. With bone crisis, a patient may have severe pain in the back or extremities, fever, and an elevated white blood cell count. Radiographs may show periosteal reaction or lytic lesions and are difficult to differentiate from osteomyelitis. Technetium 99 bone scan often demonstrates no increased uptake with a crisis; gallium 67 scintigraphy may be useful to differentiate the 2 conditions. The role of surgical treatment of acute osteomyelitis in Gaucher's disease remains controversial.

The medical management of Gaucher's disease with enzyme replacement (alglucerase) is offered to patients with at least moderate disease symptoms. Recent reports support 3 times weekly dosing with satisfactory clinical results and few side effects. The annual cost of treatment is approximately $100,000.

Fanconi's Anemia

Fanconi's anemia is a rare condition with congenital hypoplastic or aplastic anemia. It is inherited as an autosomal recessive trait and is associated with diverse developmental abnormalities (ie, clinical heterogeneity; variable phenotype). Diagnosis on clinical manifestations is difficult. Other disorders (vertebral, anal, cardiac, tracheal, esophageal, renal, and limb; Baller-Gerold syndrome; Bloom syndrome) may be phenotypic variations of the same disease. Fanconi's anemia is often associated with short stature, skin dyspigmentation, microcephaly, micrognathia, microphthalmia, and beak nose. Anomalies of the upper extremity usually involve the preaxial aspect of the upper limb. Lower extremity deformities similar to those in thrombocytopenia with absent radii (TAR) syndrome may occur. Progressive bone marrow failure may or may not be present during the first year of life. Anemia, granulocytopenia, and thrombocytopenia may become severe. A predisposition to malignancy (especially acute leukemia) is also seen. The diagnosis is usually made by demonstrating chromosomal fragility. Treatment of the anemia usually requires oxymetholone (an androgen) and low dose corticosteroids (to keep physes open). Transfusion is used as necessary. Bone marrow transplant is occasionally needed for those with severe hypoplastic or aplastic anemia. Prenatal diagnosis is now possible.

Thrombocytopenia With Absent Radii

Thrombocytopenia with absent radii (TAR) is a rare, autosomal recessive, congenital syndrome. It is currently believed to be an inherited impaired DNA repair syndrome (radiation sensitivity). Upper extremity deformity usually consists of complete absence of the radii, with intact thumbs, giving the typical appearance of a radial club hand. Various ulnocarpal stabilization procedures have been described. Lower extremity deformities include genu varum with tibial torsion and knee varus and flexion with any joint contracture attributed to an intra-articular knee dysplasia. Progressive deformity may be treated with braces, surgery, or both. Occult hip dysplasia may be present; screening radiographs should be done once the child reaches walking age. Hematologic findings are hypomegakaryocytic thrombocytopenia, periodic leukemoid reactions, and eosinophilia. Resolution of the thrombocytopenia usually occurs after 1 year of age but may require transfusion support before this time. Cardiac abnormalities include tetralogy of Fallot and atrial septal defect. Of affected individuals, 7% have mental retardation secondary to intracranial hemorrhage or cerebral dysgenesis. Cow's milk allergy is also common. Prenatal diagnosis and subsequent treatment with umbilical platelet transfusion is being evaluated.

Annotated Bibliography

Hemophilia

Connelly S, Kaleko M: Gene therapy for hemophilia A. *Thromb Haemost* 1997;78:31–36.

The authors cover current state of the art gene therapy for patients with hemophilia.

DiMichele D: Hemophilia 1996: New approach to an old disease. *Pediatr Clin North Am* 1996;43:709–736.

This is a recent overview of hemophilia.

Greene WB, McMillan CW, Warren MW: Prophylactic transfusion for hypertrophic synovitis in children with hemophilia. *Clin Orthop* 1997;343:19–24.

This is a review of prophylactic transfusions for hypertrophic synovitis in 19 children with severe hemophilia. Results are mixed.

Ribbans WJ, Giangrande P, Beeton K: Conservative treatment of hemarthrosis for prevention of hemophilic synovitis. *Clin Orthop* 1997;343:12–18.

This review supports early and aggressive prophylactic treatment for children with hemophilia.

Rodriguez-Merchan EC: Pathogenesis, early diagnosis, and prophylaxis for chronic hemophilic synovitis. *Clin Orthop* 1997;343:6–11.

This is another review. Much of this volume is devoted to the treatment of children with hemophilia.

Shopnick RI, Brettler DB: Hemostasis: A practical review of conservative and operative care. *Clin Orthop* 1996;328:34–38.

This is another review supporting early and aggressive prophylactic treatment for children with hemophilia. Both conservative and surgical care are reviewed.

Sickle Cell Disease

Bookchin RM, Lew VL: Pathophysiology of sickle cell anemia. *Hematol Oncol Clin North Am* 1996;10:1241–1253.

The authors review the current understanding of the pathophysiology of sickle cell anemia.

Dalton GP, Drummond DS, Davidson RS, Robertson WW Jr: Bone infarction versus infection in sickle cell disease in children. *J Pediatr Orthop* 1996;16:540–544.

Osteoarticular bacterial infection is uncommon in children with SCD admitted to the hospital for musculoskeletal complaints (1.6% of 247 admissions in this series). Aspiration remains the diagnostic procedure of choice in diagnosing infection.

Ohene-Frempong K, Smith-Whitley K: Use of hydroxyurea in children with sickle cell disease: What comes next? *Semin Hematol* 1997;34(suppl 3):30–41.

This is an update on the potential use of hydroxyurea in children with SCD.

Smith JA: Bone disorders in sickle cell disease. *Hematol Oncol Clin North Am* 1996;10:1345–1356.

This is an excellent review of dactylitis, bone infarction, aseptic necrosis and infection in children with SCD.

Vichinsky EP, Haberkern CM, Neumayr L, et al: A comparison of conservative and aggressive transfusion regimens in the perioperative management of sickle cell disease: The Preoperative Transfusion in Sickle Cell Disease Study Group. *N Engl J Med* 1995;333:206–213.

A randomized multicenter study found that a conservative transfusion regimen was as effective as an aggressive regimen in preventing perioperative complications, and the conservative approach resulted in only half as many transfusion-associated complications.

Walters MC, Patience M, Leisenring W, et al: Barriers to bone marrow transplantation for sickle cell anemia. *Biol Blood Marrow Transplant* 1996;2:100–104.

Barriers to bone marrow transplantation for patients with sickle cell anemia are discussed in this multicenter retrospective review.

Leukemia

Bizot P, Witvoet J, Sedel L: Avascular necrosis of the femoral head after allogenic bone-marrow transplantation: A retrospective study of 27 consecutive THAs with a minimal two-year follow-up. *J Bone Joint Surg* 1996;78B:878–883.

This is a retrospective study of 27 patients treated with total hip arthroplasty for ON after allogenic bone marrow transplantation.

Gallagher DJ, Phillips DJ, Heinrich SD: Orthopedic manifestations of acute pediatric leukemia. *Orthop Clin North Am* 1996;27:635–644.

Heinrich SD, Gallagher D, Warrior R, Phelan K, George VT, MacEwen GD: The prognostic significance of the skeletal manifestations of acute lymphoblastic leukemia of childhood. *J Pediatr Orthop* 1994;14:105–111.

Retrospective analysis of 83 children suggests that children without radiographic skeletal abnormalities at presentation have an aggressive form of leukemia.

Meehan PL, Viroslav S, Schmitt EW Jr: Vertebral collapse in childhood leukemia. *J Pediatr Orthop* 1995;15:592–595.

At the time of initial presentation, 10% of children have normal peripheral blood counts. Appendicular skeletal involvement occurs in ~ 50% of cases.

Gaucher's and Niemann-Pick Disease

Ming JE, Mazur AT, Kaplan P: Gaucher disease and Niemann-Pick disease, in Altschuler S, Liacouras CA (eds): *Clinical Pediatric Gastroenterology.* Philadelphia, PA, WB Saunders, 1998.

This excellent review of Gaucher's and Neimann-Pick disease includes clinical course, newer treatment, and outcomes.

Zimran A, Elstein D, Levy-Lahad E, et al: Replacement therapy with imiglucerase for type 1 Gaucher's disease. *Lancet* 1995; 345:1479–1480.

The authors report on low-dose imiglucerase (Cerezyme, Genxyme), the placental recombinant human-derived beta glucocerebrosidase enzyme replacement therapy for type 1 Gaucher's disease.

Fanconi's Anemia

Giampietro PF, Adler-Brecher B, Verlander PC, Pavlakis SG, Davis JG, Auerbach AD: The need for more accurate and timely diagnosis in Fanconi anemia: A report from the International Fanconi Anemia Registry. *Pediatrics* 1993;91:1116–1120.

The Fanconi anemia phenotype is more variable than recognized previously, and a more timely diagnosis in the preanemic phase is needed to implement appropriate therapy.

252   Systemic Disorders

Murer-Orlando M, Llerena JC Jr, Birjandi F, Gibson RA, Mathew CG: FACC gene mutations and early prenatal diagnosis of Fanconi's anaemia. *Lancet* 1993;342:686.

Prenatal diagnosis of Fanconi's anemia is reviewed.

Thrombocytopenia With Absent Radii

Moir JS, Scotland T: Thrombocytopenia absent radius syndrome and knee deformity. *J Pediatr Orthop* 1995;4B:222–225.

This review of lower extremity manifestations of a child with TAR is presented with review of lower extremity deformity and treatment.

Classic Bibliography

Alter BP: Arm anomalies and bone marrow failure may go hand in hand. *J Hand Surg* 1992;17A:566–571.

Bennett OM, Namnyak SS: Bone and joint manifestations of sickle-cell anaemia. *J Bone Joint Surg* 1990;72B:494–499.

Bilchik TR, Heyman S: Skeletal scintigraphy of pseudo-osteomyelitis in Gaucher's disease: Two case reports and a review of the literature. *Clin Nucl Med* 1992;17:279–282.

Giardina PJ, Hilgartner MW: Update on thalassemia. *Pediatr Rev* 1992;13:55–62.

Section 3
Upper Extremity

American Academy of Orthopaedic Surgeons

Chapter 24
Shoulder and Arm: Pediatric Aspects

Congenital Anomalies and Acquired Disorders

Brachial Plexus Injuries

The incidence of brachial plexus injuries is between 0.1% and 0.4% of all live births. Risk factors, which are similar to those for perinatal clavicular fractures, include increased birth weight, maternal diabetes, shoulder dystocia, prolonged and/or instrumented delivery, and breech presentation. Brachial plexus injuries vary in severity, ranging from transient neurapraxia to complete avulsion of cervical roots from the spinal cord.

Any neonate with a suspected brachial plexus palsy must be examined carefully to assess the extent of neurologic injury, and any associated abnormality should be documented. The infant will not move the extremity normally and may posture in a manner reflective of the motor imbalance present. Clinical examination and appropriate radiographic studies, including shoulder ultrasound, may be useful. Pseudoparalysis resulting from clavicular or humeral fractures generally resolves in 7 to 10 days, and these patients will have an intact Moro's reflex, which will be absent in a true plexopathy. Clavicular fractures occur concurrently with brachial plexus injuries in 7% to 13% of reported cases.

Early perinatal care of patients with brachial plexus palsy includes documentation of neurologic status and initiation of a therapy program. Nonsurgical care should be continued for at least 3 months while awaiting potential spontaneous recovery. The role of electrodiagnostic studies is not clear. Prior to surgical intervention, magnetic resonance imaging may be of value in distinguishing postganglionic ruptures from preganglionic root avulsions in patients with inconsistent physical findings.

Questions remain regarding the natural history of brachial plexus palsy. Studies have shown that most patients, particularly those with upper lesions, recover spontaneously. However, a standard system for assessing these patients does not exist, and debate continues as to what constitutes a good result, specifically regarding active and passive motion of the shoulder. Traditionally, return of biceps function has been

considered the primary indicator of brachial plexus recovery, and patients without biceps return at 3 months were believed to have a poor prognosis with nonsurgical management. However, in 1 study the return of biceps function alone at 3 months had a 12% failure rate in determining a good or poor result. When elbow flexion was combined with wrist and digital extension, this failure rate was decreased to 5%.

Criteria for microsurgical intervention in patients with brachial plexus palsy continue to evolve, and include total plexus involvement without return of biceps contraction by 3 months of age, as well as upper trunk injuries with failure of biceps return at 3 to 6 months. A scoring system for surgical indications has been proposed based on active shoulder abduction, elbow flexion, wrist extension, and digital extension. A more conservative approach has been advocated by others who believe that spontaneous recovery will occur in the majority of patients and that secondary reconstructive procedures are available for any residual functional deformity. A recent study from Finland, which followed up nonsurgically treated patients, showed good results only in C-5 and C-6 lesions. The authors recommended surgical intervention in all cases in which biceps function was not regained within 12 weeks. At this time, there have been no studies that have prospectively randomized patients with brachial plexus palsy to evaluate the results of early surgical intervention versus delayed reconstructive procedures.

Specific procedures are dictated by the intraoperative findings. In the case of postganglionic ruptures, neuroma resection and sural nerve grafting are recommended. Direct repair is rarely performed. If the injury involves preganglionic avulsions, nerve transfers using thoracic intercostal nerves or branches of the spinal accessory nerve may be indicated. In general, upper plexopathies tend to be postganglionic, except those C-5 to C-6 lesions resulting from breech delivery, which have a higher rate of preganglionic injury. Lower plexus injuries are more likely to be preganglionic.

Progressive glenohumeral deformity, as well as infantile shoulder dislocation, have been reported in patients with persistent shoulder muscle imbalance. It has been suggested that infants with marked limitations of external rotation

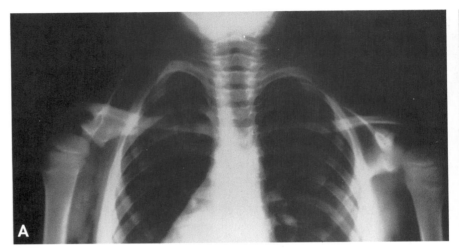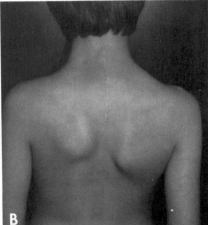

Figure 1

Sprengel's deformity. A, Chest radiograph shows elevation and rotation of left scapula. B, Appearance after Woodward procedure.

undergo subscapularis release. Pectoralis major release and posterior transfer of the latissimus dorsi/teres major to the rotator cuff or greater tuberosity are indicated in patients younger than 7 years of age without significant glenohumeral flattening. Once severe humeral head flattening and adjacent glenoid deformity are present, only a derotational osteotomy of the humerus will improve external rotation.

Sprengel's Deformity

Interruption of the normal caudal migration of the scapula during fetal development leads to congenital elevation of the scapula, or Sprengel's deformity (Fig. 1). This is the most common congenital anomaly of the shoulder. An omovertebral connection, either bony or fibrous, between the medial border of the scapula and the cervical spine, may be present in a third of cases. Glenohumeral instability has been reported in patients with Sprengel's deformity, possibly as the result of repetitive capsular stretching to compensate for limited scapulothoracic motion.

Sprengel's deformity is often a cosmetic problem with little functional limitation. Mild cosmetic deformity can be corrected by excision of the superior medial angle of the scapula, but this will not improve shoulder motion. In patients with significant cosmetic concerns and/or marked functional limitations, surgical reconstruction may be required. The Green and Woodward procedures lower the scapula and may increase shoulder abduction by up to 60°. Patients appear to retain improved range of motion when followed up until skeletal maturity. When indicated, most authors recommend surgical intervention in patients younger than 6 years of age.

Congenital Pseudarthrosis of the Clavicle

Congenital pseudarthrosis of the clavicle (CPC) is primarily unilateral and generally involves the right side. However, it may be bilateral in 10% to 15% of cases. CPC is present from birth and can be differentiated from an acute neonatal fracture in that union does not occur. CPC is usually an isolated entity, but it may occur in conjunction with cleidocranial dysostosis and may have familial inheritance patterns. Unlike congenital pseudarthrosis of the tibia, there is no correlation between congenital pseudarthrosis of the clavicle and neurofibromatosis.

Patients with pseudarthrosis of the clavicle generally present with a painless mass over the middle third of the right clavicle that may enlarge with skeletal growth. The lesion is usually asymptomatic, but there may be pain with lifting and overhead activities as the patient matures. Radiographs reveal a pseudarthrosis that may be either atrophic or hypertrophic.

Indications for surgical management include pain or significant cosmetic deformity. Generally, treatment is limited to patients older than 5 to 6 years of age and consists of pseudarthrosis excision, autogenous bone grafting, and compression plating. Intramedullary fixation has been reported with some success. Younger patients have responded to pseudarthrosis excision and reapposition of the bone ends within the preserved periosteal sleeve.

Epiphysiolysis of the Proximal Humerus

Adolescents involved with repetitive athletic activities that stress the upper extremities may present with proximal humeral pain. This is most common in teenage baseball

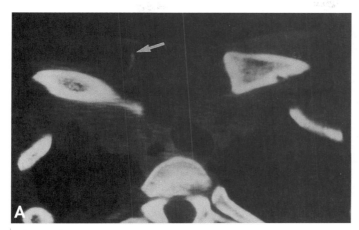
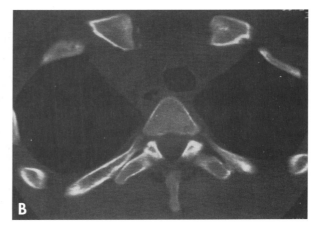

Figure 2

A physeal fracture of the medial end of the left clavicle with posterior displacement in a teenager, before (A) and after closed reduction (B). This injury can be mistaken for a posterior sternoclavicular dislocation clinically, but computed tomography is useful in establishing the diagnosis (arrow indicates epiphyseal fragment). (Reproduced with permission from Kasser JR (ed): *Orthopaedic Knowledge Update 5*. Rosemont, IL, American Academy of Orthopaedic Surgeons, 1996, p 241.)

pitchers, but has been reported in adolescent gymnasts. Plain radiographs are diagnostic, and reveal widening of the proximal humeral physis consistent with a stress fracture. Minimal displacement of the physis has been reported, and the similarity of this Salter I-type injury to slipped capital femoral epiphysis has been noted. Management includes symptomatic care and limiting stressful activities. Patients may gradually resume activities when asymptomatic, but are at risk of recurrence until physeal closure.

Traumatic Injuries

Fractures of the Medial End of the Clavicle
Fractures of the medial clavicle are rare, accounting for less than 5% of all clavicular trauma. The medial clavicular physis is the last to close in the body, often remaining open until 22 to 25 years of age. The combination of relative physeal weakness and strong capsular attachments at the sternoclavicular joint leads to physeal fractures rather than true joint dislocations. Displacement of the clavicular fragment may be anterior or posterior to the sternum, and anteriorly displaced fracture separations are most common. Standard anteroposterior radiographs of the region may not be sufficient because of overlapping ribs and sternum. An apical lordotic view with the X-ray tube centered at the manubrium and angled 50° cephalad is valuable. A computed tomography scan of the area that shows both sternoclavicular joints and both medial clavicles will often provide definitive diagnostic information.

Management of injuries involving the medial end of the clavicle varies depending on the direction of displacement. Anteriorly displaced fractures often reduce spontaneously, and even those with significant displacement require only sling immobilization and support. Because approximately 80% of clavicular growth occurs at the medial physis, remodeling potential is great. Little residual deformity and minimal functional disability are expected in most cases.

Posteriorly displaced fractures are more serious injuries (Fig. 2). The displaced fragment may result in respiratory distress, dysphagia, vascular compromise, and/or brachial plexus injury. Basic principles of trauma management must be followed, and a secure airway must be ensured. Upper extremity circulation must be carefully examined, and appropriate diagnostic studies should be obtained as required. In patients with significant symptoms or displacement, closed reduction should be performed in an operating room setting, and a vascular or thoracic surgeon should be available for repair of any injured vessels. A figure-of-8 dressing will maintain reduction in most cases, and internal fixation is rarely necessary. Metal implants, especially pins, should never be used because of the risk of migration. Chronic posterior fractures or dislocations without evidence of associated mediastinal injury are best treated symptomatically.

Clavicular Fractures
Fractures of the middle third of the clavicle in children are extremely common. In the perinatal period, clavicular fractures resulting from birth trauma may be discovered during the evaluation of an apparently flail or "pseudoparalyzed"

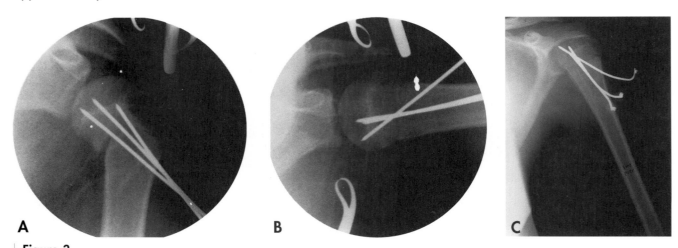

Figure 3

Intraoperative anteroposterior (A) and lateral (B) radiographs of a 13-year-old girl after closed reduction and percutaneous pin fixation of an unstable proximal humeral fracture. C, One month status after fixation demonstrates maintenance of alignment and healing fracture.

upper extremity. However, many birth-related clavicular fractures are diagnosed only when healing callus appears. Fracture management in neonates requires little more than stabilization of the arm against the chest. Older children may benefit from sling and/or figure-of-8 immobilization.

Surgical treatment is rarely necessary in children. Indications include open fractures, those with such severe displacement that the overlying skin is compromised, and painful fracture nonunions. In fractures requiring surgical intervention, open reduction with low profile plate fixation is recommended, and autogenous iliac crest bone graft should be used in cases of non-union. Intramedullary fixation must be used with caution because of reports of asymptomatic, but potentially dangerous, migration of smooth pins around the shoulder.

Fractures of the Lateral End of the Clavicle
Injuries of the lateral clavicle in children generally involve a fracture through the lateral clavicular physis, rather than an acromioclavicular dislocation typically seen in adults. The clavicular shaft fragment, constituting the proximal portion of the physeal fracture, herniates through the periosteum, leaving the distal physeal fragment in place within the remaining periosteal sleeve.

Management of most of these injuries in children is non-surgical, requiring only supportive immobilization. The remaining periosteal sleeve allows rapid healing and provides excellent remodeling. Older adolescents with buttonholed fragments or stripping of the trapezius and/or deltoid from the clavicle may require open repair secondary to instability,

deformity, and/or potential compromise of the overlying skin. Although uncommon, fractures with inferior displacement of the proximal fragment may require open reduction and soft-tissue repair.

Fractures of the Proximal Humerus
Fractures of the proximal humerus are uncommon in infants, and child abuse must be suspected when seen in this age group. Radiographic studies of the proximal humerus must be closely evaluated for evidence of metaphyseal lesions that are distinctive findings associated with intentional injury. Similar fractures may be the result of birth trauma. Ultrasound evaluation may be useful in neonates to assess the possibility of physeal fracture.

Generally, proximal humeral fractures can be managed nonsurgically with sling and swath immobilization. Because of the excellent remodeling potential of these fractures, relatively large amounts of displacement and angulation are acceptable, particularly in younger patients. Guidelines for adequate reduction of these fractures vary depending on patient age. In patients with less than 2 years of growth remaining, criteria are similar to those for a skeletally mature adult.

Surgical intervention is required when an adequate closed reduction cannot be attained or maintained, and in the rare open fracture necessitating debridement. Percutaneous pinning, using multiple smooth or partially threaded pins, is often used in these situations with good success (Fig. 3, A and B). Fixation is required until callus is apparent radiographically (usually 2 to 4 weeks) (Fig. 3, C). The potential for pin migration is minimized by bending the pins at the skin surface or using locking pinballs.

Humeral Shaft Fractures

Humeral shaft fractures increase in incidence with age as sport and motor vehicle related injuries become more common. Fractures seen in patients younger than 3 years of age are highly correlated with child abuse in most reports; however, a recent review revealed only 18% of humeral shaft fractures in a group of patients younger than 3 could be classified as probable abuse.

The vast majority of humeral shaft fractures may be treated nonsurgically with immobilization. Significant angulation is acceptable in younger children because of the excellent remodeling potential of the humerus. If angulation cannot be controlled with simple immobilization, a hanging arm cast may be used. Functional bracing may be used in adolescents after the acute postfracture period.

Humeral shaft fractures may be associated with radial nerve abnormalities. The majority of radial nerve injuries associated with a fracture resolve within 3 to 4 months. Internal fixation of humeral shaft fractures is rarely indicated in pediatric patients. Patients with open fractures, multiple extremity involvement, associated vascular injury, severe head trauma, or those with a "floating elbow" fracture pattern may benefit from internal fixation. External fixation may be necessary in fractures associated with severe adjacent soft-tissue injuries.

Annotated Bibliography

Obstetric Brachial Plexus Palsy

al-Qattan MM, Clarke HM, Curtis CG: Klumpkeís birth palsy: does it really exist? *J Hand Surg* 1995;20B:19–23.

A review of 235 consecutive brachial plexus injuries revealed no cases of lower plexus palsies (Klumpke's palsy). However, only 6 of 233 vaginal deliveries were breech, the position historically related to lower plexus injury.

Geutjens G, Gilbert A, Helsen K: Obstetric brachial plexus palsy associated with breech delivery: A different pattern of injury. *J Bone Joint Surg* 1996;78B:303–306.

The authors retrospectively reviewed 36 infants with obstetric brachial plexopathy after breech delivery, and found that 81% had avulsion injuries of the upper roots. They recommend caution in breech deliveries, especially in low birth weight/premature infants.

Lindell-Iwan HL, Partanen VS, Makkonen ML: Obstetric brachial plexus palsy. *J Pediatr Orthop* 1996;5B:210–215.

A retrospective review of 46 conservatively managed patients found that C-5 to C-6 injuries may be treated nonsurgically with good results. However, if biceps function is not apparent at 3 months, microsurgical treatment should be initiated.

Michelow BJ, Clarke HM, Curtis CG, Zuker RM, Seifu Y, Andrews DF: The natural history of obstetrical brachial plexus palsy. *Plast Reconstr Surg* 1994;93:675–680.

Sixty-six patients with obstetric brachial plexus palsy were reviewed; 92% recovered spontaneously. Attempts were made to predict outcome. Elbow flexion alone at 3 months incorrectly predicted outcome at 12 months in 12.8% of cases. When using a scoring system combining elbow flexion and wrist and digital extension, incorrect predictions were lowered to 5.2%.

Waters PM: Obstetric brachial plexus injuries: Evaluation and management. *J Am Acad Orthop Surg* 1997;5:205–214.

This review article covers the diagnosis, natural history, and management of patients with obstetric brachial plexus injuries. It includes extensive discussion of reconstructive techniques to address resultant secondary shoulder, forearm, and hand deformities.

Sprengel's Deformity

Borges JL, Shah A, Torres BC, Bowen JR: Modified Woodward procedure for Sprengel deformity of the shoulder: Long-term results. *J Pediatr Orthop* 1996;16:508–513.

Fifteen patients with Sprengel's deformity were followed up for an average of 8 years after modified Woodward procedures. Postoperative improvements in abduction were maintained, and 86% of patients were satisfied with the results.

Hamner DL, Hall JE: Sprengel's deformity associated with multidirectional shoulder instability. *J Pediatr Orthop* 1995;15:641–643.

The authors report 2 cases of multidirectional shoulder instability in patients with Sprengel's deformity. They hypothesize that repetitive attempts at active shoulder abduction in the face of limited scapulothoracic motion may lead to instability.

Proximal Humeral Epiphysiolysis

Dalldorf PG, Bryan WJ: Displaced Salter-Harris type I injury in a gymnast: A slipped capital humeral epiphysis? *Orthop Rev* 1994;23:538–541.

The authors report an injury similar to little leaguer's elbow in a female gymnast. This physeal stress fracture was minimally displaced. The authors note the similarities to slipped capital femoral epiphysis and recommend activity limitation and symptomatic care.

Traumatic Injuries

Fisher NA, Newman B, Lloyd J, Mimouni F: Ultrasonographic evaluation of birth injury to the shoulder: *J Perinatol* 1995;15:398–400.

This case report illustrates the utility of ultrasound in the assessment and diagnosis of a proximal humerus fracture in the neonatal period.

Kleinman PK, Marks SC Jr: A regional approach to the classic metaphyseal lesion in abused infants: The proximal humerus. *Am J Roentgenol* 1996;167:1399ñ1403.

The authors analyze the radiographic and histologic patterns of metaphyseal lesions found in the proximal humerus that are associated with child abuse injuries. Seven such lesions were found in 31 infants who died of abuse. They recommend close radiographic evaluation of the proximal humeral metaphysis in cases of suspected abuse.

Many A, Brenner SH, Yaron Y, Lusky A, Peyser MR, Lessing JB: Prospective study of incidence and predisposing factors for clavicular fracture in the newborn. *Acta Obstet Gynecol Scand* 1996;75:378–381.

Three thousand and thirty newborns delivered vaginally were evaluated for clavicle fractures. Fractures were associated with higher birth weight, older maternal age, instrumented delivery, and shoulder dystocia. Despite these associations, they were not predictive for subsequent birth injury.

Shaw BA, Murphy KM, Shaw A, Oppenheim WL, Myracle MR: Humerus shaft fractures in young children: Accident or abuse? *J Pediatr Orthop* 1997;17:293–297.

In this retrospective review of 34 humeral shaft fractures in children younger than 3 years of age, only 18% of the injuries were classified as the result of probable child abuse. Although suspicion should remain high, this fracture pattern does not appear to be pathognomonic for abuse in this age group.

Chapter 25
Shoulder and Elbow Injuries in the Overhead Athlete

Shoulder Injuries

Overhead athletes, including swimmers and baseball, tennis, and volleyball players, have a unique predilection for shoulder injuries because of repetitive use at the extremes of shoulder motion. Often, subtle anteroinferior instability is the underlying etiology for shoulder problems in the younger, competitive athlete, whereas subacromial impingement and rotator cuff disease are more common in the older, recreational athlete. Advances in diagnostic and surgical arthroscopy have led to the identification of superior labral and biceps anchor pathology (superior labral anterior and posterior, or SLAP lesions) and to the description of a new concept, "internal impingement."

Pathomechanics

Although the various overhead sports involve characteristic shoulder motions, all are very similar to throwing from a biomechanical standpoint (Fig. 1). The throwing motion requires a delicate balance of dynamic, coordinated muscle activities and static ligamentous restraints performed at the extremes of glenohumeral motion. Humeral angular velocities approaching 7,000°/second and rotational torques exceeding 14,000 inch pounds contribute to the accumulated repetitive trauma over the course of a season and career. The rotator cuff, biceps tendon, and parascapular muscles may all participate in dynamic stabilization of the throwing shoulder. It is postulated that most shoulder injuries in overhead athletes are related to chronic fatigue of these dynamic stabiliz-

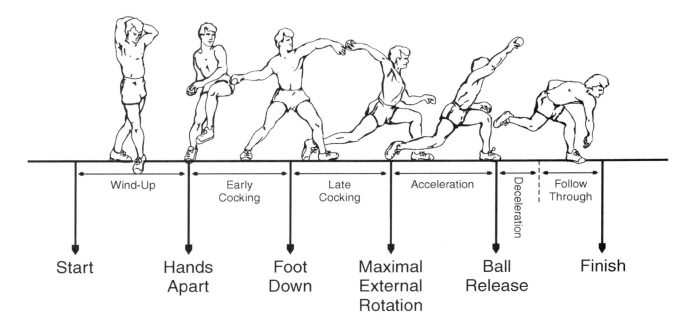

| Wind-Up | Early Cocking | Late Cocking | Acceleration | Deceleration | Follow Through |

| Start | Hands Apart | Foot Down | Maximal External Rotation | Ball Release | Finish |

Figure 1

The phases of the throwing motion: wind-up, early cocking, late cocking, acceleration, deceleration, and follow-through. (Reproduced with permission from DiGiovine NM, Jobe FW, Pink M, et al: An electromyographic analysis of the upper extremity in pitching. *J Shoulder Elbow Surg* 1992;1:15–25.)

ers. Without optimum dynamic stabilization, excessive repetitive stresses are placed on the static stabilizers of the shoulder, which may eventually lead to stretching and plastic deformation of the anteroinferior glenohumeral ligaments. With continued throwing, pathologic anterior subluxation of the humeral head may then occur during the late cocking and early acceleration phases of throwing. The excessive external rotation and humeral extension associated with the overhead throwing motion, possibly combined with anterior subluxation, causes impingement of the undersurface of the rotator cuff tendon on the posterosuperior glenoid labrum, a mechanism termed internal impingement (Fig. 2). In addition, symptomatic subacromial impingement and inflammation may occur from fatigue of the rotator cuff and its inability to stabilize the humeral head.

There is biomechanical and clinical evidence to suggest a mechanism for the occurrence of SLAP lesions in overhead athletes. Electromyographic studies have shown increased activity in the biceps after ball release, suggesting that the large forces on the biceps tendon during the deceleration phase of throwing may create SLAP lesions. A relationship between shoulder instability and superior labral/biceps anchor pathology was supported by a biomechanical study, which showed that lesions that destabilize the biceps anchor lead to increased translation of the glenohumeral joint. In another cadaveric study, it was found that a superior labral lesion decreased the shoulder's resistance to torsion and placed greater strain on the interior glenohumeral ligament. A number of recent clinical series have also documented a subset of patients with SLAP lesions who have concomitant pathologic findings of shoulder instability.

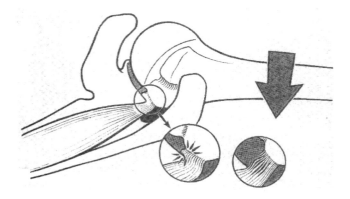

Figure 2

Internal impingement (illustration of mechanism). (Reproduced with permission from Walch G, Boileau P, Noel E, Donell ST: Impingement of the deep surface of the supraspinatus tendon on the posterosuperior glenoid rim: An arthroscopic study. *J Shoulder Elbow Surg* 1992;1:238-245.)

Clinical Evaluation

The clinical evaluation of shoulder pain in the throwing athlete begins with a careful history. It should address whether the initial onset of symptoms was sudden or gradual, which phase(s) of throwing is/are symptomatic, and whether there are any mechanical or dead arm symptoms. The physician should also inquire about the athlete's training regimen, throwing mechanics, and performance expectations.

There usually are differences in active and passive motion between the dominant and nondominant shoulders, and it should not necessarily be assumed that decreased internal rotation of the dominant shoulder is pathologic. In a large group of asymptomatic professional baseball players, the average external rotation with the arm in 90° of abduction was statistically greater, and the average internal rotation was statistically less, when comparing dominant to nondominant shoulders. Pitchers were found to have a greater degree of inferior laxity than players in other positions.

Suprascapular Neuropathy On examination, careful assessment should be made of shoulder symmetry. The presence of parascapular muscle atrophy is not uncommon and has been seen in baseball pitchers and volleyball players. A study of 96 top level asymptomatic volleyball players found that 12 had an isolated suprascapular neuropathy with atrophy of the infraspinatus of the dominant shoulder. During the throwing motion, the suprascapular nerve may be stretched as it passes around the spinoglenoid notch. Ganglion cysts may cause compression of the suprascapular nerve. Usually symptomatic suprascapular neuropathy in the absence of a well-defined nerve compression lesion responds well to nonsurgical management. In those cases resistant to nonsurgical treatment that have a spinoglenoid notch ganglion cyst causing compression of the suprascapular nerve, treatment of the often associated intra-articular glenoid labral injury and arthroscopic or open decompression of the ganglion are indicated.

Shoulder Instability A number of provocative tests can help clarify the etiology of the shoulder pain. Neer's impingement sign may be positive, but it is imperative to rule out subtle underlying instability as the cause of the apparent subacromial pain. It is unusual to have isolated subacromial impingement syndrome with or without rotator cuff pathology unless the overhead athlete is older (eg, recreational tennis player or golfer). This is supported by reports of less than satisfactory results of anterior acromioplasty in young overhead athletes with anterior shoulder pain. These athletes will often have pain, but rarely experience true apprehension with instability maneuvers. The relocation test has proven to be useful in the setting: first, the arm is placed in the abducted and externally rotated position, while applying an anteriorly-directed force to the humeral head. If this reproduces the patient's symptoms, a posteriorly directed force is then applied to the humeral head (Fig. 3). If the symptoms are eliminated, the presence of subtle anterior subluxation, perhaps also with internal impingement, is suggested. However, the specificity of the relocation test for instability is reduced if pain and not true apprehension is elicited.

SLAP Lesion A number of physical examination tests have been described to help in the detection of SLAP lesions. The clunk or "compression rotation test" is performed with the patient in the supine position, the shoulder abducted 90°, and the elbow flexed 90°. A compression force is applied through the arm to the glenohumeral joint as the arm is rotated and a catch or clunk is elicited. A variation known as the "crank" test used for detecting glenoid labral tears is performed by loading and rotating the arm in a position of maximal forward flexion. The O'Brien test may be the most specific for identifying superior labral pathology. This test is performed with the elbow extended, the shoulder flexed 90° and adducted 30° to 45°, and the arm internally rotated with the thumb pointing down. This position places the biceps under tension and in direct contact with the anterosuperior labrum. The examiner then resists the patient's attempts to elevate the arm from this position. Deep anterior shoulder pain and weakness, which is relieved as this maneuver is carried out with the arm in this position but externally rotated, is highly suggestive of anterosuperior labral or biceps anchor injury.

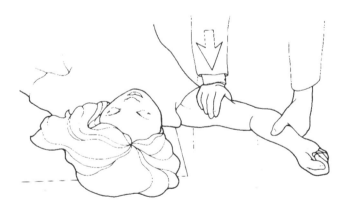

Figure 3

The relocation test. During the apprehension maneuver, posteriorly directed force on the humerus reduces the symptoms. (Reproduced with permission from Poss R (ed): *Orthopaedic Knowledge Update 3*. Park Ridge, IL, American Academy of Orthopaedic Surgeons, 1990, pp 293–302.)

Acromioclavicular Joint The possibility of acromioclavicular (AC) joint disease must be entertained. The physical finding of point tenderness on the AC joint and the anterosuperior pain at the AC joint with horizontal adduction of the arm across the body are sometimes difficult to distinguish from the physical findings of impingement and SLAP lesions. Differential lidocaine injections into the AC joint and subacromial space can be helpful in this regard.

Radiographs are often normal in young patients, but findings of a type III acromial morphology, os acromiale, bone excrescences on the greater tuberosity, or AC joint degenerative changes may be significant in the older population. Magnetic resonance imaging (MRI) may show signal intensity changes consistent with rotator cuff or labral pathology, but these findings must be corroborated with the clinical presentation. A study of MRIs of dominant and nondominant shoulders of asymptomatic professional and collegiate level tennis players and baseball pitchers has been performed in an attempt to define the prevalence of these findings. Dominant shoulders were found to have a 40% prevalence of signal intensity changes consistent with partial- or full-thickness cuff tears as compared to 0% in nondominant shoulders. Thus, an abnormal MRI without supportive clinical findings should not be used in isolation as an indication for surgery in this patient population. The use of MRI with gadolinium is thought to increase the sensitivity and specificity for identifying SLAP lesions, but quite often the definitive diagnosis is not made until the time of arthroscopy.

Superior Labrum/Biceps Anchor Lesions

The identification of lesions involving the superior glenoid labrum and the origin of the long head of the biceps tendon has been an important development that deserves special attention. SLAP lesions are relatively uncommon; they were found in only 6% of a large series of symptomatic shoulders evaluated arthroscopically. A common mechanism of injury described is an acute traumatic superior compressive force on the shoulder, usually caused by a fall on an outstretched arm, which shears the labrum and biceps anchor off the superior glenoid. Others suggest an inferior traction mechanism, either on the basis of a sudden traumatic inferior pull on the arm or from the instability that occurs with the repetitive microtrauma of overhead sports activity. Symptoms include deep anterior shoulder pain with overhead use, accompanied by intermittent popping or catching sensations. Patients may misinterpret these sensations as their shoulder sliding in and out of place. The physical findings in patients with SLAP lesions are variable, and can easily be confused with AC joint pain or impingement. Provocative tests designed to precipitate entrapment of the superior labral complex between the humeral head and glenoid are useful in making the diagnosis.

One of the most variable areas of glenohumeral anatomy is the anterosuperior labrum, extending from the biceps anchor to the middle glenohumeral notch. Along the superior glenoid, the hyaline cartilage extends over the superior edge into a small recess or synovial reflection just below the biceps insertion on the superior glenoid tubercle. The sublabral foramen is a normal opening or hole between the labrum and glenoid rim that may vary in size from only a few millimeters to spanning the entire anterior/superior quadrant. This normal separation, as well as other anatomic variants such as a "cord-like" middle glenohumeral ligament, must be recognized and not misinterpreted as pathologic. SLAP lesions have been classified into 4 types based on arthroscopic findings (Fig. 4). A type I lesion has degenerative fraying of the superior labral edge with the biceps anchor remaining firmly attached to the glenoid. In type II lesions, the superior labrum and attached biceps tendon are stripped off the superior glenoid, thus destabilizing the biceps anchor. Type III lesions involve a bucket-handle tear of the superior labrum, which displaces into the joint. The peripheral edge of the labrum and biceps anchor remain intact. In type IV lesions, a bucket-handle tear is present, as in type III, but the tear extends into the biceps tendon itself. Other investigators have described variations of SLAP lesions, which are often combinations of 2 or more of the basic types. Additionally, SLAP lesions have occurred with a Bankart lesion in patients with concomitant traumatic instability.

The recommended treatment depends on the type of lesion encountered. Type I labral fraying is debrided and type III bucket-handle tears are excised. Biceps anchor detachment must be firmly secured back to the glenoid, because debridement alone of these lesions has proven to be unsuccessful. If more than 50% of the biceps tendon is torn, a biceps tenodesis is recommended. Absorbable tack and suture anchor fixation methods have been equally effective, achieving successful clinical results in 80% to 90% of patients.

Rehabilitation

Once the diagnosis has been established, a comprehensive physician-directed nonsurgical rehabilitation program is instituted. The initial phase of this program, focused on the alleviation of pain and inflammation, is accomplished by a brief period of selective rest, ice, nonsteroidal anti-inflammatory medications, and therapeutic modalities. Emphasis is placed on posterior capsular stretching to equalize anterior and posterior laxity, as well as strengthening and endurance training for the rotator cuff and scapular stabilizers. Electromyographic analysis of shoulder rehabilitative exercises has shown that a number of specific exercises—forward elevation in internal rotation, prone horizontal abduction in external rotation, and press-ups—are particularly effective in strengthening the muscles needed by the overhead athlete. Proprioceptive neuromuscular facilitation (PNF) drills are helpful in developing synchronous function of the rotator cuff and scapulothoracic musculature. Plyometric training, which is characterized by a rapid stretch of the muscle before it contracts (eg, catching and throwing back a weighted ball), may be helpful and is focused on eccentric strengthening of

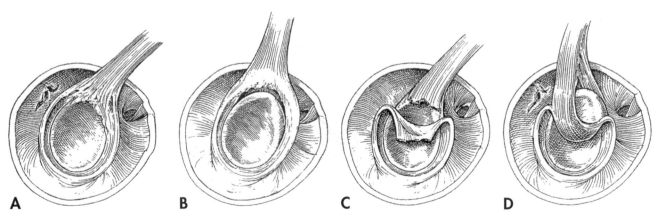

A   **B**   **C**   **D**

Figure 4

Classification system for pathology of the superior labrum anterior and posterior lesions (SLAP lesions). A, Type I, degenerative fraying of the superior labrum edge with the biceps anchor remaining firmly attached to the glenoid; B, type II, superior labrum and attached biceps tendon stripped off the superior glenoid; C, type III, bucket-handle tear of superior labrum, peripheral edge of labrum and biceps anchor remain intact; D, type IV, bucket-handle tear as in type III, but the tear extends into the biceps tendon. (Reproduced with permission from Snyder SJ, Karzel RP, Del Pizzo W, et al: SLAP lesions of the shoulder. *Arthroscopy* 1990;6:274–279.)

the posterior cuff in the latter stages of rehabilitation. The importance of eccentric muscle strengthening is emphasized by a recent study of collegiate baseball players that showed eccentric strength of the shoulder muscles was 114% that of concentric strength, and that the eccentric strength of elbow muscles averaged 33% higher than concentric strength. Finally, sports-specific exercises are gradually introduced in preparation for return to competition.

Surgical Management

The indication for surgery is failure of an appropriate supervised rehabilitation program. The specific surgical procedure should be tailored to the pertinent shoulder pathology identified through the history, physical examination, examination under anesthesia (EUA), and diagnostic arthroscopy. The expected differences in shoulder motion and laxity between the dominant and nondominant shoulders in the overhead athlete should be remembered while performing an EUA. Arthroscopic assessment confirms any subtle underlying instability and can identify associated undersurface rotator cuff tears, posterosuperior labral tears, and SLAP lesions. The diagnosis of internal impingement is usually made with the arthroscope in the anterosuperior portal. Placing the arm in abduction and external rotation may demonstrate impingement of the articular surface of the rotator cuff against the posterosuperior glenoid rim. The rotator cuff pathology of internal impingement is usually not at the leading edge of the supraspinatus next to the biceps tendon, but is more posterior where direct contact of the cuff and labrum occur. Inspection of the superior labrum and biceps anchor is necessary to rule out the presence of a SLAP lesion. The surgeon should be prepared not only to distinguish normal anatomic variance from pathology, but also to debride labral fraying and stabilize the biceps anchor as indicated.

The management recommendations for partial rotator cuff tears in young overhead athletes continue to evolve. A recent study of this subject identified 2 primary groups: one group had acute, traumatic subacromial bursitis without increased glenohumeral translation or labral lesions, and the other group had an insidious atraumatic etiology to their shoulder pain and associated findings of subluxation. The first group had 86% satisfactory postoperative results with arthroscopic subacromial decompression. The other group with evidence of shoulder instability fared worse, achieving only 66% satisfactory results. If a small full-thickness rotator cuff tear is encountered, it is usually amenable to repair via an arthroscopic-assisted, mini-open technique designed to preserve the deltoid origin.

Successful surgical management of shoulder pain in the overhead athlete often depends on the recognition and surgical correction of the subtle anterior instability. Arthroscopic findings suggestive of anterior subluxation include glenoid chondromalacia, anteroinferior labral fraying, and posterior humeral head chondromalacia, in conjunction with abnormal anteroinferior humeral head translation from inferior glenohumeral ligament complex insufficiency. Open capsular plication procedures are recommended in this clinical setting. Current literature does not support the use of arthroscopic stabilization techniques, because consistently reliable results have not been achieved.

The anterior capsulolabral reconstruction (ACLR) has been specifically developed to address recurrent anterior subluxation in the throwing athlete. The capsulorrhaphy is accomplished through a subscapularis splitting approach that minimizes the morbidity of the procedure and allows for early aggressive rehabilitation (Fig. 5). The underlying capsule is separated from the subscapularis muscle and mobilized. The capsular redundancy is obliterated using a horizontal capsulotomy and shifting the inferior flap superiorly and the superior flap inferiorly in pants-over-vest fashion. The medial capsule or labrum is secured to the glenoid rim using suture anchors. In a review of 75 athletes who underwent this surgery for recurrent subluxation or dislocation, 100% of collegiate and 75% of professional pitchers returned to their previous level of pitching. Overall results were 77% excellent, 15% good, 3% fair, and 5% poor. The inferior capsular shift procedure is recommended in patients

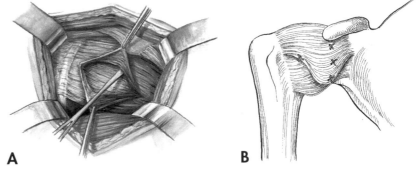

A   **B**

Figure 5

Technique of anterior capsulolabral reconstruction. A, Subscapularis split. B, Horizontal capsulorrhaphy. (Reproduced with permission from Elattrache NS, Mulholland JB, McMahon PJ: Capsulolabral reconstruction for anterior glenohumeral instability, in Fu FH, Ticker JB, Imhoff AB (eds): *An Atlas of Shoulder Surgery*. London, England, Martin Dunitz, 1998, pp 15–22.)

with a multidirectional component to their instability. Care should be taken with either procedure to avoid excessive medialization or overtightening of the capsule because even minimal loss of external rotation will compromise the delicate balance between restoration of stability and maintenance of function in the overhead athlete.

Elbow Injuries

Elbow injuries are common in the overhead athlete, affecting participants at virtually all levels of competition. Repetitive motion and enormous angular velocities associated with many overhead sports create a circumstance in which proper technique, conditioning, and appropriate rest may be the only factors separating the injured observer from the healthy participant.

Biomechanics

The biomechanics of many overhead sports are similar to those of pitching in baseball. The baseball pitch is divided into 6 phases: windup, early cocking, late cocking, acceleration, deceleration, and follow-through (Fig. 1). The valgus moment across the elbow is greatest in late cocking and acceleration. The medial collateral ligament (MCL) is the primary stabilizer against valgus forces about the elbow. The anterior band of the MCL is functionally the most important part of the MCL in resisting valgus forces. After ball release, the elbow flexors and extensors work together to decelerate the forearm.

Valgus Extension Overload

Excessive repetitive stress as seen in pitching can create overuse-related osteoligamentous injuries that roughly fall into 1 of 3 categories: tension overload of the medial structures, compression injuries of the lateral structures, and posterior compartment extension overload (Fig. 6). These processes commonly overlap, and in many ways, they are all part of a common problem that can develop in throwing.

Excessive valgus forces progressively damage the MCL. While large tensile forces are being generated in the medial aspect of the joint, compressive forces are seen at the lateral aspect of the joint. As the MCL becomes less capable of resisting these forces, the compressive force in the lateral aspect of the joint increases. This increase can lead to osteochondral injury, synovitis, and degenerative changes at the radio-capitellar joint. Commonly seen in throwing athletes, such pathology is also reported in gymnasts, along with abnormalities of the capitellum (including osteochondritis dissecans), radial head, radial neck, and olecranon epiphysis.

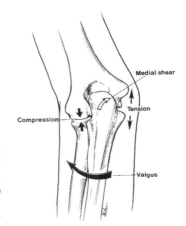

Figure 6

Valgus extension overload. Tension overload on the medial stabilizing structures, compressive forces in the lateral compartment, and extension overload of the posterior compartment can be present in the overhead athlete. (Reproduced with permission from Harner CD, Bradley JP, McMahon PJ, Kocher MS: Baseball, in Fu FH, Stone DA (eds): *Sports Injuries: Mechanisms, Prevention, and Treatment.* Baltimore, MD, Williams & Wilkins, 1994, pp 191-207.)

During the deceleration phase of the throw, the kinetic energy of the forearm must be dissipated. Although the elbow flexors and extensors bear much of this responsibility, the articulation between the olecranon and the olecranon fossa often becomes the final decelerator. This process can create a spectrum of injury, which includes posteromedial osteophytes, hypertrophic olecranon spurs, loose bodies, scar formation in the olecranon fossa, triceps tendon strain, and even avulsion of the olecranon tip.

In a series of 72 baseball players who underwent elbow surgery, the most common diagnoses were posteromedial olecranon osteophytes (65%), MCL injury (25%), and ulnar neuritis (15%). Patients who underwent only removal of posteromedial olecranon osteophytes had the highest rate of reoperation, often requiring a later MCL reconstruction. This suggests that MCL injuries were likely underdiagnosed at the index operation, and treatment was focused on secondary pathology. This series also shows that athletes who have had an MCL reconstruction have a high rate of return to play.

A surgical alternative to flexor-pronator detachment and ulnar nerve transposition for MCL reconstruction has been described. A split is made through the flexor-pronator muscle mass beginning at the medial humeral epicondyle and extending to a point distal to the coronoid tubercle to access the ulna. Cadaveric dissection demonstrated that a neurovascular "safe zone" exists from the medial epicondyle to 1 cm distal to the MCL insertion at the ulnar tubercle. Theoretical advantages of a muscle splitting approach include less trauma to the tendinous origin of the flexor-pronator mass, reduced manipulation of the ulnar nerve, and decreased time in surgery.

Arthroscopy

In a population of overhead athletes, arthroscopy is of particular benefit as a tool for diagnosis and minimally invasive treatment. In throwing athletes, arthroscopy is useful to remove loose bodies in the joint (both anteriorly and posteriorly); debride and/or drill osteochondral injuries; and debride synovitis, scar, and posterior osteophytes. Awareness of the possibility of medial elbow instability must be maintained, because if present, treatment focused on these secondary pathologies alone may fail.

Despite its benefits, elbow arthroscopy is not effective in consistently visualizing the various parts of the MCL. Although the posterior band can be completely seen, the anterior band of the MCL cannot consistently be visualized, regardless of flexion angle and portal used.

Tendinitis

Lateral epicondylitis, while commonly referred to as tennis elbow, is a pathologic process that can occur with virtually any activity requiring repetitive wrist extensor activity. Current information suggests that lateral epicondylitis begins as a microtear, most commonly at the extensor carpi radialis brevis origin. Histologically, hyaline degeneration and vascular proliferation are often seen. Nonsurgical management is focused on relieving pain and promoting healing of the involved tissues. For failed nonsurgical management, surgery may be performed. Although a variety of less invasive techniques, including arthroscopy, are surfacing, the most widely used technique remains an open, extra-articular approach to lateral epicondylitis. Basic principles include excision of pathologic tissue, decortication or drilling the lateral epicondyle, and repair of the extensor mechanism.

Valgus forces at the elbow seen in overhead sports can create stress in the flexor/pronator origin as well as in the MCL. These valgus forces are at the root of the pathophysiology of medial epicondylitis, which is less common than but equally painful to its lateral counterpart. Macroscopic tearing of the flexor/pronator origin is usually in the pronator teres and the flexor carpi radialis. In a series of 48 patients with medial epicondylitis who failed nonsurgical management, histologic assessment of involved tissue showed angiofibroblastic tendinosis and fibrillar degeneration of collagen. Resection and repair universally improved the patients' level of pain and dynamometer strength testing. Despite this, 10 of 48 did not return to their previous sporting or occupational activity. Another recent series suggests that 12% of patients with medial epicondylitis will fail nonsurgical management and eventually require surgery. This is to be compared with a 4% failure rate for lateral epicondylitis over the same period. Basic principles of surgery for medial epicondylitis include excision of the reactive fibrous tissue in the flexor pronator mass with care to preserve the origin's integrity. Alternatively, firm reattachment of the flexor/pronator origin is required, if distal reflection of the origin is performed.

Elbow Injuries in Skeletally Immature Athletes

The term "little league elbow" describes many different conditions of the skeletally immature athlete's elbow. These include apophysitis of the medial epicondyle and olecranon, osteochrondrosis of the radiocapitellar joint, and more serious conditions, such as osteochondritis dissecans of the capitellum. Because of the propensity for the young athlete's elbow to develop overuse-related pathology, it is important for the physician, coach, and parent to be mindful of this possibility. Suggestions such as using a "pitch count" to ensure that the athlete does not throw too much can be of use. Similar techniques can be applied to other adolescent athletic endeavors. Consideration of a short-term position change with less throwing may be reasonable.

Recently, persistence of the olecranon physis has been described as a cause of elbow pain in the adolescent baseball player. Symptoms will often improve with rest. However, if the symptoms persist and the contralateral growth plate has closed, internal fixation has occasionally been recommended. Adolescent gymnasts can also develop chronic stress-related injuries to the olecranon, including physeal irregularities, epiphyseal fragmentation, and stress fractures. The same population of athletes has also been reported to develop osteochondritis dissecans in the lateral condyle of the humerus.

Annotated Bibliography

Shoulder Injuries

Bigliani LU, Codd TP, Connor PM, Levine WN, Littlefield MA, Hershon SJ: Shoulder motion and laxity in the professional baseball player. *Am J Sports Med* 1997;25:609–613.

In a study of 148 professional baseball players, average external rotation with the arm in 90° of abduction was statistically greater and average internal rotation was statistically less in dominant shoulders than in nondominant shoulders. The degree of inferior laxity was significantly greater in pitchers than in position players.

Bigliani LU, Kurzweil PR, Schwartzbach CC, Wolfe IN, Flatow EL: Inferior capsular shift procedure for anterior-inferior shoulder instability in athletes. *Am J Sports Med* 1994;22:578–584.

Sixty-three patients (including 31 throwing athletes) with anteroinferior glenohumeral instability underwent a laterally based capsular shift procedure, combined with repair of a Bankart lesion when present (31%). Satisfactory results were achieved in 94%, and 92% returned to sports (75% at the same level). The rate of recurrent instability was 3%.

Davidson PA, Elattrache NS, Jobe CM, Jobe FW: Rotator cuff and posterior-superior glenoid labrum injury associated with increased glenohumeral motion: A new site of impingement. *J Shoulder Elbow Surg* 1995;4:384–390.

These authors discuss internal impingement as direct contact between the posterior-superior labrum and articular side of the rotator cuff when the shoulder is in 90° of abduction and maximum external rotation. The relocation test is recommended for diagnosis.

Maffet MW, Gartsman GM, Moseley B: Superior labrum-biceps tendon complex lesions of the shoulder. *Am J Sports Med* 1995;23:93–98.

The authors present a series of 84 patients with superior labral and biceps tendon lesions, noting that 75% had a preoperative diagnosis of impingement. They emphasized that an inferior traction pull on the shoulder is a common mechanism of injury. Forty-three percent of shoulders had increased humeral head translation, suggesting concomitant instability. Additional subtypes for the SLAP lesion classification system are proposed.

Martin SD, Warren RF, Martin TL, Kennedy K, O'Brien SJ, Wickiewicz TL: Suprascapular neuropathy: Results of non-operative treatment. *J Bone Joint Surg* 1997;79A:1159–1165.

This retrospective review of 15 patients documented suprascapular neuropathy, suggesting that, in the absence of a well-defined lesion producing mechanical compression of the suprascapular nerve, this condition should be treated nonsurgically.

Mikesky AE, Edwards JE, Wigglesworth JK, Kunkel S: Eccentric and concentric strength of the shoulder and arm musculature in collegiate baseball pitchers. *Am J Sports Med* 1995;23:638–642.

This study assesses eccentric and concentric muscular strength of the shoulder's external and internal rotator muscles and the elbow's flexor and extensor muscles in collegiate baseball pitchers. Eccentric strength of both the shoulder and elbow was found to be greater than concentric strength; these findings have implications for the rehabilitation and conditioning of throwing athletes.

Moore TP, Fritts HM, Quick DC, Buss DD: Suprascapular nerve entrapment caused by supraglenoid cyst compression. *J Shoulder Elbow Surg* 1997;6:455–462.

The authors describe the association of supraglenoid ganglion cyst compression of the suprascapular nerve with intra-articular glenoid labral pathology. Recommendations based on this study are to perform SLAP lesion debridement or repair as well as ganglion decompression (arthroscopic or open) in patients recalcitrant to nonsurgical management.

Pagnani MJ, Deng XH, Warren RF, Torzilli PA, Altchek DW: Effect of lesions of the superior portion of the glenoid labrum on glenohumeral translation. *J Bone Joint Surg* 1995;77A:1003–1010.

This biomechanical cadaveric study shows that superior labral lesions that destabilize the biceps anchor resulted in significant increases in glenohumeral translations, thereby suggesting a relationship between SLAP lesions and shoulder instability.

Pagnani MJ, Speer KP, Altchek DW, Warren RF, Dines DM: Arthroscopic fixation of superior labral lesions using a biodegradable implant: A preliminary report. *Arthroscopy* 1995;11:194–198.

Twenty-two patients with type II and type IV SLAP lesions were stabilized using a biodegradable tack. At 2-year average follow-up, satisfactory results were obtained in 86% of patients with no complications.

Payne LZ, Altchek DW, Craig EV, Warren RF: Arthroscopic treatment of partial rotator cuff tears in young athletes: A preliminary report. *Am J Sports Med* 1997;25:299–305.

Two groups were identified in this study. Group A had acute, traumatic injuries with inflamed subacromial bursas and rarely had increased glenohumeral translation and/or labral lesions. Group B had insidious, atraumatic shoulder pain. Arthroscopic subacromial decompression and tear debridement gave 86% satisfactory results in group A compared to 66% in group B. The diagnosis and treatment of associated subtle instability in group B was emphasized.

Rodosky MW, Harner CD, Fu FH: The role of the long head of the biceps muscle and superior glenoid labrum in anterior stability of the shoulder. *Am J Sports Med* 1994;22:121–130.

Data from a dynamic cadaveric shoulder model indicated that a superior labral lesion decreased the shoulder's resistance to torsion and placed greater strain on the inferior glenohumeral ligament.

Snyder SJ, Banas MP, Karzel RP: An analysis of 140 injuries to the superior glenoid labrum. *J Shoulder Elbow Surg* 1995;4:243–248.

Analysis of the largest series in the literature on superior glenoid labral injuries found that only 28% of cases were isolated lesions of the superior labrum. Partial or full-thickness tearing of the rotator cuff accompanied 40% of the injuries, and 22% had an anterior Bankart lesion.

Williams MS, Snyder SJ, Buford D: The Buford complex: The "cord-like" middle glenohumeral ligament and absent anterosuperior labrum complex: A normal anatomic capsulolabral variant. *Arthroscopy* 1994;10:241–247.

Two hundred shoulder arthroscopies were reviewed to study the anatomy of the anterior superior glenoid quadrant. Normal anatomic variants were described and their incidence noted, including: sublabral foramen (12%), "cord-like" middle glenohumeral ligament (9%), and "Buford complex" (1.5%). Inappropriate fixation of these anatomic variants will cause painful restriction of rotation and elevation.

Elbow Injuries

Andrews JR, Timmerman LA: Outcome of elbow surgery in professional baseball players. *Am J Sports Med* 1995;23:407–413.

Patients who underwent MCL reconstruction had the highest rate of return to play. The incidence of MCL injuries was likely underestimated in this group of athletes, with initial treatment directed at secondary injuries instead of the primary MCL injury.

Field LD, Callaway GH, O'Brien SJ, Altchek DW: Arthroscopic assessment of the medial collateral ligament complex of the elbow. *Am J Sports Med* 1995;23:396–400.

This study shows that the arthroscope is of limited value in visualizing the MCL complex. Further, direct pressure is placed on the ulnar nerve when the arthroscope is advanced into the posteromedial gutter in contact with the posterior bundle of the MCL.

Lowery WD Jr, Kurzweil PR, Forman SK, Morrison DS: Persistence of the olecranon physis: A cause of "little league elbow." *J Shoulder Elbow Surg* 1995;4:143–147.

This article presents a series of 3 adolescent pitchers with a painful persistence of the olecranon physis. Symptoms may improve with rest. However, if symptoms persist and the contralateral growth plate has closed, internal fixation is suggested.

O'Dwyer KJ, Howie CR: Medial epicondylitis of the elbow. *Int Orthop* 1995;19:69–71.

In a series of 95 cases of medial epicondylitis, 12% failed nonsurgical management and required surgery. This is compared to a 4% surgery rate for lateral epicondylitis over the same period.

Ollivierre CO, Nirschl RP, Pettrone FA: Resection and repair for medial tennis elbow: A prospective analysis. *Am J Sports Med* 1995;23:214–221.

Fifty cases of intractable medial tennis elbow were treated by excising the injured tendon and closing the defect. All patients noted improvements in pain level, and dynamometer testing showed improvements in strength. Despite this, 10 patients did not return to their sporting or occupational activities.

Smith GR, Altchek DW, Pagnani MJ, Keeley JR: A muscle-splitting approach to the ulnar collateral ligament of the elbow: Neuroanatomy and operative technique. *Am J Sports Med* 1996;24:575–580.

In performing a muscle-splitting approach to the MCL, a safe zone exists from the medial epicondyle to 1 cm past the ulnar tubercle. Further, using this approach is effective and may minimize trauma to the flexor-pronator muscle mass.

Classic Bibliography

Andrews JR, Carson WG Jr, McLeod WD: Glenoid labrum tears related to the long head of the biceps. *Am J Sports Med* 1985;13:337–341.

Bigliani LU, Kimmel J, McCann PD, Wolfe I: Repair of rotator cuff tears in tennis players. *Am J Sports Med* 1992;20:112–117.

Blackburn TA, McLeod WD, White B, Wofford L: EMG analysis of posterior rotator cuff exercises. *Athletic Training* 1990;25:40–45.

Chan D, Aldridge MJ, Maffulli N, Davies AM: Chronic stress injuries of the elbow in young gymnasts. *Br J Radiol* 1991;64:1113–1118.

Conway JE, Jobe FW, Glousman RE, Pink M: Medial instability of the elbow in throwing athletes: Treatment by repair or reconstruction of the ulnar collateral ligament. *J Bone Joint Surg* 1992;74A:67–83.

Cordasco FA, Steinmann S, Flatow EL, Bigliani LU: Arthroscopic treatment of glenoid labral tears. *Am J Sports Med* 1993;21:425–430.

DiGiovine NM, Jobe FW, Pink M, Perry J: An electromyographic analysis of the upper extremity in pitching. *J Shoulder Elbow Surg* 1992;1:15–25.

Feltner M, Dapena J: Dynamics of the shoulder and elbow joints of the throwing arm during a baseball pitch. *Int J Sport Biomech* 1986;2:235–259.

Ferretti A, Cerullo G, Russo G: Suprascapular neuropathy in volleyball players. *J Bone Joint Surg* 1987;69A:260–263.

Field LD, Savoie FH III: Arthroscopic suture repair of superior labral detachment lesions of the shoulder. *Am J Sports Med* 1993;21:783–790.

Gugenheim JJ Jr, Stanley RF, Woods GW, Tullos HS: Little League survey: The Houston study. *Am J Sports Med* 1976;4:189–200.

Jackson DW, Silvino N, Reiman P: Osteochondritis in the female gymnast's elbow. *Arthroscopy* 1989;5:129–136.

Jobe FW, Stark H, Lombardo SJ: Reconstruction of the ulnar collateral ligament in athletes. *J Bone Joint Surg* 1986;68A:1158–1163.

Morrey BF, An KN: Functional anatomy of the ligaments of the elbow. *Clin Orthop* 1985;201:84–90.

Nirschl RP, Pettrone FA: Tennis elbow: The surgical treatment of lateral epicondylitis. *J Bone Joint Surg* 1979;61A:832–839.

Poehling GG, Ekman EF: Arthroscopy of the elbow, in Jackson DW (ed): *Instructional Course Lectures 44.* Rosemont, IL, American Academy of Orthopaedic Surgeons, 1995, pp 217–223.

Regan W, Wold LE, Coonrad R, Morrey BF: Microscopic histopathology of chronic refractory lateral epicondylitis. *Am J Sports Med* 1992;20:746–749.

Rubenstein DL, Jobe FW, Glousman RE, Kvitne RS, Pink M, Giangarra CE: Anterior capsulolabral reconstruction of the shoulder in athletes. *J Shoulder Elbow Surg* 1992;1:229–237.

Sisto DJ, Jobe FW, Moynes DR, Antonelli DJ: An electromyographic analysis of the elbow in pitching. *Am J Sports Med* 1987;15:260–263.

Snyder SJ, Karzel RP, Del Pizzo W, Ferkel RD, Friedman MJ: SLAP lesions of the shoulder. *Arthroscopy* 1990;6:274–279.

Tibone JE, Elrod B, Jobe FW, et al: Surgical treatment of tears of the rotator cuff in athletes. *J Bone Joint Surg* 1986;68A: 887–891.

Tibone JE, Jobe FW, Kerlan RK, et al: Shoulder impingement syndrome in athletes treated by an anterior acromioplasty. *Clin Orthop* 1985;198:134–140.

Townsend H, Jobe FW, Pink M, Perry J: Electromyographic analysis of the glenohumeral muscles during a baseball rehabilitation program. *Am J Sports Med* 1991;19:264–272.

Walch G, Boileau P, Noel E, Donell ST: Impingement of the deep surface of the supraspinatus tendon on the posterosuperior glenoid rim: An arthroscopic study. *J Shoulder Elbow Surg* 1992;1:238–245.

Vangsness CT Jr, Jobe FW: Surgical treatment of medial epicondylitis: Results in 35 elbows. *J Bone Joint Surg* 1991;73B: 409–411.

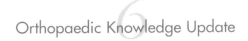

Chapter 26
Shoulder Trauma: Bone

Proximal Humeral Fractures

Proximal humeral fractures represent approximately 4% to 5% of all fractures. Because of the increasing elderly population, they are being seen with increasing frequency. Approximately 85% of proximal humeral fractures are minimally displaced. Much of the controversy over diagnosis and treatment rests with the other 15%.

Proximal humeral fractures frequently result from falls and involve osteoporotic bone. Dual photon absorptiometry and bone mineral analysis studies have confirmed that the humeral neck is the weakest region of the proximal humerus. This region has one half the bone mineral density and one third the mechanical strength of the humeral head. Younger patients, however, often sustain more severe trauma with concomitant soft-tissue and neurovascular injury. Electrical shock and convulsion may result in a fracture-dislocation.

Blood supply to the proximal humerus is important in determining survival of the humeral head. The anterior humeral circumflex artery contributes the major blood supply to the humeral head through the ascending anterolateral branch, which enters the proximal aspect of the bicipital groove. Other contributions include vessels entering the tuberosities through the rotator cuff insertions and direct branches of the circumflex vessels.

Classification of proximal humeral fractures is based on the 4-part system of Neer. Identification of the commonly occurring anatomic fragments—humeral head, greater tuberosity, lesser tuberosity, and humeral shaft—and determination of displacement > 1 cm or angulation > 45° is used to classify these fractures. Applying this classification system to routine radiographs or computed tomography (CT) scans yields fair to poor interobserver reliability and intraobserver reproducibility. Therefore, these imaging studies should not be used alone to determine fracture classification for evaluation of prognosis, treatment options, and functional outcome of proximal humeral fractures. Intraoperative evaluation of the fracture may improve the reliability of this classification system.

Despite the advances in radiographic imaging, the trauma series remains the standard for evaluating proximal humeral fractures. Quality scapular anteroposterior (AP), lateral, and axillary radiographs are necessary to evaluate the fracture pattern. Recent studies have found the AP and axillary radio-

graphs to be the most useful. CT scans are useful adjuvants to evaluate fracture fragment size and glenoid fractures.

The treatment of proximal humeral fractures is based on many factors including patient age, bone quality, medical comorbidities, other concurrent injuries, and fracture type. Younger patients with good bone quality may have a better outcome with humeral head salvage, in contrast to elderly patients with osteoporotic bone or degenerative changes in the rotator cuff or glenohumeral joint. In a recent biomechanical study, 10 different fixation types loaded in shear on fresh frozen and embalmed specimens were compared. Plate and screw fixation and Ender nails with figure-of-8 tension band were the strongest constructs in surgical neck fractures. Tension band techniques alone with nonabsorbable suture or wire were the weakest fixation as a result of cut-out of the proximal humerus. In another study, Ender nails were found to increase the torsional strength of a figure-of-8 construct for surgical neck fractures by 1.5 times.

Nonsurgical treatment with early passive motion remains the treatment of choice for minimally or nondisplaced fractures. However, a recent report indicated that functional outcome was inferior to previously reported results. Of 104 minimally displaced fractures, only 77% resulted in good or excellent results. Although all fractures healed, and 90% of patients had little or no pain, functional recovery was incomplete. If physical therapy was started within 14 days, the percentage of good and excellent results increased as well as the amount of external rotation. Early passive motion within 14 days is recommended for stable fractures. Active range of motion is started at 4 to 6 weeks when healing is evident.

Two-part fractures of the surgical neck represent the most common displaced proximal humeral fracture. Mode of treatment depends on the stability of the fracture. If a stable closed reduction cannot be maintained, the addition of percutaneous pins is warranted. Open treatment is reserved for fractures that cannot be reduced closed. Ender nails with figure-of-8 tension banding (Fig. 1) or plate and screw fixation appear to be the most biomechanically sound.

Surgical reconstruction of nonunions of the surgical neck remains challenging. A significant improvement in pain can be expected with fracture union, but improvement in active motion and function often is only modest. A recent study of 20 surgically reconstructed surgical neck nonunions revealed

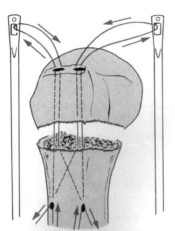 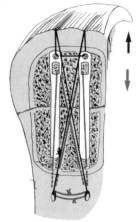 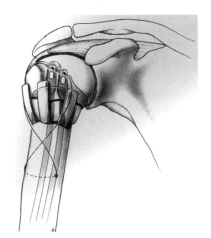

Figure 2

Open reduction and internal fixation with modified Ender rods and figure-of-8 wire for surgical neck nonunion. Nonunion site is bone grafted. (Reproduced with permission from Duralde XA, Flatow EL, Pollock RG, Nicholson GP, Self EB, Bigliani LU: Operative treatment of nonunions of the surgical neck of the humerus. *J Shoulder Elbow Surg* 1996;5:169–180.)

Figure 1

Technique of open reduction and internal fixation of 2- and 3-part fractures of the surgical neck using modified Ender rods. The superior hole is used for the figure-of-8 tension band. Additional sutures through the rods and secured through drill holes beyond the fracture site preclude the rods from migrating into the subacromial space. (Reproduced with permission from Norris TR: Fractures of the proximal humerus, in *Skeletal Trauma.* Philadelphia, PA, WB Saunders, 1992, vol 2, p 1248.)

only 25% excellent, 30% satisfactory, and 45% unsatisfactory results. Reconstruction was obtained with either Ender nails and figure-of-8 wire with bone graft or humeral head replacement with bone graft (Fig. 2). Newer fixation devices, such as contoured blade plates, have been developed in an effort to improve union.

Two-part fractures of the greater tuberosity commonly occur in conjunction with a glenohumeral dislocation. It is important to rule out an associated surgical neck fracture before attempting reduction, to avoid displacing the surgical neck fracture. After closed reduction of the glenohumeral dislocation, the tuberosity may return to its anatomic position. If superior or posterior displacement > 5 to 10 mm persists, open reduction and fixation of the tuberosity fragment with repair of the rotator cuff tear is considered. Untreated residual displacement > 5 mm can cause impingement of a superiorly displaced tuberosity against the acromion in elevation or abutment of a posteriorly displaced tuberosity against the glenoid in external rotation. Fixation of the tuberosity usually is achieved with intraosseous sutures incorporating the cuff insertion (Fig. 3). Occasionally, if the tuberosity is a single large piece, screw fixation may be used. An acromioplasty can be performed at the time of open reduction and internal fixation (ORIF) to prevent postoperative impingement from healing tissues such as scar and callus.

Displaced lesser tuberosity fractures are rare and can be associated with posterior shoulder dislocations. If the fragment is widely displaced, loss of active internal rotation may occur, and ORIF with a screw or sutures and repair of the rotator interval tear may be considered.

The treatment of 3- and 4-part fractures of the proximal humerus remains controversial. In a recent multicenter study, the functional results in anatomically reduced 3-part fractures were significantly better than in fractures with residual displacement. Figure-of-8 tension band technique combined with Ender nails is a common method of fixation. However, recent reports of good results with percutaneous reduction and screw fixation raise the question of possibly improved results with minimal osteosynthesis (Fig. 4). This technique is ideally suited for an attempt to save the humeral head in young patients with good bone quality and no osteoarthritis. Percutaneous fixation is technically demanding but results from experienced surgeons have been promising. Postoperative motion usually is delayed several weeks until the pins are removed, but stiffness does not appear to be common. This technique can also be done under direct visualization (open reduction) as long as soft-tissue stripping is avoided.

Four-part fractures usually are treated with humeral head replacement. Preserving the humeral head is an option, especially in the valgus-impacted fracture in young patients with good bone quality. In this fracture pattern, the medial periosteal hinge remains intact with the accompanying blood supply to the humeral head. The reported rate of osteonecrosis in these fractures treated with minimal osteosynthesis has been relatively low (9% to 11%). Anatomic reconstruction is paramount because it correlates directly with the functional results.

Primary prosthetic replacement historically has resulted in better functional scores when compared to either conservative treatment or ORIF. Late prosthetic replacement for failed conservative or open reduction treatment of 3- and 4-part

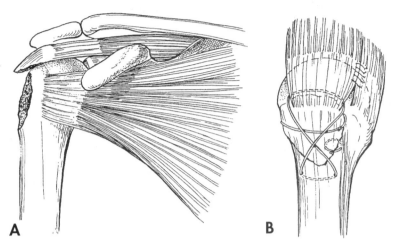

Figure 3

A, Isolated greater tuberosity fracture with superoposterior displacement. B, Reduction of the greater tuberosity and internal fixation using transosseous horizontal sutures and vertical figure-of-8 sutures. (Reproduced with permission from Warner JJP, Iannotti JP, Gerber C: *Complex and Revision Problems in Shoulder Surgery.* Philadelphia, PA, Lippincott-Raven, 1997.)

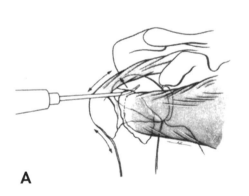
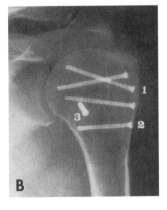

Figure 4

Percutaneous fixation of 3- and 4-part fractures of the proximal humerus. A, When the head is raised the periosteum on the medial side acts like a hinge, and the greater tuberosity returns to its anatomic position as a result of the inferior pull of the periosteum and the superior pull of the rotator cuff. B, The correct location of the screws in the tuberosities is demonstrated: (1) through the greater tuberosity into the head; (2) through the greater tuberosity into the shaft; (3) through the lesser tuberosity into the head. (Reproduced with permission from Resch H, Povacz P, Frolich R, Wambacher M: Percutaneous fixation of three and four part fractures of the proximal humerus. *J Bone Joint Surg* 1997;79B:295-300.)

of treatment of 4-part fractures, especially in the elderly. Fixation of the tuberosities to the fin of the prosthesis and to the humeral shaft is necessary to restore functional integrity of the rotator cuff. Despite optimal fixation, the recovery of function and range of motion is less predictable in humeral head replacement for fracture than in that for arthritis. In a study of 26 humeral head replacements for acute 3- and 4-part fractures, 73% of patients had difficulty with some functional task such as lifting, carrying a weight, or using the hand at or above shoulder level.

Fractures of the Clavicle

Clavicular fractures account for 4% to 15% of all fractures and 35% of fractures about the shoulder. Eighty-five percent involve the middle third of the clavicle. Associated injuries occur in less than 3% of clavicular fractures. Direct trauma is the usual mechanism of injury followed by the indirect mechanism of a fall onto the outstretched hand.

In displaced middle third fractures, the sternocleidomastoid and trapezius muscles pull the medial fragment superior and posterior while the weight of the arm and pectoralis major pull the lateral fragment inferomedially. AP and cephalic tilt radiographs are obtained to evaluate superoinferior and AP displacement, respectively. Most middle third fractures are treated nonsurgically with a figure-of-8 bandage or sling for 6 weeks or until healing is evident. Shortening and a residual painless deformity, which commonly do not interfere with shoulder function, may result. Indications for surgical treatment include open fractures, neurovascular injury/compromise, and displaced fractures with impending skin compromise (Fig. 5). Recent studies have suggested that ORIF be considered for widely displaced midclavicular fractures. In one review, 29 fractures that healed with a mean of 11.1 mm of shortening (range, 8.2 to 14.0 mm) in patients older than 15 years had the same mobility, strength, and functional rating as the uninjured side at 5-year

fractures has had inferior results. In a study of 23 patients with late prosthetic replacements, only 53% could perform activities above shoulder level. Late arthroplasty can substantially reduce pain, although improvements in motion and function are usually more modest.

Humeral head replacement remains the preferred method

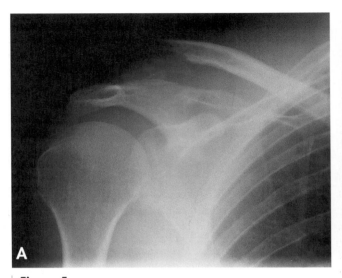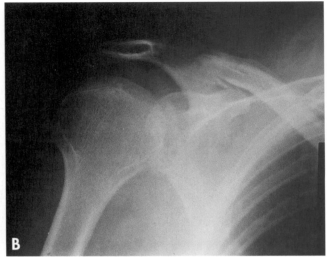

Figure 5
A, Comminuted type II fracture of the distal clavicle. B, Reconstruction of coracoclavicular ligaments with distal fragment excision because of comminution and articular surface involvement.

follow-up. A review of 52 completely displaced middle third fractures in adults (mean age 34 years) indicated that shortening at the fracture of ≥ 20 mm at the time of injury was a risk factor for the development of nonunion ($p < 0.0001$). The authors recommend ORIF for severely displaced fractures of the middle third of the clavicle in adult patients. Plate and screw fixation and intramedullary devices have been used with good results. Bone grafting should be considered for comminuted fractures.

Lateral third fractures are subclassified according to the location of the coracoclavicular ligaments relative to the fracture. Type I fractures are minimally displaced interligamentous fractures between the conoid and trapezoid or between the coracoclavicular and coracoacromial ligaments. Type II fractures are displaced secondary to a fracture medial to the coracoclavicular ligaments, and type III fractures involve the articular surface of the lateral clavicle with no ligamentous injury. An AP view of both shoulders with weights strapped to the wrists may aid in evaluating the coracoclavicular ligament's integrity by comparing the distance from the coracoid to the medial fragment. Anterior and posterior 45° oblique views assist in viewing the fracture in the AP plane.

Type I fractures are stable and treated in the same manner as middle third fractures. In type II fractures, the medial fragment is disconnected from the remaining shoulder girdle, creating an unstable situation. Muscle forces elevate the medial fragment while the weight of the upper extremity pulls the small lateral fragment downward through its connection with the coracoclavicular ligaments, possibly creating

a large gap between the fracture fragments, predisposing to nonunion. Treatment for the unstable type II fractures remains controversial. The original recommendation to operate was based on a 30% nonunion rate after nonsurgical treatment. However, many authors advocate nonsurgical treatment. In general, the more displacement at the fracture site, the higher the risk of nonunion and the greater the indication for surgical reduction and internal stabilization. Intramedullary devices and coracoclavicular stabilization techniques with either nonabsorbable sutures or screws have been described, with the primary goal being to reconstruct the coracoclavicular ligaments in order to resuspend the upper extremity from the axial skeleton.

If the distal fragment is small, necrotic, or there is articular damage and ORIF cannot be achieved, excision of this fragment (in conjunction with coracoclavicular ligament reconstruction) is an option. However, all attempts should be made to achieve osseous healing of the fracture because the attached acromioclavicular ligaments will help the overall stability of the construct. One recent series described 9 type II fractures treated with Dacron suture to reconstruct the coracoclavicular ligaments and #5 nonabsorbable sutures between the fracture ends. All healed with good clinical results. Type III fractures can be adequately managed nonsurgically although ORIF may be indicated if a large fragment resulting in significant articular step-off is present. Distal clavicle resection is the procedure of choice if symptomatic degenerative disease occurs.

Complications after clavicular fractures are uncommon and

include nonunion, malunion, neurovascular sequelae, and postoperative degenerative disease of either the acromioclavicular or sternoclavicular joint. The incidence of nonunion has been reported to be 0.9% to 4.0%. Eighty-five percent of nonunions occur in the middle third. Predisposing factors include inadequate immobilization, significant displacement, severity of initial trauma, soft-tissue interposition, refracture, and primary ORIF. No treatment is necessary unless asymptomatic nonunion is present. ORIF in the form of compression plating or intramedullary fixation and bone grafting should be considered if pain, shoulder dysfunction, or neurovascular compromise are present. For atrophic nonunions with large gaps, tricortical iliac crest interposition graft with AO dynamic compression plating has been used with good results (Fig. 6).

Fracture displacement may rarely cause an acute laceration of the subclavian vessels or brachial plexus injury. Delayed neurovascular complications can occur from compression by exuberant callus or a mobile nonunion. Malunion is common and rarely symptomatic but can cause an unacceptable prominence. Surgical intervention to improve cosmesis may result in an ugly scar or a painful nonunion. Posttraumatic arthritis can result from intra-articular fractures of either end of the clavicle. Resection of the lateral or medial end may be necessary if the patient is sufficiently symptomatic.

Fractures of the Scapula

Fractures of the scapula account for only 0.5% to 1% of all fractures and 3% to 5% of reported shoulder fractures. They occur most frequently in men between 35 and 45 years of age. High-energy trauma is required to cause a scapular fracture because of protection by the surrounding muscles and chest wall. Associated injuries may be severe and life-threatening. As a result, many scapular fractures are overlooked on the initial patient examination. The most common associated injury is the ipsilateral rib fracture with resulting hemopneumothorax (27% to 54%) followed by clavicular fracture (17% to 38%), closed head injury (11% to 57%), injury to the face and skull (10% to 24%), and brachial plexus disruption (3% to 8%). The combination of a scapular fracture and first rib fracture is particularly serious because of the risk of pulmonary and neurovascular compromise.

True scapular AP and lateral views and an axillary view (trauma series) are necessary to identify glenoid, neck, body, and acromion fractures. The West Point axillary view helps identify acromial and glenoid rim fractures, whereas the cephalic tilt or Stryker notch view can aid in identifying coracoid fractures. Because of the complex bony anatomy in this region, CT can assist in detecting and defining the extent and/or displacement of intra-articular fractures as well as the degree of any humeral head displacement. A chest radiograph also should be considered an essential part of the evaluation because of the high incidence of associated injuries that involve the thoracic structures.

Scapular fractures are commonly classified according to the anatomic location. Fractures of the body and spine are common (50%), followed by scapular neck (25%), glenoid (10%), acromion (7%), and coracoid process (3%) fractures. Many fractures are combinations of these different types. Also, avulsion fractures at musculotendinous and ligamentous attachment sites can occur with indirect forces, and fatigue or stress fractures occasionally are seen. Recently, the epidemiology of scapular fractures, with special reference to intra-articular glenoid fractures, was reviewed in a prospec-

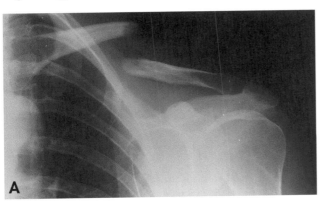
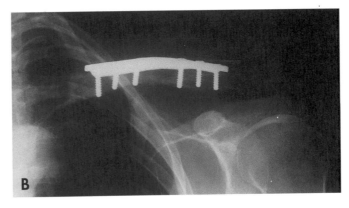

Figure 6

A, Atrophic nonunion of midshaft clavicular fracture with significant displacement. B, Open reduction and internal fixation with 3.5-mm dynamic compression plating and bone graft led to union.

tive study over a 10-year period. Annual incidence was 10 per 100,000, of which 30% affected the glenoid cavity. This figure was higher than previously reported, and the difference was believed to be related to the inclusion of "chip" fractures seen in association with dislocations.

Of all scapular fractures, body fractures have the highest incidence of associated injury. Even when scapular fractures are severely comminuted and displaced, treatment generally is symptomatic and nonsurgical; no reduction is attempted. Short-term immobilization in a sling and swathe bandage for comfort and early progressive range of shoulder motion exercises are begun as pain subsides. In one study, long-term results (10- to 20-year follow-up) after fracture of the scapular body were analyzed; only 3 of 7 scapular body fractures with > 10 mm displacement had good results while 29 of 34 with < 10 mm displacement had good results.

Glenoid neck fractures extend from the suprascapular notch area across the neck to the lateral border of the scapula without involvement of the articular surface. The fracture is often displaced but stable if the clavicle and coracoclavicular ligaments remain intact. Further displacement is rare and treatment is nonsurgical. Surgery has been suggested if the glenoid fragment is displaced > 1 cm or angulated ≥ 40° in either the transverse or coronal plane because shoulder pain and dysfunction can be caused by altered bony relationships and musculotendinous dynamics. The goals of surgery are to prevent glenohumeral dysfunction and glenohumeral instability. Glenoid neck fractures are approached posteriorly with superior extension if necessary. The glenoid fragment is reduced and internally fixed as anatomically and securely as possible.

Intra-articular glenoid fractures have been classified into 6 types. Type I fractures involve the glenoid rim. Anatomic reduction and internal fixation is considered for fragments involving 25% of the anterior glenoid or 33% of the posterior glenoid with fracture displacement > 10 mm. The goal is to reestablish osseous stability, thus preventing chronic glenohumeral instability. Type II fractures are transverse or oblique fractures through the glenoid fossa, producing a free inferior triangular fragment. Type III fractures exit the mid-superior border of the scapula and involve the superior third of the glenoid, including the coracoid. They often are associated with acromioclavicular dislocation or fracture. Type IV fractures exit through the medial border of the scapula, type V fractures combine types II and IV fracture patterns, and type VI is a severely comminuted glenoid fracture. Because these fractures are rare, no large series or controlled studies are available to guide treatment. Suggested indications for ORIF of types II through VI include: (1) subluxation of the humeral head with a major fragment; (2) ≥ 5 mm intra-artic-

ular step-off, especially with the superior glenoid displaced laterally; and (3) severe separation between the glenoid fragments. The goal of surgical treatment is to prevent posttraumatic glenohumeral osteoarthritis, chronic glenohumeral instability, and nonunion.

Most fractures of the acromion are minimally displaced and can be treated with supervised therapy, avoiding resisted deltoid function until fracture union. ORIF is indicated in depressed acromial fractures that encroach on the subacromial space and interfere with rotator cuff function. Isolated coracoid fractures can be managed nonsurgically because anatomic alignment is not necessary for adequate function or healing. Indications for surgical intervention include associated acromioclavicular separation, significant fracture displacement, brachial plexus compression, and suprascapular nerve paralysis with fracture in the suprascapular notch area. In a recent study, 64 coracoid fractures were classified into 2 types according to the relationship of the fracture site to the coracoclavicular ligaments. Fifty-three type I fractures were posterior to the attachment of the ligaments and thus potentially unstable, while 11 type II fractures were anterior to the ligaments and were considered stable. The authors recommended surgical treatment for unstable type I fractures.

The complexity of scapular fractures increases when a combination of injuries renders the shoulder girdle unstable. The concept of a superior shoulder suspensory complex (SSSC) has been proposed to help understand and unite a group of difficult to treat injuries that previously have been described in isolation. The SSSC is a bone and soft-tissue ring (composed of the glenoid process, coracoid process, coracoclavicular ligaments, distal clavicle, acromioclavicular joint, and acromial process) at the end of superior (the middle clavicle) and inferior (the lateral scapular body) bony struts. Single disruptions of the SSSC, which do not disrupt the overall integrity of the complex, tend to be minimally displaced with nonsurgical treatment often sufficient. A double disruption may compromise the integrity of the complex, increasing the likelihood that significant displacement at either or both sites will cause possible adverse healing and/or functional consequences. ORIF is indicated for double disruption of the SSSC if 1 or both injury sites have unacceptable displacement. Often surgical stabilization at 1 site will reduce and stabilize the other disruption indirectly and satisfactorily (Fig. 7).

A fracture of the coracoid process and a grade III disruption of the acromioclavicular joint is a double disruption of the SSSC. A combined fracture of the middle third clavicle and glenoid neck has been termed a "floating shoulder." In isolation, each fracture may be managed nonsurgically. In combination, however, they constitute a double disruption of the SSSC. The clavicular fracture often allows significant dis-

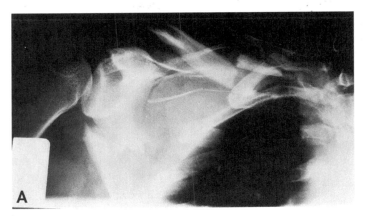
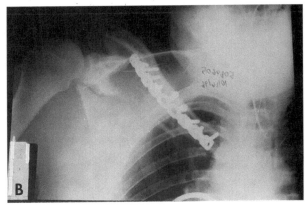

Figure 7

A, Double disruption of the superior shoulder suspensory complex (SSSC) demonstrated by both comminuted midshaft clavicular and scapular neck fractures with significant displacement.
B, Surgical stabilization of the clavicle was performed alone with acceptable scapular alignment achieved indirectly.

placement of the glenoid neck fracture, and the glenoid neck fracture frequently leads to unacceptable displacement at the clavicular fracture site. Most of these injuries may be treated by surgical stabilization of the clavicle or acromioclavicular joint alone, but some investigators recommend ORIF of both the clavicle (or the acromioclavicular joint) and scapula, although results of this treatment are rarely reported in the literature. One report noted good results in 12 cases treated with osteosynthesis of the clavicular injury alone.

Injuries associated with scapular fractures cause the most significant complications. Complications associated with the scapular fracture itself are relatively uncommon. Malunion of fractures of the body usually are well tolerated, although painful scapulothoracic crepitus may occur. Nonunion is extremely rare because the extensive soft-tissue cover provides an excellent blood supply for healing. Suprascapular nerve injuries can occur in association with body, neck, or coracoid fractures involving the suprascapular notch. Electromyography (EMG) helps confirm this diagnosis. Surgical exploration and decompression should be considered. Glenohumeral degenerative joint disease can occur from inadequately reduced glenoid cavity fractures. Significantly displaced glenoid neck (angulatory displacement) and rim fractures can lead to instability. Translational displacement of the glenoid neck may cause glenohumeral dysfunction as a result of altered mechanics of the surrounding soft tissues.

Scapulothoracic dissociation is a rare, often fatal, closed injury manifested by lateral displacement of the scapula with associated neurovascular injury and either acromioclavicular or sternoclavicular separation or clavicular fracture. A severe direct force over the shoulder accompanied by traction applied to the upper extremity is the mechanism of injury, which is often referred to as a "closed, traumatic forequarter amputation." Severe soft-tissue damage may occur to the supporting muscles, especially those that run from the chest wall to the scapula or the chest wall to the humerus. Vascular disruption usually occurs at the level of the subclavian vessels and can result in a pulseless extremity. The associated brachial plexus injury is usually complete.

Scapulothoracic dissociation should be considered in any patient who sustained massive trauma to the upper extremity associated with a neurovascular deficit. Massive soft-tissue swelling over the shoulder girdle may be the only external sign. Significant lateral displacement of the scapula seen on a non-rotated chest radiograph is pathognomonic. An immediate evaluation of the ipsilateral vascular structures or angiography is mandatory to avoid fatal internal hemorrhage. ORIF of the clavicular fracture or acromioclavicular disruption should be considered to stabilize the scapulothoracic articulation.

Once the vascular lesion is delineated, surgical exploration to restore vascularity to the ischemic limb is performed, and severity of the brachial plexus injury is assessed. Also, a careful neurologic examination including EMG testing, if indicated, helps determine the level and degree of injury once the patient is hemodynamically stable. Early above-elbow amputation and shoulder fusion are considered for complete brachial plexus injuries with root avulsions because they result in a flail limb with no potential for neurologic recovery. Patients with partial plexus injuries may achieve complete recovery or regain functional use of the extremity. Nerve repair or grafting may be considered if portions of the plexus are intact. Late reconstructive efforts are guided and dictated by the degree of neurologic return.

Humeral Shaft Fractures

Humeral shaft fractures account for approximately 3% of all fractures; these injuries can result from either direct or indirect forces. A direct load to the side of the arm usually causes a short oblique fracture with a lateral butterfly fragment; a fall onto the flexed elbow causes a long oblique fracture; and an indirect torque causes a spiral fracture. Elderly patients who have humeral shaft fractures as a result of a fall generally have less comminuted fracture patterns.

Evaluation

Patients with humeral shaft fractures usually have arm pain, swelling, and deformity. The arm is shortened, with motion and crepitus on gentle manipulation. In humeral shaft fractures that result from high-energy trauma, the physician should have a high index of suspicion for other more serious associated injuries. Physical examination should include a systematic inspection of the entire limb. The neurovascular status of the limb must be assessed. Doppler pulse and compartment pressure measurements should be made if indicated.

Imaging

The standard radiographic examination of the humerus includes AP and lateral orthogonal views. The shoulder and elbow joint should be included on each view. The radiographs are obtained by moving the patient rather than by rotating the injured limb through the fracture. When considering intramedullary (IM) nailing, the physician must ascertain that the fracture does not extend into the anticipated nail entry point. In highly comminuted or severely displaced fractures, traction radiographs may allow better definition of the fragments, and comparison radiographs of the contralateral humerus may be helpful for preoperative determination of length.

Nonsurgical Treatment

Most closed humeral shaft fractures and fractures caused by low-energy handgun wounds can be managed nonsurgically with closed reduction and application of a coaptation splint or hanging arm cast followed by a functional fracture brace at 1 to 2 weeks. Indications for use of the hanging arm cast include displaced midshaft fractures with shortening, particularly oblique or spiral fractures. In some cases, a functional brace can be applied initially without prior use of a cast or splint. The brace, which consists of an anterior and a posterior plastic shell, held together with Velcro straps (Fig. 8), effects fracture reduction through soft-tissue compression. It is to be tightened as swelling decreases. Over-the-shoulder extensions are avail-

able, but are seldom necessary. Such extensions restrict shoulder motion and are most often used for comminuted fractures of the proximal humerus. Contraindications to use of the functional brace include: (1) massive soft-tissue or bone loss; (2) an unreliable or uncooperative patient; and (3) an inability to obtain or maintain acceptable fracture alignment. Regardless of the initial fracture treatment, the patient is instructed to remain upright, initially either standing or sitting in a semireclining position, and not lean on the elbow for support. The patient is encouraged to perform shoulder pendulum exercises and range of motion exercises of the elbow, wrist, and hand. Assisted range of motion exercises for the shoulder are started as soon as tolerated.

Fractures of the humeral shaft caused by low-energy handgun wounds behave the same as closed fractures with respect to healing and infection, and, except for debridement of the skin at the entry (and exit) sites and a single dose of prophylactic antibiotics, they may be treated as if they were closed fractures.

Surgical Treatment

The indications for surgical treatment of humeral shaft fractures are listed in Outline 1. Open humeral fractures, except those caused by low-energy handgun wounds, require immediate debridement before fracture stabilization to reduce the incidence of infection. If there is associated vascular injury, the fracture is best fixed to protect the vascular repair. The floating elbow (ipsilateral fractures of the humerus and radius/ulna) is best treated by internal fixation of the fractures followed by early range of elbow motion. Surgical treatment of a segmental humeral fracture reduces the high risk of nonunion at 1 or both fracture sites. Pathologic fractures and

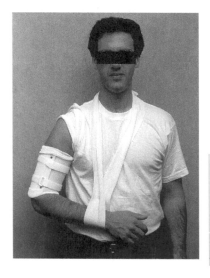

Figure 8

A humeral functional brace effects fracture reduction through soft-tissue compression; it consists of an anterior and posterior shell held together with Velcro straps.

impending fractures should be fixed internally to maximize patient comfort and upper limb function. Surgical stabilization of bilateral humeral fractures is necessary to allow patient self-care. The semisitting position necessary for nonsurgical fracture treatment often is unreasonable for the polytrauma patient, and surgical stabilization of the humerus may allow early use of crutches or other aids to ambulation. Neurologic loss after humeral fracture caused by lacerating injury is an indication for nerve exploration. Neurologic loss after manipulation or reduction of a humeral fracture is an indication for nerve exploration, although this has become controversial recently.

Fractures that cannot be maintained in acceptable alignment should be surgically stabilized. Up to 20° of anterior or posterior angulation, 30° of varus or valgus angulation, and 3 cm of shortening may be well tolerated. Varus or valgus angulation is better tolerated proximally, near the very mobile shoulder joint than a similar angulation more distally. More angulation may be tolerated by an obese patient. Fractures in obese patients and women with large pendulous breasts are at increased risk of varus angulation if treated nonsurgically. Considerable malrotation is well tolerated because of compensatory shoulder motion. Finally, fractures of the humeral shaft with displaced intra-articular fracture extension require surgical treatment.

Surgical Fixation Using Plates and Screws Use of plates and screws allows direct fracture reduction and stable fixation of the humeral shaft without violation of the rotator cuff or elbow. Indications for use of plates and screws include humeri with small medullary canals or preexisting deformity, proximal and distal fractures not amenable to IM nailing, fractures with intra-articular extension, fractures that require exploration for evaluation and treatment of an associated neurologic or vascular lesion, and nonunions (Fig. 9).

The surgical approach for plating the humerus depends on the fracture level and the need to expose the radial nerve. The anterolateral approach is preferred for proximal third fractures; the anterolateral and posterior approaches are both adequate for midshaft and distal third fractures.

The surgeon should avoid excessive soft-tissue stripping and take care not to devitalize butterfly fragments. A 4.5-mm broad dynamic compression plate is usually selected for midshaft humeral fractures; a 4.5-mm narrow dynamic compression plate may be used in smaller patients. Proximal and distal fractures require use of other types of implants (single or double reconstruction plates, T plates). If the fracture pattern permits, the plate should be applied in compression. Lag screws should be inserted whenever possible. The surgeon should obtain 5 to 6 cortices of fixation both proximal and

---

Outline 1

Indications for surgical management of humeral shaft fractures

Open fracture, except low-energy handgun wound

Associated vascular injury

Floating elbow

Segmental fracture

Pathologic fracture

Bilateral humeral fractures

Humeral fracture in polytrauma patient

Neurologic loss after lacerating injury

Neurologic loss during closed fracture alignment

Inability to maintain acceptable alignment

Displaced intra-articular fracture extension

---

distal to the fracture. The surgeon must assess fixation stability prior to closure. The need to bone graft is determined by the amount of comminution and soft-tissue stripping.

Intramedullary Fixation IM nails offer certain biologic and mechanical advantages over plates and screws; IM nails can be inserted without direct fracture exposure, thus minimizing soft-tissue scarring. Because the IM nail is closer to the mechanical axis than the usual plate position on the external surface of the bone, IM nails are subjected to smaller bending loads than plates and are less likely to fail by fatigue. IM nails can act as load-sharing devices in fractures that have cortical contact if the nail is not statically locked. Finally, stress shielding with resultant cortical osteopenia, commonly seen with plates and screws, is minimized with IM implants. However, an increasing number of authors have reported a high incidence of shoulder pain after antegrade humeral nailing. Indications for use of IM nails include segmental fractures in which plate placement would require considerable soft-tissue dissection, fractures in osteopenic bone, pathologic fractures, and humeral shaft fractures in polytrauma patients who may need to use the injured arm for mobilization and ambulation.

Two general types of IM devices are available for use in the humeral shaft: flexible and interlocked nails. Flexible IM devices available for use in the management of humeral fractures include Ender pins, Hackethal nails, and Rush rods (Fig. 10). Multiple flexible pins are required to achieve adequate

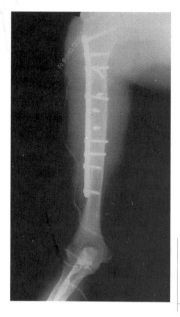

Figure 9

Humeral shaft fracture with proximal fracture extension, stabilized with a compression plate and lag screws.

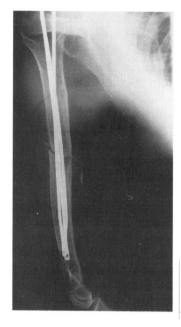

Figure 10

Retrograde flexible Ender nails used to stabilize a humeral shaft fracture.

fracture stability. These devices can be inserted retrograde from the distal humerus or antegrade through the rotator cuff. The best results using flexible implants were obtained using retrograde insertion through an entry portal proximal to the olecranon fossa. Flexible IM nails do not prevent fracture shortening nor do they provide significant rotational control. Therefore, they should be reserved for humeral shaft fractures with minimal comminution. Use of a functional fracture brace to prevent fracture displacement should be considered after flexible IM nailing.

Locked IM nails are able to maintain alignment of unstable fracture patterns and prevent fracture shortening and malrotation (Fig. 11). Interlocked nails can be used to stabilize fractures from 2 cm distal to the surgical neck to 3 cm proximal to the olecranon. Most of these nails rely on proximal and distal screw fixation to provide stability. They can be inserted antegrade through the rotator cuff or retrograde proximal to the olecranon fossa, with or without prior reaming.

Reaming increases the length along which the nail contacts the endosteal surface of the IM canal, thereby providing better fracture stability. Reaming decreases the risk of nail incarceration and permits placement of a larger diameter (and thus stronger) nail. Reaming results in the production of morcellized bone chips, which ought to induce new bone formation; however, the few studies available have not shown much beneficial effect on healing produced by reaming in the human humerus.

Reaming may obliterate the nutrient artery and endosteal blood supply. Excessive endosteal reaming may thin the cortex and result in increased fracture comminution and has been shown to be associated with subsequent nonunion.

With antegrade insertion, the surgeon must bury the humeral nail below the rotator cuff to prevent nail impingement under the acromion. An increasing number of authors have reported a high incidence of shoulder pain after antegrade nail insertion, despite seating of the nail below the rotator cuff. However, loss of shoulder motion has also been reported with plate and screw fixation and with retrograde nails, so some of the shoulder problems may be caused by the injury itself. Oblique proximal locking screws inserted from proximal lateral to distal medial may result in subacromial impingement if the screws are located proximal to the equator of the humeral head. The axillary nerve may be at risk during proximal locking screw insertion. The distal locking screws can be inserted anterior to posterior, posterior to anterior, or lateral to medial by an open technique and may endanger the radial, median, or musculocutaneous nerves.

Complications

Radial Nerve Injury Up to 18% of humeral shaft fractures have an associated radial nerve injury. Although the Holstein-Lewis fracture (oblique, distal third) is best known for its association with neurologic injury, radial nerve palsy is most commonly associated with middle third humeral fractures. Most nerve injuries are a neurapraxia or axonotmesis; 90% will resolve in 3 to 4 months. Electromyography and nerve conduction studies can help to determine the degree of nerve injury and monitor the rate of nerve regeneration. Indications for early radial nerve exploration after humeral fracture are radial nerve palsy associated with a lacerating wound or a deterioration in nerve function believed to be iatrogenically caused during fracture manipulation. Development of a radial nerve palsy after manipulation of a closed humeral shaft fracture was an absolute indication for surgical fracture treatment with radial nerve exploration. More recently, some authors have recommended nonsurgical fracture treatment with surgical exploration 3 or 4 months after injury if there is no evidence of neurologic recovery.

In a recent study, 9 of 14 patients (64%) with an associated radial nerve palsy after open humeral shaft fracture were found to have a radial nerve that was either lacerated or interposed between the fracture fragments. The incidence of radial nerve laceration and entrapment was equal between types I, II, and III open fractures. Epineural radial nerve repair, done primarily or secondarily, provided a satisfactory return of radial nerve function at a minimum of 1-year follow-up. The authors concluded that patients who have a radial nerve palsy in association with an open humeral fracture should have a nerve exploration at the time of initial fracture surgery.

Vascular Injury Although uncommon, laceration or other injury to the brachial artery can be associated with fracture of the humeral shaft. Mechanisms of injury include gunshot wound, stab wound, vessel entrapment between the fracture fragments, and occlusion after hematoma or swelling in a tight retinacular compartment. Risk for injury of the brachial artery is greatest in the proximal and distal thirds of the arm. The role of arteriography in evaluation of long-bone fractures with associated vascular compromise remains controversial. Unnecessary delays for studies of equivocal value are imprudent in the management of an ischemic limb. Arterial flow should be emergently reestablished in cases approaching an ischemic time of 6 hours. At surgery, the vessel should be explored and repaired and the fracture stabilized. If limb viability is not in jeopardy, the surgeon may provide osseous stability prior to vascular repair. If there is significant ischemic time without distal limb perfusion, the vascular surgeon can place a temporary intraluminal vascular shunt before the fracture is stabilized.

Nonunion The nonunion rate following humeral shaft fracture is approximately 7%. The proximal and distal humerus are at greatest risk of nonunion. Patterns associated with nonunion include a transverse fracture pattern as might be expected, but also, paradoxically, a long oblique fracture pattern. Other factors associated with nonunion include fracture

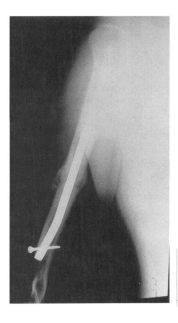

Figure 11

Retrograde locked intramedullary nail used to stabilize a midshaft humeral fracture.

distraction, soft-tissue interposition, obesity, alcohol abuse, and inadequate immobilization. Limitation of shoulder motion also increases the risk of humeral nonunion. With loss of normal shoulder motion, increased stresses occur at the fracture. Other factors that may predispose to nonunion include older age, poor nutritional status, use of steroids, anticoagulation, previous radiation, and fractures underlying a burn.

Compression plating is the treatment of choice for most established humeral nonunions. The surgeon must obtain osseous stability, eliminate nonunion gap, maintain or restore osseous vascularity, and eradicate infection. Compression plating combined with cancellous bone grafting to treat humeral nonunions has been effective in 2 recent series. In one series, union was successful in 24 of 25 (96%) aseptic nonunions of the humerus. In the other, there was a 97% healing rate with 1 surgical procedure in 32 humeral nonunions treated with plates and screws.

Pathologic Fractures The humeral shaft is commonly involved by metastatic disease, and pathologic fracture may result. Surgical stabilization of pathologic humeral fractures has been found to be the best way to relieve patient pain, facilitate nursing care, and maximize patient independence. An interlocked nail is the implant of choice for these fractures; it provides stable fixation, immediate pain relief, and prompt restoration of upper extremity function. An interlocked nail can be augmented with adjunctive polymethylmethacrylate (PMMA) in patients who have a large tumor defect.

Results and Outcomes

In a series of 233 humeral shaft fractures treated using a prefabricated functional brace, 170 were available for follow-up (range 5 weeks to 48 months). Of these, 43 fractures were open, and 127 were closed; 167 (96%) united with an average time to union of 9.5 weeks for closed fractures and 13.6 weeks for open fractures. At follow-up, varus-valgus angulation averaged 5°, anteroposterior angulation averaged 3°, and shortening averaged 4 mm. Results were good to excellent with nearly full range of shoulder and elbow motion in 158 patients.

In a series of 85 extra-articular comminuted distal third humeral fractures treated with a functional brace, 15% were open fractures and 18% had initial radial nerve injury. Seventy-two fractures were available for follow-up; 69 fractures (96%) united. There were no infections. All nerve injuries resolved or were improved at the latest examination. At union, 56 fractures had varus deformity (average, 9°). The most affected shoulder motion was external rotation; 45% of patients lost between 5° and 45°.

In a series of 39 humeral shaft fractures stabilized with plates and screws, 33 of 34 fractures (97%) available for follow-up united primarily. Shoulder and elbow motion at follow-up was excellent. Complications included 1 nonunion, 1 fixation failure, and 1 infection. There were no instances of permanent nerve damage.

All of a series of 102 humeral shaft fractures stabilized with plates and screws united at 1-year minimum follow-up, and 89 patients (87%) had full functional recovery of their upper extremities. There were 2 transitory postoperative radial nerve palsies, 5 early failures of internal fixation because of technical error, 2 nonunions, and 4 postoperative infections.

In a series of 58 fractures of the humeral shaft stabilized with IM flexible rods or nails, 55 (94%) united at an average of 10.5 weeks after surgery. Both antegrade and retrograde entry portals were used as well as insertion through the distal humeral epicondyles. Antegrade nailing was associated with excellent functional results if the entry portal did not violate the rotator cuff. Symptoms of subacromial impingement required early hardware removal in 7 patients. All fractures that had retrograde nail insertion through the epicondyles had a poor result, but retrograde insertion with the entry portal proximal to the olecranon fossa was associated with excellent results.

A series of 19 humeral shaft fractures was stabilized using the Seidel interlocking nail. All nails were inserted after reaming. All fractures united at an average of 2 months after

surgery, and no infections or secondary radial nerve injuries occurred. Eighteen patients regained full shoulder motion by 6 weeks. Return to work varied from 4 to 10 weeks.

A series of 41 humeral shaft fractures were stabilized using a modified Grosse-Kempf reamed tibial nail. Eleven nails were inserted antegrade and 30 retrograde. Twenty of 21 acute fractures united. At 6 weeks, all patients with antegrade nail insertion had significant restriction of active shoulder flexion.

In a prospective series of 51 consecutive humeral nailings with an interlocked IM nail, 41 patients were available for 6-month minimum follow-up. Union was achieved in all acute fractures and 8 of 10 nonunions; all pathologic fractures united or were asymptomatic. Complications included 3 transient brachial plexus neurapraxias, 2 infections, 3 cases of nail impingement, and 2 intraoperative fractures.

Annotated Bibliography

Proximal Humerus Fractures

Bernstein J, Adler LM, Blank JE, Dalsey RM, Williams GR, Iannotti JP: Evaluation of the Neer system of classification of proximal humeral fractures with computerized tomographic scans and plain radiographs. *J Bone Joint Surg* 1996;78A: 1371–1375.

The intraobserver and interobserver reliability of the Neer classification system was assessed on plain radiographs and CT scans. Twenty fractures were reviewed by 2 senior residents and 2 shoulder surgeons. The addition of CT scans did not improve the reliability, nor did use of a simplified classification system ignoring displacement and angulation.

Duralde XA, Flatow EL, Pollock RG, Nicholson GP, Self EB, Bigliani LU: Operative treatment of nonunions of the surgical neck of the humerus. *J Shoulder Elbow Surg* 1996;5:169–180.

Twenty patients who underwent surgical reconstruction for nonunion of the surgical neck of the humerus were reviewed at an average follow-up of 51 months. Significant improvement in pain was obtained but the improvement in active motion and function was modest.

Goldman RT, Koval KJ, Cuomo F, Gallagher MA, Zuckerman JD: Functional outcome after humeral head replacement for acute three- and four-part proximal humeral fractures. *J Shoulder Elbow Surg* 1995;4:81–86.

Twenty-six hemiarthroplasties performed for acute 3- and 4-part proximal humeral fractures were reviewed an average of 30 months after surgery. Functional recovery and range of motion were found less predictable in arthroplasties performed for fracture compared to those performed for arthritis.

Koval KJ, Gallagher MA, Marsicano JG, Cuomo F, McShinawy A, Zuckerman JD: Functional outcome after minimally displaced fractures of the proximal part of the humerus. *J Bone Joint Surg* 1997;79A:203–207.

One hundred four minimally displaced fractures of the proximal humerus were reviewed more than 1 year after fracture. All were found to unite without further displacement; however, only 77% had good or excellent results. The percentage of good and excellent results was significantly greater in patients who had started physical therapy within 14 days after fracture.

Koval KJ, Blair B, Takei R, Kummer FJ, Zuckerman JD: Surgical neck fractures of the proximal humerus: A laboratory evaluation of ten fixation techniques. *J Trauma* 1996;40:778–783.

A biomechanical cadaveric study was performed to evaluate strength of 10 fixation devices for surgical neck fractures. Ender nails with tension band or T-plate with screws provided significantly stronger fixation than other methods. Tension band fixation alone was the weakest.

Norris TR, Green A, McGuigan FX: Late prosthetic shoulder arthroplasty for displaced proximal humerus fractures. *J Shoulder Elbow Surg* 1995;4:271–280.

Twenty-three patients treated with prosthetic arthroplasty after failed treatment for 3- and 4-part fractures were reviewed. Despite 95% improvement in pain, only 53% could perform activities above shoulder level. Late arthroplasty for proximal humeral fractures demonstrated inferior results compared to acute humeral head replacement.

Resch H, Povacz P, Frohlich R, Wambacher M: Percutaneous fixation of three- and four-part fractures of the proximal humerus. *J Bone Joint Surg* 1997;79B:295–300.

Twenty-seven 3- and 4-part fractures treated with percutaneous reduction and screw fixation were reviewed at an average follow-up of 24 months. All 3-part fractures showed good to excellent results. Osteonecrosis occurred in only 11% of 4-part fractures, and results were good for valgus-impacted 4-part fractures; 4-part fractures with lateral displacement of the head had much poorer results.

Resch H, Beck E, Bayley I: Reconstruction of the valgus-impacted humeral head fracture. *J Shoulder Elbow Surg* 1995;4:73–80.

Twenty-two valgus-impacted 4-part fractures were treated with open reduction and minimal osteosynthesis with pins and sutures. At an average follow-up of 36 months, only 2 patients (9%) developed osteonecrosis. When anatomic reconstruction was achieved, the functional result was similar to the uninjured side.

Saitoh S, Nakatsuchi Y, Latta L, Milne E: Distribution of bone mineral density and bone strength of the proximal humerus. *J Shoulder Elbow Surg* 1994;3:234–242.

Dual photon absorptiometry and bone mineral analysis were used to confirm that the top part of the humeral head had the greatest amount of bone mineral. The humeral neck had only one half the bone mineral density and one third the mechanical strength of the humeral head.

Sidor ML, Zuckerman JD, Lyon T, Koval K, Schoenberg N: Classification of proximal humerus fractures: The contribution of the scapular lateral and axillary radiographs. *J Shoulder Elbow Surg* 1994;3:24–27.

Fifty proximal humeral fractures were evaluated using trauma series radiographs to determine the contribution of scapular lateral and axillary radiographs. It was found that the axillary radiograph contributed significantly more to fracture classification with the Neer system than did the scapular lateral.

Williams GR Jr, Copley LA, Iannotti JP, Lisser SP: The influence of intramedullary fixation on figure-of-eight wiring for surgical neck fractures of the proximal humerus: A biomechanical comparison. *J Shoulder Elbow Surg* 1997;6:423–428.

Ten fresh-frozen human cadaver shoulders were used to test the torsional resistance of a surgical neck fracture fixed with figure-of-8 wire alone versus figure-of-8 wire supplemented with intramedullary Ender rods. Ender rods were found to statistically improve the mean maximal torsional load by 1.5 times.

Clavicular Fractures

Boyer MI, Axelrod TS: Atrophic nonunion of the clavicle: Treatment by compression plate, lag-screw fixation and bone graft. *J Bone Joint Surg* 1997;79B:301–303.

Seven clavicular pseudarthroses were successfully reconstructed by primary excision of the nonunion, lag-screw fixation, compression plating using the AO technique, and cancellous grafting with iliac-crest bone graft. The consequent narrowing of the shoulder girdle (range, 0 to 2 cm) was functionally and cosmetically acceptable.

Goldberg JA, Bruce WJ, Sonnabend DH, Walsh WR: Type 2 fractures of the distal clavicle: A new surgical technique. *J Shoulder Elbow Surg* 1997;6:380–382.

Nine patients with type II fractures of the distal clavicle were successfully treated with coracoclavicular ligament reconstruction using Dacron suture between the clavicle and coracoid and nonabsorbable suture between the fractured bone ends.

Hill JM, McGuire MH, Crosby LA: Closed treatment of displaced middle-third fractures of the clavicle gives poor results. *J Bone Joint Surg* 1997;79B:537–539.

Fifty-two completely displaced midclavicular fractures in adults treated nonsurgically were evaluated. Eight (15%) fractures developed nonunion and 16 patients (31%) reported unsatisfactory results. Initial shortening at the fracture of ≥ 20 mm had a highly significant association with nonunion ($p < 0.0001$) and the chance of an unsatisfactory result. Final shortening of ≥ 20 mm was associated with an unsatisfactory result, but not with nonunion.

Nordqvist A, Petersson C: The incidence of fractures of the clavicle. *Clin Orthop* 1994;300:127–132.

The authors determined the age and gender-specific incidences in 2,035 clavicular fractures. Of the fractures, 76% were midclavicular, with a median patient age of 13 years; 21% were lateral clavicular, with a median age of 47 years; and 3% were medial clavicular, with a median age of 59 years. All groups had a significant preponderance of men.

Nordqvist A, Redlund-Johnell I, von Scheele A, Petersson CJ: Shortening of clavicle after fracture: Incidence and clinical significance, a 5-year follow-up of 85 patients. *Acta Orthop Scand* 1997;68:349–351.

Eighty-five patients were reexamined 5 years after either a mid or lateral clavicular fracture treated with sling immobilization. The authors found that permanent shortening of the clavicle is common after fracture, but has no clinical significance.

Scapular Fractures

Blue JM, Anglen JO, Helikson MA: Fracture of the scapula with intrathoracic penetration: A case report. *J Bone Joint Surg* 1997;79A:1076–1078.

This article presents a case of a fracture of the body of the scapula with penetration of the thoracic cavity by a fracture fragment in a 13-year-old boy. A general review of scapular fractures is presented.

Damschen DD, Cogbill TH, Siegel MJ: Scapulothoracic dissociation caused by blunt trauma. *J Trauma* 1997;42:537–540.

The authors present 4 of their own cases of scapulothoracic dissociation and review 54 other cases adequately described in the literature. They believe scapulothoracic dissociation represents a spectrum of musculoskeletal, neurologic, and vascular injuries caused by lateral distraction or rotational forces applied to the shoulder, and they propose a more inclusive clinical classification system and management pathway.

Ideberg R, Grevsten S, Larsson S: Epidemiology of scapular fractures: Incidence and classification of 338 fractures. *Acta Orthop Scand* 1995;66:395–397.

This prospective study over a 10-year period evaluated 338 scapular fractures with 100 intra-articular glenoid fractures classified into 5 main types. The annual incidence was 10 per 100,000, of which 30% affected the glenoid cavity.

Ogawa K, Yoshida A, Takahashi M, Ui M: Fractures of the coracoid process. *J Bone Joint Surg* 1997;79B:17–19.

The authors classified 64 coracoid fractures into 2 types—type I, posterior to the coracoclavicular ligament's attachment site and type II, anterior—based on stability of the surrounding osseous structures. Type I fractures with associated shoulder injuries were considered unstable; type II fractures were considered relatively stable, and most were treated nonsurgically.

Rikli D, Regazzoni P, Renner N: The unstable shoulder girdle: Early functional treatment utilizing open reduction and internal fixation. *J Orthop Trauma* 1995;9:93–97.

In this retrospective review of 12 patients with unstable shoulder girdles (clavicular fracture or acromioclavicular dislocation with scapular neck fracture) treated with osteosynthesis of the clavicle only and indirect reduction of the scapular neck, functional results were excellent.

Humeral Shaft Fractures

Amillo S, Barrios RH, Martinez-Peric R, Losada JI: Surgical treatment of the radial nerve lesions associated with fractures of the humerus. *J Orthop Trauma* 1993;7:211–215.

Twelve patients had delayed surgical repair of a radial nerve injury associated with a humeral shaft fracture. The mean interval between the injury and surgical repair was 6 months. Excellent to good results were obtained in 91% of cases. The authors recommended surgical exploration if there are no clinical or electrophysiologic signs of nerve recovery after 3 months.

Crolla RM, de Vries LS, Clevers GJ: Locked intramedullary nailing of humeral fractures. *Injury* 1993;24:403–406.

A Seidel nail was used to stabilize 30 acute humeral shaft fractures, 9 humeral nonunions, and 7 pathologic fractures. All 27 acute fractures available for follow-up united within 4 months; 18 patients had an excellent functional result, 3 had a satisfactory result, 2 had an unsatisfactory result, and 4 had a poor result (all attributable to a preexisting condition). Six nonunions united within 6 months. All 7 patients who had a pathologic fracture were pain free while alive.

Foster RJ, Swiontkowski MF, Bach AW, Sack JT: Radial nerve palsy caused by open humeral shaft fractures. *J Hand Surg* 1993;18A:121–124.

The authors report 14 open humeral shaft fractures with an associated radial nerve injury. In 9 patients (64%) the radial nerve was either lacerated or interposed between the fracture fragments. Incidence of radial nerve laceration versus entrapment was equal regardless of the degree of soft-tissue injury (grade I, II, or III). Epineural radial nerve repair, performed primarily or secondarily, provided satisfactory return of radial nerve function at a minimum of 1-year follow-up.

Heim D, Herkert F, Hess P, Regazzoni: Surgical treatment of humeral shaft fractures: The Basel experience. *J Trauma* 1993;35:226–232.

The authors report 127 patients with humeral shaft fractures stabilized using plates and screws. Fractures in 102 patients available for 1-year follow-up had united. Eighty-nine patients (87%) had full functional recovery of their upper extremity; 2 had a transient postoperative radial nerve palsy; 4 had a postoperative infection; 5 were considered fixation failures; and 2 developed a nonunion.

Ingman AM, Waters DA: Locked intramedullary nailing of humeral shaft fractures: Implant design, surgical technique, and clinical results. *J Bone Joint Surg* 1994;76B:23–29.

Forty-one humeral shaft fractures were stabilized using a modified 9-mm reamed interlocked tibial nail. The first 11 nails were inserted antegrade through the rotator cuff; the remainder were inserted retrograde through a portal proximal to the olecranon fossa. Ninety-five percent of acute fractures and 80% of nonunions united; all 7 pathologic fractures available for 3-month follow-up united.

McKee MD, Miranda MA, Riemer BL, et al: Management of humeral nonunion after the failure of locking intramedullary nails. *J Orthop Trauma* 1996;10:492–499.

In a multicenter retrospective study of humeral nonunions, initial "excessive" reaming was found to be a predictor of subsequent nonunion.

Redmond BJ, Biermann JS, Blasier RB: Interlocking intramedullary nailing of pathological fractures of the shaft of the humerus. *J Bone Joint Surg* 1996;78A:891–896.

The authors performed a retrospective study of 16 pathologic humeral fractures secondary to metastatic disease that were stabilized using an interlocking nail; 15 nails were inserted using a closed technique. Fourteen extremities had nearly full return of function within 3 weeks of surgery; pain relief was rated as good or excellent in 15 patients. The fracture united in all 7 patients who survived for a minimum 3 months and had radiographs available.

Robinson CM, Bell KM, Court-Brown CM, McQueen MM: Locked nailing of humeral shaft fractures: Experience in Edinburgh over a two-year period. *J Bone Joint Surg* 1992;74B:558–562.

The authors report their experiences using a locked nail for stabilization of 30 humeral shaft fractures. Frequent technical difficulties were encountered at surgery, particularly involving the locking mechanism. Nail protrusion above the greater tuberosity in 12 patients resulted in shoulder pain and poor shoulder function. Poor shoulder function in 5 patients without evidence of nail protrusion was attributed to local rotator cuff damage during nail insertion.

Rodriguez-Merchan EC: Compression plating versus hackethal nailing in closed humeral shaft fractures failing nonoperative reduction. *J Orthop Trauma* 1995;9:194–197.

In a prospective study, compression plating was compared to retrograde Hackethal nailing for stabilization of humeral shaft fractures in 40 patients. Fractures united in 19 of 20 patients who had either IM fixation or compression plating. Patients who had IM fixation required prolonged fracture bracing; 19 patients with IM fixation required removal of hardware secondary to nail prominence. There was no difference in functional outcome between the 2 groups.

Rommens PM, Verbruggen J, Broos PL: Retrograde locked nailing of humeral shaft fractures: A review of 39 patients. *J Bone Joint Surg* 1995;77B:84–89.

Thirty-nine humeral shaft fractures were stabilized with closed retrograde insertion of a locked Russell-Taylor humeral nail. All fractures united at an average of 13.7 weeks. At latest follow-up, 92.3% of patients had excellent shoulder function, and 87.2% had excellent elbow function. One patient had a postoperative radial nerve palsy, which recovered spontaneously within 3 months.

Classic Bibliography

Ada JR, Miller ME: Scapular fractures: Analysis of 113 cases. *Clin Orthop* 1991;269:174–180.

Balfour GW, Mooney V, Ashby ME: Diaphyseal fractures of the humerus treated with a ready-made fracture brace. *J Bone Joint Surg* 1982;64A:11–13.

Barquet A, Fernandez A, Luvizio J, Masliah R: A combined therapeutic protocol for aseptic nonunion of the humeral shaft: A report of 25 cases. *J Trauma* 1989;29:95–98.

Bell MJ, Beauchamp CG, Kellam JK, McMurtry RY: The results of plating humeral shaft fractures in patients with multiple injuries: The Sunnybrook experience. *J Bone Joint Surg* 1985;67B: 293–296.

Brumback RJ, Bosse MJ, Poka A, Burgess AR: Intramedullary stabilization of humeral shaft fractures in patients with multiple trauma. *J Bone Joint Surg* 1986;68A:960–969.

Ebraheim NA, An HS, Jackson WT, et al: Scapulothoracic dissociation. *J Bone Joint Surg* 1988;70A:428–432.

Flemming JE, Beals RK: Pathologic fracture of the humerus. *Clin Orthop* 1986;203:258–260.

Foster RJ, Dixon GL Jr, Bach AW, Appleyard RW, Green TM: Internal fixation of fractures and non-unions of the humeral shaft: Indications and results in a multi-center study. *J Bone Joint Surg* 1985;67A:857–864.

Goss TP: Fractures of the glenoid cavity. *J Bone Joint Surg* 1992;74A:299–305.

Habernek H, Orthner E: A locking nail for fractures of the humerus. *J Bone Joint Surg* 1991;73B:651–653.

Hall RF Jr, Pankovich AM: Ender nailing of acute fractures of the humerus: A study of closed fixation by intramedullary nails without reaming. *J Bone Joint Surg* 1987;69A:558–567.

Healey WL, White GM, Mick CA, Brooker AF Jr, Weiland AJ: Nonunion of the humeral shaft. *Clin Orthop* 1987;219: 206–213.

Hems TE, Bhullar TP: Interlocking nailing of humeral shaft fractures: The Oxford experience 1991 to 1994. *Injury* 1996;27:485–489.

Herscovici D Jr, Fiennes AG, Allgower M, Ruedi TP: The floating shoulder: Ipsilateral clavicle and scapular neck fractures. *J Bone Joint Surg* 1992;74B:362–364.

Holm CL: Management of humeral shaft fractures: Fundamental nonoperative techniques. *Clin Orthop* 1970;71:132–139.

Holstein A, Lewis GB: Fractures of the humerus with radial-nerve paralysis. *J Bone Joint Surg* 1963;45A:1382–1388.

Hunter SG: The closed treatment of fractures of the humeral shaft. *Clin Orthop* 1982;164:192–198.

Jensen CH, Hansen D, Jorgensen U: Humeral shaft fractures treated by interlocking nailing: A preliminary report on 16 patients. *Injury* 1992;23:234–236.

Kavanagh BF, Bradway JK, Cofield RH: Open reduction and internal fixation of displaced intra-articular fractures of the glenoid fossa. *J Bone Joint Surg* 1993;75A:479–484.

Kettlekamp DB, Alexander H: Clinical review of radial nerve injury. *J Trauma* 1967;7:424–432.

Leung KS, Lam TP: Open reduction and internal fixation of ipsilateral fractures of the scapular neck and clavicle. *J Bone Joint Surg* 1993;75A:1015–1018.

Lewallen RP, Pritchard DJ, Sim FH: Treatment of pathologic fractures or impending fractures of the humerus with Rush rods and methylmethacrylate: Experience with 55 cases in 54 patients, 1968–1977. *Clin Orthop* 1982;166:193–198.

Naver L, Aalberg JR: Humeral shaft fractures treated with a ready-made fracture brace. *Arch Orthop Trauma Surg* 1986;106:20–22.

Neer CS II: Fractures of the distal third of the clavicle. *Clin Orthop* 1968;58:43–50.

Nordqvist A, Petersson C: Fracture of the body, neck, or spine of the scapula: A long-term follow-up study. *Clin Orthop* 1992;283:139–144.

Nordqvist A, Petersson C, Redlund-Johnell I: The natural course of lateral clavicle fracture: 15 (11-21) year follow-up of 110 cases. *Acta Orthop Scand* 1993;64:87–91.

Pollock FH, Drake D, Bovill EG, Day L, Trafton PG: Treatment of radial neuropathy associated with fractures of the humerus. *J Bone Joint Surg* 1981;63A:239–243.

Rosen H: The treatment of nonunions and pseudarthroses of the humeral shaft. *Orthop Clin North Am* 1990;21:725–742.

Sarmiento A, Horowitch A, Aboulafia A, Vangsness CT Jr: Functional bracing for comminuted extra-articular fractures of the distal third of the humerus. *J Bone Joint Surg* 1990;72B:283–287.

Sarmiento A, Kinman PB, Galvin EG, Schmitt RH, Phillips JG: Functional bracing of fractures of the shaft of the humerus. *J Bone Joint Surg* 1977:59A:596–601.

Stern PJ, Mattingly DA, Pomeroy DL, Zenni EJ Jr, Kreig JK: Intramedullary fixation of humeral shaft fractures. *J Bone Joint Surg* 1984;66A:639–646.

Wright TW, Cofield RH: Humeral fractures after shoulder arthroplasty. *J Bone Joint Surg* 1995;77A:1340–1346.

Zagorski JB, Latta LL, Zych GA, Finnieston AR: Diaphyseal fractures of the humerus: Treatment with prefabricated braces. *J Bone Joint Surg* 1988;70A:607–610.

Chapter 27
Shoulder Instability

287

Natural History

The most common sequela of traumatic anterior shoulder instability is recurrence. Classic studies have stratified the recurrence rate as inversely proportional to patient age with rates over 90% for those 11 to 20 years of age. More recently, large studies have documented recurrence rates averaging between 55% and 66%. In a recent study of United States military cadets, 47 of 55 patients (87%) had recurrent instability after nonsurgical treatment that included closed reduction, a brief period of immobilization (3 to 6 weeks), and activity restriction followed by a supervised physical therapy program.

Traumatic anterior shoulder dislocation in the skeletally immature individual frequently is associated with the development of a Bankart lesion (labral detachment of the inferior glenohumeral ligament complex, IGHLC). This problem has been associated with a recurrence rate ranging from 64% to 100% at 3- to 5-year follow-up. Length of immobilization, avoidance of overhead activity, and supervised physical therapy had no effect on outcome in this population with open physes.

Although patients over 40 years of age have a lower redislocation rate, 2 recent studies showed that symptoms may persist. Neurologic injury and rotator cuff tears were more frequent in this group than in younger patients. In 1 study, 11 of 12 patients over age 40 years with recurrent dislocations had a subscapularis and capsular tear from the lesser tuberosity. Careful evaluation is necessary for these associated injuries in the older patient.

Biomechanics

A mismatch of articular curvature between the glenoid and humeral head has been traditionally referred to as a source of shoulder joint instability. However, many older studies used radiography to determine congruence, evaluating bony and not articular cartilage geometry. A recent study showed that the glenoid cartilage is thicker peripherally, so that the glenoid subchondral bone is flatter than that of the humerus even though the true articular cartilage surfaces are highly conforming. Furthermore, radiographic studies may overestimate translations of the humeral head, because they track the geometric center of the humeral subchondral bone rather than the center of the articular (cartilage) surface. Therefore, other imaging modalities, especially magnetic resonance imaging (MRI), may provide a better representation of glenohumeral congruence by visualizing articular cartilage and thus a more accurate depiction of in vivo shoulder mechanics. The major reason for the decreased importance of glenohumeral congruence for stability of the articulating surfaces in the shoulder compared to the hip is the fact that the glenoid has a much smaller surface area than the humeral head. Factors that disrupt normal congruence, such as glenoid hypoplasia, or reduce even further glenoid surface area, including glenoid wear or fracture, may predispose towards instability.

The superior glenohumeral ligament (SGHL) and coracohumeral ligament (CHL) are often described together because they run a parallel course and constitute the rotator interval region between the anterior border of the supraspinatus and the superior border of the subscapularis. A recent study found that the cross-sectional area of the CHL is 4 times greater than that of the SGHL. The CHL is more than twice as stiff as the SGHL and can sustain 3 times its ultimate load to failure. Although individual variations occur, the CHL and SGHL resist inferior translation in forward flexion, adduction, and internal rotation. For comparison, the overall strength of the SGHL and CHL is less than 15% that of the anterior cruciate ligament.

The middle glenohumeral ligament (MGHL) is absent or poorly defined in 40% of all specimens. It appears to limit anterior translation in lower ranges of abduction (60° to 90°). Glenohumeral stability in these ranges is greatly enhanced by the dynamic actions of the rotator cuff and the concavity-compression mechanism of the articular surface and labrum, when the majority of the capsular ligaments are lax.

The IGHLC, composed of a superior band and anterior and posterior pouch regions, is the primary restraint to anterior and posterior translation in external and internal rotation, respectively, at greater degrees of abduction. Furthermore, in abduction, it serves as a secondary restraint to inferior translation. A recent study found that the superior band had the greatest stiffness, and the anterior pouch had the highest strain to failure. The tissue near the insertion sites exhibited more viscoelastic behavior with capsular avulsions (Bankart lesions), whereas midsubstance tissue had near elastic behavior (capsular stretch).

A kinematic investigation noted that, in a cadaver model, an

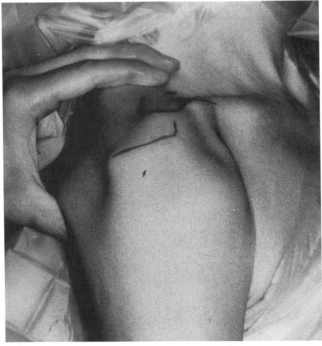

Figure 1

Sulcus sign of the right shoulder. Note the dimple between the humeral head and the acromion.

overly tight anterior capsulorrhaphy caused posterior translation of the humeral head throughout the entire range of motion. This resulted in a decrease in the contact area between the humeral head and the glenoid, suggesting a mechanism for articular surface degeneration (particularly the posterior glenoid) after overly tight anterior repairs. In another biomechanical study, the technique of capsular shift with a simulated Bankart lesion was evaluated. A 5-mm medial shift was compared to a superior shift of 5 mm on the glenoid. Restraint to anterior translation was equivalent for both reconstructions; however, a 5-mm superior shift significantly decreased translation more than a 5-mm medial shift for posterior and inferior translation with the arm in 45° abduction.

Although articular conformity and capsuloligamentous structures play a key role in glenohumeral stability, dynamic factors must not be overlooked. As the rotator cuff muscles center the humeral head on the glenoid, they simultaneously "dynamize" the capsule and are critical in maintaining joint stability. The capsuloligamentous structures provide afferent feedback for reflexive muscular control of the rotator cuff and biceps to modulate excessive translations and rotations, which may cause injury. In a recent study on proprioception

it was found that joint position sense was impaired in patients with untreated instability. This difference was not apparent in healthy volunteers and those who had undergone stabilization procedures.

Patient Evaluation

History Although a history of a single traumatic event with the arm in abduction and external rotation with a resultant dislocation is classically associated with anterior instability, many patients may present solely with the complaint of shoulder pain with activities and may not experience any sensation of instability. Furthermore, symptoms of fatigue, loss of pitch velocity, and pain during late cocking may predominate athlete's complaints resulting from subluxation. Assessment of provocative arm positions as well as of training habits is important in evaluating the unstable shoulder. Anterior instability is more symptomatic during the late cocking phase, whereas symptoms of posterior instability are typically seen during follow-through.

Physical Examination The physical examination should include a thorough neurovascular examination, with particular attention to the brachial plexus and axillary nerve, especially in patients with a history of a traumatic dislocation. A careful range of motion must be documented and specific attention must be paid to the rotator cuff and deltoid for symptoms of pain and for discrepancies between active and passive range of motion. An evaluation for ligamentous laxity should be performed in all patients.

Specific provocative tests, namely the apprehension/relocation test and sulcus sign test (Fig. 1), are helpful in the diagnosis of instability. Pain without true apprehension during a forced abduction and external rotation maneuver is nonspecific; only when a sensation of true subluxation or dislocation occurs is the accuracy of this test greater than 80%. Furthermore, the appearance of a sulcus sign (a dimple in the area between the humeral head and acromion with inferior translation of the humeral head) with the arm in neutral rotation that persists despite external rotation may indicate a rotator interval lesion. Excessive external rotation with the arm at the side may indicate deficiency of the rotator interval (SGHL and CHL) and the MGHL, with resultant multidirectional hyperlaxity.

A posterior directed force on the humerus with the shoulder in 90° flexion, adduction, and internal rotation may elicit a sensation of subluxation or posterior translation. This maneuver, designed to demonstrate posterior instability, may be particularly difficult in muscular patients.

Throwing athletes may present with posterior capsular

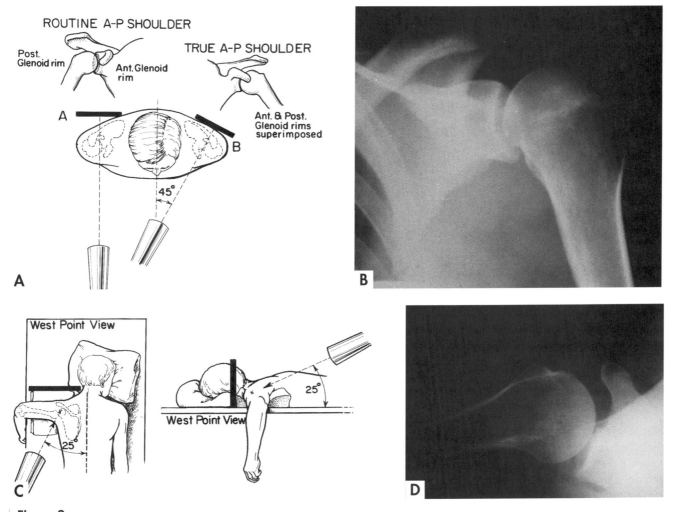

Figure 2

A, Schematic diagram of a true anteroposterior radiograph of shoulder. (Reproduced with permission from Rockwood CA, Szalay EA, Curtis RJ, et al: X-ray evaluation of shoulder problems, in Rockwood CA, Matsen FA III (eds): *The Shoulder.* Philadelphia, PA, WB Saunders, 1990.) B, True anteroposterior view. C, Schematic diagram of West Point view (axillary). D, Axillary view.

tightness, pain, or impingement signs, all of which may be sequelae of instability. Furthermore, transient neurologic symptoms may occur provoking a "dead arm" sensation, particularly in contact sports. Impingement in throwing athletes may be secondary to loss of internal rotation.

Imaging Radiographic analysis should include a true anteroposterior radiograph in the plane of the scapula, a lateral scapular image (Y-view), and an axillary view (Fig. 2). A West Point axillary view may demonstrate an anteroinferior glenoid fracture better than a standard axillary view.

Imaging studies of the soft tissues that provide the best information about capsular volume or labral injury are computed tomography (CT) arthrogram or MRI (with or without gadolinium contrast). The presence of altered glenoid anatomy, particularly hypoplasia and excessive retroversion, is best visualized with CT studies (Fig. 3). Several recent studies correlating MRI arthrogram with surgical findings demonstrated an 88% sensitivity and 100% specificity in diagnosing tears of the inferior glenohumeral ligament (IGHL) (Fig. 4). Recently, sensitivity and specificity rates for anterior and superior labral injuries were reported to be greater than 86% and 95% using unenhanced MRI imaging with high resolution fast-spin and gradient echo images.

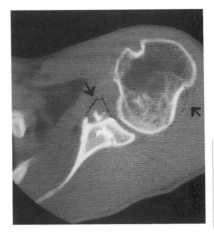

Figure 3

Computed tomography scan of glenohumeral joint with significant anterior bone loss and presence of Hill-Sachs lesion.

Treatment

Anterior Instability

Nonsurgical Treatment The initial treatment for primary anterior shoulder dislocation is nonsurgical. Confirmed

Examination Under Anesthesia and Arthroscopy When the office history or physical examination is limited, examination under anesthesia (EUA) may confirm the diagnosis as well as influence surgical technique (Fig. 5). Moreover, in obese or muscular patients who are especially difficult to examine, the EUA can help to elucidate the degree and direction of instability.

Arthroscopy can provide detailed information about associated pathology. Classically, anterior labral detachment (ie, Bankart lesion), capsular injury (with increased capsular volume), and the presence of a posterosuperior humeral head impression fracture (Hill-Sachs lesion) are associated with anterior instability. Recently, several investigators have reported their findings during arthroscopic evaluation after a first time dislocation. In a recent study, the arthroscopic findings of 212 patients with instability of varying duration and frequency were prospectively evaluated. Bankart lesions were identified in 184 of these 212 patients (87%); 168 (79%) exhibited capsular insufficiency, 144 (68%) had Hill-Sachs lesions, and 116 (55%) were found to have glenohumeral ligament insufficiency.

Although Bankart's "essential lesion" with detachment of the labrum from the anterior inferior glenoid is the most common finding in anterior instability, it is apparent that a wide spectrum of pathology is associated with this disorder. Moreover, capsular laxity in the absence of a Bankart lesion is a common finding in many large series of traumatic anterior instability.

A recent biomechanical study demonstrated that the creation of a Bankart lesion alone is insufficient to permit shoulder dislocation. Thus, some capsular injury or elongation of the IGHLC must occur for instability to be present. The value of arthroscopy is that it allows delineation of the injury pattern to direct further open or arthroscopic management

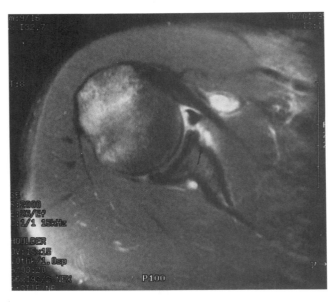

Figure 4

Magnetic resonance image with arthrogram of large Bankart lesion.

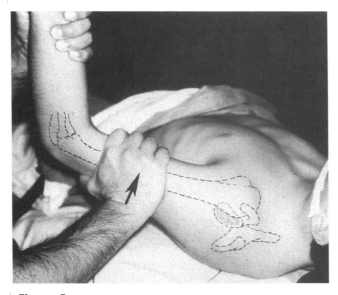

Figure 5

Examination under anesthesia demonstrating anterior instability.

closed reduction, a brief period of immobilization, and activity modification with a supervised rehabilitation program (with specific rotator cuff and periscapular stabilizing exercises) are indicated. Acute stabilization may occasionally be considered in young athletes returning to contact sports but is not indicated in most cases.

Once recurrent episodes of instability occur, nonsurgical treatment emphasizes avoidance of at-risk activities and positions and strengthening of the stabilizing musculature. Such a program can be effective for recurrent subluxation, but is usually less helpful for recurrent dislocations unless the patient is willing and able to drastically restrict activities. The use of a harness or brace to limit abduction and external rotation in contact sports appears to decrease the episodes of instability, although a randomized, prospective study has yet to be published. Once conservative treatment has failed, surgical treatment is considered. Procedures that restore the normal glenohumeral anatomy are favored over historic procedures. The repair of an avulsion of the capsular tissue (Bankart lesion) or reduction of excessive capsular laxity/redundancy is the goal of reconstructive surgery.

Arthroscopic Surgery A variety of arthroscopic techniques have been performed for anterior instability. The earliest techniques used staple capsulorraphy; high complication rates resulting from recurrence, staple loosening or migration, and articular surface injury caused by staple penetration have led to near abandonment of this technique. Transglenoid suture repair of Bankart lesions has demonstrated varying success rates. Failure rates between 4.5% and 48% have been reported. In a recent retrospective study of 41 consecutive patients, 19% demonstrated recurrent instability, all within 2 years of surgery; the absence of a true Bankart lesion was associated with a higher redislocation rate. In another recent study, recurrence rate was stratified with labral injury. In those with single detachment without significant other lesions, redislocation occurred in 1 of 22 patients (4.5%). If significant degeneration of the anterior inferior labrum was found, 13 of 15 (87%) experienced recurrence. Passage of transosseous sutures poses a particular risk to the suprascapular nerve, and injury to this structure has been reported.

Fixation of anteroinferior labral lesions with cannulated bioabsorbable tacks has also enjoyed variable success. In a recent series of over 50 patients with at least 2-year follow-up, 11 patients (21%) developed recurrent instability, often without trauma. At open stabilization, 7 of these 11 patients were noted to have complete healing of the Bankart lesion with a patulous capsule requiring capsulorraphy. Another recent study using strict selection criteria (excluding hyperlaxity, multidirectional instability, poor capsular tissue, and atrau-

matic or volitional instability) documented a redislocation rate of 71% at 4-year follow-up. By using meticulous patient selection and reserving this device for unidirectional instability without a significant capsular injury, the success of this technique may be improved. Synovitis from the bioabsorbable material has been sporadically reported.

Recently, procedures involving suture anchors have become popular, but few long-term follow-up data are available. In 1 recent study 40 patients were followed for 1.5 to 3 years after arthroscopic instability repairs using suture anchors, and 93% remained stable.

Currently, there is much interest in thermal techniques of capsular shrinkage. No long-term follow-up data have been reported. Biomechanical studies have noted shortening of cadaver capsule when heated, perhaps in association with some degradation of material properties. The effect of the healing response has not been fully elucidated.

Open Surgical Procedures Open surgical stabilization has historically been associated with a 95% or greater reduction in redislocation. Early procedures, such as the Magnuson-Stack and Putti-Platt, markedly limited external rotation and created functional limitation by restriction of motion. Recent modifications to open stabilization, designed to reduce loss of external rotation, include anteroinferior capsular shifts, T-plasty Bankart repair, and subscapularis splitting approaches. These techniques permit repair of the Bankart lesion and plication of a large pouch if necessary without mediolateral shortening, which would limit motion.

Modifications of capsular plication to prevent excessive capsular tightening have recently been proposed. In a recent study in which selective capsular tightening was performed, varying arm position to avoid overtightening each region of the capsule, there was a very low recurrence rate with symmetric motion in 11 of 18 patients (Fig. 6). Only 1 patient in this series had greater than 10° loss of external rotation in abduction.

An enlarged rotator interval was found to be the major lesion in a recent series of 15 patients. Isolated closure or imbrication of this defect was successful in treating instability; however, the population was clearly distinct from classic anterior instability.

Posterior Instability

As with anterior instability, the initial treatment of posterior instability is nonsurgical. Whereas surgical treatment of anterior instability is well accepted, posterior stabilization procedures remain controversial. If a lengthy conservative treatment program has failed, surgical repair is considered.

The rationale of glenoid osteotomy to prevent posterior dis-

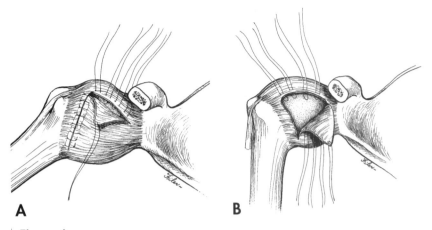

Figure 6

Selective capsular tightening. A, The inferior capsule is tightened with the arm in 10° flexion, 60° abduction, and 45° to 60° external rotation. B, The superior capsule is tightened with the arm in 0° abduction and 45° external rotation.

placement is to increase glenoid anteversion. An opening wedge osteotomy is typically performed, often near the articular margin. However, a recent study of 12 patients found 2 (19%) had persistent clinical instability after osteotomy, and 3 others (25%) had pain. Postoperative evaluation documented unpredictable changes in anteversion, and the authors concluded glenoid osteotomy should be used with considerable caution. This is especially true because most studies have not found altered anteversion or other bone abnormalities in shoulders with posterior instability.

Posteroinferior capsular shift, with or without posterior labral repair, has been successful in reducing capsular volume and instability. Isolated unidirectional posterior instability is rare. There is usually a component of inferior instability present as well. Moreover, many patients with multidirectional instability demonstrate primarily posterior instability; this population may have a higher recurrence rate following surgery than those with anterior instability. In a recent study of 34 patients who underwent posteroinferior capsular shift, 6 were classified as unidirectional, 7 were bidirectional (posterior and inferior), and 22 multidirectional. Overall, 28 of 35 (80%) had a good or excellent result, with 6 of 7 failures occurring in those patients who had a previous surgical procedure. Therefore, posteroinferior capsular shift has been recommended as the standard approach for posterior instability, with bony procedures reserved for rare cases of glenoid deficiency.

Multidirectional Instability

After failure of a prolonged course of therapy directed at the rotator cuff, deltoid, and periscapular stabilizers, surgery should be considered for multidirectional instability. It is important to identify the voluntary dislocators, because they are poor candidates for surgical stabilization. Furthermore, specific attention should be directed at whether there is a predominant direction to the instability, which may either be more symptomatic or demonstrate greater translation. Once appropriate patient selection is completed, success rates of over 90% in this population may be expected.

The inferior capsular shift is designed to globally reduce capsular volume. By approaching from the most symptomatic side, this area obtains reinforcement; the inferior and opposite sides are tightened by reducing the volume of the capsule by advancing the inferior pouch, obliterating this space. This maneuver tightens the opposite side; thus, the inferior shift will tension the opposite side of the joint. The critical steps in this technique are adequate capsular take down and overlap of the capsular flaps. Postoperative immobilization is usually maintained by a brace for 6 weeks, with gentle range of motion exercises until 12 weeks; progressive strengthening is then initiated. Long-term follow-up (up to 11 years) has demonstrated generally successful outcomes with a low recurrence of instability.

Acromioclavicular Instability

The typical mechanism of acromioclavicular (AC) joint injuries is a direct fall on the point of the shoulder at the lateral edge of the acromion, usually in contact sports or falls off bicycles. Tenderness at the AC joint is always present, along with possible skin abrasions at the site of contact with the ground. If there is a dislocation of the AC joint, characteristic prominence of the distal clavicle is evident on inspection. The classic Allman-Tossy classification of these injuries has been expanded by Rockwood, and this expanded classification is extremely helpful in determining appropriate treatment (Fig. 7).

In the Rockwood classification, a type I injury is a sprain of the AC joint without displacement of the clavicle. A type II injury includes partial rupture of the AC ligaments and the coracoclavicular ligaments with subluxation of the AC joint. A type III injury is a dislocation of the AC joint with complete disruption of the coracoclavicular and AC ligaments. A type IV injury is a dislocation of the AC joint with posterior displacement of the clavicle into or through the trapezius muscle. A type V injury is a dislocation of the AC joint with marked superior displacement of the clavicle greater than twice the normal coracoclavicular distance. The type VI injury is an extremely uncommon inferior dislocation of the AC joint with subcoracoid displacement of the clavicle.

Initial treatment of types I and II AC joint injuries is nonsurgical. A sling is used until pain at the AC joint subsides and ice to the shoulder and nonsteroidal anti-inflammatory drugs are used as necessary. Range of motion and strengthening of the shoulder begin when pain in the shoulder subsides, typically within 2 weeks. Nonsurgical treatment of types I and II injuries leads to good results in over 90% of cases. Failure of this treatment is usually related to the development of symptomatic degenerative joint disease of the AC joint.

The treatment of type III injuries remains controversial. No study has proven that surgical management of type III injuries is superior to nonsurgical treatment. However, not all patients with type III injuries do well. These patients may have pain with activities of the shoulder in the overhead position, especially when performing manual work. The specific patient group that will benefit from surgical management remains unclear. Furthermore, although 1 study of surgical treatment of acute and chronic AC dislocations showed no statistical difference in results between these 2 groups, there was a definite trend that patients with chronic injuries treated surgically did not have as good a result as those patients treated acutely. Nevertheless, the literature currently supports the initial nonsurgical treatment of most patients with type III injuries. Surgical treatment has often been recommended for acute injuries in laborers or high demand overhead athletes, and for chronic injuries in which initial nonsurgical treatment fails. There is currently little support for treating type III injuries with closed reduction using straps and braces owing to poor compliance using these devices and the potential for skin pressure necrosis.

Because of the severe displacement of the clavicle in types IV, V, and VI AC joint injuries, initial surgical management of these injuries is considered. Several options are available for surgical stabilization of the AC joint. These include AC fixation with pins or plates and coracoclavicular fixation with nonabsorbable suture or metallic screws. The current trend is toward coracoclavicular fixation using nonmetallic implants, obviating the need for subsequent hardware removal. A recent report described a modification of the classic Weaver-Dunn technique in which coracoclavicular fixation is achieved with nonabsorbable suture passed around the base of the coracoid and through drill holes in the clavicle (Fig. 8). Minimal distal clavicle resection with transfer of the coracoacromial ligament is used in chronic cases in which healing of the coracoclavicular ligaments cannot be assured. Careful

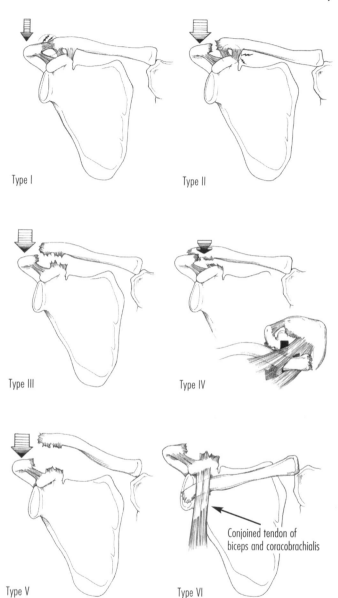

Figure 7

Rockwood classification of ligamentous injuries to the acromioclavicular joint. (Reproduced with permission from Rockwood CA, Williams GR, Young DC: Shoulder instability, in Rockwood CA, Green DP, Bucholz RN, Heckman JD (eds): *Rockwood and Green's Fractures in Adults.* Philadelphia, PA, Lippincott-Raven, 1996, vol 2, p 1354.)

closure of the deltotrapezial fascia is important. Patients treated surgically should use a sling for the first 6 weeks after surgery to protect the surgical construct, because failures will result from too early active use of the involved extremity. Range of motion and strengthening of the shoulder begin at

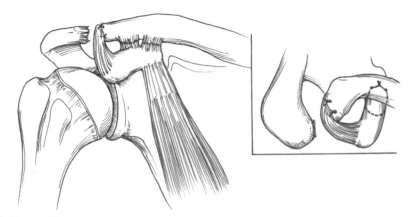

Figure 8

Schematic drawing of the modified Weaver-Dunn procedure demonstrating coracoclavicular fixation with 2 heavy No. 5 nonabsorbable sutures combined with transfer of the coracoacromial ligament to the distal clavicle. A minimal (5 to 7 mm) resection of the distal clavicle has been performed. (Reproduced with permission from Weinstein DM, McCann PD, McIlveen SJ, Flatow EL, Bigliani LU: Surgical treatment of complete acromioclavicular dislocations. *Am J Sports Med* 1995;23:324–331.)

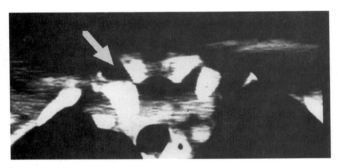

Figure 9

Computed tomography scan (axial view) demonstrating a posterior dislocation of the right sternoclavicular joint.

6 weeks postoperatively. Full activity of the shoulder is permitted at 6 months.

Sternoclavicular Instability

Sternoclavicular joint instability is extremely uncommon and can be divided into anterior and posterior dislocations. Posterior dislocation of the sternoclavicular joint is the more serious injury and is often associated with high-energy collisions and multiple trauma. Anterior dislocation of the sternoclavicular joint is more common and may present atraumatically or with minimal trauma. Diagnosis of sternoclavicular instability is difficult on physical examination, and radiographs of the sternoclavicular joint often are nondiagnostic. The most consistent diagnostic modality is CT, which clearly delineates the pathology.

Anterior dislocations of the sternoclavicular joint are usually managed nonsurgically with activity modification and reassurance. Posterior dislocations may require treatment because of the proximity of major neurovascular structures and the airway (Fig. 9). A closed reduction of the posterior dislocation is performed with the patient under general anesthesia in the operating room and with a chest surgeon available to address any potential vascular or airway catastrophe associated with injuries to the mediastinum. Successful closed reduction of a posterior sternoclavicular joint is usually stable. Internal fixation should be avoided in sternoclavicular instability because of the likelihood of hardware migration and possible injury to the mediastinal structures. If closed reduction of the posterior dislocation is unsuccessful, open reduction is indicated. Treatment following reduction of the sternoclavicular joint includes the placement of a figure-of-8 splint and the use of a sling for a 6-week period, followed by stretching and strengthening exercises. Recurrent instability of the sternoclavicular joint is uncommon.

Annotated Bibliography

Natural History

Neviaser RJ, Neviaser TJ: Recurrent instability of the shoulder after age 40. *J Shoulder Elbow Surg* 1995;4:416–418.

Of 12 patients with recurrent instability (onset after age 40), 11 had anterior instability, and 1 had a posterior dislocation. All patients with anterior instability had ruptured the subscapularis and anterior capsule, whereas the posterior dislocator had torn the infraspinatus and upper teres minor with the posterior capsule. Stability was restored in all cases by reattaching the ruptured tendons and capsule to the tuberosities.

Biomechanics

Boardman ND, Debski RE, Warner JJ, et al: Tensile properties of the superior glenohumeral and coracohumeral ligaments. *J Shoulder Elbow Surg* 1996;5:249–254.

Tensile properties of the SGHL and CHL with bone-ligament-bone complexes from fresh-frozen shoulders were studied with uniaxial tensile testing. The coracohumeral ligament is an important capsuloligamentous structure with significantly greater cross-sectional area, stiffness, and ultimate load to failure than that of the superior glenohumeral ligament.

O'Brien SJ, Schwartz RS, Warren RF, Torzilli PA: Capsular restraints to anterior-posterior motion of the abducted shoulder: A biomechanical study. *J Shoulder Elbow Surg* 1995;4: 298–308.

Twenty-three cadaveric shoulders were tested biomechanically to quantitate the contribution of specific capsular structures to restricting anteroposterior (AP) translation of the abducted shoulder. The primary AP stabilizer of the abducted shoulder is the IGHLC. The anterior band is the primary stabilizer in 30° of horizontal extension and at 0° (neutral). The posterior band is the primary stabilizer in 30° of horizontal flexion.

Ticker JB, Bigliani LU, Soslowsky LJ, Pawluk RJ, Flatow EL, Mow VC: Inferior glenohumeral ligament: Geometric and strain-rate dependent properties. *J Shoulder Elbow Surg* 1996;5:269–279.

Bone-to-bone strain was always greater than midsubstance strain, indicating that when the IGHL is stretched, the tissue near the insertion sites will experience much greater strain than the tissue in the midsubstance. Insertion failures were more likely at slower strain rates, and ligamentous failures were predominant at the fast strain rate. This superior band and anterior axillary pouch viscoelastic stiffening effect suggests that these two regions may function to restrain the humeral head from rapid abnormal anterior displacement.

Warner JJ, Lephart S, Fu FH: Role of proprioception in pathoetiology of shoulder instability. *Clin Orthop* 1996;330:35–39.

The authors evaluated proprioception in individuals with normal shoulders, unstable shoulders, and after surgical stabilization, by assessing threshold to detection of passive motion and the ability to passively reposition the arm in space. In normal shoulders, there is no difference between the dominant and nondominant shoulder; in unstable shoulders, there is a significantly decreased proprioceptive ability.

Patient Evaluation

Chandnani VP, Gagliardi JA, Murnane TG, et al: Glenohumeral ligaments and shoulder capsular mechanism: Evaluation with MR arthrography. *Radiology* 1995;196:27–32.

MR arthrograms were evaluated retrospectively in 46 patients with a history of shoulder instability, impingement syndrome, or pain and correlated with surgical observations. In diagnosis of tears of the SGHL, MGHL, and IGHL, MR arthrography had a sensitivity of 100%, 89%, and 88% and a specificity of 94%, 88%, and 100%, respectively.

Gusmer PB, Potter HG, Schatz JA, et al: Labral injuries: Accuracy of detection with unenhanced MR imaging of the shoulder. *Radiology* 1996;200:519–524.

One hundred three patients with clinically suspected shoulder injuries were prospectively examined with unenhanced MRI with surgical correlation in all patients. At surgery, 37 torn anterior, 36 torn superior, and 19 torn posterior labra were identified. The sensitivity for detection of these tears with MRI was 100%, 86%, and 74%, respectively; the specificity was 95%, 100%, and 95%, respectively.

Hintermann B, Gachter A: Arthroscopic findings after shoulder dislocation. *Am J Sports Med* 1995;23:545–551.

Arthroscopic examination was performed on 212 patients who had at least 1 documented shoulder dislocation. Of these, 184 (87%) had anterior glenoid labral tears, 168 (79%) had ventral capsule insufficiency, 144 (68%) had Hill-Sachs compression fractures, 116 (55%) had glenohumeral ligament insufficiency 30 patients (14%) had complete rotator cuff tendon tears, and 14 patients (7%) had superior labrum anterior and inferior lesions.

Wolf EM, Cheng JC, Dickson K: Humeral avulsion of glenohumeral ligaments as a cause of anterior shoulder instability. *Arthroscopy* 1995;11:600–607.

The incidence of humeral avulsion of glenohumeral ligaments (HAGL) and its role in anterior glenohumeral instability were studied. Sixty-four shoulders with a diagnosis of anterior instability were prospectively evaluated by arthroscopy, 6 shoulders (9.3%) had HAGL lesions, 11 (17.2%) had generalized capsular laxity, and 47 (73.5%) Bankart lesions.

Treatment

Bigliani LU, Pollock RG, McIlveen SJ, Endrizzi DP, Flatow EL: Shift of the posteroinferior aspect of the capsule for recurrent posterior glenohumeral instability. *J Bone Joint Surg* 1995;77A: 1011–1020.

Thirty-five shoulders were treated with a superior shift of the posteroinferior capsule for recurrent posterior subluxation and dislocation (22 MDI). At 5 years postoperatively, 17 of the 35 were rated as excellent; 11, as good; 1, as fair; and 6, as poor. Four shoulders became unstable again. Six of the 7 patients with unsatisfactory results had had previous attempts at stabilization.

DeBerardino TM, Arciero RA, Taylor DC: Arthroscopic stabilization of acute initial anterior shoulder dislocation: The West Point experience. *J South Orthop Assoc* 1996;5:263–271.

Seventy-two military cadets were treated surgically for acute initial shoulder dislocation with 3 separate arthroscopic techniques (arthroscopic abrasion/staple repair, transglenoid sutures, or bioabsorbable tack). Recurrence rates of 22% (2 of 9), 14% (3 of 21), and 10% (4 of 39) were obtained respectively.

Field LD, Warren RF, O'Brien SJ, Altchek DW, Wickiewicz TL: Isolated closure of rotator interval defects for shoulder instability. *Am J Sports Med* 1995;23:557–563.

Fifteen patients noted at surgery to have an isolated rotator interval defect (averaging 2.7 × 2.3 cm) underwent closure of the defect as an isolated procedure for recurrent instability. At 3.3 years' follow-up, all patients achieved either a good or excellent result.

Green MR, Christensen KP: Arthroscopic Bankart procedure: Two- to five-year followup with clinical correlation to severity of glenoid labral lesion. *Am J Sports Med* 1995;23:276–81.

Transglenoid suture technique was used arthroscopically in 47 consecutive shoulders. One of 22 cases (4.5%) of simple detachment of the labrum (type II labrum) failed; 13 of the 15 cases (87%) with significant or complete degeneration of the glenoid labrum-inferior glenohumeral ligament complex (types IV or V labra) failed. Redislocation rate correlated directly with the degree of glenoid labrum-IGHLC lesion.

Hovelius L, Augustini BG, Fredin H, Johansson O, Norlin R, Thorling J: Primary anterior dislocation of the shoulder in young patients: A 10-year prospective study. *J Bone Joint Surg* 1996;78A:1677–1684.

Among 245 patients (age 12 to 40 years) followed up for 10 years after nonsurgical treatment, 58 shoulders (23%) required surgical treatment. The type and duration of the initial treatment had no effect on the rate of recurrence, but a Hill-Sachs lesion was associated with a significantly worse prognosis. At 10 years, radiographs indicated that 23 shoulders (11%) had mild arthropathy and 18 (9%) had moderate or severe arthropathy.

Morrison DS, Lemos MJ: Acromioclavicular separation: Reconstruction using synthetic loop augmentation. *Am J Sports Med* 1995;23:105–110.

Fourteen patients with Rockwood grades III, IV, or V AC joint dislocations underwent surgical reconstruction using a synthetic loop passed through drill holes in the base of the coracoid and in the anterior third of the clavicle. Twelve of 14 patients had good or excellent results at an average 44-month follow-up.

Pagnani MJ, Warren RF, Altchek DW, Wickiewicz TL, Anderson AF: Arthroscopic shoulder stabilization using transglenoid sutures: A 4-year minimum followup. *Am J Sports Med* 1996;24:459–467.

Thirty-seven patients with recurrent anterior instability of the shoulder were retrospectively observed after an arthroscopic transglenoid suture stabilization; 27 patients (74%) had good or excellent results, 3 (7%) were graded as fair, and 7 (19%) developed recurrent instability with absence of a Bankart lesion associated with postoperative instability.

Speer KP, Warren RF, Pagnani M, Warner JJ: An arthroscopic technique for anterior stabilization of the shoulder with a bioabsorbable tack. *J Bone Joint Surg* 1996;78A:1801–1807.

Arthroscopically assisted repair with use of a bioabsorbable tack was performed in 50 shoulders having a Bankart lesion. Of the patients, 41 (79%) were asymptomatic and were able to participate in sports without restriction. The repair was considered to have failed in 11 (21%). Anterior stabilization of the shoulder with a bioabsorbable tack may be indicated for patients who have anterior instability but do not need a capsulorrhaphy.

Ungersbock A, Michel M, Hertel R: Factors influencing the results of a modified Bankart procedure. *J Shoulder Elbow Surg* 1995;4:365–369.

Forty-two shoulders (all with confirmed Bankart lesions) were operated on for anterior instability with follow-up of 47 months. Four shoulders had 1 or more recurrent anterior dislocations, and 4 had recurrent anterior subluxations. The presence and magnitude of a Hill-Sachs lesion did not influence the frequency of recurrence. In patients with a large Bankart lesion, the rate of recurrence was significantly higher.

Warner JJ, Johnson D, Miller M, Caborn DN: Technique for selecting capsular tightness in repair of anterior-inferior shoulder instability. *J Shoulder Elbow Surg* 1995;4:352–364.

The authors describe and present preliminary data for a modified anteroinferior capsular shift technique that tightens the inferior capsule with the shoulder positioned in abduction and external rotation and the superior capsule with the shoulder in adduction and external rotation. Of the 18 patients, 11 (61%) maintained symmetric motion; the others had minimal loss of external rotation compared with that of the contralateral shoulder.

Warner JJ, Miller MD, Marks P, Fu FH: Arthroscopic Bankart repair with the Suretac device: Part I. Clinical observations. *Arthroscopy* 1995;11:2–13.

Fifteen patients underwent a "second-look" arthroscopy to evaluate and treat pain or recurrent instability following arthroscopic Bankart repair with the Suretac device. In the 7 patients with recurrent instability, the Bankart repair was found to be completely healed in 3 (43%), partially healed in 1 (14%), and had recurred in 3 (43%); however, 6 of 7 were observed to have lax capsular tissue.

Weinstein DM, McCann PD, McIlveen SJ, Flatow EL, Bigliani LU: Surgical treatment of complete acromioclavicular dislocations. *Am J Sports Med* 1995;23:324–331.

Forty-four patients (27 acute, 17 chronic) with Allman-Tossy grade III AC dislocations were treated surgically using a modified Weaver-Dunn technique. There was a trend for better results in return to sports or heavy labor with early repairs. Overall, 39 patients (89%) achieved a satisfactory result.

Wirth MA, Blatter G, Rockwood CA Jr: The capsular imbrication procedure for recurrent anterior instability of the shoulder *J Bone Joint Surg* 1996;78A:246–259.

One hundred forty-two shoulders with recurrent anterior instability were managed with an anatomic capsular imbrication (to reduce overall capsular volume) reconstruction. The procedure included repair of the capsulolabral injury. Of the 142 shoulders, 132 (93%) had a good or excellent result at an average of 5 years, regardless of the etiology (traumatic or atraumatic).

Classic Bibliography

Allman FL Jr: Fractures and ligamentous injuries of the clavicle and its articulation. *J Bone Joint Surg* 1967;49A:774–784.

Altchek DW, Warren RF, Skyhar MJ, Ortiz G: T-plasty modification of the Bankart procedure for multidirectional instability of the anterior and inferior types. *J Bone Joint Surg* 1991;73A:105–112.

Bankart ASB: The pathology and treatment of recurrent dislocation of the shoulder-joint. *Br J Surg* 1938;26B:23–29.

Bigliani LU, Pollock RG, Soslowsky LJ, Flatow EL, Pawluk RJ, Mow VC: Tensile properties of the inferior glenohumeral ligament. *J Orthop Res* 1992;10:187–197.

Burkhead WZ Jr, Rockwood CA Jr: Treatment of instability of the shoulder with an exercise program. *J Bone Joint Surg* 1992;74A:890–896.

Lephart SM, Warner JJP, Borsa PA, Fu FH: Proprioception of the shoulder joint in healthy, unstable, and surgically repaired shoulders. *J Shoulder Elbow Surg* 1994;3:371–380.

Lippett SB, Vanderhooft JE, Harris SL, Sidles JA, Harryman DT II, Matsen FA III: Glenohumeral stability from concavity-compression: A quantitative analysis. *J Shoulder Elbow Surg* 1993;2: 27–35.

Morgan CD, Bodenstab AB: Arthroscopic Bankart suture repair: Technique and early results. *Arthroscopy* 1987;3:111–122.

Neer CS II, Foster CR: Inferior capsular shift for involuntary inferior and multidirectional instability of the shoulder: A preliminary report. *J Bone Joint Surg* 1980;62A:897–908.

Rockwood CA Jr: Part II: Subluxations and dislocations about the shoulder: Injuries to the acromioclavicular joint, in Rockwood CA Jr, Green DP (eds): *Fractures in Adults,* ed 2. Philadelphia, PA, JB Lippincott, 1984, pp 860–910.

Rowe CR: Prognosis in dislocations of the shoulder. *J Bone Joint Surg* 1956;38A:957–977.

Soslowsky LJ, Flatow EL, Bigliani LU, Mow VC: Articular geometry of the glenohumeral joint. *Clin Orthop* 1992;285:181–190.

Speer KP, Deng X, Borrero S, Torzilli PA, Altchek DA, Warren RF: Biomechanical evaluation of a simulated Bankart lesion. *J Bone Joint Surg* 1994;76A:1819–1826.

Thomas SC, Matsen FA III: An approach to the repair of avulsion of the glenohumeral ligaments in the management of traumatic anterior glenohumeral instability. *J Bone Joint Surg* 1989;71A: 506–513.

Tibone J, Sellers R, Tonino P: Strength testing after third-degree acromioclavicular dislocations. *Am J Sports Med* 1992;20: 328–331.

Tossy JD, Mead NC, Sigmond HM: Acromioclavicular separations: Useful and practical classification for treatment. *Clin Orthop* 1963;28:111–119.

Turkel SJ, Panio MW, Marshall JL, Girgis FG: Stabilizing mechanisms preventing anterior dislocation of the glenohumeral joint. *J Bone Joint Surg* 1981;63A:1208–1217.

Warner JJ, Deng XH, Warren RF, Torzilli PA: Static capsuloligamentous restraints to superior-inferior translation of the glenohumeral joint. *Am J Sports Med* 1992;20:675–685.

Weaver JK, Dunn HK: Treatment of acromioclavicular injuries, especially complete acromioclavicular separation. *J Bone Joint Surg* 1972;54A:1187–1194.

Zuckerman JD, Matsen FA III: Complications about the glenohumeral joint related to the use of screws and staples. *J Bone Joint Surg* 1984;66A:175–180.

Chapter 28
Shoulder Reconstruction

Muscular Function and Anatomy of the Glenohumeral Joint

Force analysis studies of the deltoid and rotator cuff have provided a better understanding of the mechanism for shoulder abduction. Abduction in the plane of the scapula occurs not only through action of the deltoid and supraspinatus, but also through contributions of the infraspinatus and subscapularis. In one study, it was found that internal rotation enhanced the ability of the superior portion of the infraspinatus to elevate the arm, while external rotation facilitated this ability for the superior portion of the subscapularis. This finding might explain, for example, the ability to elevate the arm even in the absence of a functioning supraspinatus tendon. Results of another study indicated that in an intact shoulder, a larger contribution of force from the supraspinatus is required near the beginning of abduction, whereas the middle deltoid becomes more important near terminal abduction in the scapular plane. Other investigators have pointed out that it is important to consider the effects of external rotation exertions on the rotator cuff as well as effects of abduction. This could lead to the design of more ergonomically efficient work and exercise programs for people with symptoms of rotator cuff disease.

The precise role of the long head of the biceps tendon as a shoulder stabilizer remains controversial. Data from one biomechanical study led to the conclusion that the long head of the biceps contributes to anterior stability of the glenohumeral joint by increasing the shoulder's resistance to torsional forces when it is in the abducted and externally rotated position. Moreover, the biceps muscle was found to diminish stresses on the inferior glenohumeral ligament. In a clinical study of 7 patients who had isolated loss of the proximal attachment of the long head of the biceps tendon, 2 to 6 mm of superior translation of the humeral head during humeral abduction was found in all patients. These translations were significantly greater than those for the contralateral control shoulder. These authors concluded that the long head of the biceps serves as a stabilizer of the humeral head. However, data from an electromyographic study of biceps activity during shoulder motion failed to demonstrate significant biceps activity in either normal shoulders or those with rotator cuff tears. Thus, the authors concluded that the biceps tendon has no active role during shoulder motion. Other recent biomechanical data suggest that the long head of the biceps may provide at least passive stability for the shoulder, especially in a rotator cuff deficient shoulder.

Effective function of the glenohumeral joint is achieved by a complex interaction between the various articular and soft-tissue restraints. The rotator cuff muscles center the humeral head in the congruent glenoid fossa through the midrange of motion, when the capsuloligamentous structures are lax. Humeral head translations on the glenoid are small (usually < 2 mm) in all 3 directions (anteroposterior, lateral-medial, and inferior-superior) during active abduction of the humerus in the scapular plane. In a biomechanical cadaver model, incongruent joints were found to have larger translations, which occur at the extremes of motion, especially with testing in external rotation. This mechanism of "concavity-compression," the maintenance of the humeral head in the concave glenoid fossa by forces from the rotator cuff muscles, demonstrates the interrelationship between the dynamic muscular stabilizers and the articular geometry in providing stability and function for the shoulder. Disturbance of this mechanism by the creation of an anteroinferior chondral-labral defect results in a reduction in stability against translations in the direction of the defect.

Recent investigations have focused on the neural anatomy of the shoulder and how proprioceptive mechanisms may mediate interactions between the muscles and capsuloligamentous structures. The presence of mechanoreceptors and free nerve endings in the glenohumeral ligaments, as well as free nerve endings in the labrum and through the subacromial bursa has been demonstrated in several studies. Specifically, classic Ruffini end organ receptors and Pacinian corpuscles were found in the capsular ligaments. Other investigators have demonstrated the existence of ligamentomuscular reflex arcs in the feline glenohumeral joint. Stimulation of branches of the axillary nerve, which terminated in the glenohumeral joint capsule, resulted in electromyographic activity in the biceps and rotator cuff muscles. Transection of these articular branches resulted in electrical silence in the rotator cuff on stimulation, demonstrating that these branches are an afferent type. The authors concluded that the existence of such ligamentomuscular reflex arcs in the gleno-

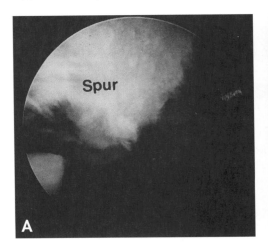

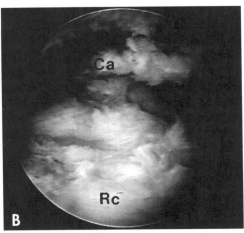

Figure 1

A, Arthroscopic view of prominent anterior acromial spur visualized from within the subacromial space. B, Arthroscopic view of bursal side partial-thickness rotator cuff tear prior to debridement. (Reproduced with permission from Hartzog CW Jr, Savoie FH III, Field LD: Arthroscopic acromioplasty and arthroscopic distal clavicle resection, mini-open rotator cuff repair: Indications, techniques, and outcome, in Iannotti JP (ed): *The Rotator Cuff: Current Concepts and Complex Problems.* Rosemont, IL, American Academy of Orthopaedic Surgeons, 1998, p 25–57.)

humeral joint suggests that ligaments and muscles function synergistically in stabilizing the shoulder.

A number of clinical reports also have focused on the significance of the perception of joint position and joint motion in the shoulder. Shoulders with anterior instability demonstrated proprioceptive deficits compared to the normal contralateral shoulder in several studies. It is speculated that injury to the capsuloligamentous structures disrupts the normal neuromuscular feedback mechanisms. These proprioceptive deficits appear to be reversible through surgical reconstruction.

Arthroscopy of the Shoulder

The use of arthroscopy and arthroscopic techniques for the diagnosis and treatment of shoulder disorders has continued to increase. As a diagnostic tool, arthroscopy has been a helpful adjunct to examination under anesthesia in selected patients for confirming the diagnosis of glenohumeral instability. Arthroscopy also has been useful in visualizing signs of superior glenoid or internal impingement (Fig. 1), with pathology involving 1 or more of 5 intra-articular structures: the superior labrum, the rotator cuff undersurface, the inferior glenohumeral ligament, the greater tuberosity, and the bony glenoid. Arthroscopy provides a better means of evaluating superior labral pathology than present imaging techniques because it allows evaluation of subacromial pathology, as well as possible concomitant intra-articular damage (eg, early osteoarthritis) in patients with impingement syndrome. Arthroscopic examination has also recently been used in painful shoulders to evaluate glenoid component loosening after prosthetic replacement.

Arthroscopic subacromial decompression has become widely accepted as an alternative to open anterior acromio-

plasty, and the results of arthroscopic and open decompression have been comparable in several series. Similarly, arthroscopic excision of the distal clavicle has been successful in treating degenerative disorders of the acromioclavicular joint, such as osteolysis and osteoarthritis. Arthroscopic and arthroscopically-assisted techniques for treating frozen shoulder and rotator cuff tears also have been advanced in recent years, and these are discussed later in this chapter.

Arthroscopic treatment of superior labral pathology also has been used, although controversy persists concerning the treatment of labral tears. Some authors have reported satisfactory results with arthroscopic debridement of anteroinferior or posterior labral flap tears, while others contend that this treatment does not yield consistent long-term results. A recent review of a large series of superior labral tears (SLAP lesions) provided useful information about the demographics and treatment of these lesions. The authors found that the average patient age was 38 years, and 91% were male. Most patients had pain, and 49% noted mechanical catching or grinding. Moreover, 40% had associated rotator cuff pathology and 22% had Bankart lesions. Treatment consisted of debridement of type I (flap) tears, debridement with abrasion of the glenoid rim and, more recently, stabilization of type II lesions with suture anchors, and either debridement or stabilization of type III and type IV lesions, depending on the extent of labral tissue disrupted.

A number of arthroscopic techniques have been developed for the repair of dislocating or subluxating shoulders. These have involved the use of staples, sutures or suture anchors, and bioabsorbable tacks for fixation of the anteroinferior labrum to the glenoid rim. Reported advantages of arthroscopic stabilization procedures include reductions in surgical time, blood loss, postoperative morbidity, and duration of hospitalization, and easier rehabilitation. While a few authors have reported low recurrence rates with arthroscopic stabilization, which equal or approach recurrence rates reported for open stabilization, others have reported failure rates as high as 40% to 50%. A steep learning curve, difficulty evaluating ligament tension arthroscopically, and diminished scarring response are some of the possible reasons for the higher recurrence rates after arthroscopic stabilization procedures. There have been few studies comparing patients with shoulder instability treated arthroscopically with those treated with an open procedure. In the few available series, open stabilization resulted in a much lower rate of recurrence.

Rotator Cuff Disease

Etiology
Rotator cuff disorders represent a spectrum of disease, including tendon inflammation, tendon and bursal fibrosis, tendon tears (partial- or full-thickness), and cuff tear arthropathy. Mechanical impingement, or compression of the supraspinatus tendon between the acromion and the greater tuberosity, and intrinsic degenerative processes within the aging tendon have both been cited as factors underlying rotator cuff disease, and debate continues as to the relative importance of the various factors contributing to these disorders.

Lateral radiographs have been used to classify the acromion into 3 morphologic patterns: flat, curved, and hooked. In cadavers and in a clinical population, a higher incidence of rotator cuff tears has been found in shoulders with a hooked acromion that compromised the subacromial space. In a recent study of 420 scapulae from cadavers of various ages it was found that basic acromial morphology (flat, curved, or hooked,) is independent of age and is a primary anatomic characteristic. However, spur formation on the anterior acromion is an age-dependent process. Thus, it appears that variations in acromial shape contribute to impingement both independent of age-related degenerative processes and through age-related degenerative spurring.

The report of another recent cadaver study covered histologic findings in the coracoacromial arch and rotator cuff. The authors found age-related degenerative changes in the coracoacromial ligament, degeneration of the acromial bone-ligament junction, and acromial spur formation. These degenerative structural changes of the coracoacromial arch were found even in the presence of a normal rotator cuff. The incidence of rotator cuff tears was greater in the group of subjects with a type III (hooked) acromion. The authors concluded that rotator cuff tears originating on the bursal side are related to acromial morphology and that changes in the coracoacromial arch, including osteophyte formation, are

caused by age-related degenerative changes, which are not dependent on the presence of a rotator cuff tear.

In a biomechanical study of the excursion of the rotator cuff under the acromion, subacromial contact during scapular elevation was studied using stereophotogrammetry. Contact started at the anterolateral edge of the acromion at 0° of elevation and shifted medially on the acromion with elevation. On the humeral side, contact shifted from proximal to distal on the supraspinatus tendon with elevation. The acromial undersurface and rotator cuff were in closest proximity between 60° and 120° of elevation. Contact was consistently more pronounced for specimens with a type III acromion. Contact was consistently centered on the supraspinatus insertion, suggesting a mechanical reason for the initiation of rotator cuff pathology in this region. Moreover, the study results suggest that some degree of contact between the rotator cuff and coracoacromial arch is normal, but a markedly increased or focused contact (such as seen in a type III acromion) may be deleterious to the tendon.

Other studies have concentrated on the intrinsic histologic and mechanical properties of the rotator cuff tendons. In one study histologic differences were found between the bursal- and joint-side layers of the supraspinatus tendon, as well as differences in their biomechanical properties. Histologically, the bursal-side layer was composed of tendon bundles with a decreasing muscular component near the insertion, while the joint-side layer was a complex of tendon, ligament, and joint capsule. The strain-to-yield point and ultimate failure stress in the bursal-side layer were twice as great as those of the joint-side layer. Because it is composed primarily of a group of longitudinal tendon bundles, the bursal-side layer generates greater resistance when loaded in tension. The thinner, interlacing fibers of the joint-side layer are believed to render it more vulnerable to a tensile load.

Impingement Syndrome
Impingement syndrome is one of the most common causes of shoulder pain. It is a clinical diagnosis, which is made on the basis of a careful history and physical examination. Radiographs, especially the supraspinatus outlet view, are helpful in demonstrating the presence of subacromial spurs and the morphology of the acromion, providing supportive evidence for the diagnosis of outlet impingement. A subacromial lidocaine injection is also quite useful in verifying this diagnosis and differentiating it from other causes of anterior shoulder pain. In some patients, especially overhead athletes, differentiating between functional impingement and subtle instability may be difficult. The relocation test and subacromial lidocaine injection are used to help make the diagnosis, but there is also overlap in this population (ie, patients with

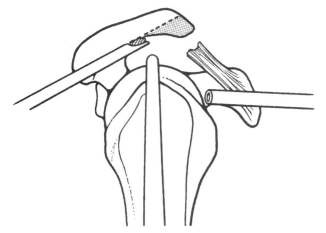

Figure 2

Line of resection for arthroscopic acromioplasty. Note portion of acromial undersurface to be resected from posterior to anterior using the posterior aspect of the acromion as a resection guide. Care must be taken to avoid amputation of bone anteriorly. (Reproduced with permission from Hartzog CW Jr, Savoie FH III, Field LD: Arthroscopic acromioplasty and arthroscopic distal clavicle resection, mini-open rotator cuff repair: Indications, techniques, and outcome, in Iannotti JP (ed): *The Rotator Cuff: Current Concepts and Complex Problems.* Rosemont, IL, American Academy of Orthopaedic Surgeons, 1998, pp 25–57.)

findings suggestive of both impingement and instability). In this subgroup, examination under anesthesia and arthroscopic examination of the glenohumeral joint and subacromial space may provide useful information about the underlying disorder(s). Likewise, arthroscopic examination may confirm the diagnosis of "internal impingement" of the undersurface of the rotator cuff on the posterior glenoid rim, another mechanism for shoulder pain in younger patients.

The efficacy of corticosteroid injections for treating subacromial impingement syndrome has been examined in a recent prospective, controlled, double-blind clinical study of 40 patients. At an average follow-up of 7 to 8 months, the patients who received a corticosteroid injection had better pain relief and greater increases in active motion, and were much more likely to have a negative impingement sign than those in the control group. The authors concluded that subacromial injection of corticosteroids is an effective short-term therapy for the treatment of subacromial impingement. They also recommend that no more than 2 subacromial cortisone injections be given and that multiple cortisone injections should be avoided in patients with a known history of a full-thickness rotator cuff tear.

The results of nonsurgical treatment of subacromial impingement syndrome with anti-inflammatory medications and a supervised program of physical therapy in a series of 616 patients have been reported recently. The physical

therapy regimen consisted of isotonic internal and external rotation exercises, performed with the arm at the side using surgical tubing and aimed at strengthening the rotator cuff. Overall, 413 patients (67%) had satisfactory results, and only 74 patients (18% of those with a successful result) had a recurrence of symptoms during the follow-up period. Patients who had symptoms for less than 4 weeks were the most likely to respond (78%). Patients with a type I acromion were more likely to respond to treatment (91%) than those with a type II or III acromion (68% and 64%, respectively). Shoulder dominance, gender, and concomitant tenderness of the acromioclavicular joint did not affect the result significantly.

If nonsurgical treatment is unsuccessful, arthroscopic acromioplasty often is used for treating subacromial impingement syndrome that occurs in the presence of an intact rotator cuff (Fig. 2). In several large series, the results of arthroscopic acromioplasty were essentially equal to those reported for open acromioplasty. One group found no statistical difference in the mean postoperative shoulder scores between those who had arthroscopic acromioplasty and those treated with an open acromioplasty, although there were more excellent results in the open acromioplasty group. The advantages of arthroscopic acromioplasty include reduced early perioperative morbidity, easier rehabilitation, decreased hospitalization time, the ability to detect and treat concomitant glenohumeral pathology, perhaps better preservation of the deltoid origin, and a smaller surgical scar. Failure of arthroscopic acromioplasty may result from improper diagnosis, inadequate bone removal, and other technical errors, such as overaggressive bone removal leading to deltoid injury or in rare cases to acromial fracture.

Rotator Cuff Tears

Partial-Thickness Tears

Partial-thickness tears of the rotator cuff are more readily diagnosed with advances in magnetic resonance imaging (MRI) and arthroscopy, but their treatment remains controversial. Many partial-thickness rotator cuff tears can be managed nonsurgically. Some authors have recommended arthroscopic anterior acromioplasty and debridement of the tear for most partial-thickness tears. The report of a recent series recommended open anterior acromioplasty with debridement of the abnormal tendon tissue and repair of the tendon to bone with sutures. In that report, 85% of patients had excellent or satisfactory results and only 15% had unsatisfactory results. At an average follow-up of nearly 5 years, none of the patients had required reoperation.

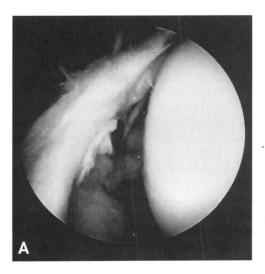
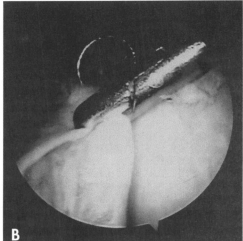

Figure 3

A, Large full-thickness rotator cuff tear "at rest" as visualized through the lateral portal. B, Determination of rotator cuff tendon quality and excursion using arthroscopic grabber positioned from the posterior portal to advance the tendon laterally to its insertion at the greater tuberosity. (Reproduced with permission from Hartzog CW Jr, Savoie FH III, Field LD: Arthroscopic acromioplasty and arthroscopic distal clavicle resection, mini-open rotator cuff repair: Indications, techniques, and outcome, in Iannotti JP (ed): *The Rotator Cuff: Current Concepts and Complex Problems.* Rosemont, IL, American Academy of Orthopaedic Surgeons, 1998, pp 25–57.)

Another recent study compared arthroscopic debridement and acromioplasty to arthroscopic acromioplasty and mini-open repair for the treatment of partial-thickness tears involving at least 50% of the thickness of the tendon. In this study, 32 patients were treated with arthroscopic debridement and 33 with mini-open repair, according to patient preference. In the debridement group, there were only 15 good results with 8 fair and 9 poor results. Three of these extended to full-thickness tears, and 3 additional patients required further surgery for persistent pain. In the mini-open repair group, there were 31 excellent or good results and only 1 fair and 1 poor result. Based on these data, the author recommends arthroscopic acromioplasty and mini-open repair for the treatment of significant partial-thickness tears.

Full-Thickness Tears

Anterior acromioplasty and rotator cuff repair remain the mainstays of surgical treatment for symptomatic full-thickness rotator cuff tears (Fig. 3). Factors to consider in decision-making about the choice of treatment (surgical, nonsurgical, and what type of surgery) include severity and duration of symptoms, functional limitations, patient demands and expectations, tear size, and tear location. Conventional open repair techniques have obtained excellent pain relief in most series for tears of all sizes, although functional results are less predictable with large tears. Surgical technique, the extent of damage to the cuff, and postoperative rehabilitation all affect the results of rotator cuff repair. A recent prospective outcome study of rotator cuff repair found 88% good or excellent results. Postoperative objective scores correlated well with patients' subjective ratings of the final result. Preoperative tear size also correlated with the quality of the tendon tissue, difficulty of tendon mobilization, and

presence of a rupture of the long head of the biceps, and these factors adversely affected postoperative function, patient satisfaction, and overall shoulder score.

Early series of arthroscopic subacromial decompression and debridement without repair of rotator cuff tears reported satisfactory results. However, in series with longer follow-up, the results of debridement without repair appeared to deteriorate over time. One group initially reported 84% satisfactory results with this method at 2-year follow-up, but then found only 68% satisfactory results at 3- to 6-year follow-up. These authors concluded that they no longer could recommend the use of decompression and debridement alone in the treatment of reparable full-thickness rotator cuff tears. In another prospective study, 87 consecutive patients were randomly assigned to either open rotator cuff repair or arthroscopic subacromial decompression and debridement groups. Surgical repair of full-thickness tears provided results superior to those of arthroscopic debridement, and the authors recommended rotator cuff repair.

Arthroscopically assisted or mini-open repair has become increasingly popular as a means of treating full-thickness rotator cuff tears (Figs. 4 and 5). The technique combines arthroscopic subacromial decompression with open tendon repair through a limited deltoid splitting incision. Advantages over traditional open repair include relative preservation of the deltoid origin, a better means of diagnosing and treating associated intra-articular pathology, shorter hospitalization, reduced early morbidity, easier and quicker rehabilitation, and a smaller scar. The results of mini-open repair have been similar to the results of open rotator cuff repair in several series. When the quality of the torn tendon(s) is poor and extensive soft-tissue releases are necessary to mobilize the tendons, or when there is subscapularis involvement,

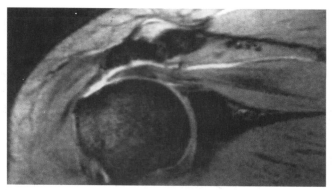

Figure 4

Magnetic resonance imaging scan of the shoulder demonstrating a full-thickness tear of the supraspinatus tendon with only mild retraction and no muscle atrophy. This type of tear is ideal for arthroscopically assisted or "mini-open" repair.

open repair may be more appropriate, because it provides wider exposure for easier mobilization and transposition of the torn tendons. Entirely arthroscopic repair techniques have been recently developed, and early results appear promising. In one report, 49 of 53 patients achieved good or excellent results at 2- to 3-year follow-up.

Surgical treatment of massive rotator cuff tears remains difficult. Surgical options that have been used include subacromial decompression and debridement, mobilization and repair of existing local tendons, transfer of a distant tendon (latissimus dorsi, teres major, or trapezius), and reconstruction using grafts or synthetic materials. Subacromial decompression with debridement has been recommended by several authors for irreparable rotator cuff tears. In one report, the overall results were satisfactory in 83%. A favorable outcome was achieved in shoulders in which both the anterior deltoid and long head of the biceps tendon were intact and no previous surgery had been performed. The authors concluded that adequate subacromial decompression and proper postoperative rehabilitation can provide pain relief and restoration of shoulder function. In another series of subacromial decompression and debridement of massive tears, 79% of patients reported improvement after surgery. There were significant decreases in pain and increases in range of motion and function, although the results were inferior to those reported for repair of torn rotator cuff tendons. Recently, the importance of the coracoacromial ligament in containing humeral head migration superiorly in shoulders with rotator cuff deficiency has been emphasized, leading some authors to caution against aggressive subacromial decompression and to advocate coracoacromial ligament preservation in patients with deficient cuff tissue.

The repair of massive tears is made difficult by the degree of

tendon retraction and scarring, as well as by the poor quality of the cuff tissue available for repair. Repair requires systematic mobilization of the retracted tendons and often requires releases between the torn tendons, such as a complete release of the rotator interval (between the supraspinatus and subscapularis tendons) and coracohumeral ligament to the base of the coracoid. The goal is to restore functional musculotendinous units to their insertions, rather than to obtain coverage of the humeral head. Some have advocated partial repair of irreparable rotator cuff tears, in which the goal is to restore the shoulder's force couples (between the anterior and posterior rotator cuff) and thus convert the massive tear to one that is biomechanically sound. By this theory, tendon transposition of intact rotator cuff tissue (eg, intact subscapularis) to cover a defect in the cuff is not recommended, because it may adversely affect the biomechanics of the shoulder.

When there is marked superior migration of the humeral head and severe atrophy and fatty degeneration of the muscles of the rotator cuff, some authors recommend the use of tendon transfers to restore strength. Transfer of the latissimus dorsi or the teres major has been described to substitute for combined infraspinatus and supraspinatus loss, whereas transfer of the pectoralis major has been reported for irreparable subscapularis tears. Other flaps involving a portion of the deltoid or trapezius also have been described for treating rotator cuff deficiency.

Other recent studies have focused on the mechanical strength of rotator cuff repair. One report indicated that nonabsorbable braided polyester is an extremely stiff material with excellent ultimate tensile strength, which maintains its strength until healing can occur. A modification of the Mason-Allen suture technique showed better holding strength than simple sutures and may be helpful, especially in the repair of larger tears in which the repair is under greater tension. Another report indicated that the strength of fixation of a rotator cuff repair can be increased by placing transosseous sutures at least 10 mm distal to the tip of the greater tuberosity and by tying them over a bone bridge that is at least 10 mm wide. Both of these reports also suggested that in osteoporotic bone, cortical augmentation with a plastic button strengthens the repair.

Prosthetic Arthroplasty

Basic Science

Shoulder replacement poses a considerable challenge: relieving pain while obtaining a desirable amount of function (strength, smoothness, mobility, stability). Shoulder motion

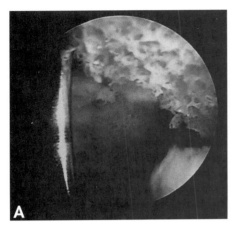 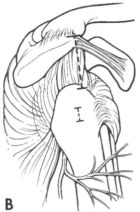 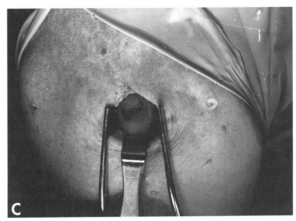

Figure 5

A, Localization of incision for mini-open rotator cuff repair using an 18-gauge spinal needle percutaneously placed at the anterolateral border of the resected acromion. B, Line of incision. This incision should not be extended beyond 4 cm from the lateral edge of the acromion to avoid risk of axillary nerve injury. C, Photograph of mini-open approach to rotator cuff repair. Rotator cuff tear is exposed within the wound. Note that incision does not extend as far laterally as the lateral portal. (Reproduced with permission from Hartzog CW Jr, Savoie FH III, Field LD: Arthroscopic acromioplasty and arthroscopic distal clavicle resection, mini-open rotator cuff repair: Indications, techniques, and outcome, in Iannotti JP (ed): *The Rotator Cuff: Current Concepts and Complex Problems.* Rosemont, IL, American Academy of Orthopaedic Surgeons, 1998, pp 25–57.)

includes that of the glenohumeral joint itself as well as of the scapulothoracic articulation. In a recent study, these motions were examined before and after arthroplasty for arthritis. A normal ratio of these motions was not restored by shoulder arthroplasty. The underlying disease process and its sequelae may continue to be factors in these patients postoperatively.

Data from recent studies suggest that humeral translation occurs with normal glenohumeral motion and thus may deviate from expected ball and socket kinematics. The question remains whether prosthetic joint surfaces should conform completely, possibly constraining the articulation more than desired and contributing to early loosening of the glenoid component, or should have a slight degree of mismatch. It appears that some degree of component mismatch results in more normal glenohumeral kinematics.

The relative "stuffing" of the glenohumeral joint with glenoid and humeral components warrants concern. The fullness of the available joint volume is critical to the length-tension relationships that are present in the capsuloligamentous structures and necessary for normal function of the rotator cuff musculature. Thus, the position and size of the glenoid and humeral components coupled with the attachments of the rotator cuff and concomitant capsular releases relate directly to the amount of motion and strength obtained when the joint is replaced. Components that are too large can lead to tightness and pain, while those that are too small can effectively disadvantage the musculature of the rotator cuff and increase the potential for instability. Optimizing soft-tissue balance appears to be a critical factor in the outcome of shoulder replacement surgery. The advent of humeral head modularity combined with an improved understanding of component positioning and appropriate releases have improved the ability to minimize the potential for problems related to the available joint volume.

Concerns about radiolucent lines and glenoid component loosening have led to renewed efforts to improve glenoid fixation. The need to compensate for posterior glenoid erosion in osteoarthritis has been emphasized. Careful glenoid preparation to conform to the glenoid component while leaving the subchondral bone intact may reduce implant failure. Results of recent studies suggest that peg fixation without metal backing may preserve bone stock, distribute stress more evenly to the underlying bone, and help decrease the frequency of component loosening.

Indications and Results

Several recent reviews evaluating hemiarthroplasty and total shoulder arthroplasty in arthritic patients document good results with both procedures. In some studies, shoulder arthroplasties that include glenoid replacement result in better pain relief and function than does a hemiarthroplasty. Still, a variety of concerns related to the glenoid component remain. One concern is the potential for polyethylene wear debris, although this has been largely theoretical and based on experience in the hip and knee, where the forces across the joint are much larger. The advantages of a hemiarthroplasty over total shoulder arthroplasty are ease of technique, decreased surgery time, and elimination of the risk of glenoid loosening. Factors important in the decision to resurface the glenoid include patient age and activity level, glenoid wear and bone stock, the status of the rotator cuff, and the type of arthritis involved.

Rheumatoid arthritis and other inflammatory arthropathies continue to present a difficult therapeutic dilemma. A recent review of 46 shoulder arthroplasties done for rheumatoid arthritis revealed that those who underwent total shoulder arthroplasty had a slightly better range of motion and overall function than those with a hemiarthroplasty. However, the total shoulder arthroplasties were limited to those shoulders without significant glenoid bone loss, massive rotator cuff tears, or severe contracture.

In rotator cuff tear arthropathy, the longevity of a glenoid replacement is severely compromised because of eccentric loading of the component by a high-riding humeral head. The trend is to use an anatomic hemiarthroplasty, replacing and smoothing the joint surface without changing the overall length-tension relationships of the soft tissues. In a recent review, 16 patients treated with hemiarthroplasty obtained relatively good pain relief, although functional gains were less reliable.

The most common application of shoulder arthroplasty is in the osteoarthritic patient. Although certain problems exist, including posterior glenoid erosion and contracture, reliably good results can be achieved. A recent review of 38 total shoulder arthroplasties done by 1 surgeon reported excellent results in most patients. Modern cementing technique was used for both the glenoid and humeral components. Comfort and functional results were good, with only a small number of follow-up radiographs revealing radiolucent lines. Implant survivorship was 97% at 5 years and 93% at 8 years.

In a recent report emphasizing the inherent problems and difficulties related to shoulder arthroplasty in patients with Parkinson's disease, 15 patients undergoing 16 unconstrained shoulder arthroplasties were reviewed. After an average of 5.3 years, pain relief was good while functional results were less reliable. The authors concluded that, particularly in patients who were 65 years of age or older, functional results were poor and complications frequent.

The results of glenohumeral arthroplasty for arthritis after previous instability surgery, or capsulorrhaphy arthropathy, are encouraging for this small subset of relatively young patients. A number of important technical considerations and methods of dealing with them are described to help improve the management of this challenging problem, which often includes severe contractures and asymmetric wear of the glenoid. Another report outlines the success of humeral head replacement for locked posterior fracture dislocations.

The treatment of young active patients with severe glenoid arthrosis is difficult. One approach, recently described, is a combination of humeral head replacement with an interposition arthroplasty with soft tissue to create a smooth glenoid surface. Early results appear promising, but this is a challenging procedure and is likely applicable to a relatively small number of patients.

Reported complications of total shoulder arthroplasty include glenoid and humeral loosening, component instability, rotator cuff tears, periprosthetic fractures, infection, nerve injuries, implant dissociation, and deltoid dysfunction.

Effectiveness

Outcomes of shoulder arthroplasties have been evaluated in a variety of ways related to different techniques, prostheses, and diagnoses. Many authors have reported that patients with arthritis of the glenohumeral joint benefit from shoulder arthroplasty, based on patient evaluation by the surgeon using criteria such as range of motion, strength, activities of daily living, overall satisfaction, and radiographic findings. Only a small amount of these data have been gathered from the patients' own perspective both before and after treatment. While the analysis and interest in the effectiveness of shoulder arthroplasty have progressed, so have the methods of determining it. A recent prospective evaluation of 29 consecutive patients treated for primary osteoarthritis of the shoulder demonstrated excellent results and improvement of both shoulder function and overall health status. Using patient self-assessment questionnaires to evaluate patients before and after shoulder arthroplasty, large gains were documented in pain relief, function, and general health parameters such as comfort and physical role function.

Glenohumeral Arthrodesis

Shoulder fusion remains a salvage procedure. Ideally, it provides a stable base from which to power an otherwise functional arm (elbow, wrist, hand) in a patient with severe glenohumeral joint destruction, instability, pain, and/or a flail or weak supporting musculature, particularly in a laborer. At present, its indications are generally limited to severe neurologic problems about the shoulder, certain tumors, recalcitrant instability, and infection.

In a recent series of 16 shoulder arthrodeses done for brachial plexus injuries with an average follow-up of almost 7 years, there was excellent restoration of function, with good strength despite less external rotation than achieved with nerve repair. The only difficulties noted included 2 nonunions requiring bone grafting and 3 humeral fractures in the first 6 months after surgery. Another review of patients with arthrodeses for infection, posttraumatic arthritis, and brachial plexus palsy noted significant improvement in pain relief and function in all but 1 of 10 patients.

The report of 1 recent study emphasized the difficulties related to the revision of a failed fusion and the importance of proper technique when performing the initial procedure. The authors used a corrective osteotomy to revise 9 maligned fusions, eliminating the patients' pain and improving their ability to perform activities of daily living. The most common errors in positioning included excessive flexion (> 15°) or abduction (> 15°), and/or an improper amount of internal rotation (< 40° or > 60°).

Adhesive Capsulitis

Frozen shoulder is a poorly defined syndrome, in which both active and passive shoulder motion is lost because of soft-tissue contracture. Adhesive capsulitis is a term for idiopathic loss of shoulder motion characterized pathologically by thickening and contracture of the joint capsule, which results in decreased joint volume. It is believed to be a benign self-limited disorder, which tends to resolve over 1 to 2 years, although patients often are left with some residual loss of motion. A variety of etiologies, including trivial trauma and immunologic, inflammatory, and endocrine disorders, have been implicated in the development of frozen shoulder. It is common in patients with diabetes mellitus and is more frequently bilateral and resistant to treatment in these patients.

In a recent histologic study, the coracohumeral ligament and rotator interval of the capsule were examined in 12 patients with resistant frozen shoulder. The pathologic process found was active fibroblastic proliferation, accompanied by some transformation to myofibroblasts. The collagen laid down appeared as thick nodular strands, similar to those seen in Dupuytren's disease of the hand. The authors suggested that primary frozen shoulder is a fibrosing condition, rather than an inflammatory one, because inflammatory cells were either absent or scanty.

Most patients with frozen shoulder respond to nonsurgical treatment with a supervised physical therapy program combined with a home program of stretching exercises. If conservative therapy is unsuccessful, manipulation under anesthesia can be done to regain motion. Manipulation should be avoided in patients with severe osteoporosis, because the risk of fracture of the humerus during manipulation is high in this group. In recent years, arthroscopic capsular release has been used for treating resistant frozen shoulder, usually in conjunction with manipulation under anesthesia. In several recent series, there were satisfactory results with arthroscopic release of the coracohumeral ligament and contracted capsule. Significant increases in range of motion and improvements in pain level and function with a low complication rate have been seen using this technique for cases of resistant frozen shoulder. When extra-articular adhesions and tissue contractures are present (such as in cases of stiffness after a Putti-Platt or Bristow repair), open release is usually required. The use of an indwelling interscalene catheter or intermittent administration of interscalene anesthesia for several days may facilitate early postoperative therapy in patients who have undergone surgical treatment for frozen shoulder.

Long Thoracic Nerve Palsy

Long thoracic nerve palsy results in weakness of the serratus anterior muscle, which presents clinically as periscapular pain, winging of the scapula, and difficulty elevating the arm above shoulder level. There are many causes for this problem, including blunt trauma or stretching of the nerve (such as in young athletes), viral infection, and iatrogenic trauma (during a mastectomy with axillary dissection or first rib resection). This palsy results in a loss of normal scapular stability and rotation, because the scapula lies retracted and its inferior pole is rotated medially (Fig. 6). Winging is increased with attempts to elevate the arm, thus compromising overhead activity. Electromyography is used to confirm the diagnosis and to follow nerve recovery.

In most patients in whom the etiology involves a closed injury or an atraumatic cause, recovery usually occurs within 12 to 18 months. Treatment in these patients includes observation and periscapular muscle strengthening. In patients with symptomatic serratus winging for longer than 1 year, who demonstrate no electromyographic or clinical evidence of recovery, surgical treatment may be considered to diminish pain and improve scapular function. A number of surgical alternatives have been described, including scapulothoracic fusion, scapulopexy (fascial sling suspension), and dynamic muscle transfers. Transfer of the sternal head of the pectoralis major with the use of autogenous fascia lata graft to reinforce the repair has become the preferred transfer to substitute for serratus function. In 1 recent series, at an average follow-up of 41 months, 10 of 11 patients had satisfactory results with this dynamic transfer. Ten of the patients had improved scapular tracking with no scapular winging or only mild winging at follow-up, and they had significant functional improvement and reduction of pain. To date, there are

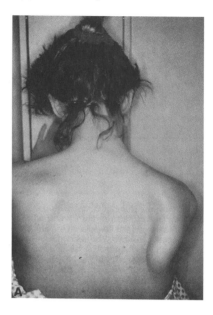

Figure 6

Patient with serratus pattern of scapular winging. Winging is increased by pushing against the wall with the arm flexed to 90°.

few data to support nerve exploration and reconstruction for long thoracic nerve palsy, and pectoralis major transfer remains the favored surgical option for symptomatic patients.

Brachial Plexus Injury

The most common causes of brachial plexus injuries are traction caused by extreme movements, such as when the head is forced laterally upon impact in a motorcycle accident, and crush lesions caused by direct trauma to the supraclavicular region and usually associated with fractures of the clavicle. A history and physical examination, including a complete neurologic evaluation and supplemented by electrodiagnostic studies, are essential in diagnosing the location, extent, and completeness of the injury. Electromyography, which includes the cervical paravertebral muscles and periscapular muscles (especially the serratus anterior and rhomboids), is helpful in establishing whether the injury is postganglionic or involves root avulsion. A computed tomography myelogram also is helpful in clarifying the issue of root avulsion, which is suggested by the presence of Horner's syndrome and a flail, anesthetic limb.

In general, supraclavicular and complete injuries have a worse prognosis than infraclavicular and incomplete lesions. Although lesions of the lower trunk of the brachial plexus are less common than upper trunk lesions, the potential for recovery of intrinsic hand function is generally poor with lower trunk lesions. With root avulsions involving the upper trunk of the plexus, the prognosis for spontaneous recovery is very poor, and involvement of the serratus anterior limits the ability to regain shoulder function with an arthrodesis of the glenohumeral joint, because the patient has inadequate scapular control. Patients with less severe injuries who demonstrate spontaneous neural recovery or have minimal signs and symptoms, are treated conservatively. Nerve reconstruction or repair is considered for more severe postganglionic lesions. It is generally believed that earlier attempts at reconstruction or repair (within the first 3 to 4 months after injury) have a better potential for functional improvement, and that delay beyond 6 months may significantly decrease the chance of success.

As microsurgical techniques have progressed, so have the overall results of nerve repair and reconstruction. A recent report assessed the efficacy of free nerve grafts in 90 patients with brachial plexus injury. Useful recovery was found in the elbow flexor and extensor muscles, as well as in the shoulder girdle muscles. However, the results in the forearm flexors and extensors and hand intrinsics were poor. Moreover, recovery of the deltoid and infraspinatus muscles was better when the injury had occurred to the axillary and suprascapular nerves rather than to the plexus itself. Intercostal nerves and the sural nerve are most commonly used for this type of grafting. Arthrodesis of the glenohumeral joint, another surgical option, is most effective with isolated loss of both the axillary and suprascapular nerves in the presence of functioning scapular muscles and good distal extremity function.

Annotated Bibliography

Muscular Function and Anatomy of the Glenohumeral Joint

Bigliani LU, Kelkar R, Flatow EL, Pollock RG, Mow VC: Glenohumeral stability: Biomechanical properties of passive and active stabilizers. *Clin Orthop* 1996;330:13–30.

Effective function of the glenohumeral articulation is achieved by a complex interaction between the articular and soft-tissue restraints. The rotator cuff muscles center the humeral head in the congruent glenoid and allow only small translations (< 2 mm) during scapular abduction. Incongruent joints have somewhat larger translations, especially at extremes of external rotation.

Lazarus MD, Sidles JA, Harryman DT II, Matsen FA III: Effect of a chondral-labral defect on glenoid concavity and glenohumeral stability: A cadaveric model. *J Bone Joint Surg* 1996;78A: 94–102.

A prime stabilizing mechanism of the glenohumeral joint is concavity-compression, by which the surrounding muscles maintain the humeral head in the glenoid fossa by compressive forces. Creation of a chondral-labral defect anteroinferiorly reduced the stability ratio by 65% for translation in the direction of the defect.

Otis JC, Jiang CC, Wickiewicz TL, Peterson MG, Warren RF, Santner TJ: Changes in the moment arms of the rotator cuff and deltoid muscles with abduction and rotation. *J Bone Joint Surg* 1994;76A:667–676.

This study demonstrates a role for the infraspinatus and subscapularis muscles in elevation of the arm in the scapular plane. Internal rotation enhances the contribution of the infraspinatus in elevation, while external rotation enhances that of the subscapularis. These data may explain how active elevation is possible in the absence of a functional supraspinatus.

Solomonow M, Guanche C, Wink C, Knatt T, Baratta RV, Lu Y: Mechanoreceptors and reflex arc in the feline shoulder. *J Shoulder Elbow Surg* 1996;5:139–146.

A reflex arc from the glenohumeral capsule to the biceps and rotator cuff muscles is demonstrated in a feline shoulder. The existence of a ligamentomuscular reflex arc suggests an interaction between the passive and active restraints in stabilizing the shoulder.

Yamaguchi K, Riew KD, Galatz LM, Syme JA, Neviaser RJ: Biceps activity during shoulder motion: An electromyographic analysis. *Clin Orthop* 1997;336:122–129.

No significant biceps activity was observed in 44 electromyographically studied shoulders (either normal or with rotator cuff tears) during active shoulder motion. Thus, the biceps doesn't appear to play an active role in shoulder stabilization.

Shoulder Arthroscopy

Flatow EL, Duralde XA, Nicholson GP, Pollock RG, Bigliani LU: Arthroscopic resection of the distal clavicle with a superior approach. *J Shoulder Elbow Surg* 1995;4:41–50.

Forty-one shoulders with acromioclavicular (AC) joint disease refractory to conservative treatment underwent arthroscopic distal clavicle resection. Results were satisfactory in 93% with AC arthritis or osteolysis of the distal clavicle, while those with previous grade II AC separations or AC hypermobility had less satisfactory results. An even resection of bone, rather than total amount of bone resection, correlated with success.

Geiger DF, Hurley JA, Tovey JA, Rao JP: Results of arthroscopic versus open Bankart suture repair. *Clin Orthop* 1997; 337:111–117.

Eighteen shoulders were treated with an open Bankart repair (group I), while 16 were stabilized arthroscopically (group II). Group I had 83% good to excellent results with no recurrent instability, while group II had only 50% good to excellent results with 7 shoulders requiring a second operation. There were no significant differences between the 2 groups in the amount of external rotation lost.

Snyder SJ, Banas MP, Karzel RP: An analysis of 140 injuries to the superior glenoid labrum. *J Shoulder Elbow Surg* 1995; 4:243–248.

Twenty-nine percent of lesions were associated with a partial-thickness rotator cuff tear, 11% with a full-thickness tear, and 22% with an anterior Bankart lesion. Type I lesions were debrided, type II lesions treated with stabilization, and type III and IV lesions treated with either debridement or stabilization, depending on the extent of damage. No preoperative imaging modality consistently identified the SLAP lesion.

Rotator Cuff Disease

Blair B, Rokito AS, Cuomo F, Jarolem K, Zuckerman JD: Efficacy of injections of corticosteroids for subacromial impingement syndrome. *J Bone Joint Surg* 1996;78A:1685–1689.

In a prospective, randomized, controlled double-blind clinical study of 40 patients, subacromial injection of corticosteroids was found to be an effective short-term treatment for symptomatic subacromial impingement syndrome. The injections were found to substantially decrease pain and increase the range of motion of the shoulder.

Flatow EL, Soslowsky LJ, Ticker JB, et al: Excursion of the rotator cuff under the acromion: Patterns of subacromial contact. *Am J Sports Med* 1994;22:779–788.

Stereophotogrammetric measurement of subacromial contact demonstrated that on the humeral surface, contact shifts from proximal to distal on the supraspinatus tendon with arm elevation. The acromial undersurface and rotator cuff are in closest proximity between 60° and 120° of elevation. Contact was more pronounced for type III acromions.

Morrison DS, Frogameni AD, Woodworth P: Non-operative treatment of subacromial impingement syndrome. *J Bone Joint Surg* 1997;79A:732–737.

A retrospective analysis was performed of 616 patients with subacromial impingement syndrome treated nonsurgically. Overall 67% had a satisfactory result with anti-inflammatory medication and a specific program of strengthening exercises for the rotator cuff. Patients who had symptoms for less than 4 weeks and those with type I acromions had the best results with nonsurgical treatment.

Rotator Cuff Tears

Baker CL, Liu SH: Comparison of open and arthroscopically assisted rotator cuff repairs. *Am J Sports Med* 1995;23:99–104.

Similar results were achieved with open and arthroscopically-assisted rotator cuff repair (80% versus 85% good-to-excellent results, respectively). The arthroscopically-assisted repair group was hospitalized 1.2 days less, and they returned to previous activity an average of 1 month earlier.

Gerber C, Schneeberger AG, Beck M, Schlegel U: Mechanical strength of repairs of the rotator cuff. *J Bone Joint Surg* 1994;76B:371–380.

Nonabsorbable braided polyester sutures demonstrated excellent strength characteristics for tendon repair and maintained strength over the 6-week early healing period. The modified Mason-Allen suture technique showed superior tendon grasping ability. The use of a 2-mm thick polylactide augmentation device was found to improve failure strength in osteoporotic bone.

Iannotti JP, Bernot MP, Kuhlman JR, Kelley MJ, Williams GR: Postoperative assessment of shoulder function: A prospective study of full-thickness rotator cuff tears. *J Shoulder Elbow Surg* 1996;5:449–457.

In a prospective study of 40 patients undergoing open rotator cuff repair of a chronic, full thickness tear, 88% achieved good or excellent results. Postoperative scores correlated most closely with preoperative tear size. Other factors influencing prognosis included quality of the tendon tissue, difficulty of tendon mobilization, and rupture of the long head of the biceps.

Montgomery TJ, Yerger B, Savoie FH III: Management of rotator cuff tears: A comparison of arthroscopic debridement and surgical repair. *J Shoulder Elbow Surg* 1994;3:70–78.

In a prospective randomized study comparing arthroscopic debridement to open tendon repair in 88 chronic full-thickness rotator cuff tears, open surgical repair provided superior results to those of arthroscopic debridement and subacromial decompression ($p = 0.0028$).

Rockwood CA Jr, Williams GR Jr, Burkhead WZ Jr: Debridement of degenerative, irreparable lesions of the rotator cuff. *J Bone Joint Surg* 1995;77A:857–866.

A modified anterior acromioplasty, subacromial decompression, and debridement of massive irreparable tears of the supraspinatus and infraspinatus tendons was performed in 57 patients. Satisfactory results were achieved in 83%. A favorable outcome was observed when the anterior deltoid and long head of the biceps tendon were intact and when no previous surgery had been performed.

Weber SC: Arthroscopic debridement and acromioplasty versus mini-open repair in the management of significant partial-thickness tears of the rotator cuff. *Orthop Clin North Am* 1997;28:79–82.

Thirty-two patients were treated with arthroscopic acromioplasty and debridement of the rotator cuff and 33 patients with arthroscopic acromioplasty and mini-open rotator cuff repair for significant partial-thickness tears (> 50% of the tendon thickness). Superior results were achieved in the mini-open repair group.

Prosthetic Arthroplasty

Bigliani LU, Weinstein DM, Glasgow MT, Pollock RG, Flatow EL: Glenohumeral arthroplasty for arthritis after instability surgery. *J Shoulder Elbow Surg* 1995;4:87–94.

The difficulties related to soft-tissue contracture and asymmetric posterior erosion with special reference to techniques of dealing with the overall problem are discussed.

Burkhead WZ Jr, Hutton KS: Biologic resurfacing of the glenoid with hemiarthroplasty of the shoulder. *J Shoulder Elbow Surg* 1995;4:263–270.

A humeral head replacement was combined with fascial resurfacing of the glenoid using either fascia lata or anterior joint capsule in 6 patients, with 5 excellent and 1 satisfactory result. It provides an encouraging alternative for a small group of patients with degenerative joint disease who are young and active or otherwise inappropriate for glenoid resurfacing.

Field LD, Dines DM, Zabinski SJ, Warren RF: Hemiarthroplasty of the shoulder for rotator cuff arthropathy. *J Shoulder Elbow Surg* 1997;6:18–23.

The authors review the results of 16 patients treated with a hemiarthroplasty for cuff tear arthropathy. Ten were considered a success while 6 were not. Pain was generally improved although functional gains were modest. An intact deltoid and coracoacromial arch were important in achieving a good result.

Karduna AR, Williams GR, Williams JL, Iannotti JP: Glenohumeral joint translations before and after total shoulder arthroplasty. A study in cadavera. *J Bone Joint Surg* 1997; 79A:1166–1174.

The authors evaluate the motion of natural and prosthetically reconstructed glenohumeral joints with varying degrees of articular conformity. Mismatched prosthetic glenohumeral joints more closely approximated normal joint motion.

Kelly IG: Unconstrained shoulder arthroplasty in rheumatoid arthritis. *Clin Orthop* 1994;307:94–102.

The author reviews the treatment of rheumatoid arthritis of the glenohumeral joint discussing patterns of involvement and their implications and describes experience with total shoulder arthroplasty, various technical considerations, and current trends in treatment.

Koch LD, Cofield RH, Ahlskog JE: Total shoulder arthroplasty in patients with Parkinson's disease. *J Shoulder Elbow Surg* 1997; 6:24–28.

The authors review 16 patients with Parkinson's disease who received an unconstrained total shoulder arthroplasty. Follow-up averaged 5.3 years with patients receiving good pain relief, although functional gains were poor and complications were more frequent.

L'Insalata JC, Pagnani MJ, Warren RF, Dines DM: Humeral head osteonecrosis: Clinical course and radiographic predictors of outcome. *J Shoulder Elbow Surg* 1996;5:355–361.

Sixty-five shoulders with osteonecrosis of the humeral head were reviewed. Only half of those treated conservatively did well, and core decompression did not appear to alter the course of stage III disease. The disease progressed in 71% with subsequent shoulder arthroplasty or severe pain and disability.

Matsen FA III: Early effectiveness of shoulder arthroplasty for patients with primary glenohumeral degenerative joint disease. *J Bone Joint Surg* 1996;78A:260–264.

Pre- and postoperative patient self-assessment questionnaires documented reliable gains in pain relief, shoulder function, and general health status.

Arthrodesis

Groh GI, Williams GR, Jarman RN, Rockwood Jr CA: Treatment of complications of shoulder arthrodesis. *J Bone Joint Surg* 1997;79A:881–887.

A reconstructive osteotomy was performed in 9 patients with malpositioned shoulder arthrodeses having too much abduction, flexion, and/or an improper amount of internal rotation. Revision resulted in improved pain relief and function.

Chammas M, Meyer zu Reckendorf G, Allieu Y: Arthrodesis of the shoulder for post-traumatic palsy of the brachial plexus: Analysis of a series of 18 cases. *Rev Chir Orthop Reparatrice Appar Mot* 1996;82:386–395.

Follow-up results after an average of almost 7 years for 16 shoulder arthrodeses performed for brachial plexus injuries are presented. Improved strength was achieved despite limited external rotation when compared with nerve repair alone. Minimal complications related to the procedure were noted.

Frozen Shoulder

Warner JJ, Allen A, Marks PH, Wong P: Arthroscopic release for chronic, refractory adhesive capsulitis of the shoulder. *J Bone Joint Surg* 1996;78A:1808–1816.

Twenty-three patients underwent arthroscopic release for idiopathic adhesive capsulitis, which had failed to respond to physical therapy or closed manipulation. At a mean follow-up of 39 months, the Constant score of these patients improved by an average of 48 points. Significant gains ($p < 0.01$) in motion were seen for all planes, and the motion at follow-up was within 7° of that for the contralateral, normal shoulder.

Long Thoracic Nerve Palsy

Connor PM, Yamaguchi K, Manifold SG, Pollock RG, Flatow EL, Bigliani LU: Split pectoralis major transfer for serratus anterior palsy. *Clin Orthop* 1997;341:134–142

Eleven patients underwent transfer of the sternal head of the pectoralis major tendon for symptomatic scapular winging due to serratus anterior palsy. At an average follow-up of 41 months, 10 of 11 patients had satisfactory results with improvement in function, reduction in pain, and no or minimal scapular winging.

Brachial Plexus Injury

Ochiai N, Nagano A, Sugioka H, Hara T: Nerve grafting in brachial plexus injuries: Results of free grafts in 90 patients. *J Bone Joint Surg* 1996;78B:754–758.

Results of free nerve grafts in 90 cases of brachial plexus nerve injury demonstrate relatively good recovery of the elbow flexor and extensor muscles and of shoulder girdle muscles. Recovery of hand and forearm muscles was poor.

Waters PM: Obstetric brachial plexus injuries: Evaluation and management. *J Am Acad Orthop Surg* 1997;5:205–214.

A review of obstetric brachial plexus injuries is presented, with algorithms for treatment of patients with incomplete recovery of neural function and with internal rotation contractures.

Classic Bibliography

Arntz CT, Jackins S, Matsen FA III: Prosthetic replacement of the shoulder for the treatment of defects in the rotator cuff and the surface of the glenohumeral joint. *J Bone Joint Surg* 1993;75A:485–491.

Bassett RW, Cofield RH: Acute tears of the rotator cuff: The timing of surgical repair. *Clin Orthop* 1983;175:18–24.

Bigliani LU, Cordasco FA, McIlveen SJ, et al: Operative repair of massive rotator cuff tears: Long-term results. *J Shoulder Elbow Surg* 1992;1:120–130.

Bigliani LU, Cordasco FA, McIlveen SJ, Musso ES: Operative treatment of failed repairs of the rotator cuff. *J Bone Joint Surg* 1992;74A:1505–1515.

Brenner BC, Ferlic DC, Clayton ML, Dennis DA: Survivorship of unconstrained total shoulder arthroplasty. *J Bone Joint Surg* 1989;71A:1289–1296.

Cofield RH: Total shoulder arthroplasty with the Neer prosthesis. *J Bone Joint Surg* 1984;66A:899–906.

Cofield RH, Briggs BT: Glenohumeral arthrodesis: Operative and long-term functional results. *J Bone Joint Surg* 1979;61A:668–677.

Ellman H, Hanker G, Bayer M: Repair of the rotator cuff: End-result study of factors influencing reconstruction. *J Bone Joint Surg* 1986:68A:1136–1144.

Friedman RJ, Thornhill TS, Thomas WH, Sledge CB: Non-constrained total shoulder replacement in patients who have rheumatoid arthritis and class-IV function. *J Bone Joint Surg* 1989;71A:494–498.

Gartsman GM: Arthroscopic acromioplasty for lesions of the rotator cuff. *J Bone Joint Surg* 1990;72A:169–180.

Gerber C: Latissimus dorsi transfer for the treatment of irreparable tears of the rotator cuff. *Clin Orthop* 1992;275:152–160.

Gerber C, Schneeberger AG, Vinh TS: The arterial vascularization of the humeral head: An anatomical study. *J Bone Joint Surg* 1990;72A:1486–1494.

Harryman DT II, Mack LA, Wang KY, Jackins SE, Richardson ML, Matsen FA III: Repairs of the rotator cuff: Correlation of functional results with integrity of the cuff. *J Bone Joint Surg* 1991; 73A:982–989.

Hawkins RJ, Neer CS II: A functional analysis of shoulder fusions. *Clin Orthop* 1987;223:65–76.

Howell SM, Imobersteg AM, Seger DH, Marone PJ: Clarification of the role of the supraspinatus muscle in shoulder function. *J Bone Joint Surg* 1986;68A:398–404.

Iannotti JP, Zlatkin MB, Esterhai JL, Kressel HY, Dalinka MK, Spindler KP: Magnetic resonance imaging of the shoulder: Sensitivity, specificity, and predictive value. *J Bone Joint Surg* 1991;73A:17–29.

Inman VT, Saunders JB dec M, Abbott LC: Observations on the function of the shoulder joint. *J Bone Joint Surg* 1944;26:1–30.

Leffert RD, Seddon H: Infraclavicular brachial plexus injuries. *J Bone Joint Surg* 1965;47B:9–22.

McLaughlin HL: Lesions of the musculotendinous cuff of the shoulder: I. The exposure and treatment of tears with retraction. *J Bone Joint Surg* 1944:26:31–51.

Narakas A: Surgical treatment of traction injuries of the brachial plexus. *Clin Orthop* 1978;133:71–90.

Neer CS II: Anterior acromioplasty for the chronic impingement syndrome in the shoulder: A preliminary report. *J Bone Joint Surg* 1972:54A:41–50.

Neer CS II: Impingement lesions. *Clin Orthop* 1983;173:70–77.

Neer CS II, Watson KC, Stanton FJ: Recent experience in total shoulder replacement. *J Bone Joint Surg* 1982;64A:319–337.

Neviaser JS: Adhesive capsulitis of the shoulder: A study of the pathological findings in periarthritis of the shoulder. *J Bone Joint Surg* 1945;27:211–222.

Neviaser RJ, Neviaser TJ: Reoperation for failed rotator cuff repair: Analysis of fifty cases. *J Shoulder Elbow Surg* 1992;1: 283–286.

Richards RR, Beaton D, Hudson AR: Shoulder arthrodesis with plate fixation: Functional outcome analysis. *J Shoulder Elbow Surg* 1993;2:225–239.

Sunderland S (ed): *Nerves and Nerve Injuries,* ed 2. Edinburgh, Scotland, Churchill Livingstone, 1978.

Wiley AM: Arthroscopic appearance of frozen shoulder. *Arthroscopy* 1991;7:138–143.

Chapter 29
Elbow and Forearm: Pediatric Aspects

Congenital Anomalies and Acquired Disorders

Development of the Elbow

Cartilaginous anlages of the humerus, radius, and ulna are present in the developing embryo by 6 weeks of gestation. Cavitation of the joint space occurs in the seventh week, at the same time that enchondral bone formation of the radius and ulna starts at the midshaft. Enchondrification of the physes occurs much later. The radial head and neck are initially the same diameter, with the head enlarging after joint formation. The annular ligament is relatively loosely attached distally. An anterior dislocation of the radial head in a 19-week fetus has been shown with a persistence of a small radial head in comparison to the neck. Presumably, contact with the capitellum is needed to induce the shape and size of the normal radial head.

Congenital Dislocation of the Radial Head

Congenital dislocation of the radial head is usually a sporadic occurrence, although reported familial cases suggest a hereditary component. This condition can also be seen in conjunction with many syndromes or congenital anomalies. It can occur unilaterally or bilaterally, and bilateral cases may not be symmetric. Congenital dislocation of the radial head often may not be diagnosed until childhood activities disclose a limitation in range of motion, particularly extension. Use of ultrasound has been reported in early diagnosis. Hallmarks of congenital dislocation include a small, rounded radial head with hypoplasia and incongruency of the capitellum. In the congenitally dislocated radial head an arthrogram will disclose an "intra-articular dislocation," that is, the radial head is still within the joint capsule. Traumatic dislocations will show disruption of the elbow capsule.

Attempts to reduce congenital radial head dislocation, even in early infancy, are not warranted. Loss of terminal elbow extension may be a functional problem for certain activities. Competitive as opposed to recreational gymnastics or other forearm loading sports should probably be discouraged, because force transfer across the forearm and elbow is altered. Symptoms in the older child are often correlated with activity and related to the extremes of range of motion of an incongruous joint.

Late treatment consists of resection of the radial head at or near skeletal maturity. Overgrowth of the radial neck may occur as a result of retained periosteum. Resection of an adequate amount of the proximal radius should improve results. Congenital posterior dislocation of the radial head is usually associated with a bowed radius. The proximal end of the radius rotates in an arc and does not pivot about a capitellar point. Impingement of the residual proximal radius during rotation may cause persistent symptoms. Resection of the radial head prior to adolescence is thought to increase the likelihood of symptoms at the distal radioulnar articulation and should be delayed until skeletal maturity.

Congenital Radioulnar Synostosis

Congenital radioulnar synostosis is a failure of normal mesodermal separation. The dysplasia of the proximal forearm involves both soft tissue and bone. The supinator muscle may be absent or small. The tissues that would normally be present between proximal ulna and radius, including the articular cartilage at the proximal radioulnar joint, periosteum, and biceps tendon, are not present or are abnormally located. Familial cases implicate autosomal dominant inheritance. The indications for surgical treatment are an unacceptable position of forearm rotation. Excessive pronation is not well compensated by shoulder abduction and may compromise function. Simple osteotomy through the synostosis is associated with a potential for neurovascular compromise unless a shortening is performed before the rotation. Subperiosteal osteotomy distal to the synostosis and corrective "malreduction" with cast or pin immobilization appears to be a less risky alternative in young children. This technique is less likely to cause neurovascular compromise, and the final position can be adjusted with manipulation and cast changes during the first several weeks following osteotomy.

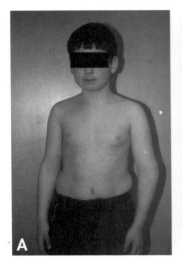 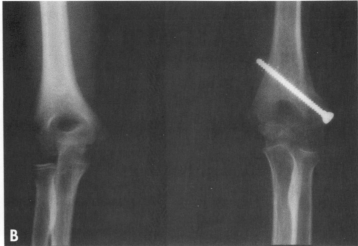

Figure 1

Cubitus varus. A, Deformity after closed treatment of a type II supracondylar humeral fracture. B, After supracondylar humeral osteotomy with screw fixation.

Osteochondritis Dissecans of the Capitellum

Osteochondritis dissecans of the capitellum affects adolescents and young adults. Prognosis is better in younger patients and those with less advanced lesions. Magnetic resonance imaging can make the diagnosis and define the stage of the lesion. Panner's disease, an osteochondrosis of the entire capitellum, occurs between age 4 and 8 years and has a different natural history, being self-limited and usually benign.

Repetitive valgus compression microtrauma in the throwing athlete is implicated in the majority of cases. The microtrauma results in breakdown and avascularity of the subchondral bone of the capitellum. A difference in the stiffness of the radial head and capitellar articular surfaces may increase strain on the softer capitellar surface leading to osteochondritis dissecans.

Treatment consists of rest and modification of the contributing activity. Lesions that have not fragmented may heal if protected from further trauma. Loose fragments are treated by arthroscopic or open debridement with or without drilling of the capitellar defect. Results of fragment fixation have been disappointing. Long-term results demonstrate improved comfort but limited elbow extension.

Trauma

Supracondylar Humeral Fracture

Supracondylar humeral fracture is the most common fracture about the elbow. The mechanism of injury is typically a fall on an outstretched hand, driving the olecranon into the posterior aspect of the distal humerus. This extension-type mechanism accounts for 98% of supracondylar humeral fractures. Only 2% of supracondylar fractures are flexion-type injuries, caused by a direct fall on the posterior aspect of the elbow. Supracondylar humeral fractures are most simply classified by severity into 3 types: undisplaced (type 1), displaced, but some cortical contact (type 2), or completely displaced (type 3). Type 1 fractures may demonstrate impaction of the medial or lateral columns, type 2 fractures may be malrotated as well as angulated, and type 3 fractures have no contact between the proximal and distal fragments.

Complications of this fracture include nerve palsy, cubitus varus (Fig. 1), vascular injury, and compartment syndrome. Injuries to the radial and median (usually the anterior interosseous branch) nerves are more common than injury to the ulnar nerve. Nerve injuries are typically the result of stretch or direct trauma at the time of fracture but can rarely be iatrogenic (entrapment during fracture reduction or impalement during pin fixation). Most nerve injuries recover spontaneously over a period of 6 to 8 weeks after fracture treatment and do not need to be acutely explored. Ischemia can occur as a complication of the fracture or its treatment. Closed reduction with immobilization of the elbow in excessive flexion (> 120°) in the face of soft-tissue swelling increases the risk of brachial artery compression and/or forearm ischemia. Malunion (cubitus varus, hyperextension) results from inadequate fracture reduction or inability to maintain reduction and is most common after nonsurgical treatment.

Treatment Closed reduction and percutaneous pin fixation has become the most common treatment for this injury. Retrograde pinning with divergent lateral or crossed (medial and lateral) Kirschner wires (K-wires) has been used for many years. Experimentally, the crossed pin configuration provides superior fracture fixation and has traditionally been favored for grossly unstable (type 3) fractures. However, the proven biomechanical superiority of crossed pins may not offer any significant clinical advantage over lateral pinning alone based on results of recent clinical studies comparing the techniques. Lateral pinning minimizes the risk of iatrogenic ulnar nerve injury when soft-tissue swelling prevents palpation of the nerve and/or bony landmarks on the medial side of the elbow. A small medial incision serves the same purpose when placing crossed pins.

Nondisplaced or minimally displaced fractures without collapse of the medial or lateral columns can be treated by immobilization in a cast or splint for approximately 3 weeks, with close observation of neurovascular status and radiographic documentation of reduction. Type 2 fractures with impaction of the medial column and all type fractures require closed reduction to restore the normal carrying angle of the elbow. The most accurate guide to correct reduction of the fracture is the contralateral Baumann's angle, which has been shown to vary less than 2° from injured to uninjured elbows. Open reduction and internal fixation (ORIF) is indicated when satisfactory closed reduction cannot be achieved, when the fracture is open, or when vascular compromise is present. An anteromedial or anterolateral approach can be used if there is no evidence of vascular injury. If vascular repair is anticipated, an S-shaped anterior approach is more utilitarian. Function following open reduction is not necessarily compromised by stiffness if satisfactory alignment and fracture union are achieved.

Complications When distal pulses are absent and vascular insufficiency (as indicated by pallor or decreased capillary refill) is present, the fracture should be reduced and stabilized immediately. If the hand remains pale and appears nonviable, the artery should be explored and pathology addressed appropriately: arteriotomy and repair with vein graft, if necessary. Any nerve injury present preoperatively should be observed.

Abnormality of the carrying angle of the elbow (cubitus varus or valgus) is usually caused by inadequate reduction of the fracture. Growth arrest and osteonecrosis are infrequent causes of angular deformity following supracondylar humeral fractures. Malalignment of more than 15° is usually noticeable from a cosmetic standpoint, although it rarely is significant from a functional perspective. Biomechanically, varus malalignment may increase the risk of a subsequent lateral condyle humeral fracture. Cubitus varus can be corrected by osteotomy of the distal humerus (Fig. 1). Although transverse (rotational) and sagittal (hyperextension) plane deformities may also be present, the primary goal is full correction of the coronal plane deformity. Techniques using a laterally based, closing-wedge osteotomy with preservation of a medial

periosteal hinge and stable fixation (internal or external) have proven to be effective in correcting deformity and relatively safe in avoiding the significant complications (nerve palsy, infection, loss of fixation, reoperation), which have historically been associated with corrective distal humeral osteotomy.

Fractures of the Lateral Humeral Condyle

Fractures of the lateral condyle are intra-articular, have a potential risk of nonunion, and usually require internal fixation. They can be graded by the amount of displacement of the metaphyseal fragment and integrity of the articular cartilage. Stage I fractures are displaced less than 2 mm and the articular cartilage is intact; stage II fractures are displaced 2 to 4 mm and the articular surface is disrupted; stage III fractures are severely displaced and rotated. Arthrography may be helpful to delineate displacement or incongruence of the articular surface in very young children or when the diagnosis is uncertain. Fractures that are minimally displaced (< 2 mm) can be treated by cast immobilization with the elbow flexed to 90°, with close radiographic follow-up (weekly) until the fracture has healed. If the fracture displaces, closed reduction and percutaneous pinning or ORIF may be necessary. Fractures that are displaced from 2 to 4 mm with an intact articular hinge and are stable to stress (varus or valgus) can be treated by closed reduction and percutaneous pinning. Unstable stage II and all stage III fractures require ORIF through a lateral approach. Posterior dissection should be limited to avoid injury to the blood supply of the ossification centers. Pin fixation can be removed at 3 to 4 weeks but adequate follow-up is indicated until radiographic union.

The most common complication of lateral condyle fractures is nonunion, which can lead to progressive cubitus valgus and tardy ulnar nerve palsy. Fractures that fail to unite by 10 weeks can be treated by bone grafting and internal fixation when there is a large metaphyseal fragment and < 1 cm of displacement. Treatment of an established nonunion by bone grafting and internal fixation has a potential risk of joint stiffness and osteonecrosis. For this reason, a painless, chronic, stable, fibrous nonunion that is in an acceptable position may best be left untreated. Cubitus valgus deformity can be corrected by varus osteotomy if the elbow is unstable or the appearance is cosmetically unacceptable. Ulnar neuropathy occurs as a late complication of valgus malalignment (average time of onset 22 years after injury) and can be treated by anterior transposition of the ulnar nerve.

Fractures of the Capitellum

Fractures of the capitellum are relatively rare injuries generally seen in adolescents (11 to 17 years). The mechanism of injury is a shearing of the capitellum by the radial head resulting from a fall on an outstretched hand and extended elbow. It is postulated that the predominantly cartilaginous nature of the capitellum in younger children effectively precludes this type of injury in the very young. Fractures of the capitellum can be difficult to identify radiographically because of the small amount of cancellous bone in the capitellar fragment. Because of the intra-articular nature of this fracture and the limitations of radiographic visualization, capitellar fractures are best treated by ORIF of large fragments and excision of smaller fragments.

Fractures of the Medial Humeral Condyle

Fractures of the medial humeral condyle account for less than 2% of elbow fractures and are frequently overlooked or misdiagnosed because they usually occur prior to ossification of the trochlea. As with fractures of the lateral condyle, classification and treatment are based on the amount of displacement. Minimally displaced (< 2 mm) fractures can be treated by cast immobilization. Fractures that are displaced > 2 mm usually require ORIF to restore joint congruity.

Medial Epicondyle Fractures

Fractures of the medial epicondyle are caused by valgus stress to the elbow, applied through the ulnar collateral ligament, or by overpull of the flexor/pronator attachment. They occur most commonly between the ages of 9 and 15 years. These injuries often accompany dislocations of the elbow, and the fracture fragment may become trapped in the joint, blocking reduction. Most fractures can be effectively treated nonsurgically even if widely displaced. Fibrous union is usually well tolerated. ORIF is indicated if the fracture fragment is incarcerated in the joint or if ulnar nerve dysfunction is present. Surgical treatment may be appropriate for fractures displaced more than 5 to 10 mm in adolescents who are engaged in activities that place repetitive, valgus loads on the elbow.

Transphyseal Injuries

Separation of the distal humeral physis is most common in children younger than 3 years of age. The typical mechanism of injury in a newborn is birth trauma and in older infants, a fall. However, child abuse is also a common cause of this injury. Transphyseal fractures are typically Salter-Harris type I or II injuries. Diagnosis is difficult because of the cartilaginous nature of the distal humerus in this young age group. These injuries must be differentiated from elbow dislocations and lateral condyle fractures. Radiographically, the normal relationship of the long axis of the radius to the center of the capitellum remains intact but is translated (together with the ulna) in a transphyseal separation. If the diagnosis is in ques-

tion, as may be the case prior to appearance of the capitellar ossification center, arthrography or ultrasonography may help determine the injury pattern. Simple immobilization is usually sufficient treatment for minimally displaced fractures in an infant. In children with displaced fractures, accurate reduction and stable pin fixation are necessary to prevent angular deformity.

Elbow Dislocation

Elbow dislocations account for only 5% of injuries about the elbow in children and are rare in children younger than 6 years. Peak incidence is during adolescence. The typical mechanism is hyperextension of the elbow with abduction. Fractures of the radial neck, medial epicondyle, lateral condyle, and coronoid process frequently accompany dislocation of the elbow. Most dislocations occur in a straight posterior direction, although anterior, lateral, medial, and divergent (disruption of the proximal radioulnar joint) dislocations can occur.

Neurologic injury is seen in about 10% of cases. The median and ulnar nerves are more frequently involved than the radial nerve. Most neuropathies spontaneously resolve following reduction of the joint unless the nerve is entrapped. Injury to the brachial artery is uncommon but more likely to occur with an open dislocation.

Most elbow dislocations can be successfully reduced by closed manipulation. If the reduction is stable, immobilization should not exceed 10 to 14 days to minimize joint stiffness. Failure of closed reduction is usually caused by an inverted osteochondral fragment or interposition of soft-tissue structures, including the ulnar nerve. Open reduction is indicated if closed reduction is unsuccessful, if the injury is open, or if there are associated fractures that require treatment or impede reduction.

Recurrent elbow dislocation is a recently described condition attributed to some or all of the following pathology: a shallow trochlear notch, instability caused by intra-articular fractures, capsular laxity, and ligamentous laxity. Posterolateral instability is the most common pattern. If the child is symptomatic, soft-tissue repair on the lateral side of the elbow with reattachment of the lateral capsule and lateral collateral ligament is recommended.

Radial Neck Fractures

Fractures of the radial neck may be metaphyseal or Salter-Harris type I or II injuries of the radial head. These injuries occur by 1 of 3 mechanisms: valgus force typically caused by a fall on an extended forearm; shearing force associated with elbow dislocation or reduction; or dislocation accompanying a forearm fracture. A fracture of the olecranon or an avulsion of the medial epicondyle often accompanies radial neck fractures caused by valgus loading.

Correction of excessive angulation and avoiding significant translocation of the radial head are the keys to successful treatment. The remodeling potential of the radial neck after fracture is considerable and the majority of these injuries can be treated nonsurgically. Fractures with < 45° angulation and < 50% translation can be treated by cast or splint immobilization for 10 to 14 days and then progressively mobilized. Fractures that are angulated > 45° or with translation > 50% should be reduced. Closed reduction is performed by extending the elbow and then applying varus force and direct thumb pressure to the radial head. Another technique of closed reduction is to wrap the forearm with an Esmarch bandage in a distal to proximal direction. When closed techniques are unsuccessful, percutaneous reduction with a K-wire or open reduction may be necessary. Once reduced, these fractures are usually stable. Unstable fractures should be fixed with 1 or 2 small oblique K-wires. The use of retrograde pin manipulation and pinning of displaced radial neck fractures has been of recent interest. Fixation across the radiocapitellar joint should be avoided. Cast and/or oblique pins should be removed by about 3 weeks and range of motion exercises started.

Joint stiffness is the most common problem after fracture of the radial neck. Loss of motion may result from overgrowth of the radial head or by radioulnar synostosis. Compartment syndrome of the volar forearm is a recently reported rare complication.

Olecranon Fractures

Isolated fractures of the olecranon in children are rare. Fractures involving the apophysis and avulsion fractures are usually hyperflexion injuries. Fractures of the metaphysis occur by a variety of mechanisms including flexion, extension, and shear. Fractures with < 5 mm of displacement are usually stable and can be treated by casting in mild flexion. Displaced and unstable fractures should be treated by ORIF. Surgical treatment yields satisfactory results in most children. Most unsatisfactory results are caused by growth abnormalities of the olecranon with loss of elbow flexion and extension.

Monteggia Fracture-Dislocations

The Monteggia lesion refers to a complex of injuries that consist of a radial head fracture or dislocation in association with an ulnar fracture. Type I injuries are characterized by anterior dislocation of the radial head; type II, by posterior dislocation; and type III, by lateral dislocation. In each type, the apical angulation of the fracture is in the same direction as the displacement of the radial head. In type IV injuries, the

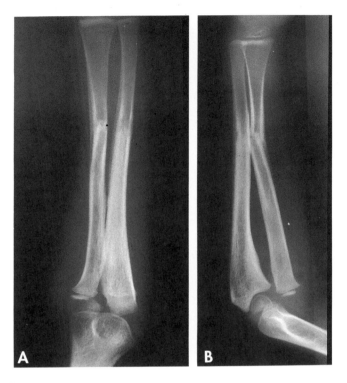

Figure 2

A and B, Type IV Monteggia fracture-dislocation. Radial head dislocation was not recognized. Note anterior angulation of ulna, anterior and lateral dislocation of radial head.

radial head dislocation is accompanied with both radial and ulnar fractures (Fig. 2). Monteggia equivalent injuries include "isolated" dislocations of the radial head and fractures of the ulnar shaft and radial neck. Type I injuries make up about 70% percent of the Monteggia lesions followed by type III (25%) and type II (< 5%).

These injuries may go undetected as a result of inadequate radiographic visualization of the elbow or failure of the clinician to recognize the elbow pathology. Most Monteggia fractures in children can be treated by closed reduction. The key to successful closed management is anatomic restoration of the ulnar fracture. Unstable fractures of the ulna should be treated primarily by ORIF. Occasionally, interposition of the annular ligament or joint capsule may block reduction of the radial head and require an open reduction. Late cases of radial head dislocation are usually associated with malunion of the ulna, which must be corrected by osteotomy prior to reduction of the joint. Open reduction and reconstruction of the annular ligament may be necessary in these cases. Chronic Monteggia legions may be successfully treated in this manner in children for up to 6 years following the original

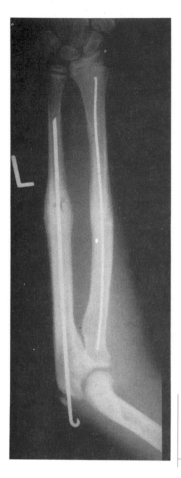

Figure 3

Both-bone forearm fracture in an 11-year-old boy was treated with flexible intramedullary rods.

injury, although radiographic results may not correlate with clinical motion. Complications of Monteggia fractures include loss of motion, recurrent dislocations, and nerve palsy. Injuries to the radial nerve are most common, but are usually transient.

Fractures of the Forearm

Fractures of the distal radial metaphysis account for 75% of all forearm fractures. The vast majority of these fractures are closed. Fractures with more than 15° to 25° of angulation are usually treated by closed reduction and long arm cast immobilization. Loss of reduction and the need for repeat closed reduction has been observed in up to one third of cases. Risk factors for loss of reduction include poor cast technique, plastic deformation of the ulna, and initial angulation greater than 30°. Angulation in the flexion/extension plane readily remodels, as does malunion in the radial/ulnar plane. For these reasons, the need for repeat reduction is lower in children younger than 10 years of age. Repeat manipulation of fractures that do not involve the physis has been performed

successfully up to 3 weeks following initial treatment. Percutaneous stabilization may occasionally be needed after reduction if the fracture is unstable; if neurovascular compromise is present; or if the fracture is initially angulated more than 30° and displaced more than 50%, or associated with a concomitant elbow fracture.

Diaphyseal fractures are classified as plastic, incomplete (torus, greenstick), and complete injuries. Displaced diaphyseal fractures tend to occur in older children and are frequently unstable. Most authors agree that up to 10° of angulation or 50° of total malrotation in children younger than 8 to 10 years old is well tolerated from both a cosmetic and functional standpoint. Closed treatment should be attempted for closed injuries. Open reduction may be necessary for fractures that cannot be adequately reduced by closed methods; fractures that are unstable; open fractures; segmental fractures; "floating elbow" injuries; and refractures. With appropriate indications, open reduction and stabilization with intramedullary fixation in juveniles (Fig. 3) and compression plating in older adolescents has been shown to be effective in several series.

Plastic deformation may occur in either the radius or ulna. In addition to cosmetic deformity, there may be limitation of rotation caused by narrowing of the interosseous space. Correction of plastic deformation should be performed if there is more than 15° of bowing in children older than 10 years or more than 20° in children between 5 and 10 years old. Closed reduction is usually successful in correcting the angulation caused by this injury.

Galeazzi Fractures

True Galeazzi injuries, defined by disruption of the distal radioulnar joint (DRUJ) in conjunction with a distal radial metadiaphyseal fracture, are rare in children. Galeazzi-equivalent fractures, in which the associated injury is a fracture of the distal ulnar physis, are more common. Anatomic reduction of the radial and ulnar fractures and of the DRUJ dislocation is required to restore normal function. In children, this goal is often achieved by closed reduction. Inability to obtain a closed reduction of the ulnar physeal fracture may be caused by interposition of the extensor tendon or periosteum and, if so, requires open reduction. Late instability is rare following the Galeazzi-equivalent fracture but premature arrest of the ulnar physis has been reported in up to 55% of cases.

In the true Galeazzi injury, the DRUJ is dislocated in pronation. Acutely, this injury requires closed reduction and immobilization with the forearm in supination. Late instability of the DRUJ is rare when the injury is recognized early and treated appropriately. Dorsal dislocation of the radiocarpal unit in supination appears to be the more common late instability pattern. Soft-tissue reconstruction with a portion of the retinaculum of the fifth and sixth dorsal extensor compartments and a distally based slip of the extensor carpi ulnaris tendon can stabilize the DRUJ. Any malunion contributing to instability of the joint should also be corrected with osteotomy.

Annotated Bibliography

Congenital Anomalies and Acquired Disorders

Bar-On E, Howard CB, Porat S: The use of ultrasound in the diagnosis of atypical pathology in the unossified skeleton. *J Pediatr Orthop* 1995;15:817–820.

Antenatal diagnosis of congenital dislocation of the radial head is reported.

Castello JR, Garro L, Campo M: Congenital radioulnar synostosis: Surgical correction by derotational osteotomy. *Ann Chir Main Memb Super* 1996;15:11–17.

Four cases treated with proximal derotational osteotomy showed improvement in function.

Dougall TW, Gibson PH: Bilateral, asymmetric congenital dislocation of radial heads in trisomy 8 syndrome. *Bull Hosp Jt Dis* 1997;56:113–114.

Asymmetry or radiographic and clinical presentation in bilateral radial head dislocation is reported.

Janarv PM, Hesser U, Hirsch G: Osteochondral lesions in the radiocapitellar joint in the skeletally immature: Radiographic, MRI, and arthroscopic findings in 13 consecutive cases. *J Pediatr Orthop* 1997;17:311–314.

Arthroscopy confirmed magnetic resonance imaging findings of site and severity of lesion.

Reichenbach H, Hormann D, Theile H: Hereditary congenital posterior dislocation of radial heads. *Am J Med Genet* 1995;55:101–104.

Radial head dislocation occurred in 3 generations of a family with evidence of autosomal dominant inheritance pattern. Bilateral or unilateral congenital dislocation resulted in mild to moderate limitation of range of motion with greater difficulty in rotation.

Rizzo R, Pavone V, Corsello G, Sorge G, Neri G, Opitz JM: Autosomal dominant and sporadic radio-ulnar synostosis. *Am J Med Genet* 1997;68:127–134.

Five cases in a Sicilian family, and 2 cases with sporadic occurrence are reviewed in this article.

Schenck RC Jr, Goodnight JM: Osteochondritis dissecans. *J Bone Joint Surg* 1996;78A:439–456.

This is a comprehensive review article on osteochondritis dissecans of the knee, elbow, and ankle with extensive bibliography.

Supracondylar Fractures of the Humerus

Brown IC, Zinar DM: Traumatic and iatrogenic neurological complications after supracondylar humerus fractures in children. *J Pediatr Orthop* 1995;15:440–443.

The incidence of neural injuries in 162 children was 12%, and the risk of neuropathy was greatest (42%) in fractures showing complete displacement. A waiting period of 6 months is suggested before considering exploration. The incidence of iatrogenic nerve injury after pinning was 3%. The ulnar nerve was most susceptible. A medial "mini" incision is recommended when soft-tissue swelling is severe.

Campbell CC, Waters PM, Emans JB, Kasser JR, Millis MB: Neurovascular injury and displacement in type III supracondylar humerus fractures. *J Pediatr Orthop* 1995;15:47–52.

Neurovascular injuries were found in 29 (49%) of 59 children with type III fractures. Median nerve injury (15 patients) was associated with posterolateral displacement and radial nerve injury (8 patients) with posteromedial displacement. Injuries to the brachial artery occurred with either type of displacement.

Copley LA, Dormans JP, Davidson RS: Vascular injuries and their sequelae in pediatric supracondylar humeral fractures: Toward a goal of prevention. *J Pediatr Orthop* 1996;16:99–103.

Initially absent radial pulses returned following fracture reduction and stabilization in 14 of 17 children with displaced supracondylar humerus fractures. Significant vascular injury was found in children with persistent absence of the radial pulse (3 patients) or progressive decline in vascularity (2 patients) following fracture reduction and stabilization.

De Boeck H, De Smet P, Penders W, De Rydt D: Supracondylar elbow fractures with impaction of the medial condyle in children. *J Pediatr Orthop* 1995;15:444–448.

This article reviews the cases of 13 children with supracondylar elbow fractures in which the medial column of the distal humerus was impacted. Subtle collapse of this structure led to significant varus deformity if not recognized and treated aggressively. Closed reduction and percutaneous pinning is recommended to prevent this complication.

Garbuz DS, Leitch K, Wright JG: The treatment of supracondylar fractures in children with an absent radial pulse. *J Pediatr Orthop* 1996;16:594–596.

Fifteen of 22 children had a well-perfused hand and normal outcome following closed reduction and K-wire fixation despite absence of the radial pulse in 5. The authors suggest that an absent radial pulse is not an absolute indication for arterial exploration in a nonischemic limb.

Hadlow AT, Devane P, Nicol RO: A selective treatment approach to supracondylar fracture of the humerus in children. *J Pediatr Orthop* 1996;16:104–106.

Selective treatment in 176 patients with supracondylar humerus fractures resulted in satisfactory outcomes in 46/75 (61%) type III fractures and in 37/48 (77%) type II fractures treated by closed reduction and casting. The authors suggest that there may still be a role for nonsurgical treatment.

Keenan WN, Clegg J: Variation of Baumann's angle with age, sex, and side: Implications for its use in radiological monitoring of supracondylar fracture of the humerus in children. *J Pediatr Orthop* 1996;16:97–98.

Based on review of 577 elbow radiographs of children aged 2 to 14 years, this study showed no significant population variation in Baumann's angle with respect to age, sex, or side.

Levine MJ, Horn BD, Pizzutillo PD: Treatment of posttraumatic cubitus varus in the pediatric population with humeral osteotomy and external fixation. *J Pediatr Orthop* 1996;16:597–601.

Voss FR, Kasser JR, Trepman E, Simmons E Jr, Hall JE: Uniplanar supracondylar humeral osteotomy with preset Kirschner wires for posttraumatic cubitus varus. *J Pediatr Orthop 1994;14: 471–478.*

These articles describe results of a variety of surgical techniques for correction of cubitus varus deformity.

Sabharwal S, Tredwell SJ, Beauchamp RD, et al: Management of pulseless pink hand in pediatric supracondylar fractures of humerus. *J Pediatr Orthop* 1997;17:303–310.

A combination of segmental pressure monitoring, color-flow duplex scanning, and magnetic resonance imaging was used to document a relatively high rate of asymptomatic reocclusion and brachial artery stenosis following early revascularization of a pulseless but otherwise well-perfused hand. The authors suggest a period of close neurovascular observation before performing exploration and vascular repair when the extremity is viable.

Topping RE, Blanco JS, Davis TJ: Clinical evaluation of crossed-pin versus lateral-pin fixation in displaced supracondylar humerus fractures. *J Pediatr Orthop* 1995;15:435–439.

The results of closed reduction and crossed pin (27 patients) versus lateral pin (20 patients) fixation of displaced supracondylar fractures were compared. No difference in maintenance of reduction was found. The authors conclude that crossed pins offer no advantage clinically over 2 laterally placed pins.

Distal Humeral Epiphyseal Separation

Abe M, Ishizu T, Nagaoka T, Onomura T: Epiphyseal separation of the distal end of the humeral epiphysis: A follow-up note. *J Pediatr Orthop* 1995;15:426–434.

Cubitus varus deformity occurred in 15 of 21 children with transphyseal fractures of the distal humerus. Analysis showed the cause to be malreduction in 12 patients and loss of reduction in 2. Accurate reduction and stable fixation is recommended to avoid this complication.

Davidson RS, Markowitz RI, Dormans J, Drummond DS: Ultrasonographic evaluation of the elbow in infants and young children after suspected trauma. *J Bone Joint Surg* 1994; 76A:1804–1813.

The authors report their experience with ultrasonography for diagnosis of fractures about the elbow in 7 infants and 1 child.

Lateral Condylar Fractures of the Humerus

Finnbogason T, Karlsson G, Lindberg L, Mortensson W: Nondisplaced and minimally displaced fractures of the lateral humeral condyle in children: A prospective radiographic investigation of fracture stability. *J Pediatr Orthop* 1995;15:422–425.

The authors identify radiographic criteria that can be used to predict potential instability and subsequent displacement of nondisplaced or minimally displaced fractures of the lateral humeral condyle.

Fractures of the Capitellum

Letts M, Rumball K, Bauermeister S, McIntyre W, D'Astous J: Fractures of the capitellum in adolescents. *J Pediatr Orthop* 1997;17:315–320.

The authors recommend accurate open reduction and internal fixation for this relatively uncommon injury.

Radial Neck Fractures

Gonzalez-Herranz P, Alvarez-Romera A, Burgos J, Rapariz JM, Hevia E: Displaced radial neck fractures in children treated by closed intramedullary pinning (Metaizeau technique). *J Pediatr Orthop* 1997;17:325–331.

The authors describe their technique of closed intramedullary pinning for reduction and stabilization in 17 children with displaced fractures of the radial neck.

Peters CL, Scott SM: Compartment syndrome in the forearm following fractures of the radial head or neck in children. *J Bone Joint Surg* 1995;77A:1070–1074.

The authors report 3 cases of volar compartment syndrome following minimally displaced fractures of the radial neck. Diagnosis within the first 12 to 24 hours and emergency fasciotomy resulted in full recovery in each case.

Monteggia Fracture-Dislocations

Rodgers WB, Waters PM, Hall JE: Chronic Monteggia lesions in children: Complications and results of reconstruction. *J Bone Joint Surg* 1996;78A:1322–1329.

Fourteen complications occurred in 7 patients following surgical treatment of chronic Monteggia lesions. All patients had some loss of forearm rotation. The authors emphasize the salvage nature of these procedures.

Fractures of the Forearm

Huber RI, Keller HW, Huber PM, Rehm KE: Flexible intramedullary nailing as fracture treatment in children. *J Pediatr Orthop* 1996;16:602–605.

The authors describe their experience with flexible (titanium rod), intramedullary fixation for forearm fractures in children between 4 and 12 years of age.

Ortega R, Loder RT, Louis DS: Open reduction and internal fixation of forearm fractures in children. *J Pediatr Orthop* 1996;16:651–654.

Wyrsch B, Mencio GA, Green NE: Open reduction and internal fixation of pediatric forearm fractures. *J Pediatr Orthop* 1996;16:644-650.

These 2 articles report excellent results in treating pediatric forearm fractures with open reduction and internal fixation using a variety of stabilization techniques. Indications for surgical treatment are discussed.

Classic Bibliography

Best TN: Management of old unreduced Monteggia fracture dislocations of the elbow in children. *J Pediatr Orthop* 1994; 14:193–199.

Davids JR, Maguire MF, Mubarak SJ, Wenger DR: Lateral condylar fracture of the humerus following posttraumatic cubitus varus. *J Pediatr Orthop* 1994;14:466–470.

Gaddy BC, Manske PR, Pruitt DL, Schoenecker PL, Rouse AM: Distal humeral osteotomy for correction of posttraumatic cubitus varus. *J Pediatr Orthop* 1994;14:214–219.

Gibbons CL, Woods DA, Pailthorpe C, Carr AJ, Worlock P: The management of isolated distal radius fractures in children. *J Pediatr Orthop* 1994;14:207–210.

Hernandez MA III, Roach JW: Corrective osteotomy for cubitus varus deformity. *J Pediatr Orthop* 1994;14:487–491.

Mintzer CM, Waters PM, Brown DJ, Kasser JR: Percutaneous pinning in the treatment of displaced lateral condyle fractures. *J Pediatr Orthop* 1994;14:462–465.

Schenck RC Jr, Athanasiou KA, Constantinides G, Gomez E: A biomechanical analysis of articular cartilage of the human elbow and a potential relationship to osteochondritis dissecans. *Clin Orthop* 1994;299:305–312.

Uhthoff HK (ed): *The Embryology of the Human Locomotor System.* Berlin, Germany, Springer-Verlag, 1990.

Zionts LE, McKellop HA, Hathaway R: Torsional strength of pin configurations used to fix supracondylar fractures of the humerus in children. *J Bone Joint Surg* 1994;76A:253–256.

Chapter 30
Elbow and Forearm: Adult Trauma

Distal Humeral Fractures

In younger adults, distal humeral fractures are usually the result of high-energy trauma from motor vehicle accidents, falls, or direct blows; up to 50% in some series are open fractures. In the elderly patient with demineralized bone, these fractures may occur from lower energy injuries.

Because of the proximity of the fractured distal humerus to the neurovascular structures about the elbow, careful evaluation of the perfusion, sensation, and motor control is mandatory. Standard anteroposterior (AP), lateral, and capitocondylar radiographs of the elbow are usually sufficient to characterize the fracture, although computed tomography (CT) may assist preoperative planning in comminuted fractures.

Historically, there have been numerous attempts to develop a classification system for fractures of the distal humerus. Recent authors have contributed a logical three-part classification with subdivisions (Outline 1 and Fig. 1).

Bicolumn fractures of the distal humerus are the most common and usually result from high-energy trauma. Single column fractures are rare in adults and probably result from an abduction or adduction force or are caused by an axial load from the olecranon in those patients with a fenestrated olecranon/coronoid fossa. Transcolumn fractures rarely occur in the skeletally mature patient.

Contemporary treatment of distal humeral fractures includes anatomic reduction and stable internal fixation to allow early motion. The olecranon osteotomy gives full exposure to the distal humerus and can be transverse, chevron shaped, or extra-articular; the chevron osteotomy offers better geometry for stable fixation. The triceps-splitting approach is used sparingly in the adult population because it does not offer much better exposure than alternatives and is accompanied by postoperative muscle fibrosis. Because of a 10% to 30% olecranon nonunion rate and compromise of the triceps with the muscle splitting approach, the triceps-sparing alternative has become popular for treatment of a wide range of distal humeral fracture patterns. This approach is particularly useful when the intra-articular

extension of the fracture is limited.

Biomechanically, plate and screw fixation is stronger than pin fixation. In an attempt to define the most stable construct for plating, a biomechanical study was conducted in which various multiple plating techniques of the distal humerus were compared. The strongest construct was defined as a medial pelvic reconstruction plate combined with a postero-

> ### Outline 1
> #### Classification of fractures of the distal humerus
>
> **Transcolumn—nonarticular fracture**
>
>   High—above the olecranon fossa
>
>   Low—through the olecranon fossa
>
> **Single column**
>
>   High—the fracture includes the majority of the trochlea and is unstable (the ulna and radius follow the displacement of the fractured column)
>
>   Low—the fracture does not exit above the olecranon fossa
>
> **Bicolumn**
>
>   High T fracture—transverse component crosses above olecranon fossa
>
>   Low T fracture—transverse component crosses below olecranon fossa
>
>   Y fracture—oblique transverse components
>
>   H fracture—fractures in medial and lateral columns along with transverse components, which renders the trochlea a free, fourth fragment
>
>   Medial lambda—medial side partially intact
>
>   Lateral lambda—lateral side partially intact

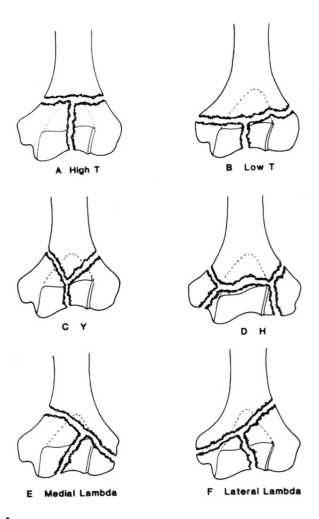

Figure 1

Bicolumn fractures of the distal humerus. (Reproduced with permission from Jupiter JB, Mehne DK: Fractures of the distal humerus. *Orthopedics* 1992;15:825–833.)

A High T

B Low T

C Y

D H

E Medial Lambda

F Lateral Lambda

Reported complications associated with distal humeral fractures and their treatment include nonunion, malunion, infection (up to 6% in type III open injuries), and ulnar nerve palsy (up to 15%).

Capitellar Fractures

Capitellar fractures are rare injuries, accounting for only 1% of all elbow fractures. They are typically the result of shear forces encountered as the radial head imparts a tangential force to the capitellum, often separating the capitellum from the lateral column of the humerus. They are associated with radial head fractures and posterior elbow dislocations.

Historically, there has been an eponymous classification for fractures of the capitellum: Hahn-Steinthal (type I) and Kocher-Lorenz (type II). Unfortunately, this binary system does not reflect the variability in the presentation of these injuries. The type I fractures are more recognizable radiographically as large fragment osteochondral injuries representing almost the entire capitellum. It is sometimes difficult to perceive the articular shell (type II) fractures. A pure cartilage delamination is rare, but the amount of bone that accompanies the cartilage fragment can range from perceptible (almost a type I) to minimal. The capitellar fragment itself can be comminuted, or a combination of injuries can be present, including fractures of the radial head and even impacted fractures of the distal humerus.

lateral dynamic compression plate. All techniques, including triple plating, were significantly less stiff than the intact distal humerus, especially in the sagittal plane.

Loss of terminal extension is frequently seen after distal humeral fracture. Exertional pain can be expected in 25% of patients. It was previously thought that younger patients do better than the elderly, but recent literature has shown good outcomes with open reduction and internal fixation (ORIF) in older patients. Selected primary total elbow arthroplasty for complex distal humeral fractures in the elderly has gained acceptance, and results in series from experienced surgeons have been good.

Closed treatment is acceptable for nondisplaced capitellum fractures, although nondisplaced fractures are rare. Manipulation and casting of displaced fractures was reported in the early literature and in at least 1 recent report, but closed treatment is unpredictable and surgical intervention is nearly universally recommended.

Displaced fractures with a generous amount of bone should be treated with ORIF. The selection of implants includes conventional miniscrews, variable pitch screws, and bioabsorbable pins. A recent report demonstrated excellent functional results with multiple 2.0-mm polyglycolide bioabsorbable pins. If fixation is secure, early postoperative motion can be initiated, although resisted or weighted elbow flexion in pronation should be avoided.

All efforts should be made to fix the fractured capitellum, yet there are some cases in which extensive comminution or lack of supporting bone will preclude fixation. Excision becomes the only logical alternative. There are no prosthetic substitutes for the excised capitellum. Additional injuries about the elbow or forearm should be recognized and treated aggressively.

Radial Head Fractures

Fractures of the radial head can result from 2 mechanisms of injury: valgus overload of the lateral elbow compartment and force transmission through the forearm axis with ultimate impact at the radiocapitellar joint. Many fractures are caused by a combination of mechanisms. Therefore, thorough examination of the elbow and forearm is imperative when radial head fracture is found. Maintaining a high index of suspicion for associated injuries is advisable.

Painful limitation of active and passive elbow motion in all planes is the usual symptom caused by the fracture itself or the accompanying hemarthrosis. Whereas displaced radial head/neck fractures can easily be seen on routine AP and lateral radiographs, minimally displaced fractures may require a radiocapitellar or capitocondylar view, which is a lateral view with the X-ray tube angled 45° toward the shoulder.

Aspiration of the acute hemarthrosis is advocated by some as a diagnostic maneuver and to promote early motion recovery. Whether aspiration is beneficial in long-term outcome remains to be proven. Nondisplaced or minimally displaced radial head fractures with stable configuration (usually less than one third of the articular surface) and no bony block to motion can be treated with early mobilization. Nondisplaced fractures involving more than one third of the articular surface are often unstable and may require immobilization for up to 2 weeks, followed by protected mobilization for another week (Fig. 2).

Fragment incongruity, comminution, or mechanical block caused by an intra-articular loose fragment necessitates surgical management. Displaced 2-part radial head fractures are amenable to open reduction and fixation with Kirschner wires (K-

wires), minifragment screws, variable pitch screws, or small plates.

Comminution in the subchondral metaphyseal region, small fragments, and limited portals for hardware placement make fixation of the fractured radial head technically challenging. Provisional fixation with K-wires can stabilize the reduction until miniscrews or a small plate can be applied. There is a 90° to 100° nonarticular "safe zone" around the circumference of the radial head. This region does not articulate with the lesser sigmoid fossa of the ulna at the proximal radioulnar joint (PRUJ) (Fig. 3). Even when implants are introduced through this zone, care must be exercised to avoid penetration through the opposite surface or into the proximal concavity that articulates with the capitellum.

In the case of an Essex-Lopresti fracture-dislocation, the fracture at the radial head is the proximal manifestation of a global forearm axis disruption including injury to the distal radioulnar joint, interosseous ligament, and radial head. In this constellation of injuries, maintaining the relationships at the PRUJ and throughout the forearm is imperative. Simple excision of the radial head can have adverse consequences in these cases, because the radius will then migrate proximally, causing significant biomechanical disturbance at the wrist and elbow. Initial fixation of the radial head is advocated. Even late excision of an incongruous radial head, after healing, has been found to be superior to early excision in the face of global injury. If salvage is impossible, consideration must

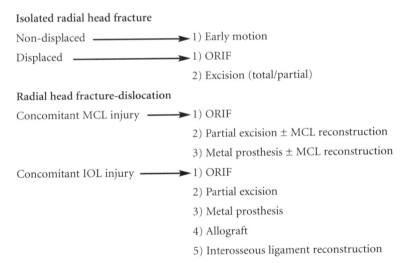

Isolated radial head fracture

Non-displaced ⟶ 1) Early motion

Displaced ⟶ 1) ORIF

   2) Excision (total/partial)

Radial head fracture-dislocation

Concomitant MCL injury ⟶ 1) ORIF

   2) Partial excision ± MCL reconstruction

   3) Metal prosthesis ± MCL reconstruction

Concomitant IOL injury ⟶ 1) ORIF

   2) Partial excision

   3) Metal prosthesis

   4) Allograft

   5) Interosseous ligament reconstruction

Figure 2

Radial head fracture treatment algorithm. ORIF, open reduction and internal fixation; MCL, medial collateral ligament; IOL, interosseous ligament.

be given to replacement of the radial head.

Several authors have shown that silicone prosthetic radial head replacements are too flexible to withstand the forces at the radiocapitellar joint for long periods. Prosthesis fragmentation, "cold flow," and the potential for "silicone synovitis" have dissuaded most surgeons from their use. Newer implanted biocompatible metals show promise. Stainless steel, titanium (Fig. 4), and even a bipolar type of prosthetic radial head have become increasingly popular with good functional results on 4.5- to 9-year follow-up. The use of size-matched radial head allografts for symptomatic proximal radius migration in a small group of patients was recently reported, with improvement of symptoms at 3-years' follow-up.

Olecranon Fractures

Fractures of the olecranon process can result from direct or indirect trauma. Experimentally produced direct load to the dorsal aspect of the flexed elbow caused olecranon fractures in the range of 60° to 135° of flexion. Falls on the outstretched hand with forceful triceps contraction can also cause olecranon fractures. Fractures through persistent olecranon physes caused by tension forces from the triceps have been described in the adult. The mechanism of olecranon stress fractures in athletes is debated.

A 3-part classification of olecranon fractures has been described, which considers fracture displacement, comminution, and the stability of the ulnohumeral articulation (Fig. 5). Type I fractures are nondisplaced or minimally displaced (< 2 to 3 mm displacement) with variable amounts of comminution; type II fractures are displaced and present as either noncomminuted (IIA) or comminuted (IIB); type III A and B olecranon fractures are associated with an unstable ulnohumeral relationship (fracture-dislocation).

Minimally displaced fractures (2 to 3 mm

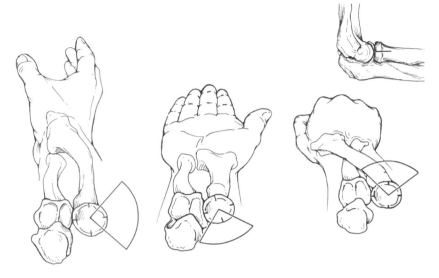

Figure 3

The safe zone for hardware placement can be found by bisecting the midline of the radial neck in neutral forearm rotation (inset). (Reproduced with permission from Hotchkiss RN: Displaced fractures of the radial head: Internal fixation or excision? *J Am Acad Orthop Surg* 1997;5:1–10.)

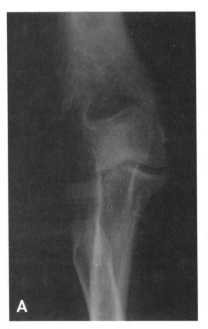
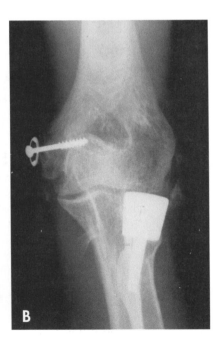

Figure 4

Forty-three-year-old man had a silicone radial head prosthesis implanted following a radial head fracture-dislocation. He had continued pain with neutral (A) radiographs that demonstrated osteolysis and valgus instability. The patient received a metal radial head prosthesis with medial collateral ligament reconstruction and regained full range of motion, relief of pain, and returned to work. Nine-year follow-up radiograph (B) demonstrates good osseous integration.

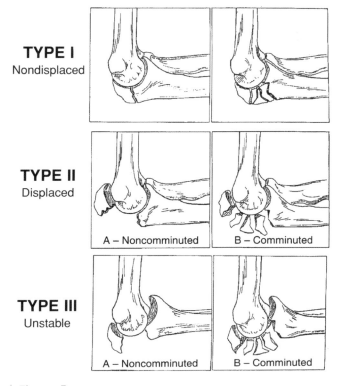

Figure 5

Three-part classification system for fractures of the olecranon. The qualifiers "A and B" reflect the amount of comminution. (Reproduced with permission from Morrey BF (ed): *The Elbow and Its Disorders*, ed 2. Philadelphia, PA, WB Saunders, 1993.)

mum, the portion of the olecranon proximal to its narrowest aspect (the nadir of the concavity) should be maintained for stability.

A variety of methods have been described for fixation of displaced olecranon fractures. The most popular options are K-wire or terminally threaded cancellous screw fixation with additional tension band wiring. Plating is usually reserved for comminuted patterns (Fig. 6). Some type IIB or IIIA fractures may require plate fixation to maintain the normal contour of the articular surface, because compression of comminuted fragments with the tension band technique may excessively narrow the ulnar semilunar notch, causing extrusion of the distal humerus. Bicortical fixation of the proximal fragment can be achieved by lateral or dorsal plating, which has been shown to be equally stable with respect to low load stability, thereby allowing early protected ROM. Dorsal plating may be

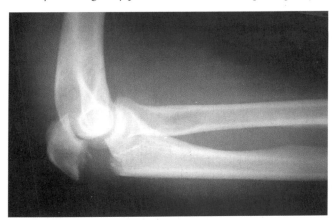

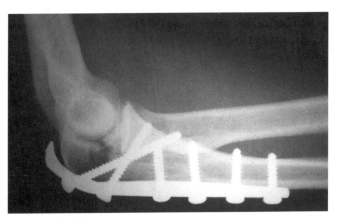

Figure 6

This comminuted olecranon fracture was treated with plate fixation. Note the small void in the nonarticular portion of the olecranon. The subcutaneous border of the ulna was the key to the reduction; care was taken to avoid altering the radius of curvature of the fossa, thus extruding the distal humerus.

displacement) may be treated with a short course of elbow immobilization in relative extension (between 45° and 90° of flexion), followed by protected active range of motion (ROM) with close radiographic follow-up to ensure the fracture does not displace.

Options for surgical treatment of displaced olecranon fractures include ORIF or olecranon fragment excision with reattachment of the triceps tendon close to the articular surface. Fragment excision is usually reserved for the comminuted fractures that occur in the elderly population. Associated ulnohumeral instability is a relative contraindication to large fragment excision. The amount of proximal olecranon that can safely be excised is not firmly established. Earlier reports documented satisfactory results with excision of up to 80% of the olecranon; however, a recent biomechanical study has shown that elbow instability may result from this large percentage of excision. Two clinical studies have shown favorable results with olecranon excision of up to 70% (with no associated elbow injury), although clinical instability following 60% excision has been reported. It is likely that, at a mini-

preferable when a displaced coronoid fragment exists that can be lagged to the plate. In 2 recent biomechanical studies, no significant difference was found between the stability of 2 different techniques of pinning with tension band wiring with respect to whether the distal aspect of the tension band was located anterior or posterior to the axial pins.

Olecranon fractures associated with ulnohumeral instability typically require olecranon fixation as well as treatment of the associated injuries: radial head fracture, coronoid fracture, or collateral ligament injury. The use of a hinged elbow fixator in addition to global treatment of other pathologies may neutralize pathologic forces and permit earlier elbow motion.

The olecranon physis occasionally may persist into adulthood. Olecranon physeal fractures may be acutely displaced after significant trauma or nondisplaced, often stress related, athletic injuries. Nondisplaced fractures through a persistent olecranon physis may resemble a typical displaced olecranon fracture. The contralateral elbow should be imaged to determine whether the persistent physis is bilateral, and if no displacement of the injured side is noted compared to the opposite side, rest may be tried. Surgical fixation of displaced fractures without bone grafting or excision of the cartilage interface will result in a stable fibrous interface with persistent lucency, but excellent results have been reported. Chronically painful, nondisplaced, physeal fractures may be successfully treated with excision of the physis with or without bone grafting, although this risks altering the normal morphology of the articular surface.

The outcome of olecranon fracture treatment has not been studied in a prospective series; however, most published reports document a 95% union rate with nonunion and ulnar nerve paresthesias as the two most common complications. The need for removal of prominent hardware after olecranon healing should not be considered a complication but a potential component of the treatment course. Patients may develop a mild flexion contracture following surgical treatment. Stable asymptomatic fibrous nonunions do not require surgical treatment; however, symptomatic nonunions may be treated with proximal fragment excision or ORIF with or without bone grafting. Degenerative changes have been reported with joint incongruity > 2 mm, but some incongruity at the articular surface is preferable to excessive narrowing of the trochlear notch.

Elbow Dislocations

Simple Elbow Dislocations

Elbow dislocations without accompanying fracture are considered "simple" dislocations and are classified according to the position of the ulna and radius with respect to the humerus: posterior, posterolateral, posteromedial, lateral, medial. In divergent dislocations, the radius and ulna are dissociated and there is a loss of congruity at the ulnohumeral joint. Acute elbow dislocations are second in frequency only to shoulder dislocations when considering all major joint dislocations. A majority are posterior or posterolateral dislocations. Medial collateral ligament (MCL) rupture has been recognized in virtually all surgical series of acute elbow dislocations. Additional injuries to supporting tissues include rupture of the lateral collateral ligament (LCL), variable injury to the flexor-pronator muscle mass, brachialis and anterior capsule avulsions, and chondral damage. Transient nerve lesions, usually of the median and ulnar nerves, have been reported in up to 20% of cases of elbow dislocation. Rupture or occlusion of the brachial artery is a rare attendant injury but should be suspected when absence of pulses or evidence of hand ischemia following elbow dislocation is seen. Vascular reconstruction with vein grafting is indicated to reestablish circulation to the forearm and hand.

Closed reduction of the simple, acute dislocation can usually be performed with intravenous sedation and gentle manipulation. Distally directed pressure may be exerted over the olecranon tip to aid in the reduction, and the patient may be placed prone with the arm hanging over the table as a gravity assist. Occasionally, if significant spasm is present, regional or general anesthesia may be required for reduction. The reduced elbow should be tested to determine the stable arc of motion and to subjectively assess the "tracking" of the joint if any incongruity or loose body is suspected. Following 5 to 7 days of immobilization, active ROM is encouraged within the limits of stability. Usually 80% of eventual motion is obtained by 3 months and full motion by 1 year following injury. Significant flexion contractures persisting beyond 6 weeks may be treated with active and active-assisted motion and a serial static splinting program. In randomized, prospective studies comparing open to closed treatment of simple elbow dislocations, results were better with closed treatment. Nonsurgical management remains the treatment of choice in routine cases.

The outcome of simple, acute elbow dislocations has been well studied. Recurrent instability is exceedingly rare; however, a flexion contracture of 10° or less is commonly encountered. Residual pain and loss of motion have been directly correlated with the period of elbow immobilization; uniformly good or excellent results are found when motion is begun within 2 weeks postinjury. Heterotopic ossification occurs in fewer than 5% of cases of simple dislocations, but the prevalence can be higher if associated with fractures of the radial head, neural axis trauma, or burns.

Complex Elbow Dislocations

Elbow dislocations with fracture are termed "complex" and constitute between 25% to 50% of all elbow dislocations. The commonly associated fractures include the medial epicondyle, radial head, and coronoid process (Fig. 7). Early elbow motion has been found to improve outcome in the complex dislocations. The use of a hinged elbow distractor as a neutralization device to permit early motion in the treatment of unstable fracture dislocations of the elbow recently has been reported to produce successful outcomes in 86% of patients, with only 1 of 7 elbows developing persistent elbow instability. Prior to using the device, results were satisfactory in only 20% of these injuries. The outcome of complex dislocations is significantly worse than that of simple dislocations; significant osteoarthritis was found in a majority of patients.

Coronoid Fractures

In addition to acting as a mechanical buttress to posterior translation of the ulna, the coronoid process is essential to elbow stability by providing the insertion sites for the anterior MCL, the anterior joint capsule, and the brachialis muscle. An anatomic study of the soft-tissue attachments of the coronoid process has found that the tip of the coronoid is intra-articular and, therefore, would be fractured by impaction, not by avulsion. Coronoid fractures are seen in up to one third of elbow dislocations. A three-part classification system of coronoid fractures is well accepted. A small fracture of the coronoid tip is classified as type I. Type II fractures involve ≤ 50% of the coronoid process. Type III injuries are basilar fractures of the coronoid process.

Treatment of isolated type I fractures is early protected ROM. Type II fractures are treated with early ROM unless the fracture is displaced and associated with an unstable ulnohumeral joint, in which case surgical fixation may be required. Type III fractures should be surgically repaired if displaced, associated with instability, or if significant comminution of the fragment exists. Coronoid reconstruction with bone graft may be necessary. Hinged elbow distraction may be used to hold the joint reduced, thus neutralizing joint reactive forces and permitting early ROM. Outcome of coronoid fracture treatment in 35 patients was satisfactory in 90% of type I fractures, 70% of type II fractures, and 20% of type III fractures.

Disorders of the Forearm Axis

General

The concept of the "forearm axis" has been developed to integrate the concepts of wrist, forearm, and elbow function and anatomy. With this comprehensive approach, diagnosis and treatment of these several conditions can be described and analyzed concurrently. The functional interdependence of the wrist, forearm, and elbow is essential to place the hand in space with the proper orientation for grasp and pinch activity. Injury to any component of the forearm axis can result in a global functional deficit.

The 3 basic stabilizers of the forearm are the tissues of the distal radioulnar joint (DRUJ), the interosseous ligament (IOL) of the forearm, and the radiocapitellar complex/proximal radioulnar joint (PRUJ) with their supporting soft tissues. Although fractures and subsequent malunions of the distal radius that affect the DRUJ or periarticular fractures of the elbow that alter PRUJ stability impact on the function of the forearm axis, this chapter will concentrate on the following entities that result in loss of function of this unique anatomy: (1) Galeazzi fractures, (2) Monteggia lesions, and (3) Essex-Lopresti fracture-dislocations.

Anatomy and Mechanics

There are 2 primary soft-tissue stabilizers of the proximal radioulnar relationship. The annular ligament, despite its name given for its near circumferential relation to the radial neck, has a broad flat insertion on the anterior ridge of the radial notch and a posterior insertion on a ridge of the proximal supinator crest. The quadrate ligament is a dense condensation of capsular tissue that inserts onto the distal and

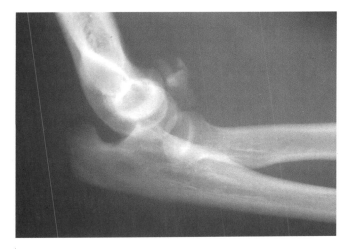

Figure 7

A complex elbow dislocation associated with a type 2 coronoid fracture. Elbow instability following closed reduction may be present in this situation.

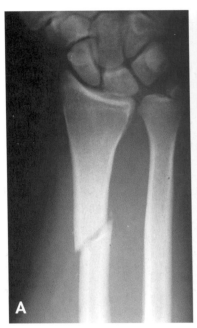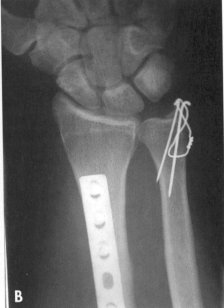

Figure 8

A, Preoperative radiograph of a Galeazzi fracture. B, Postoperative film after plating of the radius and stabilization of the basilar styloid of the fracture that destabilized the distal radioulnar joint.

The anatomic relationship of the central band, interosseous ligament, and the DRUJ along the forearm axis permits compressive loads to be accepted at the wrist level; a majority of this force is transmitted through the radius platform. In the mid-forearm, the compressive loads not only continue proximally along the radial shaft, but also develop tension in the central band of the IOL. This tension, in turn, creates distal-to-proximal compressive forces in the ulna proximal to the IOL origin. This pattern of force transmission explains why the relative contact pressures of the radius and ulna at the wrist and ulna are not equivalent.

When these force characteristics are altered by IOL rupture, forearm bone fracture, or radial head fracture/excision, the longitudinal relationship of the forearm axis is compromised. Proximal translation of the radius can have focal effects at the wrist, forearm, or elbow, but global disruption of the forearm axis is the usual result.

medial portion of the PRUJ and blends onto the surface of the ulna; its dynamic function is not clear, but it may be a static stabilizer of the proximal forearm. The lesser sigmoid fossa, a concavity of the lateral slope of the coronoid, accepts the articular surface of the radial head.

The ulna is the stable unit of the forearm; it is rigidly linked to the humerus at the highly constrained ulnotrochlear joint. The small component of counterrotation of the ulna on the humerus is confined to a short arc of 11° by the medial and lateral ligament complexes of the elbow. Therefore, forearm rotation is almost entirely the result of the radius circumscribing an arc about the stable ulna. Biomechanically, the axis of rotation of the forearm passes through a tightly defined area at the caput ulnae near the point of insertion of the triangular fibrocartilage complex (TFCC), known as the fovea. In the proximal forearm, the axis passes through the radial head/neck area.

In addition to rotation of the radius about the ulna, there is longitudinal translation of the forearm bones. Furthermore, tracing the pattern of force transmission from the wrist to the elbow is a critical exercise in understanding forearm axis mechanics. An understanding of the anatomy of the IOL and diaphyseal forearm bone structure is critical.

Specific Forearm Axis Injuries

Galeazzi Fractures A diaphyseal fracture of the radius near the junction of the middle and distal thirds accompanied by disruption of the DRUJ is known as a Galeazzi fracture (Fig. 8). In the adult, this injury is treated almost exclusively by ORIF of the radius, followed by assessment and appropriate treatment of the DRUJ lesion. Closed treatment of the joint in relative supination provides a position of stability for healing of the soft-tissue injuries at the DRUJ in most cases. Unfortunately, not all joints are reducible or stable after the radius is treated. The DRUJ component of this injury can take several forms. A fracture at the basilar region of the ulnar styloid, an ulnar-sided TFC avulsion, or a rare radial-sided disruption can all represent destabilizing injuries to the DRUJ.

After anatomic reduction and fixation of the radius, the DRUJ is tested with an anteroposterior displacement of the radius on the ulna and compared to the other side. Other indicators of persistent DRUJ disruption on radiographic assessment include ulnar styloid fracture through the fovea or basistyloid region, widening of the DRUJ on the posteroanterior view, dislocation of DRUJ on the lateral view, and more than 5 mm of radial shortening compared to the

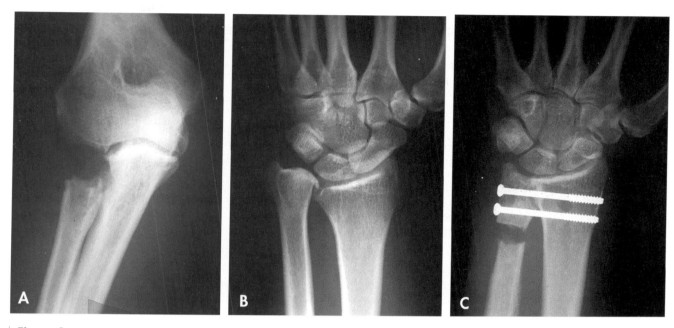

Figure 9

A, Radiograph of the elbow after excision of the radial head in an unrecognized Essex-Lopresti fracture-dislocation. B, The distal radioulnar joint (DRUJ) relationship had been altered by the proximal migration of the radius, and DRUJ degenerative change is noted. C, A Sauvé-Kapandji procedure was elected to treat this global forearm axis problem.

contralateral side. If instability is present and does not reduce with positioning in supination, then pinning or open repair of the bony and soft-tissue elements of the DRUJ disruption may be required.

Monteggia Lesion A proximal fracture of the ulna with associated injury to the lateral compartment of the elbow is termed a Monteggia lesion. The typical elbow injury is a radial head dislocation, but a variety of bony and soft-tissue injuries can fall under this heading.

Precise alignment of the length and angular relation of the ulnar fracture restores the proximal center of rotation of the forearm axis and usually relocates the radial head. After ulnar fixation, forearm rotation should be assessed with special attention to the radiocapitellar joint and the DRUJ. In a minority of cases, open treatment of the radial head dislocation will be required. A type IV Monteggia lesion manifests as an ulnar fracture and a radius fracture at the same level; fixation of both bones is usually necessary.

Essex-Lopresti Fracture-Dislocation The Essex-Lopresti frac-

ture-dislocation is a global disruption of the entire forearm axis. This lesion involves structures at the proximal and distal radioulnar joints, the radiocapitellar joint, and along the entire IOL. Radial head fracture is often the herald for more significant forearm injury although it can also result from valgus overload injuries at the elbow. Clinically, patients will have pain at the wrist and elbow in addition to tenderness to palpation and rotation throughout the forearm.

The treatment of the Essex-Lopresti lesion is predicated on recognition of the extensive nature of the injury. One of the biggest mistakes that can be made is excision of the radial head; this will result in unrestricted proximal migration of the radius (Fig. 9). Maintenance of the radial head or suitable replacement with a biologic or nonbiologic spacer is crucial to the alignment of other structures. Reconstruction at the DRUJ may also be indicated. Investigators are developing techniques to reconstruct the IOL, but more work is needed before definitive treatment can be recommended. For the chronic forearm axis disruption, treatment options range from methods to address focal pathology at each level to creation of a 1-bone forearm.

Annotated Bibliography

Distal Humerus, Capitellum, and Radial Head Fractures

Amis AA, Miller JH: The mechanisms of elbow fractures: An investigation using impact tests in vitro. *Injury* 1995;26: 163–168.

Impact loading studies on cadaveric elbows demonstrate how elbow flexion position can predict elbow fractures. Radial head and coronoid fractures followed impact up to 80°. Olecranon fractures occur by direct impact around 90°. Distal humerus fractures occurred above 110°.

Arcalis Arce A, Marti Garin D, Molero Garcia V, Pedemonte Jansana J: Treatment of radial head fractures using a fibrin adhesive seal: A review of 15 cases. *J Bone Joint Surg* 1995; 77B:422–424.

Fifteen patients with Mason II radial head fractures were treated with open reduction and Fibrin Adhesive System. At 2.3-year follow-up, all had excellent functional results, although 1 had 40° loss of extension.

Byrd JW: Elbow arthroscopy for arthrofibrosis after type I radial head fractures. *Arthroscopy* 1994;10:162–165.

Five cases of arthrofibrosis following Mason I radial head fractures were treated with arthroscopic debridement with an average 66% increase in flexion, extension, and total ROM at 24-month follow-up.

Cobb TK, Morrey BF: Acute elbow fractures treated with total elbow arthroplasty. *Orthop Trans* 1996;20:152–153.

Twenty-one acute distal humerus fractures in patients with an average of age 72 years were treated with total elbow arthroplasty. Forty-eight percent had rheumatoid arthritis. At 3.3-year follow-up, there were 15 excellent and 5 good functional results. Implant survival was 95%.

Davidson PA, Moseley JB Jr, Tullos HS: Radial head fracture: A potentially complex injury. *Clin Orthop* 1993;297:224–230.

In a series of 50 radial head fractures subjected to stress radiographs, all comminuted fractures had instability to valgus or axial stress; all displaced vertical shear type fractures had some injury to the MCL; and all minimally or nondisplaced fractures were stable.

Esser RD, Davis S, Taavao T: Fractures of the radial head treated by internal fixation: Late results in 26 cases. *J Orthop Trauma* 1995;9:318–323.

Twenty-six patients with displaced radial head fractures were evaluated 7.3 years after ORIF. Good or excellent functional results were obtained in all Mason II and III radial head fractures. Four of 6 Mason IV radial head fractures had good or excellent functional results.

Hirvensalo E, Bostman O, Partio E, Tormala P, Rokkanen P: Fracture of the humeral capitellum fixed with absorbable polyglycolide pins: 1-year follow-up of 8 adults. *Acta Orthop Scand* 1993;64:85–86.

Eight type I capitellum fractures were treated with multiple 2-mm polyglycolide pins. All healed with no hardware failures and 1 sterile synovitis that spontaneously resolved.

Hotchkiss RN: Displaced fractures of the radial head: Internal fixation or excision? *J Am Acad Orthop Surg* 1997;5:1–10.

This review article outlines the treatment of displaced radial head fractures. Type II fractures might be amenable to ORIF. Type III fractures are usually too comminuted for ORIF, but the importance of restoration of the radiocapitellar buttress is highlighted, particularly with disruption of the IOL.

Jacobson SR, Glisson RR, Urbaniak JR: A comparison of distal humerus fracture fixation: A biomechanical study. *Orthop Trans* 1995;19:425.

Biomechanical comparison of 5 methods of distal humerus fixation determined that multiple plate constructs, even triple plating, offer significantly less bending stiffness than the intact specimen, particularly in the sagittal plane.

Judet T, Garreau de Loubresse C, Piriou P, Charnley G: A floating prosthesis for radial-head fractures. *J Bone Joint Surg* 1996; 78B:244–249.

Twelve patients with Mason III radial head fractures were treated with a modular, floating, chrome-cobalt and polyethylene bipolar-like prosthesis. There were 3 excellent, 7 good, and 2 fair results at 49-month follow-up.

Knight DJ, Rymaszewski LA, Amis AA, Miller JH: Primary replacement of the fractured radial head with a metal prosthesis. *J Bone Joint Surg* 1993;75B:572–576.

Thirty-one comminuted radial head fractures were treated with Vitalium radial head prostheses. At follow-up of 4.5 years, 2 patients had proximal migration of the radius. There were no dislocations. All had functional ROM with good pain relief. Two were removed for loosening.

Koval KJ, Pereles T, Rosen H: Open reduction and internal fixation of the distal humerus: Functional outcome in the elderly. *Orthop Trans* 1995;19:163.

Nineteen distal humerus fractures in patients with a mean age of 71 years were treated with ORIF. At 3.7-year follow-up, there were 25% excellent and 75% good results.

McKee MD, Jupiter JB, Bamberger HB: Coronal shear fractures of the distal end of the humerus. *J Bone Joint Surg* 1996; 78A:49–54.

Six patients (average age 38 years) sustained a coronal shear fracture involving the capitellum and a portion of the trochlea. All were treated with ORIF. At 22-month follow-up, 3 had excellent and 3 had good functional results.

Ochner RS, Bloom H, Palumbo RC, Coyle MP: Closed reduction of coronal fractures of the capitellum. *J Trauma* 1996;40: 199–203.

Nine patients with displaced fractures of the capitellum were treated with closed reduction and splinting. All obtained functional ROM at final follow-up.

Sellman DC, Seitz WH Jr, Postak PD, Greenwald AS: Reconstructive strategies for radioulnar dissociation: A biomechanical study. *J Orthop Trauma* 1995;9:516–522.

This biomechanical study demonstrated that in forearms with disrupted interosseous membranes, reconstruction with a silicone radial head prosthesis is insufficient, but titanium radial head or interosseous membrane reconstruction restored stiffness to near normal.

Smith GR, Hotchkiss RN: Internal fixation of radial head and neck fractures: Intraoperative determination of proper hardware location. *Orthop Trans* 1995;19:33.

Cadaveric elbow dissection determined the 110° nonarticulating segment termed the "safe zone" could be estimated by marking the radial head through a lateral exposure at full pronation, neutral, and full supination. The anterior limit of the safe zone is two thirds the distance from the neutral to the supinated mark. The posterior limit is halfway between the neutral and pronated marks.

Szabo RM, Hotchkiss RN, Slater RR Jr: The use of frozen-allograft radial head replacement for treatment of established symptomatic proximal translation of the radius: Preliminary experience in five cases. *J Hand Surg* 1997;22A:269–278.

Five patients with symptomatic proximal translation of the radius after radial head excision were implanted with frozen-allograft radial heads. At 3-year follow-up, all had pain relief and improved forearm rotation and wrist motion. One required revision.

Unsworth-White J, Koka R, Churchill M, D'Arcy JC, James SE: The non-operative management of radial head fractures: A randomized trial of three treatments. *Injury* 1994;25:165–167.

Ninety-eight Mason I and II radial head fractures were randomized into 3 treatment regimens: immediate motion, immobilization in 90° cast for 2 weeks, and immobilization in extension cast for 2 weeks. At 25-month follow-up, there was no difference between immediate mobilization and 2 weeks of initial casting. Patients with 90° flexion casting had reduced ROM and more pain than those with extension casting.

Wong DK, Low W: Elbow fracture dislocations: Assessment of stability and correlation with outcome. *Orthop Trans* 1995;19: 258–259.

Seventeen elbows with radial head fractures and elbow dislocations were treated with ORIF. Two thirds of patients had satisfactory results. Five patients had instability and poor results.

Olecranon Fractures

King GJ, Lammens PN, Milne AD, Roth JH, Johnson JA: Plate fixation of comminuted olecranon fractures: An in vitro biomechanical study. *J Shoulder Elbow Surg* 1996;5:437–441.

This cadaveric study demonstrated no difference between the stability of dorsal and lateral ulnar plating; both should provide stability sufficient for early motion.

Morrey BF: Current concepts in the treatment of fractures of the radial head, the olecranon, and the coronoid. *J Bone Joint Surg* 1995;77A:316–327.

This is an excellent review of the current concepts concerning these injuries.

Paremain GP, Novak VP, Jinnah RH, Belkoff SM: Biomechanical evaluation of tension band placement for the repair of olecranon fractures. *Clin Orthop* 1997;335:325–330.

This cadaveric study confirms there is no difference between AO tension band technique and a modified AO technique with anterior placement of wire.

Simpson NS, Goodman LA, Jupiter JB: Contoured LCDC plating of the proximal ulna. *Injury* 1996;27:411–417.

In this clinical study of 37 comminuted fractures of the proximal ulna using a limited contact titanium plate applied dorsally with a 90° bend around proximal tip, there were good or excellent results in 27 patients at 2-year follow-up.

Skak SV: Fracture of the olecranon through a persistent physis in an adult: A case report. *J Bone Joint Surg* 1993;75A:272–275.

In this case report, excision of the physis and tension band repair were required to achieve successful union. The contralateral side also had a persistent physis.

Turtel AH, Andrews JR, Schob CJ, Kupferman SP, Gross AE: Fractures of unfused olecranon physis: A re-evaluation of this injury in three athletes. *Orthopedics* 1995;18:390–394.

In this review of 3 olecranon physeal fractures requiring surgical treatment, 1 patient with a chronic injury was bone grafted; a stable fibrous union was achieved in the other 2 cases following ORIF.

Elbow Dislocations

Cobb TK, Morrey BF: Use of distraction arthroplasty in unstable fracture dislocations of the elbow. *Clin Orthop* 1995;312: 201–210.

The authors report 6 of 7 cases with satisfactory results following treatment with a hinged joint distraction device for extremely unstable elbow dislocations associated with coronoid fractures. The device maintains joint reduction while allowing early motion.

334 Upper Extremity

Cole RJ, Jemison DM, Hayes CW: Anterior elbow dislocation following medial epicondylectomy: A case report. *J Hand Surg* 1994;19A:614–616.

The authors report an unusual complication following a large medial epicondylectomy for ulnar neuritis.

Kharrazi FD, Rodgers WB, Waters PM, Koris MJ: Dislocation of the elbow complicated by arterial injury: Reconstructive strategy and functional outcome. *Am J Orthop* 1995;(suppl):11–15.

Four cases of arterial injury complicating posterior dislocation of the elbow are presented. Three also had neurologic deficits and impending compartment syndromes. All extremities remained well perfused with stable joints following joint and vascular repair, but cold intolerance and persistent nerve deficits were a long-term problem. Arterial reconstruction is recommended in these cases.

Morrey BF: Acute and chronic instability of the elbow. *J Am Acad Orthop Surg* 1996;4:117–128.

This is a concise summary of the current concepts of the evaluation, diagnosis, and treatment of these injuries.

Rodgers WB, Kharrazi FD, Waters PM, Kennedy JG, McKee MD, Lhowe DW: The use of osseous suture anchors in the treatment of severe, complicated elbow dislocations. *Am J Orthop* 1996; 25:794–798.

Seventeen patients with severe dislocation or fracture-dislocation of the elbow underwent surgical soft-tissue attachment with suture anchors; 5 patients were also treated with a hinged external fixator. All elbows were stable at follow-up, with 88% good or excellent results.

Coronoid Fractures

Cage DJ, Abrams RA, Callahan JJ, Botte MJ: Soft tissue attachments of the ulnar coronoid process: An anatomic study with radiographic correlation. *Clin Orthop* 1995;320:154–158.

This cadaveric study demonstrates locations of insertion of joint capsule, MCL, and brachialis onto the coronoid process. Only in type III coronoid fractures are the brachialis and MCL insertions attached to the fragment.

Liu SH, Henry M, Bowen R: Complications of type I coronoid fractures in competitive athletes: Report of two cases and review of the literature. *J Shoulder Elbow Surg* 1996;5:223–227.

The authors describe rare cases of persistent elbow pain following type I coronoid fractures. Both responded to arthroscopic intervention.

Regan W, Morrey BF: Classification and treatment of coronoid process fractures. Orthopedics 1992;15:845–848.

The originators of the 3-part coronoid fracture classification system

Forearm Axis

Birkbeck DP, Failla JM, Hoshaw SJ, Fyhrie DP, Schaffler M: The interosseous membrane affects load distribution in the forearm. *J Hand Surg* 1997;22A:975–980.

This clinical study of load transfer from distal to proximal and from radius to ulna in 5 specimens demonstrates that the IOL has significant function when intact to transfer longitudinal load.

De Boeck H, Haentjens P, Handelberg F, Casteleyn PP, Opdecam D: Treatment of isolated distal ulnar shaft fractures with below-elbow plaster cast. *Arch Orthop Trauma Surg* 1996;115: 316–320.

Prospective analysis of 52 patients treated with below elbow immobilization for ulnar diaphysis fracture resulted in 89% primary union rate and good to excellent return of forearm motion. No identifiable cause for nonunion in 2 patients could be found from clinical criteria.

Hollister AM, Gellman H, Waters RL: The relationship of the interosseous membrane to the axis of rotation of the forearm. *Clin Orthop* 1994;298:272–276.

This anatomic study uses an axis finder instrument to assess the forearm axis both proximally and distally. The relation of the IOL is analyzed in relation to this axis of rotation.

Jupiter JB, Kour AK, Richards RR, Nathan J, Meinhard B: The floating radius in bipolar fracture-dislocation of the forearm. *J Orthop Trauma* 1994;8:99–106.

Treatment methods are described for 10 patients with various patterns of soft-tissue and bony lesions. The essential injury pattern described results in the radius "floating" away from its usual constraint of the ulna. Careful anatomic reduction of the lesion of bone and repair of the soft tissues resulted in excellent motion. The chief residual deformity was DRUJ instability in 6 patients.

Schemitsch EH, Jones D, Henley B, Tencer AF: A comparison of malreduction after plate and intramedullary nail fixation of forearm fractures. *J Orthop Trauma* 1995;9:8–16.

Eight matched pairs of forearm bones were subjected to osteotomy followed by fixation with plates, intramedullary (IM) nails, or a combination thereof. Gaps were created in some specimens with fixation. Radial bow was quantified. Plate fixation created constructs with the most exact reconstruction of radial bow; however, IM rod fixation of one bone and plating of the other gave the same indices. Minimal but measurable and significant loss of radial bow occurred when both bones were treated with IM rods.

Sellman DC, Seitz WH Jr, Postak PD, Greenwald AS: Reconstructive strategies for radioulnar dissociation: A biomechanical study. *J Orthop Trauma* 1995;9:516–522.

This laboratory study demonstrates little resistance to proximal migration of the radius when a silicone radial head is used. Titanium radial heads and a flexible IOL reconstruction provide ample longitudinal stability. An excellent anatomic description of the IOL exposure is included in this article.

Skahen JR III, Palmer AK, Werner FW, Fortino MD: The interosseous membrane of the forearm: Anatomy and function. *J Hand Surg* 1997;22A:981–985.

This is an anatomic study of 20 forearm specimens with resultant strain analysis of the central band of the IOM (IOL). Radial head removal consistently increased strain in the IOL.

Trousdale RT, Linscheid RL: Operative treatment of malunited fractures of the forearm. *J Bone Joint Surg* 1995;77A:894–902.

Corrective osteotomy in 20 patients for loss of motion associated with forearm bone malunion was studied. Correction in malunions less than 1 year old resulted in greater rotation return than later correction.

Classic Bibliography

An K-N, Morrey BF, Chao EY: The effect of partial removal of proximal ulna on elbow constraint. *Clin Orthop* 1986;209:270–279.

Anderson LD, Sisk D, Tooms RE, Park WI III: Compression-plate fixation in acute diaphyseal fractures of the radius and ulna. *J Bone Joint Surg* 1975;57A:287–297.

Bado JL: The Monteggia lesion. *Clin Orthop* 1967;50:71–86.

Broberg MA, Morrey BF: Results of delayed excision of the radial head after fracture. *J Bone Joint Surg* 1986;68A:669–674.

Bryan RS, Morrey BF: Fractures of the distal humerus, in Morrey BF (ed): *The Elbow and Its Disorders*. Philadelphia, PA, WB Saunders, 1985, pp 302–339.

Chapman MW, Gordon JE, Zissimos AG: Compression-plate fixation of acute fractures of the diaphyses of the radius and ulna. *J Bone Joint Surg* 1989;71A:159–169.

Edwards GS Jr, Jupiter JB: Radial head fractures with acute distal radioulnar dislocation: Essex-Lopresti revisited. *Clin Orthop* 1988;234:61–69.

Essex-Lopresti P: Fractures of the radial head with distal radio-ulnar dislocation: Report of two cases. *J Bone Joint Surg* 1951;33B:244–247.

Fleetcroft JP: Abstract: Fractures of the radial head: Early aspiration and mobilisation. *J Bone Joint Surg* 1984;66B:141–142.

Gartsman GM, Sculco TP, Otis JC: Operative treatment of olecranon fractures: Excision or open reduction with internal fixation. *J Bone Joint Surg* 1981;63A:718–721.

Geel CW, Palmer AK: Radial head fractures and their effect on the distal radioulnar joint: A rationale for treatment. *Clin Orthop* 1992;275:79–84.

Hotchkiss RN, An KN, Sowa DT, Basta S, Weiland AJ: An anatomic and mechanical study of the interosseous membrane of the forearm: Pathomechanics of proximal migration of the radius. *J Hand Surg* 1989;14A:256–261.

Josefsson PO, Gentz CF, Johnell O, Wendeberg B: Surgical versus non-surgical treatment of ligamentous injuries following dislocation of the elbow joint: A prospective randomized study. *J Bone Joint Surg* 1987;69A:605–608.

Josefsson PO, Johnell O, Gentz CF: Long-term sequelae of simple dislocation of the elbow. *J Bone Joint Surg* 1984;66A:927–930.

Mason ML: Some observations on fractures of the head of the radius with a review of one hundred cases. *Br J Surg* 1954;42:123–132.

Regan W, Morrey B: Fractures of the coronoid process of the ulna. *J Bone Joint Surg* 1989;71A:1348–1354.

Schemitsch EH, Richards RR: The effect of malunion on functional outcome after plate fixation of fractures of both bones of the forearm in adults. *J Bone Joint Surg* 1992;74A:1068–1078.

Wolfgang G, Burke F, Bush D, et al: Surgical treatment of displaced olecranon fractures by tension band wiring technique. *Clin Orthop* 1987;224:192–204.

Chapter 31
Elbow Reconstruction

Diagnostic Studies

A careful history and physical examination with plain radiographs are sufficient for diagnosis and treatment of most elbow disorders. Magnetic resonance imaging (MRI) has emerged as a popular adjunctive diagnostic test for elbow pathologies. It is very important to identify the exact indication for MRI to justify the high cost. Its most distinctive advantage over other imaging modalities is in evaluation of the soft tissues about the elbow. MRI is useful for detection and localization of tears of the medial collateral ligament (MCL), and it can be used for accurate detection of distal biceps tendon avulsion. In a recent clinical study, MRI of 21 patients clinically suspected to have distal biceps tendon injury showed 100% agreement with surgical findings.

Furthermore, certain bone and cartilage injuries that cannot be seen in plain radiographs or even computed tomography can be detected by MRI, which can be done in the presence of a cast without decrement of the image quality. Stress fractures of the middle third of the olecranon in throwing athletes, physeal injury, osteochondritis dissecans of the capitellum, and loose bodies can also be accurately detected and evaluated by MRI.

Biomechanics and Kinematics

The elbow is a tricompartmental joint with 2 degrees of freedom: flexion-extension and pronation-supination. The normal range of motion at the ulnotrochlear joint is

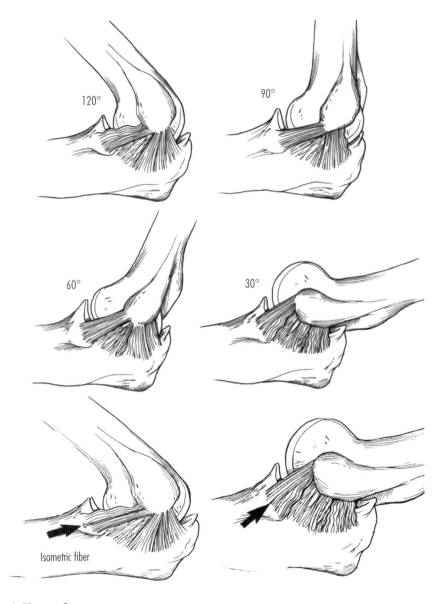

Figure 1

The anatomy of the medial collateral ligament of the elbow at 120°, 90°, 60°, and 30° of flexion. (Reproduced with permission of the Mayo Foundation, Rochester, MN.)

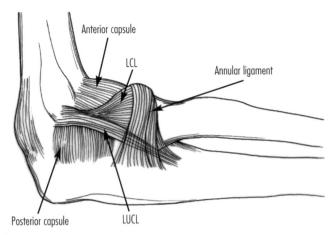

Figure 2

Lateral collateral ligament (LCL) complex of the elbow. LUCL; lateral ulnar collateral ligament. (Reproduced with permission of the Mayo Foundation, Rochester, MN.)

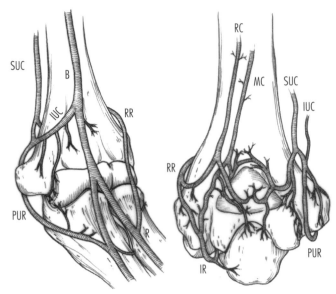

Figure 3

Vascular anatomy of the elbow. SUC, superior ulnar collateral branch; IUC, inferior ulnar collateral branch; PUR, posterior ulnar recurrent artery; B, brachial artery; RR, radial recurrent artery; IR, intraosseous recurrent artery; RC, radial collateral artery; MC, middle collateral artery. (Reproduced with permission of the Mayo Foundation, Rochester, MN.)

from 0° to 150°, while it is 75° pronation and 85° supination at the radiocapitellar joint. The elbow axis of rotation in flexion and extension lies in the line drawn from the lateral epicondyle to the anteroinferior medial epicondyle, anterior to the midline of the humerus. With the elbow in extension, 60% of joint reactive force distributes across the radiocapitellar joint while the other 40% transmits across the ulnotrochlear joint.

The MCL (medial or ulnar collateral ligament) is an important valgus stabilizer of the elbow. It is composed of anterior and posterior bundles, and a transverse ligament. The anterior bundle, which is the primary valgus stabilizer of the elbow, spans from the inferior surface of the medial epicondyle to the medial coronoid. This anterior bundle is further divided into anterior and posterior bands. The anterior band is the primary restraint to valgus stress at 30°, 60°, and 90° of flexion and is a co-primary restraint at 120° of flexion (Fig. 1). An electromyographic analysis of the muscles of the flexor-pronator group showed no increase in activity in pitchers with MCL deficiency. Thus, dynamic contribution of the flexor-pronator mass to the medial stability of the elbow is questionable.

The lateral collateral ligament (LCL) complex plays a major role in elbow instability, especially in the presence of rotational stresses. This complex is composed of the radial collateral ligament (or LCL), the lateral ulnar collateral ligament (LUCL), the annular ligament, the accessory collateral ligament, and the elbow capsule. Incompetence of the LUCL has been implicated in the development of posterolateral rotatory instability (Fig. 2). When the contribution of the LUCL was compared to that of the LCL in a cadaveric study, isolated sectioning of the LUCL alone produced only minor laxity. Hence, it is likely that the LCL complex provides elbow stability as a constellation of structures rather than as discreet bands that are easily separated anatomically or functionally.

Anatomy/Vascular Approaches

The extraosseous vascular anatomy about the elbow can be organized into 3 vascular arcades. A medial arcade is formed from the superior and inferior ulnar collateral branches of the brachial arteries, which form an anastomosis with the posterior and anterior ulnar recurrent arteries. A lateral arcade is formed from the radial collateral, radial recurrent, and intraosseous recurrent arteries, while a posterior arcade is formed from the medial and lateral arcades and middle collateral arteries. The olecranon is well vascularized from both medial and lateral vessels. The radial head depends on a single branch of the radial recurrent artery. The capitellum and lateral trochlea are supplied primarily by posterior vessels from the radial arcade. Posterior dissection on the lateral distal humerus may compromise osseous blood supply, whereas posterior dissection on the medial side is less likely to have vascular consequences (Fig. 3).

Surgical Exposures

The posterior approach has proven to be a safe and comprehensive surgical exposure for most reconstructive procedures. After posterior skin incision, a posteromedial or posterolateral arthrotomy can be performed to gain access to the joint. The elbow joint can be exposed by several different routes of deep dissection. A triceps-sparing approach elevates the triceps and varying amounts of the lateral extensor mass off the proximal ulna from medial to lateral. This approach can be used for nearly all intra-articular pathologies of the elbow with the exception of anterior neurovascular obstruction. Access to the anterior aspect of the joint can be gained by medial, lateral, or transhumeral (Outerbridge-Kashiwagi ulnohumeral arthroplasty) routes. More limited access for focal pathology can be obtained medially with the "over the top" exposure, or laterally with the "column approach." The medial approach exploits the interval between the flexor carpi ulnaris and the remainder of the flexor-pronator mass anteriorly; the ulnar nerve is easily controlled, yet access to the radial head is limited through the "over the top" approach. The "column" exposure is a more limited lateral arthrotomy made after either a posterior or direct lateral skin incision. The extensor carpi radialis longus and brevis origins are released from the lateral supracondylar ridge and dissection is carried medially between the joint capsule and deep surface of the brachialis to expose the anterior compartment of the elbow joint. Both these limited exposures can be converted to a full triceps-sparing approach if necessary. The Kocher lateral approach can still be used for more limited pathology of the lateral elbow, including radial compartment problems and limited capsulectomy.

A muscle-splitting approach has been proposed for repair or reconstruction of the MCL. The traditional approach has been to elevate the common flexor origin from the medial epicondyle. The site of the muscle-splitting is at the raphe between the flexor carpi ulnaris and palmaris longus muscles superficially and the flexor carpi ulnaris and flexor digitorum superficialis muscles slightly deeper. The distal extension of incision should be less than 1 cm from the sublime tubercle (insertion of MCL) to minimize the risk of injury to the branches of the ulnar and median nerves. In 22 patients who underwent surgical repair or reconstruction of the MCL, no patient had any clinical evidence of neuropathy. It is thought that this approach is less traumatic than the dissection about the flexor-pronator origin (Fig. 4).

The vulnerability of the posterior interosseous nerve (PIN) is well recognized during surgical approaches to the proximal forearm and elbow. The average distance between the PIN and the most prominent point of the bicipital tuberosity of the radius was 2.3 cm (range, 1.8 to 3.2 cm). This distance was not affected by forearm rotation. Therefore, palpation of the bicipital tuberosity is a reliable guide to the position of the PIN.

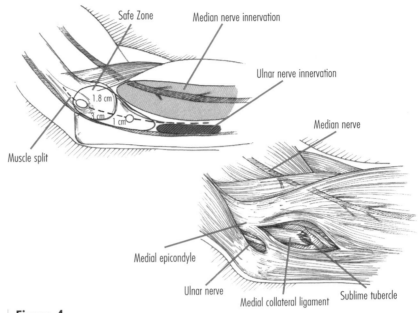

Figure 4

The muscle-splitting approach to the medial collateral ligament. The safe zone for the approach is shown. (Reproduced with permission of the Mayo Foundation, Rochester, MN.)

Arthroscopy

The role of elbow arthroscopy has been expanded not only as a valuable diagnostic tool, but also as a minimally invasive primary treatment modality for various pathologies. The indications for arthroscopy of the elbow include diagnosis of intra-articular pathology, removal of loose bodies and osteophytes, debridement of osteochondritis dissecans and synovitis, olecranon tip excision for impingement, limited assisted open reduction and internal fixation, radial head excision, arthroscopic ulnohumeral arthroplasty, and capsular release.

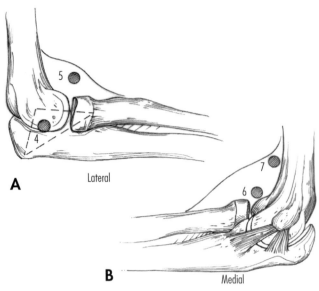

Figure 5

Arthroscopy portals. A, Lateral view shows the anterior superior lateral portal (5) located directly over the radial capitellar joint approximately 2 cm anterior to the lateral epicondyle. An additional portal, the proximal anterior lateral site (not shown in this figure) is positioned 2 cm proximal and 1 cm anterior to the lateral epicondyle and allows the greatest safe distance from the radial nerve. The straight lateral portal (4) lies at the center of a triangle between the olecranon tip, radial head, and lateral epicondyle. B, A medial view shows the proximal anterior medial portal (7) lying 2 cm proximal to the medial epicondyle and just anterior to the intermuscular septum. The anterior medial portal (6) is positioned 2 cm distal and 2 cm anterior to the medial epicondyle. (Reproduced with permission of the Mayo Foundation, Rochester, MN.)

A thorough understanding of portal anatomy is crucial to avoid injury to neurovascular structures (Fig. 5). Medial approaches, such as the proximal anteromedial and the anteromedial portals, lie close to the ulnar nerve and the medial antebrachial cutaneous nerve, respectively. Three lateral portals have been described. When these lateral portals were compared in a cadaveric study, the proximal anterolateral portal, located 2 cm proximal and 1 cm anterior to the lateral epicondyle, had the farthest safe distance from the radial nerve (7.9 mm in extension and 13.7 mm in flexion).

The arthroscopic release of posttraumatic arthrofibrosis has been examined in recent studies. One study showed an average 30° (from 41° to 11°) increase in extension after arthroscopic release. Adequate elbow distension and a position of flexion increase the margin of safety; however, arthrofibrosis limits capsular extensibility and reduces the interval distance to neurovascular structures. Thus, when the capsule is closer to the bony anatomy as seen in arthrofibrosis, the corresponding safe distance is dramatically reduced. It can be as little as 6 mm for both the median and radial nerves. The

arthroscopic debridement of anterior adhesions has resulted in at least 1 reported case of median nerve injury.

Elbow Instability

Medial Collateral Ligament Injury/Insufficiency

Soft-tissue injury to the medial aspect of the elbow typically results from a valgus stress injury. The association between lateral compartment elbow pathology, particularly radial head fracture, and medial collateral injury is well recognized. Careful examination of the MCL must accompany recognition of radial head/capitellar fracture. Repair or reconstruction of the lateral compartment injury is usually sufficient to promote healing of the MCL insufficiency.

Lateral Collateral Ligament Complex Injury/Insufficiency

Acute isolated injury to the LCL complex due to a supination, axial compression stress injury is rare and can typically be treated nonsurgically. Long arm immobilization in relative forearm pronation for 3 weeks is recommended, followed by protected flexion and extension in a hinged splint.

There is an emerging appreciation of chronic posttraumatic incompetence of the LUCL resulting in posterolateral rotatory instability. Physical examination may show tenderness over the lateral aspect of the joint and a mechanical element with apprehension when the lateral pivot shift test is executed. The lateral elbow pivot shift maneuver is difficult to perform, especially in the awake patient; examination under anesthesia may be necessary to confirm the diagnosis. For chronic, symptomatic posterolateral rotating instability, the reconstruction of the LUCL with a palmaris longus tendon graft through specifically designed drill holes is recommended for the treatment. The Kocher's approach is used for the exposure, and the tendon graft is placed from the base of the tubercle of the crista supinatoris to the isometric point of the lateral epicondyle. The tendon graft is secured through the bone tunnels created in both ends and sutured with the elbow in 30° of flexion. Postoperative care is similar to the treatment for the acute injury. The procedure has restored stability in 90% of patients. However, the satisfaction from the surgery can be affected by the presence or absence of degenerative changes in the elbow.

Contracture and Ankylosis

The elbow is one of the most constrained joints in the body. Any alteration of the bony or soft-tissue anatomy has the potential to compromise elbow motion. Contractures of the elbow are classified as intrinsic or extrinsic. Extrinsic contractures result from periarticular soft-tissue contracture, heterotopic bone formation, or extra-articular bony deformity. Intrinsic contractures result from intra-articular pathology, including articular adhesions, or intra-articular deformity and degenerative changes. Extra-articular contractures typically accompany intrinsic contractures. The articular surface is generally spared in the extrinsic type, even when extra-articular heterotopic ossification eliminates elbow motion.

The most effective treatment of contractures is preventing their occurrence. Early motion requires stability of the elbow, a congruous articular relationship, and adequate pain relief. If pain precludes early motion, intermittent regional anesthesia or an indwelling catheter is helpful in managing pain and allowing early motion. In the motivated patient, a home therapy program of active and active-assisted exercises is usually sufficient to regain a functional arc of motion. If passive motion is instituted, it must be gentle and focused. Motion loss identified early (3 to 12 months) can be improved with adjustable flexion-extension splints. Most meaningful improvements in motion come in the first 6 months.

Splinting programs for stiffness take advantage of the viscoelastic properties of tissue. Dynamic splints apply a constant load to tissues and take advantage of tissue creep to achieve their desired effect. They require extended periods of time and can be painful for the patient to wear. This continued stress might actually inflame contracted tissues and worsen the stiffness cycle. Conversely, serial static elbow splints use the principles of stress relaxation to achieve their effect (Fig. 6). Contracted tissues held stationary at a point of mild tissue tension will accommodate this lengthened position. These splints are well tolerated by the patient. Loss of forearm rotation is much more problematic and difficult to treat both nonsurgically and surgically.

Surgical management of the stiff elbow depends on the degree and etiology of intrinsic and extrinsic contractures. Preoperative evaluation includes a careful history, physical examination (to record motion arcs, end-point quality, and a contralateral comparison), and radiographic evaluation. Special radiographic studies including tomography or MRI scans are very useful in assessing the extent of heterotopic bone and the degree of articular damage. When a surgical course is selected, the approach for release depends on the etiology of contracture, the location of the pathology, and additional factors related to tissue quality, location of old scars, and prior procedures.

A posterior skin incision is a utilitarian approach for most releases, including access to the medial and lateral sides of the elbow. A limited lateral approach is often adequate for limited anterior and posterior capsulectomy and surgery on the radiocapitellar joint. A medial exposure provides access to the ulnar nerve and coronoid process, in addition to the anterior and posterior capsules. A transhumeral approach to decompression of the olecranon and coronoid fossae, the Outerbridge-Kashiwagi ulnohumeral arthroplasty, is an innovative way to perform posterior and anterior surgery through a single posterior approach.

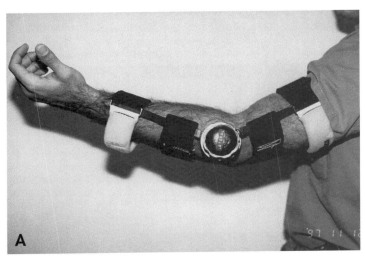
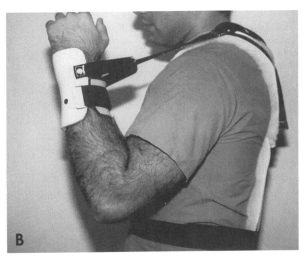

Figure 6

Static flexion-extension splints use stress relaxation of tissue to achieve their desired effect. An alternating stretching program in flexion and extension achieves the desired result. A, Obtaining flexion above 90° with the flexion extension brace is limited by the design of the brace. A hyperflexion brace (B) uses a forearm-based splint attached to a chest harness to gain flexion.

Arthroscopic capsular release for stiffness has shown promise in several studies but is a technically demanding procedure that requires extensive skill with arthroscopy of the elbow. Capsular volume is significantly reduced and is accompanied by a periarticular scar that can alter the normal anatomic relationship. Capsular release from the anterior humeral shaft minimizes risk to the neurovascular structures about the elbow. Dissection against the capsule can result in inadvertent violation of the capsule, placing the neurovascular structures at risk.

Arthritis

Osteoarthritis

Primary osteoarthritis of the elbow is a rare condition compared to posttraumatic degenerative arthritis, accounting for 1% to 2% of all patients presenting with elbow arthritis. Primary osteoarthritis typically occurs in men between the third and eighth decades who have a history of heavy manual labor or repetitive use of the extremity.

The earliest sign of primary osteoarthritis of the elbow is a mild flexion contracture. Pain, not loss of motion, typically prompts consultation with a physician. Pain at the extremes of motion is typical, especially at the limit of extension. Motion through the majority of the flexion-extension arc is not painful, because impingement at the limits is the typical etiology of the discomfort and limitation. Rarely, osteophytes from the medial aspect of the ulnohumeral joint can encroach on the ulnar nerve resulting in nerve compression.

The surgical management of primary osteoarthritis of the elbow depends on the degree of articular involvement and condition of the ulnar nerve. The Outerbridge-Kashiwagi ulnohumeral arthroplasty can be used for a posterior triceps splitting or triceps reflecting approach to remove osteophytes from the olecranon process, open the narrowed olecranon fossa, and remove the coronoid process osteophyte through the olecranon fossa with the elbow in extreme flexion (Fig. 7). It is easier to address ulnar nerve pathology through the posterior approach used for this procedure. If the ulnar nerve is not involved, debridement can be conducted through a lateral column approach to the anterior and posterior aspect of the elbow joint. The ulnar nerve must be located, particularly when debriding the posterior compartment. If the safety of the ulnar nerve cannot be guaranteed, a separate medial incision is suggested.

Posttraumatic Arthritis

All 3 articulations of the elbow (the ulnotrochlear, radiocapitellar, and proximal radioulnar) can manifest degenerative change after trauma. The most common posttraumatic arthritis of the elbow involves the ulnotrochlear joint following intra-articular fractures of the distal humerus. Damage to the articular surface is often accompanied by intrinsic and extrinsic contracture.

The treatment of advanced arthritis of the elbow in the young patient is an unsolved problem. The alternatives available tend to fall short in stability, pain relief, or longevity, especially in this population predominantly composed of young males. Two surgical alternatives that have been used are interposition arthroplasty and elbow replacement.

Interposition arthroplasty of the elbow with fascia, cutis, or allograft material is used when extensive articular destruction causes pain and limited motion. The concomitant soft-tissue

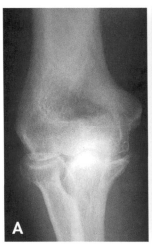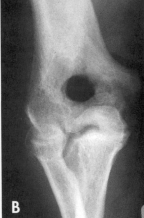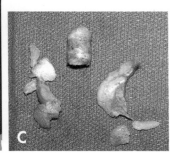

Figure 7

A, Anteroposterior view of an elbow with fracture deformity in the distal humeral shaft with near obliteration of the olecranon and coronoid fossae by osteophytosis and a posterior loose body. B, After performance of the Outerbridge-Kashiwagi (OK) ulnohumeral arthroplasty, the fossae are open to permit flexion and extension without impingement. C, The excised bone from a typical OK arthroplasty includes peripheral osteophytes, the tips of the coronoid and olecranon and a cylinder of bone from the area of the fossae. Note the thickness of this cylinder (middle, top) and recall that this aperture is typically thin or fenestrated.

releases required to mobilize and resurface the joint can result in instability. Application of a hinged elbow distractor allows early motion while providing joint alignment and stability after surgery.

Total elbow arthroplasty (TEA) for posttraumatic conditions of the elbow has traditionally been reserved for patients older than 60 years because of wear and loosening issues. Recent reports indicate that in carefully selected nongeriatric patients, TEA for posttraumatic destruction of the elbow joint can result in an excellent outcome.

Rheumatoid Arthritis

The elbow is involved in 20% of patients with rheumatoid arthritis. If optimal medical support and nonsurgical management of the rheumatoid elbow fail to control the patient's symptoms, surgery is considered. The options for surgical care include arthroscopic or open synovectomy, radial head resection, ulnohumeral resection arthroplasty, interposition arthroplasty, and TEA.

The role of synovectomy in the treatment of rheumatoid arthritis of the elbow has diminished as the success of TEA for this condition has improved. Synovectomy is useful in the early stages of rheumatoid arthritis for pain relief and slowing of joint destruction. Radial head excision can be combined with synovectomy when the lateral compartment and proximal radioulnar joints are major sources of pain. Open synovectomy through a single lateral incision allows access to the radial head as well as the anterior and posterior compartments of the joint.

Arthroscopic synovectomy allows full visualization of the joint and a more complete synovectomy. The risk of injury to neurovascular structures may limit the ability to perform a complete synovectomy. Transient nerve injuries have been reported following arthroscopic synovectomy. The short-term results of arthroscopic synovectomy are comparable to those of open techniques, but the results deteriorate over time. The success of TEA in patients with rheumatoid arthritis has resulted in its application in patients with advanced disease (stage III and IV).

Resection arthroplasty and interposition arthroplasty should be considered when advanced destruction of the ulnotrochlear joint exists. Resection arthroplasty can diminish pain, but it can also result in instability. Interposition arthroplasty is a variation on the joint resection that carries a similar risk-benefit profile.

The most common indication for TEA is rheumatoid arthritis. Experience with handling the changes associated with inflammatory arthropathy has been successful, especially since the advent of cemented semiconstrained prostheses.

Total Elbow Arthroplasty

Indications

Traditionally, TEA has been reserved for patients older than 60 years of age. The success of TEA in the elderly rheumatoid population has expanded the indications to carefully selected younger patients and those with posttraumatic disorders, including nonunion of the distal humerus, instability of the elbow, and acute comminuted fractures of the distal humerus in elderly patients with osteopenic bone. The only absolute contraindication for TEA is the presence of active infection.

Juvenile rheumatoid arthritis (JRA) patients have a predilection for stiffness, and severe bony deformities accompany their articular disease. TEA is technically challenging in this group of patients. Cemented semiconstrained implants have performed well without the need for custom implants. Pain relief is excellent, but improvement in motion is less predictable.

Implant Selection

Two general types of implants are available for TEA: unlinked, nonconstrained resurfacing implants and linked semiconstrained implants. Highly constrained implants have been abandoned as a result of a high incidence of loosening and implant failure. Bone loss, gross instability, stiffness (ankylosis), and need for extensive soft-tissue releases preclude the use of unlinked resurfacing implants. Semiconstrained implants offer more latitude for their use. They can be used for elbow replacement in any patient group, and they even perform well when extensive bone loss or soft-tissue compromise is present. The semiconstrained design has diminished the incidence of loosening, while motion and stability have been recovered even in cases of extreme elbow destruction.

Clinical Results

Excellent pain relief can be expected after TEA in over 90% of patients. Functional improvement can be equally dramatic when compared to preoperative levels. Achieving a functional range of motion should be expected following TEA, even in patients with significant preoperative limitations. Motion tends to be better following TEA with linked semiconstrained implants compared to unlinked resurfacing implants because the former allow aggressive soft-tissue release and rehabilitation without concern for instability.

Instability (recurrent dislocation and subluxation) as a postoperative complication of TEA is primarily isolated to the unlinked resurfacing implants. The rate of instability has been lower in recent reports (approximately 5% to 10%). Previous surgery on the elbow may influence the rate of instability following TEA with an unlinked resurfacing design. In a recent report of capitellocondylar (resurfacing) TEA, 22% of patients with previous open synovectomy experienced instability compared to none of the patients without previous surgery. This difference could be because of the aggressiveness of the disease process or the extent of prior soft-tissue dissection.

Linked semiconstrained implants eliminate the possibility of dislocation by physically coupling the humeral and ulnar components. Rotational and varus-valgus laxity allow the soft tissues to absorb the forces that tend to loosen the implant. In a study of semiconstrained TEA in patients with rheumatoid arthritis, there was no mechanical loosening at an average follow-up of 3.8 years.

The success of TEA has resulted in its application to younger patients. TEA should be considered in selected young patients only after all other nonsurgical and alternative surgical options have been considered. Experience is expanding with elbow replacement in the younger patient, because newer designs and fixation techniques may allow expansion of this procedure to this population of patients.

Complications

Complications of TEA include loosening, instability, ulnar nerve injury, triceps insufficiency, and problems with wound healing. Improved implant design and surgical technique have diminished the incidence of these complications. The application of TEA to younger patients with complex pathology and greater functional demands has resulted in a shift in the types of complications encountered. Increased physical demands on the implant and reliance on the prosthesis to align the unstable extremity have resulted in an increase in reports of mechanical failure.

A greater number of revision surgeries for prosthetic loosening with or without infection, periprosthetic fracture, mechanical failure of the implant, and implant instability are anticipated as the indications change to include the younger patient. Traditionally, failed TEA has been treated with resection arthroplasty or arthrodesis. Revision TEA for aseptic causes of failure has had good success but highlighted the demanding nature of this procedure and the potential for significant complications. Infection following TEA is a devastating complication. Management depends on the causative organism and fixation of the implants. Implant removal, aggressive debridement, and intravenous antibiotics should be used for all loose implants. The timing of staged reimplantation depends on the causative organism and demonstrated eradication of the infection. Removal of well-fixed implants can result in destruction of bone stock, making reimplanta-

tion difficult or impossible. In a recent study, no implants infected by *Staphylococcus epidermidis* were successfully salvaged by incision and drainage whereas 7 of 10 implants infected by other causative organisms were successfully salvaged.

Annotated Bibliography

Adolfsson L: Arthroscopy of the elbow joint: A cadaveric study of portal placement. *J Shoulder Elbow Surg* 1994;3:53–61.

The posterior antebrachial cutaneous nerve was found an average of 7 mm from the direct lateral and the anterolateral portal. The radial nerve was an average of 12 mm in the sagittal plane and 7 mm in the frontal plane from the anterolateral portal. The median antebrachial cutaneous nerve was an average of 4 mm from the low anteromedial and 6 mm from the high anteromedial portal. The combination of the low posterolateral, the direct lateral, and the high anteromedial portals provided the largest visualized area.

Byrd JW: Elbow arthroscopy for arthrofibrosis after type I radial head fractures. *Arthroscopy* 1994;10:162–165.

Arthroscopic debridement for arthrofibrosis after type I radial head fractures was performed in 5 patients with average follow-up of 24 months. When the arthroscopy was performed an average of 6 months postinjury, an average gain in extension was 30°.

Callaway GH, Field LD, Deng XH, et al: Biomechanical evaluation of the medial collateral ligament of the elbow. *J Bone Joint Surg* 1997;79A:1223–1231.

Anatomic and biomechanical evaluation of the MCL was performed in 10 fresh-frozen cadaveric elbows. The anterior bundle of the MCL should be examined carefully with the elbow flexed in 90°. The tendon graft for the reconstruction procedures should be placed from the inferior aspect of the medial epicondyle to the area of the sublimis tubercle to anatomically reproduce the anterior bundle of the MCL.

Field LD, Altchek DW: Evaluation of the arthroscopic valgus instability test of the elbow. *Am J Sports Med* 1996;24:177–181.

Complete release of the MCL led to significant increases in medial joint opening (4 to 10 mm). The medial opening was best visualized with the elbow flexed at 60° to 75°. The entire anterior bundle must be sectioned before measurable and reproducible valgus instability is noted.

Fitzgerald SW, Curry DR, Erickson SJ, Quinn SF, Friedman H: Distal biceps tendon injury: MR imaging diagnosis. *Radiology* 1994;191:203–206.

Complete tears of the distal biceps tendon were characterized by complete disruption of tendon fibers, increased intratendinous signal intensity, and peritendinous fluid and hematoma in axial images. Variable amounts of biceps tendon retraction were observed in the sagittal MRIs.

Gallagher MA, Cuomo F, Polonsky L, Berliner K, Zuckerman JD: Effects of age, testing speed, and arm dominance on isokinetic strength of the elbow. *J Shoulder Elbow Surg* 1997;6:340–346.

In 60 right hand-dominant men, the strength of active flexion-extension and supination-pronation was measured isokinetically. While significant differences were observed between the young and older groups in flexion and extension, no differences were found in supination and pronation.

Kelley JD, Lombardo SJ, Pink M, Perry J, Giangarra CE: Electromyographic and cinematographic analysis of elbow function in tennis players with lateral epicondylitis. *Am J Sports Med* 1994;22:359–363.

Electromyographic activities of forearm muscles in 8 tennis players with lateral epicondylitis were compared to those in 14 players with normal upper extremities. The significantly greater activity was measured in wrist extensors and pronator teres of the injured players. The faulty mechanics in stroke may lead to the increased wrist activity.

Kim SJ, Kim HK, Lee JW: Arthroscopy for limitation of motion of the elbow. *Arthroscopy* 1995;11:680–683.

Arthroscopic debridement was performed in 25 patients with limited motion of the elbow joint caused by various intra-articular pathology. At the mean 25-month follow-up, 23 patients were satisfied with the results. Elbow extension was improved from 21° to 14° and flexion from 113° to 130°. Transient median nerve palsy, which recovered completely 4 weeks after the operation, occurred in 2 cases.

Lee BP, Morrey BF: Arthroscopic synovectomy of the elbow for rheumatoid arthritis: A prospective study. *J Bone Joint Surg* 1997;79B:770–772.

Fourteen arthroscopic synovectomies of the elbow in 11 patients with rheumatoid arthritis were evaluated at an average follow-up of 42 months. Only 57% maintained excellent or good results. Transient neurapraxia of the ulnar and radial nerves occurred in 1 case each. Four patients (4 elbows) subsequently required TEA for pain.

Lonner JH, Stuchin SA: Synovectomy, radial head excision, and anterior capsular release in stage III inflammatory arthritis of the elbow. *J Hand Surg* 1997;22A:279–285.

Pain was eliminated or improved in 12 rheumatoid elbows with stage III inflammatory arthritis. Average flexion arc improved from 93° to 116° with flexion contracture improving 13°. Total arc of forearm rotation increased from 95° to 145°. Serial postoperative radiographs showed no significant disease progression over time.

Miller CD, Jobe CM, Wright MH: Neuroanatomy in elbow arthroscopy. *J Shoulder Elbow Surg* 1995;4:168–174.

The distance from the nerves to the capsule and bones of the elbow was studied in 6 pairs of cadaveric elbows. After 20 ml of saline solution insufflation into the elbow joint, the nerve-to-bone distance was increased to 12 mm for the median nerve and to 6 mm for the radial nerve. This insufflation did not change capsule-to-nerve distance. Extension eliminated the protective effects of insufflation and brought the nerve closer to the bone.

Ogilvie-Harris DJ, Gordon R, MacKay M: Arthroscopic treatment for posterior impingement in degenerative arthritis of the elbow. *Arthroscopy* 1995;11:437–443.

Arthroscopic debridement and removal of loose bodies were performed in 21 patients with posterior impingement associated with degenerative elbow arthritis. At an average follow-up of 35 months, significant improvement of pain and function were observed.

Olsen BS, Sojbjerg JO, Dalstra M, Sneppen O: Kinematics of the lateral ligamentous constraints of the elbow joint. *J Shoulder Elbow Surg* 1996;5:333–341.

The role of the LCL complex was studied in 30 cadaveric elbows. Transection of the LCL (radial collateral ligament) induced more significant laxity. Total transection of LCL complex caused the maximal laxity.

Strauch RJ, Rosenwasser MP, Glazer PA: Surgical exposure of the dorsal proximal third of the radius: How vulnerable is the posterior interosseous nerve? *J Shoulder Elbow Surg* 1996;5:342–346.

The average distance between the posterior interosseous nerve and the most prominent point of bicipital tuberosity of the radius was 2.3 cm with intracadaver variation of 1.3 mm.

Timmerman LA, Andrews JR: Arthroscopic treatment of posttraumatic elbow pain and stiffness. *Am J Sports Med* 1994; 22:230–235.

Nineteen patients with posttraumatic arthrofibrosis of the elbow were treated with arthroscopic debridement and manipulation. At an average follow-up of 29 months, 79% of the patients had good-to-excellent overall result with extension improvement from 29° to 11° and flexion from an average of 123° to 134°.

Contracture and Ankylosis

Bonutti PM, Windau JE, Ables BA, Miller BG: Static progressive stretch to reestablish elbow range of motion. *Clin Orthop* 1994;303:128–134.

Twenty patients with established contractures of the elbow that were unresponsive to other treatment modalities used a static progressive stretching program. The average increase in motion averaged 31° after 1 to 3 months of brace treatment. All patients were satisfied and none experienced deterioration at 1-year follow-up.

Jones GS, Savoie FH III: Arthroscopic capsular release of flexion contractures (arthrofibrosis) of the elbow. *Arthroscopy* 1993;9: 277–283.

Twelve patients with flexion contractures were treated with arthroscopic anterior capsular release and posterior compartment debridement. The flexion contracture decreased from 38° preoperatively to 3° following surgery. Forearm rotation also improved following surgery. One patient experienced a permanent posterior interosseous nerve injury.

Arthritis

Ljung P, Jonsson K, Larsson K, Rydholm U: Interposition arthroplasty of the elbow with rheumatoid arthritis. *J Shoulder Elbow Surg* 1996;5:81–85.

Interposition arthroplasty was performed in 35 elbows with rheumatoid arthritis. Pain relief was adequate in most patients but stability and motion were fair. The results were inferior when compared to TEA. The authors concluded that primary TEA is the treatment of choice for advanced rheumatoid arthritis of the elbow.

Total Elbow Arthroplasty

Cobb TK, Morrey BF: Total elbow arthroplasty as primary treatment for distal humeral fractures in elderly patients. *J Bone Joint Surg* 1997;79A:826–832.

Primary TEA for comminuted distal humeral fractures was performed in 21 elbows between 1982 and 1992. Considerations for TEA included extensive comminution in elderly patients when a suitable alternative was absent. Several patients had preexisting rheumatoid arthritis, which influenced the treatment decision. All patients had a satisfactory result at 3.3-year follow-up.

King GJ, Itoi E, Niebur GL, Morrey BF, An KN: Motion and laxity of the capitellocondylar total elbow prosthesis. *J Bone Joint Surg* 1994;76A:1000–1008.

The motion and laxity of 17 cadaveric elbows were evaluated after implantation of a capitellocondylar unconstrained TEA using a passive elbow model with simulated muscle loads. Stability of the prosthesis was found to depend on proper component position and the integrity of the MCL and LCL. The MCL attachment to the ulna was found to be at risk from improper component placement of the ulnar component.

Schemitsch EH, Ewald FC, Thornhill TS: Results of total elbow arthroplasty after excision of the radial head and synovectomy in patients who had rheumatoid arthritis. *J Bone Joint Surg* 1996;78A:1541–1547.

Twenty-three patients with primary capitellocondylar TEA were compared to 23 patients with capitellocondylar TEA following previous synovectomy and radial head excision. Six of 23 patients (26%) with previous surgery experienced postoperative instability; none of the patients with primary TEA had instability.

Schneeberger AG, Adams R, Morrey BF: Semiconstrained total elbow replacement for the treatment of post-traumatic osteoarthrosis. *J Bone Joint Surg* 1997;79A:1211–1222.

Forty-one patients with posttraumatic osteoarthritis treated with a noncustom semiconstrained TEA were evaluated at 5 years 8 months. Satisfactory results were obtained in 34 patients (83%). Mechanical failure of the implant (breakage and bushing wear) was the principal cause of failure. Infections occurred in 2 patients.

Chapter 32
Wrist and Hand: Pediatric Aspects

Congenital Differences

Successful treatment of the patient with a congenital difference of the hand requires an integrated team involving the surgeon, the therapist, and the parents. Except for the thalidomide disaster in the 1950s, the incidence of congenital hand anomalies has remained stable, occurring in 6% to 7% of full-term births. Only 10% are pronounced enough to require surgical treatment. Approximately 25% result from gene mutations or chromosomal abnormalities. Environmental teratogenic influences account for approximately 10%; however, the majority (65%) are idiopathic. The development of the upper extremity is simultaneous with that of other major organ systems; therefore, the presence of concomitant cardiovascular, craniofacial, musculoskeletal, genitourinary, and neurologic anomalies is common. It is incumbent on the orthopaedic surgeon to recognize the potential for anomalies associated with congenital hand differences. Consultation with pediatric specialists and a thorough systemic workup are suggested.

Surgical timing is a critical issue to maximize outcome. Few congenital disorders require immediate reconstruction (eg, ischemia resulting from constriction bands). Some anomalies exert a pathologic influence on adjacent tissue (eg, complete, complex syndactyly) and should be reconstructed in the first year. A majority of differences can be addressed between the first year and the start of formal schooling (eg, hypoplastic thumb). Certain reconstructions, such as tendon transfers that require patient cooperation, are best delayed until the child can intellectually participate in the rehabilitation process.

The classification system developed by The International Federation of Societies for Surgery of the Hand (IFSSH) separates congenital differences into 7 groups: (1) failure of formation of parts; (2) failure of differentiation of parts; (3) duplication; (4) overgrowth; (5) undergrowth; (6) constriction band syndrome; and (7) generalized skeletal abnormalities. Although some congenital hand differences, such as the polysyndactylies, may demonstrate features of more than 1 group, this scheme assists the surgeon treating and reporting on these problems.

Failure of Formation

Failure of formation may be complete or partial, and is further subdivided into transverse or longitudinal.

Transverse Arrest In transverse arrest, there is complete absence of the structures distal to a certain point; it may occur at any level from the shoulder to the fingertips. This anomaly should not be confused with an intrauterine amputation caused by congenital constriction bands. The below-elbow amputation remains the most common deficiency, seen in 1 in 20,000 live births. The more proximal upper arm amputation occurs in 1 in 270,000 live births.

The etiology of congenital below-elbow deficiencies remains unknown and most likely represents a sporadic mutation, although an autosomal-recessive form has been described. Two thirds of the children have a concomitant radial head dislocation. The direction of the dislocation is usually related to the length of the forearm; an anterior dislocation usually accompanies the shortest forearms. There are limited indications for surgery in this population, and prosthetic fitting is the usual method of treatment.

When the infant can sit (approximately 6 months), a passive prosthetic device is prescribed to enable the development of spatial orientation with 2 limbs of similar length. Between 18 and 36 months of age, fitting with an initial hook, then graduation to a body-powered, voluntary closing terminal device is recommended. In the adolescent or in the young child who demonstrates early facile use of the prosthesis, a myoelectric prosthesis may be indicated. A prosthesis usually requires a proximal residual limb of 6 to 8 cm. Surgical lengthening through osteotomy with gradual distraction can lengthen the residual limb and improve the lever arm for better prosthetic fitting (Fig. 1). Residual limb revision (removing prominent bone or bursae) may be needed to improve prosthetic fit.

With a transverse deficiency at the digital level, procedures to improve both pinch and grasp are indicated. If an adequate soft-tissue envelope is present, then transfer of a nonvascularized toe phalanx will provide potential pinch posts. Continued growth of the transferred bone may occur. For the best chance of continued growth of the nonvascularized phalanx, surgery should be performed before 18 months of age.

Surgical procedures for the older child with transverse digital deficiencies include lengthening, "on-top plasty," intercalary bone graft, or microvascular toe transfer. Lengthening requires bony elements long enough for placement of a mini-external fixator device. Incremental lengthening can permit equilibration of the soft tissues and regenerate bone formation. Maturity of the new bone can be assessed by radiographs or ultrasound methods. One-stage lengthening can also be performed with intercalated bone grafting to achieve desired length. Between 5% and 30% of length can be obtained with this single-stage method. Advantages of one-stage intercalary bone grafting include the avoidance of the external fixator; however, distraction lengthening proponents believe that increased length can be achieved with fewer soft-tissue complications.

Microvascular toe transfer in the patient with complete absence of digits or in the monodactylic hand can provide pinch and cylindrical grasp. Caution is advised in these procedures because the possible presence of hypoplastic or anomalous vasculature may preclude a successful transfer.

Radial-Longitudinal Deficiency The longitudinal deficiencies are characterized by hypoplasia or aplasia that is concentrated on either the preaxial or postaxial side of the upper extremity, although more global involvement to some degree is not uncharacteristic. The incidence ranges from 1 in 30,000 to 1 in 100,000 live births. It is usually sporadic, although familial patterns, radiation, and other teratogens have been

implicated in its etiology. Radial deficiency can encompass the entire preaxial upper extremity and may involve the shoulder to the fingertips. This difference is often associated with cardiac (Holt-Oram syndrome), hematologic (Fanconi's anemia or thrombocytopenia absent radius, TAR), or other skeletal anomalies. The frequent association of radial-sided hypoplasia is with a constellation of deficiencies termed VATER syndrome, which includes vertebral, anal, tracheoesophageal, and renal abnormalities. All preaxial structures are affected to variable degrees, and even muscles arising from the postaxial border may have poor distal differentiation. Neurovascular aberrations, such as absence of the radial artery and superficial radial nerve, are common. Sensation to the radial side of the hand is often supplied by a branch of the median nerve and is very susceptible to inadvertent surgical damage at the time of centralization or radialization of the wrist. Skeletal deficiencies include absence of the scaphoid, trapezium, and trapezoid; stiffness of the remaining radial fingers; and varying degrees of thumb hypoplasia.

Radial deficiency is bilateral in 50% of cases and is classified as follows: type I, short radius with delayed distal physeal

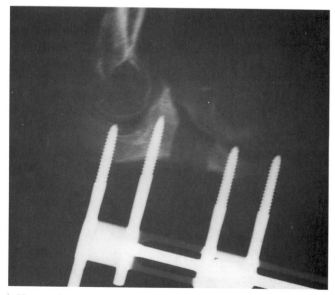

Figure 1

Example of limb lengthening with an external fixator in a patient with a short below-elbow amputation, midway through the course.

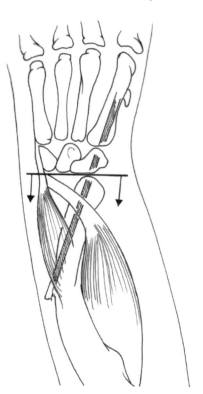

Figure 2

Radialization.(Reproduced with permission from Buck-Gramcko D: Radialization as a new treatment for radial club hand. *J Hand Surg* 1985;10A:964-968.)

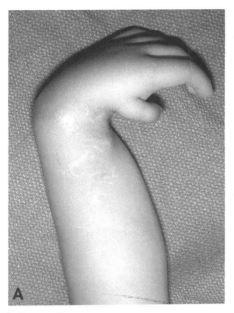
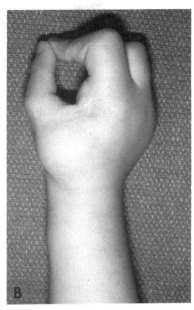

Figure 3

A and B, Patient with a significant radial deviation deformity and a pouce flottant (floating thumb). The patient has already had an unsuccessful attempt at realigning the hand-forearm unit.

growth; type II, radius in "miniature" with defective proximal and distal physeal growth; type III, partial absence of the radius, usually distal; and type IV, which is most common, complete absence of the radius.

There are several considerations when treating a patient with radial deficiency. First, ascertain the patient's response to nonsurgical (manipulation, splinting) measures started in the neonatal period. Determine the functional status of the elbow; poor elbow function is a relative contraindication for heroic reconstruction of the hand and wrist. Select a reconstructive plan for comprehensive restoration of upper extremity function, including wrist balancing and thumb reconstruction as needed. Last, it must be decided whether the patient's overall health status is compatible with safe surgical conduct; patients with TAR and Fanconi's anemia or congenital heart anomalies have special perioperative risks.

Surgical balancing of the wrist can take one of two forms, radialization or centralization. In radialization, the carpal elements are spared, as an attempt to balance the scaphoid (or radial carpus) over the ulna is made (Fig. 2). Transfer of the radial-sided tendons, flexor and extensor carpi radialis, to the ulnar aspect of the carpus improves the vector of force and turns deforming tendons into aids in ulnocarpal balance. Diaphyseal osteotomy of the ulna often accompanies the work done at the wrist level. Pinning through the radial-most metacarpal stabilizes the balanced construct. Conversely, cen-

tralization usually requires central carpal resection to accommodate the distal ulna. Varying amounts of bone excision are needed to create a balance that minimizes compressive forces at the distal ulnar physis. Failed radializations are salvaged with centralization.

Recently described strategies for radial deficiency include the use of external fixation for bony lengthening in adolescence or adulthood. Complication rates remain high with this reconstruction. Progress in microvascular surgery has made epiphyseal transfer an option in treating radial deficiency. Transfer of the vascularized proximal fibular epiphysis to reconstruct the deficient radial epiphysis demonstrates open physes at follow-up in 82%, with 1 cm per year of growth. Longer follow-up is needed before this can be recommended. Most but not all patients with radial deficiency will manifest some degree of thumb hypoplasia. The anatomic characteristics of the hypoplastic thumb include gracile bony elements, a contracted first web space, thenar muscle insufficiency, abnormal tendon insertions, and variable levels of stability of the osteoarticular column (Fig. 3). Further definition of hypoplastic thumb variations has emerged. These important distinctions have treatment implications (Table 1).

Ulnar Longitudinal Deficiency Ulnar longitudinal deficiency is 5 to 10 times less prevalent than radial deficiency. Most often occurrence is sporadic; it is often associated with musculoskeletal differences in contrast to the pattern of visceral organ system involvement seen with radial deficiencies. The hand is usually stable at the wrist with varying degrees of ulnar deviation. The elbow is often unstable. Classification is based on the degree of ulnar deficiency: type I, hypoplasia; type II, partial absence of the ulna; type III, total absence of the ulna; and type IV, total absence of the ulna with radiohumeral synostosis. Type II is the most common. Classification of a type III deficiency should be reserved until 1 year of age, because the proximal portion of the ulna may not ossify until that time. Types II and IV each have been associated with a fibrous anlage that tethers the carpus to the foreshortened ulna. The anlage has the potential to accentuate the ulnar deviation of the carpus and the bowing of the radius. Progressive bowing may even result in late radial head dislocation.

Table 1
Classification of the hypoplastic thumb

Type	Anatomic Characteristics
I	Minimal shortening of the thumb
II	First web-space narrowing
	Thenar muscle hypoplasia
	MP joint instability
IIIA	Type II features
	Extrinsic tendon abnormalities
	Metacarpal hypoplasia
	Stable CMC joint
IIIB	Type II features
	Extrinsic tendon abnormalities
	Partial metacarpal aplasia
	Unstable CMC joint
IV	Floating thumb (pouce flottant)
V	Absent thumb

*CMC, carpometacarpal: MP, metacarpalphalangeal.

(Reproduced with permission from Graham TJ, Louis DS: A comprehensive approach to surgical management of the type IIIA hypoplastic thumb. *J Hand Surg* 1998;23A:3–13.)

Proponents recommend excision of the ulnar anlage if ulnar deviation of the carpus exceeding 30° is present for more than 6 months. Others believe that the ulnar anlage does not potentiate the deformity and that its excision does not halt deformity progression. The functional result without resection has been reported to be excellent. Surgical reconstruction to improve hand position by osteotomy through the radiohumeral synostosis (type IV) is accepted; the upper extremity is positioned at 60° to 90° of flexion and neutral pronation-supination. Rotation osteotomies of border digits and syndactyly release are worthwhile to improve pinch and grasp. The severe type II deformity with an unstable forearm-

hand unit may be improved by creation of a 1-bone forearm.

Ulnar deficiency has recently been classified based on the thumb web space deficiency. This newer classification takes into account the high percentage of radial-sided anomalies that accompany ulnar-sided suppression. The spectrum of thumb changes seen with ulnar longitudinal deficiency ranges from the completely normal thumb, includes varying degrees of hypoplasia, and extends to the completely absent thumb.

Central Longitudinal Deficiency/ Symbrachydactyly
Changes in nomenclature have been used in an attempt to clarify the types of cleft hands and better take into account the true anatomic abnormalities. The terms "cleft hand" and "symbrachydactyly" now are used to characterize the differences that are readily recognizable as central deficiencies of the "typical" and "atypical"varieties. The incidence of typical cleft hand is 1 in 90,000 live births. The V-shaped central cleft is created by varying degrees of absence of the long ray. It usually presents bilaterally, is transmitted by an autosomal dominant mode, and is associated with lower extremity musculoskeletal differences (Fig. 4). Syndactyly in the remaining digits is common, and other associated anomalies such as cleft lip and palate have been reported.

Symbrachydactyly, in contrast, is usually unilateral and involves several central deficient rays. The wider cleft is U-shaped, with a sporadic pattern of presentation. Syndactyly is uncommon and there are usually no other associated organ systems anomalies. Both cleft hand and symbrachydactyly have functionally normal forearms and wrists. In the typical cleft hand, treatment is directed toward increasing prehension by allowing opposition of the radial and ulnar components. This is achieved by release of the syndactyly of the border digits and closure of the cleft in one of many described procedures. If syndactyly is present, it usually is released at the age of 6 to 12 months, and the cleft is closed 6 to 12 months later. However, some patients rely on the cleft to adequately oppose the border digits and further closure may only impair prehension. Careful functional analysis through observation is needed because the typical cleft is usually a very functional hand although it is abnormal in appearance.

The treatment goal for symbrachydactyly is functional pinch and grasp. Nonfunctional digits are removed because they are unstable and compromise grasping of the border digits. Rotational osteotomies of the border digits are often performed along with tendon transfers to help restore opposition and pinch. In the severe form of a single-digit hand, microvascular or toe-phalanx transfers may create a post for opposition.

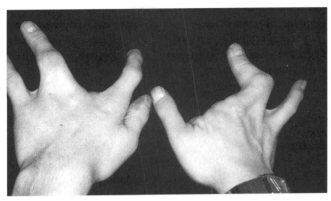

Figure 4

Example of an adult patient with bilateral central ray deficiencies. The left hand appears to be an expression of the symbrachydactyly variant, while the right hand is more of a typical cleft hand.

Failure of Differentiation

Syndactyly Syndactyly results from failure of programmed cell necrosis between the digits occurring at 7 weeks of gestation. Its incidence is 1 in 2,000 live births, and it can be inherited by an autosomal dominant pattern, although sporadic occurrence accounts for almost 80% of the cases. It is more common in whites than blacks. Syndactyly is designated as complete when the webbing of the fingers extends to the fingertips. It is designated simple if only the skin is involved and complex if the bones of adjacent fingers have not separated. An additional category, designated complicated complex syndactyly, includes features of syndactyly combined with additional anomalies, such as clinodactyly, camptodactyly, symphalangism, or associated anomalies, such as Poland's, Apert's, and amniotic band syndromes.

The incidence of syndactyly is highest between the middle and ring fingers, followed in decreasing order of frequency by the ring-small web, index-middle web, and thumb-index web. Surgical release is usually pursued because functional improvement can be realized, and the cosmetic advantage is undisputed. Many techniques have been described, but all involve creation of a web space and separation of conjoined structures. The commissure is created by release and local flap transposition to recreate the normal web contour. Skin grafting is almost always required except in the mild, simple, incomplete syndactyly. Full-thickness grafts from the groin are superior to split-thickness skin grafts because they prevent further contractile scarring (creep) and hyperpigment minimally. Distal fusion of the nail plate and eponychium (synonchia) necessitates reconstruction using local rotation flaps or composite skin grafts; nail bed grafts from the toe are sometimes needed. However, simple narrowing of the remaining separate nail beds and allowance for closure by secondary intention will provide a satisfactory digit tip. In complex syndactyly, an anomalous vascular supply is often present. Even in simple syndactyly, the usual distal bifurcation of the common digital artery may be anomalous. The common digital nerve can be separated proximally by intrafascicular dissection.

Surgical reconstruction is directed first at border digits because the unequal length may promote angular deformity if not released during the first year. Similarly, complex syndactylies are usually treated between 6 and 12 months of age. However, syndactyly involving the middle-ring fingers can be delayed to approximately 2 to 3 years of age, but should be reconstructed before the child enters school. It is wise to warn the parents that even in simple syndactyly, there is a 30% chance that later revision will be required as the hand grows. Web creep remains an inherent problem. Techniques for diminishing the potential of web creep include careful insetting to the appropriate proximal volar position, specialized flaps that diminish the opportunity for transitional scars, and the liberal use of skin grafting for the donor defects in the adjacent digits.

Newer developments have been directed at release of the syndactyly in the neonatal period using simple longitudinal incisions; proponents claim this may avoid the need for skin grafting. Early recurrence, however, has been seen and this procedure remains controversial. Similarly, the use of tissue expanders to increase available skin is attractive, yet an unacceptably high complication rate still accompanies this technique. Treatment of the acrosyndactyly often seen with Apert's syndrome is a technical challenge (Fig. 5). Creation of a 3-digit hand in 2 or more stages is the typical strategy for reconstruction. Dissection on both sides of any digit at the same surgical sitting is contraindicated because of the potential for bilateral neurovascular compromise. The first stage is typically directed to creation of a thumb and adequate first web space, and initial ulnar digit separation. The second stage focuses on separation of one of the digital masses to provide a 4-membered hand.

Carpal Coalitions Failure of segmentation of the cartilaginous carpal precursor results in carpal coalition. The lunotriquetral (LT) coalition is the most common, with a 1.6% prevalence in the general population; the capitohamate is second in prevalence. Although associated with many syndromes, this condition remains an incidental finding on many radiographs, with few if any symptoms reported by the patients with this anomaly. It is found in approximately 0.1% of the white population, 1.5% of the American black popula-

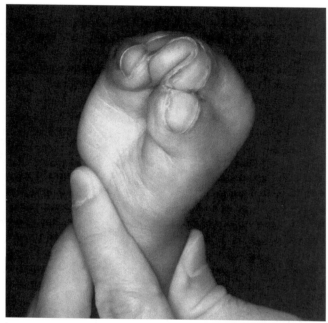

Figure 5

Typical appearance of the hand in a patient with acrocephalosyndactyly or Apert's syndrome. Note the confluence of the nail or "synonychia" and the cleft or pit between the radial digits.

tion, and has an 8% incidence in West African blacks and in the South African Bantu. Recently, symptomatic degenerative changes of the wrist, believed to be related to carpal coalition, have been reported. In all cases, symptoms were believed to result from incomplete coalitions at the lunotriquetral joint predisposing to excessive stress and accelerated degenerative changes that would not have been seen if the coalition was complete. Successful treatment of an acute separation of an LT synchondrosis or degenerative LT changes in the incomplete coalition is by arthrodesis of the LT joint.

Camptodactyly Camptodactyly, from the Greek for "bent finger," maintains the typical posture of mild hypertension of the metacarpophalangeal (MCP) joint with flexion contracture of the proximal interphalangeal (PIP) joint. Its incidence is approximately 1% to 2% of the population, with the small finger most commonly involved. Two thirds of cases are bilateral, and 3 different presentations have been described: infantile, adolescent, and more recently, a severe form that involves all the triphalangeal digits. Much overlap exists, and many believe that the adolescent variant is a progression of the infantile form. Progression occurs during the major growth spurts in approximately 80% of cases (between 1 and 3 years of age, 10 and 13 years of age).

The underlying abnormality is usually an imbalance of pull or static tether between the flexor and extensor mechanisms. The most commonly accepted theory is that an anomalous insertion of the lumbrical muscle into the flexor tendon sheath causes the abnormality, but a single unifying theory or focal anatomic aberration is not consistently identified.

Dynamic or serial static splinting may be beneficial, especially during times of rapid growth. Surgical treatment is unpredictable with some series reporting improvement in only 35% of cases. The young child who shows progressive deformity with adequate nonsurgical treatment may be a candidate for surgical intervention, especially when PIP flexion exceeds 60°. Surgery is designed to correct the PIP joint flexion deformity through release or transfer of the abnormal tethering structures. Transferring a flexor to the extensor mechanism can negate the intrinsic minus position. If an anomalous insertion of the lumbrical muscle is present, resection or transfer may be elected (Fig. 6). In extreme cases, osteotomy after skeletal maturity may improve the position of the phalangeal head, or PIP joint fusion can be used to combat the soft-tissue forces. New techniques, such as a

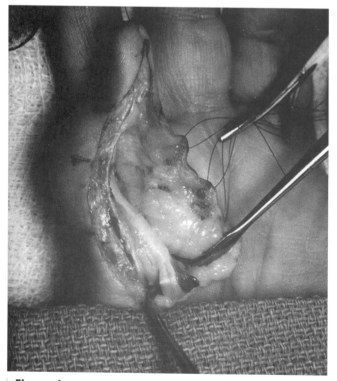

Figure 6

The Ragnel retractor is placed around the lumbrical muscle, with its anomalous insertion into the flexor tendon sheath. Retraction of it accentuates the deformity in campodactyly.

hinged PIP distraction device, may allow for correction of the contraction and minimize the need for extensive reconstructive surgery; more experience and long-term follow-up are needed before this can be recommended.

Clinodactyly Clinodactyly is an angular deformity of the finger in the radioulnar plane. The distal interphalangeal (DIP) joint is deviated radially in the most common form. The small finger is most frequently involved, and the anomaly is usually bilateral. It can be seen in up to 80% of children with Down syndrome. It is sporadically inherited by an autosomal dominant pattern.

Small amounts of angulation (10° to 20°) result in minimal functional loss. Progressive clinodactyly, especially when seen with a delta middle phalanx, can cause significant angulation and interfere with functional grasp. Correction of the angulation is best accomplished by a closing osteotomy of the middle phalanx. Other options include an opening wedge osteotomy or a reversed wedge osteotomy. More recent surgical reconstruction has been directed at the "C-shaped" physis or bracketed epiphysis seen in the delta phalanx. Osteotomies and resection of the abnormal portion with interposition of fat have been described.

Duplication

General Concepts Polydactyly of the human hand is universal and frequent. For this reason, it is likely that all orthopaedic surgeons will encounter one of its manifestations at some time in their career. Because of confusion with classification and reporting, true incidence data of polydactyly in general, and the specific subtypes, are lacking. However, general trends can be appreciated, and certain polydactylies in specific racial or gender populations may be a herald for systemic anomalies. Although there are emerging descriptive classification systems that separate thumb duplication, index duplication, central ray polydactyly, and polydactyly of the ulnar hand, the accepted separation of preaxial and postaxial duplication remains widely used.

Preaxial Polydactyly Preaxial polydactyly is nearly evenly distributed between the white and black populations with an incidence of between 1 and 3 occurrences per 1,000 live births. It is seen with slightly greater frequency in Native Americans and some Asian populations. One of the most common presentations of preaxial polydactyly is the duplicated thumb. The designation bifid thumb is slightly inaccurate because there are rarely 2 normal thumbs because both duplicates are hypoplastic (Fig. 7). Almost all types interfere with prehensile activity. The Wassel classification system has

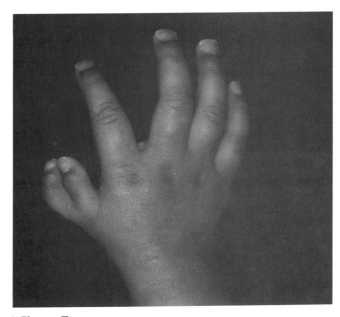

Figure 7
Duplicated thumbs.

been widely used to describe the duplicated thumb. It is based on the level of duplication and the completeness of the separation. The metacarpal or phalanges can be bifid or completely duplicated. The most common type, Wassel IV, is manifested as a duplicated proximal phalanx with a broadened metacarpal proximally and separate distal phalanges.

Almost all infants born with a bifid thumb require reconstruction to: (1) ablate the most hypoplastic thumb, usually the radial; (2) combine structures from both thumbs to create a stable MCP joint; (3) align all bony units and centralize tendinous structures; (4) optimize range of motion of the reconstructed thumb; and (5) create a sensate pulp for pinch and prehensile activity. For the rare type I (bifid) and II (duplicated) distal phalanx, a Bilhaut-Clouquet, reduction-combination can be considered. Removal of central elements, including bone and nail tissue, followed by an attempt to create a symmetric single thumb is intellectually appealing. However, this reconstruction is technically arduous and problems with angular deformity and nail growth disturbance plague the reconstruction.

Removal of the radial hypoplastic component with preservation of the thenar musculature and transfer to the ulnar component is a sound surgical option. A periosteal capsular sleeve from the radial component helps reconstruct the radial collateral ligament on the preserved ulnar component. A radial closing wedge osteotomy is often needed at the metacarpal level to better align the thumb and may be combined with a phalangeal osteotomy. Centralization of the tendinous structures is often needed to avoid a "zig-zag" deformity.

Repeat operation is needed in over 30% of patients after duplicate thumb reconstruction; inherent stiffness is often present in the reconstructed thumb. The zig-zag deformity discussed above is most commonly caused by the imbalanced pull of the flexors and extensors at their DIP insertion. Other causes include radial longitudinal scarring, inadequate reconstruction of the radial thenar musculature, inadequate reconstruction of the MCP radial collateral ligament, and failure to adequately osteotomize the metacarpal or centralize tendinous structures. A small subset of patients born with a rudimentary radial component and treated with suture ligature have also developed this deformity. Treatment of the zig-zag deformity includes revision of the longitudinal scar, proper transfer of the thenar musculature, reconstruction of the MCP radial collateral ligament, and repeat osteotomy and tendon realignment as needed (Fig. 8).

Postaxial Polydactyly Postaxial polydactyly is the second most common congenital difference behind syndactyly. When the ulnar-sided duplicate is well-formed, with all digital elements included, the incidence in the black and white populations is roughly equivalent. Conversely, when the duplicate is rudimentary, postaxial polydactyly is 10 times more common in blacks than in whites. It has a strong autosomal dominant pattern in blacks, whereas in whites it is rare

enough to alert the clinician to look for associated anomalies (Ellis-van Creveld, Laurence-Moon, and Bardet-Biedl syndromes). Several classifications have been proposed, yet the elements remain relatively similar; the duplicate can range from a vestigial skin tag to a well-developed supernumerary digit that has a separate articulation with the fifth metacarpal (or more rarely, its own additional metacarpal). Simple suture ligation of the "skin-tag" has been the historic treatment, which often was done by the pediatrician in the newborn nursery. Inferior results with this minimalistic approach have ranged from unsightly tissue prominence to exsanguination. Excision of the entire remnant under local anesthesia may become more standard. Reconstruction of a well-developed duplicate includes tissue excision, collateral ligament transfer, and possibly ablation of a duplicated or widened metacarpal physis and epiphysis.

Overgrowth

Macrodactyly is one of the rarest congenital differences, with an incidence of 0.9%. One classification divides macrodactyly into primary or true macrodactyly, in which all the tissues are enlarged, and secondary macrodactyly, which results from disorders such as neurofibromatosis, hemangioma, lymphangioma, arteriovenous malformations, fibrous dysplasia, and lipoma. The classification system proposed is: type I, digital gigantism with lipofibromatous hamartoma; type II, digital gigantism with neurofibromatosis; and type III, hyperostotic digital gigantism. Although there remains some overlap between the 3 types, the most common expressions of overgrowth are types I and II, which accompany nerve enlargement and have been characterized as nerve territory oriented macrodactyly. These 2 types of macrodactyly can be either static (an enlarged digit at birth that grows proportionally to the other digits) or progressive (a digit that continues to grow at an accelerated rate throughout childhood). It is usually unilateral, found on the radial side of the hand, and most commonly affects the index finger. All of the phalanges of the involved digits are enlarged both in the transverse and longitudinal plane, with the metacarpals being less commonly involved.

There is not only a marked increase in bone volume but also in subcutaneous fat, digital artery caliber, and digital nerve size and tortuosity. Surgical reconstruction is almost always desired by the patient and

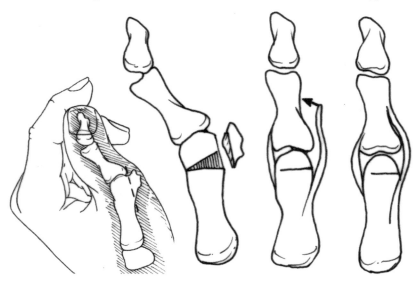

Figure 8

Reconstruction of the zig-zag deformity. (Reproduced with permission from Lourie GM, Costas BL, Bayne LG: The zig-zag deformity in pre-axial polydactyly: A new cause and its treatment. *J Hand Surg* 1995;20B:561-564.)

may become necessary as a result of vascular "steal" causing ischemia of adjacent digits. Reduction of the enlarged digit is usually performed in 2 stages, with each stage involving removal of half of the soft tissue. The convex side is usually approached first. The phalanges are also narrowed by removing up to 25% of each side of the phalanx. If the digit has already grown to the size of the similar digit found in the parent, then epiphysiodesis is performed. Other intricate procedures have been described, such as phalangeal reduction osteotomies to shorten the macrodactylous digit. All these procedures also have a high complication rate, including skin necrosis, stiffness, pain, and residual or recurrent deformity. Uncontrolled growth is most frequently handled by ray resection; unfortunately, this can lead to accelerated growth in neighboring digits, and parents should be warned of this possibility.

Congenital Constriction Band Syndrome

Congenital constriction bands occur between 1 in 5,000 to 1 in 15,000 births; male-female distribution is equal. The index, middle, and ring fingers are involved in roughly equal proportion, although the latter is slightly more common; the thumb and small finger are rarely involved. This syndrome is more often seen in first pregnancies and premature births. Amniotic rupture with reduction in the fluid volume inducing uterine contraction is postulated to produce amniotic bands. Annular grooves produced by the constriction bands vary from mild skin depression to deep involvement affecting nerves, vessels, and bone. Treatment is directed at release of the circumferential band to reestablish venous and lymphatic drainage in the distal portions, and release of any associated syndactyly. Surgery is typically done in 2 stages on a single digit to prevent vascular compromise from a circumferential dissection. Some case reports do advocate single-stage reconstruction, but caution should be exercised. Multiple Z-plasties release the band. Recent refinements to the technique have emphasized mobilizing the subcutaneous fat as a separate layer and placing the Z-plasty in a midlateral position; this reduces the significant indentation resulting from the constriction band and gives a much improved appearance.

Wrist and Hand Fractures

Epidemiology

Radius and ulna fractures are the most common long-bone fractures in children, accounting for 45% of all childhood fractures and 62% of upper extremity fractures. Approximately 75% to 84% of these forearm fractures occur in the distal third, with 15% to 18% occurring in the middle third,

and less than 5% in the proximal third. Much less commonly, children will sustain injuries to their distal radioulnar joint or carpal bones. Intercarpal ligament injuries are rare in childhood. The most common carpal bone fracture is the scaphoid and yet, it accounts for only 0.45% of all pediatric upper extremity fractures. By comparison, the hand is the most common body part injured in a child. Approximately 75% of pediatric finger fractures are stable and can be treated with simple, brief immobilization. However, the problem fractures need to be recognized, appropriately reduced, and stabilized to prevent long-term complications.

Distal Radial Physeal Fractures

Most distal radial physeal fractures are Salter-Harris type II injuries that occur in the adolescent. Displacement is typically dorsal with apex volar angulation. Atraumatic closed reduction and long arm cast immobilization is indicated for fractures with more than 10° to 20° malangulation and 50% displacement. The most significant complications with these fractures are acute neurovascular compromise and growth arrest. The incidence of associated nerve injuries may be as high as 8% in displaced fractures. Patients with signs or symptoms of median nerve injury at the time of presentation may be managed by immediate closed reduction and percutaneous pin fixation rather than cast immobilization to lessen the risk of forearm compartment syndrome or acute carpal tunnel syndrome that may require release. A single oblique smooth Kirschner wire (K-wire) inserted from the radial styloid and directed proximally to the ulnar aspect of the radial metaphysis provides sufficient fixation. Care must be taken to avoid the radial sensory nerve during pin insertion.

Patients with redisplacement of the fracture or late presentation should not undergo aggressive closed reduction after 7 to 10 days to avoid possible physeal injury. Late open reduction should be avoided for the same reason. Because these fractures displace in the plane of motion of the wrist joint and are juxtaphyseal, there is tremendous potential for remodeling of a malunion in the younger adolescent. If the malunion does not remodel with growth, a dorsal opening wedge osteotomy with bone graft and internal fixation may be performed at skeletal maturity (Figure 9). Growth arrest rarely occurs after distal radial physeal fractures. Patients with displaced physeal fractures should be examined 1 to 2 years after fracture to rule out growth disturbance. Those patients with significant growth arrest of the radius may develop ulnar overgrowth. This can lead to ulnocarpal impaction, distal radioulnar joint incongruity, or a triangular fibrocartilage complex (TFCC) tear. These patients may develop wrist pain and loss of forearm and wrist motion. If these are disabling, surgical alternatives usually reserved for

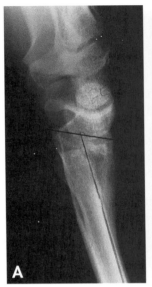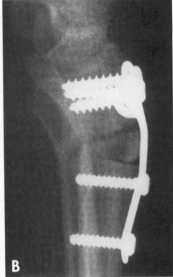

Figure 9

A, Lateral radiograph of a malunited distal radial physeal fracture that failed to remodel with growth. B, Corrective osteotomy with dorsal iliac crest bone graft and internal fixation immediately after surgery.

the adult, such as ulnar shortening, radial osteotomy, or repair of a torn TFCC, can be performed.

Salter-Harris type III and IV fractures of the hand and wrist are rare but require anatomic reduction to restore articular and physeal congruity. Open reduction or arthroscopic percutaneous reduction is indicated for those fractures that fail closed reduction. Wrist arthroscopy has been used sparingly in adolescent distal radial fractures to assess the intra-articular alignment after reduction and percutaneous fixation.

Carpal Injuries

Scaphoid Fractures Most scaphoid fractures in the skeletally immature patient are fractures or avulsions of the distal pole. These heal readily with thumb spica cast immobilization of 4 to 8 weeks with minimal risk of nonunion or osteonecrosis. Scaphoid waist fractures, however, carry the same risks of nonunion and osteonecrosis in a child as they do in an adult. Scaphoid waist fractures may be assessed with tomography for fracture displacement. If displaced more than 1 to 2 mm, then open reduction and internal fixation (ORIF) is indicated as in the adult. If the fracture is not displaced, thumb spica cast immobilization is indicated for 3 to 6 months until healing can be confirmed. The issue of whether acute fractures of the scaphoid should be immobilized in long or short arm plaster remains unresolved, yet recent evidence appears to

support enhanced rates of healing with above-elbow immobilization for displaced fractures.

An established nonunion in a child or adolescent should be treated with open reduction, bone grafting, and, usually, internal fixation. Variable pitch, double-threaded screws have been used in children both with acute displaced waist fractures and established nonunions. Proximal pole fractures have recently been observed in children and adolescents, with the risk of osteonecrosis and nonunion approaching 100%. If the small proximal pole fracture fails to heal with immobilization, both nonvascularized bone graft and vascularized radial bone graft have been used. The issue of whether a bipartite scaphoid, even if bilateral, is congenital or posttraumatic is still debated, although a traumatic etiology is supported by most authors. However, if a bipartite scaphoid is symptomatic, it should be treated as a nonunion with open reduction and bone grafting.

Triangular Fibrocartilage Complex Tears Ulnar-sided wrist pain in a child or adolescent must be thoroughly investigated. It should be recalled that degenerative perforation of the triangular fibrocartilage has not been seen in patients in the first 3 decades of life. The presence of an ulnar styloid nonunion in an adolescent with persistent ulnar-sided wrist pain after radial and ulnar fractures may represent ulnocarpal impaction and a peripheral TFCC tear. In patients who fail nonsurgical therapy, excision of the nonunion and repair of the TFCC tear are helpful.

Diagnostic wrist arthroscopy has led to an appreciation that unresolved ulnar-sided wrist pain may indicate an unrecognized TFCC tear. Wrist arthrography and magnetic resonance imaging (MRI) scans have both been shown to have an unacceptably high rate of false negative results when compared with wrist arthroscopy in prospective studies comparing multiple imaging techniques. The development of the 2.5- to 3.0-mm diameter arthroscopes and small instruments has offered easy access to the radiocarpal, midcarpal, and radioulnar joints. Isolated tears of the TFCC are now being diagnosed in adolescents. In children and adolescents, peripheral tears are most common (1B lesions) and respond well to open or arthroscopic surgical repair. Tears at the attachment of the TFCC to the radius (1D lesions) are the next most common lesion in this age group. These tears are more difficult to repair, requiring reattachment of the TFCC to the radius. Ulnar shortening may lessen the tension of these repairs in this avascular region and improve healing.

Hand Fractures

The hand is the most commonly injured body part in the child. The most common pattern of injury is a Salter-

Harris type II fracture; the most commonly injured single digit is the small finger. In toddlers and young children, the most common pattern of injury is a distal phalangeal fracture associated with a nail bed laceration or distal tip amputation from a crush injury.

Phalangeal Fractures Deformities of the distal interphalangeal (DIP) joint may result from extensor disruption or physeal separation. The mallet deformity in a young child or adolescent often results from physeal separation rather than rupture of the terminal extensor from its epiphyseal insertion on the distal phalanx. These injuries may be associated with interposition of germinal matrix between the fracture fragments (Fig. 10). Complete epiphyseal dislocation is rare but needs to be ruled out in a mallet finger, especially if the epiphysis is unossified. Treatment of the physeal separation involves open repair of the germinal matrix laceration and pin fixation or splinting of the distal phalanx in a reduced position for 3 weeks. Chronic mallet fingers are rare in young children and are often secondary to a missed extensor tendon laceration. When splinting fails, these may be successfully treated with soft-tissue imbrication or dermodesis. Treatment of soft tissue and bony mallet fingers in the older child follows standard adult treatment. DIP joint subluxation needs to be reduced, but can be controlled with splinting or by percutaneous pinning of the joint. Open reduction is rarely indicated, even in the presence of a large fracture fragment. The complication of open reduction is subsequent loss of flexion. Most patients prefer a mild extension lag to a loss of DIP flexion.

Phalangeal neck fractures occur through the bone of the subcondylar fossa and are associated with significant potential complications from displacement and bony overgrowth. Displacement of the fracture into extension and malrotation is common. The distal fragment is tethered by the collateral ligaments as it rotates dorsally up to 90° (Fig. 11). The fracture is unstable and often will displace after closed reduction. Pin fixation is usually required. In a young child, fixation may be accomplished with a single oblique pin. If open reduction is necessary, the collateral ligaments should not be dissected from the distal fragment. Collateral dissection increases the risk of osteonecrosis. Frequently, patients present late with an impending malunion because a satisfactory reduction was not achieved or maintained. Open reduction at this stage is challenging. On occasion, immature callus can be broken down by use of a percutaneous pin as a lever in the fracture site from the dorsum. This step allows for anatomic reduction and percutaneous pin fixation. Alternatively, the fracture should be allowed to heal, and a late subcondylar fossa reconstruction is performed if there is a bony block to flexion. An

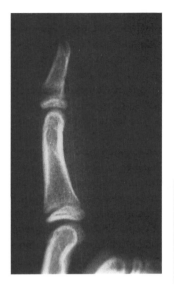

Figure 10

Lateral radiograph of a patient presenting 1 week after crush injury. The patient's germinal matrix was interposed in the physis requiring surgical extraction and repair.

average of 90° of proximal interphalangeal (PIP) joint flexion can be obtained with re-creation of the subcondylar fossa. Spontaneous remodeling of a malunited fracture is rare because of the significant distance from the physis and the potential rotational deformity that is present.

Intercondylar fractures of the proximal phalanx are complex injuries to diagnose and treat. Often concealed on the anteroposterior radiograph, this injury is inferred on the lateral view by the appearance of 2 articular surfaces, or a "double density" shadow. Often, the best image on which to diagnose the intercondylar fracture is the oblique film.

Intercondylar fractures in young children have a high risk of nonunion, malunion, and osteonecrosis. These displaced intra-articular fractures need to be treated aggressively with open reduction while preserving the collateral ligament attachments to the fragment to reduce the risk of osteonecrosis. Despite meticulous surgical handling and careful reduc-

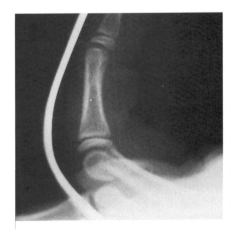

Figure 11

Displaced phalangeal neck fracture with unsuccessful closed reduction and splinting. The subcondylar fossa is obliterated by the proximal metaphyseal bone blocking flexion.

tion, motion recovery is not guaranteed. In the adolescent, treatment of intercondylar fractures is similar to that in adults. Anatomic reduction and pin or screw fixation are necessary to restore the joint surface and to prevent loss of reduction that can occur with this unstable fracture. In some cases, this procedure can be performed closed, using distraction and a sterile percutaneous towel clip to obtain reduction. Open reduction is generally performed through a dorsal approach but volar or midaxial approaches can be used. Rigid fixation and early mobilization are important to minimize PIP joint stiffness.

Diaphyseal level phalangeal fractures are more common in the teenager. The major concern is malrotation, which may be most apparent with digital flexion. Frequently, children will not actively move their finger in the acute setting to allow for accurate assessment of digital rotation. However, passive wrist flexion and extension will cause enough digital motion by tenodesis to allow for an accurate assessment. If closed treatment is chosen, secure the injured finger to the adjacent digits to lessen the risk of loss of reduction. If the finger is malrotated and unstable, reduction with pin or screw stabilization may be necessary.

Physeal fractures make up 30% to 70% of pediatric finger fractures. A Salter-Harris type II fracture of the small finger, the "extra octave fracture," is the most common. Closed reduction of the fracture is performed in metacarpophalangeal (MCP) flexion to lessen the restraint of the more distal web space. Postreduction stability is maintained in an ulnar gutter splint or a short arm mitten cast for 3 weeks. Less common type III physeal fractures require open reduction if there is greater than 2 mm of displacement or intra-articular incongruity. Physeal fractures that appear benign on radiographs can have significant clinical malrotation. Test for malrotation with both active flexion and passive wrist tenodesis.

Metacarpal Fractures   Fractures of the metacarpal neck, "boxer's fractures," are common in adolescents. Closed reduction and cast immobilization with 3-point fixation for 3 weeks are preferred for displaced fractures. Often these patients will not seek medical attention until there is significant healing. Fortunately, the fracture is adjacent to the distal metacarpal physis, and the flexion malunion will remodel if there is sufficient growth remaining. Late open reduction carries the risk of physeal injury and should be avoided. Diaphyseal fractures of the fifth metacarpal have a higher risk of rotational malunion that will not remodel. Closed reduction and percutaneous pinning or ORIF is the treatment of choice if the deformity is severe and closed methods fail to control the fracture. Corrective osteotomy may be necessary in the severe, malunit-

ed diaphyseal fracture. The osteotomy is performed either through the fracture or at the proximal metaphysis.

Thumb Fractures   Two unique fractures of the thumb in the skeletally immature are Salter-Harris type III fractures of the proximal phalanx and metacarpal base fractures. A type III physeal fracture of the thumb proximal phalanx is the equivalent of an adult ulnar collateral ligament disruption (Fig. 12). These fractures require ORIF to restore joint stability and physeal alignment. The ulnar collateral ligament is usually intact so that after reflection of the adductor aponeurosis, the MCP joint should be exposed through the fracture site rather than by inadvertent incision of the ligament. Long-term results of anatomic open reductions are excellent.

Metaphyseal fractures at the base of the thumb metacarpal often displace and are unstable. Immobilization and observation, even with displaced fractures, are appropriate because the malunited dorsal-radial prominence will remodel over the ensuing 6 to 12 months. Severe displacement can be treated with closed reduction and percutaneous pinning. A displaced Bennett's fracture requires anatomic alignment of the intra-articular component; pin fixation of the thumb metacarpal to the adjacent second metacarpal and carpus is suggested.

Dislocations
Traumatic injuries to the joints in children are usually stable PIP joint volar plate injuries with minimal Salter-Harris type

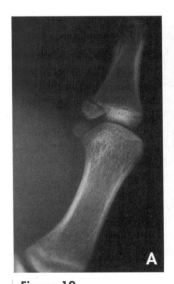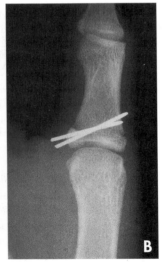

Figure 12

A, Displaced Salter-Harris type III proximal phalangeal thumb fracture. B, Open reduction and internal fixation restores articular congruity.

III middle phalangeal physeal avulsions. Treatment should be brief immobilization for comfort followed by buddy taping until asymptomatic. This will prevent the PIP joint stiffness that can occur with prolonged immobilization. True interphalangeal dislocations are usually dorsal and occur far more commonly at the PIP joint than the DIP joint. Closed reduction with distraction and dorsal to volar manipulation are generally successful in restoring the articular relationship. Rarely, a displaced epiphysis, flexor or extensor tendon, or interposed volar plate can block reduction and will require open reduction. A dorsal blocking splint and active motion in the stable range can be initiated soon after reduction.

MCP joint dislocations of the thumb or fingers can be simple or complex. Those dislocations that are irreducible by closed means are considered complex and usually have an interposed volar plate blocking reduction. Radiographs often reveal widening of the joint space as well as "bayonet" alignment or "parallelism" of the proximal phalanx and metacarpal. Open reduction can be performed through either a volar or dorsal approach. Because the radial neurovascular bundle is tented just beneath the skin by the metacarpal head, extreme caution is necessary with the volar skin incision in order to prevent a nerve laceration. For that reason, the dorsal approach is favored by most surgeons. Regardless of approach, the volar plate must be extracted from the joint to allow reduction and anatomic realignment of the flexor tendons and collateral ligaments. Postoperative treatment includes early protected motion with extension block splinting. Chronic instability is rare, but limited MCP motion is not. Any digital nerve dysfunction secondary to the dislocation is usually transient in this age group.

Amputations

Fingertip trauma is very common in children. Incomplete amputations may involve the sterile or germinal matrices and require meticulous closure with 6-0 absorbable suture. Complete fingertip amputations that have spared the distal phalanx can be treated with nonadherent dressing changes. Local coverage with advancement flaps, skin grafts, composite grafts, or pedicle flaps is rarely necessary and should be reserved for significantly exposed bone or an older adolescent. Composite grafting has been used in very young children and is most successful in patients younger than age 2 years. Defatting of the graft increases survival. Because the physis of the distal phalanx is proximal to the level of injury in most cases, skeletal growth will continue and eventually compensate for any shortening that resulted from the injury in a toddler or preschool-age child. Longitudinal studies have found that nail deformity (hook or parrot's beak nail), digital foreshortening, and loss of sensibility are rare in children

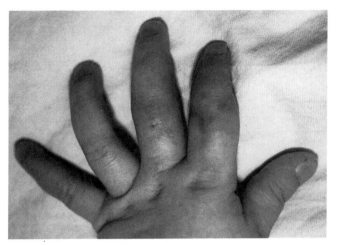

Figure 13

Three-year-old child 1 month after an index finger replant. Original injury was a crush amputation from an exercise bicycle.

regardless of the method of treatment for tip amputation.

Treatment of more proximal, complete digital amputations with replantation in children as young as 1 year of age is now standard. In children, the indications for replantation are more liberal than in adults and include single digit amputations in zones I and II and multiple digit, thumb, midpalm, hand, and distal forearm amputations. Crush amputations from doors, heavy objects, or bicycle chains (Fig. 13) have a peak incidence at age 5 years while sharp amputations occur more commonly in adolescents. Digital survival rates from replantation range from 69% to 89% in pediatric series. More favorable digital survival was seen in sharp amputations, body weight greater than 11 kg, more than 1 vein repaired, bone shortening, intraosseous wire fixation, and vein grafting of arteries and veins. Vessel size generally exceeds 0.8 mm in digital replants in children and is technically feasible. Index and long finger replants have done better than small finger replants in children. A survival rate of 95% occurred in children if prompt reperfusion was seen after arterial repair, with at least 1 successful venous anastomosis, compared with poor survival if 1 or both of these were absent. Neural recovery rates far exceed those cited in adults, with near universal return of 2-point discrimination less than 5 mm. Tenolysis may be necessary after tendon repair. Two-stage flexor tendon reconstruction in children has a higher rate of complications than in adults. Growth arrest and subsequent deformity are more common if there is a crush component to the amputation. Microvascular toe to thumb transfer is a very successful alternative to pollicization following a failed thumb replant in a young child.

Annotated Bibliography

Cole RJ, Manske PR: Classification of ulnar deficiency according to the thumb and first web. *J Hand Surg* 1997;22A:479–488.

These authors present a newer classification based on the frequently seen deficient thumb and first web. This excellent new classification focuses the surgeon's attention on these deficiencies and proposes surgical reconstruction based on them.

Gallant GG, Bora FW Jr: Congenital deformities of the upper extremity. *J Am Acad Orthop Surg* 1996;4:162–171.

An excellent review of the more common congenital differences of the upper extremity and recent publications devoted to it is presented.

Lamb DW, Scott H, Lam WL, Gillespie WJ, Hooper G: Operative correction of radial club hand: A long-term follow-up of centralization of the hand on the ulna. *J Hand Surg* 1997;22B:533–536.

This long-term follow-up of 21 centralizations for radial longitudinal deficiency in 17 patients is reviewed a mean of 27 years after surgery. Although the ulna remained short, there were no premature fusions of the distal ulnar physis and function was satisfactory. Many of the cases with poor results initially presented with fixed deformities greater than 90°, prompting the push for earlier referral and treatment.

Lourie GM, Costas BL, Bayne LG: The zig-zag deformity in preaxial polydactyly: A new cause and its treatment. *J Hand Surg* 1995;20B:561–564.

This article reviews the zig-zag deformity seen as a complication in preaxial polydactyly reconstruction and describes a new cause and its treatment. The surgeon and pediatrician should be alerted to this presentation to expedite referral. Eight cases are presented and the principles of reconstruction outlined.

Manske PR, Halikis MN: Surgical classification of central deficiency according to the thumb web. *J Hand Surg* 1995;20A:687–697.

This excellent new classification proposes a newer scheme based on the severity of the thumb web contracture and helps direct the surgeon with reconstruction.

Nanchahal J, Tonkin MA: Preoperative distraction lengthening for radial longitudinal deficiency. *J Hand Surg* 1996;21B:103–107.

This article documents the success achieved with preoperative soft-tissue distraction in correction of patients with radial longitudinal deficiency. It not only helps to achieve preoperative correction of the deformity, but also in short-term follow-up seems to maintain the correction achieved with centralization.

Classic Bibliography

Baker GL, Kleinert JM: Digit replantation in infants and young children: Determinants of survival. *Plast Reconstr Surg* 1994;94:139–145.

Dixon GL Jr, Moon NF: Rotational supracondylar fractures of the proximal phalanx in children. *Clin Orthop* 1972;83:151–156.

Gibbons CL, Woods DA, Pailthorpe C, Carr AJ, Worlock P: The management of isolated distal radius fractures in children. *J Pediatr Orthop* 1994;14:207–210.

Letts M, Rowhani N: Galeazzi-equivalent injuries of the wrist in children. *J Pediatr Orthop* 1993;13:561–566.

Mani GV, Hui PW, Cheng JC: Translation of the radius as a predictor of outcome in distal radial fractures of children. *J Bone Joint Surg* 1993;75B:808–811.

Mintzer CM, Waters PM, Simmons BP: Nonunion of the scaphoid in children treated by Herbert screw fixation and bone grafting: A report of five cases. *J Bone Joint Surg* 1995;77B:98–100.

O'Connell SJ, Moore MM, Strickland JW, Frazier GT, Dell PC: Results of zone I and zone II flexor tendon repairs in children. *J Hand Surg* 1994;19A:48–52.

Proctor MT, Moore DJ, Paterson JM: Redisplacement after manipulation of distal radial fractures in children. *J Bone Joint Surg* 1993;75B:453–454.

Waters PM, Kolettis GJ, Schwend R: Acute median neuropathy following physeal fractures of the distal radius. *J Pediatr Orthop* 1994;14:173–177.

Chapter 33
Wrist and Hand Trauma

Fractures of the Distal Radius

Distal radial fractures are among the most common orthopaedic injuries. The incidence is approximately 1 in 500 people, with a bimodal age distribution. One peak reflects high-energy injuries in adolescents and young adults. A second peak is associated with fractures in postmenopausal elderly women. Advances in technology and technique, coupled with increasing patient expectations, have caused the orthopaedic community to reexamine the outcome from this injury and to place a greater emphasis on restoration of anatomy and return of function. New classifications have been developed to characterize the fracture line extensions, amount of comminution, and fragment displacement. Despite enhanced imaging capabilities and increasing sophistication on the part of surgeons and radiologists, there is still a high rate of disagreement in inter- and intraobserver studies. This fact explains, at least in part, why a universally useful classification scheme with important predictive value still does not exist. The evaluation of distal radial fractures requires good quality posteroanterior (PA), lateral, and oblique radiographs. A knowledge of the standard radiographic parameters for the geometry of the radius platform remains important. Comparison to the accepted standards and imaging of the contralateral wrist will provide the basic information to determine the extent of fracture deformity. The articular surface should be evaluated on all 3 views to determine fracture fragment gap and step-off.

There has been interest in which radiographic parameters, if any, play a role in determining the functional outcome of distal radial fractures. The effect of residual dorsal tilt on range of motion (ROM) and carpal alignment was investigated in 30 patients with extra-articular fractures. Increasing dorsal tilt of the radial platform resulted in the intercalated segment adopting a dorsal posture, similar to dorsal intercalated segment instability (DISI), but without intercarpal ligament rupture. Adverse clinical results were noted when dorsal tilt was greater than 10°, and signs of midcarpal instability occurred when dorsal tilt averaged 30°. In another study, computer-simulated analysis of radiocarpal stress demonstrated that increasing dorsal angulation shifted stress concentration dorsally from a more physiologic palmar position. Results of this study support previous work, which indicated

that dorsal angulation of more than 30° was associated with an increased incidence of radiocarpal degenerative arthrosis.

In another laboratory study, the effects of 4 common types of radial deformity on distal radioulnar joint (DRUJ) mechanics were investigated. Radial shortening caused the greatest disturbance in kinematics and the most distortion of the triangular fibrocartilage; loss of volar tilt and radial inclination had a moderate effect, and anteroposterior (AP) translation had little deleterious effect. Ulnocarpal abutment occurred when shortening was greater than 6 mm, and loss of radial inclination beyond 10° increased load at the lunate fossa. The effect of intra-articular incongruity on the development of degenerative arthritis also has been examined. In a review of 47 patients 30 or more years after intra-articular fractures, as little as 1 mm of joint incongruity significantly increased the presence of radiographic degenerative changes in both the radiocarpal joint and the DRUJ. Based on data from these laboratory studies and clinical observations, criteria for an acceptable reduction of the radius platform have evolved (Table 1).

In recent clinical studies, investigators have attempted to correlate adequacy of the reduction with subjective out-

Table 1
Radiographic criteria for acceptable healing of a distal radial fracture

Radiographic Criterion	Acceptable Measurement
Radioulnar length discrepancy	Radial shortening of < 5mm at DRUJ compared with contralateral wrist
Radial inclination	Inclination on posteroanterior film ≥ 15°
Radial tilt	Sagittal tilt on lateral projection between 15° dorsal tilt and 20° volar tilt
Articular incongruity	Incongruity of the intra-articular fracture is ≤ 2 mm at radiocarpal joint

(Reproduced with permission from Graham TJ: Surgical correction of malunited fractures of the distal radius. J Am Acad Orthop Surg 1997;5:273–274.)

comes. In a retrospective study involving 76 patients who were reviewed 27 to 36 years after treatment of their distal radial fractures, clinical outcome was compared with radiographic parameters. The results revealed a weak correlation between degenerative changes in the radiocarpal joint and DRUJ, and clinical outcome. In another retrospective study, displaced intra-articular fractures in young adults were evaluated an average of 7.1 years after open reduction. Two independent "blinded" observers assessed plain radiographs and computed tomography scans. A strong association was found between the presence of radiographic signs of osteoarthritis and residual displacement of articular fragments at the time of osseous union. However, the functional status, as determined by physical examination and response to outcome questionnaires, did not correlate with the magnitude of step-off and gap displacement at the time of fracture healing. The authors concluded that surgical treatment of intra-articular malunion in young adults should be based on clinical findings rather than on radiographic evidence of osteoarthritis. However, in another retrospective study, 2 radiographic factors had a significant association with poorer functional results: radiographic evidence of osteoarthritis and reversal of the normal volar tilt of the distal radius.

Currently, most surgeons believe that anatomic reduction is critical even though the precise clinical consequences of displacement, especially articular incongruity, have not been determined. Therefore, in active healthy patients aggressive treatment measures are warranted to achieve and maintain stable reduction, but in elderly or physically compromised individuals, the risks and long-term benefits of aggressive management must be carefully considered.

In addition to closed reduction and casting, options available for the treatment of distal radial fractures include external fixation, percutaneous pinning (including intrafocal pinning), plate fixation, arthroscopically-assisted reduction, and various forms of bone defect filling. Each of these can achieve a specific desired effect, and the use of multiple complementary techniques is sometimes necessary (Fig. 1).

Percutaneous pinning following closed reduction is a time-honored method of stabilizing large distal radial fragments. Recent mechanical testing of extra-articular distal radial fractures stabilized with percutaneous pins demonstrated that the most stable construct in both torsion and cantilever bending uses 3 Kirschner wires (K-wires). Two K-wires are placed through the radial styloid and the other through the dorsal ulnar corner of the radius.

Intrafocal or transfracture pinning has been widely used in Europe. Unlike the treatment regimens used by most North American surgeons, unprotected early motion is allowed after the intrafocal fracture treatment. The original indication for intrafocal fixation was an unstable extra-articular fracture in a young adult. However, indications have been extended to include elderly patients and intra-articular fractures with large fragments. Relative contraindications include significant intra-articular involvement, volar comminution, and advanced osteopenia. In a prospective study comparing

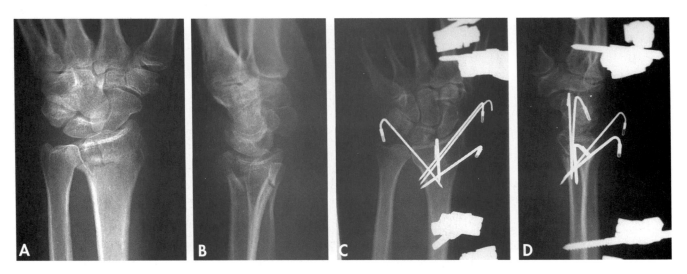

Figure 1

A and B, Radiographs showing an intra-articular, moderately comminuted fracture of the distal radius. C and D, This fracture was treated by a combination of Kapandji or intrafocal pinning and standard transfragment percutaneous pinning and neutralized by an external fixator.

transstyloid K-wire fixation and intrafocal pin fixation, pain and reflex sympathetic dystrophy occurred more frequently after intrafocal fixation and early mobilization. Although initial ROM was better in the intrafocal group, the difference became statistically insignificant after 6 weeks.

External fixators provide and maintain fracture reduction through ligamentotaxis. Radial height and inclination can be preserved, but orthopaedists report that palmar tilt often is lost. In a study of 26 patients with severe distal radial fractures, functional outcome was adversely affected in proportion to the amount and duration of distraction applied by the external fixator. In another study, 40 patients with severely comminuted intra-articular distal radial fractures were followed up for an average of 2.3 years. All fractures were treated with 3 weeks of external fixation using distraction, followed by 3 weeks of external fixation in neutral traction. ROM approximated 80% of the uninjured side, with an overall 82.5% of the patients showing good or excellent results.

External fixation also has been coupled with other methods of fracture treatment (Fig. 2). In a retrospective study the results were evaluated of treating combined internal and external fixation of highly comminuted distal radial fractures through palmar and dorsal surgical approaches. Ten of 12 patients followed up for an average of 27 months had good or excellent wrist function. External fixation also has been used in conjunction with percutaneous pin fixation; this is termed augmented external fixation. The goals of plate or pin fixa-tion combined with external fixation are to obtain a better reduction and to decrease the duration of distraction frame wear required to achieve and maintain a stable reduction.

Another adjunct to external fixation is the use of bone graft or bone void filler in fractures with severe comminution. In a prospective study of 32 unstable fractures treated by external fixation and dorsal cancellous bone grafting, the results were encouraging. Overall grip strength was 95% of normal, and radial height was maintained in all but 5 patients. The duration of the external fixation was only 5 weeks, and there were no reported nonunions. Many new graft substitutes and allografts have been used successfully as bone void fillers.

Use of "pins-and-plaster" has declined in the past decade. Unlike earlier reports in which infection was a primary problem, a more recent retrospective analysis identified residual stiffness of the wrist and fingers as the most common complication. There was 1 pin track infection in the 73 patients treated.

Open reduction with plating is indicated for displaced palmar intra-articular fractures and palmar margin fractures (Smith type II or volar Barton's fractures). Studies have demonstrated that these fractures cannot be reduced by ligamentotaxis alone. Such fracture types require open reduction and internal fixation (ORIF) using a palmar approach and buttress fixation.

Dorsal plating has been associated with frequent complications (tendon irritation and rupture, prominent hardware).

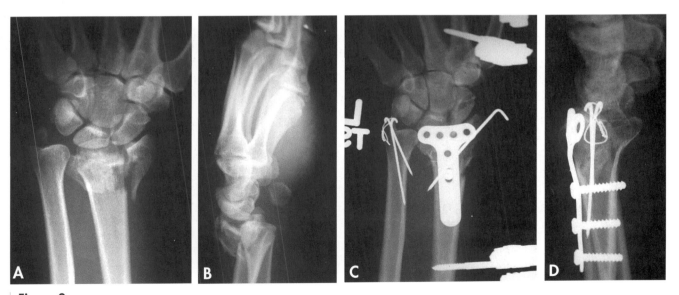

Figure 2

A and B, Radiographs of a highly complex fracture of the distal radius with additional fracture at the base of the ulnar styloid. C and D, This fracture required a combination of internal and external fixation. The basistyloid fracture was stabilized with tension-band technique.

Therefore, dorsal displacement usually is treated by pins or external fixation and grafts (if comminution is significant). Lower profile dorsal plates have been developed and may become popular if additional studies confirm their safety and reliability.

Arthroscopically-assisted reduction of distal radial fractures followed by bone graft is an option when there is significant central comminution of the articular surface. Subcortical pins, bone grafts, and/or an external fixator are required for additional support. As an alternative to arthroscopy, some surgeons make a dorsal arthrotomy and reduce the fragments under direct vision. General recommendations for the selection of treatment methods for distal radial fractures are emerging (Table 2).

Table 2
Classification and treatment recommendations for distal radial fractures

Classification	Treatment*
Extra-articular	
Nondisplaced or reduced	CR, splint/cast
Displaced	
Dorsal	
Large Fragments	CRPP
Small fragments (comminution)	Ex-fix, ICBG
Palmar	
Large fragments	CRPP
Vertical shear	Palmar plate
Small fragments	Palmar plate + ICBG
Intra-articular	
Nondisplaced or reduced	CR & splint/cast
Displaced	
Radial styloid†	CRPP
Dorsal fragments	
Large fragments	CRPP
Small fragments	Ex-fix + ICBG
Palmar fragments	Palmar plate
Dorsal and palmar fragments	
Large dorsal fragments	Palmar plate + dorsal K-wires
Small dorsal fragments	Palmar plate + ex-fix + ICBG
Central depression	Open or arthroscopic reduction + (PP or ex-fix) + ICBG

*CR, closed reduction; PP, percutaneous pinning; ex-fix, external fixator; ICBG, iliac crest bone graft
†Can combine with next 3 intra-articular categories (treat additively)

Injuries About the Distal Ulna

Injuries to the triangular fibrocartilage complex (TFCC) and acute disorders of the DRUJ have often been considered separate lesions. Recently, there has been an increasing awareness of the interdependence of these structures in this region.

The DRUJ is composed of a convex distal "seat," two thirds of which is covered by articular cartilage, around which rotates a concave radial sigmoid notch. The ulnar "pole" is separated from the carpus by the triangular fibrocartilage. The differential radius of curvature of the radius and ulna at the DRUJ permits the composite motions of rotation and translation. Pronation is associated with palmar translation of the radiocarpal unit, whereas supination is associated with dorsal translation of the radius. Additionally, in pronation, the radius migrates proximally relative to the ulna, whereas in supination the radius migrates distally. There has been much controversy regarding which of the distal radioulnar ligaments (palmar or dorsal) tighten in pronation and supination. Both contribute to DRUJ stability.

The TFCC is made up of several components: the articular disk, the dorsal and palmar radioulnar ligaments, the extensor carpi ulnaris subsheath, and the ulnolunate and ulnotriquetral ligaments. The central fibrocartilage disk does not provide stability to the DRUJ but acts primarily as a cushion between the carpus and the DRUJ. The remaining components of the TFCC do impart stability to the DRUJ. Of clinical significance is the fact that most of the stabilizing TFCC structures have a confluent attachment to the base (fovea) and proximal third of the ulnar styloid. Large fractures of the styloid can, therefore, destabilize the DRUJ (Fig. 3).

Functionally, the TFCC suspends the distal radius and the carpus from the distal ulna. When the TFCC is incompetent, the radiocarpal complex moves away from the distal ulna. Biomechanically, this move disrupts the arc of motion that the radius and carpus circumscribe around the distal ulna, resulting in limited prosupination and pain.

The treatment of TFCC lesions is predicated, in part, on the availability of a blood supply. The central portion of the TFCC is avascular, and, therefore, is not amenable to primary repair; debridement is recommended. The peripheral 40%

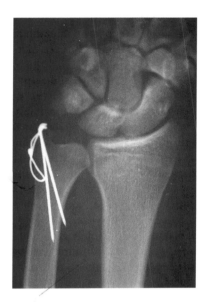

Figure 3

The radial fracture was stable but instability at the distal radioulnar joint was caused by the ulnar styloid fracture, which required fixation.

struction of peripheral TFCC tears were assessed in 45 patients with clinical instability of the DRUJ secondary to trauma. Only 15 of the 41 wrists had definitive diagnoses before surgery. Four of the 45 wrists had associated distal radial fractures, and 2 of the 45 wrists had associated ulnar styloid fractures. The remaining injuries were determined at arthroscopy. Peripheral tears that were arthroscopically

of the TFCC is vascular; therefore, healing after primary repair is possible.

Injuries to the TFCC have been classified as either traumatic (class I) or degenerative (class II), and within these 2 broad categories, specific injuries are classified by the portion of the TFCC affected (Fig. 4). Depending on their location and severity, injuries of the TFCC can affect stability of the DRUJ. Therefore it is logical to classify these injuries based upon their destabilizing effect (Outline 1).

Although careful historic information gathering and physical examination are the cornerstone of diagnosis of problems about the ulnar wrist, imaging modalities play a critical role in defining pathology. Wrist arthrography has many advocates, but all acknowledge that there are large numbers of false negatives and false positives. TFCC tears can be diagnosed accurately with good quality magnetic resonance imaging (MRI). In a recent study involving 31 wrists evaluated by 3-dimensional gradient recalled echo sequences and arthroscopy, the MRI sequence was highly sensitive and specific for diagnosing TFCC tears. Low sensitivity and specificity were found for injuries of the TFCC that involved the ulnocarpal ligaments. Regardless of the results of MRI or arthrography, those patients recalcitrant to conservative care are candidates for arthroscopy. In a study involving 22 patients with central (type IA) tears of the TFCC who were treated by arthroscopic debridement and followed up for 1 year, there was return to full activity in 12 weeks with no residual stiffness or persistence of pain in the wrist. Data from a recent study demonstrate that type ID lesions can be repaired using an arthroscopically-assisted technique.

In a multicenter study, the results of arthroscopic recon-

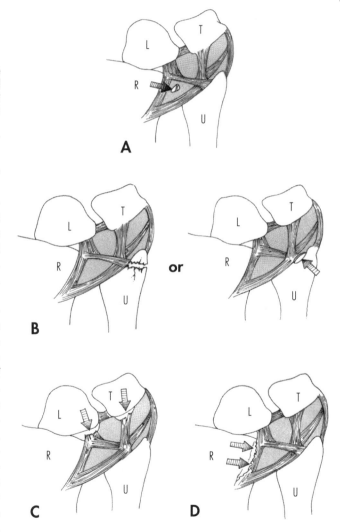

Figure 4

Diagrammatic drawing of traumatic, or class 1, abnormalities of the triangular fibrocartilage complex. A, Class 1A, central perforation (arrow). B, Class 1B, ulnar avulsion (arrow), with or without distal ulnar fracture. C, Class 1C, distal avulsion (arrows). D, Class 1D, radial avulsion (arrows), with or without sigmoid notch fracture. L = lunate; R = radius; T = triquetrum; U = ulna. (Reproduced with permission from Palmer AK: Triangular fibrocartilage complex lesions: A classification. *J Hand Surg* 1989;14A:594–606.)

Outline 1
Classification of carpal instabilities

Carpal instability dissociative (CID)
   Dorsiflexion (DISI)
   Palmarflexion (VISI)
Carpal instability nondissociative (CIND)
   Radiocarpal
   Midcarpal
   Ulnar translocation
Carpal instability complex (CIC)
   Dorsal perilunate volar lunate dislocation
   Transscaphoid perilunate fracture dislocation
Carpal instability longitudinal (CIL)
   Axial ulnar (AU)
   Axial radial (AR)
   Axial ulnar-radial combined (AUR)
Severity of instability grade
   Dynamic instability (normal plain radiographs; diagnosis
      made on stress or motion studies or cineradiographs)
   Static (fixed) instability (seen on routine radiographs)
   Dislocation or fracture dislocation

(Reproduced with permission from Amadio PC: Carpal kinematics and instability: A clinical and anatomic primer. *Clin Anat* 1991;4:1–12)

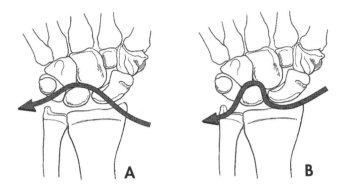

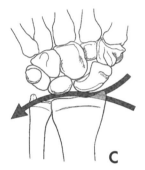

Figure 5

A, The "greater arc" injury is a transverse carpal injury with fractures of the wrist bones, with or without fracture of the radial styloid. B, Force transmission in the "lesser arc" injury is through the intercarpal ligaments. C, In the "inferior arc" injury, the forces are transmitted through the radiocarpal level. (Adapted with permission from Weber ER, Chao EV: An experimental approach to mechanism of scaphoid fractures. *J Hand Surg* 1978;2: 142–148.)

repaired using an inside-out technique had the most good results.

Carpal Instability

In an effort to standardize diagnostic and treatment modalities, wrist investigators have recommended that all carpal instability patterns be classified into 6 categories describing (1) chronicity, (2) consistency, (3) etiology, (4) location, (5) direction, and (6) pattern of instability (Outline 1). The pattern of instability that is produced is correlated to the anatomic structures injured. For example, a DISI deformity will result when the scapholunate (SL) ligament or both the SL and lunotriquetral (LT) ligaments are ruptured. A volar intercalary segment instability (VISI) pattern occurs with

injury to the LT ligaments as well as with the laxity of the midcarpal support structures.

The typical fall on an outstretched hand results in wrist dorsiflexion, ulnar deviation, and intercarpal supination. These forces enter the radiocarpal unit from the lateral or radial side then progress ulnarward—a "transverse" instability pattern. The path of energy across the wrist is variable and is determined by many factors (wrist position at time of fall, patient's weight and previous wrist status, direction of body weight forces). The pathologic forces typically follow 1 of 3 paths known as the "greater, lesser, and inferior arcs" (Fig. 5). The path of the greater and lesser arc injuries are similar; the distinction indicates that the injury complex involves bones or soft tissues for the greater and lesser arcs, respectively. The important deflector of forces in these injuries is the radio-lunotriquetral ligament (long radiolunate ligament). In the lesser arc injury, for example, this stout structure directs the force through the path of least resistance, the SL interosseous ligament (SLIL; stage I). The space of Pourier dissipates the energy at the midcarpal joint in most injuries (stage II), but in some injuries, the forces are of sufficient magnitude to also rupture the LT interosseous ligament (stage III). In the ultimate expression of this transverse instability, the lunate is dislocated (stage IV) (Fig. 6). The greater arc pattern resembles this path of force transmission except that the energy travels through bone, as in a transstyloid fracture or fracture-dislocation.

The "inferior arc" is another transverse instability in which the forces are transmitted from radial to ulnar at the radiocarpal level. Often, this injury is accompanied by fractures of the radial and ulnar styloids, or volar and dorsal ligament avulsions from the margin of the radius platform (Fig. 5, B and C). The most severe injury in the inferior arc spectrum is radiocarpal dislocation.

An understanding of the transverse pattern of force transmission allows accurate identification of the location of injury, even in complex carpal disruptions. SL dissociation (stage I) is the prototype of carpal instability. SL instability can occur in association with acute scaphoid fracture, but most commonly is caused by an isolated ligament injury. Anatomically, the SLIL is a C-shaped fibrocartilage complex divided into a palmar component, a proximal membranous

component, and a dorsal component. Dorsally and palmarly, stout fibrous connections run between the scaphoid and lunate bones and attach to the strong radiocarpal ligaments. Histologic and anatomic studies suggest that the dorsal fibrous segment of the SLIL is a primary stabilizer.

A provocative test used to demonstrate SL instability is the scaphoid shift test. For the test to be considered positive, a painful clunk must be produced as the wrist is brought from ulnar to radial deviation with dorsally directed pressure on the scaphoid tubercle. The specificity of this test has been questioned by data from recent investigations. In one study, a positive shift was elicited in 32% of asymptomatic patients without SL instability.

The plain radiograph is the single most important study for patients with suspected SL injury. Bilateral comparison radiographs are often necessary. An AP view may show loss of SL articular parallelism, SL diastasis of more than 3 mm, and the presence of a scaphoid cortical ring sign. The ring to proximal pole distance is decreased (less than 3 mm) with acute scaphoid flexion. From a true lateral radiograph, the radioscaphoid, SL, and the capitolunate angles are determined. A radioscaphoid angle of more than 80°, a capitolunate angle of more than 20°, and an SL angle of more than 70°, all representing flexion of the scaphoid and extension of the lunate (DISI), are indicative of an SL dissociation.

Triple injection wrist arthrography is often the next step in the workup, but the validity of this test has been questioned. Triple injection arthrography and wrist arthroscopy were

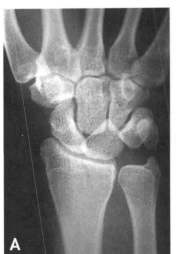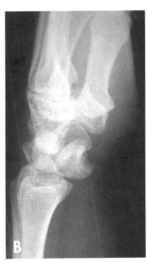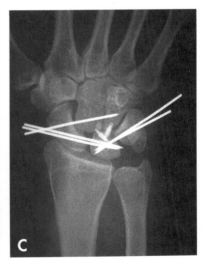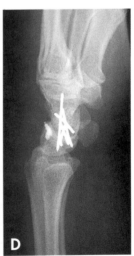

Figure 6

A and B, Radiographs of a lunate dislocation. C and D, The lunate is reduced back to its position on the radius and the remaining carpal bones relocated. The intercarpal ligaments are repaired and the construct stabilized with pins during healing.

compared in 50 consecutive patients who had a history of clinical findings consistent with an internal derangement of the wrist. The sensitivity, specificity, and accuracy of triple injection cinearthrography in detecting tears of the SL ligament, LT ligament, and triangular fibrocartilage as a group were 56%, 83%, and 60%, respectively. A negative arthrographic study does not rule out the possibility of an internal derangement.

The role of diagnostic and therapeutic wrist arthroscopy is evolving. Wrist arthroscopy is considered by some to be the standard for diagnosing SL injuries. It allows visual examination of both the radiocarpal and midcarpal joints to establish the integrity of the SL and other intercarpal ligaments, as well as treatment of certain intra-articular injuries. Several studies have confirmed the benefit of arthroscopic debridement of torn SL ligaments. In a retrospective study of 128 patients with internal derangement of the wrist, arthroscopy allowed accurate diagnosis and successful treatment in 52%. In 20% of patients, wrist arthroscopy provided definitive diagnoses
• where pathologies were previously undiagnosed. It was estimated that 50% of patients avoided wrist arthrotomy as a result of the judicious use of arthroscopy. In a recent study, intercarpal soft-tissue lesions were evaluated in 60 patients with displaced intra-articular radial fractures treated with arthroscopically-assisted reduction and internal fixation. Injury to the intercarpal ligaments was most frequently associated with radial fractures involving the lunate facet.

The goals of SL ligament reconstruction are stable reduction of the SL joint and correction of the corresponding carpal collapse. If possible, the dorsal (and proximal) SLILs are directly repaired. K-wires are placed across the reduced SL joint, and left in place for approximately 8 weeks. The results of repairing the SLIL (12 patients) were compared to those of open reduction and pinning without ligament repair (20 patients) in 32 patients with perilunate dislocations. Patients who had better radiographic intercarpal relationships had better function. This study suggests that even after 4 weeks, ligament repair should be attempted. If sufficient dorsal interosseous ligament is not present, dorsal capsulodesis can be performed. In a retrospective study, 15 of 17 patients with capsulodesis returned to their original occupations, but all patients demonstrated a loss of palmar flexion.

Acute SL injury in a young, active individual should be treated by direct repair or capsulodesis to prevent scapholunate advanced collapse (SLAC). However, for a chronic injury, other reconstructive options such as proximal row carpectomy, scaphotrapeziotrapezoid (STT) fusion, and other limited intercarpal arthrodeses may be selected.

In perilunate dislocation, the lunate remains located on the radius and the remaining carpal bones translocate dorsally. In palmar lunate dislocation, the remaining carpus is colinear with the radius and the lunate is extruded into the carpal canal or volar forearm. Treatment of perilunate injuries typically consists of closed reduction, followed by dorsal ligament repair and interosseous pinning (radiocarpal fixation is used in some circumstances). A volar approach usually is reserved for chronic perilunate dislocations and lunate dislocations that cannot fail by closed means or are associated with median nerve compression. In 1 series, combined volar and dorsal approaches were used to treat 11 perilunate dislocations and fracture-dislocations. Volar ligament tears were repaired directly followed by dorsal reduction of the SL joints. Grip strength, ROM, radiographs, and patient satisfaction were assessed at an average of 5 years after treatment. Overall, 10 of the 11 patients were satisfied with these results and 1 developed radiographic signs of SLAC arthritis and was not satisfied with the result.

Twenty-nine transscaphoid perilunate dislocations treated with open reduction and Herbert screw fixation of the scaphoid along with ligament repair and supplemental K-wire stabilization were evaluated an average of 24 months after injury. The scaphoid fractures united in all patients with proper carpal alignment. There were no signs of SLAC wrist and most patients were satisfied with their clinical outcomes.

Acute, isolated LT instability is much less common than SL instability. The static radiographic pattern most commonly associated with this lesion is VISI. Recent cadaveric studies have demonstrated that injury to the LT interosseous ligament alone is not enough to establish the clinical deformity. Disruption of the dorsal radiotriquetral ligament must also occur. The pathogenesis of this type of deformity has been postulated to be an ulnar to radial progression of ligamentous disruption, possibly caused by a blow on the hypothenar eminence when the hand is outstretched. Positive ulnar variance has been suggested as another predisposing factor. LT instability can also develop after perilunate dislocation when the LT injury was not reconstructed.

Treatment of acute LT injuries is directed by the severity of the injury. In a suspected acute tear with normal radiographs, wrist immobilization for 3 to 5 weeks is the treatment of choice. If symptoms persist after closed treatment, arthroscopic confirmation and debridement of the torn LT ligament can be performed. If radiographs show a static VISI deformity initially, open or closed reduction and pinning are indicated. LT injuries associated with ulnar positive variance may be part of an ulnar abutment syndrome. In that case, ulnar shortening osteotomy can be done as part of the reconstruction.

Palmar midcarpal instability was described in a series of patients with palmar sag on the ulnar side of the wrist and a history of a painful clunk at the midcarpal joint with ulnar deviation. This is the most common form of carpal instability nondissociative (CIND). Anatomic studies demonstrate that the ulnar arm of the palmar arcuate ligament and the dorsal radiotriquetral ligament often are attenuated in patients with palmar midcarpal instability. Palmar midcarpal instability is a dynamic condition, best seen on videofluoroscopy. This study shows the characteristic sudden dorsiflexion of the proximal row (catch-up clunk) as the wrist achieves full ulnar deviation.

Palmar midcarpal instability often is treated successfully by avoidance of aggravating activities and intermittent splinting. Surgical treatment for palmar midcarpal instability is midcarpal fusion. Stabilization by reinforcement of the attenuated ligaments is under investigation.

The remaining carpal instability patterns are less frequently encountered. The extreme expression of the inferior arc injury, radiocarpal dislocation, is detected by observing the ulnar translocation of the carpus and accompanying fractures of the radial and/or ulnar styloids. Open reduction, ligament repair and bone fixation, and radiocarpal balancing with external fixation are often needed for these complex injuries. The so-called "longitudinal" or "axial" instabilities refer to high-energy injuries. The term axial is likely a misnomer because most of these injuries occur as a result of crushing mechanisms; thus, the carpus is likely exploded from the standpoint of hoop stresses rather than longitudinal transfer of forces along the rays. Hand fasciotomies and nerve releases often are needed in addition to fracture reduction and stabilization.

Fractures of the scaphoid are the most common fractures of the carpus. Some are radiographically apparent from initial evaluation, but in many a fracture line is not visible until bony resorption at the fracture advances. Debate still exists as to the superiority or necessity of long-arm immobilization over short arm casting for the fractured scaphoid. Some clinical and mechanical evidence supports the neutralization of elbow and forearm motion in promoting stability of the fractured scaphoid. Although repeat radiographs and bone scanning have traditionally been used for the diagnosis of occult scaphoid fractures, MRI may be useful in detecting subtle fracture lines and bone edema at an even earlier stage.

Treatment of nondisplaced fractures of the scaphoid consists of immobilization until clinical or radiographic healing occurs. Acceptable reduction of scaphoid fractures allows no more than 10° of angular deviation and 1 mm of displacement; these strict criteria indicate the frequency of nonunion of scaphoid fractures. Displaced fractures are treated by open reduction and pinning or compression screw fixation. The volar approach is typically selected for its greater margin of safety with regard to the critical dorsal blood supply. However, the dorsal approach is useful for exposing fractures in the proximal third of the scaphoid. With the expanding knowledge of local perfusion territories of the radius, new vascularized bone flaps from the radius have been described. These pedicled bone islands can favorably change the biology and provide structural support for scaphoid reconstruction in nonunion.

Thumb Metacarpophalangeal Joint Collateral Ligament Injuries

At the thumb metacarpophalangeal (MCP) joint, the ulnar collateral ligament (UCL) provides stability against radially directed stress and resists volar subluxation and supination of the proximal phalanx. The proper collateral ligament is the primary joint stabilizer when the MCP joint is flexed. The accessory collateral ligament provides stability with the joint in full extension. It is contiguous with the proper collateral ligament, originating from its volar surface and inserting into the volar plate.

UCL failure occurs most often at the proximal phalangeal insertion. The tear may be incomplete or complete with variable amounts of proximal ligament retraction. For gross instability to result, the proper and the accessory collateral ligaments must both be ruptured. An intact accessory collateral ligament will prevent retraction of a ruptured proper collateral ligament.

Identification of a complete and retracted UCL tear is based on physical examination. A palpable mass over the ulnar aspect of the MCP joint may represent the retracted ligament stump displaced proximal and dorsal to the adductor aponeurosis (Stener's lesion). Ligament integrity is evaluated by valgus stress testing, with the joint anesthetized and placed in 30° of flexion and in extension. More than 35° of joint laxity, or 15° more laxity than is present in the uninjured thumb in both flexed and extended joint positions, is consistent with a complete UCL rupture and probable retraction (89% of the time). Radiographic findings of proximal phalanx volar subluxation and radial deviation may indicate complete ligament disruption.

Arthrography, ultrasound, and MRI have been used to identify complete tears. However, these tests add cost and provide little additional information. Careful stress examination is still the optimal method for determining ligament integrity.

For incomplete tears, a period of immobilization or protected mobilization will predictably yield good results.

Complete ligament tears require surgical repair (Table 3). A variety of surgical methods have been advocated including repair using suture anchors and arthroscopic reduction of Stener's lesions. Almost any method of anatomic repair performed within 3 weeks of injury will achieve good or excellent results in 90% of patients. If a fracture constituting a large portion of the articular surface is rotated or displaced or if the joint is unstable, open reduction and internal fixation are indicated. Small or comminuted fractures can be excised and the ligament advanced into the bony defect. Even nondisplaced fractures may coexist with complete ligament tears.

Chronic instability can result in loss of pinch strength, pain, and posttraumatic arthrosis. Despite ligament retraction and fibrosis, chronic UCL instability usually can be reconstructed with local tissues. If local tissue is inadequate, joint stability can be restored using a free tendon graft. In patients with arthrosis and pain resulting from long-standing instability, arthrodesis is the treatment of choice.

Radial collateral ligament injuries are less common and surgical indications less well defined. Acute injuries are best managed by immobilization. Often patients present late with symptoms of pain and instability. In 1 series of 18 patients, there was no significant difference in outcome between acute and chronic repairs.

Table 3
Treatment of thumb ulnar collateral ligament injuries

Valgus Instability With MCP* Joint Flexed 30°	Valgus Instability With MCP Joint Extended	Palpable Stener's Lesion or Proximal Phalanx Volar Subluxation	Displaced or Rotated Avulsion Fracture or >10% Articular Involvement	Treatment†
Yes	No	No	No	Immobilization (4 weeks)
Yes/No	No	Yes	No	Immobilization (reexamination in 5 to 7 days)
Yes/No	Yes/No	Yes/No	Yes	ORIF or ligament advancement
Yes	Yes	Yes/No	Yes/No	Ligament reconstruction

*MCP = Metacarpophalangeal

†ORIF = Open reduction and internal fixation

Metacarpal and Phalangeal Fractures

Most tubular bone fractures in the hand are treated nonsurgically. Surgical indications must be individualized but include: (1) the inability to obtain or maintain an acceptable reduction using closed means; (2) displaced articular fractures; (3) open fractures and those with bone loss; (4) fractures that may displace during care for associated soft-tissue injuries; (5) multiple hand or wrist fractures; and (6) fractures in the polytraumatized patient.

Patients tolerate sagittal plane angulation better than coronal plane angulation and fracture rotation. However, the shortening created by sagittal plane angulation of phalangeal fractures may upset the balance between flexion and extension forces. In 2 separate cadaveric studies, this was true for metacarpal (MC) fractures as well. More than 30° of apex dorsal MC shaft angulation significantly lessened flexion force. Both flexion and extension force decreased if MC shortening exceeded 3 mm. Despite these laboratory findings, clinical reviews continue to document excellent functional results even with 50° of residual angulation in fifth MC neck fractures.

Coronal plane angulation and malrotation of MC and phalangeal fractures may lead to digital overlap. Rotational malalignment is difficult to determine on radiographs and is best assessed by physical examination. With flexion, there should be no digital scissoring, and the injured finger should point to the scaphoid tuberosity. Contralateral comparison is always advised.

Fracture stability is based on fracture pattern, fracture displacement, and supporting structures. Displaced oblique, spiral, and articular fractures tend to be unstable after reduction, particularly when comminuted. For example, unicondylar and bicondylar proximal phalangeal fractures usually require surgical stabilization. Third and fourth MC fractures often are stable despite unstable fracture patterns due to the support of the adjacent MCs and their intermetacarpal ligaments.

Whenever possible, closed reduction and percutaneous fix-

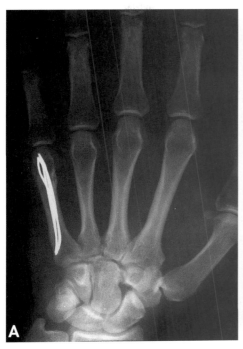
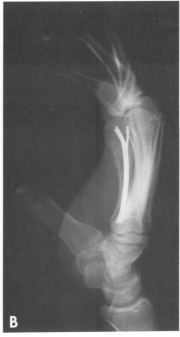

Figure 7

A and B, Radiographs of a fifth metacarpal neck fracture treated by "bouquet" pinning.

is significantly higher and ROM is worse following minifragment plate fixation for open injuries and for phalangeal fractures than for MC fractures. In 53 patients with 68 MC and phalangeal articular and peri-articular fractures fixed with minicondylar plates, there were 67 complications in 29 patients. Again MC fractures had a significantly higher percentage of excellent results.

Malunion is the most common bony complication. An MC osteotomy at the proximal metaphysis can correct approximately 20° of malrotation of the index, long, and ring fingers and 20° to 30° of malrotation of the small finger. In a review of 59 corrective phalangeal osteotomies for a variety of phalangeal malunions, satisfactory correction was found in 76% of patients with no nonunions. Active ROM was increased in 89% of patients. Ninety-six percent of those patients requiring only correction of the bone obtained good or excellent results.

ation using K-wires or screws are done. When an acceptable reduction cannot be obtained closed or when fixation cannot be achieved using percutaneous techniques, open reduction is required. K-wires alone and combined with other forms of fixation remain the most widely used and versatile stabilization devices for both MC and phalangeal fractures. Long oblique and spiral fractures (fracture length exceeds twice the bone diameter) can be fixed using interfragmentary compression screws. The fracture fragments should be at least 3 times the outer diameter of the screw in order to avoid splintering. Screws also are effective for stabilizing minimally comminuted articular fractures, particularly condylar phalangeal fractures. Unstable transverse and short oblique fractures with minimal comminution can be treated by K-wire fixation, interosseous wiring, composite wiring using a tension band technique, and intramedullary fixation ("bouquet" pinning) (Fig. 7). In the MCs these fractures are amenable to plate fixation.

In general, plates are indicated for fractures characterized by displacement, comminution, or bone loss. Anatomic restoration, rigid fixation, and early active motion are the goals of surgical intervention in indicated situations. Immobilization longer than 3 to 4 weeks promotes digital stiffness and poor functional outcomes. The major complication rate

Thumb Metacarpal Base Fracture-Dislocations

Nondisplaced Bennett's fractures without joint instability are treated with a thumb spica cast carefully molded to counteract the deforming forces. Most displaced Bennett's fractures can be reduced closed but require internal fixation. Reduction is accomplished with traction, mild pronation, and downward pressure over the dorsal radial base of the extended, palmarly abducted thumb MC. T- or Y-shaped intra-articular fractures (Rolando's fractures) frequently require ORIF. Oblique longitudinal traction or external fixation with or without limited internal fixation and bone grafting are beneficial in fractures with extensive comminution.

Anatomic reduction of Bennett's fractures is important to avoid painful carpometacarpal instability and posttraumatic arthrosis. Eighteen patients with surgically treated Bennett's fractures were followed up for a mean of 10.5 years. The severity of osteoarthritis determined radiographically correlated with the accuracy of reduction. However, almost all patients had evidence of joint degeneration despite exact fracture reduction, and there was no correlation between arthritis and symptoms. The results of this and previous studies bring into question the benefit of extreme measures in obtaining anatomic reduction of Bennett's fractures.

Proximal Interphalangeal Joint Fracture-Dislocations

Proximal interphalangeal (PIP) joint fracture-dislocations most often involve the base of the middle phalanx and are caused by axial loading or hyperextension forces (Fig. 8). Avulsion injuries at the insertions of the volar plate, collateral ligaments, and central slip may result in loss of the volar or dorsal buttress, allowing joint dislocation.

Dorsal fracture-dislocations involving 30% or less of the volar articular surface are usually stable when treated by closed reduction and extension block splinting. Stability must be assessed both clinically and radiographically. Frequently, when more than 40% to 50% of the volar articular surface is fractured, either reduction cannot be achieved by closed methods or excessive flexion is needed to prevent dorsal dislocation. The volar buttress can be reestablished by ORIF of large fracture fragments or volar plate arthroplasty. Advancement of the volar plate is highly effective when comminution precludes internal fixation and in neglected fractures. If more than 60% of the volar joint surface is involved, surgical results are less predictable. One treatment option is fracture reduction, juxta-articular bone grafting, and dynamic external fixation. Chronic injuries have been reconstructed by osteotomy, distraction, or implant arthroplasty, and salvaged by arthrodesis.

The treatment of severe fracture-dislocations continues to evolve. Controversy exists regarding the relative value of indirect joint reduction with dynamic external fixators and ORIF and bone grafting. Dynamic external fixation combines the concepts of ligamentotaxis and continuous passive motion to restore articular symmetry, enhance nutrition, stimulate healing of articular cartilage, and avoid joint contracture (Fig. 9). Dynamic traction can be used in conjunction with open reduction of the joint surface. Impressive remodeling has been reported in fractures when dynamic traction has been used.

Fourteen patients with dorsal and volar fracture-dislocations and pilon injuries were treated using a dynamic digital traction device applied in an office setting. Motion exercises were started immediately. Despite articular disruption averaging 80%, the 10 patients with isolated PIP joint injuries obtained 95° of motion at the PIP joint. Radiographs taken an average of 2 years after surgery revealed joint remodeling with maintenance of the joint space and no posttraumatic arthritis or recurrent dislocation. Central articular depression was not improved by this procedure but did not seem to affect the results. Similar results have been obtained with open reconstruction of the depressed articular surface. Twelve patients treated by ORIF and bone grafting were followed an average of 2.1 years. Cerclage wiring achieved fracture and joint reduction. Motion was initiated by postoperative day 4. Final radiographs revealed minor degenerative changes in only 1 patient. Active PIP motion averaged 89° with an 8° flexion contracture.

Because of the lack of soft-tissue attachments, dynamic external fixation cannot achieve indirect reduction of depressed central articular fragments. In general, these impacted articular fragments should be elevated, supported by bone graft, and, if possible, stabilized as long as this can be done without extensive soft-tissue dissection.

Extensor Tendon Injuries

The investment of the common extensor tendon is from both the superficial and deep layers of the sagittal band. Spontaneous dislocations of the extensor tendons may be caused by rupture of the thin superficial layer and detachment from the deeper thick layer; the direction of tendon displacement typically is ulnarward. Tearing of the deep sagittal band layer accompanies traumatic subluxations. If treated within 2 weeks after injury, these tendon subluxations may be managed effectively by splinting the MCP joint in full extension and radial deviation for 6 weeks. When diagnosed more than 2 to 3 weeks after injury these symptomatic subluxations are considered chronic and frequently require surgical management. Primary sagittal band repair may be possible; however, reinforcement techniques are commonly necessary, especially for spontaneous dislocations. Sections of juncic tendinae, slips of the common extensor tendons, or even free grafts anchored or routed in various ways have been used

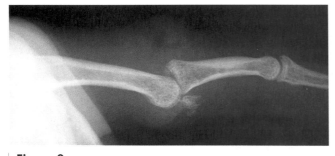

Figure 8

A dorsal fracture-dislocation of the proximal interphalangeal joint, including a central depressed articular segment.

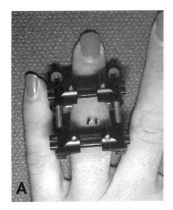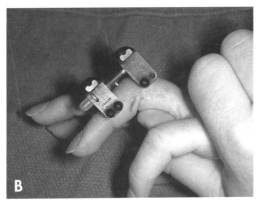

Figure 9

A, A comminuted intra-articular fracture of the proximal interphalangeal joint was treated with dynamic external fixation and percutaneous pinning of a volar fragment. B, Early motion is permitted by the fixator.

when the sagittal band is deficient or absent. No recurrent dislocations occurred in 27 recently reported fractures, 21 of which required direct repair, reefing, or common extensor tendon augmentation of the sagittal band.

Extensor tendon injuries distal to the MCP joints are particularly troublesome, especially those directly over the PIP joints and the proximal phalanges, zones III and IV, respectively (Fig. 10). Traditional treatment with 4 weeks of PIP joint immobilization in full extension may result in loss of flexion from PIP joint capsular contracture and periosteal-skin adherence. A short arc motion (SAM) program reduces these complications by immediately permitting 0° to 30° of active PIP joint motion and progressively allowing more flexion. In a comparison of SAM to a traditional immobilization program there were more favorable outcomes with SAM. The maximum improvement in PIP joint flexion was realized by 6 weeks postoperatively, and the resultant extensor lag was less in the SAM program. Moreover, the final arcs of motion were more functional in the SAM program (3° to 88°) than in the standard immobilization program (13° to 77°).

After surgical repair, thumb and digital extensor tendon lacerations at and proximal to the MCP joint level can be treated effectively by functional static splinting. Dynamic splints are cumbersome, expensive, difficult to make, and foster noncompliance. Molded thermoplastic splints keeping wrists in 30° of extension and MCP joints in 20° to 30° of flexion have been

found to achieve 86% good or excellent results. Early interphalangeal motion is encouraged, and limited use of the hand is possible during the 6 weeks of splint wear.

Traumatic extensor tendon ruptures at the musculotendinous junction occur when forceful flexion forces are applied to actively extended digits. Complete ruptures require either side-to-side tenorrhaphy or tendon transfers. In a recent report of 10 patients with extensor avulsions at the musculotendinous junction, good to excellent results were obtained in 9. One patient treated by transfer of a radial wrist extensor tendon had an inferior result, likely because of excursion mismatch. Extensor pollicis longus tendon ruptures are most commonly treated by extensor indicis proprius (EIP) tendon transfer. Donor site deficits can be minimized by sectioning the EIP tendon just proximal to the extensor hood. Independent extension of the index finger is not lost after EIP harvest. Most patients tolerate an extensor lag and some independent extensor weakness without difficulty.

Flexor Tendon Injuries

Digital and thumb flexor tendon injury zones correspond to the well-defined retinacular structures of the hand. Poor

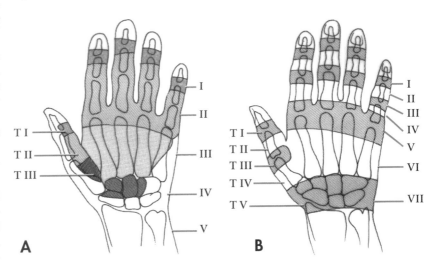

Figure 10

A, Flexor tendon zones. B, Extensor tendon zones. (Reproduced with permission from Kleinert HE, Schepel S, Gill T: Flexor tendon injuries. *Surg Clin North Am* 1981;61:267–286.)

prognostic factors, such as fractures, skin loss, joint damage, and neurovascular injuries, require special treatment considerations, and outcomes even from isolated sharp zone II flexor tendon lacerations are not uniformly successful.

Flexor tendon repair strength during the first several weeks depends primarily on the repair technique and the number of suture strands crossing the repair rather than the biologic healing response. Digital swelling after injury or repair increases the tensile demands placed on the normal flexor digitorum profundus (FDP) tendon, which vary from 900 g during passive motion to 9,000 g during tight index tip pinch. Light grip requires 1,500 g, and 5,000 g is required for tight grip. Moreover, reduction in the initial repair strength of 10% to 50% during the first 5 to 21 days after repair further underscores the importance of the initial suture repair and biologically based rehabilitation regimens. The ability of various suture linkages of severed tendon ends to provide appropriate tendon gliding and strength has been the focus of numerous in vitro efforts (Fig. 11). The repair strength depends on the number of strands that cross the repair site; addition of locking loops has not been found to provide additional strength. Among commonly used repair techniques evaluated biomechanically, a 4-strand technique was found to have properties suitable for early active motion (Fig. 12). In other well-designed studies, newer modifications to epitenon and core suture techniques have been evaluated to determine the efficacy of early active motion rehabilitation programs. Testing to failure of several suture techniques showed that core suture placement in the dorsal portion of

the tendon increased tensile strength, decreased the work of flexion, and did not appear to have a deleterious effect on tendon healing caused by compromise of the dorsal vascular supply. Other investigators have supported this finding and reported that the mean strength of the dorsal half of the FDP tendon is 58.3% greater than that of the palmar half. In another laboratory study, the depth of the epitenon stitch also correlated with repair strength. A 6-0 monofilament polypropylene stitch placed deeply provided a repair that was 80% stronger in mean failure than a more superficially placed epitenon suture.

Full activity after zone II flexor tendon repairs has routinely been avoided for 10 to 12 weeks because of fear of tendon repair ruptures. Results of a randomized study of 91 flexor tendon lacerations (82 patients) with no concomitant bone, joint, soft-tissue, or neurovascular injury indicated that full activity could be allowed at 8 weeks after repair. All tendons were repaired within 24 hours of injury, and a passive flexion and active extension program was administered for the first 6 weeks postoperatively. Because no ruptures were found 7 weeks after repair, the authors concluded that absence from work could be reduced by 2.1 weeks with the early mobilization program. In another series of 233 patients, no flexor tendon ruptures occurred later than 8 weeks after repair. Digital tendon rupture rates of 5.8% and thumb flexor tendon rupture rates of 16.6% were reported for repairs in zones I and II. All ruptures occurred within the first 5 weeks after surgery, and most occurred within the first 2 weeks.

Rehabilitation of pediatric patients with flexor tendon injuries varies from complete immobilization to early active mobilization programs. Outcomes of zone I and II flexor tendon lacerations in 78 patients younger than 16 years of age were reported in a multicenter study. Complete immobilization for less than 4 weeks gave total active motion (TAM) equal to early mobilization programs (77% normal TAM). The final results deteriorated when immobilization was longer than 4 weeks (41% to 62% normal TAM). Although no tendon ruptures were reported in this series, 3 of 38 patients in another patient population (age 7 months to 13 years) had zone II ruptures. Repeat repairs resulted in good outcomes. No tenolyses were required in either of these 2 series.

The aperture of the A2 pulley is narrow and rigid and is where the flexor digitorum superficialis (FDS) bifurcates and the FDP is relatively avascular. Repair of FDP and FDS lacerations in this region is difficult. Inferior repair results prompted a randomized prospective clinical study of injuries beneath the A2 pulley (Tang zone 2C injuries). TAM of 204° when only the FDP was repaired compared to 187° when both tendons were repaired has led these authors to routine-

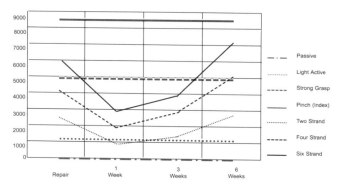

Figure 11

Estimated strength measured in grams for 2-, 4-, and 6-strand flexor tendon repairs performed without the use of epitendinous sutures. Light active grasp should be permissible with the 4-strand epitendinous suture technique. (Reproduced with permission from Strickland JW: Flexor tendon injuries: I. Foundations of treatment. *J Am Acad Orthop Surg* 1995;3:44–54.)

ly excise the adult FDS when both tendons are lacerated. Despite the results of this study, most hand surgeons believe that both tendons should be repaired when possible.

Nerve Injuries

Digital nerve lacerations are the most common nerve injuries of the hand. Under the ideal conditions of a sharp transection in a young, healthy patient, a timely primary repair consistently produces good to excellent sensory recovery. Extended proximal and distal dissection along the neurovascular bundle promotes mobilization of the nerve ends before repair. The optimal surgical technique requires proper high power loupe or microscopic magnification and precise epineural approximation. Tension across the repair site during gentle passive finger ROM is assessed. A protective hand position is maintained in a splint or cast for 3 weeks following most digital nerve repairs. The immobilization period varies according to the postoperative protocol for associated injuries, such as flexor tendon lacerations or phalangeal and MC fractures.

Reconstruction of major peripheral nerve injuries of the upper extremity has continued to stimulate clinical research in the fields of direct repair, conventional nerve grafts, and tubular substitutes. In an experimental study, it was shown that when a prosthetic interposition tubular graft was used, malalignment of the proximal and distal ends of a severed nerve increased axonal dispersion, which occurred without sign of neurotropic interactions to promote correction of growth. These findings were more apparent with larger gaps; therefore, in the clinical setting, traditional nerve grafting was recommended for major mixed peripheral nerve reconstruction.

The importance of alignment of the proximal and distal nerve fibers was confirmed in another review of experimental

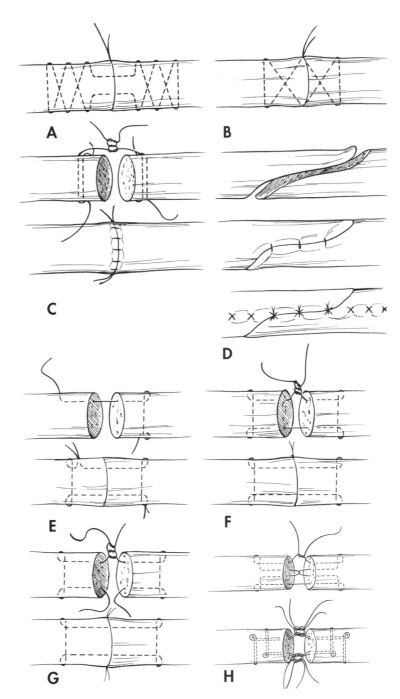

Figure 12

Commonly used techniques for end-to-end tendon suture. A, Conventional Bunnell stich. B, Crisscross stitch. C, Mason-Allen (Chicago) stitch. D, Becker bevel (overlapped) repair. E, Kessler grasping stitch. F, Modified Kessler stitch with single knot at the repair site. G, Tajima modification of the Kessler stitch with double knots at the repair site. H, Four-strand techniques. (Reproduced with permission from Strickland JW: Flexor tendon injuries: I. Foundations of treatment. *J Am Acad Orthop Surg* 1995;3:44–54.)

repair with correctly aligned and malaligned fibers within a 5-mm collagen tube. Similar alignment variation was tested with a 5-mm gap within a 10-mm collagen tube. Recovery was optimal in the well-aligned repair regardless of a small gap. Malalignment of nerve fibers adversely influenced motor restoration with direct repair, whereas corrective realignment was noted within the small gap model. In theory, a prosthetic conduit may be of clinical benefit when a persistent gap is present in a mixed peripheral nerve with the potential for malalignment.

In a clinical study, 18 patients were randomized to either tubulization with a 3- to 4-mm gap or conventional microsurgical repair of median and ulnar nerve injuries. Although there was improved sensory recovery for the tubulization group at 3 months, follow-up evaluation at 1 year revealed no difference in motor or sensory recovery between the 2 groups. Correct nerve alignment for either direct repair and tubulization is essential to improve final results. Definitive clinical evaluation of either conduit nerve repair or laser-assisted neuroanastomosis has yet to be completed in a comprehensive prospective multicenter study.

Fingertip Injuries

Fingertip injuries are one of the most common problems seen in the emergency room setting. Distal partial amputations often result in loss of soft-tissue pulp substance, sterile or germinal matrix tissue, portions of the distal phalanx, and terminal digital nerve branches. Soft-tissue coverage for fingertip amputations depends on the age and general medical health of the patient, the affected digit, the size and orientation of the amputation, and associated injuries. Younger patients often can tolerate the necessary immobilization associated with thenar flap or cross finger flap coverage, whereas PIP joint stiffness is a significant concern in older patients managed in similar fashion. When applicable, a local soft-tissue transfer from part of the injured digit (homodigital flap) can avoid the complications associated with more distant tissue transfers. The Hueston flap, a commonly used homodigital flap, was recently reviewed in 41 patients with isolated fingertip amputations. At a mean follow-up of 3 years, 30 patients were satisfied overall with their recovery and results of treatment. Modification of the flap design potentially avoids the need for supplemental skin grafting to the donor site and prevents distal tissue overlap. Wire fixation of the flap also has been advocated to provide nail bed support. Chronic cold intolerance was the main complaint encountered at final follow-up.

Another variation of the homodigital flap has been described with sufficient follow-up evaluation. Sixteen patients with isolated digital volar-oblique pulp loss of 1.5 cm or less were treated with dorsal lateral neurovascular island flaps. Evaluation 2 years after injury revealed satisfactory results in 88% of the patients, with regained protective sensation and a functional arc of motion.

Because of its distinct anatomy and function, the thumb requires special considerations after tip amputation. Advancement and neurovascular pedicle flaps are well suited for thumb tip volar surface amputations. Although small defects of less than 1 cm without exposed bone can heal by secondary intention with excellent predictable results, larger defects require various coverage procedures. Depending on the orientation of the defect, a 2-cm oblique amputation can be covered by an advancement flap with slight flexion of the interphalangeal joint. A defect larger than 2.5 cm requires modification by a proximal flap transverse incision or V-Y closure. Defects of more than 75% of the volar surface cannot be covered by advancement flaps and, therefore, are optimally treated by an index cross finger flap, a neurovascular island flap, or pedicled transfer from the ulnar aspect of the ring finger.

Infections

Management of hand infections is based on the depth and location of the condition, the affecting organism, proximal involvement through direct spread or lymphatic drainage, and the underlying medical condition of the patient. Most uncomplicated cellulitis of the hand is well controlled by oral antibiotics and elevation. Adequate surgical decompression and mechanical debridement are the cornerstone for successful treatment of deeper infections and abscesses involving localized compartments of the hand, tendon, bone, or articular structures.

Over the past several years, a growing number of human immunodeficiency virus (HIV)- and acquired immunodeficiency syndrome (AIDS)-related hand infections have been encountered, necessitating a heightened awareness of the unique complications related to these conditions. Most important is the increased suspicion for the more frequent occurrence of atypical infections such as *Mycobacteria*, *Candida*, and *Nocardia* organisms. In a study of HIV-positive patients with hand-related injuries, septic HIV patients required more surgical intervention and prolonged hospitalization than septic non-HIV patients. With an increasing survival rate in patients with AIDS and associated conditions, a growing number of HIV-positive patients are likely to require treatment for related hand infections. The immunosuppression of organ transplant patients also puts them at risk for opportunistic or severe hand infections.

Equally challenging is the treatment of diabetic patients with hand infections. In a review of 25 diabetic patients with hand infections, multiple organisms were encountered in most, with gram-negative organisms in 73% of the positive cultures. Surgical debridement, combined parenteral antibiotics, strict diabetic control, and limb elevation consistently resulted in successful recovery without recurrence.

The correct diagnosis and treatment of conditions simulating hand infections can be confusing because of overlapping signs and symptoms. Patients who have acute calcific tendinitis, gout, pseudogout, and foreign body reactions can have erythema, pain, and dysfunction, which mimic infection. Brown recluse spider bites, pyogenic granulomas, pyoderma gangrenosum, metastatic lesions, factitious diseases, and rheumatoid arthritis can all produce ambiguous clinical and radiographic findings that need to be considered when treating a patient with a suspected hand infection.

Burns

The need for a complete and comprehensive program for burns of the hand has been well identified in the medical literature and emphasized by the success of regional burn centers throughout the world. In a large study of over 1,000 burns of the hand in 659 patients during a 10-year period, most patients with superficial and deep injuries regained normal hand function after protective splinting and passive motion of the affected articulations, in conjunction with sheet autograft wound care and various surgical procedures. A guarded prognosis was directly related to involvement of the extensor tendon, joint capsule, or bone in deeper injuries.

Palmar burns in young children are seen with an increased frequency once ambulation begins. The cause of these burns is direct contact with a hot object or boiling water in most patients. The treatment of choice is early eschar excision followed by serial debridements under general anesthesia or sedation, along with protective medicated bandages. In a study of 81 children younger than 3 years of age, nearly 80% had uncomplicated healing at 1-year follow-up after this method of management. The most common residual loss requiring surgery was first web space contracture treated by local flap reconstruction. Overall, palmar burns in children are associated with a good prognosis in comparison to similar conditions in adults.

High-Pressure Injection Injuries

High-pressure injection injuries of the hand and digits frequently are overlooked because of the innocuous appearance of the entry site and the lack of initial appreciation for the magnitude of the underlying pathology (Fig. 13). Often the clinical presentation is that of a small puncture wound in the skin and modest pain and swelling. Oil-based solvents such as grease, paint, and paint thinner are particularly hazardous. Factors associated with poor outcome include high-injection pressures, large volume injections, delays in treatment, and secondary infection. Acute tissue necrosis has been described in a recent report of paint injection injuries in 2 patients. Prompt surgical debridement of the injected paint along the affected compartment or flexor sheath is essential to diminish the adverse soft-tissue response to this foreign matter. Despite optimal management, soft-tissue necrosis may prevail if digital vessel involvement is present. It should be recognized that amputation is a potential outcome.

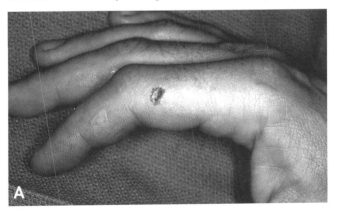
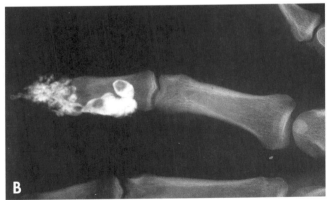

Figure 13
A, The innocuous entry site belies the severity of the injury. B, A paint injection with the radio-opaque material easily seen.

Replantation and Microsurgery

Microsurgery, which is entering its fourth decade of clinical use, has been applied in nearly every surgical field. The impact of microsurgery on orthopaedics occurs primarily in the areas of replantation surgery, soft-tissue transfer, and peripheral nerve repair.

Replantation

A multivariate analysis of parameters related to function after digit replantation revealed that in every possible setting the most significant measure of success and patient satisfaction was the quality of sensory return. The role of rehabilitation was explored by comparing patients entered into a formal sensory education program with patients who received no postreplantation therapy. Approximately 1 year postoperatively, 2-point discrimination and the Semmes-Weinstein pressure threshold test were statistically better in the group receiving therapy. Similarly, digital motion was better when patients received formal training.

Persistent cold intolerance after replantation continues to be problematic and poorly understood. Measurement of digital blood flow in replanted digits demonstrated that even when resting pressure and flow returned to normal, cold stimulus led to an exaggerated and persistent decrease in blood flow. Previously it was believed that with time and return of sensation, cold-induced vasospasm would improve. Although this may be true in the first months after replantation, an evaluation of patients 2 and 12 years after replantation indicated that improvement beyond 2 years appears to reflect personal adaptation rather than physiologic recovery. Uniformly, those patients with the fewest symptoms pursued lifestyles that led to the least cold exposure. The possibility of unrelenting cold intolerance should be discussed with patients before undertaking replantation.

The best indications for replantation of digits in adults, general health and compliance permitting, include thumb amputations, multiple digit amputations, or single-finger amputations in patients with specialized needs, such as a musician. The indications in children are much more liberal, and are predicated mostly on the ability to identify reparable structures.

In their report of 46 patients with isolated thumb replantations or revascularizations, surgeons in Ljubljana, Slovinia, identified the socioeconomic implications of thumb replantation and defined subjective and objective outcome parameters. Their data demonstrated that the more distal the amputation and the more isolated the trauma (ie, laceration or narrow crush versus broad crush or avulsion injuries), the better the functional results of successful replants. Contrary to results of previous series, there was no significance to patient age or whether the injury was an amputation or just required revascularization, as long as the thumb survived. The fact that all of the patients who were employed at the time of injury continued to be employed after successful replantation or revascularization may be a function of the patient population, but more likely reflects the critical role the thumb plays in occupational hand functions.

One hundred twenty children with 73 replantations and 81 revascularizations were placed in 1 of 3 levels of injury: level I, injuries distal to the insertion of the flexor digitorum superficialis; level II, injuries proximal to the flexor digitorum superficialis insertion and distal to the radiocarpal joint; and level III, proximal to the wrist. The survivorship of level I replantations was similar to that reported in adult replantations at this level, but survivorship at level II was disappointing. The authors suggest that this may be explained by the tendency to undertake replantation in a child of a part that would otherwise be discarded in an adult. They did not find any relationship between the age of the patient and the rate of survival of the injured part after revascularization; however, there was a significantly higher rate of survival after replantation in children younger than 9 years old when compared to their older counterparts. Among the patients with incomplete amputations, no replant failed when the injury resulted from a laceration, whereas one fourth of the digits failed when the injury resulted from crushing. Functional outcome reflects location and degree of injury, as it does in the adult thumb study mentioned above, but also reflects age. Children younger than 9 years old had better 2-point discrimination than older children.

In a separate study, 12 children with 13 amputated parts were followed up into adulthood to determine the effect of replantation on skeletal growth. Growth was affected in all patients, but the effect was significant only when physes were within the immediate zone of injury. In light of these studies, the difficult and time-consuming efforts to replant thumbs in all patients and any digit in a child remain worthwhile.

Replantation of amputations at or distal to the germinal matrix can obtain excellent cosmetic and functional recovery. Repair or grafting of venous outflow is a critical indication of viability. Operating room time is less when compared to more proximal replantation attempts, and several groups advocate performing the extremely distal replant as an outpatient procedure, which is more cost-effective.

Free Tissue Transfer

Timely wound closure of open fractures, especially those involving the tibia, decreases infection and speeds fracture union. Expedient wound closure depends on meticulous debridement of all doubtfully viable tissue. With the current understanding of local muscle, local fasciocutaneous flaps, and free tissue transfer, the argument that a surgeon should be reluctant to remove marginal tissues to prevent the creation of wounds that are difficult to close or cover is no longer valid. It is often the tissue at the margin of the injury zone that serves as the nidus for acute and chronic infection, thus judicious mechanical debridement should favor excision in questionable circumstances.

The enabling factor for this aggressive approach to debridement is the ability to reliably perform free tissue transfer to reconstruct resulting defects. The concept of immediate (less than 3 to 7 days after injury) free tissue transfer is controversial, with detractors suggesting that the microsurgical success rates, infection rates, and patient morbidity are all compromised by this overzealous approach. Advocates of immediate free tissue transfer, after review of results in both upper and lower extremity injuries, argue otherwise. In a recent review, the donor and recipient site morbidity, the required number of secondary operations, the length of hospital stay, and the functional results were equal to or better than those obtained with delayed coverage methods. Two well-accepted indications for immediate microsurgical tissue transfer are the salvage of a functional knee or elbow by transferring skin or a muscle from an unreplantable part and the coverage of an exposed neurovascular reconstruction. The long-term consequences of lower limb reconstruction have been questioned for the last 15 years, prompting the creation of scoring systems to assist with determining which patients would best be treated by immediate amputation and which would benefit from extensive reconstruction. An emerging appreciation for the cosmetic and functional status of the donor site has resulted from critical outcome analysis in microsurgery.

Surprisingly, the large-sized latissimus dorsi flap, often used to cover extensive defects, results in acceptable donor site morbidity. The most common sequelae immediately after surgery include seroma formation, shoulder stiffness, and shoulder weakness. In 1 study, the development of seromas was investigated in relation to the method by which the flap was raised and the various methods by which the donor site was closed. Scalpel dissection, suture ligation of perforating vessels, and tacking the skin flaps to underlying structures lead to the lowest rate of seroma formation; use of electrocautery for flap evaluation and performing simple skin closure resulted in the highest rate of formation.

An early study of shoulder function after harvesting latissimus dorsi pedicle and free flaps indicated that initial mild to moderate shoulder weakness and loss of shoulder motion improved with vigorous ROM and strengthening exercises. More recently, a group of patients were evaluated at regular intervals for shoulder strength and ROM after latissimus dorsi harvest. Patients had little problem regaining motion and subjectively regaining strength despite having a 30% decrease in shoulder extension strength in the early postoperative period. Despite this measurable loss of power, the only consistent patient complaints were those related to the surgical scar and a shallow posterior axillary fold.

Harvesting the gracilis muscle was found to be accompanied by an 11% decrease in leg adduction strength. Similar to the findings for the latissimus dorsi, most patients are not aware of the initial deficiency, which in all resolved within months. More than 50% of patients had no complaints, whereas 40% identified tolerable hypesthesias in the cutaneous distribution of the obturator nerve. For a few patients, the donor site appearance was bothersome, especially when a combined myofasciocutaneous flap had been harvested.

The rectus abdominis muscle is an appealing donor because it is easily dissected and its vascular supply, the inferior epigastric artery, is consistent. The rectus abdominis is most frequently used for breast reconstruction, but is also used for coverage of moderate size extremity defects. Donor site morbidity is of considerable concern because weakening of abdominal wall integrity accompanies removal of this muscle. In a study comparing the donor site morbidity of this muscle either as a free flap or a pedicle flap in healthy and chronically ill patients, complication rates were similar. Three hernias among the 50 patients reviewed were believed to be unavoidable, with the author concluding that the benefit of this flap far outweighs the risk. However, with reliable alternatives to the rectus abdominis, this donor site is much less appealing, especially in women who require breast reconstruction after undergoing mastectomy for cancer treatment.

Free fasciocutaneous flaps have advantages over flaps containing muscle in that skin grafts at the recipient sites are not necessary, and there have been no objective functional deficits reported in the 4 most common donor sites: the groin, scapula, radial forearm, and lateral arm flap. The disadvantages of fasciocutaneous flaps are limited size, limited ability to fill dead space, relatively decreased perfusion, and greater difficulty in harvesting the flap. This last concern is particularly true of the groin flap, which is unfortunate, because the groin is the least conspicuous donor site in all of free tissue transfer. The most obvious and unsightly donor sites are created when harvesting radial forearm and lateral arm flaps. In a review of patient perspectives after lateral arm free flaps, although there was no functional deficit, patients frequently were dissatisfied with the appearance, especially if skin grafts were required to close the donor defect. No studies specifically concern the donor site morbidity of scapular/parascapular flaps; however, it is likely that because this is a fasciocutaneous flap there would be no motor weakness and the patient's attitude toward the surgical scar would be similar to that of patients with latissimus dorsi muscle transfer.

Nerve Repair

Results of nerve repair are adversely affected by advanced age, delays before reconstruction, tension across repair sites, significant gaps, and compromised healing environment. The positive effects of youth are seen in the results of replantation discussed earlier and in a recent study of 9 children with segmental sciatic nerve or peroneal nerve defects who were treated with interposition grafting. Whereas minimal functional gains would be anticipated in adult patients, protective sensation returned in each pediatric patient. Four children had sufficient return of motor strength to significantly decrease the need for full-time bracing.

The impact of delayed treatment was reported in 2 studies of radial nerve injuries. In 1 study of 14 patients with open humeral fractures and radial nerve deficits, exploration revealed 8 nerve contusions, 5 completely transsected nerves, and 2 partially lacerated nerves. After wound debridement and rigid fracture fixation, the nerve lacerations were repaired. Seven of the 8 contused nerves and 5 of the 7 repaired nerves had complete return of motor function; 1 patient was lost to follow-up, and the remaining 2 patients had no significant recovery. In contrast, a review of 20 patients who had nerve grafting for chronic nerve deficits noted that patients treated within 6 months of injury fared significantly better than those treated later. No patient grafted 12 months after injury recovered any useful function. Patient age and graft length did not affect the results.

Tension across nerve repairs is believed to affect outcome. Supporting this hypothesis is an evaluation of 2-point discrimination in 90 complete digital nerve injuries seen 1 year after repair. Primary repairs of simple lacerations fared better than primary repairs for mild crush or saw injuries. Nerves reconstructed with primary grafting had significantly better results than those repaired end-to-end under some degree of tension. The length of digital nerve gap that warrants grafting is unknown. In a cadaver study correlating digit motion and the amount of nerve resection, digital nerves were divided at the PIP joint and then repaired, mobilized, and inspected. If the resection was no greater than 2.5 mm, all repairs were resistant to disruption even when the digits were moved through a complete ROM including hyperextension. When the resection length was 1 cm, all repairs were disrupted. Results of these 2 studies seem to suggest that any gap beyond 3 mm is best treated with grafting.

The prospect that nerve gaps could be managed by placing the cut of nerves in chambers or tubes has received considerable attention. It has been proposed that the chambers retain key neurotrophic agents such as nerve growth factor, brain-derived neurotrophic factor, and ciliary neurotrophic factor. These factors would then promote healing across gaps and direct the nerve buds emanating from the proximal nerve end of a mixed nerve to find their appropriate counterparts in the distal cut end. Gaps as large as 3 cm have been bridged in laboratory animals but until recently the ability of peripheral nerves in humans to be directed in growth by a biologic or synthetic conduit has been unproven. Laboratory and clinical trials have indicated that conduits may provide acceptable results, but this technique has not been carefully compared with conventional repairs. Other areas of inquiry include the development of bioabsorbable tubes and production of templates to influence the orientation of regenerating fascicles.

Annotated Bibliography

Distal Radial Fractures

Andersen DJ, Blair WF, Steyers CM Jr, Adams BD, el-Khouri GY, Brandser EA: Classification of distal radial fractures: An analysis of interobserver reliability and intraobserver reproducibility. *J Hand Surg* 1996;21A:574–582.

This is a comparative study of the Frykman, Malone, Mayo, and AO classification systems to determine reliability and reproducibility. The results demonstrated that inter- and intraobserver reliability is low for all systems. However, reduction of the AO system to only 3 substantial types improved intra- and interobserver reliability.

Baratz ME, Des Jardins JD, Anderson DD, Imbriglia JE: Displaced intra-articular fractures of the distal radial: The effect of fracture displacement on contact stresses in a cadaver model. *J Hand Surg* 1996;21A:183–188.

Contact stresses in the wrist were measured after simulating displaced fractures of the lunate fossa in the distal radius with 8 human cadaver arms. Maximum stress is significantly increased with step-offs of more than 2 mm. As the magnitude of fracture displacement increased, there was a shift in focus of the maximum stress toward the fracture line, thus simulating the mechanism of a die punch injury.

Bass RL, Blair WF, Hubbard PP: Results of combined internal and external fixation for the treatment of severe AO-C3 fractures of the distal radius. *J Hand Surg* 1995;20A:373–381.

In this study of 12 patients followed up for an average of 27 months, wrist motion averaged 60° of flexion and 45° of extension. The injured extremity had a mean grip strength of 83% of the uninjured side. Follow-up radiographs showed a dorsal tilt of 1°, radial inclination of 18°, and radial length of 12 mm.

Cannegieter DM, Juttman JW: Cancellous grafting and external fixation for unstable Colles' fractures. *J Bone Joint Surg* 1997; 79B:428–432.

In this prospective study, 32 unstable Colles' fractures were treated by combined external fixation and cancellous bone grafting. The external fixator was maintained for 5 weeks. Results were good or excellent in 27 patients and 5 malunions were present. Overall, grip strength was 95° of the normal side.

Catalano LW III, Cole RJ, Gelberman RH, Evanoff BA, Gilula LA, Borrelli J Jr: Displaced intra-articular fractures of the distal aspect of the radius: Long-term results in young adults after open reduction and internal fixation. *J Bone Joint Surg* 1997;79A: 1290–1302.

In this retrospective study, long-term functional and radiographic outcome was evaluated in a series of young adults with acute displaced intra-articular fractures treated with ORIF. There was a strong association between the development of osteoarthritis of the radiocarpal joint and residual displacement of the articular fragment at 7-year follow-up. Functional status at the most recent follow-up did not directly correlate with these radiographic findings.

Kihara H, Palmer AK, Werner FW, Short WH, Fortino MD: The effect of dorsally angulated distal radial fractures on distal radioulnar joint congruency and forearm rotation. *J Hand Surg* 1996;21A:40–47.

In this biomechanical cadaver study, the most dramatic changes occurred when more than 20° of dorsal angulation of the distal radius was present. This corresponded to approximately 10° of dorsal tilt of the articular surface of the radius, as measured on X-ray film.

Lenoble E, Dumontier C, Goutallier D, Apoil A: Fracture of the distal radius: A prospective comparison between trans-styloid and Kapandji fixations. *J Bone Joint Surg* 1995;77B:562–567.

In this prospective study of 96 patients with extra-articular or intra-articular fractures of the distal radius, 42 patients (mean age, 57) were treated with transstyloid K-wire fixation and 44 (mean age, 57.7) had intrafocal fixation and immediate immobilization according to the original protocol. Pain and reflex sympathetic dystrophy were more frequent and ROM was better initially in intrafocal fixation and early mobilization. Overall, the clinical results for both groups were similar at 2 years.

Parry BR: Collesí fracture: Efficacy of pins and plaster. *Am J Orthop* 1997;26:45-50.

In this retrospective analysis of 73 patients (average age, 64.7 years) with distal radial fractures treated with pins and plaster, the complication rate was 55%. The most common complication was some degree of residual finger and wrist stiffness; pin tract infections were rare.

Injuries About the Distal Ulna

Adams BD, Samani JE, Holley KA: Triangular fibrocartilage injury: A laboratory model. *J Hand Surg* 1996;21A:189–193.

A potential injury mechanism for triangular fibrocartilage tears and ulnar styloid fractures was investigated using cadaver specimens. The authors found that DRUJ distraction can cause avulsion of the triangular fibrocartilage. However, ulnar styloid fractures and tears within the disk are more likely caused by injury mechanisms that include shear or compressive forces.

Geissler WB, Fernandez DL, Lamey DM: Distal radioulnar joint injuries associated with fractures of the distal radius. *Clin Orthop* 1996;327:135–146.

This article provides treatment options, arthroscopic treatment techniques, and a soft-tissue injury grading system as well as a treatment algorithm for evaluating distal radial fractures and associated DRUJ injuries.

Mikic ZD: Treatment of acute injuries of the triangular fibrocartilage complex associated with distal radioulnar joint instability. *J Hand Surg* 1995;20A:319–323.

In this study, 100 patients who had an injury to the TFCC with DRUJ instability all were treated surgically. The TFCC injury with DRUJ instability occurred as an isolated lesion in 20 patients; the avulsion was from the ulnar styloid in 19 patients. Postoperatively, all patients were immobilized in a long arm cast in neutral rotation for 6 weeks.

Carpal Instability

Geissler WB, Freeland AE, Savoie FH, McIntyre LW, Whipple TL: Intracarpal soft-tissue lesions associated with an intra-articular fracture of the distal end of the radius. *J Bone Joint Surg* 1996; 78A:357–365.

Patients who had a displaced intra-articular fracture of the distal radius were managed with manipulation and internal fixation performed under both fluoroscopic and arthroscopic guidance. Forty-one of 60 patients had soft-tissue injuries of the wrist. A staging system for soft-tissue injury is offered.

Hodge JC, Gilula LA, Larsen CF, Amadio PC: Analysis of carpal instability: II. Clinical applications. *J Hand Surg* 1995;20A: 765–776.

An analytic scheme for carpal instability patterns has been described to help standardized reporting of these conditions. Examples have been presented; usefulness of this scheme has yet to be proven.

Patterson R, Viegas SF: Biomechanics of the wrist. *J Hand Surg* 1995;8:97–105.

The results of the studies of radiocarpal instability and fractures have demonstrated an increased load in areas where degenerative arthritis is seen, and in these conditions have furnished the means by which biomechanical efficiency of certain surgical treatments can be measured.

Short WH, Werner FW, Fortino MD, Palmer AK, Mann KA: A dynamic biomechanical study of scapholunate ligament sectioning. *J Hand Surg* 1995;20A:986–999.

Sectioning the SLIL caused increased scaphoid flexion, scaphoid pronation, and lunate extension in fresh cadaver forearms. Pressure in the radiocarpal and ulnocarpal joints was redistributed following ligament sectioning.

Weiss AP, Akelman E, Lambiase R: Comparison of the findings of triple-injection cinearthrography of the wrist with those of arthroscopy. *J Bone Joint Surg* 1996;78A:348–356.

When compared to arthroscopy, the sensitivity, specificity, and accuracy of triple injection cinearthrography in detecting tears of the scapholunate, lunotriquetral, and triangular fibrocartilage ligaments as a group were 56%, 83%, and 60%, respectively. A negative arthrography does not necessarily rule out the possibility of internal derangement.

Winman BI, Gelberman RH, Katz JN: Dynamic scapholunate instability: Results of operative treatment with dorsal capsulodesis. *J Hand Surg* 1995;20A:971–979.

Nineteen patients who underwent 20 dorsal capsulodeses for dynamic scapholunate instability were followed for a mean of 34 months. Objective evaluation by physical examination revealed a significant improvement in wrist stability is determined by a scaphoid shift test and an average loss of 12° of wrist flexion.

Carpal Fracture-Dislocations

Inoue G, Imaeda T: Management of trans-scaphoid perilunate dislocations: Herbert screw fixation, ligamentous repair and early wrist mobilization. *Arch Orthop Trauma Surg* 1997;116:338–340.

In this retrospective review, overall results demonstrated scaphoids united with proper alignment of the carpal bones. This study seems to indicate that Herbert screw fixation is a useful adjunct in the treatment of these transscaphoid perilunate dislocations.

Sotereanos DG, Mitsionis GJ, Giannakopoulos PN, Tomaino MM, Herndon JH: Perilunate dislocation and fracture dislocation: A critical analysis of the volar-dorsal approach. *J Hand Surg* 1997;22A:49–56.

In this retrospective evaluation, results demonstrated that a combined volar dorsal approach can be used safely and effectively to restore normal intercarpal relationships and provide fixation for the accompanying fractures.

Thumb Metacarpophalangeal Joint Collateral Ligament Injuries

Heyman P: Injuries to the ulnar collateral ligament of the thumb: Metacarpophalangeal joint. *J Am Acad Orthop Surg* 1997;5:224–229.

This comprehensive review focuses on the diagnosis and treatment of ulnar collateral ligament injuries of the thumb MCP joint.

Ryu J, Fagan R: Arthroscopic treatment of acute complete thumb metacarpophalangeal ulnar collateral ligament tears. *J Hand Surg* 1995;20A:1037–1042.

Stener's lesions were reduced arthroscopically in 8 thumbs. Time in surgery averaged 47 minutes. At an average follow-up of 39 months, the authors found excellent recovery of pinch and grip strength and ROM in "most all patients." There were no reports of pain or functional limitation. Only 1 patient exhibited mild laxity with stress testing at their final examination.

Weiland AJ, Berner SH, Hotchkiss RN, McCormack RR Jr, Gerwin M: Repair of acute ulnar collateral ligament injuries of the thumb metacarpophalangeal joint with an intraosseous suture anchor. *J Hand Surg* 1997;22A:585–591.

Thirty patients were evaluated an average of 11 months after anatomic repair of a complete UCL tear using an intraosseous suture anchor. At final follow-up, motion was 15° less at the interphalangeal joint and 10° less at the MCP joint compared with the contralateral thumb. There was no instability and no significant complications.

Metacarpal and Phalangeal Fractures

Buchler U, Gupta A, Ruf S: Corrective osteotomy for post-traumatic malunion of the phalanges in the hand. *J Hand Surg* 1996;21B:33–42.

Fifty-seven patients with 59 phalangeal malunions underwent corrective osteotomy. Surgical correction was achieved in 76% with bony union in all. Outcomes were good or excellent in 96% of patients with bony malunion only and in 64% of patients with multiple structure involvement.

Foucher G: "Bouquet" osteosynthesis in metacarpal neck fractures: A series of 66 patients. *J Hand Surg* 1995;20A:S86–S90.

In this retrospective review of 66 patients with 68 MC neck fractures treated by closed reduction and internal fixation using multiple prebent K-wires, the average preoperative angulation measured 58°. There were 8 incomplete reductions with an average residual angulation of 18°. At final follow-up (average 4.5 years) all patients were pain-free and had returned to all activities.

Low CK, Wong HC, Low YP, Wong HP: A cadaver study of the effects of dorsal angulation and shortening of the metacarpal shaft on the extension and flexion force ratios of the index and little fingers. *J Hand Surg* 1995;20B:609–613.

This biomechanical study evaluated flexion and extension force after osteotomy of the second and fifth MCs. Beyond 30° of dorsal apex angulation, flexion force significantly decreased and extension force increased.

Ouellette EA, Freeland AE: Use of the minicondylar plate in metacarpal and phalangeal fractures. *Clin Orthop* 1996;327:38–46.

Sixty-eight articular and periarticular metacarpal and phalangeal fractures were stabilized using the minicondylar plate and followed up for an average of 17 months. There were no nonunions or malunion; however, there were 67 complications associated with 40 fractures.

Timmenga EJ, Blokhuis TJ, Maas M, Raaijmakers EL: Long-term evaluation of Bennett's fracture: A comparison between open and closed reduction. *J Hand Surg* 1994;19B:373–377.

Seven patients with Bennett's fractures underwent closed reduction and K-wire fixation and 11 underwent ORIF. The authors noted that at 10.7 years follow-up all had some decrease in strength with minimal symptoms and no loss of motion. Arthrosis correlated with the quality of reduction but was present even in patients with an exact reduction.

Proximal Interphalangeal Joint Fracture-Dislocations

Morgan JP, Gordon DA, Klug MS, Perry PE, Barre PS: Dynamic digital traction for unstable comminuted intra-articular fracture-dislocations of the proximal interphalangeal joint. *J Hand Surg* 1995;20A:565–573.

Fourteen patients treated by closed reduction and dynamic digital traction applied in the office were followed up for an average of 2 years. The average articular involvement was 80%. The final active arc of motion was 89°. Joint remodeling and joint space preservation were noted on final radiographs.

Weiss AP: Cerclage fixation for fracture dislocation of the proximal interphalangeal joint. *Clin Orthop* 1996;327:21–28.

A volar cerclage wiring technique was combined with early ROM. Twelve patients were followed up for an average of 2.1 years; only 1 had evidence of mild arthrosis. Final arc of motion averaged 89°.

Extensor Tendon Injuries

Evans RB: Immediate active short arc motion following extensor tendon repair. *Hand Clin* 1995;11:483–512.

Rationale for initiation of an immediate active motion postoperative program for extensor tendon injuries is outlined. Earlier and more functional results were realized in comparison to traditional immobilization in 64 digits with zone III and IV injuries.

Noorda RJ, Hage JJ, de Groot PJ, Bloem JJ: Index finger extension and strength after extensor indicis proprius transfer. *J Hand Surg* 1994;19A:844–849.

An extensor lag persisted in 24 of 34 patients (5° to 105°) at 8-year follow-up. Despite this lag and decreased extensor strength, 30 perceived no limitation of activities of daily living. The authors recommend sectioning the EIP tendon proximal to the dorsal aponeurosis.

Slater RR Jr, Bynum DK: Simplified functional splinting after extensor tenorrhaphy. *J Hand Surg* 1997;22A:445–451.

Treatment of extensor tendon lacerations in Verdan zones V to VIII (thumb TIII to TV) with static splinting resulted in no residual functional impairment. Molded splints with wrists in 30° extension and MCP joints in 20° to 30° of flexion (thumbs in neutral position) permitted interphalangeal joint motion. This functional splinting technique had no tenorrhaphy failures and 86% good or excellent results.

Vaccaro AR, Kupcha P, Schneider LH: The operative repair of chronic nontraumatic extensor tendon subluxations in the hand. *Hand Clin* 1995;11:431–440.

The authors report a technique in which they use half of the extensor digitorum communis tendon as a tether on the central extensor tendon, recentralizing it over the MCP joint.

Flexor Tendon Injuries

Adolfsson L, Soderberg G, Larsson M, Karlander LE: The effects of a shortened postoperative mobilization programme after flexor tendon repair in zone 2. *J Hand Surg* 1996;21B:67–71.

In a prospective, randomized study, tendons of 91 digits in 82 patients were repaired within 24 hours of injury and unrestricted use was allowed at 8 or 10 weeks There were no significant differences in functional results, rupture rates, grip strength, or subjective assessment of the patient groups.

Elliot D, Moiemen NS, Flemming AF, Harris SB, Foster AJ: The rupture rate of acute flexor tendon repairs mobilized by the controlled active motion regimen. *J Hand Surg* 1994;19B:607–612.

All 203 patients with 317 divided tendons in 224 finger injuries in zones I and II and 30 patients with 30 complete divisions of the flexor pollicis longus tendon in zones I and II were mobilized postoperatively in a controlled active motion regimen. Thirteen fingers (5.8%) and 5 thumbs (16.6%) suffered tendon rupture.

Grobbelaar AO, Hudson DA: Flexor tendon injuries in children. *J Hand Surg* 1994;19B:696–698.

Thirty-eight children (22 boys and 16 girls) with a mean age of 6.7 years were treated for flexor tendon injuries by primary suture and controlled mobilization. Repair of both FDS and FDP was better than repair of FDP alone, even in zone II.

O'Connell SJ, Moore MM, Strickland JW, Frazier GT, Dell PC: Results of zone I and zone II flexor tendon repairs in children. *J Hand Surg* 1994;19A:48–52.

All profundus repairs in zone I returned to excellent function. Isolated profundus and combined profundus and superficialis repairs in zone II achieved comparable results when managed with an early passive motion program or following immobilization for 3 or 4 weeks. Immobilization for longer than 4 weeks resulted in an appreciable deterioration of function.

Strickland JW: Flexor tendon injuries: I. Foundations of treatment. *J Am Acad Orthop Surg* 1995;3:44–54.

The basic science for flexor tendon repair is reviewed and the rationale for repair methods contrasted. A 4-strand core suture with a strong running epitendinous suture appears to allow early light active motion.

Tang JB: Flexor tendon repair in zone 2C. *J Hand Surg* 1994;19B:72–75.

A randomized prospective clinical study was carried out in 33 patients (37 fingers) with lacerations of both FDS and FDP tendons in the area covered by the A2 pulley (zone IIC). Both lacerated tendons were repaired in 19 fingers and only the FDP was repaired with regional excision of the FDS in 18 fingers. The fingers with suture of both tendons showed a higher rate of reoperation due to adhesions or rupture of repair.

Nerve Injuries

Brushart TM, Mathur V, Sood R, Koschorke GM: Dispersion of regenerating axons across enclosed neural gaps. *J Hand Surg* 1995;20A:557–564.

This experiment demonstrated the dependence of axonal regeneration on appropriate alignment of the proximal and distal nerve ends and minimal length of the gap to be crossed, without evidence of specific neurotropic interactions to promote correct reinnervation.

Lundborg G, Rosen B, Dahlin L, Danielsen N, Holmberg J: Tubular versus conventional repair of median and ulnar nerves in the human forearm: Early results from a prospective, randomized, clinical study. *J Hand Surg* 1997;22A:99–106.

Eighteen patients with median or ulnar nerve lacerations were randomized into either direct repair or tubulization. After 1-year follow-up, no significant difference in motor or sensory recovery was seen between groups.

Wang WZ, Crain GM, Baylis W, Tsai TM: Outcome of digital nerve injuries in adults. *J Hand Surg* 1996;21A:138–143.

Sixty-seven adults with 90 digital nerve lacerations were evaluated 1 year postoperatively. Mild crush or saw injuries have a significantly worse prognosis compared to simple lacerations. Younger patients and a tension-free repair site are identified as good prognostic indicators.

Fingertip Injuries

Foucher G, Dallaserra M, Tilquin B, Lenoble E, Sammut D: The Hueston flap in reconstruction of fingertip skin loss: Results in a series of 41 patients. *J Hand Surg* 1994;19A:508–515.

Forty-three Hueston flaps in 41 patients were completed with a high degree of overall patient satisfaction at long-term follow-up. Modifications of the technique are described in attempt to avoid a donor site skin graft, distal dog ear overlap, and nail horn deformity.

Hynes DE: Neurovascular pedicle and advancement flaps for palmar thumb defects. *Hand Clin* 1997;13:207–216.

This article reviews the options for thumb tip volar soft-tissue amputations and describes the surgical technique for each procedure. The author's preference of treatment is based on the size of the thumb defect after debridement of nonviable tissue.

Tsai TM, Yuen JC: A neurovascular island flap for volar-oblique fingertip amputations: Analysis of long-term results. *J Hand Surg* 1996;21B:94–98.

Sixteen patients with volar oblique fingertip amputations were treated by a new neurovascular island homodigital flap. Satisfactory motion and protective sensation were restored in the majority of cases (88%), with the highest complication of cold intolerance seen in 6 patients.

Infections

Ching V, Ritz M, Song C, De Aguir G, Mohanlal P: Human immunodeficiency virus infection in an emergency hand service. *J Hand Surg* 1996;21A:696–699.

Twenty-four of 500 patients seen by the emergency hand service tested positive for the HIV virus. Among patients seen for infections, the HIV-positive patients required a more complex management program of prolonged antibiotics and more surgical procedures.

Kann SE, Jacquemin JB, Stern PJ: Simulators of hand infections. *J Bone Joint Surg* 1996;78A:1114–1128.

This is a comprehensive review of conditions that can be mistaken for infections of the hand. Clinical and radiographic findings of each of the simulators are discussed.

Kour AK, Looi KP, Phone MH, Pho RW: Hand infections in patients with diabetes. *Clin Orthop* 1996;331:238–244.

This article discusses the findings in 25 hand infections in patients with diabetes. Specific attention is directed to the multiple organisms identified and suggestions for comprehensive management. Gram-negative organisms were present in the majority of patients.

Burns

Sheridan RL, Hurley J, Smith MA, et al: The acutely burned hand: Management and outcome based on a 10-year experience with 1047 acute hand burns. *J Trauma* 1995;38:406–411.

In a large series of patients with burns of the hand treated at a single burn center with uniformly good functional recovery, success is attributed to a multidisciplinary approach to soft-tissue coverage, skeletal fixation, and joint mobilization.

Vasseur C, Martinot V, Pellerin P, Herbaux B, Debeugny P: Palmar burns of the hand in children: 81 cases. *Ann Chir Main Memb Super* 1994;13:233–239.

Palmar burns in children generally have a better prognosis than similar injuries in adults. This large study of similar burns shows good functional recovery with early serial debridement. Soft-tissue reconstructive procedures (Z-plasty, skin grafts, or flaps) were needed for those patients with residual contractures.

High-Pressure Injection Injuries

Failla JM, Linden MD: The acute pathologic changes of paint-injection injury and correlation to surgical treatment: A report of two cases. *J Hand Surg* 1997;22A:156–159.

Two patients with similar injuries to the digits with high-pressure paint injections showed similar soft-tissue necrotic response. Early surgical debridement of the paint resulted in a good functional result in 1 patient, whereas a delay in treatment required amputation in the other.

Replantation

Carr MM, Manktelow RT, Zuker RM: Gracilis donor site morbidity. *Microsurgery* 1995;16:598–600.

Donor site morbidity after gracilis free tissue transfer was examined. There was a significant difference between adults and children. More than half the respondents had no complaints. Children complained more of immediate sensitivity, tightness, noticeability, and ugliness of the scar. Fifteen percent of patients reported temporary reduction of leg strength.

Chiu HY, Shieh SJ, Hsu HY: Multivariate analysis of factors influencing the functional recovery after finger replantation or revascularization. *Microsurgery* 1995;16:713–717.

The younger the patient, the smaller the zone of injury; the more distal the amputation, the better the functional recovery after replantation or revascularization.

Foster RJ, Swiontkowski MF, Bach AW, Sack JT: Radial nerve palsy caused by open humeral shaft fractures. *J Hand Surg* 1993;18A:121–124.

In a series of 14 patients with radial nerve palsy caused by an open humeral shaft fracture, 9 (64%) had a radial nerve that was either lacerated or interposed between the fracture fragments. Nerve exploration, wound debridement, rigid fracture fixation, and nerve repair in that order are recommended by these authors.

Graham B, Adkins P, Scheker LR: Complications and morbidity of the donor and recipient sites in 123 lateral arm flaps. *J Hand Surg* 1992;17B:189–192.

The lateral arm flap donor and recipient sites may produce an assortment of relatively minor complaints in a large proportion of patients. After reviewing 123 cases, the authors concluded that the lateral arm flap should be limited to males and cases in which the resulting donor site can be closed primarily.

Janezic TF, Arnez ZM, Solinc M, Zaletel-Kragelj L: Functional results of 46 thumb replantations and revascularizations. *Microsurgery* 1996;17:264–267.

The functional results of 46 patients with isolated thumb replantations and revascularizations were evaluated. Eighty-five percent had the same employment as before injury. All the patients had economically suitable employment. All but 8 patients experienced cold intolerance. Three of 8 women were not pleased with the appearance of their hands, whereas only 3 of 38 men voiced similar feelings.

Nunley JA, Saies AD, Sandow MJ, Urbaniak JR: Results of interfascicular nerve grafting for radial nerve lesions. *Microsurgery* 1996;17:431–437.

Age of the patient and length of the nerve graft did not seem to influence outcome. Time from initial injury to nerve grafting did affect outcome, with 85% of patients grafted within 6 months obtaining M3 or better recovery. No patient grafted 12 months after injury recovered any useful function.

Povlsen B, Nylander G, Nylander E: Cold-induced vasospasm after digital replantation does not improve with time: A 12-year prospective study. *J Hand Surg* 1995;20B:237–239.

The authors concluded that after replantation digital flow may reach normal levels at room temperature but cold-induced discomfort and a normal blood flow response to cold never return.

Salmi A, Tuominen R, Tukiainen E, Asko-Seljavaara S: Morbidity of donor and recipient sites after free flap surgery: A prospective study. *Scand J Plast Reconstr Surg Hand Surg* 1995;29: 337–341.

This study shows that measurable shoulder extension strength decreased after part of the latissimus dorsi muscle had been removed even though subjective morbidity was minimal. Morbidity at the recipient site decreased significantly with time.

Classic Bibliography

Chuang DC, Jeng SF, Chen HT, Chen HC, Wei FC: Experience of 73 free groin flaps. *J Plast Surg* 1992;45B: 81–85.

Hallock GG: Identical rectus abdominis donor-site morbidity in compromised and healthy patients. *J Reconstr Microsurg* 1994; 10:339–343.

Ishizuki M: Traumatic and spontaneous dislocation of extensor tendon of the long finger. *J Hand Surg* 1990;15A:967–972.

Kleinert HE, Verdan C: Report of the Committee on Tendon Injuries. *J Hand Surg* 1983;8A:794–798.

Minami A, Kaneda K: Repair and/or reconstruction of scapholunate interosseous ligament in lunate and perilunate dislocations. *J Hand Surg* 1993;18A:1099–1106.

Rettig ME, Amadio PC: Wrist arthroscopy: Indications and clinical applications. *J Hand Surg* 1994;19B:774–777.

Schuind F, Garcia-Elias M, Cooney WP III, An KN: Flexor tendon forces: In vivo measurements. *J Hand Surg* 1992;17A:291–298.

386 Upper Extremity

Saies AD, Urbaniak JR, Nunley JA, Taras JS, Goldner RD, Fitch RD: Results after replantation and revascularization in the upper extremity in children. *J Bone Joint Surg* 1994;76A:1766–1776.

Trumble TE, Schmitt SR, Vedder NB: Factors affecting functional outcome of displaced intra-articular distal radial fractures. *J Hand Surg* 1994;19A:325–340.

Wang WZ, Crain GM, Baylis W, Tsai TM: Outcome of digital nerve injuries in adults. *J Hand Surg* 1996;21A:138–143.

Chapter 34
Wrist and Hand Reconstruction

Nerve Compression Syndromes

External pressure of 20 to 30 mm Hg impairs venous flow, slows axonal transport, and causes changes in intraneural blood vessel permeability. At higher pressures an acute conduction block may occur and, eventually, rapid deterioration of nerve function. The greatest changes take place in the superficial regions and at the junction of uncompressed and compressed nerve segments. The absolute magnitude and the duration of pressure are important. Nerves with underlying problems (diabetes mellitus, other compression sites) are more susceptible to injury. The early stages of nerve dysfunction caused by compression are the result of ischemia and respond to nonsurgical treatment. In advanced cases with epineural fibrosis, decompression may not relieve all symptoms.

Peripheral nerves have considerable motion; therefore adhesions that cause traction and limit motion can compromise nerve function. Compression on one part of a nerve lowers the threshold for occurrence of another compression at another location along the nerve. This is the concept of "double crush." The most common double crush is coexistent cervical radiculopathy and carpal tunnel syndrome. The results of treatment may be suboptimal unless both sites are treated.

The diagnosis of a compressive neuropathy is based on a complete physical examination and history, including previous trauma, recreational activities, work history, and prior treatment. Conditions that can affect nerve function include diabetes mellitus, hypothyroidism, pregnancy, gout, alcoholism, dialysis, trauma, exposure to neurotoxic chemicals, rheumatoid arthritis, and mucopolysaccharidosis. The physical examination should include the neck, shoulders, and both upper extremities. The assessment includes evaluation for cervical radiculopathy and thoracic outlet syndrome, when indicated. Tinel's percussion test and compression tests can be done at any level to provoke sensory symptoms. Each nerve should be palpated through its entire length. Sensibility testing can evaluate the fiber type (slowly or quickly adapting), threshold (single fiber), and innervation density. Threshold testing is more sensitive for nerve compression. Radiographs are indicated if there is a history of significant trauma, fracture, deformity, or loss of motion. They can be

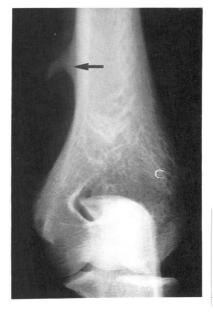

Figure 1

A supracondylar process (arrow), which with its attached ligament of Struthers may compress the median nerve proximal to the elbow.

helpful to evaluate for cervical ribs and other bone abnormalities associated with nerve compression, such as the rare supracondylar process attached to the ligament of Struthers (Fig. 1). A chest radiograph to rule out a Pancoast's tumor is obtained if ulnar nerve symptoms are present in a patient who smokes, especially if there is also shoulder pain. Cross-sectional imaging, magnetic resonance imaging (MRI), or computed tomography (CT) scan can be a valuable diagnostic aid when used judiciously.

Electrophysiologic (EPS) testing should include nerve conduction velocity (NCV) and electromyography (EMG). EPS testing is indicated if there is a question regarding the diagnosis or when surgery is being considered. Comparison to previous testing can help localize the lesion. In the many early stages of entrapment, electrical testing may be negative even when symptoms are evident. Nonsurgical treatment, including splinting in a relaxed position, avoiding provocative activities, avoiding pressure on the nerve, optimizing work station design (ergonomics), and patient education, can be helpful in mild to moderate cases. Surgery is considered if the nonsurgical protocol does not relieve the symptoms, especially if there is loss of motor strength or atrophy. The prognosis after surgery depends on the clarity of the diagnosis, the reliabili-

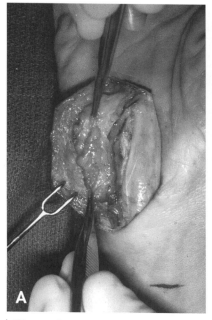
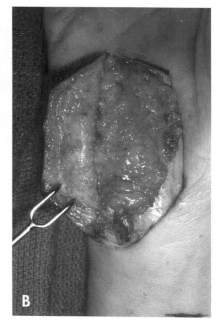

Figure 2

The pedicled hypothenar fat pad flap. A, The carpal tunnel and Guyon's canal are released. The perineural scarring about the median nerve is dissected carefully, and the transverse carpal ligament excised, as the fat pad is liberated from the skin overlying the hypothenar eminence. B, The fat pad is secured to the radial pillar of the carpal tunnel as coverage for its contents. The release of Guyon's canal prevents significant traction on the ulnar neurovascular bundle.

ty of the surgical treatment, and the degree of nerve damage. When the diagnosis is not clear and there is symptom magnification, other factors, such as thoracic outlet syndrome, reflex sympathetic dystrophy, or systemic polyneuropathy, should be investigated.

Carpal Tunnel Syndrome

Carpal tunnel syndrome is the most common and well-described upper extremity nerve entrapment syndrome. The cornerstone of therapy remains accurate diagnosis and appropriate nonsurgical treatment. Despite this regimen, persistent symptoms require surgical intervention in some patients. Night pain is the most reliably relieved symptom after decompression and, therefore, is an excellent indication for surgery. Routine transverse carpal ligament reconstruction, release of Guyon's canal, flexor tenosynovectomy, and internal neurolysis have not been shown to enhance results over simple release. Good clinical results can be obtained with decompression using minimal incisions. Reconstruction of the transverse carpal ligament may be considered in selected young workers who have high manual impact occupations.

When there is tenderness and dysesthesias resulting from perineural fibrosis or atrophic scarred skin, some have recommended padding the nerve with muscle, fat, or synovium. Free fat, local pedicled fat flaps, and vascular rotational forearm fat and fascia flaps, and abductor digiti quinti and palmaris brevis rotational flaps have been used. Theoretically, these vascularized flaps protect the median nerve and provide additional blood supply to the scarred nerve. When the volar skin coverage is adequate, neurolysis and coverage with a pedicled hypothenar fat pad flap (based on the ulnar artery in Guyon's canal) is an excellent alternative (Fig. 2).

Proximal nerve entrapment, such as pronator syndrome, thoracic outlet syndrome, or cervical radiculopathy, should be ruled out when symptoms persist. The most common cause of unrelieved symptoms is incomplete release of the transverse carpal ligament, although failure may be related to the degree of initial median nerve involvement, duration of the entrapment, and advanced age.

Symptoms also recur in patients with systemic diseases that cause an increase in flexor tenosynovium. When reoperation is performed, a limited biopsy of the tenosynovium is recommended to rule out pathologies such as amyloidosis and crystalline arthropathy. Volar subluxation of the flexor tendons is uncommon but also can be associated with persistent symptoms and pain. This is best evaluated intraoperatively by asking the patient to actively flex the fingers. If the flexor tendons subluxate over the hook of hamate, reconstruction of the transverse carpal ligament should be considered.

Reoperation is most commonly performed through the same incision, which is extended proximally and distally, crossing the wrist crease in an oblique fashion. The median nerve is mobilized from adjacent tissues, and coverage is provided as needed. Early postoperative mobilization of the wrist and fingers helps prevent recurrent adhesions. The results of reoperation are not as good as those of primary surgery and vary with the cause and indications for the reoperation. A retrospective study found that 53% were improved and 28% of the patients who were previously employed returned to work. Poor outcome after repeat carpal tunnel surgery was associated with workers' compensation, repetitive hand use, and normal EPS testing.

Anterior Interosseous Nerve Compression Syndrome

The anterior interosseous nerve (AIN) is a pure motor branch of the median nerve. It arises from the posterior lateral surface of the median nerve 5 to 8 cm distal to the medial epicondyle. Compression of the AIN results in anterior forearm pain and weakness or paralysis of the flexor pollicis longus (FPL), flexor digitorum profundus (FDP) to the index and middle fingers, and the pronator quadratus (PQ).

This is an uncommon compression neuropathy with varied presentations. Isolated involvement of the FDP to the index finger or that of the FPL can be seen. There can be variable weakness of the interphalangeal (IP) joint of the thumb and distal IP (DIP) joint weakness of the index and middle fingers. When attempting tip-to-tip pinch, the distal joints collapse (hyperextend) with pinch creating pulp-to-pulp contact (Fig. 3). The status of the PQ is best evaluated by flexing the elbow to relax the humeral head of the pronator teres (PT), which supplies 75% of the strength of the PT, requiring the PQ to supply more power of pronation. Pronation is weaker than the opposite side if an AIN palsy is present.

Anatomic variations do occur and influence the presentation. The AIN may innervate the whole FDP or just the index finger and, rarely, some of the flexor digitorum superficialis (FDS). If a Martin-Gruber connection is present, the communication often runs in the AIN, so the intrinsic muscles of the hand may be "cross-innervated." The differential diagnosis of AIN palsy includes tendon rupture, proximal compression (cervical compression, partial median nerve), or a brachial neuritis. Any sensory involvement suggests other diagnoses, and the EMG is typically abnormal.

Structures that can compress the AIN include the lacertus fibrosis, pronator teres, and FDS, as well as various fibrous bands and vascular structures. Although trauma, anomalous structures, and viral entities have been implicated in the evolution of AIN palsy, more than a third of cases are idiopathic. Exploration is indicated if there is no improvement, clinically or electrically, in 12 weeks. If a brachial neuritis is suspected then a more prolonged nonsurgical treatment of up to 6 months is warranted. When exploration is done, a longitudinal extensile exposure of the entire AIN is indicated. Most symptoms improve after decompression.

Pronator Syndrome

Pronator syndrome is a proximal entrapment of the median nerve. The common sites of compression are the ligament of Struthers (associated with a supracondylar process), lacertus fibrosis, PT (fibrous bands), and the FDS fibrous arch. It is more common in women and in the fifth decade. This is an uncommon nerve entrapment but must be considered in

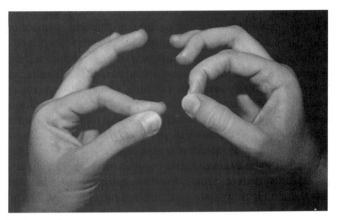

Figure 3
Position of the hand (left) with a complete anterior interosseous nerve palsy demonstrating pulp-to-pulp contact.

patients with vague forearm and distal arm pain; the finding of numbness or paresthesias in the median nerve distribution is distinctly rare. The condition often is dynamic and symptoms occur during active use of the extremity; the examination may need to be done after exertion. Palpation proximal to the medial epicondyle may reveal a supracondylar process. When nonsurgical treatment fails (approximately 50%) and the clinical diagnosis is clear (even with normal EPS testing), surgical release is indicated.

Ulnar Nerve

Compression of the ulnar nerve can occur in the arm and forearm (cubital tunnel syndrome) or at the wrist (Guyon's canal, ulnar tunnel syndrome). Compression in either location can cause paresthesias or numbness in the small and ulnar half of the ring finger, whereas compression only at the elbow causes sensory symptoms in the dorsal ulnar aspect of the hand. Clawing, if present, is more pronounced when the FDP is not involved (low ulnar palsy).

Cubital Tunnel Syndrome

The cubital tunnel is a fibro-osseous canal formed by the medial epicondyle and proximal ulna with a fibrous roof (Osborne's band). The cubital tunnel changes shape and volume with elbow motion. With elbow flexion the tunnel changes from an oval to an ellipse with 55% narrowing. With combined elbow flexion, wrist extension, and shoulder abduction, the intraneural pressure increases 6 times. Any swelling or mass in the cubital tunnel, thickening of its borders, or tethering of the nerve can impair longitudinal excursion. The term cubital tunnel syndrome describes ulnar nerve entrapment from the arcade of Struthers and medial intramuscular septum proximally to the fasciae of the flexor carpi ulnaris and sublimus arcade distally. Osteophytosis, ganglia, and anomalous structures, such as the anconeus epitrochlearis, can cause nerve entrapment.

Sensory symptoms usually predate motor findings because the sensory fibers are more superficial and vulnerable to compression. Evidence of ulnar nerve subluxation should be sought but is not usually the sole indication for surgery. Even in more advanced cases with denervation on the EMG, the NCV may be normal.

In mild ulnar nerve entrapment, nonsurgical treatment with night extension splinting is usually successful. If symptoms persist or advance, surgical treatment may involve in situ decompression, medial epicondylectomy, or anterior transposition with eventual positioning of the ulnar nerve in a subcutaneous, intramuscular, or submuscular position. Nerve kinking or secondary compression must be avoided when anterior transposition is done.

Complications include cutaneous neuromas, elbow flexion contracture, medial epicondylitis, elbow instability, and unrelieved or recurrent symptoms. Early motion and awareness of the possibility of a flexion contracture are helpful, and surgery rarely is needed for correction. Cutaneous injury to the medial brachial or antebrachial terminal branches is minimized by keeping the incision relatively posterior. The most common findings at reoperation for recalcitrant symptoms are perineural scarring, inadequate decompression within the cubital canal, or tethering at the medial intermuscular septum or deep fascia of the flexor carpi ulnaris (FCU). Submuscular transposition is preferred for revision of a failed primary ulnar nerve surgery, and decreases symptoms in approximately 80% of patients. Internal neurolysis does not improve results. For a reoperation to be successful, the ulnar nerve must be examined and all potential levels of compression must be appropriately released. EMG evidence of denervation and previous submuscular transposition have been associated with a poor outcome in patients older than 50 years.

Ulnar Tunnel Syndrome

Ulnar nerve entrapment at the wrist is uncommon. The ulnar tunnel extends from the proximal aspect of the transverse carpal ligament to the fibrous arch of the hypothenar muscles. This area has been divided into three zones. Zone 1 is proximal to the bifurcation of the nerve, zone 2 surrounds the motor branch, and zone 3 surrounds the superficial branch. Symptom presentation can be related to these specific anatomic regions. Provocative testing includes nerve percussion, nerve compression test, Allen's test, and Phalen's sign. Causes of compression include acute or chronic repetitive trauma, ganglia, lipomas, ulnar artery aneurysms or thrombosis, hook of hamate fracture, pisiform fractures and arthritis. Ganglion cyst has been implicated as the most common cause of focal ulnar nerve impairment in Guyon's canal, although fibrous septi, sequelae of arthrosis or fracture, and arterial thrombosis or dilation appear to be the most logical etiologies.

When surgical intervention is indicated, all 3 zones must be explored. In 40% of patients the origin of the hypothenar muscles is thickened and fibrotic. All masses are excised, fibrous septi are released, and, if needed, the hook of the hamate or pisiform is excised. Thrombosis or aneurysmal dilation of the ulnar artery can be treated by resection and ligation in most patients who maintain a clinically complete arch or by reconstruction with a reverse vein graft. Preoperative and intraoperative perfusion tests are critical in the decision-making.

Radial Nerve

Compression of the radial nerve in the proximal forearm has been divided into 2 syndromes, posterior interosseous nerve (PIN) compression syndrome and radial tunnel syndrome. PIN compression syndrome causes motor weakness but no pain. Radial tunnel syndrome is compression of the PIN that causes pain without weakness. Whether these are 2 separate entities is controversial. Isolated compression of the dorsal sensory branch of the radial nerve at the brachioradialis tendon in the distal forearm (Wartenburg's syndrome) also causes pain and occasionally sensory loss.

Posterior Interosseous Nerve Compression Syndrome

PIN compression syndrome is essentially a low radial nerve palsy. Paralysis may affect any of the PIN-innervated muscles. Because the extensor carpi radialis, brevis, and supinator usually are innervated proximal to the arcade of Frohse and are not involved, the wrist is radially deviated and active finger metacarpophalangeal (MCP) extension is limited. The nerve can be compressed by a vascular leash, the arcade of Frohse, tumors (lipoma), ganglia, or elbow synovitis, or the compression may be idiopathic. EPS testing will confirm the clinical presentation. The sensory action potential from the cutaneous portion of the radial nerve should be normal. Tendon rupture or primary joint pathology must be ruled out.

Occasionally, nonsurgical treatment (for 4 to 12 weeks) may be successful for a partial nonprogressive lesion, but surgery usually is required if there is no sign of improvement for 4 to 12 weeks. Decompression of the PIN from the radial recurrent vessels (leash of Henry) proximal to the arcade of Frohse to the distal end of the supinator will relieve all potential areas of compression (radial recurrent vessels, fibrous edge of the extensor carpi radialis brevis, arcade of Frohse, distal edge of supinator). Full recovery may take up to 18 months.

Radial Tunnel Syndrome (Posterior Interosseous Nerve Pain Syndrome)

Radial tunnel syndrome is believed to be a dynamic compression of the PIN in the region of the elbow. It often occurs with lateral epicondylitis. Provocative testing for either entity is not reliable. Differential injections can help distinguish the 2 pathologies. The differential diagnosis includes lateral epicondylitis, extensor tendinitis, lateral elbow instability, or cervical radiculopathy. In many patients it is difficult to determine a clear diagnosis, because symptoms and signs of other diagnoses overlap and there are few confirmatory tests. EPS studies usually are negative in radial tunnel syndrome. Nonsurgical management is appropriate for most patients. If decompression is done, the PIN is completely released as described. A recent review found only 67% good or excellent results after decompression of the radial tunnel.

Radial Sensory Nerve Entrapment

Radial sensory nerve entrapment (Wartenberg's syndrome) may be related to closed direct trauma, laceration, tight bands (such as watch bands), or a mass. it also may be associated with repetitive ulnar deviation and pronation causing compression between the tendons of the brachioradialis and extensor carpi radialis longus in the distal third of the forearm. The significance of this problem is not the sensory loss but the associated pain. The physical examination reliably demonstrates a positive Tinel's sign (96%). Wrist flexion and ulnar deviation and pronation place traction on the nerve and increase symptoms. The forearm pronation test (hyperpronation of the forearm with the wrist in neutral) may be positive. The Finkelstein test places traction on the nerve and may increase symptoms. EPS testing may document the problem and is indicated if symptoms persist after nonsurgical treatment and surgery is being considered or if the diagnosis is in doubt. The sensory action potential, conduction velocity, and amplitude are decreased. Motor testing is normal. Differential diagnosis includes de Quervain's disease, thumb carpometacarpal arthritis, lateral antebrachial cutaneous nerve compression, and C-6 radiculopathy. The forearm pronation test is not positive in these diagnoses. The lateral antebrachial cutaneous nerve can have considerable overlap with the sensory radial nerve in 75% of patients. Differential lidocaine nerve blocks as well as EPS testing help differentiate lesions of these nerves.

Nonsurgical treatment can be successful (37% to 71%), but often the nerve must be decompressed, starting at the fascia between the brachioradialis and extensor carpi radialis longus and continuing distally past any area of injury. The sharp dorsal edge of the brachioradialis usually is excised. Results are excellent or good in 86%. Hypertrophy of the scar can be treated with pressure pads and topical steroid cream. Hypersensitivity of the nerve may last 3 months and is treated with desensitization.

Scaphoid Nonunion

Critical analysis of the literature regarding the natural history of scaphoid nonunion has exposed the limited value of these studies from an epidemiologic viewpoint. Although the biases of these investigations are recognized, the overwhelming message from the literature appears to be that scaphoid nonunion is associated with the dorsal intercalary segment instability and subsequent degenerative arthrosis noted radiographically in all nonunions of more than 10 years' duration. One study emphasized the rapid progression of degenerative changes in patients with greater displacement of bone fragments. The value of CT as well as MRI scanning has been documented for determining fracture displacement, comminution, alignment, and the presence of vascular compromise. Almost all methods of bone grafting have been reported to achieve favorable results. Iliac crest bone grafting through a palmar approach combined with internal fixation remains the standard, with a high rate of union (92%). Success using bone graft harvested from the adjacent volar distal radius also has been reported. Satisfactory results have been reported for various fixation techniques, including Kirschner wires (K-wires), Herbert screws, cannulated screws, and staples. Each device has associated complications that must be recognized by the surgeon. Although most authors report the use of a palmar approach, the dorsal approach may have some advantages in exposure of the proximal scaphoid and preservation of the palmar ligaments. Correction of angular deformity through the waist of the scaphoid is difficult through a dorsal approach.

Correction of the malalignment of the scaphoid through the pseudarthrosis is of utmost importance because an increased intrascaphoid angle has been shown to be associated with reduced range of motion (ROM), the development of posttraumatic arthrosis, and diminished strength. Authors have reported that patients may function well and be satisfied with surgery despite diminished strength and ROM.

Detailed studies of regional vascular anatomy have led to the use of vascularized bone grafts and of vascular bundle implantation as other methods for treating scaphoid nonunion. Although these were originally reserved for

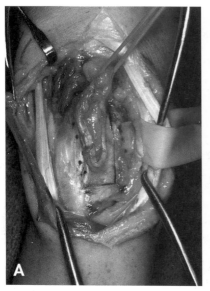 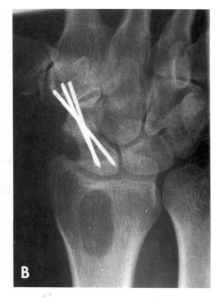

Figure 4

The Zaidenberg vascularized graft for scaphoid nonunion. A, The bone flap territory on the dorsal radius is elevated and careful marginal dissection at the articular margin of the radius frees the pedicled transfer. B, Radiograph soon after the vascularized bone graft with the construct stabilized with Kirschner wires.

osteonecrosis or failed bone grafting, they currently are being done as primary procedures. Vascular anatomy of the distal radius has been well-described, and vascular grafts from the distal radius have been shown to have an acceptable rate of healing, with the potential to revascularize avascular segments of bone (Fig. 4). The use of an implanted vascular bundle based on the second dorsal intermetacarpal artery combined with cortical cancellous bone graft has been successful in gaining union in 90% of patients with proximal pole nonunions.

Salvage procedures for failed scaphoid nonunion surgery include scaphoid excision and limited intercarpal fusion, proximal row carpectomy, and total wrist arthrodesis. These are discussed in the section on wrist reconstruction.

Wrist Reconstruction: Kienböck's Disease

Kienböck's disease or lunatomalacia is a rare diagnosis that is often made by exclusion of more common etiologies for dorsal wrist pain. The disease can present insidiously, without a history of significant wrist trauma. It is debated whether osteonecrosis of the lunate results from a single insult or from repetitive microtrauma.

The patient's anatomy may be a predisposing factor for development of osteonecrosis of the lunate. A relative radial positive-ulnar negative relationship at the distal radioulnar joint has been implicated, as well as the intraosseous vascular pattern of the lunate. Three-fourths of lunates have both a dorsal and a volar extraosseous blood supply (Fig. 5).

Classification of Kienböck's disease has evolved to include description of normal appearing lunates with evidence of vascular compromise found only on advanced imaging tests (bone scan and MRI). In stage I disease, the lunate appears normal on plain radiographs, but trispiral or computed tomography reveals microfractures, or the MRI demonstrates the inhomogeneity characteristic of vascular compromise (Fig. 6). Lunate sclerosis becomes radiographically evident in stage II disease, although collapse has not occurred. Stage III is characterized by collapse of the lunate without carpal disruption (III A) and collapse accompanied by static rotatory subluxation of the scaphoid (III B). In stage IV, degenerative arthrosis is present in the adjacent articulations of the lunate (Fig. 7).

The treatment of Kienböck's disease is based on the degree of lunate involvement, the relative relationship of the distal radius and ulna, and the status of the surrounding carpus. Some consider symptomatic treatment such as immobilization to be acceptable for the earlier stages, whereas others maintain that surgery is necessary. Early external fixation to provide symptom relief and, potentially, to decrease stress on the compromised lunate is being investigated. Treatment options include joint leveling, revascularization, intracapsular wrist procedures including carpal bone excisions or fusions, and total wrist arthrodesis. A suggested surgical treatment plan is summarized in Table 1.

Chronic Scapholunate Instability

Chronic scapholunate instability has been treated by a number of different procedures including direct repair, dorsal capsulodesis, tendon grafting or transfer, and intercarpal fusion. Dorsal capsulodesis has been shown to be beneficial for dynamic scapholunate instability with improvement in

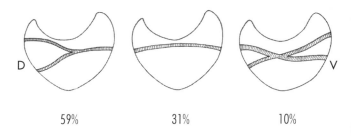

Figure 5

The patterns of intraosseous vascular anastomoses. D, dorsal; V, volar. (Adapted with permission from Williams CS, Gelberman RH: Vascularity of the lunate. *Hand Clin* 1993;9:395.)

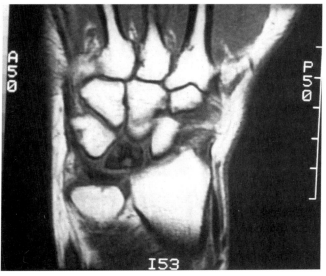

Figure 6

Magnetic resonance imaging scan demonstrating the low signal intensity on T1-weighted images that reflect the avascular status of the lunate in Kienböck's disease.

subjective symptoms, such as clunking and wrist pain; however it has been associated with loss of wrist flexion with minimal effect on other wrist motions. Investigators continue to report results of transfer of tendons such as the flexor carpi radialis as a means of preventing malrotation of the scaphoid. Other long-term studies are needed to define the role of soft-tissue procedures for scapholunate dissociation.

Limited wrist arthrodeses involving the scaphocapitate (SC), scaphotrapezial-trapezoidal (STT), and capitolunate joints all have been used as a treatment for scapholunate dissociation. While the initial reports of STT fusion were promising, a number of complications have been noted, with an overall complication rate of 50% or more in large series. STT and SC fusions affect wrist motion in a similar fashion and have comparable clinical results. In both techniques, proper maintenance of the lunate position is of utmost importance, and failure to properly reduce the lunate assures a poor result. Almost all limited wrist fusions have shown a high percentage of nonunions. Recent reports of capitolunate arthrodesis as well as SLAC wrist reconstruction or 4-corner fusion (scaphoid excision combined with arthrodesis of the capitate-lunate-triquetrum-hamate) have supported the usefulness of these procedures in scaphoid nonunion because they may allow preservation of approximately 50% of normal wrist motion.

Proximal row carpectomy (PRC) has gained favor when compared to scaphoid excision and 4-corner fusion. In 1 study with intermediate follow-up, all patients undergoing PRC reported less pain and greater motion and strength than patients undergoing 4-corner fusion. The long-term fate of the radiocapitate articulation remains in question, but these intermediate reports are promising. The ultimate salvage procedure for advanced degenerative changes in the wrist is total arthrodesis with plate and screw fixation.

Degenerative Arthrosis of the Small Joints

Thumb Carpometacarpal Joint

Although the use of silicone prostheses once was commonplace, the awareness of silicone synovitis has significantly reduced the use of this material at the carpometacarpal (CMC) joint. Most current techniques have maintained the concept of tendon interposition arthroplasty, but have used autogenous tendon. CMC joint fusion also is an alternative for selected patients with CMC arthrosis. In young female patients with excessive thumb CMC joint laxity, reefing and/or tendon augmentation of the CMC joint capsule can provide symptomatic relief. If evidence of advanced degenerative change in the cartilage is noted, these patients may be candidates for soft-tissue arthroplasty reconstruction.

Although specific techniques differ, almost all soft-tissue reconstructions for basilar thumb arthrosis include trapezium excision, tendon interposition, and suspensionplasty by tendon transfer. Recent anatomic studies defining the importance of the deep palmar ligament for ultimate stability of the thumb metacarpal have led to the development of techniques involving sling suspension of the thumb metacarpal in an attempt to maintain metacarpal height and avoid subsidence. Clinical studies have demonstrated excellent overall functional outcome using these soft-tissue reconstruction tech-

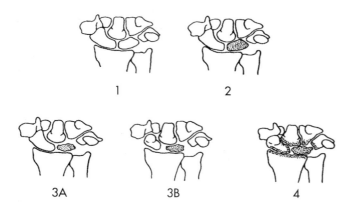

Figure 7

Radiographic classification of Kienböck's disease according to the method of Lichtman and associates, modified by Weiss and associates. Stage 1: no change visible in the lunate; stage 2: sclerosis of the lunate; stage 3A: sclerosis and fragmentation of the lunate; stage 3B: stage 3A with proximal migration of the capitate or fixed rotation of the scaphoid; stage 4: stage 3A or B combined with degenerative changes at adjacent intercarpal joints. (Reproduced with permission from Weiland AJ: Avascular necrosis of the corpus, in American Society for Surgery of the Hand: *Hand Surgery Update.* Rosemont, IL, American Academy of Orthopaedic Surgeons, 1996, pp 85–91.)

Table 1	
Treatment of Kienböck's disease by stage	
Stage	**Treatment**
Stage I, II, IIIA	
Ulnar positive	Joint leveling
Ulnar negative	Revascularization or medial closing wedge osteotomy of radius
Stage IIIB	Limited intercarpal fusion
Stage IV	
Lunate fossa/ capitate intact	Proximal row carpectomy
Strength desired over motion	Wrist arthrodesis

(Reproduced with permission from Gerwin M, Weiland AJ: Avascular necrosis of the carpals. *Hand Clin* 1993;761.)

niques and patient satisfaction approaching 90%. Long-term comparison of patients who had interposition arthroplasty with those who had ligament reconstruction is still lacking. Both techniques have similar patient satisfaction profiles. New techniques of implant arthroplasty have revived interest in this procedure for the thumb CMC joint, but no long-term results are available yet.

Because soft-tissue reconstruction has the potential for some loss of stability and strength, the use of these techniques in manual laborers has been questioned. Thumb CMC fusion to provide a stable fulcrum for the use of the thumb has been shown to be quite effective in pain relief and maintenance of strength. The drawbacks include decreased thumb adduction and inability to flatten the hand. The indications for each of these techniques are evolving, although well-controlled comparative studies are still lacking. Recent reports, however, indicate good patient satisfaction regardless of the method of treatment for degenerative arthrosis of the CMC joint of the thumb.

Metacarpophalangeal Joint

In patients with rheumatoid arthritis, silicone implant arthroplasty remains the treatment of choice for painful or dislocated MCP joints. Several studies demonstrated excellent pain reduction, correction of deformity, and improved

function. In general, a functional arc of motion is maintained, although some deterioration in maximum flexion as well as extensor lag occurs during the first 5 years of follow-up. The use of silicone implant arthroplasty in patients with significant osteoarthritis remains controversial. This group usually has sustained isolated trauma and demands a far greater activity level than patients with rheumatoid arthritis. The use of implants in the nonborder digits is generally accepted, although the longevity of these implants can be limited. Less optimal results have been found when replacing the index finger MCP joint with a silicone implant. Although motion is lost, fusion of the index finger MCP joint provides predictable stability and pain relief.

The use of vascularized whole joint transfers from the toes as a replacement for the MCP joint has been advocated, but most studies have not been encouraging with regard to the final ROM obtained by the use of these free joint transfers. Overall motion obtained is generally no better than that with silicone implant arthroplasty, and the morbidity of free joint transfer is substantially greater. In addition, the technical aspects of free joint transfer are far more complicated than those of implant arthroplasty.

Proximal Interphalangeal Joint

Arthrodesis of the proximal interphalangeal (PIP) joint is still the most commonly performed procedure for advanced arthrosis. Union is extremely predictable regardless of the methods used, although a recent large study demonstrated the best union rate with the use of intramedullary screws, an intermediate union rate using tension band wires, and the lowest union rate using K-wire fixation. The primary non-union rate was highest in patients with psoriatic arthritis, intermediate in patients with rheumatoid arthritis, and lowest in patients with arthrosis secondary to acute trauma or post-traumatic reconstruction. Nonunion in osteoarthritic patients was rare regardless of fixation technique. The inherent initial stability obtained with intramedullary screws also has reduced the requirement for external protection during the early postoperative period. Nevertheless, because complications can occur, especially at the proximal screw fixation point in the distal portion of the proximal phalanx, this technique has less room for error than methods using tension band or K-wire fixation.

Alternative methods of treatment for advanced PIP destruction include volar plate interposition and silicone replacement arthroplasty. A recent study of 69 PIP joint arthroplasties using a volar approach demonstrated excellent pain relief, although overall total active motion was not increased and deformities in the coronal plane were not corrected. Long-term follow-up of PIP joint silicone arthroplasties is still lacking. The volar approach is preferred to the dorsal approach except in patients who require concomitant extensor tendon rebalancing.

Distal Interphalangeal Joint

Degenerative arthrosis of the DIP joint is most frequently treated symptomatically with splints or surgically by debridement or arthrodesis. An intramedullary screw provides excellent intrinsic stability immediately after surgery and has significantly reduced the incidences of infection and hardware loosening. A recent study demonstrated greater inherent strength of intramedullary screw fixation compared to tension band wiring techniques. Nevertheless, in patients with a small distal phalanx (most commonly females), care to avoid violation of the nail bed by the screw threads is essential. The advantage of using K-wire techniques for arthrodesis is that the fusion angle can be altered from the neutral posture required by the use of an intramedullary screw. Silicone joint replacement of the DIP joint is not advocated.

A recent large study examining the surgical treatment of mucous cysts formed secondary to degenerative arthritis at the DIP joint showed excellent functional outcome and minimal recurrence rate as long as debridement of the DIP joint osteophytes was undertaken simultaneously with cyst excision (Fig. 8). Appropriate excision of the cyst and debridement of the DIP joint generally allow spontaneous resolution of the nail deformity associated with the cyst.

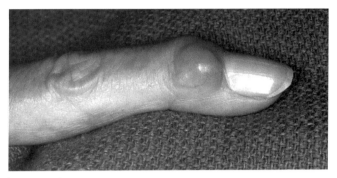

Figure 8

Classic appearance of a mucous cyst at the distal interphalangeal joint. The attenuated skin over the cyst is fragile, and the longitudinal nail deformity is indicative of pressure on the germinal matrix.

Rheumatoid Wrist Reconstruction

Arthrodesis of the rheumatoid wrist is a reliable surgical procedure that corrects deformity, imparts stability, and relieves pain. Radiocarpal fusion (radioscaphoid, radiolunate, or radioscapholunate) has been used to diminish ulnar translation of the carpus and preserve some motion at the midcarpal joint. Total wrist arthroplasty may have a role in patients who already have or will likely need a contralateral wrist arthrodesis; maintaining 1 mobile wrist may have a positive overall functional result.

Total wrist arthroplasty is a consideration for limited to low demand rheumatoid arthritis (RA) patients with intact wrist extensor and flexor tendons. Wrist arthroplasty has been suggested to provide a distinct advantage over wrist arthrodesis in RA patients who prefer to maintain motion. The bone stock of the distal radius and metacarpals must be relatively preserved to perform the arthroplasty.

Silicone wrist spacers are still in use. A recent study of 50 silicone wrist replacements followed for a mean of 8 years showed substantial functional improvements in daily living activities (90%). However, 11 implants fractured at the junction of the middle column and the distal stem. Several were painful, requiring reoperation between 3 and 8 years later. All follow-up radiographs showed some degree of carpal collapse, usually on both sides of the radiocarpal joint.

Total wrist arthroplasty with metal and plastic components continues to evolve. Most common complications have been related to distal component subsidence and dislocation. In a recent series of 50 prostheses followed for an average of 4.5 years after surgery, results were excellent in 24, good in 12, fair in 5, and poor in 9 wrists. The authors emphasized the technical challenge of accurate placement of wrist components. Radiographs identified malposition of carpal components in 11 wrists, with 8 showing signs of loosening that required surgical revision. These results are comparable to those of previous studies.

Salvage after failed total wrist arthroplasty is one of the most challenging procedures in hand surgery. Arthrodesis of the wrist is the salvage solution to this clinical problem. A recent study reviewed 12 failed wrist implant arthroplasties, including 8 silicone implants and 4 metal/plastic total wrist implants. The surgical method involved a tricortical iliac crest bone graft and an intramedullary Steinman pin. There were 7 excellent results, 4 good results, and 1 poor result. Seven patients had solid fusions and 5 had pseudarthroses. Four pseudarthroses occurred at the graft-metacarpal junction and 1 occurred at the graft-radius junction. All patients who had solid fusions had excellent results; however, there were 17 complications in 9 patients. The authors recommended using more rigid fixation techniques and generous bone grafting in patients with failed wrist arthroplasty.

Distal Radioulnar Joint

Synovitis of the distal radioulnar joint (DRUJ) leads to erosion about the distal ulna and instability of the joint. With the volar translation of the radiocarpal unit, the irregular distal ulna appears prominent dorsally. Attrition of the extensor tendons on the eroded distal ulna can lead to rupture, characteristic of the Vaughn-Jackson syndrome. Resection of the distal end of the ulna has been implicated in promoting ulnar subluxation of the carpus. Several techniques have been described for surgical treatment of the distal ulna in rheumatoid disease. The Sauvé-Kapandji procedure has been recommended to provide radioulnar and ulnocarpal stability and to prevent deformity and extensor tendon rupture caused by prominence of the ulnar stump. A recent study evaluated a modified Sauvé-Kapandji procedure in 28 patients, 19 of whom had DRUJ subluxation caused by RA. Twenty-seven of the 28 had little or no pain at the DRUJ after the procedure.

Another study investigated the long-term functional outcome in patients who had unilateral distal ulna resection, the Darrach procedure or its modifications. Radiographs of the surgically treated and untreated hands were compared 4 to 9 years after surgery with respect to ulnocarpal distance, ulnar translation of the carpus, and radialization of the ulna. The results showed a mean ulnar translation in the treated wrists of 5.3 mm, which was significantly larger than the 3.7 mm in the untreated wrists, indicating that radiocarpal stabilization should be considered in conjunction with unlar column ablation procedures.

Metacarpophalangeal Joint Arthroplasty

Silicone implants have been used since the 1960s to treat MCP joint subluxation and ulnar deviation secondary to RA. Silicone implants have been reported to be stable and long lived and to have a low rate of complications. Despite success with the traditional implant, new designs have been introduced to increase the digital extensor moment arm, to duplicate the center of rotation of the MCP joint, and to reduce the potential for palmar bony impingement. In a review of 168 new silicone MCP joint arthroplasty implants in patients with RA, 20% of the implants were fractured at an average of 27 months after surgery. The number rose to 45% after 3 years. Because of a higher implant fracture incidence at a relatively shorter follow-up period, the authors noted that they had abandoned the use of this new implant.

Proximal Interphalangeal Joint Arthroplasty

Patients with rheumatoid disease at the PIP joint level experience a significant loss of function. Symptoms range from stiffness to instability; loss of grip and pinch strength are the consequences. Some PIP joint deformities have been treated with silicone implant arthroplasty. In a large study of patients with PIP implant arthroplasty for systemic inflammatory arthritis, digits with boutonnière deformities and previous or concurrent MCP joint silicone arthroplasties had much more successful outcomes than those without. The authors indicated that MCP joint arthroplasties done concurrently with PIP joint arthroplasties more closely restored extrinsic and intrinsic muscular balance. They believe that flexible silicone implants should not be used in joints that are ankylosed before surgery and in digits with swan neck deformities.

In a recent review of a new technique using the volar approach to the PIP joint for silicone PIP joint replacement arthroplasty, the authors suggested that the volar approach to the PIP joint allowed preservation of the central slip and initiation of immediate postoperative motion in 47 patients with 87 joints treated using this approach.

Tenosynovitis

In RA, tenosynovitis circumferentially involves the entire flexor tendon structure. Stenosing tenosynovitis in patients with RA causes limited digital motion secondary to mechanical catching at multiple pulley sites. An A1 pulley release in RA patients can exasercbate ulnar drift of the fingers as the flexor tendon moment, a deforming force, is increased. A recent article reviewed these important anatomic and biomechanical factors and recommended tenosynovectomy between pulley windows without release of specific pulleys. Large flexor tendon nodules should be treated by excising a slip of the flexor digitorum superficialis, a reduction tenoplasty.

Wrist Imaging

Multiple algorithms have been published to guide the investigation of wrist disorders. Wrist arthroscopy and MRI have added greatly to anatomic knowledge. Arthroscopy has become the recognized standard for the diagnosis of intra-articular soft-tissue injuries of the wrist. However, MRI offers the potential for minimizing the need for invasive procedures such as arthrography or arthroscopy.

The complex osseous and soft-tissue anatomy of the wrist makes it challenging to determine which studies offer useful clinical information. For example, oblique views of the wrist are part of the standard radiographic examination in many hospitals, but have been found to rarely add information that changes the treatment course.

A bone scan is a highly sensitive test; a negative bone scan practically rules out overt osseous pathology. Wrist arthroscopy is highly specific with the capability of confirming a triangular fibrocartilage complex (TFCC) tear more reliably than MRI or an arthrogram.

Radiography

Although plain films remain valuable in wrist imaging, they have significant limitations. Radiographs of lunate morphology have been shown to be only 66% accurate in predicting the presence of a type II lunate with a medial or hamate facet. Because this problem frequently is associated with hamate arthrosis and ulnar wrist pain, reliance on plain radiographs may miss this cause of wrist pain.

Films of the opposite wrist are reliable indicators of carpal height and carpal angle reference, but provide no better reference for ulnar variance, palmar tilt, and radial inclination of the radius platform than general age and sex stratified databases.

In evaluating distal radial fractures, intra-articular displacement is poorly measured on plain films, even by experienced physicians. Ulnar variance, palmar tilt, and radial shift are reliably measured. Because of the importance of articular congruity in distal radial fractures, CT scanning is more helpful for evaluation of complex distal radial fractures than plain radiographs.

Arthrography

Arthrography is a well-established tool for investigation of intra-articular wrist pathology. Although single injection radiocarpal arthrography has been shown to have significant limitations, triple injection arthrography has a high degree of accuracy. Digital subtraction arthrography alone has a high false-negative rate, but combining it with standard 3-compartment arthrography increases the accuracy.

Compared to arthroscopy, 3-compartment arthrography was shown to have a sensitivity of 56% and a specificity of 83%. Arthrography was most accurate in identifying TFCC lesions, but commonly missed intercarpal injuries. With high specificity and low sensitivity, a normal arthrogram did not rule out pathology: in 80% of patients with normal arthrograms, arthroscopy revealed intra-articular pathology. Arthrography does not quantify the size or type of the TFCC perforation or interosseus ligament rupture, so an extensive tear and a small perforation have the same arthrographic appearance. Furthermore, a high rate of false-positive results has been reported in the asymptomatic wrists of patients in whom bilateral wrist arthrography was done to investigate unilateral pathology. In over half the patients, findings at the TFCC and interosseous ligaments were symmetrical, even in the absence of bilateral symptoms.

Magnetic Resonance Imaging

Wrist TFCC and Interosseous Ligament Injuries MRI is a noninvasive diagnostic tool that can effectively image the wrist. Recent work has shown that MRI can distinguish partial thickness TFCC degeneration from complete perforation. Sensitivity rates for diagnosis of TFCC tears vary from 72% to 93%, which is comparable to 3-compartment arthrography. MRI may produce false-negative images, but generally produces only a few false positives, which are due to irregularities of the central portion of the TFCC.

Complete scapholunate ligament tears can be imaged on MRI with a sensitivity of up to 90%. Partial scapholunate ligament tears are poorly seen with current technology. Assessment of triquetrolunate (TL) ligament tears with MRI is more difficult than scapholunate ligament injuries because of the small size and the oblique orientation of the ligament. The reported sensitivity of MRI in TL ligament tears ranges from 23% to 50%.

A weakness of MRI is the inability to detect the cartilage erosions often associated with TFCC tears. Studies have shown that MRI is able to visualize only 10% of cartilaginous lesions later seen at arthroscopy.

Flexor Tendons MRI has recently been shown to have a high accuracy in detecting postoperative flexor tendon ruptures. MRI was shown to differentiate rupture from adhesions with a 100% accuracy rate.

Fractures MRI has an extremely high sensitivity, specificity, and interobserver agreement for scaphoid fracture detection, even when plain radiographs are considered negative. Fractures are typically identified on a combination of STIR and T1 images by appreciation of bone edema and imaging of the occult fracture line, in some cases.

Infections MRI has been used successfully for evaluation of acute soft-tissue infections of the hand, although it offers little advantage over clinical assessment for establishing the necessity of surgical intervention. However, MRI has been shown to be of value in the diagnosis of osteomyelitis. It is extremely sensitive and has been shown to be superior to indium-111 white cell scans, gallium-67 scans, or technetium-99 scans in detecting bone infections.

Kienböck's Disease MRI has been established as the investigation of choice for assessment of the vascularity of the lunate and the proximal pole of the scaphoid. It is more sensitive than bone scintigraphy in diagnosing Kienböck's disease.

Tumors MRI is also the current investigation of choice for assessment of soft-tissue tumors of the hand and wrist. Although excellent for defining the extent of the tumor, it is not diagnostic for tumor type. However, it can be diagnostic for hemangiomas, lipomas, giant cell tumor of tendon sheath, and ganglia.

Computed Tomography
CT scanning is currently the test of choice for imaging osseous pathology about the hand and wrist. Although plain tomography and CT have the same theoretical resolution, the reduced blur and enhanced contrast of CT make diagnosis easier. Additional information is provided because CT images can be obtained in more planes (axial, sagittal, and coronal) than plain tomography (PA and lateral). The value of CT in evaluation of distal radial fractures has been shown for assessment of the DRUJ as well as for the radiocarpal joint. CT has a clear advantage over plain radiographs in assessing fracture displacement and comminution. In one study, CT scans showed increased displacement of more than 2 mm when compared to plain films in 13 of 18 fractures involving the lunate facet and showed greater comminution in 17 of 18 fractures. It is estimated that 30% of plain radiographs under or over estimate displacement compared to CT. CT scans also can provide better assessment of rotational malalignment than plain films, with a described interobserver reliability correlation of 0.94.

Ultrasound
Ultrasound has been shown to be of great value in detecting occult ganglia, with a sensitivity of 96%, as well as documenting the extent and origin of the ganglion. This sensitivity and specificity for cystic structures has been shown to be equal to MRI, and ultrasound should be the initial screening procedure for ganglia.

Ultrasound has proven useful in the detection of nonradiopaque foreign bodies. High sensitivities and specificities for detection of foreign bodies as small as 1 × 4 mm have been reported. It has also been useful in assessing the integrity of tendon repairs; a sensitivity of 88% and an accuracy of 85% in detecting ruptures have been shown.

Another use has been to detect the presence of plantaris tendons as a source for tendon graft harvest. Ultrasound has been shown to have a sensitivity of 95% for detecting a tendon suitable for grafting. All patients with positive studies had a plantaris tendon, a specificity of 100%. Finally, ultrasound is a poor screening tool for nonspecific wrist pain and should be used to answer specific questions.

Bone Scintigraphy
Bone scans have been shown to have a sensitivity of 100% and a specificity of 98% for the diagnosis of occult scaphoid fractures if performed at least 72 hours after the injury. Three-phase bone scans have been used for the diagnosis of reflex sympathetic dystrophy, with a specificity of over 90%; however, the sensitivity appears to be only 50%. This diagnosis remains a clinical one.

Wrist Arthroscopy

Anatomy
Wrist arthroscopy portals are named in relation to the extensor tendon compartments. Standard landmarks for establishing the portals are well-established. Evolving knowledge of the local anatomy assists the arthroscopist in safely establishing portals without injury to tendons or cutaneous nerves.

Interosseous Ligament and TFCC Injuries
In spite of improvement in MRI scanning, arthroscopy remains the standard for diagnosis of intercarpal ligament injuries. It provides the best evaluation of the ligaments and joint surfaces and allows the surgeon to view these joints while performing provocative maneuvers. The treatment of interosseous ligament tears remains controversial. Arthroscopic reduction and internal fixation may have a role in acute injuries but healing is unpredictable. Arthroscopic debridement alone has been shown to provide pain relief over the short term (2 years) in patients with complete tears as well as incomplete tears. The long-term results of this treatment have not been determined.

Fractures of the Distal Radius

Arthroscopically assisted reduction and internal fixation of carpal and distal radial fractures has been used to obtain anatomic reduction with minimal soft-tissue disruption. However, after anatomic reduction and stable fixation of fractures, results for distal radial fracture were suboptimal. Recent studies in which wrist arthroscopy was used in patients with fractures of the radius and carpus showed that many had sustained concomitant injuries to the soft-tissue elements about the wrist. TFCC tears were found in 53% of extra-articular fractures and 35% of intra-articular radial fractures. Scapholunate ligament injuries accompanied 21.5% of intra-articular radial fractures. TL ligament injuries with instability were present in 13.3% of extra-articular fractures. Preoperative plain radiographs correlated with TFCC injuries but had poor predictive value for scapholunate and TL ligament injuries. In extra-articular fractures with an ulnar variance of more than 3 mm, 73% of patients had TFCC tears demonstrated on arthroscopy.

Chronic Wrist Pain

Chronic wrist pain remains a difficult diagnostic problem. Conventional studies including MRI often fail to delineate the problem. Recent work has shown that up to 34% of patients with chronic wrist pain may have chondral lesions, which are poorly seen on MRI, with only 10% being found in one series. Arthroscopy can be a valuable tool in evaluating chronic wrist pain of a mechanical nature (crepitus, locking, activity-associated change in symptoms), but has little use in evaluating vague wrist discomfort without suspected anatomic derangement.

Combined ligamentous and cartilage injuries are seen with arthroscopy in 70% to 96% of patients. Although arthroscopy is a valuable tool in the evaluation of patients with wrist pain, correlation of the arthroscopic findings with the clinical symptoms is critical.

Cerebral Palsy in the Upper Extremity

Typical postures in spastic cerebral palsy include increased elbow flexion, forearm pronation, wrist flexion, thumb adduction or thumb-in-palm deformity, and finger flexion. Many children require reconstructive or palliative surgery to increase function or for hygiene in advanced cases. Surgical management is directed toward removing deforming muscle forces, releasing contracted joints, and transferring voluntary muscles to balancing insertions. Transfer of hypertonic muscles without voluntary control often leads to a different and often antagonistic imbalance. Lengthening or release of tendons and ligaments or muscle origin and musculotendinous fractional lengthening are valuable surgical variations that alter muscle forces and joint deformation. Although patients with suboptimal sensation should not be excluded from reconstructive efforts, those with 10 mm 2-point discrimination or better have the best surgical outcomes. Intellectual development and coordination (assessed by the rapidity of performance of alternating movements) have been suggested as potential positive indicators of surgical outcome.

Shoulder internal rotation and adduction contracture may not be disabling in all children, but this posture is cosmetically and functionally unacceptable to many patients and families. Correction of the posture by release of the shoulder capsule, the subscapularis, and the pectoralis major has been classic (L'Episcopo procedure), although osteotomy of the humerus is regaining favor to provide external rotation.

Elbow flexion contracture sometimes requires release by Z-lengthening of the biceps, brachialis, and brachioradialis and release of the anterior elbow capsule. Care should be taken to avoid overstretching the median nerve and brachial artery in postoperative cast correction. Progressive bending is preferred. A desirable posture for function and appearance places the elbow at 45° of flexion with the wrist in neutral to 30° of extension and the forearm slightly pronated.

Finger flexor tightness is improved by fractional lengthening of tight flexor digitorum sublimis and profundus. Severe contractures and minimally functioning muscles are lengthened by sublimis to profundus transfer.

Thumb adduction contractures caused by adductor pollicis contracture may benefit from a precise palmar muscle slide and web space deepening. Thumb-in-palm deformity increases with wrist extension if the flexor pollicis longus is tight. When a flexed wrist is being repositioned in a more extended posture, lengthening the digital and thumb flexors usually is necessary. Rerouting the extensor pollicis longus may simplify thumb balance when combined with MCP arthrodesis and muscle release. Deforming forces, such as the flexor carpi ulnaris, can be released and transferred to the extensor carpi radialis brevis to maintain wrist extension. Unless sufficient voluntary wrist flexion moment from the flexor carpi radialis or palmaris longus is present, wrist extension deformity, essentially an overcorrection, can result. Dynamic EMG, botulinum toxin, and phenol injections of nerve and muscle may help the long-term effects of surgical treatment.

Table 2
ASIA classification and International classification

ASIA (grade 3)*	Group	Muscles functioning (grade 4)*
C5 biceps	0	Weak BR (≤ grade 3*)
	I	BR (≥ grade 4*)
C6 wrist extension	II	BR, ECRL
	III	BR, ECRL, ECRB
C7 triceps	IV	BR, ECRL, ECRB, PT
	V	BR, ECRL, ECRB, PT, FCR
	VI	BR, ECRL, ECRB, PT, FCR, EDC
	VII	BR, ECRL, ECRB, PT, FCR, EDC, EPL
C8 EDQ*	VIII	Lack only intrinsics

* Medical Research Council grade; BR, brachioradialis; ECRB, extensor carpi radialis brevis; ECRL, extensor carpi radialis longus; FCR, flexor carpi radialis; PT, pronator teres; EDC, extensor digitorum communis; EDQ, extensor digiti quinti; EPL, extensor pollicis longus

Tetraplegia

Model spinal injury centers provide care from the time of injury through rehabilitation. About 2,000 new spinal cord injury patients are seen each year. Treatment at specialized facilities has been shown to improve survival and ultimate functional level. Shortened average hospital length of stay has led to less rehabilitation before return to home and an increasing dependence on community based ambulatory care. One third of patients have American Spinal Injury Association (ASIA) level C-5 and C-6 tetraplegia (Table 2).

In C-1 to C-4 tetraplegia, weakness and loss of sensation curtail independent hand function. Attendant care and substitution using environmental control devices are needed to sustain functionality. Respiratory insufficiency may limit endurance and mobility.

Patients with C-5 tetraplegia have voluntary deltoid and elbow flexor function at grade 3. They require active attendant care for most activities of daily living and transfers, use motorized wheelchairs, and wear splints adapted for specific activities such as eating or writing. Patients with preserved elbow flexion benefit from transfer of a grade 4 brachioradialis to the extensor carpi radialis brevis for wrist extension and tenodesis finger movements. Tenodesis of flexor pollicis longus (Moberg) allows key pinch. Split flexor pollicis longus tenodesis stabilizes the thumb interphalangeal joint. Alternatively, the flexor pollicis longus can be attached to the brachioradialis transfer for active pinch.

Patients with C-6 tetraplegia maintain wrist extension. Tenodesis splints can produce mechanical palmar prehension. Posterior deltoid transfer restores elbow stability or extension. One wrist extensor can be transferred for finger flexion and the brachioradialis can be transferred to the flexor pollicis longus for pinch. Extensor tenodeses to the radius may allow finger extension. Dressing, personal activities of daily living, self-catheterization, and manual wheelchair propulsion are possible.

For C-5 to C-6 level patients, a combination of tendon transfers and functional electric stimulation shows promise. An implanted neuroprosthesis can control up to 8 upper motor neuron innervated muscles in the forearm and hand to provide elbow extension, phalangeal flexion and extension, adduction and abduction, intrinsic control, pronation, or sensory feedback.

Patients with a C-7 level usually are independent in activities of daily living. The presence of triceps function allows strong wheelchair propulsion and transfers. Hand functions in grasp and release can be enhanced with transfers. Patients with C-8 tetraplegia lack only intrinsic function and seldom need extensive reconstruction except for intrinsicplasty because finger flexion is present.

Brachial Plexus Injuries

Brachial injuries are often devastating, variable, and complex. The anatomic lesions can include avulsion axon loss, partial and complete nerve injury, absent or incomplete regeneration, and muscle degeneration or fibrosis. The clinical results range from compromise of sensation, strength, and joint movement to a "flail arm." The goal of surgical intervention is for patients to achieve grade 3 elbow flexion recovery by nerve repair, graft, neurotization, or tendon transfer surgery. Each technique has literature support.

The early recognition of nerve root avulsion is important to the staging and decision making regarding repair, neurotization, and reconstruction. In a study comparing intradural explorations to preoperative studies, CT myelography was better (85%) at this stage than MRI alone (52% accurate). Accuracy of MRI myelography is improving.

Early exploration of traction injuries with intra-operative assessment of viability of the damaged nerve or root is essential. Biopsy of the proximal nerve or root and histologic stains for live axons is the most reassuring method to demonstrate root continuity. Somatosensory evoked potentials can demonstrate electrical conductivity through a neuroma in continuity. The number of surviving fibers is less certain without quantitative axon counts. Axons have been restored to the most functional muscle groups, usually the elbow flexors in proximal (C-5, C-6) injuries, using free vascular and cable grafts and using neurotizations with intercostal, spinal accessory, pectorals, phrenic, or thoracodorsal nerves.

Evidence suggests that early intervention is better for the recovery of elbow flexion. Patients treated after 9 months from injury have progressively less successful recovery of muscle after reinnervation. Neurotization and free tissue transfer after regrowth of the axons is gaining acceptance for late treatment. Electrical stimulation of paralyzed muscle and cross-innervation from the contralateral plexus are under continuing investigation. Tendon transfer surgery for elbow flexion provides predictable strength when donor muscles are available. Transfers of pectoralis, latissimus dorsi, or the flexor-pronator origin to the proximal anterior humerus can provide satisfactory power.

Stabilization of the shoulder by arthrodesis provides stabile alignment for the arm. In the absence of scapular stabilizers, however, the proximal thoracic instability is worse than glenohumeral paralysis. Shoulder arthrodesis is among the final procedures elected.

Vascular Disorders

A history of nontraumatic vascular insufficiency with discoloration, mottling, pallor, numbness, tingling, pain, skin ulceration, and skin thickening should prompt a search for an anatomic or physiologic diagnosis. Raynaud's phenomenon, direct vascular trauma, connective tissue diseases, occupational exposure to vibration and cold, nicotine addiction, vascular injection injuries, reflex sympathetic dystrophy, renal insufficiency, and psychiatric illness are among common diagnoses. Differential diagnosis should exclude proximal occlusion, such as vascular steal syndromes, and compression disorders of nerve and vessels at the wrist, elbow and shoulder, and thoracic outlet. A positive cold stress test points to vasospastic disease. Medical management has improved diagnosis and treatment, although connective tissue diseases and scleroderma remain serious threats to digital survival. Currently, calcium channel blockers, steroids, chemotherapy agents, anti-inflammatory medications, regional blocks, systemic anticoagulants, counseling, biofeedback, and alternative medical treatments are used. Intravenous prostaglandin infusion may have additional promise.

A trial of regional anesthetic nerve, stellate ganglion, or local sympathetic blockade may reduce vasospasm and suggest that digital sympathectomy is indicated. Exclusion of digital occlusive disease by digital subtraction angiography with intra-

arterial vasodilators is important in staging exploration. Active digital artery vasculitis has a poor prognosis, and biopsy may be indicated if the patient has symptoms elsewhere. Systemic medications may be required to suppress vasculitis.

Digital and palmar arch sympathectomy has been shown to reduce pain and allow ulcers to heal. Adventitial stripping and excision and grafting around occlusive disease may be combined. Noting evidence of distal runoff is necessary, and avoiding damage to collateral circulation is important. It is difficult to predict the longevity of the benefit and the rate of progression of the disease in most patients. Recent animal studies demonstrated preservation of distal adrenergic innervation in spite of perivascular adventitial resection.

Tumors of the Hand

Although malignant lesions below the elbow are rare, all masses of the hand should be treated as potentially dangerous. The most common mass in the hand is a ganglion cyst, a fluid-filled simple cyst that often communicates with wrist joint fluid at the junction of the membranous and fibrous portion of the scapholunate ligament. In children spontaneous remission is frequent, but in adults these cysts usually are persistent. Aspiration for diagnosis is warranted, but excisional biopsy with excision and scarification of the origin is indicated for recurrence.

The most common hand malignancy is squamous cell carcinoma, which is increased in incidence by solar and radiation exposure. Metastases to regional and axillary nodes should be sought on physical examination and biopsy. Increased solar exposure has recently raised concern about an increased incidence of melanoma on the hand.

The most common soft-tissue sarcoma of the hand is epithelioid sarcoma. Characterized by subtle changes in the quality of skin and tissue, it may involve a diffuse area with skin ulceration. It masquerades as other benign reactive tissues including Dupuytren's contracture, resembling a fibrous mass. It recurs relentlessly and requires wide local barrier tissue excision or amputation for cure. Hematogenous metastases, regional lymphatic spread, and spread along tissue planes are common. In general, MRI helps define disease-free barrier tissues.

In children, rhabdomyosarcoma is the most common histologic diagnosis of a solid soft-tissue mass. Treatment should rely on oncologic consultation to consider chemotherapy protocols.

The most common benign bone tumor in the hand is an enchondroma. The most common bone malignancy is a metastatic tumor, often from renal cell or lung, and may be a presenting finding of the primary disease. Giant cell tumors of bone in the hand can be aggressive lesions; if inadequately excised they may metastasize to the lungs. Wide local excision is indicated, and even amputation may be necessary.

Principles and Concerns of Hand Tumor Surgery

Biopsy should be done by the clinician responsible for anatomic definition and definitive care. Planning of incisions is as important as the plan for excision, reconstruction, or amputation. Gravity exsanguination is prudent. Tourniquets should not be used in such a way that tumor cells can be spread through veins or lymphatics by applied pressure.

Surgical equipment, gowns, gloves, and drapes used for biopsy should be replaced for subsequent reconstruction to avoid contamination of clean donor sites and healthy tissues. Imprudent harvest of a graft or flap for coverage may contaminate the donor site.

Reconstructive surgeons must creatively manage the tissue deficits created by adequate tumor removal. The alternatives of amputation versus limb salvage must be balanced by experienced musculoskeletal oncologists and upper extremity surgeons.

Annotated Bibliography

Nerve Compression Syndromes

Terrono AL, Millender LH: Management of work-related upper-extremity nerve entrapments. *Orthop Clin North Am* 1996;27: 783–793.

Diagnostic labels should not be given unless the physician is sure of the diagnosis. A detailed evaluation of the worker, job, and medical and psychosocial conditions must be performed. Understanding "at risk" patients and managing them carefully can decrease disability and improve results following treatment.

Carpal Tunnel Syndrome

Cobb TK, Amadio PC, Leatherwood DF, Schleck CD, Ilstrup DM: Outcome of reoperation for carpal tunnel syndrome. *J Hand Surg* 1996;21A:347–356.

Most patients improve after reoperation; persistent symptoms are likely, and failure is more frequent than after primary carpal tunnel surgery. Risk factors for failure include the presence of an active workers' compensation claim, pain in the ulnar nerve distribution, and a normal EMG.

Strickland JW, Idler RS, Lourie GM, Plancher KD: The hypothenar fat pad flap for management of recalcitrant carpal tunnel syndrome. *J Hand Surg* 1996;21A:840–848.

The hypothenar fat pad flap interposes adipose tissue from the hypothenar eminence between the median nerve and overlying tissue. It is a reliable local source of well-vascularized adipose tissue used for coverage of the median nerve during re-exploration of carpal tunnel syndrome.

Pronator Syndrome

Olehnik WK, Manske PR, Szerzinski J: Median nerve compression in the proximal forearm. *J Hand Surg* 1994;19A:121–126.

Fifty-three percent of the patients had prior ipsilateral carpal tunnel releases. The most common physical finding was a positive pronator compression test, followed by median nerve hypesthesia. Thirty percent had abnormal nerve conduction tests.

Radial Tunnel Syndrome

Jebson PJ, Engber WD: Radial tunnel syndrome: Long-term results of surgical decompression. *J Hand Surg* 1997;22A: 889–896.

Outcome for 67% was rated as good/excellent. The majority of patients were satisfied and felt helped. Complete pain relief and return to activities following radial tunnel surgery is not as predictable as previous studies have indicated.

Scapholunate Instability

Wyrick JD, Stern PJ, Kiefhaber TR: Motion-preserving procedures in the treatment of scapholunate advanced collapse wrist: Proximal row carpectomy versus four-corner arthrodesis. *J Hand Surg* 1995;20A:965–970.

Results of proximal row carpectomy were compared to those of scaphoid excision and 4-bone fusion. Overall, patients undergoing proximal row carpectomy preserved a greater ROM, were able to achieve greater grip strength, and had reduced rates of revision surgery. After follow-up of 27 months for the arthrodesis and 37 months for proximal row carpectomy, the authors concluded that proximal row carpectomy may have significant advantages in terms of patient outcome with less complications than 4-bone fusion.

Degenerative Arthrosis of the Small Joints

Leibovic SJ, Strickland JW: Arthrodesis of the proximal interphalangeal joint of the finger: Comparison of the use of the Herbert screw with other fixation methods. *J Hand Surg* 1994;19A: 181–188.

A review of 224 PIP joint arthrodeses demonstrated that the primary nonunion rate was highest using K-wires, intermediate using tension band wires, and lowest using Herbert screws.

Lin HH, Wyrick JD, Stem PJ: Proximal interphalangeal joint silicone replacement arthroplasty: Clinical results using an anterior approach. *J Hand Surg* 1995;20A:123–132.

Sixty-nine PIP joint silicone arthroplasties were reviewed. The total active motion did not significantly increase, but pain relief was obtained in 67 of 69 digits. Five implants fractured. The anterior approach allows preservation of the central slip insertion.

Rheumatoid Wrist

Bass RL, Stern PJ, Nairus JG: High implant fracture incidence with Sutter silicone metacarpophalangeal joint arthroplasty. *J Hand Surg* 1996;21A:813–818.

This retrospective view of a new MCP joint arthroplasty for RA evaluated 168 implants. The authors show a significantly higher implant fracture incidence at a relatively shorter follow-up period.

Beer TA, Turner RH: Wrist arthrodesis for failed wrist implant arthroplasty. *J Hand Surg* 1997;22A:685–693.

These authors review 13 wrist arthrodeses for failed wrist implant arthroplasty. Based on their results, they recommend using more rigid fixation techniques in patients with failed wrist arthroplasty.

Della Santa D, Chamay A: Radiological evolution of the rheumatoid wrist after radiolunate arthrodesis. *J Hand Surg* 1995;20B:146–154.

These authors show that although radiolunate arthrodesis prevents dislocation of the unstable wrist, it does not prevent collapse, ulnar translation, intercarpal instability, or tilt of the lunate.

Rothwell AG, O'Neill L, Cragg K: Sauve Kapandji procedure for disorders of the distal radioulnar joint: A simplified technique. *J Hand Surg* 1996;21A: 771–777.

These authors describe a simplified technique for the Sauvé-Kapandji procedure. They report excellent results with a shortened operating time.

Van Gemert AM, Spauwen PH: Radiological evaluation of the long-term effects of resection of the distal ulna in rheumatoid arthritis. *J Hand Surg* 1994;19B:330–333.

A retrospective review was made to see if resection of the distal ulna causes long-term functional limitations. The authors feel that long-term changes in the wrist secondary to distal ulna resection, including ulnar translation, are the consequence of the RA itself and not ulna resection.

Plain Radiographs

Schuind F, Alemzadeh S, Stallenberg B, Burny F: Does the normal contralateral wrist provide the best reference for x-ray film measurements of the pathologic wrist? *J Hand Surg* 1996;21A: 24–30.

Poor correlation was seen between affected and unaffected wrists for values other than carpal height and angles.

Diagnostic Value of Wrist Arthrography

Cantor RM, Stern PJ, Wyrick JD, Michaels SE: The relevance of ligament tears or perforations in the diagnosis of wrist pain: An arthrographic study. *J Hand Surg* 1994;19A:945–953.

In patients with radial TFCC tears, 88% were symmetrically bilateral. In patients with TL tears, 59% were bilateral, and 57% of scapholunate tears were bilateral. Care must be taken to correlate clinical findings with arthrographic defects.

Weiss AP, Akelman E, Lambiase R: Comparison of the findings of triple-injection cinearthrography of the wrist with those of arthroscopy. *J Bone Joint Surg* 1996;78A:348–356.

Triple injection arthrography was only 56% sensitive and 83% specific in detecting scapholunate (SL), LT, and TFCC injuries. Sensitivity was best for LT at 93% but was only 60% for SL and TFCC injuries.

MRI

Pretorius ES, Epstein RE, Dalinka MK: MR Imaging of the wrist. *Radiol Clin North Am* 1997;35:145–161.

Sensitivity of MRI for scapholunate injuries is reported at 50% to 93% with a specificity of 86% to 100%. For the LT ligament sensitivities are reported as 40% to 56% with specificities of 45% to 100%. TFCC tears are better visualized with sensitivities of 72% to 100% and specificities of 89% to 100%.

Computed Tomography

Pruitt DL, Gilula LA, Manske PR, Vannier MW: Computed tomography scanning with image reconstruction in evaluation of distal radius fractures. *J Hand Surg* 1994;19A:720–727.

CT scan showed increased displacement > 2 mm when compared to plain films in 13 of 18 cases involving the lunate facet and showed greater comminution in 17 of 18 cases.

Ultrasound

Read JW, Conolly WB, Lanzetta M, Spielman S, Snodgrass D, Korber JS: Diagnostic ultrasound of the hand and wrist. *J Hand Surg* 1996;21A:1004–1010.

A sensitivity of 96% and a specificity of 100% was found in using ultrasound for diagnosis of wrist ganglia. In diagnosing tendon ruptures, sensitivity was 88% and specificity was 100%. For foreign bodies, sensitivity was 75% and specificity was 100%.

Wrist Arthroscopy

Arthroscopic Anatomy

Abrams RA, Petersen M, Botte MJ: Arthroscopic portals of the wrist: An anatomic study. *J Hand Surg* 1994;19A:940–944.

The 1-2, 6R and 6U portals are in close proximity to the radial artery, dorsal radial and dorsal ulnar nerves, respectively. These are the portals at highest risk for soft-tissue injury.

Arthroscopy for Interosseous Ligament and TFCC Injuries

Ruch DS, Poehling GG: Arthroscopic management of partial scapholunate and lunotriquetral injuries of the wrist. *J Hand Surg* 1996;21A:412–417.

In patients with chronic pain (> 6 months) and partial ligament injuries, excellent results were reported in 13 of 14 patients with debridement alone.

Weiss AP, Sachar K, Glowacki KA: Arthroscopic debridement alone for intercarpal ligament tears. *J Hand Surg* 1997;22A: 344–349.

At an average follow-up of 27 months, the authors showed pain relief in 66% of complete scapholunate ligament (SL) tears and 85% of partial SL tears.

Arthroscopy for Radius Fractures

Geissler WB, Freeland AE, Savoie FH, McIntyre LW, Whipple TL: Intracarpal soft-tissue lesions associated with an intraarticular fracture of the distal end of the radius. *J Bone Joint Surg* 1996; 78A:357–365.

Sixty-eight percent of patients had intracarpal injuries; 43% had TFCC tears, 31% had scapholunate ligament injuries, and 15% had lunotriquetral ligament injuries.

Arthroscopy for Chronic Wrist Pain

Vanden Eynde S, De Smet L, Fabry G: Diagnostic value of arthrography and arthroscopy of the radiocarpal joint. *Arthroscopy* 1994;10:50–53.

Arthroscopy found lesions in 89% of patients with chronic wrist pain, including 34% with chondral lesions. An arthroscopic diagnosis was made in 92% of cases with negative arthrography.

Tetraplegia

Keith MW, Kilgore KL, Peckham PH, Wuolle KS, Creasey G, Lemay M: Tendon transfers and functional electrical stimulation for restoration of hand function in spinal cord injury. *J Hand Surg* 1996;21A:89–99.

This is a summary of methods, procedures, and device designs that permit C-5 and C-6 spinal injured patients to achieve greater pinch and grasp strength than possible with tendon transfer surgery alone at these levels.

Waters RL, Sie IH, Gellman H, Tognella M: Functional hand surgery following tetraplegia: *Arch Phys Med Rehabil* 1996;77: 86–94.

This thorough review of the surgical literature outlines the multiple diverse approaches needed to address the neurologic variability, issues of timing, cost reduction, and surgical efficiency.

Brachial Plexus Injuries

Carvalho GA, Nikkhah G, Matthies C, Penkert G, Samii M: Diagnosis of root avulsions in traumatic brachial plexus injuries: Value of computerized tomography myelography and magnetic resonance imaging. *J Neurosurg* 1997;86:69–76.

CT myelography is more accurate than MRI in diagnosing root avulsions.

Emmelot CH, Nielsen HK, Eisma WH: Shoulder fusion for paralyzed upper limb. *Clin Orthop* 1997;340:95–101.

Shoulder arthrodesis is superior to flail shoulder in compared cases.

Vascular Disorders

Koman LA, Smith BP, Pollock FE Jr, Smith TL, Pollock D, Russell GB: The microcirculatory effects of peripheral sympathectomy. *J Hand Surg* 1995;20:709–717.

Patients undergoing digital sympathectomy experienced improved nutrition and pain relief, although total blood flow as indicated by temperature was not increased.

Hand Tumors

Athanasian EA, Wold LE, Amadio PC: Giant cell tumors of the bones of the hand. *J Hand Surg* 1997;22A:91–98.

Giant cell tumors of the hand are rare; 79% recur after intralesional excision, and only 36% recur after wide resection or amputation.

Upton J, Kocher MS, Wolfort FG: Reconstruction following resection of malignancies of the upper extremity. *Surg Oncol Clin N Am* 1996;5:847–892.

Resection is a separate task from reconstruction.

Warso M, Gray T, Gonzalez M: Melanoma of the hand. *J Hand Surg* 1997;22A:354–360.

Melanomas of the hand are relatively rare, but serious misleading lesions.

Classic Bibliography

Condit DP, Idler RS, Fischer TJ, Hastings HH: Preoperative factors and outcome after lunate decompression for Kienbock's disease. *J Hand Surg* 1993;18A:691–696.

Fernandez DL: Anterior bone grafting and conventional lag screw fixation to treat scaphoid nonunions. *J Hand Surg* 1990; 15A:140–147.

Fuss FK, Wurzl GH: Radial nerve entrapment at the elbow: Surgical anatomy. *J Hand Surg* 1991;16A:742–747.

Gabel GT, Amadio PC: Reoperation for failed decompression of the ulnar nerve in the region of the elbow. *J Bone Joint Surg* 1990;72A:213–219.

Gelberman RH, Eaton R, Urbaniak JR: Peripheral nerve compression. *J Bone Joint Surg* 1993;75A:1854–1878.

Kasdan ML, Stallings SP, Leis VM, Wolens D: Outcome of surgically treated mucous cysts of the hand. *J Hand Surg* 1994;19A:504–507.

Kleinman WB, Carroll C IV: Scapho-trapezio-trapezoid arthrodesis for treatment of chronic static and dynamic scapholunate instability: A 10-year perspective on pitfalls and complications. *J Hand Surg* 1990;15A:408–414.

Lee GW, Weeks PM: The role of bone scintigraphy in diagnosing reflex sympathetic dystrophy. *J Hand Surg* 1995;20A:458–463.

Mack GR, Bosse MJ, Gelberman RH, Yu E: The natural history of scaphoid non-union. *J Bone Joint Surg* 1984;66A:504–509.

O'Malley MJ, Evanoff M, Terrono AL, Millender LH: Factors that determine reexploration treatment of carpal tunnel syndrome. *J Hand Surg* 1992;17A:638–641.

Ritts GD, Wood MB, Linscheid RL: Radial tunnel syndrome: A ten-year surgical experience. *Clin Orthop* 1987;219:201–205.

Ruby LK, Stinson J, Belsky MR: The natural history of scaphoid non-union: A review of fifty-five cases. *J Bone Joint Surg* 1985;67A:428–432.

Tiel-van Buul MM, van Beek EJ, Borm JJ, Gubler FM, Broekhuizen AH, van Royen EA: The value of radiographs and bone scintigraphy in suspected scaphoid fracture: A statistical analysis. *J Hand Surg* 1993;18B:403–406.

Weiss AP, Weiland AJ, Moore JR, Wilgis EF: Radial shortening for Kienbock disease. *J Bone Joint Surg* 1991;73A:384–391.

Wilgis EF: Evaluation and treatment of chronic digital ischemia. *Ann Surg* 1981;193:693–698.

Zaidemberg C, Siebert JW, Angrigiani C: A new vascularized bone graft for scaphoid nonunion. *J Hand Surg* 1991;16A:474–478.

Ritts GD, Wood MB, Linscheid RL: Radial tunnel syndrome: A ten-year surgical experience. *Clin Orthop* 1987;219:201–205.

Ruby LK, Stinson J, Belsky MR: The natural history of scaphoid non-union: A review of fifty-five cases. *J Bone Joint Surg* 1985;67A:428–432.

Tiel-van Buul MM, van Beek EJ, Borm JJ, Gubler FM, Broekhuizen AH, van Royen EA: The value of radiographs and bone scintigraphy in suspected scaphoid fracture: A statistical analysis. *J Hand Surg* 1993;18B:403–406.

Weiss AP, Weiland AJ, Moore JR, Wilgis EF: Radial shortening for Kienbock disease. *J Bone Joint Surg* 1991;73A:384–391.

Wilgis EF: Evaluation and treatment of chronic digital ischemia. *Ann Surg* 1981;193:693–698.

Zaidemberg C, Siebert JW, Angrigiani C: A new vascularized bone graft for scaphoid nonunion. *J Hand Surg* 1991;16A:474–478.

Section 4
Lower Extremity

Chapter 35
Hip, Pelvis, and Femur: Pediatric Aspects

Congenital Disorders

Developmental Dysplasia of the Hip

Developmental dysplasia of the hip (DDH) encompasses a group of related disorders: neonatal hip instability, subluxation, dislocation, and acetabular dysplasia. These disorders typically occur after birth, hence the term developmental rather than congenital. All can be bilateral, but are more frequently on the left side when unilateral. Causes can be both genetic and environmental. Risk factors include positive family history (generalized ligamentous laxity), gender (female), intrauterine position (breech), and increased birth weight. Teratologic dislocations occur prior to birth, are therefore congenital, and are not considered with DDH.

Diagnosis Clinical examination of the newborn is the best method for detection of DDH. Neonatal hip screening has proven very successful. This is best performed at birth and again between 2 and 3 months of age. Three clinical tests (Barlow's test, Ortolani test, and hip abduction) are the most useful. Hip "clicks," a common finding, are rarely due to DDH.

Radiographs are usually not beneficial in an infant younger than 3 months of age, although sometimes they can be clearly abnormal in the neonate or in the infant with a teratologic hip dislocation. Ultrasound is sensitive and currently very popular. It requires an experienced ultrasonographer and is more costly than radiography. Ultrasound may be helpful in screening high-risk infants older than 6 weeks of age (positive family history, breech), in infants who have an inconclu-

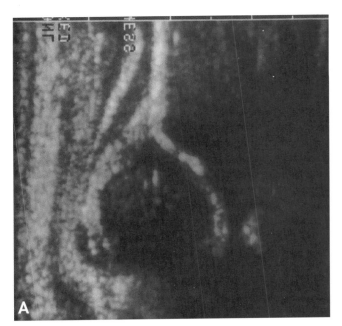
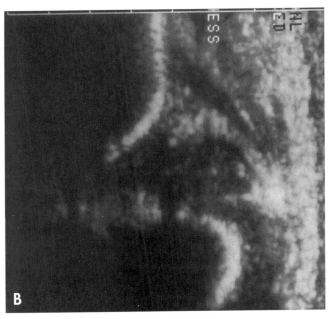

Figure 1
Ultrasound evaluation of developmental dysplasia of the hip. A, Coronal view demonstrates reduction of right femoral head in acetabulum. B, Femoral head dislocated in the left hip.

sive clinical examination, and to confirm hip reduction and monitor treatment in a Pavlik harness (Fig. 1). Anteroposterior (AP) radiographs are used to assess the hips in infants 4 months of age and older and to follow the results of treatment.

Treatment The goal in neonatal DDH is to obtain gentle, atraumatic concentric reduction, confirm it, and maintain it by flexion and abduction positioning until capsular laxity resolves and the hip is stable. Treatment in older infants and young children depends on age at diagnosis: most infants 4 months of age or younger can be satisfactorily treated with a Pavlik harness; children 4 to 18 months of age, by closed or open reduction; and those over 18 to 24 months, with open reduction and pelvic and/or femoral osteotomy. It has recently been shown that males may not respond as well as females to standard treatment regimens and, therefore, represent a high-risk group. All patients must be followed until near the end of growth. Any residual acetabular dysplasia or subluxation should be corrected to ensure maximal function and to minimize the risk of degenerative osteoarthritis as an adult.

Pavlik Harness The most common method for achieving reduction in infants is the Pavlik harness, which allows successful spontaneous reduction of dislocated hips within 2 to 4 weeks in up to 90% of cases. Subluxatable hips and hips with a positive Ortolani test are most likely to respond favorably. Failures are more frequent in bilateral dislocations, Ortolani negative dislocations, and infants older than 2 to 3 months of age.

The Pavlik harness must be properly applied. The chest strap should cross the nipples, and the anterior foot straps should maintain 100° to 110° of flexion; conversely, too much flexion can cause reversible femoral neuropathy. The posterior straps should achieve full passive abduction, but not be too tight because this can cause osteonecrosis (ON). Pavlik treatment is most successful in infants younger than 7 weeks of age, but may effect reduction up to 6 months of age.

If Pavlik harness treatment does not effect a concentric reduction after 4 to 6 weeks of proper use, or if the child is over 6 months of age, closed or open reduction should be considered. It is unwise to persist with the harness because it can cause posterior acetabular deformation or "Pavlik harness disease" that makes future treatment more difficult.

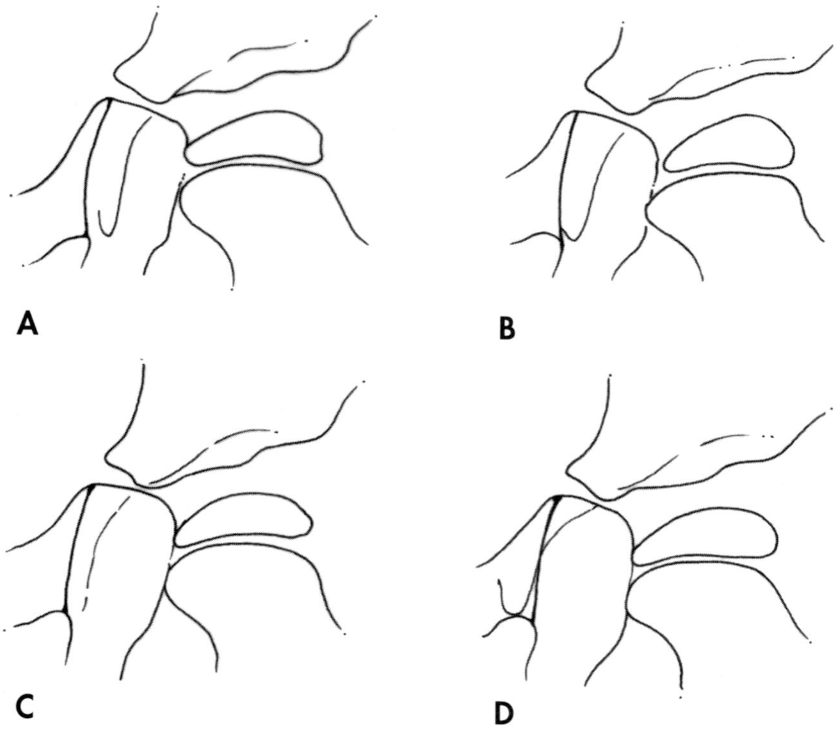

Closed Reduction Closed reduction is done with the child under general anesthesia. The hip must be stable with an acceptable "safe zone," with flexion of 100° to 110° and abduction in flexion of 45° to 60°. If the adductor muscle is tight, adductor tenotomy can be performed. Forced abduction and internal rotation must be avoided because this will increase intracapsular pressure and the risk of ON. The value of preliminary traction, either at home or in the hospital, with respect to success of closed reduction and the incidence of ON is controversial. Intraoperative hip arthrography is helpful to evaluate reduction and stability. Postreduction computed tomography (CT) scan can confirm the reduction and position of the femoral head. Hip-abduction angles > 55° are associated with a 20% prevalence of ON. The spica cast may be changed every 6 to 8 weeks under anesthesia until the joint is stable (usually 12 to 16 weeks). The appearance of a normal radiographic teardrop figure (Fig. 2) within 6 months of reduction is strongly associated

Figure 2

Schematic diagram of the radiographic types of acetabular teardrops: open (A), closed (B), crossed (C), and reversed (D). (Reproduced with permission from Albiñana J, Morcuende JA, Weinstein SL: The teardrop in congenital dislocation of the hip diagnosed late: A quantitative study. *J Bone Joint Surg* 1996;78A:1048–1055.)

with a favorable long-term outcome. A V-shape, rather than a U-shape teardrop, 2 years following treatment is predictive of residual acetabular dysplasia. Also, the center-head distance discrepancy at 1 year following treatment has been shown to be a good predictor of outcome.

Open Reduction and Osteotomies The upper age limit for closed reduction is approximately 18 months. Open reduction can be performed through an anterolateral, medial, or anteromedial approach. The choice of approach varies with surgical training and experience. The anterolateral approach avoids the medial circumflex vessels, and allows a capsulorrhaphy and other procedures, such as acetabuloplasty or pelvic osteotomy, to be performed concomitantly.

Pelvic (Pemberton, Salter) osteotomy or femoral shortening derotation osteotomy, with or without varus, are generally

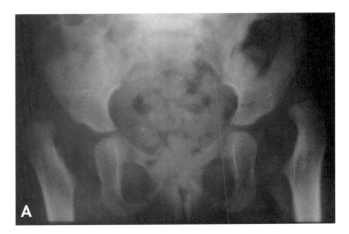

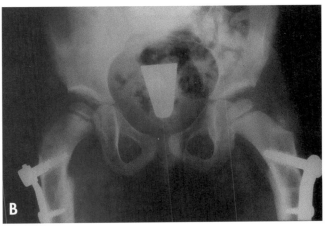

Figure 3

A, Untreated bilateral developmental dysplasia of the hip in a 3-year-old child. B, After bilateral anterolateral open reduction and primary femoral shortening.

indicated at the time of open reduction in children 18 to 36 months of age or older to stabilize the reduction and to correct acetabular dysplasia, excessive femoral anteversion, or both (Fig. 3). If the reduction is unstable, a pelvic osteotomy will improve stability. If reduction requires excessive force (compression), especially after a pelvic osteotomy, then femoral shortening is appropriate. Limited varus and derotation can be performed if necessary. The negative effects of a varus osteotomy usually resolve within 5 years. Children 3 years of age or older usually require both a pelvic and a femoral osteotomy.

Isolated pelvic or femoral osteotomies are useful for management of residual acetabular dysplasia. In general, a pelvic osteotomy (Pemberton, Salter, Steel) is the procedure of choice. Children with an enlarged acetabulum may benefit from an osteotomy that reduces the capacity of the acetabulum while rendering its superior roof more horizontal (Pemberton). Salter osteotomy requires a concentric open reduction. Femoral osteotomies are useful only in children younger than 4 years of age. Between ages 4 and 8 years, acetabular response to femoral osteotomy is variable. In children older than 8 years of age, there is no role for isolated femoral osteotomy as treatment for residual acetabular dysplasia.

The treatment of asymptomatic acetabular dysplasia and early degenerative changes in adolescents and young adults is controversial. Most surgeons avoid major redirectional reconstructive procedures based on radiographic changes alone in the absence of pain. Others, however, have recommended these procedures to postpone symptomatic degeneration. Reconstruction or salvage procedures are indicated for painful residual acetabular dysplasia. Three-dimensional CT can be very beneficial in preoperative planning. With adequate joint space, acetabular reorientation, sometimes combined with femoral osteotomy, can improve femoral head coverage and joint mechanics and relieve pain. If complex reorientation to a concentric hip is impossible, a Chiari osteotomy or acetabular shelf (Staheli) procedure can reduce pain and improve bone stock for later total joint arthroplasty.

ON may complicate any stage of treatment, including the Pavlik harness. It may be mild, transient (radiographic only), and of little importance, although late growth arrest is possible. More frequently, ON leads to femoral head collapse and deformity as well as failure of capital femoral epiphyseal growth. A combination of collapse and residual subluxation should be treated by continued abduction bracing or pelvic osteotomy, despite the fact that results are compromised by the presence of ON. However, early Salter osteotomy has been shown to enhance femoral head remodeling and produce better clinical and radiographic results. Leg-length inequality can be managed by contralateral femoral epiphysiodesis at the appropriate age. If a Trendelenberg gait is present at that time, distal and lateral transfer of the greater trochanter is recommended.

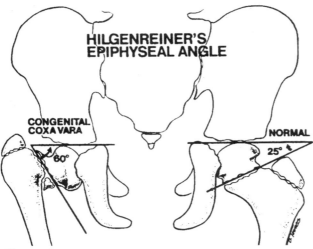

Figure 4

Determination of the Hilgenreiner-epiphyseal angle using Hilgenreiner's line as the horizontal axis and a line through the defect adjacent to the metaphysis axis. (Reproduced with permission from Weinstein JN, Kuo KN, Millar EA: Congenital coxa vara: A retrospective review. *J Pediatr Orthop* 1984;4:70–77.)

Congenital Coxa Vara

Congenital coxa vara is an anomaly of the proximal femur characterized by a decreased neck-shaft angle and an ossification defect in the femoral neck, usually associated with a triangular fragment of bone located at the inferior physeal-metaphyseal junction. It is usually a unilateral deformity, and the sex ratio is equal. Children typically present with a Trendelenberg or waddling gait (bilateral involvement) and increased lumbar lordosis. Pain is rarely present. Other findings may include leg-length discrepancy, limited hip abduction and internal rotation, and increased hip external rotation.

Radiographically, the neck-shaft angle is decreased and the Hilgenreiner-epiphyseal (HE) angle increased (Fig. 4). Valgus osteotomy is recommended for hips with an HE angle > 60°; hips with an angle of < 45° generally correct spontaneously. Hips with an HE angle between 60° and 45° should be observed. If the angles increase with growth, a subtrochanteric valgus osteotomy should be performed. The surgical goal is to obtain an HE angle of ≤ 35° and a neck-shaft angle of ≥ 135° (Fig. 5). This will minimize the risk for recurrent deformity. The proximal femoral retroversion that is always present should be corrected concomitantly. The most important aspect in treatment is removing the shear stress from the abnormal physeal area. Recurrence is more likely in children younger than 5 years of age and with inadequate correction. Concomitant greater trochanteric apophyseodesis may be considered for younger patients. Because the proxi-

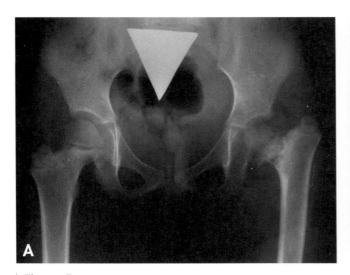
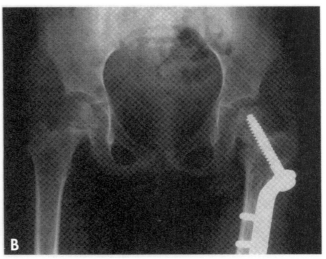

Figure 5

A, Congenital coxa vara in a 5-year-old child. B, After valgus subtrochanteric osteotomy with compression-screw fixation. (Reproduced with permission from Kasser JR (ed): *Orthopaedic Knowledge Update 5*. Rosemont, IL, American Academy of Orthopaedic Surgeons, 1996, pp 351–364.)

mal femoral physis frequently fuses after successful surgery, long-term follow-up and treatment for associated leg-length discrepancy are necessary.

Bladder and Cloacal Exstrophy
Epispadias, bladder exstrophy, and cloacal exstrophy are a spectrum producing the exstrophy complex. Epispadias refers to failure of tubularization of the urethra and may occur close to or with bladder exstrophy. Bladder exstrophy is a defect in the lower abdominal wall exposing an open protruding bladder. It occurs in one in 30,000 live births. Cloacal exstrophy is an even rarer, more severe abnormality that involves prolapse of the intestines between the halves of the exstrophied bladder. Pelvic deformities in the 2 latter disorders, as demonstrated by CT, include external rotation of the posterior aspect of the pelvis, acetabular retroversion, and external rotation and shortening of the pubic rami, as well as the pubic diastasis. The pubic diastasis often requires bilateral pelvic osteotomy to facilitate abdominal wall closure, to decrease postoperative wound dehiscence, and to assist in urinary reconstruction. These osteotomies previously were performed posteriorly, just lateral and parallel to the sacroiliac joint from the superior ilium into the sciatic notch. Newer techniques, however, include superior pubic ramomotomy, innominate osteotomy (the standard Salter, modified by an internal rotation maneuver, pin fixation, and without a wedge bone graft), and, most recently, an oblique osteotomy that is equidistant between the posterior and Salter osteotomies. These osteotomies are not necessary for normal hip function or gait in later childhood or adolescence. The external rotation gait in early childhood, caused by acetabular retroversion, improves as a result of the development of increased femoral anteversion.

All children should have spinal radiographs because of an increased incidence of spinal deformities. Those with cloacal exstrophy have a 100% incidence of spina bifida, often associated with a lipomeningocele, tethered spinal cord syndrome, and lower extremity paralysis. There is also an increased incidence of congenital spinal deformity, foot deformities (clubfoot), and congenital hip dysplasia. Children with bladder exstrophy have an increased incidence of scoliosis, but the risk for progression is low.

Congenital Femoral Anomalies
Congenital femoral anomalies include proximal femoral focal deficiency (PFFD) and congenital short femur.

Proximal Femoral Focal Deficiency PFFD is characterized by shortening of the femur and a defect in the proximal femur, which is either unossified cartilage or a true discontinuity.

Several different radiologic classifications exist; unfortunately, these are difficult to apply in infancy. The most widely used classification is that of Aitken (Fig. 6). In type A, there is a radiographic gap (cartilaginous) between the proximal femur and shaft, but it eventually ossifies by maturity. The femur is short with varus deformity between the neck and subtrochanteric region. In type B, the gap fails to unite, and the acetabulum and femoral head are hypoplastic. In type C, the femoral head is absent or hypoplastic, and the acetabulum is markedly dysplastic; the distal femur migrates progressively proximally. In type D, both the acetabulum and femoral head are absent, and the distal femur consists primarily of the metaphysis and epiphysis.

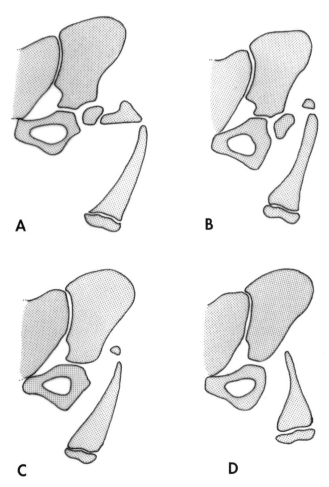

Figure 6

Aitken classification of proximal femoral focal deficiency. (Reproduced with permission from Kasser JR (ed): *Orthopaedic Knowledge Update 5*. Rosemont, IL, American Academy of Orthopaedic Surgeons, 1996, pp 351–364.)

The etiology of this condition is unknown. Because the lower leg and foot are often abnormal as well, it may be a multifocal teratogenic process. The only known teratogen is thalidomide. On physical examination, the affected proximal limb is flexed, abducted, and externally rotated. Approximately 15% of patients have bilateral involvement, and over 50% have anomalies distal to the femur, especially paraxial fibular hemimelia, absence of lateral rays of the foot, and tarsal coalition (talocalcaneal).

Radiographic features vary with age. Portions of the proximal cartilage anlage ossify late, especially in types A and B. The presence of an acetabulum usually indicates that a cartilaginous femoral head is present. Ultrasound in infants and magnetic resonance imaging (MRI) in older children may help delineate the pathoanatomy. Fixation of the femoral head in the acetabulum may be indicated by a supra-acetabular bump, increased diameter of the obturator foramen, and a horizontal roof of the acetabulum. MRI is also useful in defining the soft-tissue anatomy. The muscles are present, but may be abnormal. The sartorius is hypertrophied and may contribute to the flexed-abducted-externally rotated position of the proximal limb. The obturator externus is also enlarged and may function as a depressor of the femur. Several other muscles, especially the hip adductors and abductors, form a cuff to stabilize the proximal femur and probably contribute to the stability of the dysplastic proximal fragment.

Treatment must correct as many of the 4 functional defects in PFFD as possible: (1) leg-length inequality (if unilateral); (2) pelvic-femoral instability; (3) malrotation of the lower extremity, including hip flexion-abduction-external rotation and knee flexion contracture; and (4) proximal hip muscle weakness.

For most patients with unilateral PFFD, treatment is primarily prosthetic. Axis correction and joint stabilization procedures may be beneficial in selected patients. Only occasionally is lengthening an option. A proximal femoral valgus osteotomy may be beneficial to decrease coxa vara in type A and to achieve union in type B. This procedure is followed by knee fusion and a van Nes rotationplasty or a Syme or Boyd amputation, depending on the length of the limb, structure of the foot, and patient preference. The Syme or Boyd amputation allows fitting as an above-knee amputee, while the rotationplasty allows fitting as a below-knee amputee. Recent studies have shown that rotationplasty leads to a more normal quality of gait and decreased oxygen consumption during gait, with no measurable decrease in self-image.

Recently, it has been demonstrated that hip immobilization in infancy may result in healing of the femoral neck lesion in types A and B. If there is residual coxa vara and retroversion, this is corrected surgically. Preliminary results of this regimen

have shown some restoration of relatively normal growth of the proximal femur.

Types C and D PFFD may be treated with Syme or Boyd amputation and prosthesis. In selected patients, pelvic-femoral fusion is performed to gain hip stability to allow for rotationplasty, with the true knee functioning as the hip joint. Patients with bilateral PFFD usually are most functional without any prosthesis. When increased standing height is desirable, an extension prostheses may be constructed to wear fitted below the shoe, with the ankle at knee level.

Congenital Short Femur This sporadic disorder represents primary shortening of the femur with a relatively normal hip. It is frequently considered part of a spectrum with PFFD, but the treatment implications are different. Usually, the shortening is 5 to 10 cm at maturity. Physical findings include bowing of the femoral shaft in the direction of flexion-abduction-external rotation and distal femoral valgus caused by condylar hypoplasia. The latter may not be obvious because of the external rotation. CT has recently been shown to be helpful in evaluating the external rotation deformity. The femoral head and neck may be slightly small. The knee often has AP laxity, which is indicated on radiographs by flattening of the intercondylar notch. MRI is indicated prior to lengthening procedures for patients with both positive Lachman's and anterior drawer tests. The lower leg may also be short, because there is an increased incidence of fibular deficiency.

The femoral growth inhibition is proportionate throughout development. Many patients are best treated with limb lengthening for difference > 5 cm, depending on the status of the ipsilateral hip, knee, and foot. Proximal lengthening has less risk of knee stiffness, but some believe that the regenerate bone formed is not as abundant as in a normal femur. Concomitant correction of the distal femoral valgus, external rotation, and length may require a 2-level osteotomy. Knee subluxation during lengthening is a frequent complication, which is due to the cruciate laxity present in many of these patients.

Acquired Disorders

Transient Synovitis of the Hip

Transient synovitis is a common, self-limited disorder characterized by hip or knee pain, limp, unwillingness to walk, decreased hip motion, and normal radiographs. It usually affects children younger than 6 years of age, often following an upper respiratory infection. Although there have been

Table 1
Common bacterial organisms in septic hip

Age	Organism
Neonate	Group B Streptococcus
	Staphylococcus aureus
	Gram-negative bacteria
Children to age under 4	Group A Streptococcus
	Staphylococcus aureus
	Haemophilus influenza B
	(if child not HIB immunized)
Children over 4 years	*Staphylococcus aureus*
Adolescents	*Staphylococcus aureus*
	Gonococcus

attempts to link it to a viral etiology, it is generally considered to be noninfectious. It is important to differentiate transient synovitis from a septic hip, which can occasionally be difficult if the latter has been modified by previous antibiotic treatment. If there is any suspicion, aspiration must be performed.

Transient synovitis is a uniformly benign condition with no sequelae. Follow-up radiographs are unnecessary if the patient has no symptoms and a normal hip examination. Because early Legg-Calvé-Perthes disease (LCPD) may present with synovitis, there may be confusion between the 2 disorders, but subsequent examinations will establish the correct diagnosis. There is little evidence that transient synovitis itself causes or progresses into LCPD.

Septic Arthritis

Septic arthritis of the hip results either from hematogenous inoculation of the synovium or from extension of osteomyelitis of the intracapsular femoral neck into the joint space. It frequently follows an upper respiratory or distant infection. The presence of bacteria in the joint stimulates an aggressive white cell response, with enzyme release that can rapidly erode articular cartilage. Edema, thrombosis, and increased intra-articular pressure rapidly occlude the tenuous blood supply to the proximal femoral epiphysis, leading to ON with serious life-long growth and joint problems.

Septic hip is a true surgical emergency. A rapid workup with examination, radiographs, and hip aspiration should be followed by empiric antibiotic administration and prompt surgical drainage. The usually clear diagnosis can be altered by previous antibiotic use. Neonates may show no clinical or laboratory evidence of sepsis and can develop advanced disease before detection. Bone scans are nonspecific and usually delay, rather than establish, the diagnosis. Ultrasound will demonstrate effusion in confusing cases. The aspiration should be sent for culture, Gram stain, and cell count. Negative aspiration should be confirmed flouroscopically or by ultrasound. Initial antibiotics should cover appropriate likely organisms (Table 1). Antibiotics should be changed according to the culture, but negative cultures in 30% of cases may require long-term empiric treatment.

The anterior surgical approach is preferred, because there is less danger to the posterior vascular supply of the femoral head and the risk of postoperative subluxation is lower. However, a surgeon inexperienced in this approach may use a posterior approach, with careful dissection at the femoral head-acetabulum margin and postoperative spica cast or traction to minimize subluxation. An open capsulotomy should be created, and placement of a drain is optional depending on surgical findings. Some surgeons drill the femoral neck to drain potential osteomyelitis, but others feel this is probably unnecessary unless radiographs reveal metaphyseal lucency requiring debridement, especially in children older than 18 to 24 months. In neonates, contiguous osteomyelitis is more common and has a poorer prognosis.

Asymptomatic mild coxa magna may occur in successfully treated septic hips. Early sequelae of subluxation and dislocation can be controlled by casting. Re-debridement may be required for persistent sepsis. Late ON, growth arrest, joint narrowing and erosion, and complete resorption of the proximal femur may require late reconstructive procedures, although clinical results in joints destroyed by infection are frequently best when surgery is avoided.

Legg-Calvé-Perthes Disease

LCPD is a poorly understood disorder of the hip. It typically affects boys 4 to 8 years of age most frequently, but may be seen as early as 18 months (usually asymptomatic) or as late as 12 years. It is thought to be an ON of the femoral epiphysis, but there is some evidence that several sequential episodes of interference to blood supply occur. The etiology is unknown, although recent studies have theorized a link with transient or permanent hypercoagulation states of various types, particularly protein-C and protein-S deficiency. LCPD patients tend to be of small stature, with delayed bone age, and may be hyperactive.

Radiography LCPD affects varying amounts of the femoral head; greater degrees of epiphyseal involvement in older children have a worse prognosis. The Catterall classification of extent remains useful; some surgeons prefer the lateral pillar

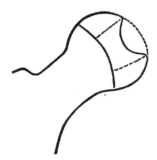

Figure 7

Lateral pillar classification derived from lines of demarcation between central sequestrum and remainder of epiphysis on AP radiograph. (Reproduced with permission from Herring JA, Neustadt JB, Williams JJ, et al: The lateral pillar classification of Legg-Calvé-Perthes disease. J Pediatr Orthop 1992;12:143–150.)

classification (Fig. 7), which links extent of necrosis with lateral collapse of the femoral head. The natural history of LCPD is one of progressive collapse of the necrotic fragment; reossification begins during the first year after onset and continues for several years with the possibility of late remodeling. Deformity of the femoral head during this time can be caused by mechanical collapse, hyperemic overgrowth of peripheral epiphysis, heterotopic ossification of overgrown cartilage, and subluxation of the head. Prognosis is worse in older children (bone age > 6 years) and those with extensive lesions, although poor results can be seen in treated young children and good results in untreated older children. Serial radiographs are usually sufficient to diagnose and follow up cases of LCPD; bone scans and MRI add little to the clinical management.

Treatment All treatment methods are controversial, and each has advocates. The natural history is relatively benign in 60%

to 70%. Crutches do not change collapse and are useful only for symptom control. Maintaining motion is the mainstay of all treatment, and the use of traction or abduction casts should be considered if progressive abduction loss is documented early, particularly with hip subluxation. Abduction bracing often is difficult if the hip is contracted, and compliance may be a problem. In children older than 8 to 9 years, some surgeons recommend femoral varus osteotomy, acetabular osteotomy (Salter), or acetabular shelf augmentation, which may have an effect on mild subluxation or on the late remodeling environment, and thus alter the natural history.

After reossification, there is still potential for remodeling, especially in young children. The role of osteotomy or acetabular shelf augmentation in this circumstance is highly controversial, but some surgeons believe that such procedures sufficiently alter the mechanical environment that late remodeling (and ultimate outcome) can be improved. In addition, hinging of an extruded but remodeled femoral head may limit abduction and cause pain; treatment with valgus osteotomy may improve function and symptoms.

Slipped Capital Femoral Epiphysis

Slipped capital femoral epiphysis (SCFE) is the most common disorder of the hip in early adolescence. It is most often seen in overweight children, and more often in boys. It is thought to be caused by a combination of excessive mechanical shear, retroversion (seen in obesity), and biologic susceptibility of the adolescent physis. It is also seen in endocrinopathies (hypothyroidism, exogenous growth hor-

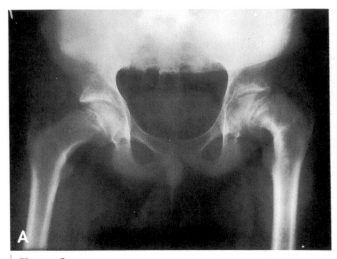
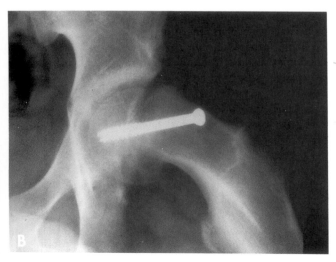

Figure 8

A, Bilateral slipped capital femoral epiphysis in a 13-year-old boy: grade 1, chronic, stable slip on right; grade 2, chronic, stable slip on left. B, Left hip after single cannulated screw fixation of slip.

mone treatment), and thyroid studies have been advocated by some in children younger than 11 years with SCFE.

Approximately 35% of cases will be bilateral (Fig. 8); a third of these are detectable at presentation, but the remaining cases usually develop contralateral symptoms or displacement within 18 months. Frequent radiographic monitoring of the opposite hip is appropriate. More than 90% of SCFEs are chronic and stable with symptoms and limp of several months' duration; acute, unstable SCFEs with < 3 weeks of symptoms have sudden displacement of the femoral epiphysis and potential for the serious complication of ON. It is useful to classify acute slips as "stable" (where the child can bear weight) and "unstable" (where the child is unable to bear weight). Stable acute SCFE can safely be treated in a similar manner to chronic SCFE, but the unstable acute slip has a guarded prognosis due to the increased incidence of ON.

Standard treatment of the chronic, stable SCFE is surgical, by prompt fixation using percutaneous cannulated screw fixation inserted under fluoroscopic control. The incision is anterolateral in the thigh, and the device is directed posteromedially to enter the center of the femoral epiphysis perpendicular to the physis in the AP and lateral planes. By triangulation, the screw can be inserted very atraumatically; most surgeons use a single screw for stable SCFE and 1 or 2 screws for unstable SCFE. The screw should avoid the superior quadrant of the femoral epiphysis because of potential interference with the intraosseous blood supply. Central placement makes it easier to avoid persistent penetration into the joint (the primary iatrogenic cause of chondrolysis), but the surgeon should determine range of motion of the hip under live fluoroscopy after insertion to be certain that penetration has not occurred. There is still controversy about management of acute, unstable slips. Many surgeons advocate fixing the epiphysis in situ without additional reduction; however, reduction may occur with anesthesia and positioning. Others advocate careful partial reduction by internal rotation before fixation. In addition, traction or early fixation has been used in some centers, while others have postponed fixation of acute, unstable slips until the synovitis resolves in an attempt to encourage biologic stability and decrease the risk of ON. Current research focuses on the effect of time to reduction, type of reduction, and technique of fixation on the incidence of ON.

Although chondrolysis is occasionally present at the time of diagnosis of SCFE, it is usually associated with persistent implant penetration that is avoidable by careful surgical technique. ON has no specific early treatment other than symptomatic use of analgesics and crutches; reossification takes approximately 2 years in this age group. After healing, some patients without pain may be treated with reorientation osteotomy if their range of motion is nonfunctional. Painful adolescent hips with extensive ON may require arthrodesis or total joint arthroplasty in young adulthood.

After moderate or severe slips, the anterior metaphyseal prominence may impact against the anterior acetabulum, causing aching with sitting and external rotation gait. If symptoms persist for 1 to 2 years, realignment osteotomy can correct the impingement and external rotation gait. Cuneiform osteotomy at the level of the deformity is anatomically direct but has higher rates of ON. Intertrochanteric osteotomy is safer and technically more familiar to most surgeons, but corrects the problem at a distance from the actual anatomic deformity. Basilar neck osteotomy splits these differences.

Traumatic Disorders

Pelvic Fractures

Children generally sustain pelvic ring trauma in high-energy motor vehicle accidents or as pedestrians struck by cars. Significant pelvic ring fractures are often associated with multiple injuries that may be life threatening but do not typically result in exsanguinating hemorrhage.

Pelvic fractures in children have been classified by Torode and Zieg (Fig. 9). A type I avulsion fracture usually occurs as a result of sudden forceful muscle pull in an adolescent athlete. Typically, a portion of the apophysis is pulled off the crest or 1 of the anterior iliac spines. If the apophysis is ossified, plain radiographs will reveal the injury. Unossified avulsion may be identified by ultrasound. Symptomatic treatment is generally associated with a full recovery.

Type II fracture results from a direct blow to the ilium that injures the apophysis or causes a linear fracture of the ilium. Symptomatic treatment is sufficient.

Type III simple ring fractures are anterior ramus fractures or symphysis disruptions without posterior disruption. Specifically, there may be sacroiliac injury but no posterior instability. These fractures may result from AP compression, lateral compression, or vertical shear. Reduction is usually unnecessary, and conservative treatment is sufficient. Hemipelvic rotation and symphysis disruption will often incompletely remodel but late symptoms are unusual.

Type IV fractures occur by mechanisms similar to those in type III injury. These injuries include bilateral pubic ramus fractures, anterior ramus or symphysis disruption with concomitant posterior disruption, and anterior ramus or symphysis disruption with fracture into the acetabulum. Type IV fractures are more serious, have a higher incidence of associated injury, and are more likely to have permanent sequelae. An attempt to realign the pelvis with external fixation or internal fixation of a displaced acetabular fracture may benefit the patient. Surgical treatment has not shown long-term benefit in children but should be considered in cases with expanding intrapelvic hematoma, uncontrolled bleeding from the pelvis, gross instability that precludes movement or handling of the patient, gross displacement that is disfiguring or unlikely to remodel or heal, or to stabilize open injuries, unstable fracture patterns, and intra-articular hip and triradiate fractures.

Complications of pelvic fracture can include pain, limp, malunion with pelvic obliquity, sacroiliac joint changes, hip degeneration, leg-length discrepancy, and pelvic outlet obstruction. Injury to the triradiate physeal cartilage is rare but may lead to arrested acetabular growth, which may require late acetabular reconstruction.

Hip Dislocation

Hip dislocation is uncommon but can occur in falls, motor vehicle accidents, sports, and recreation. Posterior dislocation is most frequently seen. Traumatic dislocation usually is seen between ages 7 and 10 years. The child's pliable cartilaginous acetabulum and relative ligamentous laxity enable hip dislocation even from trivial trauma. Associated vascular and nerve injuries and fracture of the ipsilateral femur should be identified prior to attempts at reduction.

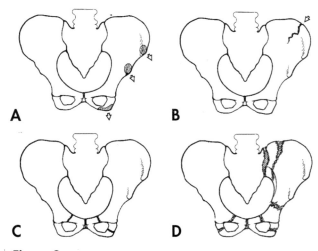

Figure 9

Torode and Zieg four-part classification system for children's pelvic fractures. A, Type I, Apophyseal avulsion from pelvis. B, Type II, fracture of iliac spine. C, Type III, simple ring fracture without instability of another segment of pelvis. D, Type IV, ring disruption in two places creating an unstable segment in between. (Reproduced with permission from Torode I, Zieg D: Pelvic fractures in children. *J Pediatr Orthop* 1985;5: 76–84.)

Reduction is effected by traction in line with the femur. If a concomitant femoral fracture precludes a traction maneuver, insertion of a Steinmann pin proximal to the fracture may help with reduction. Otherwise, open hip reduction or stabilization of the femoral fracture must be undertaken. If the hip is not reducible, soft-tissue interposition is usually the cause. Open reduction is indicated from the disrupted capsule side of the original dislocation.

Postreduction radiographs should confirm concentric reduction. If the joint space appears widened, a CT scan may show intra-articular loose bodies or soft-tissue interposition that requires surgical removal. Minimal widening may also be caused by hemarthrosis, generally resolving in a few days without treatment. Crutch ambulation, bed rest, traction, and spica casting have all been used until pain and irritability subside.

ON complicates about 10% of hip dislocations in children and usually is associated with a high-energy injury. Prompt reduction is encouraged but may not reduce the incidence of ON, which may present as late as 2 years after injury. Recurrent dislocations may occur, are usually posterior and in children younger than 7 years of age, and have been associated with children with associated connective tissue disorders. Postreduction immobilization has no effect on redislocation. A posterior capsular defect is the usual cause and may require capsulorrhaphy. If childhood hip dislocations are followed up to maturity, up to 36% will have clinical or radiographic signs of degenerative joint disease. This is most likely a result of joint surface trauma and is not preventable. The dislocated hip diagnosed late should have an attempt at reduction by skeletal traction or an open reduction, but the prognosis is guarded.

Hip Fractures

Hip fractures are relatively rare in children and usually occur as a result of high-energy trauma. Complications are frequent as a result of the precarious nature of the blood supply to the capital femoral epiphysis, and the proximity of the physis.

At birth, the entire proximal femur including head, neck, and greater trochanter are cartilaginous. The blood supply to the femoral head is from the medial and lateral circumflex arteries. By age 4 years the major blood supply to the capital femoral epiphysis is by the posterosuperior and posteroinferior retinacular vessels. These retinacular vessels are at risk in femoral neck fracture.

Traumatic epiphysiolysis can occur in the newborn as a result of a difficult delivery. The limb will appear motionless but sensation will be intact and passive motion of the limb will be painful. Because the femoral head is cartilaginous at this age, arthrography, ultrasound, or MRI will be required to confirm the diagnosis. Closed reduction and immobilization are sufficient treatment. Healing and vigorous remodeling are usual even for markedly displaced fractures or those recognized late.

For older children, the classification system described by Delbet is useful (Fig. 10). Type I fractures tend to occur in young children and may be associated with dislocation of the capital femoral epiphysis from the acetabulum. The risk of ON is high as a result of tearing of the retinacular vessels and is increased with dislocation or displacement. Treatment in the older child should consist of closed manipulation or open reduction, and fixation with smooth pins in the young child or cannulated screws that must cross the physis in order to achieve adequate fixation.

Type II (transcervical) fractures are the most common femoral neck fracture in children. ON may occur in up to 50% of these fractures and is more common after significant displacement. Varus displacement requires immediate reduction and internal fixation. Unstable fractures should be reduced and internally fixed. In small children, pins can stabilize the

fracture. In larger children, cannulated screws can be used.

Type III (cervicotrochanteric) fractures are not as common as type II. ON may complicate up to 25% of these fractures and is more likely after displacement. Treatment is the same as for type II.

Type IV (intertrochanteric) fractures have a small risk of ON and tend to heal readily. Stable fractures that are well aligned can be immobilized in a cast. For unstable or displaced fractures, open reduction and internal fixation can be undertaken or traction can be applied followed by spica casting when the fracture is sticky.

Stress fracture of the femoral neck can occur in children and adolescents. These fractures can result from abnormal or unaccustomed stress applied to normal bone or physiologic stress applied to deficient bone. Pain may not be severe enough to preclude usual activities. If plain films are not diagnostic, bone scanning or MRI may be necessary to make the diagnosis. A stress lesion may present as a sclerotic reactive lesion, undisplaced fracture, or displaced fracture of the femoral neck. Treatment for undisplaced fractures along the inferior femoral neck should be immediate preclusion from weightbearing until pain subsides and full motion returns. Superior femoral neck stress fractures are best treated by cannulated screw fixation. Undisplaced fractures that progress or fail to heal should be fixed. Displaced fractures should be reduced and internally fixed.

Complications of hip fractures in children can be difficult to manage. ON is the most feared complication because there is no reliable treatment. Prompt reduction and evacuation of intracapsular hematoma have been postulated but have not been proven to be effective in preventing ON. For established ON, containment of the hip and maintaining range of motion are short-term goals. Osteotomies to maintain coverage or relieve stress in involved portions of the femoral head may be helpful for some patients. Premature physeal closure may occur and is usually associated with ON. It is not clear if the incidence of physeal closure is increased by the use of pins or screws across the physis. Treatment for leg-length discrepancy should be according to the patient's needs.

Coxa vara can occur from late fracture displacement or as a result of growth derangement of the capital femoral physis. Varus that does not remodel or is unlikely to remodel should be corrected with a valgus femoral osteotomy.

Nonunion can occur and results from inability to obtain or maintain reduction of the femoral neck fracture. Fixation of the fracture with implants in the femoral head should take priority over the risk of physeal closure and leg-length discrepancy. Rigid compression fixation, bone graft, or valgus osteotomy to improve fracture mechanics should be used to treat established nonunions.

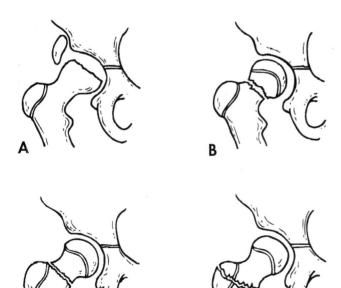

Figure 10

Delbet 4-part classification system for fracture of the head and neck of children's femurs. A, Type I, epiphyseal separation with or without femoral head dislocation. B, Type II, transcervical fracture. C, Type III, cervicotrochanteric fracture. D, Type IV, intertrochanteric fracture. (Reproduced with permission from Hughes LO, Beaty JH: Fractures of the head and neck of the femur in children. *J Bone Joint Surg* 1994;76A:283–292.)

Femoral Shaft Fractures

Fracture of the femur is common in children and adolescents; it occurs as a result of trivial to very high energy trauma. Gun shot wounds that involve the femoral shaft unfortunately are becoming more commonplace. In very young children, abuse or neglect is often implicated. The result of femoral shaft fracture in children and adolescents generally is benign, with solid healing occurring in the majority of cases. In children younger than age 10 years, limb overgrowth is common but not entirely predictable. Minimizing the cost of treatment and residual impairment has become important in considering treatment options.

Satisfactory results have been obtained after traction, traction followed by spica casting, traction followed by cast bracing, home traction, immediate spica casting, spica casting incorporating a traction pin, external fixation, flexible intramedullary nailing, locked intramedullary nailing, and plating. The choice of appropriate treatment depends on several factors including age, associated injury, associated medical conditions, open wounds, bone stock, and social issues.

Treatment is variable and is often best described according to age. In infants, immediate spica casting is the mainstay of treatment. The use of the Pavlik harness has been advocated in children younger than 3 to 6 months of age, but motion at the fracture site may result in pain until callus starts to form. For the very ill child, cloth bolsters and careful handling may be sufficient treatment. Residual deformity or leg-length discrepancy are unusual.

For children aged 6 months to 6 years, closed reduction followed by immediate spica casting with the patient under an anesthetic is the usual treatment of choice for low enery fractures. Reduction to within 20° of angulation in the coronal plane, 30° in the sagittal plane, and 20° of rotation will generally assure a good result. Shortening of 0.5 to 1.5 cm is accepted in anticipation of a similar amount of overgrowth. Fractures that can be telescoped > 3 cm are likely to shorten in the cast and should be treated in an alternative manner.

For children aged 6 to 10 years, traction followed by spica casting has fallen out of favor because of prolonged hospitalization and immobility. Immediate spica casting can be used for patients with a stable fracture and a negative telescope test but does not enable ambulation. Surgical treatment, such as external fixation or flexible intramedullary fixation, is gaining popularity. Problems with external fixation include pin tract irritation, scarring, and recent concerns about delayed union and refracture. Flexible pinning may not provide good control of rotation or maintain length in the comminuted fracture. Incorporating a traction pin in a spica cast may control shortening and enable a short hospital admission but will not enable ambulatory treatment. Cast bracing will allow ambulatory treatment but may not provide good control of fracture alignment.

For the child older than 10 to 12 years of age, casting becomes less practical because of prolonged immobility. Internal fixation with a locked intramedullary nail has been advocated for isolated femoral fracture in this age group, but recent reports of ON of the proximal femoral epiphysis and growth abnormalities of the proximal femur have tempered enthusiasm. The risk of these adverse effects can be decreased by using the tip of the greater trochanter as an entry portal until skeletal maturity. External fixation, flexible intramedullary nails inserted from distal to proximal, and compression plating remain viable options in this age group.

While uncomplicated femoral shaft fractures in children should not be treated overaggressively, there are indications for surgical fixation at any age. Fractures that shorten excessively in a cast can be relengthened by skeletal traction or conversion to external fixation. Patients with fractures complicated by open wounds, burns, polytrauma, ipsilateral fractures, or head injury may benefit from surgical femoral stabilization if the care of these associated lesions would be compromised by the presence of a cast or traction.

Complications of femoral shaft fracture include malunion, leg-length discrepancy, and refracture. These can be treated by routine methods. Nonunion and joint stiffness are not usual after femoral fracture in children.

Annotated Bibliography

Developmental Dysplasia of the Hip

Albiñana J, Morcuende JA, Weinstein SL: The teardrop in congenital dislocation of the hip diagnosed late: A quantitative study. *J Bone Joint Surg* 1996;78A:1048–1055.

The V-shaped medial teardrop following treatment of DDH is due to widening of its superior width and thickening of the acetabular floor and is predictive of residual acetabular dysplasia.

Bar-On E, Huo MH, DeLuca PA: Early innominate osteotomy as a treatment for avascular necrosis complicating developmental hip dysplasia. *J Pediatr Orthop* 1997;6B:138–145.

The authors studied 25 children with ON complicating DDH; 7 had an innominate osteotomy 1 to 3 years following ischemia, 8 at 5 to 10 years after ischemia, and 10 had no osteotomy. All were followed up for more than 10 years. The early osteotomy group had the best clinical and radiographic results.

Borges JL, Kumar SJ, Guille JT: Congenital dislocation of the hip in boys. *J Bone Joint Surg* 1995;77A:975–984.

The authors studied 55 boys with 78 dislocated hips and found that they did not respond well to standard treatment regimens and, therefore, constituted a high-risk group.

Camp J, Herring JA, Dworezynski C: Comparison of inpatient and outpatient traction in developmental dislocation of the hip. *J Pediatr Orthop* 1994;14:9–12.

There was no difference in the incidence of ON in 72 children (83 hips) treated with home or in-hospital traction without attention to the radiographic hip station.

Chen I-H, Kuo KN, Lubicky JP: Prognosticating factors in acetabular development following reduction of developmental dysplasia of the hip. *J Pediatr Orthop* 1994;14:3–8.

The best predictor of success in unilateral DDH was the center-head distance discrepancy (CHDD) at 1-year follow-up. A CHDD ≤ 6% had a 96% satisfactory result; those hips with a CHDD > 6% had 75% unsatisfactory results using the Severin classification.

Davids JR, Benson LJ, Mubarak SJ, McNeil N: Ultrasonography and developmental dysplasia of the hip: A cost-benefit analysis of 3 delivery systems. *J Pediatr Orthop* 1995;15:325–329.

Office based ultrasound in the orthopaedic office is convenient, accurate, and cost-effective.

Harding MG, Harcke HT, Bowen JR, Guille JT, Glutting J: Management of dislocated hips with Pavlik harness treatment and ultrasound monitoring. *J Pediatr Orthop* 1997;17:189–198.

The authors demonstrate the efficacy of ultrasound monitoring in the management of infants with DDH being treated with a Pavlik harness.

Kim HT, Wenger DR: The morphology of residual acetabular deficiency in childhood hip dysplasia: Three-dimensional computed tomographic analysis. *J Pediatr Orthop* 1997;17: 637–647.

The authors classified acetabular and femoral head deformity into 4 groups based on 3-dimensional CT. They also produced a contact map that replicates the contact area between the acetabulum and femoral head. These data allow more accurate preoperative planning.

Malvitz TA, Weinstein SL: Closed reduction for congenital dysplasia of the hip: Functional and radiographic results after an average of thirty years. *J Bone Joint Surg* 1994;76A: 1777–1792.

The authors studied the clinical and radiographic results in 119 patients with 152 DDH followed up for a mean of 30 years after treatment. Any residual subluxation was associated with poorer function and increased degenerative changes.

Morcuende JA, Meyer MD, Dolan LA, Weinstein SL: Long-term outcome after open reduction through an anteromedial approach for congenital dislocation of the hip. *J Bone Joint Surg* 1997;79A:810–817.

The authors studied 93 developmentally dislocated hips treated by open reduction through an anteromedial approach. They found 66 hips (71%) had an excellent or good result according to the Severin classification; 22 hips had ON.

Porat S, Robin GC, Howard CB: Cure of the limp in children with congenital dislocation of the hip and ischaemic necrosis: Fifteen cases treated by trochanteric transfer and contralateral epiphysiodesis. *J Bone Joint Surg* 1994;76B:463–467.

Trendelenberg gait and leg-length discrepancy were corrected by greater trochanteric advancement and contralateral epiphysiodesis in 15 patients who had ON following DDH.

Sangavi SM, Szöke G, Murray DW, Benson MK: Femoral remodelling after subtrochanteric osteotomy for developmental dysplasia of the hip. *J Bone Joint Surg* 1996;78B:917–923.

The proximal femur neck-shaft angle returned to normal in approximately 5 years postoperatively in 40 children.

Schoenecker PL, Anderson DJ, Capelli AM: The acetabular response to proximal femoral varus rotational osteotomy: Results after failure of post-reduction abduction splinting in patients who had congenital dislocation of the hip. *J Bone Joint Surg* 1995; 77A:990–997.

There was a mean improvement of 16° in the acetabular index in 25 patients (33 hips) who failed closed or open reduction and then were treated with an abduction splint. At 7 years following a proximal femoral varus osteotomy, 29 of 33 hips had an acetabular index within normal limits.

Schoenecker PL, Dollard PA, Sheridan JJ, Strecker WB: Closed reduction of developmental dislocation of the hip in children older than 18 months. *J Pediatr Orthop* 1995;15:763–767.

Twenty-six of 38 hips in 32 patients ≥ 18 months of age underwent a successful closed reduction. Three had loss of reduction requiring open reduction and 12 required a later pelvic or femoral osteotomy. Younger children (< 22 months) had better results.

Smith BG, Millis MB, Hey LA, Jaramillo D, Kasser JR: Postreduction computed tomography in developmental dislocation of the hip: Part II. Predictive valve for outcome. *J Pediatr Orthop* 1997;17:631–636.

Postreduction CT scan can confirm reduction, but none of the measurements were predictive of residual hip dysplasia. ON (20%) was associated with hip-abduction angles > 55°.

Smith JT, Matan A, Coleman SS, Stevens PM, Scott SM: The predictive value of the development of the acetabular teardrop figure in developmental dysplasia of the hip. *J Pediatr Orthop* 1997;17:165–169.

The appearance of the radiographic acetabular teardrop suggested a favorable long-term outcome.

Stans AA, Coleman SS: Colonna arthroplasty with concomitant femoral shortening and rotational osteotomy: Long-term results. *J Bone Joint Surg* 1997;79A:84–96.

The results are described of Colonna arthroplasty in 22 deformed hips in 20 patients older than 5 years of age. Thirteen hips in 12 patients had concomitant femoral shortening and derotation osteotomy, and more developed ON.

Tumer Y, Ward WT, Grudziak J: Medial open reduction in the treatment of developmental dislocation of the hip. *J Pediatr Orthop* 1997;17:176–180.

The authors report 98% excellent or good results in 56 hips (37 patients) following medial open reduction without preliminary traction at a mean age of 11 months (range, 2 to 25 months). Five hips (9%) developed ON.

Ward WT, Vogt M, Grudziak JS, Tumer Y, Cook PC, Fitch RD: Severin classification system for evaluation of the results of operative treatment of congenital dislocation of the hip: A study of intraobserver and interobserver reliability. *J Bone Joint Surg* 1997;77A:656–663.

Intraobserver and interobserver reliability was unacceptable in using the Severin classification to rate the postoperative radiographs of 37 children (56 hips) with DDH.

Wingstrand H: Intracapsular pressure in congenital dislocation of the hip. *J Pediatr Orthop* 1997;6B:245–247.

Intracapsular hip joint pressure increases with decreasing flexion and increasing degrees of internal rotation. Forced internal rotation should be avoided during closed reduction of DDH to decrease the risk of ON.

Bladder and Cloacal Exstrophy

Kantor R, Salai M, Ganel A: Orthopaedic long term aspects of bladder exstrophy. *Clin Orthop* 1997;335:240–245.

Pelvic osteotomies in bladder or cloacal exstrophy facilitated closure of the abdominal wall and urinary reconstruction. Function or gait were invariably normal in late childhood and adolescence with or without pelvic osteotomy.

Nordin S, Clementson C, Herrlin K, Hägglund G: Hip configuration and function in bladder exstrophy treated without pelvic osteotomy. *J Pediatr Orthop* 1996;5B:119–122.

Nine children with bladder exstrophy treated without a pelvic osteotomy were evaluated at a mean age of 13 years (range, 9 to 16 years). All had normal hip function and only 2 had a slight waddling gait. Retroversion of the acetabulum becomes balanced by increased femoral anteversion.

Sponseller PD, Bisson LJ, Gearhart JP, Jeffs RD, Magid D, Fishman E: The anatomy of the pelvis in the exstrophy complex. *J Bone Joint Surg* 1995;77A:177–189.

Describes the pelvic deformity seen on CT in 24 patients with bladder exstrophy compared with age-matched controls.

Sutherland D, Pike L, Kaufman K, Mowery C, Kaplan G, Romanus B: Hip function and gait in patients treated for bladder exstrophy. *J Pediatr Orthop* 1994;14:709–714.

Gait analysis in 15 patients showed that pelvic osteotomy is not necessary to improve hip function or gait, but only to assist in abdominal wall closure and the results of urinary reconstruction.

Wakim A, Barbet J-P, Lair-Milan F, Dubousset J: The pelvis of fetuses in the exstrophy complex. *J Pediatr Orthop* 1997;17:402–405.

The authors discuss the role of CT in preoperative planning for children with bladder and cloacal exstrophy.

Proximal Femoral Focal Deficiency

Court C, Carlioz H: Radiological study of severe proximal femoral focal deficiency. *J Pediatr Orthop* 1997;17:520–524.

The authors describe 3 criteria of fixation of the femoral head in the acetabulum in children younger than 2 years of age with PFFD: supraacetabular bump, increased diameter of the obturator foramen, and a horizontal acetabular roof.

Fowler E, Zernicke R, Setoguchi Y, Oppenheim W: Energy expenditure during walking by children who have proximal femoral focal deficiency. *J Bone Joint Surg* 1996;78A:1857–1862.

The authors demonstrated decreased mean oxygen cost (energy per unit of body mass expended per distance walked) in patients with a van Nes procedure (9 patients) compared with a Symes amputation (7 patients).

Goddard NJ, Hashemi-Nejad A, Fixsen JA: Natural history and treatment of instability of the hip in proximal femoral focal deficiency. *J Pediatr Orthop* 1995;4B:145–149.

The author studied 78 affected femurs in 67 patients and found that radiographs at 12 to 15 months of age could predict the development of hip instability, pseudoarthrosis, or failure of hip development.

Grissom LE, Harcke HT: Sonography in congenital deficiency of the femur. *J Pediatr Orthop* 1994;14:29–33.

Sonography was accurate in delineating hip position and morphology in 15 infants (19 hips) with PFFD and was a helpful adjunct to radiography.

Grogan DP, Holt GR, Ogden JA: Talocalcaneal coalition in patients who have fibular hemimelia or proximal femoral focal deficiency: A comparison of the radiographic and pathological findings. *J Bone Joint Surg* 1994;76A:1363–1370.

Incidence of talocalcaneal tarsal coalitions was increased in children with fibular hemimelia, PFFD, and, especially both.

Saleh M, Goonatillake HD: Management of congenital leg-length inequality: Value of early axis correction. *J Pediatr Orthop* 1995;4B:150–158.

The authors recommend early axis correction and joint stabilization prior to lengthening procedures.

Sanpera I Jr, Sparks LT: Proximal femoral focal deficiency: Does a radiologic classification exist? *J Pediatr Orthop* 1994;14: 34–38.

The authors compare the various radiologic classifications and demonstrate the difficulties with their use and accuracy, especially in infancy.

Tönnis D, Stanitski DF: Early conservative and operative treatment to gain early normal growth in proximal femoral focal deficiency. *J Pediatr Orthop* 1997;6B:59–67.

Hip immobilization in 3 infants with PFFD with femoral neck defects and instability resulted in healing, but with residual coxa vara and retroversion. Later surgical correction resulted in relatively normal growth of the proximal femur. The authors feel that this approach may alter the "natural history" of PFFD.

Congenital Short Femur

Sanpera I Jr, Fixsen JA, Sparks LT, Hill RA: Knee in congenital short femur. *J Pediatr Orthop* 1995;4B:159–163.

The authors analyzed 25 knees associated with a congenital short femur in 24 patients. Valgus was common, but not all had AP instability. Seven knees were Lachman positive and 15 had a positive anterior drawer test. The authors recommend preoperative MRI when both the Lachman and anterior drawer tests are positive.

Stanitski DF, Kassab S: Rotational deformity in congenital hypoplasia of the femur. *J Pediatr Orthop* 1997;17:525–527.

The authors quantitate the clinical and radiographic (CT scan) external rotation deformity in 8 patients with congenital short femur.

Transient Synovitis of the Hip

Kesteris U, Wingstrand H, Forsberg L, Egund N: The effect of arthrocentesis in transient synovitis of the hip in the child: A longitudinal sonographic study. *J Pediatr Orthop* 1996;16:24–29.

Aspiration of hip in transient synovitis consistently reduced the size of effusion as measured by ultrasonography, although there was some reaccumulation in all patients. This provides some justification to those who choose to aspirate hip effusions for the possible beneficial effect of decreasing intra-articular pressure.

Septic Arthritis

Jaramillo D, Treves ST, Kasser JR, Harper M, Sundel R, Laor T: Osteomyelitis and septic arthritis in children: Appropriate use of imaging to guide treatment. *Am J Roentgenol* 1995;165: 399–403.

This review article covers imaging options, techniques, and limitations in evaluation and management of septic arthritis.

Tuson CE, Hoffman EB, Mann MD: Isotope bone scanning for acute osteomyelitis and septic arthritis in children. *J Bone Joint Surg* 1994;76B:306–310.

When scintigraphy is used for detection of skeletal infection in difficult cases, "hot" scans have 81% predictive value and "cold" (decreased uptake) scans have 100% predictive value for localization.

Unkila-Kallio L, Kallio MJ, Peltola H: The usefulness of C-reactive protein levels in the identification of concurrent septic arthritis in children who have acute hematogenous osteomyelitis: A comparison with the usefulness of the erythrocyte sedimentation rate and the white blood-cell count. *J Bone Joint Surg* 1994;76A: 848–853.

This study compared serial white blood cell counts, erythrocyte sedimentation rates, and C-reactive protein levels in patients with osteomyelitis, some of whom also had septic arthritis. The C-reactive protein rose most dramatically and fell more slowly than the other studies in those children who had associated septic arthritis. Guidelines are given to help detection of patients who might have both infections simultaneously in a confusing clinical setting.

Legg-Calvé-Perthes Disease

Glueck CJ, Brandt G, Gruppo R, et al: Resistance to activated protein C and Legg-Perthes disease. *Clin Orthop* 1997;338: 139–152.

Glueck CJ, Crawford A, Roy D, Freiberg R, Glueck H, Stroop D: Association of antithrombotic factor deficiencies and hypofibrinolysis with Legg-Perthes disease. *J Bone Joint Surg* 1996;78 A: 3–13.

These two articles highlight some of the potential hypercoagulation defects that have recently been implicated as possible causes of LCP. The work is from the group in Cincinnati, and has yet to be be fully investigated or duplicated by other centers.

Herring JA: The treatment of Legg-Calve-Perthes disease: A critical review of the literature. *J Bone Joint Surg* 1994;76A: 448–458.

This is an excellent review of a complicated subject by a knowledgeable and unbiased orthopaedic surgeon.

Herring JA, Williams JJ, Neustadt JN, Early JS: Evolution of femoral head deformity during the healing phase of Legg-Calve-Perthes disease. *J Pediatr Orthop* 1993;13:41–45.

This study documents the continued progressive changes in femoral head contour in LCP during the 4 years following treatment and reossification. The majority of the hips improved in roundness with time. Older children, or those with extensive disease, often had progressive flattening.

Kim HT, Wenger DR: "Functional retroversion" of the femoral head in Legg-Calve-Perthes disease and epiphyseal dysplasia: Analysis of head-neck deformity and its effect on limb position using three-dimensional computed tomography. *J Pediatr Orthop* 1997;17:240–246.

Beneath some confusing descriptive nomenclature, this article has interesting and informative 3-D reconstructions of the evolution of deformity in LCP.

Ritterbusch JF, Shantharam SS, Gelinas C: Comparison of lateral pillar classification and Catterall classification of Legg-Calve-Perthes' disease. *J Pediatr Orthop* 1993;13:200–202.

Herring's lateral pillar classification of LCP is used in many pediatric orthopaedic centers. The lateral pillar classification was found to have greater interobserver reliability than the Catterall classification in this study. Unfortunately, fragmentation stage is necessary to accurately apply this classification.

Slipped Capital Femoral Epiphysis

Aronsson DD, Loder RT: Treatment of the unstable (acute) slipped capital femoral epiphysis. *Clin Orthop* 1996;322:99–110.

This excellent general review of clinical management of the patient with acute SCFE includes discussion of useful classification, debate of the value of traction versus bedrest, and a detailed description of surgical management from transfer to the fracture table to insertion of the screw.

Jerre R, Billing L, Karlsson J: Loss of hip motion in slipped capital femoral epiphysis: A calculation from the slipping angle and the slope. *J Pediatr Orthop* 1996;5B:144–150.

The authors report a long-term late study of patients with SCFE treated by in situ pinning, no treatment, or primary osteotomy. In the untreated or in situ group, only loss of internal rotation could be correlated with degree of slip angle. Other motion was relatively normal. This was a select group (no osteoarthrosis) but, in this group, excellent results were found without the need for reorientation osteotomy.

Jerne R, Hansson G, Wallin J, Karlsson J: Long-term results after realignment operations for slipped upper femoral epiphysis. *J Bone Joint Surg* 1996;78B:745–750.

This relatively small Swedish series examined patients an average of 44 years after realignment osteotomy for SCFE. The procedures were performed as primary treatment, not as late treatment for selected patients. The results at follow-up were felt to reflect the expected natural history; osteotomy or manipulative reduction was not recommended as primary treatment for SCFE.

Kallio PE, Mah ET, Foster BK, Paterson DC, LeQuesne GW: Slipped capital femoral epiphysis: Incidence and clinical assessment of physeal instability. *J Bone Joint Surg* 1995;77B:752–755.

Of 55 patients with SCFE, 5% were found to have some degree of epiphyseal shift or reduction at the time of surgery. These included 91% of children unable to bear weight (the 'unstable' acute slip) and 93% of those who had effusion on sonography. The combination of effusion and inability to bear weight was 100% sensitive and 46% selective in predicting physeal instability. The authors believe that effusion is an underappreciated sign in SCFE that should be assessed.

Kibiloski LJ, Doane RM, Karol LA, Haut RC, Loder RT: Biomechanical analysis of single- versus double-screw fixation in slipped capital femoral epiphysis at physiological load levels. *J Pediatr Orthop* 1994;14:627–630.

In a bovine model, the value of single-screw fixation in preventing mechanical creep behavior under shear force loading was demonstrated. There was no statistical difference between 1 and 2 screws. This correlates well with clinical experience in humans.

Loder RT, Hensinger RN: Slipped capital femoral epiphysis associated with renal failure osteodystrophy. *J Pediatr Orthop* 1997; 17:205–211.

SCFE associated with renal failure is the result of secondary hyperparathyroidism, and is far more likely in nondialyzed children. Medical correction of secondary hyperparathyroidism generally causes the slip to stabilize; if medical correction cannot be achieved in 1 to 2 months, surgical fixation (bilateral) with a single central screw will stabilize the slip.

Loder RT, Richards BS, Shapiro PS, Reznick LR, Aronson DD: Acute slipped capital femoral epiphysis: The importance of physeal stability. *J Bone Joint Surg* 1993;75A:1134–1140.

Fifty-five patients with "classic" acute SCFE (duration of symptoms < 3 weeks) were divided into stable (able to bear weight) and unstable (unable to bear weight) groups. Unanticipated reduction occurred in 26 of 30 unstable hips, but only 2 of 25 stable hips. All of the ON occurred in the unstable group. This classification is generally used for prognostic and treatment considerations in acute SCFE.

Loder RT, Wittenberg B, DeSilva G: Slipped capital femoral epiphysis associated with endocrine disorders. *J Pediatr Orthop* 1995;15:349–356.

In this large series of patients with SCFE and endocrine disorders, including hypothyroidism (40%), growth hormone deficiency (25%), and panhypopituitarism, the hypothyroid and growth hormone patients tended to be younger, and 61% bilaterality suggests that bilateral fixation is appropriate at the initial surgery, including 'prophylactic' treatment of radiographically normal hips.

Stasikelis PJ, Sullivan CM, Phillips WA, Polard JA: Slipped capital femoral epiphysis: Prediction of contralateral involvement. *J Bone Joint Surg* 1996;78A:1149–1155.

This retrospective review of SCFE patients examined the relationship between contralateral slip and skeletal maturity (measured with the Oxford method, using pelvic maturity landmarks). There was a linear relationship between risk and the Oxford score. Age in boys was a significant risk factor; boys younger than 11 years 7 months had a high risk of contralateral slip. There was no such association in the relatively small number of girls studied.

Traumatic Disorders

Blasier RD, Aronson J, Tursky EA: External fixation of pediatric femur fractures. *J Pediatr Orthop* 1997;17:342–346.

One hundred thirty-two children with 139 femur fractures were treated with external fixation. All fractures healed. Complications were not uncommon but were manageable.

Buehler KC, Thompson JD, Sponseller PD, Black BE, Buckley SL, Griffin PP: A prospective study of early spica casting outcomes in the treatment of femoral shaft fractures in children. *J Pediatr Orthop* 1995;15:30–35.

Based on a prospective study of 50 patients, the authors conclude that patients aged 2 to 10 years with uncomplicated femoral shaft fractures with a negative telescope test (shortening of less than 30 mm on gentle manual testing) can be safely treated with early spica casting with a 95% chance of successful outcome without excessive shortening.

Corry IS, Nicol RO: Limb length after fracture of the femoral shaft in children. *J Pediatr Orthop* 1995;15:217–219.

Scanograms were performed on 50 children with femur fractures at union and a mean of 3.9 years later to determine overgrowth. Overgrowth averaged 6.9 mm. The greatest overgrowth occurred in children aged 4 to 7 years. The authors suggest allowing for less shortening than is usually recommended.

Curtis JF, Killian JT, Alonso JE: Improved treatment of femoral shaft fractures in children utilizing the pontoon spica cast: A long-term follow-up. *J Pediatr Orthop* 1995;15:36–40.

Twenty-one patients treated with conventional spica casts were compared with 70 patients treated with the pontoon spica cast. Authors found many advantages of the pontoon cast.

Davison BL, Weinstein SL: Hip fractures in children: A long-term follow-up study. *J Pediatr Orthop* 1992;12:355–358.

Nineteen patients were followed long-term after childhood hip fracture. ON complicated 47% of cases; 78% of patients with ON required further surgical procedures.

Gonzalez-Herranz P, Burgos-Flores J, Rapariz JM, Lopez-Mondejar JA, Ocete JG, Amaya S: Intramedullary nailing of the femur in children: Effects on its proximal end. *J Bone Joint Surg* 1995;77B:262–266.

Thirty percent of 34 children studied after intramedullary nailing of the femur developed abnormality of the proximal femur. Abnormalities were most frequently seen after nail insertion through the piriform fossa.

Hughes BF, Sponseller PD, Thompson JD: Pediatric femur fractures: Effects of spica cast treatment on family and community. *J Pediatr Orthop* 1995;15:457–460.

Families of 23 consecutive children treated with a spica for isolated femur fracture were questioned regarding the impact on the home and child. Many adaptations were necessary. Recovery was unremarkable.

Ismail N, Bellemare JF, Mollitt DL, DiScala C, Koeppel B, Tepas JJ III: Death from pelvic fracture: Children are different. *J Pediatr Surg* 1996;31:82–85.

Data from 2 trauma registries were analyzed to compare outcomes of pelvic fractures in children with those of adults. Pelvic fractures were half as common in children as in adults. The mortality was 5% for children and 17% for adults.

Lazovic D, Wegner U, Peters G, Gosse F: Ultrasound for diagnosis of apophyseal injuries. *Knee Surg, Sports Traumatol, Arthrosc* 1996;3:234–237.

Apophyseal avulsions may be demonstrated by ultrasound in cases where no ossification center is visible in the apophysis by radiographs.

Rieger H, Brug E: Fractures of the pelvis in children. *Clin Orthop* 1997;336:226–239.

Fifty-four cases of pediatric pelvic fracture were reviewed; 87% had associated injuries, 14.8% died, 70% were treated by conservative

means, and 30% had surgical stabilization. In 35 patients followed up long-term, sequelae were rare. It is recommended that management should not differ from that of adults.

St. Pierre P, Staheli LT, Smith JB, Green NE: Femoral neck stress fractures in children and adolescents. *J Pediatr Orthop* 1995;15:470–473.

Five new cases and 7 cases from the literature were reviewed. All resulted from repetitive activity. Most fractures healed uneventfully. No serious complication occurred.

Trousdale RT, Ganz R: Posttraumatic acetabular dysplasia. *Clin Orthop* 1994;305:124–132.

Five cases of posttraumatic acetabular dysplasia are reported after triradiate cartilage injury. The radiographic appearance is distinct from that of developmental dysplasia.

Classic Bibliography

Aitken GT (ed): Proximal femoral focal deficiency: Definition, classification and management, in *Proximal Femoral Focal Deficiency: A Congenital Anomaly.* Washington, DC, National Academy of Sciences, 1969, pp 1–22.

Desai SS, Johnson LO: Long-term results of valgus osteotomy for congenital coxa vara. *Clin Orthop* 1993;294:204–210.

Gabuzda GM, Renshaw TS: Reduction of congenital dislocation of the hip. *J Bone Joint Surg* 1992;74A:624–631.

Greene WB, Dias LS, Lindseth RE, Torch MA: Musculoskeletal problems in association with cloacal exstrophy. *J Bone Joint Surg* 1991;73A:551–560.

Harcke HT, Kumar SJ: The role of ultrasound in the diagnosis and management of congenital dislocation and dysplasia of the hip. *J Bone Joint Surg* 1991;73A:622–628.

Offierski CM: Traumatic dislocation of the hip in children. *J Bone Joint Surg* 1981;63B:194–197.

Schmidt AH, Keenen TL, Tank ES, Bird CB, Beals RK: Pelvic osteotomy for bladder exstrophy. *J Pediatr Orthop* 1993;13:214–219.

Torode I, Zieg D: Pelvic fractures in children. *J Pediatr Orthop* 1985;5:76–84.

Weinstein JN, Kuo KN, Millar EA: Congenital coxa vara: A retrospective review. *J Pediatr Orthop* 1984;4:70–77.

Chapter 36
Pelvis and Acetabulum: Trauma

Pelvic Fractures

Evaluation

The evaluation begins with a history of the accident and determination of the patient's hemodynamic status in the field. The initial physical examination is directed at identifying associated injuries, including soft-tissue (open and closed), urologic, neurologic, and skeletal injuries, and hemorrhage. Because many patients with unstable pelvic injuries require early intubation, the physical examination begins with a carefully documented neurologic and vascular assessment of the lower extremity and perianal region. If this is delayed, the opportunity for a baseline prereduction evaluation may be missed, leading to later uncertainty. The integument is examined next to rule out open injury. The patient is "log rolled" to examine the posterior soft tissues. Large hematomas may be found, indicating significant direct injury or displacement of fractures. The perianal region, including the genitalia as well as the rectum, should be examined carefully. In male patients, the scrotum is often swollen and careful palpation is necessary to evaluate testicular injury or displacement. The penile meatus is examined for blood, although the absence of blood does not rule out urologic injury. Rectal examination may reveal a high prostate, blood, or exposed bony edges. In female patients, lacerations to the genitalia may involve the urethra or vagina. In addition to external evaluation, a bimanual examination is performed, and when the patient can be sedated, a gynecologic examination may be performed in suspected vaginal or rectal injury.

Concomitant urologic injury occurs in approximately 15% of pelvic fractures. It is more common in men than in women, and the lower urinary tract usually is affected. Blood at the meatus and a high prostate are the most common physical findings of urethral disruption. If the patient can urinate, hematuria is also indicative of injury, most commonly to the bladder. The incidence of bladder injuries in both men and women correlates with the number of pubic rami fractured. In hemodynamically stable male patients, a retrograde urethrogram is performed before foley catheter placement. In unstable male patients, an experienced team member makes a single attempt to pass a catheter. Because the female urethra is very short, catheter placement may be attempted in female patients without a urethrogram. If uro-

logic injury is present, its definitive management requires a multidisciplinary approach and is influenced by the planned orthopaedic treatment of the pelvic injury.

The anteroposterior (AP) radiograph of the pelvis may indicate complete instability, eliminating the need for manual examination of pelvic stability. If stability of the pelvis is in question, then a physical examination of the pelvic ring should be performed by an experienced team member. Although gross instability may be perceptible by manual examination, subtle instability requires stress radiographs. These examinations should be done once because repeated manipulation of an unstable injury may displace clots, lead to greater blood loss, or cause neurologic injury.

Radiographic evaluation begins with an AP view of the pelvis as part of the trauma evaluation. Pelvic injuries are then further evaluated with inlet, outlet, and Judet views (45° obliques) of the pelvis. The AP view gives the best overall assessment of the injury pattern and of vertical instability. The inlet view demonstrates the greatest displacement of the pelvis in the vast majority of cases and gives the most information about the posterior ring and sacral fractures. Complete disruption of the sacroiliac (SI) joint is demonstrated by posterior displacement of the ilium as opposed to injuries affecting only the anterior SI ligaments in which the ilium is simply rotated externally but not displaced posteriorly. The outlet view demonstrates sagittal plane rotational deformities. The Judet views are obtained only in stable patients and are useful to evaluate the acetabulum and the iliac wings. The iliac oblique view demonstrates the size of the intact iliac fragment in patients with fracture dislocations of the SI joint.

Axial computed tomography (CT) scans are routinely used in the evaluation of pelvic ring injuries. They are usually obtained in conjunction with the trauma scan and should include 5-mm cuts through the sacrum and SI joints if possible. In addition to identifying the location of pelvic hematomas, the bony windows of the scan clarify the bony injuries and displacements. The exact pattern and displacements of the posterior pelvic ring are easy to discern, allowing for proper classification of the injury. In particular, sacral fractures, posterior iliac fractures, avulsions, and the degree of posterior displacement are best seen on the CT scan. The lower lumbar spine can also be visualized and coincident

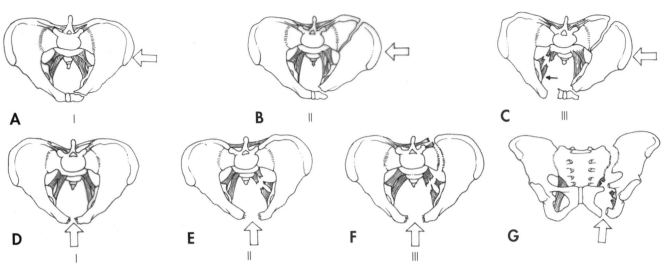

Figure 1

The Young and Burgess classification of pelvic injuries. The arrows indicate the direction of the force causing the injury. The top row (A through C) represents lateral compression (LC) injuries. Type I is a stable injury which includes rami fractures. Further displacement results in a type 2 injury with hemipelvic instability usually from a fracture dislocation posteriorly. If the force continues across the body, a type III injury with an opening of the contralateral pelvis occurs. D through F depict the increasing injury to the ligaments of the pelvis with anteroposterior compression (APC) injuries. A type I injury is stable with only the symphysis disrupted. As the force and displacement increases, the sacrospinous and sacrotuberous ligaments rupture allowing rotational instability, a type II injury. Last, the posterior sacroiliac ligaments fail creating a completely unstable hemipelvis, a type III injury. G shows a vertical shear (VS) injury, which ruptures the pelvis anteriorly and posteriorly.

injuries recognized. Sagittal reconstructions will demonstrate transverse sacral fractures.

Classification

Pelvic ring injuries can be classified by the anatomic location of the injuries (Letournel), stability (Bucholz, Tile), or mechanism of injury (Young and Burgess) (Fig. 1). Each of these systems has advantages and disadvantages; therefore, they should be used together. The anatomic system allows for a clear understanding of bony and ligamentous structures injured, assessment of the rotational and vertical stability of the pelvic ring helps to determine what immediate and definitive treatment may be required, and the mechanism of injury classification helps most in the acute phase with injury pattern recognition and prediction of blood loss. If internal fixation is to be performed, the anatomic classification is invaluable in determining the treatment plan and surgical approach.

Initial Treatment

Resuscitation/Hemorrhage Resuscitation begins on admission during the initial trauma evaluation. In addition to standard advanced trauma life support protocols and fluid infusion, blood replacement is often needed in patients with

major pelvic fractures. Patients presenting in shock (systolic blood pressure < 90 mm Hg) have mortality rates up to 10 times that of normotensive patients. Thus, hemodynamic instability should be considered an ominous sign requiring an aggressive resuscitation effort while simultaneously identifying the sources of bleeding. Frequently, hypothermia and coagulopathy play a role in continued blood loss, should be avoided when possible, and treated aggressively when they occur.

Sites of hemorrhage include the thoracic, abdominal, and retroperitoneal (including pelvis) cavities as well as external sites. External bleeding is controlled by direct pressure. The thoracic cavity is evaluated by a chest radiograph to detect any hemothorax. The abdominal cavity can be evaluated using a mini-open supraumbilical tap and lavage (SDPL), a CT scan, or an abdominal ultrasound (US). SDPL is most commonly used in hemodyamically unstable patients and CT scanning or US in hemodynamically stable patients. With these other areas of potential hemorrhage excluded, further blood loss is likely to be from the pelvic injury.

The most common direct causes of mortality in patients with pelvic fractures are head and thorax injuries. However, in accident victims with pelvic fractures, hemorrhage from pelvic injuries is considered to be a significant contributing factor to mortality. Most pelvic bleeding is venous and can be controlled by avoiding coagulopathy and providing a tamponade. However, severe bleeding resulting from arterial injury may require angiographic control. Although there is some controversy, most surgeons use early external fixation for bony stabilization and reduction of pelvic volume in the acute phase followed by angiography if blood loss continues.

External Treatment Initial external treatment may be applied in the field by the emergency services personnel. This may consist of sandbags and straps, beanbags, or military antishock trousers (MAST). MAST do stabilize the pelvis, but have been associated with significant complications, including decreased ventilatory ability, significant delay in transport time, and compartment syndromes of the lower extremities. The deflation of the device must be gradual to avoid a sudden increase in the intravascular space which can cause shock or lead to cardiac arrest.

Once in the hospital, external fixation of the pelvis is the fastest and most effective method of early skeletal stabilization and can be performed in the emergency department or in the operating room. The goal of the external frame is to reestablish the pelvic ring and thus, the pelvic volume. This decreases blood loss by providing a tamponade, opposing bleeding fracture edges, and limiting motion of the soft tissues. External fixation should be considered part of the resuscitation effort and is the best method to stabilize the pelvis for the purpose of patient mobilization and transport.

Two basic types of external fixation are available. The standard anterior fixator uses iliac crest pins and a trapezoidal frame. These devices can be used in all types of unstable pelvic injuries because compression or distraction can be applied. Although they do not provide rigid stability of the posterior pelvis, they can maintain temporary stability during the resuscitation effort. The use of traction in conjunction with an anterior frame can aid in controlling vertical displacement. Newer devices that apply a compressive force through percutaneously placed spiked pins attached to a C-shaped frame recently have been described. These can be placed anteriorly to reduce open book injuries (Fig. 2) or posteriorly to compress the posterior pelvis. Intrapelvic protrusion has been reported with posterior application, leading to the recommendation by some to use this device only under radiographic control.

Contraindications to external fixation include stable fracture patterns and unstable fracture patterns in which the pelvic volume cannot be controlled, such as those with a floating iliac wing. Acetabular fractures are a relative contraindication because pin sites may limit the types of exposures that can be used.

External fixation has been shown to reduce the mortality

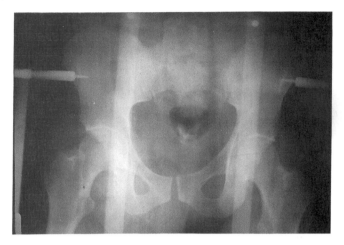

Figure 2

Use of a percutaneously placed pelvic clamp to stabilize an unstable right hemipelvic fracture (APC II).

rate of patients with unstable pelvic injuries to that of patients with stable injuries and to decrease transfusion requirements. If emergent laparotomy is required, the frame should be placed prior to the procedure and then tilted out of the surgical field. This will prevent further destabilization of the pelvis with release of the skin and abdominal muscles.

Angiography A small percentage of patients with pelvic fractures have significant arterial injuries and will benefit from angiography with selective embolization. These patients are identified by a process of elimination. Candidates for angiography include patients who have stable pelvic fractures or unstable pelvic fractures that have been stabilized with external fixation and in whom other sources of bleeding in the chest, abdomen, and retroperitoneum have been eliminated. In one series of hemodynamically unstable patients with pelvic fractures in whom no skeletal stabilization was used and all other sources of bleeding were ruled out, only 30% of the patients with continued blood loss had angiographically treatable arterial injuries. This finding supports the belief that the majority of blood loss in pelvic injuries is venous, even in hemodynamically unstable patients.

Successful embolization of arterial bleeding has been reported in 70% to 90% of cases. However, the procedure can be quite time consuming, taking 3 to 5 hours even in experienced hands. Thus, angiography has an important role to play, but is most useful after bony stabilization and complete evaluation for abdominal and thoracic injury. Other retroperitoneal and abdominal sources of bleeding, such as renal

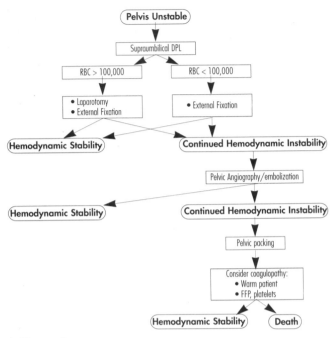

Figure 3

Algorithm for management of patients with an unstable pelvic injury and hemodynamic instability.

fractures and liver lacerations, may also be controlled with selective embolization, making this an excellent choice in selected cases with objective abdominal findings and continued blood loss. One successful algorithm for resuscitation in patients with pelvic fracture is given in Figure 3.

Fracture Treatment

Nonsurgical management is indicated for patients with stable pelvic injuries (Tile type A). Because most pelvic fractures are caused by a lateral compression mechanism that results in pubic rami fractures and stable sacral impaction, this group makes up the majority of pelvic fractures. Stable impacted sacral fractures with less than 1 cm of displacement can be observed if there is no neurologic deficit. In fact, displaced impacted sacral fractures may be difficult to disimpact if reduction is attempted. Nonsurgical management includes immediate mobilization with progressive ambulation. Repeat radiographs of the pelvis (AP and inlet) are obtained within the first week to detect further displacement. Surgical stabilization is reserved for skeletally unstable pelvic injuries.

External Fixation External fixation is an effective management for rotationally unstable injuries (Tile type B) because good control of the anterior pelvic ring can be obtained. An example of this is a lateral compression injury with pubic rami fractures and a sacral impaction injury. However, failures have been reported in obese patients as a result of difficulty in application and loss of reduction. Unstable posterior ring injuries (Tile type C) are not well controlled by external fixators. Union of bony posterior injuries will generally occur in an external fixator, but in a displaced malunited position. External fixation may also be used to control the anterior ring in some situations after internal fixation of the posterior ring is performed.

Internal Fixation Internal fixation of the pelvic ring is the most stable form of stabilization. Many successful methods of fixation have been described, but the main emphasis should be on obtaining an accurate reduction. The risks of pelvic internal fixation, including neurologic injury, vascular injury, infection, wound complications, nonunion, malunion, and loss of reduction, must also be considered.

Anterior Injury Anterior pelvic ring injuries can occur as symphysis disruptions, rami fractures, or a combination of both. Open reduction and internal fixation (ORIF) of symphyseal disruptions using single, double, and right angle plates for symphysis disruptions have all been successful. The simplest method seems to be the use of a single 6-hole 3.5-mm curved reconstruction plate placed via a rectus splitting approach (Fig. 4). This procedure uses the least soft-tissue dissection and can be done simultaneously with emergent laparotomy or lower urinary tract procedures. Fixation of rami fractures is rarely indicated unless the fracture is located medial to the pubic tubercle. One study demonstrated that in cases of unstable posterior ring injuries associated with rami fractures, properly performed posterior fixation alone is sufficient. However, if a significant gap remains at the site of a ramus fracture after posterior internal fixation, then fixation of the ramus is recommended with external as another option.

Posterior Injury The anatomic location of the pelvic injury determines the surgical approach and type of fixation used. Unstable posterior pelvic ring injuries can be classified anatomically as one of four types: sacral fractures, SI dislocations, SI fracture dislocations, and iliac wing fractures. Neurologic injuries are associated with displaced posterior pelvic ring injuries and have been reported in as high as 60% of patients. A careful examination must be performed before undertaking reduction maneuvers or surgery.

One of the current controversies regarding pelvic fracture management is the use of closed reduction and percutaneous fixation. Advocates of this method have demonstrated a very low soft-tissue complication rate because no open reduction

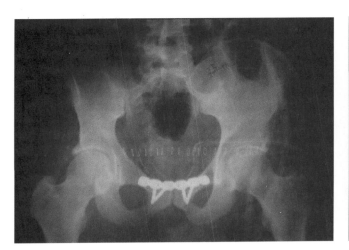

Figure 4

Stabilization of the symphysis with a 6-hole curved 3.5-mm plate.

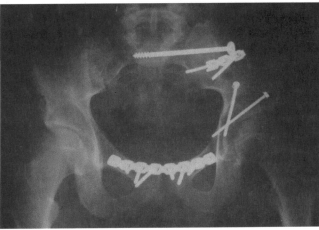

Figure 5

Postoperative anteroposterior radiograph of a patient with an APC III pelvic injury combined with a minimally displaced transverse acetabular fracture. Reduction and fixation were achieved via a simultaneous anterior approach to the symphysis and sacroiliac joint.

is used. This technique is applicable only if the posterior injury is addressed early, because delays may prohibit acceptable closed reduction, and only if the injury is amenable to iliosacral screw fixation. However, percutaneous screw fixation carries with it significant risks and should be used only if the posterior injury is unstable (Tile type C). This technique is best for posterior ring disruptions that have concomitant soft-tissue injury and are addressed within the first few days after injury. ORIF of posterior pelvic ring injuries results in extremely accurate reductions, but there is a higher risk of wound complications than when closed methods are used. Recent work by experienced surgeons has demonstrated infection rates < 3%. However, significant soft-tissue injury should be considered a relative contraindication to open reduction. The act of reducing unstable posterior injuries also presents a risk of neurologic injury. Several authors have recommended intraoperative neurologic monitoring in an attempt to avoid iatrogenic neurologic injury.

Iliac wing fractures are usually minimally displaced stable injuries and can be treated nonoperatively. ORIF is indicated only for iliac fractures that are significantly displaced. Reduction is not generally difficult and fixation can be with plates and/or lag screws.

Sacroiliac Joint Injury SI joint dislocations may be completely unstable, with no ligamentous support remaining (Tile type C), or rotationally unstable, with the posterior SI ligaments intact and only the anterior ligaments disrupted (Tile type B). Type B injuries are most commonly associated with symphyseal disruption. ORIF of the symphysis is all that is required in these cases because the intact posterior SI liga-

ments will support the posterior pelvis after anterior reduction and fixation. Type C injuries have no remaining ligamentous support and should be fixed anatomically. The SI joint may be approached and fixed from anterior, posterior, or by percutaneous techniques. The anterior approach allows for direct visualization of the superior portion of the joint, but excessive traction places the L5 nerve root at risk. Fixation is accomplished using plates with screws in the ilium and the lateral sacrum. Fractures of the sacral ala constitute a contraindication to this technique. Additionally, care must be taken not to overreduce the superior SI joint because this may cause an abduction deformity of the hemipelvis. The posterior approach allows visualization of the posterior SI joint, palpation of the anterior SI joint, and multiple opportunities for placement of reduction clamps. Fixation is achieved with iliosacral lag screws placed under fluoroscopic control, or less commonly with transiliac bars or plates. Closed reduction is possible in some cases and, if obtained, percutaneously placed iliosacral screws can be used for fixation. In all cases, the reduction must be carefully evaluated on the three views of the pelvis to confirm accuracy before fixation is placed.

Iliosacral lag screw placement is technically demanding and the surgeon must have an excellent 3-dimensional (3-D) anatomic and radiographic understanding of the pelvis and sacrum before attempting this procedure (Fig. 5). Common bony abnormalities such as lumbarization of S1, sacralization of L5, and hypoplastic sacral deformities should be recognized. One study showed that the average distance from iliosacral lag screws to the S1 neural foramen was only 3 mm, highlighting the need for precise placement. It has been suggested that the use of an oscillating drill bit may be safer than cannulated screw guidewires because it improves proprioceptive feedback when a bony cortex is encountered. In experienced hands, the complication rate for iliosacral screw placement ranges from 1% to 7%, with the L5 nerve root most commonly affected. Errant screws have been described in the S1 foramen, in the gluteal vasculature, anterior to the sacrum, and into the fifth lumbar vertebral body.

Fracture dislocations of the SI joint are a combination of an iliac fracture and a partial SI joint injury. The smaller the intact iliac fragment is, the more the injury acts like a pure dislocation, and the larger it is, the more similar it is to an iliac fracture. If the intact iliac fragment is large enough to maintain the integrity of the posterior SI ligaments, then fixation of the ilium is all that is required. This injury is referred to as a crescent fracture. Posterior ligamentous injury may occur through avulsions of the sacrum or ilium, indicating the need for iliosacral fixation.

Sacral fractures are the most common posterior pelvic injury. The majority of these fractures are stable and occur from a lateral compression mechanism. These can be managed nonsurgically. In displaced and unstable (type C) fractures, open reduction is recommended by most authors, but closed reduction and percutaneous fixation has also been described. Open reduction allows for debridement of the fracture site and decompression of the neural foramina before fixation. If bony fragments remain in the foramen during compression of the fracture then iatrogenic neurologic injury may occur. If an open anatomic reduction is obtained, then the fracture may be fixed with lag screws without the risk of overcompression. Intrasacral plate fixation has also been described, but has not yet met with enthusiasm in the United States. Percutaneous reduction and fixation has also been recommended. One author reported that a reduction to within 1 cm of anatomic was obtained in 94% of cases. The incidence of fixation failure was 10% although most were due to patient noncompliance. The nonunion rate was 3.5% and occurred only in transforaminal fractures. Fixation of the anterior ring first facilitates percutaneous reduction of the sacrum. In contradistinction, another report demonstrated more accurate reductions with ORIF than with percutaneous techniques despite greater initial displacement. In cases of unilateral injury with extreme comminution, transiliac bars or plates may be used to stabilize the sacrum.

Outcome

Many studies have examined the outcome of pelvic ring injuries. It is clear from these reports that the overall outcome of patients, determined using health profiles, functional scores, and outcome variable analysis, depends more on the associated injuries than on the pelvic fracture. One study found a 14% physical and a 5% mental impairment after surgically treated pelvic injuries. With increasing instability of the initial injury, the clinical results seem to decline. Good or excellent results after fixation of rotationally unstable type B injuries ranges from 80% to 96%. For type C injuries, only 27% to 66% have acceptable results. Pain in the region of the pelvis has been associated with residual displacement in some studies, but not confirmed in others unless the displacement was greater than 1 cm. However, the reason for the fair and poor results is rarely pelvic pain. Associated neurologic, urologic, and lower extremity injuries are the most common reasons for impairment, pain, and loss of function. Neurologic injury may affect gait, diminish sexual function, and cause referred pain. One recent report with 3-year follow-up of surgically treated patients demonstrated a 53% resolution of neurologic impairment caused by the initial injury. The L5 nerve root, however, was the least likely to return. Significant attention has also been devoted to the sequelae of genitourinary (GU) injury. Several authors have demonstrated significant sexual dysfunction in women after pelvic fracture, with dyspareunia seen in 43% of those with ≥ 5 mm of residual displacement. GU complications in men include urethral strictures in as many as 60% of patients after urethral tear. Early realignment procedures may help to minimize this problem, but impotence still occurs in up to 36%. Impotence may also occur in the absence of other GU injury. It is a serious complication and has been reported in as many as 11% of male patients after pelvic injury. One recent report has implicated disruption of the cavernosal nerves as the cause of impotence, citing an 89% success rate after injection with vasoactive agents. Finally, concomitant lower extremity fractures, particularly of the foot and ankle, remain a significant source of impairment.

Postpartum Symphyseal Separation

Several recent reports have highlighted the occurrence of symphyseal separation during childbirth. Although pelvic mobility is increased at the time of delivery, the symphysis does not generally widen more than 1 cm. Symphyseal injury may be caused by several factors, including forceful abduction of the legs in association with epidural anesthesia. An audible snap may be heard, and the abdomen may appear flattened. Nonsurgical management with a pelvic binder is usually effective. However, if pain persists for longer than 2 months or the diastasis is > 1.5 cm, then symphyseal plating may be indicated. Diastasis of > 4 cm is indicative of greater instability and failure of nonsurgical measures. In these cases, ORIF of the symphysis has been recommended.

Acetabular Fractures

Fractures of the acetabulum are considered high-energy injuries. The fracture occurs from force transmitted through the femoral head. The position of the leg with respect to the pelvis and the location of the impact determine the fracture pattern.

Evaluation

The initial evaluation of acetabular fractures is much the same as that in pelvic fractures. A detailed neurologic evaluation is necessary, particularly when the posterior acetabulum is affected or the hip is dislocated because the sciatic nerve may be damaged in up to 20% of these cases. The peroneal division of the nerve is most at risk and should be specifically evaluated for motor and sensory findings. Significant displacement into the sciatic notch is associated with superior gluteal artery injury, which can be diagnosed and treated angiographically; this should be undertaken in the presence of unexplained blood loss. Other associated injuries include hip dislocation, femoral head fracture, pelvic fracture, lower urinary tract injury, neurologic injury, thoracic injury, and abdominal injury. Hip dislocations should be reduced emergently to reduce the risk of osteonecrosis. Skeletal traction may be applied in selected patients to maintain the hip reduced or to distract the femoral head if it is abutting a fracture edge or against an incarcerated fragment.

Soft-tissue degloving injuries over the greater trochanter are referred to as Morel-Lavallee lesions and can complicate management of the acetabular fractures. Although difficult to recognize early, these lesions become more apparent several days after the injury, with the visualization of a large ecchymotic region and fluctuance upon palpation.

Standard radiographic evaluation includes AP, Judet (45° obliques), inlet, and outlet views of the pelvis as well as CT scans. The definitive CT scan can be performed on a delayed basis in multiply injured patients. However, the use of newer spiral CT machines allow for rapid and continuous information gathering. Multiple 2-dimensional (2-D) and 3-D reconstructions are easily obtained with most software packages. Although 3-D reconstructions provide information about the rotational displacements of the fragments, they underestimate minimally displaced fractures and are of little value in making treatment decisions. Sagittal and coronal 2-D reconstructions have been said to improve the visualization of

incarcerated fragments, better assess the size of marginal impaction, and aid in the determination of secondary congruence. Despite these findings, the most valuable information needed to make treatment decisions is available on the plain radiographs and routine axial CT scans.

Classification

As opposed to the controversy over the classification schemes for many fractures, acetabular fractures are universally classified by the system of Letournel and Judet (Fig. 6). There are 5 elemental and 5 associated types. Although each type has variations that affect treatment, this classification is extremely useful for planning treatment and for evaluating results. Some recent comprehensive fracture classification schemes have been described that are based on the Letournel classification with the addition of multiple subtypes. These are useful research tools, but have not yet been proven useful in any large clinical studies.

Definitive Treatment

Nonsurgical Management Displaced acetabular fractures should be considered a surgical problem unless specific criteria are met. The objective criteria for nonsurgical management are based on the plain radiographs and axial CT. The first is that the femoral head must be congruent with the acetabulum on the AP and Judet views of the pelvis. Any subluxation is unacceptable. If the hip is congruent, then the weightbearing surface of the acetabulum should be unaffected by the fracture. This is defined as having intact 45° roof arcs on the AP and Judet views of the pelvis, and intact 10-mm subchondral axial CT arc. Additionally, less than 50% of the posterior wall should be affected. If these criteria are met, then the results of nonsurgical management are equal to those of surgical management.

These criteria, however, may not apply to isolated posterior wall fractures. Even fractures that affect < 50% of the posterior wall can create instability and subsequent posttraumatic arthritis. A posterior wall fracture making up only 33% of the posterior articular surface has been shown to increase the contact stress in the roof compared to the normal hip in a simulated single leg stance model. One recent cadaveric study has suggested that a medial roof arc greater than 60° may be necessary to ensure a stable hip in transverse fractures, but this has not been verified in the clinical setting. One final specific case that may warrant separate evaluation is that of a both column fracture. In this fracture pattern, the acetabular surface is completely free floating, allowing the fragments to remain congruent with the head in some cases, but in a medially displaced position referred to as secondary congruence.

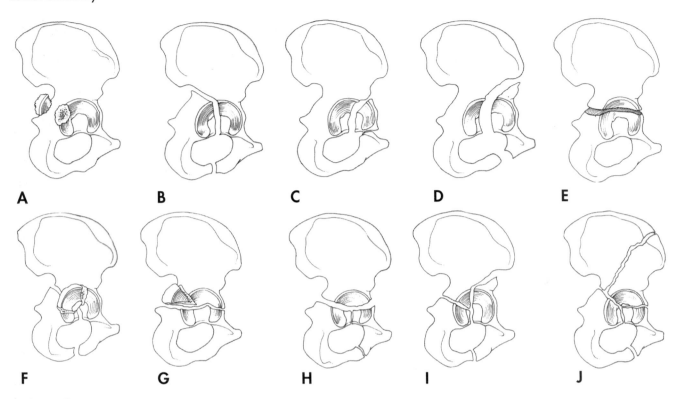

Figure 6

Letournel and Judet classification of acetabular fractures. A, Posterior wall. B, Posterior column. C, Anterior wall. D, Anterior column. E, Transverse. F, Posterior column and posterior wall. G, Transverse and posterior wall. H, T-shaped. I, Anterior and posterior hemi-transverse. J, Complete both-column. (Reproduced with permission from Letournel E, Judet R: *Fractures of the Acetabulum.* New York, NY, Springer-Verlag, 1981.)

The results in cases with good secondary congruence, although not as good as for an anatomic reduction, are better than for other displaced fractures affecting the roof. For this reason, some have recommended nonsurgical management in both column fractures of this type, particularly in the older age group.

The criteria listed for nonsurgical management are objective and related to the fracture pattern. Other factors, in particular the age and physiologic status of the patient, must also be taken into account. Although high rates of success have been reported for the surgical management of acetabular fractures in older patients, the option of hip replacement is available in this patient population. Because this option exists, nonsurgical treatment of the acetabular fracture with a planned total hip replacement if symptomatic posttraumatic arthritis occurs is not unreasonable. This method is most appropriate in both column fractures and when the hip is minimally or not subluxed. In unusual circumstances, a total hip replacement may be performed primarily in conjunction with acetabular fracture fixation.

Nonsurgical treatment should include early bed to chair mobilization followed by toe touch ambulation (20 lbs) on the affected leg. Full weightbearing should be delayed until union, usually by 3 months. Femoral traction is rarely used as definitive treatment for displaced acetabular fractures.

Surgical Management ORIF of displaced acetabular fractures is a technically demanding procedure with many potential complications. The goal of surgery is to reduce and fix the acetabulum in an anatomic position while avoiding the many possible complications. Unfortunately, much attention is paid to the approaches and fixation techniques used in acetabular fracture surgery when the truly difficult and challenging part of this surgery is obtaining an anatomic reduction. Even in the most experienced hands, truly anatomic reductions (≤ 1 mm displacement) are obtained in only 55% to 75% of large series. The rate of anatomic reduction declines with increasing complexity of the fracture, age of the patient, and the interval from the injury to the surgery. In one recent report, 96% of the elemental but only 64% of

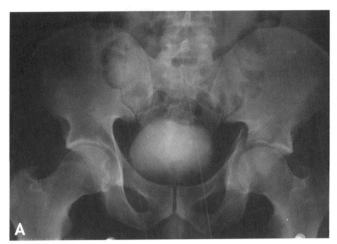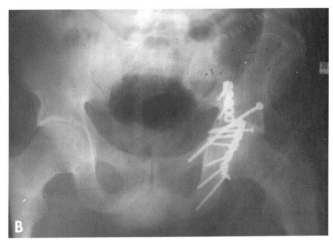

Figure 7

A, Anteroposterior (AP) view of a 28-year-old man who presented 22 days after sustaining a T-shaped acetabular fracture. The computed tomography scan demonstrated significant anterior impaction as a separate fragment. The fracture was reduced and fixed through an extended iliofemoral approach. This approach allowed the anterior impaction to be reduced under direct vision. B, Postoperative AP radiograph demonstrates an anatomic reduction.

the associated types were anatomically reduced. Another large study of fracture fixation that was delayed beyond 21 days reported anatomic reductions in 52% of cases, despite posterior wall fractures making up nearly half of the study. The most difficult are fractures that have poor reductions after an initial surgery, with 44% manifesting chondral damage of the femoral head and only 42% with acceptable results at a mean of 4.2 years after re-operation.

Surgical procedures are performed on a radiolucent table to allow for intraoperative fluoroscopy. Many surgeons use specially designed traction tables to assist with the reduction. Blood loss is reduced by using a hypervolemic, hypotensive anesthetic technique. The use of a cell saver may also reduce transfusion requirements. Sequential compression devices may be used throughout the procedure to minimize the risk of thrombosis.

The surgical approach used for fractures affecting only one column and/or wall is consistent among most surgeons. The ilioinguinal approach is used for anterior pathology (anterior column or wall) and some transverse fractures with significant anterior displacement. A Kocher-Langenbeck approach is used in cases primarily affecting the posterior acetabulum, including posterior wall, posterior column, posterior column plus posterior wall, and transverse fractures with significant posterior displacement. Although single column fractures are completely accessible through one approach, their reduction is not always easy. Special clamps, tools, and techniques are needed to manipulate the fracture fragments and maintain the reduction while fixation is placed. Even posterior wall

fractures, which some consider the simplest pattern, may be complicated by marginal impaction requiring elevation and grafting to reconstruct the joint. The use of a femoral distractor or traction table to remove incarcerated fragments and confirm the reduction of the joint may be necessary.

Options for more complex patterns include using an approach to 1 column and attempting an indirect reduction of the other, using 2 approaches (1 for each column), or using a single extensile approach. The use of simultaneous approaches is helpful in some fractures and can be facilitated by two teams of experienced surgeons. Most acute fractures can be addressed using a single nonextensile exposure to one column with an indirect reduction of the other. Both column and anterior column plus posterior hemitransverse fractures are usually treated through an ilioinguinal approach. Transverse plus posterior wall and many T-shaped fractures can be managed through a posterior approach. If a nonextensile exposure is chosen, a second sequential exposure can be used if the indirect reduction of the distant column cannot be obtained. This tactic is most useful in T-shaped, both column, and anterior column plus posterior hemitransverse fractures.

Associated patterns with significant comminution or anterior marginal impaction and those in which surgery has been delayed past 3 weeks may be best approached through an extensile approach such as the extended iliofemoral. This approach allows enough exposure to take down the callus, mobilize all elements of the fracture, and to reduce the articular surface under direct vision (Fig. 7). It should be noted that a theoretical risk exists in using this approach if the superior gluteal artery is not patent, but in many large series in which this approach was used, angiography has not been routinely performed and flap complications have been minimal.

Two recently described additional approaches may be useful in specific instances. The extended ilioinguinal approach uses a floppy lateral position and adds a subperiosteal dissection of the gluteus maximus off the outer table. It has been described for use in both column fractures in which the intercolumn fracture extends into the sciatic buttress or SI joint. The other recently described approach has been referred to as the ilioanterior or modified Stoppa approach. It is an extension of a Pfannensteil approach that allows excellent intrapelvic exposure by a dissection posterior to the iliac vessels, psoas, and femoral nerve. Ligation of anastamotic vessels between the iliac and obturator systems, which are present in more than 70% of cases, allows for exposure of the quadrilateral surface, psoas gutter, and pelvic brim from the symphysis pubis to the SI joint. Exposure of the iliac wing requires an extrapelvic subperiosteal dissection of the iliacus from the inner table. This approach is useful when buttressing of the quadrilateral surface is needed.

After reduction of the acetabulum, fixation is achieved using plates and lag screws. One recent trend is to use more lag screw fixation without plates for column fractures. However, buttress plates should be used for wall fractures to ensure stability. Special techniques involving the use of spring plates, push plates, cerclage wiring, and percutaneous screws have also gained in popularity. Fluoroscopy is used in the operating room to confirm the reduction and detect intra-articular hardware.

Postoperative management includes immediate mobilization of the patient with toe touch ambulation on the affected limb (20 lbs). Continuous passive motion machines may aid in regaining hip motion, especially after posterior approaches. The use of antithrombotic medication and mechanical compression devices is generally indicated. Active motion is deferred for 8 weeks and full weightbearing is begun at 12 weeks.

Late Reconstruction of Acetabular Fractures Late reconstruction of acetabular fractures may result from delay in primary surgery, a loss of reduction, or surgical malreduction. Although all 3 of these problems are difficult to manage, previous surgery makes the reconstruction more difficult because there is more scar formation and fewer opportunities for plate and lag screw placement. In cases of late reconstruction, the articular surface of the femoral head is more likely to have significant chondral injury, and the fracture is incompletely healed. An extensile exposure is necessary for all associated patterns because even if the initial fracture lines can be

found, an indirect reduction of the joint is not possible. The articular surface must be reduced under direct vision. The results of these procedures are usually inferior to results of early management of acute fractures.

Complications

The major surgical complications after acetabular fixation include thrombosis, neurologic injury, heterotopic ossification (HO), infection, osteonecrosis (ON) of the femoral head or acetabular segments, and arthritis.

Venous thrombosis may be more common than previously recognized. Venous doppler examination has documented the preoperative deep venous thrombosis (DVT) rate to be between 5% and 15% depending on the time from the injury. However, recent work using magnetic resonance imaging (MRI) has revealed a 33% incidence of asymptomatic thrombi. Of these, 46% occurred in veins proximal to the femoral vein or on the contralateral extremity. The clinical importance of these thrombi is not known because their natural history has not been defined and most surgeons do not use this technique for diagnosis. One major study demonstrated postoperative DVT and pulmonary embolism (PE) rates of 3% and 1%, respectively, without any fatal PE. The protocol used in this study included venous Doppler screening for patients transferred after injury. If there was no preoperative thrombosis, then mechanical (compression devices) and chemical prophylaxis (Warfarin at 1.3 to 1.4 international normalized ratio) was used for 4 weeks postoperatively. In patients with preoperative thrombi, a history of thrombosis or PE, and in those with a contraindication to anticoagulation, a caval filter is recommended to reduce the risk of PE.

Neurologic injury occurs in as many as 25% of acetabular fractures at the time of injury. Fractures associated with posterior hip dislocations and displacement in the sciatic notch most frequently affect the sciatic nerve. Resolution of these injuries can be expected to a satisfactory degree in the tibial nerve distribution. The peroneal division, however, if severely affected, is not likely to return. Iatrogenic injury to the sciatic nerve (most commonly the peroneal division) has been reported in 2% to 15% of fractures reduced and stabilized through a posterior approach. Intraoperative neurologic monitoring using sensory and/or motor pathways has been shown to provide an early warning in the operating room when the nerve is under too much tension and attempts to decrease the incidence of iatrogenic injury. Many experienced acetabular surgeons have reported rates as low as 2% without monitoring, however.

Some degree of HO occurs in up to 80% of patients after ORIF via a posterior approach. Most cases are mild and have no restriction of hip motion. Factors that have been associated with HO include extensile approaches, extensive cartilage damage, T-shaped fractures, associated injuries to the abdomen and chest, male gender, and trochanteric osteotomy. The use of indomethicin, radiation, and a combination of the two have all been recommended to decrease the incidence of clinically significant HO. Radiation with one dose of 700 Gy given on postoperative day 1 in combination with indomethicin 25 mg/day was reported to eliminate clinically significant HO. However, many surgeons are hesitant to use radiation in younger individuals, regardless of the dosage. Indomethicin is the most common method of prophylaxis used and, in several studies, has been shown to decrease the incidence of clinically significant HO. However, most of these studies are not randomized and a recent prospective randomized study did not confirm the efficacy of indomethicin. Although controversy exists, many surgeons continue to recommend indomethicin for 6 weeks. If clinically significant HO forms, then it may be resected after it is mature, followed by radiation and indomethicin to prevent recurrence. The use of Judet views in addition to the AP view has been recommended in assessing HO.

Infection after acetabular surgery occurs in 2% to 5% of most large series. The presence of a Morel-Lavallee lesion, the closed soft-tissue degloving injury centered over the trochanter, is a risk factor for infection. The liquefied collection found in these injuries are culture positive for bacteria in 46% of cases. Treatment of this injury should include surgical evacuation of the hematoma and irrigation of the region. Acetabular fixation should be delayed until the skin appears in better condition, usually 1 week later.

ON is a well recognized complication affecting the femoral head after dislocation, but it can also occur in acetabular segments. In particular, posterior wall fractures that are comminuted and devoid of soft tissue may necrose. Some preliminary investigations indicate that MRI evaluation of the femoral head may have some role in predicting ON after dislocation or fracture. Regardless of the side of the joint affected, in advanced cases the radiographic findings will be a loss of joint space followed by arthritic changes. Femoral head wear, caused by continued motion against a malreduced acetabulum or by minimal subluxation of the joint is more common than ON of the femoral head. This problem may be under-recognized and can be easily misdiagnosed as ON.

The most common complication after acetabular fracture is posttraumatic arthritis. Radiographic evidence of arthritis is present in 15% to 45% of acetabular fracture followed up for 5 years or more. The quality of the initial reduction correlates with the ultimate radiographic evaluation. Arthritis is more common after an incomplete or unacceptable reduction

(45%) than after an anatomic reduction (16%). Additionally, arthritis after an excellent reduction usually is diagnosed more than 10 years after fixation as opposed to after incomplete reduction when 80% of arthritic changes are noted within 10 years.

Clinical Outcomes

Many large series of acetabular fractures treated surgically have been reported in the past 4 years. The most consistent finding is that intermediate and long-term clinical results correlate closely with the quality of the reduction and the congruence of the hip. If anatomic or near anatomic reduction is obtained, then a good or excellent result may be expected in approximately 75% to 85% of patients. If the residual displacement is > 3 mm, then the clinical outcome is significantly worse with 50% to 68% good or excellent results.

The fracture pattern also appears to have some association with outcome. The percentage of excellent clinical results is lowest in the T-shaped and transverse plus posterior wall patterns. These findings are not surprising, however, because these fractures are the most difficult to reduce anatomically. Other factors that have been identified as negative predictors of clinical outcome include increasing age, femoral head articular injury, increased interval from injury to surgery, significant HO, ON, femoral head wear, arthritis, and infection. Examination of the results of the simplest pattern, the posterior wall fracture, demonstrates satisfactory clinical results in only 75% to 80% despite anatomic reductions in 90% to 100% of cases. These results highlight the importance of cartilage injury and vascular changes in the femoral head and acetabulum that affect the long-term outcome of acetabular fractures. The strongest predictor of clinical outcome after acetabular fractures remains the quality of the reduction.

Annotated Bibliography

Pelvic Fractures

Cole JD, Blum DA, Ansel LJ: Outcome after fixation of unstable Posterior pelvic ring injuries. *Clin Orthop* 1996;329:160–179.

A carefully followed group of 52 patients with unstable posterior ring injuries demonstrates that the clinical results based on several scoring systems were negatively affected by associated injuries including GU, neurologic, and lower extremity fractures. Of 38 patients who were full-time employees at the time of injury, 55% returned to full-time work and 16% to part-time work. The average pain score at rest was 2.8/10 and with ambulation was 4.1/10.

Copeland CE, Bosse MJ, McCarthy ML, et al: Effect of trauma and pelvic fracture on female genitourinary, sexual, and reproductive function. *J Orthop Trauma* 1997;11:73–81.

A careful evaluation of 255 women manifested an increased incidence of urinary complaints, cesarean section, and dyspareunia after pelvic fracture compared with a group of similar trauma patients without pelvic fracture. Residual displacement of > 5 mm was associated with the highest incidence of complaints.

Gruen GS, Leit ME, Gruen RJ, Garrison HG, Auble TE, Peitzman AB: Functional outcome of patients with unstable pelvic ring fractures stabilized with open reduction and internal fixation. *J Trauma* 1995;39:838–844.

One year after ORIF, 77% of patients had mild and 23% moderate disability; 62% returned to work without job modification.

Heini PF, Witt J, Ganz R: The pelvic C-clamp for the emergency treatment of unstable pelvic ring injuries: A report on clinical experience of 30 cases. *Injury* 1996;27(suppl 1):S-A38–45.

The pelvic C-clamp was hemodynamically effective in 10 of 18 patients who presented with pelvic and hemodynamic instability.

Matta JM: Indications for anterior fixation of pelvic fractures. *Clin Orthop* 1996;329:88–96.

A series of 127 patients demonstrates that fixation of ramus fractures lateral to the tubercle is not necessary after properly done posterior fixation. Fixation of symphyseal disruptions and medial ramus fractures is recommended.

Matta JM, Tornetta P III: Internal fixation of unstable pelvic ring injuries. *Clin Orthop* 1996;329:129–140.

This description of the surgical reduction and fixation of 107 unstable pelvic fractures describes a grading system for rating the reduction. The greatest displacement on the injury films was always seen on the inlet view. Ninety-five percent of all reductions were excellent or good; 70% of reductions done within 21 days were graded as excellent, compared with 55% if the surgery was delayed > 21 days.

Miranda MA, Riemer BL, Butterfield SL, Burke CJ III: Pelvic ring injuries: A long term functional outcome study. *Clin Orthop* 1996;329:152–159.

This interesting study demonstrates that even type A stable injuries have significant long-term sequelae.

Moed BR, Karges DE: Techniques for reduction and fixation of pelvic ring disruptions through the posterior approach. *Clin Orthop* 1996;329:102–114.

An excellent reduction was obtained in 25/26 unstable posterior ring injuries using open techniques. There was only one minor wound complication.

Pohlemann T, Gansslen A, Schellwald O, Culemann U, Tscherne H: Outcome after pelvic ring injuries. *Injury* 1996;27(suppl 2):B31–B38.

This series demonstrated significantly better results in type B injuries (79% good/excellent) as compared with type C injuries (27% good/excellent) despite 50% anatomic reductions and 80% with < 5 mm displacement in the type C injuries.

Reilly MC, Zinar DM, Matta JM: Neurologic injuries in pelvic ring fractures. *Clin Orthop* 1996;329:28–36.

Neurologic injury was present in 21% of a large series of unstable pelvic ring injuries; 37% had only sensory deficits whereas 63% had motor and sensory deficits. At a minimum of 2 years at least 1 grade of muscle function returned and 53% of the patients had a complete recovery. The L5 nerve root was the least likely to resolve completely.

Routt ML, Simonian PT, Defalco AJ, Miller J, Clarke T: Internal fixation in pelvic fractures and primary repairs of associated genitourinary disruptions: A team approach. *J Trauma* 1996;40:784–790.

This excellent review demonstrates the current problems and possible solutions to a challenging problem.

Templeman D, Goulet J, Duwelius PJ, Olson S, Davidson M: Internal fixation of displaced fractures of the sacrum. *Clin Orthop* 1996;329:180–185.

This multicenter study demonstrated slightly more accurate reductions after ORIF than with closed reduction and percutaeous screw placement in a nonrandomized series.

Tornetta P III, Matta JM: Outcome of operatively treated unstable posterior pelvic ring disruptions. *Clin Orthop* 1996;329:186–193.

In a series of 48 unstable pelvic injuries treated surgically, 67% of patients returned to work, 63% had no or only minimal pain, and 63% ambulated without restriction. Neurologic injury was most common after pure SI dislocation. Residual functional disability at follow-up was primarily related to associated injuries.

Tornetta P III, Dickson K, Matta JM: Outcome of rotationally unstable pelvic ring injuries treated operatively. *Clin Orthop* 1996;329:147–151.

Of 29 patients with vertically stable but rotationally unstable injuries, 96% had minimal or no pain and ambulated without restriction.

Acetabular Fractures

Helfet DL, Anand N, Malkani AL, et al: Intraoperative monitoring of motor pathways during operative fixation of acute acetabular fractures. *J Orthop Trauma* 1997;11:2–6.

Motor pathways were found to provide earlier detection of noxious stimuli affecting the sciatic nerve than sensory pathways.

Chapter 37
Hip: Trauma

Introduction

Fractures and dislocations of the proximal femur, particularly those occurring in the elderly, are a medical, social, and economic challenge. The number of hip fractures occurring each year is increasing in an older and more frail population. Advances in anesthetic techniques, medical management, and fracture fixation have decreased the incidence of postoperative complications, but continued improvements are needed to improve patient functional outcomes. As health care resources become more limited and their usage more closely scrutinized, functional outcome measures have been used increasingly to examine cost-effective intervention strategies for the clinical problems encountered. This chapter discusses hip dislocations, risk factors associated with hip fractures, and the treatment principles and expected functional outcome after femoral neck, intertrochanteric, and subtrochanteric fractures.

Hip Dislocations

Hip dislocations result from high-energy trauma, most commonly in a motor vehicle accident. Unrestrained occupants are at a significantly higher risk for sustaining a hip dislocation than passengers wearing restraint devices. Severe associated injuries are common and usually involve the craniofacial, chest, abdominal, or musculoskeletal systems. In one series, 95% of individuals who sustained a hip dislocation had an associated injury that required hospitalization. It is essential to obtain radiographs of the pelvis and entire femur to identify the most commonly associated musculoskeletal injuries: ipsilateral femoral head, neck, and shaft fractures; pelvic fractures; and acetabular fractures (Fig. 1).

Hip dislocations are most frequently posterior and anterior types according to the direction of dislocation, which is determined by the position of the leg and the direction of the applied force, as well as by the anatomy of the proximal femur. Anterior hip dislocations result from abduction and external rotation; the rare superior (inguinal) dislocations occur in extension, and inferior (obturator) dislocations occur in flexion. Approximately 90% of hip dislocations are posterior, resulting from an axial force applied to the flexed

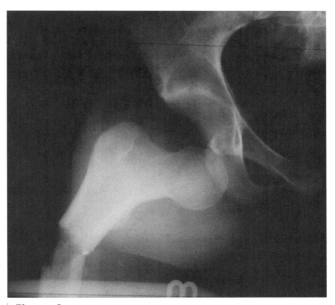

Figure 1

Anterior dislocation of the hip with an associated subtrochanteric femoral fracture.

knee. If the hip is in a neutral or adducted position, a simple dislocation occurs; if the hip is abducted, a posterior wall fracture-dislocation is likely.

In the absence of an associated femoral or tibial shaft fracture, the position of the injured lower extremity is the key to the clinical diagnosis of a hip dislocation. With an anterior dislocation, the lower extremity is externally rotated with varying amounts of hip flexion and abduction; with a posterior hip dislocation, the lower extremity is internally rotated with hip adduction and flexion. The hip dislocation should be apparent on an anteroposterior (AP) pelvic radiograph. With an anterior dislocation, the femoral head appears larger in diameter than the contralateral side because of the increased distance of the femoral head from the radiographic cassette; with a posterior dislocation, the femoral head will appear smaller than the contralateral side. An oblique or cross-table lateral radiograph can be used to confirm the direction of dislocation.

Treatment of hip dislocation should include: (1) careful clinical and radiographic evaluation to detect associated injuries; (2) immediate gentle closed or, if necessary, open reduction followed by assessment of hip stability; and (3) careful radiographic evaluation for congruency of reduction and any associated femoral head or acetabular fracture. On the AP radiograph, the joint space should be concentric and the distance from the femoral head to the ilioischial line equal to that on the uninjured side. The need for computed tomography (CT) evaluation after apparent concentric reduction of the dislocated hip remains controversial. Although most authors report that CT evaluation is essential to verify a concentric reduction and detect intra-articular fragments, authors of a recent study concluded that standard radiographs may be adequate to assess the quality of reduction after hip dislocation without associated fracture; this study, however, was based on a small number of patients.

If a concentric, stable reduction is obtained, the patient should be mobilized with protected weightbearing for 4 to 6 weeks. Approximately 5% to 10% of hip dislocations cannot be reduced by closed techniques because of either buttonholing of the femoral head through the hip capsule or soft-tissue interposition. An irreducible hip dislocation requires immediate open reduction. A nonconcentric reduction, resulting from either intra-articular osteochondral fragments, interposed soft tissue, or malreduction of an associated fracture also requires open reduction and joint exploration, but not on an emergent basis; the extremity should be placed in skeletal traction while awaiting surgery. Treatment of an associated femoral head or acetabular fracture depends on the size and location of the fragments and the stability of the hip. Small osseous fragments located in the acetabular fovea that do not impinge on the femoral head do not require excision; these fragments result from avulsion of a small portion of the femoral head by the ligamentum teres. Arthroscopy has been advocated for removal of small incarcerated intra-articular osseous fragments; this technique may be associated with less morbidity than open arthrotomy and can be used to diagnose and treat associated labral tears. An arthrotomy is necessary for removal of larger incarcerated fragments.

Femoral artery and nerve injuries are uncommon and are associated with anterior dislocations. Sciatic nerve injury occurs in approximately 10% of posterior dislocations. Osteonecrosis (ON) can occur up to 5 years after injury; the risk of ON increases with a delay of more than 6 to 12 hours before reduction. The role of magnetic resonance imaging (MRI) for determining the risk of ON after hip dislocation remains controversial. A recent report noted that MRI was not reliable for assessing marrow changes in the femoral head within 1 week of injury, nor was it helpful in predicting which patients were at risk for developing ON of the femoral head.

Anterior Dislocations

Anterior dislocations are rare and are classified as either superior or inferior. Closed reduction can be accomplished by traction in line with the femur, followed by hip extension and internal rotation. Associated femoral head fractures are classified as either transchondral or indentation types. Displaced transchondral fractures that result in a nonconcentric reduction require open reduction and either excision or internal fixation, depending on the fragment size and location. Indentation fractures, typically located on the superior aspect of the femoral head, require no specific treatment; fracture size and location have prognostic implications.

Ten percent of anterior dislocations develop ON. Risk factors include a time delay in reduction and repeated reduction attempts. The risk factors for posttraumatic degenerative arthritis include transchondral fracture, indentation fracture deeper than 4 mm, and ON.

Posterior Dislocations

Posterior dislocations account for over 90% of all hip dislocations and are classified according to the presence or absence of an associated acetabular or femoral head fracture. Closed reduction can be performed by traction on the adducted and flexed hip. Postreduction radiographs should be evaluated carefully for concentricity of reduction, intra-articular fragments, and associated fractures. If closed reduction in the emergency room with the patient sedated is unsuccessful, a closed reduction with the patient under general anesthesia with muscle paralysis should be performed; a percutaneous Schanz pin placed at the subtrochanteric level can be used as a joystick to manipulate the proximal femur. If a closed reduction is still unsuccessful or nonconcentric, an open reduction is needed; a CT may be helpful for preoperative planning.

Hip stability must be evaluated after either closed or open reduction; simple dislocations are inherently stable. CT can be used to help determine stability after reduction of posterior wall fracture-dislocations. Stability is inversely related to the size of the posterior wall fragment; cadaveric CT studies have indicated that fragments involving < 20% to 25% of the acetabular wall do not affect hip stability, whereas those involving > 40% to 50% result in instability. The status of the posterior capsule may determine stability for fragments of transitional size.

An acetabular depression fracture, the so-called "marginal impaction" fracture of Letournel, is a rotated, impacted, osteocartilaginous fragment of the posteromedial acetabulum that occurs as a result of a posterior hip fracture-dislocation. This fracture, with a reported 23% incidence using CT evaluation, should be elevated and bone grafted.

ON of the femoral head occurs after 10% of simple posterior dislocations and after as many as 50% of posterior fracture-dislocations; in a recent series of 83 posterior fracture-dislocations of the hip, 5 (6%) developed ON. The risk of ON has been related to the severity of the injury, delay in reduction (> 6 to 12 hours), and repeated closed reduction attempts. The risk factors for posttraumatic degenerative arthritis include higher energy initial injury, presence of a nonconcentric reduction, a femoral head indentation fracture, time delay between injury and reduction, and the development of ON.

Posterior Dislocations Associated With a Femoral Head Fracture

Approximately 7% of posterior dislocations have associated fractures of the femoral head or neck. Femoral head fractures are caused by an axial force applied to the flexed knee with the hip adducted and flexed less than 50°. These fractures have been categorized by Pipkin into 4 types:

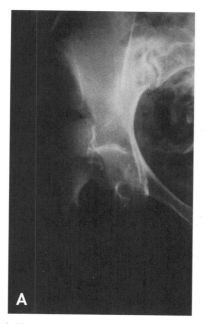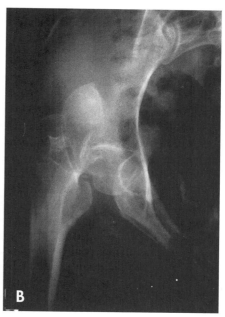

Figure 2

A, Posterior hip dislocation with a femoral head fracture and nondisplaced femoral neck fracture. B, A closed reduction was attempted with displacement of the femoral neck fracture.

type I, fracture of the femoral head caudad to the fovea; type II, fracture of the femoral head cephalad to the fovea; type III, type I or II associated with a femoral neck fracture; and type IV, type I, II, or III associated with a fracture of the acetabulum.

Identification and sizing of the femoral head fragment is difficult with standard radiographs; CT scanning can provide this important information. As with isolated hip dislocation, a gentle closed reduction should be attempted for Pipkin types I, II, and IV; type III injuries require open reduction (Fig. 2). Postreduction radiographs, including CT scanning, should be evaluated for concentricity and reduction of the femoral head fragment.

An unsuccessful or nonconcentric closed reduction (including under general anesthesia) mandates an open reduction. Pipkin types I and II fractures generally require open reduction from an anterior approach and internal fixation with well recessed cancellous or Herbert screws. A recent study comparing the efficacy of anterior and posterior approaches for Pipkin types I and II fractures reported improved fracture exposure and fixation with the anterior approach. Type III fractures in young active patients should be treated with open reduction and internal fixation of the femoral neck fracture, followed by internal fixation of the femoral head fracture. In elderly or low functional demand

patients, prosthetic replacement is indicated. Treatment of type IV injuries depends on the acetabular fracture pattern and the stability and concentricity of the reduction. If the hip is unstable or the reduction nonconcentric, open reduction with fixation of the femoral head and posterior acetabular fracture is indicated.

Posterior hip dislocations with an associated femoral head fracture are at high risk for developing ON and posttraumatic degenerative arthritis. The prognosis for these injuries varies. Pipkin types I and II are reported to have the same prognosis as a simple dislocation. Pipkin type IV injuries seem to have roughly the same prognosis as acetabular fractures without a femoral head fracture. Pipkin type III injuries have a poor prognosis with a 50% rate of posttraumatic ON.

Hip Fractures: General Considerations

Risk Factors

The incidence of hip fracture increases with increasing age, doubling for each decade beyond 50 years of age. Women are more commonly affected by a ratio of 2.5 to 1. The incidence in white women is 2 to 3 times higher than that reported for black and Hispanic women. Additional risk factors include urban dwelling, smoking, excessive alcohol and caffeine intake, physical inactivity, previous hip fracture, use of psychotropic medication (hypnotics-anxiolytics, tricyclic antidepressants, and antipsychotics), and senile dementia. Weight history has recently been implicated as a risk factor for sustaining a hip fracture; in a series of 3,683 white women followed up for 8 years, weight loss of 10% or more beginning at age 50 years significantly increased the risk for subsequent hip fracture while weight gain provided borderline protection. The contribution of osteoporosis and osteomalacia to the incidence of hip fracture has been studied extensively. In general, osteoporosis should not be considered the cause of hip fractures in the elderly, but rather a potential contributing factor along with the other risk factors described. Osteomalacia has not been shown to be a risk factor for hip fracture. The hip axis length (the distance from the greater trochanter to the inner pelvic brim) has been demonstrated to be predictive of hip fracture independent of patient age and bone mineral density. Coxarthrosis of the ipsilateral hip is rarely associated with an intracapsular femoral neck fracture, whereas intertrochanteric fractures are associated with the presence of degenerative changes.

Approximately 90% of hip fractures in the elderly result from a simple fall. In a laboratory study comparing age-related changes in femoral strength as a component of risk for hip fracture, the proximal femora from older individuals were found to be half as strong as those from younger persons and they absorbed a third as much energy before fracture. Estimated impact forces on the hip during a fall from a standing position exceeded the strength of the femora in older individuals but were less than the strength of the femora in younger individuals.

Fall characteristics (ie, poor protective responses) and body habitus have been implicated as factors influencing the risk of hip fracture in a fall. Age-related changes in neuromuscular function may increase the likelihood that a fall will result in a hip fracture. These changes include decreased speed of ambulation, which makes it more likely that the point of impact from a fall will be near the hip, and decreased reaction time, which limits the potential for a protective response. Recent work has suggested that use of external hip protectors may decrease the risk of hip fracture in the elderly, especially the nursing home population.

Studies have been performed to determine whether the demographic profile for patients who sustain a femoral neck fracture differs from those who sustain an intertrochanteric hip fracture. In a recent report, women who sustained an intertrochanteric fracture were more likely to be older, more dependent in activities of daily living (ADL), and a home dependent in activities of daily living (ADL), and a home

ambulator before hip fracture than those who sustained a femoral neck fracture; there were no demographic predictors of hip fracture type in men.

Mortality

The current overall 1-year mortality after hip fracture in the elderly ranges from 12% to 36%, which is in excess of age-matched controls. There is general agreement that the highest risk of mortality occurs within the first 4 to 6 months after fracture. After 1 year, the mortality rate approaches that of age- and sex-matched controls. The lowest mortality rates have been reported in community dwelling, cognitively intact elderly; a recent study reported a 1-year mortality rate of 12.6% in this patient population. In this report, factors associated with increased mortality included advanced age, poorly controlled systemic disease, male sex, institutionalized living, and psychiatric illness. Although the effect of delayed surgery on mortality after hip fracture remains controversial, it appears that a delay is appropriate only to permit stabilization of existing medical problems. A recent prospective study evaluated the effect of surgical delay on 1-year mortality in 367 geriatric hip fracture patients; a surgical delay was defined as more than 2 calendar days from hospitalization to surgery. Surgical delay approximately doubled the risk of the patient dying before the end of the first postoperative year when the factors of age, sex, and number of medical comorbidities were controlled.

Choice of anesthetic technique has not been shown to affect the mortality rate after hip fracture. The influence of nutrition on mortality and morbidity after hip fracture is well documented. Serum albumin level has been found to closely correlate with mortality. A recent study reported the value of lymphocyte counts as a prognostic indicator of survival following femoral neck fracture.

Treatment Principles

The primary goal of fracture treatment is to return the patient to the prefracture level of function. There is near universal agreement that in patients who sustain a hip fracture, this can best be accomplished with surgery. Historically, nonsurgical management resulted in an excessive rate of medical morbidity and mortality, as well as malunion and nonunion. Nonsurgical management is appropriate only in selected nonambulators who experience minimal discomfort from the injury. These patients, however, should be rapidly mobilized to avoid the complications of prolonged recumbency such as decubiti, atalectasis, urinary tract infection, and thrombophlebitis.

In an elderly patient who sustains a hip fracture, it is essential that all comorbid medical conditions be evaluated and corrected before surgery. Most patients can undergo surgery within 24 hours of injury. Several studies have evaluated the efficacy of preoperative skin traction in patients who sustained a femoral neck or intertrochanteric hip fracture. No difference in pain control was found between patients treated with skin traction and those whose injured leg was placed on a pillow.

Postoperative management should be directed at early patient mobilization. The ability to walk within 2 weeks after surgery has been shown to correlate with living at home 1 year after surgery. Because it is difficult for elderly patients to limit their weightbearing and there are no reported negative effects of full weightbearing after either internal fixation or prosthetic replacement, elderly patients should be allowed to bear weight as tolerated.

Thromboembolic Disease

In hip fracture patients who do not receive thromboprophylaxis, the reported incidence of lower extremity deep-vein thrombosis and fatal pulmonary embolism ranges widely from 40% to 83% and 4% to 38%, respectively. In a recent prospective study of 133 hip fracture patients who had venography on hospital admission, 13 (10%) had evidence of a deep-vein thrombosis; patients who had a delay of more than 2 days from injury to hospital presentation were at significantly increased risk for deep-vein thrombosis: 55% versus 6% in those who did not have a delay in presentation.

The standard thromboprophylaxis is warfarin sodium; the simplest way to use this medication is to administer 10 mg orally the night before surgery and then give an appropriate dose to maintain an International Normalized Ratio (INR) between 2 and 3. Use of warfarin sodium, however, can be problematic if there is a surgical delay. Dextran alone, or in combination with dihydroergotamine, has also been shown to be effective for thromboprophylaxis. However, use of dextran requires administration of a large amount of fluid, which increases the risk of fluid overload in elderly patients, especially in the presence of preexisting cardiopulmonary problems. Low-dose subcutaneous heparin has not been shown to be effective. Subcutaneous injection of low-molecular-weight heparin recently has been shown to be effective prophylaxis in patients undergoing total joint and hip fracture surgery. Aspirin generally is not recommended for thromboprophylaxis after hip fracture. Intermittent external pneumatic compression is effective, but the cost of specialized equipment and the need for recumbency may limit its usefulness. Generally, thromboprophylactic medications are continued until hospital discharge; however, with the recent push toward early discharge, consideration should be given to continuing them at home.

Imaging Studies

Most hip fractures can be identified on standard radiographs, but occult hip fractures require additional imaging studies. Bone scintigraphy may not be positive for 2 to 3 days in an elderly patient with a hip fracture. MRI has been shown to be more accurate and cost-effective than bone scanning in identification of occult fractures of the hip and can be done within 24 hours of injury (Fig. 3). MRI within 48 hours of fracture does not, however, appear to be useful for assessing femoral head vascularity or predicting the development of ON or healing complications.

Functional Recovery

Evaluation of functional recovery after hip fracture has become increasingly important as it is recognized that treatment success is considered by patients to be recovery of their prefracture level of function. Of elderly hip fracture patients, 40% to 60% are able to return directly home after hospitalization. Factors predictive of a hospital to home discharge are younger age, prefracture and early postfracture independent ambulation, ability to perform ADL, and the presence of another person at home. Within 1 year after fracture, 40% to 60% of patients regain their prefracture ambulatory status. The factors associated with regaining prefracture ambulatory status after hip fracture include younger age, male sex, and the absence of preexisting dementia. In a recent prospective study of 336 community dwelling ambulatory hip fracture patients, 92% remained ambulatory at latest follow-up; 41% regained their prefracture level of ambulation, and 59% lost some degree of ambulatory ability. Patients younger than 85 years of age who had an American Society of Anesthesiologists (ASA) rating of operative risk I or II or who had an intertrochanteric fracture were more likely to regain their prefracture ambulatory status at 1 year than patients who were 85 years or older, had an ASA rating of III or IV, or had a femoral neck fracture.

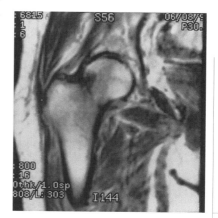

Figure 3

Nondisplaced femoral neck fracture in a 75-year-old woman visible on magnetic resonance imaging within 24 hours of injury. (Reproduced with permission from Dee R, Hurst LC, Gruber MA, Kotlmeier SA: *Principles of Orthopaedic Practice*, ed 2. New York, NY, McGraw-Hill, 1997, p 467.)

Functional independence involves the ability to perform certain ADLs. Of those who were independent in ADLs before fracture, only 20% to 35% regain their prefracture ADL independence. The factors reported to be predictive of recovery of ADLs are younger age, absence of dementia or delirium, and greater contact with a social network. The functions necessary for community dwelling have been identified as basic ADLs (BADLs) and instrumental ADLs (IADLs). BADLs include feeding, bathing, dressing, and toileting, whereas IADLs include food shopping, food preparation, banking, laundry, housework, and use of public transportation. Patients are more likely to regain independence in performance of BADLs than in IADLs.

Stress Fractures

Stress fractures of the femoral neck are relatively uncommon injuries that usually occur in military recruits and athletes. These fractures are classified as either tension or compression fractures. Tension fractures occur on the superior aspect of the femoral neck, are potentially unstable, and require surgical stabilization; these are more common in young athletes. Compression fractures occur on the inferior aspect of the femoral neck, are more stable than tension fractures, can be treated nonsurgically, and are more common in elderly patients; treatment should consist of a short period of rest followed by protected weightbearing. Nonsurgical treatment must include frequent serial radiographs to detect any changes in fracture pattern or displacement. Radiographic evidence of fracture widening or disruption of both cortices is an indication for internal fixation.

Pathologic Fractures

The proximal femur is a common site for metastatic lesions that result in pathologic fractures or impending fractures. The indications for stabilization of impending fractures include a lesion more than 2.5 cm in diameter, destruction of 50% or more of the cortex of a long bone, and mechanical pain. Patients treated prophylactically for impending fractures have less surgical mortality, fewer complications, fewer stabilization failures, and more successful rehabilitation than those undergoing surgery for displaced pathologic fractures. In addition, stabilization of an impending fracture is easier and spares the patient the pain and disability associated with fracture. Life expectancy has been used as an indication for surgical treatment. Some have recommended at least a 90 day life expectancy, while others have used 30 days. Although there is no universal agreement, surgical treatment of impending and pathologic fractures is indicated in patients whose quality of life will be enhanced, regardless of the anticipated life expectancy. Surgical management provides pain relief and allows improved patient mobilization.

Preoperative evaluation and preparation of the patient must be meticulous because these patients often are quite debilitated. Particular attention should be given to serum calcium levels, because hypercalcemia is common. Metastatic lesions that are radiosensitive should have radiotherapy preoperatively or immediately after stabilization of the fracture. Radiotherapy has not been shown to decrease soft-tissue healing, but does interfere with incorporation of bone graft. Methyl methacrylate is an important adjunct for stabilization of pathologic fractures. It is used to fill defects that remain after tumor removal and to improve implant fixation. Surgical management usually consists of internal fixation using adjunctive methyl methacrylate or prosthetic replacement. The choice depends on location, size of the lesion, and sensitivity to radiotherapy.

Hip Fractures in Young Adults

Hip fractures in young adults usually are caused by high-energy trauma. It is essential to carefully evaluate these patients for head, neck, chest, abdominal, and other long bone or pelvic injuries. Immediate stabilization of orthopaedic injuries in these frequently multiply injured patients is essential. Early attention must be given to the treatment of the hip fracture to minimize the risk of systemic and fracture complications. Internal fixation is nearly always appropriate with use of multiple screws for femoral neck fractures and a fixed angle or sliding hip screw for basicervical and intertrochanteric fractures; these same devices or a cephalomedullary interlocked nail can be used for fractures with subtrochanteric extension.

Femoral Neck Fractures

The Garden classification of femoral neck fractures is used most commonly in the literature; however, difficulty in differentiating the four types of fractures is shown by studies of interobserver reliability. Therefore, it may be more accurate to classify femoral neck fractures as impacted or nondisplaced (Garden types I and II) or displaced (Garden types III and IV).

Impacted and nondisplaced femoral neck fractures should be internally stabilized using multiple lag screws placed in parallel. Most authors report successful use of 3 or 4 screws for both nondisplaced and displaced fractures. One screw should be placed adjacent to the inferior aspect of the femoral neck to resist varus, and one screw adjacent to the posterior aspect of the femoral neck to resist posterior displacement of the femoral head. Nonunion and ON are uncommon after nondisplaced fractures, with nonunion occurring in fewer than 5% of patients, and ON in fewer than 10%.

Treatment of displaced femoral neck fractures remains controversial. Most authors advocate closed or open reduction and internal fixation in younger active patients, and primary prosthetic replacement in older, less active patients. There is general agreement that when internal fixation is chosen, anatomic reduction is the most important factor in avoiding healing complications. An acceptable reduction may have up to 15° of valgus angulation and less than 10° of anterior or posterior angulation. If a closed reduction is not acceptable, open reduction through an anterolateral or anterior approach is required. Urgent reduction with capsulotomy has been consistently shown to be of benefit in terms of optimizing femoral head blood flow in laboratory models. This benefit, however, has not been conclusively demonstrated in clinical studies of adequate design and statistical power. Although capsular distention with increased intracapsular pressure has been implicated as a possible cause of posttraumatic ON, the clinical utility of immediate capsulotomy or joint aspiration following femoral neck fracture remains unclear. Nonunion and ON continue to be problems after displaced fractures. The incidence of nonunion has ranged from 10% to 30% and that of ON from 15% to 33%. The need for reoperation after internal fixation of displaced fractures has been variable. Approximately 33% of patients with ON require additional surgery; approximately 75% of patients with nonunion or early fixation failure require additional surgery.

Postoperative bone scintimetry has been used to predict healing complications after femoral neck fracture. In a series of 46 patients who had femoral neck fractures that were internally stabilized, healing complications were associated with decreased uptake in early and 2-month scintimetry, but the specificity was only 50%. With normal uptake, uncomplicated union was predicted with 90% to 100% sensitivity. MRI in the first 2 weeks after femoral neck fracture has not been shown to be predictive for the development of postraumatic ON.

Prosthetic replacement should be used for the treatment of displaced femoral neck fractures in older and less active patients. In general, the results with methyl methacrylate are superior to those with noncemented prosthetic replacement. Progressive acetabular erosion has been found to be a problem in some series of cemented unipolar hemiarthroplasties; the factors that have best correlated with the severity of acetabular erosion are patient activity level and duration of follow-up.

The bipolar prosthesis (a prosthesis with an inner bearing) was designed to decrease the incidence of acetabular erosion. Results with use of the bipolar endoprosthesis have generally been quite satisfactory. Early results demonstrated that they were at least as good as unipolar designs. Although dislocation rates are similar, the bipolar design makes closed reduc-

tion much more difficult. Several studies have challenged whether or not bipolar motion actually occurs after insertion, claiming that inner bearing motion is rapidly diminished. Considering the higher cost of the bipolar prosthesis, some authors now advocate use of a cemented modular unipolar endoprosthesis, particularly in patients with low functional demands.

Despite improved function when compared with endoprostheses, the results of primary cemented total hip replacement after femoral neck fracture have been disappointing. In one uncontrolled study, at an average follow-up of 56 months, 18 of 37 patients (49%) younger than 70 years of age who had a primary total hip replacement after femoral neck fracture had undergone or were waiting for revision surgery. Another 4 (11%) had definitive radiologic signs of loosening. Increased activity level correlated with early failure. The results of secondary total hip replacement after failed internal fixation of a femoral neck fracture are comparable to the results obtained after primary arthroplasty for femoral neck fracture.

Young Adults

A femoral neck fracture in a young person is an orthopaedic emergency that requires prompt evaluation and definitive management. Nondisplaced fractures should be stabilized with multiple lag screws placed in parallel. Care should be taken to maintain reduction during the surgical procedure. Nonunion and ON are uncommon after nondisplaced fractures, except when the fracture was not identified initially; intracapsular hematoma may be the pathophysiologic mechanism, so capsulotomy or joint aspiration should be considered. Successful treatment of displaced fractures is related to achieving an anatomic reduction and stable internal fixation as soon as possible after the injury. A gentle, closed reduction should be attempted. If the reduction is unacceptable, an open reduction should be done, followed by multiple lag screw fixation.

Special Problems

Neurologically impaired patients include those with Parkinson's disease, previous stroke, and severe dementia. For patients with Parkinson's disease both internal fixation and prosthetic replacement have been recommended for femoral neck fractures. The choice of treatment in these patients should be based on patient age, fracture type, and severity of disease. All of these patients require meticulous medical and nursing care to avoid complications. If prosthetic replacement is chosen, correction of a hip adduction contracture by tenotomy and an anterior surgical approach should be considered. Both measures may decrease the risk of dislocation. Patients who have had a stroke are at increased risk for hip fracture, primarily because of residual balance and gait problems and osteoporosis of the paretic limb. Treatment depends on fracture type and functional status. When the fracture occurs within 1 week of the stroke, poor functional recovery can be anticipated. If prosthetic replacement is chosen, hip contractures should be corrected with tenotomy; an anterior approach may be preferred.

Institutionalized patients with severe dementia present a particular challenge. In-hospital mortality has been reported to be as high as 50%. Nondisplaced fractures should be treated by internal fixation. Displaced fractures that require prosthetic replacement should be treated through an anterior approach to decrease the risk of dislocation and infection from wound contamination in incontinent patients. In nonambulatory patients with severe dementia who do not experience significant discomfort from the injury, nonsurgical management with early bed to chair mobilization should be considered.

Femoral neck fractures are uncommon in patients with underlying osteoarthritis of the hip. When they do occur, total hip arthroplasty is indicated. Femoral neck fractures in patients with rheumatoid arthritis are associated with an increased incidence of complications. In general, nondisplaced fractures can be successfully treated by internal fixation. Total hip arthroplasty is recommended for displaced femoral neck fractures in patients with joint space loss.

Femoral neck fractures (nondisplaced and displaced) in patients with chronic renal disease or hyperparathyroidism are at increased risk for complications of internal fixation because of the associated metabolic bone disease. In these patients, cemented primary prosthetic replacement or total hip arthroplasty is recommended.

Femoral neck fractures in patients with Paget disease should be carefully evaluated because of the potential for pre-existing acetabular degeneration and deformity of the proximal femur. Nondisplaced fractures can be treated with internal fixation. For displaced fractures, prosthetic replacement is preferred. Prefracture symptoms of hip pain in the presence of acetabular degeneration are an indication for total hip arthroplasty; if acetabular deformity or degeneration is not present, cemented hemiarthroplasty should be done. Deformity of the proximal femur and the tendency for excessive bleeding are frequent technical difficulties.

Intertrochanteric Fractures

Intertrochanteric fractures occur with approximately the same frequency as femoral neck fractures in patients with similar demographic characteristics. The most important aspect of fracture classification is determination of stability.

Stability is provided by an intact posteromedial cortical buttress. Unstable fracture patterns include those with loss of the posteromedial buttress, intertrochanteric fractures with subtrochanteric extension, and reverse obliquity fractures.

Internal Fixation

A sliding hip screw is the implant of choice for the treatment of both stable and unstable intertrochanteric fractures. Sliding hip screw sideplate angles are available in 5° increments from 130° to 150°. The 135° plate is most commonly used because it is easier to insert in the desired central position of the femoral head and neck than higher angle devices. In addition, the insertion point is in metaphyseal bone, which produces less of a stress riser than the diaphyseal insertion point required for the 150° plate. Clinical studies have not shown a significant difference in the amount of sliding and impaction between these two plate angles.

The most important aspect of sliding hip screw insertion is secure placement of the screw within the proximal fragment. This requires insertion of the screw to within 1 cm of the subchondral bone. A central position within the femoral head and neck is most commonly recommended. Anterosuperior positions should be avoided because the bone is weakest in this area, thereby increasing the likelihood of superior screw cut-out. Because of the suggestion that shortening and trochanteric displacement affect gait and mobility, techniques to preserve proximal femoral anatomy while obtaining firm fixation are under active investigation.

With use of a sliding hip screw, medial displacement osteotomy is not necessary. Because the sliding hip screw allows controlled fracture collapse, unstable fractures anatomically reduced can be expected to impact into a stable pattern, which often is medially displaced. This usually results in less shortening of the extremity than a formal medial displacement osteotomy. Clinical studies comparing medial displacement to anatomic reduction for unstable fractures have found no advantage of medial displacement over anatomic reduction.

Use of a sliding hip screw for intertrochanteric fracture stabilization is associated with a 4% to 12% incidence of loss of fixation, most commonly in unstable fractures. Most fixation failures can be attributed to technical problems involving poor fracture reduction and screw placement. The tip-apex distance (the sum of the distance from tip of the lag screw to the apex of the femoral head on the AP and lateral views, corrected for magnification) has been shown to be predictive of screw cut-out after intertrochanteric fracture. In a series of 198 intertrochanteric fractures stabilized with compression hip screws, no lag screw cut-out occurred when the tip-apex distance was ≤ 25 mm; there was a strong statistical relationship between increasing tip-apex distance and the rate of lag screw cut-out, regardless of all other variables related to the fracture.

Although a sliding hip screw allows postoperative fracture impaction, it is essential to obtain an impacted reduction at the time of surgery to avoid excessive postoperative collapse that may exceed the sliding capacity of the device. If screw sliding brings the screw threads in contact with the plate barrel, additional impaction is not possible and the device becomes the biomechanical equivalent of a rigid nail-plate. The minimum amount of available screw/barrel slide necessary to reduce the risk of fixation failure with use of a compression hip screw has been estimated to be 10 mm. In a recent study, intertrochanteric fractures stabilized with compression hip screws with < 10 mm of available slide had 3 times as much risk of fixation failure as those stabilized with ≥ 10 mm slide.

The Medoff plate is a modification of the compression hip screw that may reduce the incidence of fixation failure after unstable intertrochanteric fractures (Fig. 4). It uses the same lag screw as the compression hip screw to allow compression along the axis of the femoral neck, but the side plate has been replaced with a sliding component that allows the fracture to impact parallel to the longitudinal axis of the femur. This combined, controlled biaxial compression has had good reported results when used to stabilize unstable peritrochanteric fractures.

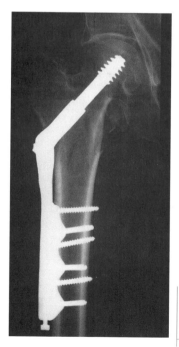

Figure 4

Unstable intertrochanteric fracture stabilized with a Medoff plate.

Intramedullary Devices

Intramedullary hip screws (IMHS) and Gamma nails are intramedullary nail/sliding hip screw devices used for the treatment of intertrochanteric hip fractures. Their theoretical advantages are both technical (limited exposure, "closed insertion," reduced operating room time, decreased blood loss) and mechanical (shorter lever arm and bending moment on the device due to its intramedullary design) compared to the sliding hip screw. Most studies comparing these devices to sliding hip screws have found no differences with respect to surgical time, duration of hospital stay, infection rate or wound complications, implant failure, screw cut out, or screw sliding. Patients treated with an intramedullary hip screw, however, are at increased risk for femoral shaft fracture at the nail tip and the insertion sites of the distal locking bolts. These devices may be best used in the treatment of comminuted intertrochanteric fractures with subtrochanteric extension, reverse obliquity fractures, and high subtrochanteric fractures.

Prosthetic Replacement

Prosthetic replacement for intertrochanteric fractures has been used successfully to treat postoperative loss of fixation when repeat open reduction and internal fixation were not possible or advisable. A calcar replacement prosthesis is necessary because of the level of the fracture. Primary prosthetic replacement for comminuted, unstable fractures has also been used successfully in a limited number of patients. The disadvantages include a larger and more extensive surgical procedure and the potential for dislocation. The indication for prosthetic replacement for acute intertrochanteric fractures is generally considered to be severe comminution in a highly osteoporotic patient.

Subtrochanteric Fractures

Subtrochanteric fractures account for approximately 15% of all proximal femoral fractures. These fractures start at or below the lesser trochanter and involve the proximal femoral shaft. They generally occur in 3 groups of patients: (1) young patients who are involved in high-energy trauma; (2) older patients with weakened bone whose fractures occur as a result of a minor fall; and (3) older patients with pathologic or impending pathologic fractures from metastatic disease. Some of the highest biomechanical stresses in the body occur at the subtrochanteric area. The medial and posteromedial cortex is a site of high compressive forces, while the lateral cortex experiences high tensile stresses. This stress distribution has important implications for fracture fixation and healing.

Many classification systems have been proposed for sub-

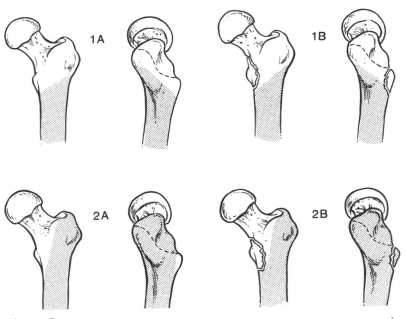

Figure 5

The Russell-Taylor classification of subtrochanteric fractures. Type 1 fractures have an intact piriformis fossa. In type 1A, the lesser trochanter is attached to the proximal fragment while in type 1B, the lesser trochanter is detached from the proximal fragment. Type 2 fractures have fracture extension into the piriformis fossa. Type 2A has a stable medial cortical buttress while type 2B has comminution of the piriformis fossae and lesser trochanter, associated with varying degrees of femoral shaft comminution. (Reproduced with permission from Dee R, Hurst LC, Gruber MA, Kotlmeier SA: *Principles of Orthopaedic Practice*, ed 2. New York, NY, McGraw-Hill, 1997, p 476.)

trochanteric fractures. The key determinant of fracture stability is an intact or reconstructible posteromedial cortical buttress. The Russell-Taylor classification divides subtrochanteric fractures into stable and unstable types and can be used to select the appropriate intramedullary implant for fracture stabilization (Fig. 5). Type 1 fractures have an intact piriformis fossa. In type 1A, the lesser trochanter is attached to the proximal fragment; this fracture type can be stabilized with standard antegrade nailing using a first generation interlocked nail. In type 1B, the lesser trochanter is detached from the proximal fragment; this fracture type can be treated with intramedullary nailing but requires a second generation interlocked nail (ie, reconstruction nail) in which the nail has screw fixation into the femoral head and neck. Type 2 fractures have fracture extension into the piriformis fossa. Type 2A has a stable medial cortical buttress, while type 2B has comminution of the piriformis fossa and lesser trochanter, associated with varying degrees of femoral shaft comminution; these fracture types are very difficult to stabilize with an intramedullary implant and may be best treated with a sliding hip screw or 95° fixed angle plate.

High rates of union have been reported in large series of subtrochanteric femoral fractures stabilized with interlocked intramedullary nails. Favorable mechanical characteristics of interlocked nails have eliminated the requirement of surgically reconstituting the medial femoral cortex. Conventional (first generation) interlocked nails are inserted through the piriformis fossa and have transverse or oblique proximal locking bolts that are directed into the subtrochanteric region; they therefore require that the lesser trochanter be attached to the proximal fragment for adequate fracture stabilization (Fig. 6). Cephalomedullary (second generation) interlocked nails have fixation into the femoral head with 1 or 2 screws and can be used to stabilize proximal fractures that do not have an intact posteromedial support, as well as ipsilateral femoral neck and shaft fractures when the femoral neck fracture is nondisplaced (Fig. 7).

Excellent subtrochanteric femoral stabilization has been reported with the use of a 95° fixed angle device, the condylar blade plate or dynamic condylar screw; these implants act as a lateral tension band if the medial cortex is intact or reconstituted. Both devices allow 2 or more cortical screws to be inserted through the proximal aspect of the plate into the calcar, providing additional fixation of the proximal fracture fragment. Technically, the dynamic condylar screw is easier to insert than the condylar blade plate; the compression screw is cannulated and is inserted over a guidewire after its channel is reamed and tapped. However, the dynamic condylar screw does not provide as much control of the proximal fragment as does the condylar blade plate, and it requires insertion of an additional screw through the plate into the proximal fragment for rotational stability. Complication rates approaching 20% have been reported with use of these fixed angle devices, usually related to an inability to restore the medial femoral cortex. It may be possible to minimize the risk of complications through use of indirect reduction techniques. If significant medial cortical comminution or soft-tissue stripping is present, bone grafting should be done.

The sliding hip screw has also been used for subtrochanteric fracture fixation. For this device to function optimally, the

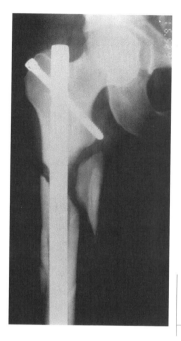

Figure 6

Russell-Taylor type 1A fracture stabilized with a first generation interlocked nail.

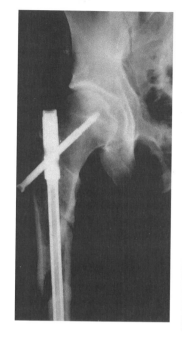

Figure 7

Russell-Taylor type 1B fracture stabilized with a cephalomedullary (second generation) interlocked nail.

sliding component of the device must cross the fracture site. This criterion can really be fulfilled only by subtrochanteric fractures with intertrochanteric extension, but in actual practice, sliding hip screws are often used to stabilize other types of subtrochanteric fractures because the surgeon is familiar with this device; in one series there was a 95% union rate when sliding hip screws were used to stabilize low energy subtrochanteric fractures in elderly patients. If a sliding hip screw is used to stabilize a distal or comminuted subtrochanteric fracture, the posteromedial cortical buttress should be reconstructed to minimize the risk of varus displacement and implant failure.

Postoperative management depends on the fracture pattern, the age and medical status of the patient, and the method of fixation. For subtrochanteric or intertrochanteric fractures treated with a sliding hip screw that allows fracture impaction, early weightbearing can be allowed. Stable fractures treated with intramedullary devices also can be treated with early weightbearing. Subtrochanteric fractures with medial or segmental comminution must be protected, regardless of the device used, for at least 6 to 8 weeks until early healing is evident.

Annotated Bibliography

Hip Dislocations

Frick SL, Sims SH: Is computed tomography useful after simple posterior hip dislocation? *J Orthop Trauma* 1995;9:388–391.

Twenty-three patients who sustained a hip dislocation without an associated fracture that had a concentric reduction on plain radiographs, and had a subsequent CT scan were identified over a 4 year period. CT scanning confirmed the reduction in all patients; 3 occult fractures but no occult intra-articular loose bodies were identified. The CT findings did not alter the treatment plan in any patients and the authors concluded that CT scanning was not useful.

Poggi JJ, Callaghan JJ, Spritzer CE, Roark T, Goldner RD: Changes on magnetic resonance images after traumatic hip dislocation. *Clin Orthop* 1995;319:249–259.

Fourteen patients who sustained a traumatic hip dislocation had serial MRI and radiographic studies from the time of injury through 24 months after injury. Eight hips had abnormal marrow signals within 6 weeks of injury; these changes progressed in 3 patients, resulting in radiographically evident ON. In the remaining 5 patients, however, the marrow changes were transient and resolved within 3 months in 4 patients.

Hip Fractures

Aharonoff GB, Koval KJ, Skovron ML, Zuckerman JD: Hip fractures in the elderly: Predictors of one year mortality. *J Orthop Trauma* 1997;11:162–165.

Six hundred and twelve ambulatory and home dwelling elderly who sustained a nonpathologic hip fracture were followed up to determine the predictors of 1-year mortality following fracture. Twenty-four patients (4%) died during hospitalization; 78 patients (12.7%) died within 1 year of fracture. Factors predictive of mortality were patient age ≥ 85 years, preinjury dependency in BADL, a history of malignancy other than skin cancer, ASA rating of surgical risk 3 or 4, and the development of 1 or more in-hospital postoperative complications.

Hinton RY, Lennox DW, Ebert FR, Jacobsen SJ, Smith GS: Relative rates of fracture of the hip in the United States: Geographic, sex, and age variations. *J Bone Joint Surg* 1995;77A:695–702.

Medicare data for 687,850 hip fractures that occurred in the United States between 1984 and 1987 were studied. The rates of femoral neck, intertrochanteric, and subtrochanteric fracture as well as the overall rate of hip fracture at any of the 3 levels increased with patient age, were greater for women than men, and were higher in the southern part of the country. The ratio of femoral neck to intertrochanteric fracture decreased from 1.5 in women who were age 65 to 69 years to 0.8 in women who were age 85 years or older; this ratio stayed at approximately 1.0 in the corresponding age groups in men.

Langlois JA, Harris T, Looker AC, Madans J: Weight change between age 50 years and old age is associated with risk of hip fracture in white women aged 67 years and older. *Arch Intern Med* 1996;156:989–994.

The association between weight change and hip fracture risk was studied in 3,683 community dwelling white women age 67 years and older. Weight loss greater than 10% or more beginning at age 50 years was associated with a significantly increased risk of subsequent hip fracture. This risk was greatest among women in the lowest and middle tertiles of body mass index at age 50. Weight gain of 10% or more provided borderline protection.

Treatment

Hefley FG Jr, WF, Nelson CL, Puskarich-May CL: Effect of delayed admission to the hospital on the preoperative prevalence of deep-vein thrombosis associated with fractures about the hip. *J Bone Joint Surg* 1996;78A:581–583.

Thirteen (10%) of 133 patients who had venography on hospital admission after hip fracture had evidence of deep-vein thrombosis (8 distal and 5 proximal thrombi). Seven of the 122 patients (6%) who presented within 2 days after fracture had evidence of thrombosis versus 6 of 11 patients (55%) who had a delay greater than 2 days between fracture and hospital presentation ($p < 0.001$).

Koval KJ, Skovron ML, Aharonoff GB, Meadows SE, Zuckerman JD: Ambulatory ability after hip fracture: A prospective study in geriatric patients. *Clin Orthop* 1995;310:150–159.

Three hundred and thirty-six community dwelling, ambulatory, geriatric hip fracture patients were followed up for at least 1 year to determine ambulatory ability. Of these, 137 (40.8%) maintained their prefracture ambulatory ability; 134 (39.9%) remained either community or household ambulators but became more dependent on assistive devices; 39 (11.6%) became household ambulators; and 26 (7.7%) became nonfunctional ambulators. Multiple logistic regression analysis comparing those patients who regained their preinjury level of ambulation with those who did not showed significant differences for patient age, prefracture ambulatory ability, ASA rating of surgical risk, and fracture type.

Femoral Neck Fractures

Broeng L, Bergholdt Hansen L, Sperling K, Kanstrup IL: Postoperative Tc-scintimetry in femoral neck fracture: A prospective study of 46 cases. *Acta Orthop Scand* 1994;65:171–174.

Forty-six patients who sustained a femoral neck fracture (8 nondisplaced, 38 displaced) treated with open reduction and internal fixation had Tc-scintimetry performed within 1 to 3 weeks after surgery, at 2 months, and at 2 years. Nine fractures had loss of fracture reduction and 5 developed ON with segmental collapse. Healing complications were associated with decreased uptake compared to the contralateral side in the early and 2 month scintimetry, but the specificity was 50%. With normal or increased uptake, uncomplicated healing was predictable with 90% to 100% sensitivity.

Calder SJ, Anderson GH, Jagger C, Harper WM, Gregg PJ: Unipolar or bipolar prosthesis for displaced intracapsular hip fractures in octogenarians: A randomised prospective study. *J Bone Joint Surg* 1996;78B:391–394.

A prospective randomized study was performed in 250 patients older than 80 years to compare a cemented unipolar versus a cemented bipolar hemiarthroplasty after displaced femoral neck fracture. Two years after surgery, there was no difference in the complication rates between the 2 groups of patients. After adjusting for confounding variables, the return to preinjury function was significantly greater with use of the unipolar prosthesis.

Intertrochanteric Fractures

Baumgaertner MR, Curtin SL, Lindskog DM, Keggi JM: The value of the tip-apex distance in predicting failure of fixation of peritrochanteric fractures of the hip. *J Bone Joint Surg* 1995;77A:1058–1064.

A radiographic measurement is described, the tip-apex distance, which is the sum of the distance from the tip of the lag screw to the apex of the femoral head on both the AP and lateral radiographs, corrected for magnification. Of 198 peritrochanteric fractures stabilized using a sliding hip screw, 19 fractures had loss of fixation, 16 of which were secondary to lag screw cut-out. The average tip-apex distance was 24 mm for the fractures that united uneventfully, compared to 38 mm in those with lag screw cut-out ($p = 0.0001$). No fracture had lag screw cut-out when the tip-apex distance was ≤ 25 mm. There was a strong statistical relationship between increasing tip-apex distance and the rate of lag screw cut-out, regardless of all other variables related to the fracture.

Gundle R, Gargan MF, Simpson AH: How to minimize failures of fixation of unstable intertrochanteric fractures. *Injury* 1995;26:611–614.

One hundred consecutive patients who sustained an unstable intertrochanteric fracture were stabilized using a sliding hip screw and were followed-up for 2 years after surgery. In fractures stabilized with less than 10 mm of available slide and in those in which the lag screw was positioned in the superior quadrant of the femoral head, the risk of failure was increased by factors of 3.2 and 5.9, respectively. Based on the Synthes DHS lag screw and sideplate specifications, the authors advocated use of a short barrel side plate when using lag screws of 85 mm or less.

Lunsjo K, Ceder L, Stigsson L, Hauggaard A: Two-way compression along the shaft and the neck of the femur with the Medoff sliding plate: One-year follow-up of 108 intertrochanteric fractures. *J Bone Joint Surg* 1996;78B:387–390.

One hundred and eight consecutive displaced intertrochanteric fractures stabilized using the Medoff sliding plate and configured to allow sliding both along the femoral neck and shaft were followed-up for 1 year. All fractures united; in most fractures, there was combined sliding along both the femoral neck and shaft. One fracture had lag screw penetration; in this patient, the lag screw had been poorly positioned.

Stappaerts KH, Deldycke J, Broos PL, Staes FF, Rommens PM, Claes P: Treatment of unstable peritrochanteric fractures in elderly patients with a compression hip screw or with the Vandeputte (VDP) endoprosthesis: A prospective randomized study. *J Orthop Trauma* 1995;9:292–297.

Ninety patients 70 years of age or older who sustained an unstable peritrochanteric fracture were randomized to either open reduction and internal fixation using a sliding hip screw or cemented hemiarthroplasty. The patients were followed-up for 3 months after surgery. No difference between the 2 treatment groups was found with respect to surgical time, wound complications, or short-term mortality; however, patients treated with prosthetic replacement had higher transfusion requirements. Severe fracture collapse or loss of fixation occurred in 26% of patients treated with the sliding hip screw, 2 of whom required additional surgery. One patient treated with prosthetic replacement required revision surgery secondary to recurrent dislocation.

Subtrochanteric Fractures

Kang S, McAndrew MP, Johnson KD: The reconstruction locked nail for complex fractures of the proximal femur. *J Orthop Trauma* 1995;9:453–463.

Thirty-seven patients who sustained complex proximal femur fractures, 31 of which involved the subtrochanteric region, were stabilized using a Reconstruction locked femoral nail. The overall union rate was 92%. Excellent results were achieved in pure subtrochanteric fractures with 1 nonunion and subsequent nail breakage. Subtrochanteric fractures with intertrochanteric extension had more limited success and were associated with higher complication rates, particularly in patients in whom an anatomic reduction was not achieved.

Classic Bibliography

Aune AK, Ekeland A, Odegaard B, Grogaard B, Alho A: Gamma nail vs compression screw for trochanteric femoral fractures: 15 reoperations in a prospective, randomized study of 378 patients. *Acta Orthop Scand* 1994;65:127–130.

Blair B, Koval KJ, Kummer F, Zuckerman JD: Basicervical fractures of the proximal femur: A biomechanical study of 3 internal fixation techniques. *Clin Orthop* 1994;306:256–263.

Desjardins AL, Roy A, Paiement G, et al: Unstable intertrochanteric fracture of the femur: A prospective randomised study comparing anatomical reduction and medial displacement osteotomy. *J Bone Joint Surg* 1993;75B:445–447.

Dreinhofer KE, Schwarzkopf SR, Haas NP, Tscherne H: Isolated traumatic dislocation of the hip: Long-term results in 50 patients. *J Bone Joint Surg* 1994;76B:6–12.

Gebhard JS, Amstutz HC, Zinar DM, Dorey FJ: A comparison of total hip arthroplasty and hemiarthroplasty for treatment of acute fractures of the femoral neck. *Clin Orthop* 1992;282:123–131.

Gehrchen PM, Nielsen JO, Olesen B: Poor reproducibility of Evans' classification of the trochanteric fracture: Assessment of 4 observers in 52 cases. *Acta Orthop Scand* 1993;64:71–72.

Kinast C, Bolhofner BR, Mast JW, Ganz R: Subtrochanteric fractures of the femur: Results of treatment with the 95 degrees condylar blade-plate. *Clin Orthop* 1989;238:122–130.

Leung KS, So WS, Shen WY, Hui PW: Gamma nails and dynamic hip screws for peritrochanteric fractures: A randomised prospective study in elderly patients. *J Bone Joint Surg* 1992;74B:345–351.

Moed BR, Maxey JW: Evaluation of fractures of the femoral head using the CT-directed pelvic oblique radiograph. *Clin Orthop* 1993;296:161–167.

Mullaji AB, Thomas TL: Low-energy subtrochanteric fractures in elderly patients: Results of fixation with the sliding screw plate. *J Trauma* 1993;34:56–61.

Rizzo PF, Gould ES, Lyden JP, Asnis SE: Diagnosis of occult fractures about the hip: Magnetic resonance imaging compared with bone-scanning. *J Bone Joint Surg* 1993;75A:395–401.

Swiontkowski MF, Thorpe M, Seiler JG, Hansen ST: Operative management of displaced femoral head fractures: Case-matched comparison of anterior versus posterior approaches for Pipkin I and Pipkin II fractures. *J Orthop Trauma* 1992;6:437–442.

Wiss DA, Brien WW: Subtrochanteric fractures of the femur: Results of treatment by interlocking nailing. *Clin Orthop* 1992;283:231–236.

Chapter 38
Hip and Pelvis: Reconstruction

Evaluation of the Hip

Clinical Assessment

Evaluation of the hip requires determining whether the patient's problem is an intra-articular or extra-articular process, or is manifested at the hip but originates at a distant source. Intra-articular discomfort can come from arthritis, osteonecrosis (ON) of the femoral head, synovitis, labral pathology, or loose bodies. Extra-articular discomfort can be caused by bursitis, tendinitis, muscular discomfort, or bony pathology, such as fracture or tumor of the proximal femur or pelvis. Sources of referred discomfort that may be felt in the hip area include the back (either mechanical or resulting from spinal stenosis), the sacroiliac joint, neurogenic pain, and vascular insufficiency.

Most problems can be diagnosed by careful history, physical examination, and plain radiographs. The most important features of the history include a description of the quality of the symptoms (pain versus a mechanical problem such as clicking), the location of the symptoms, and the circumstances under which the symptoms occurred. Pain located in the groin is particularly suggestive of hip pathology, whereas buttock discomfort is less specific and may be referred from the sacroiliac joint or spine. Pain with weightbearing is typical of arthritis or fracture; discomfort at rest suggests an active synovitis or a tumor-related problem. Trochanteric bursitis is common, typically felt over the lateral greater trochanteric area, and reproduced by pressure in that region. A history of catching or locking of the hip suggests labral pathology or a loose body. A family history of hip dysplasia should alert the physician to the possibility of acetabular dysplasia, just as a history of oral corticosteroid use or heavy ethanol intake should alert the physician to the possibility of ON of the femoral head. If surgery is contemplated, a detailed evaluation should include information about pain severity, frequency, location, impact on sleep, and impact on ability to work and to take part in recreational activities. The patient should be queried as to the functional effect on walking capacity, the ability to climb stairs, and ability to put on shoes and socks.

A Duchenne sign during gait (the patient leans to the affected side while in stance phase) suggests hip pathology. Significant loss of hip motion suggests an intra-articular or juxta-articular process. Pain with combined flexion and internal rotation of the hip and pain with hip abduction are commonly associated with arthrosis. Patients with active synovitis may hold the hip in a partially flexed, externally rotated position. Pain caused by tendinitis may be exacerbated by stretching the musculotendinous complex in question, and pain caused by bursitis may be reproduced by pressure over the affected bursa. Labral pathology and labral tears may cause a palpable click when the hip is brought from an internally rotated, flexed, adducted position to an externally rotated, abducted, extended position or visa versa. Most snapping hips occur as a result of subluxation of tendons over bony prominences. Subluxation of the iliotibial band over the greater trochanter typically is identified with the patient standing and is reproduced by rotation of the adducted hip in the stance phase. Snapping of the iliopsoas tendon over the iliopectineal eminence typically is reproduced as the hip is brought from a flexed to an extended position with the patient supine. Pain referred from the sacroiliac joint or spine, or caused by vascular insufficiency may be identified by system specific evaluation. Particularly when surgical treatment is planned, a detailed examination should include careful measurement of range of hip motion, measurement of true and apparent leg lengths, tests of abductor muscle strength, and detailed documentation of the neurovascular status of the limb. When femoral osteotomy is considered, the hip joint should be positioned in the proposed position of correction to determine whether a position of comfort exists.

Radiographic Assessment

Radiographic evaluation should include an anteroposterior (AP) radiograph of the pelvis and AP and lateral radiographs of the hip and proximal femur. Radiographic magnification markers are useful when total hip arthroplasty is planned to allow more accurate preoperative planning. A frog-lateral view of the hip is especially helpful when ON of the femoral head is suspected. When acetabular dysplasia is suspected, a false profile view helps determine the degree to which the anterior femoral head is uncovered (Fig. 1). If proximal femoral osteotomy is being considered, abduction and adduction views of the proximal femur to determine joint congruency and femoral head coverage in the proposed position of correction are useful.

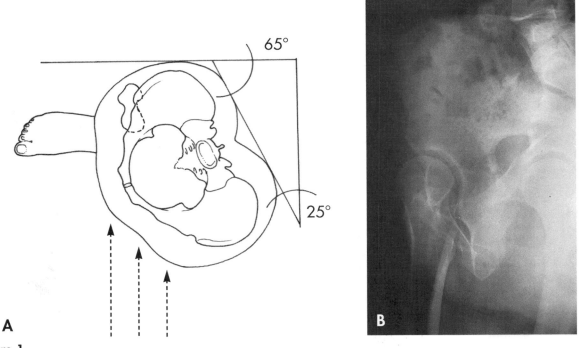

Figure 1

A., Method of obtaining false profile radiograph of the hip. (Reproduced with permission from the Mayo Foundation, Rochester, MN.) B, A false profile radiograph of the hip demonstrating acetabular dysplasia and poor anterior femoral head coverage.

Magnetic resonance imaging (MRI) of the hip is the test of choice to diagnose ON of the femoral head. Care should be taken not to misinterpret an MRI as showing osteonecrosis when, in fact, the diagnosis is ON of the hip with cyst formation in the femoral head. MRI is also a valuable test to identify stress fractures of the femoral neck and transient osteoporosis of the hip. T2-weighted MRI images readily demonstrate hip joint effusions, while T1-weighted images can identify synovitis or synovial pathology. Routine MRI often fails to identify labral pathology. The best methods of identifying a torn labrum presently are MRI with intra-articular gadolinium or computed tomography (CT) arthrography. Technetium bone scans are useful to identify occult stress fractures, as a screening test for tumors, and to identify early degenerative disease not visible on plain radiographs. Intra-articular injection under fluoroscopy with a local anesthetic is an extremely valuable diagnostic test to determine whether pain felt in the hip area or in the knee originates in the hip joint. Injection should be performed with a long-acting anesthetic, and the patient should be asked to report both the degree to which symptoms are relieved after injection and the duration of symptom relief.

Alternatives to Total Hip Arthroplasty

Arthroscopy

While arthroscopy has become an essential tool for evaluation and treatment of many joints, its role around the hip remains limited. The procedure may identify the source of intra-articular discomfort in difficult diagnoses and may be useful to treat specific conditions of the hip without an open procedure. Arthroscopy is most useful in the diagnosis of labral pathology, loose bodies, and limited chondral lesions of the acetabulum or femoral head (Fig. 2). In 2 recent studies, arthroscopy identified labral tears and loose bodies, even when they were not identified by other preoperative studies, including MRI. The indications for therapeutic hip arthroscopy include symptomatic labral tears, loose bodies, and synovial chondromatosis. The technique involves traction on the hip followed by creation of arthroscopy portals. Because the hip is difficult to distract and is far from the skin surface, and joint geometry makes visualization of the entire joint difficult, hip arthroscopy is considerably more challenging than arthroscopy of most joints. Complications of

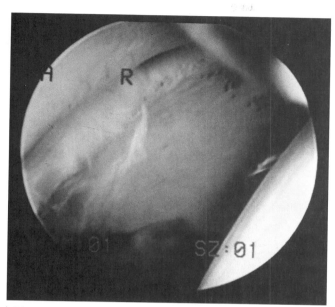

Figure 2

Arthroscopic view of the hip joint.

hip arthroscopy may occur as a result of patient positioning and traction: one report found a neurapraxia in 8 of 60 patients treated with arthroscopy (4 femoral nerve, 4 pudendal nerve).

Hip Arthrodesis

Hip arthrodesis remains a valuable procedure but in the age of successful total hip arthroplasty is less frequently accepted by patients than once was the case. The primary indication for hip arthrodesis is destruction of a single hip joint in a young active patient. Contraindications include significant associated spinal pathology, ipsilateral knee pathology, and bilateral hip disease. Although many techniques of arthrodesis have been described, present consensus suggests a technique should be chosen that preserves the anatomy necessary for a subsequent successful joint replacement. Thus, arthrodesis should cause minimal distortion of the femur and pelvis and should preserve the trochanter and abductor muscles. Preferred methods include use of a cobra plate with trochanteric reattachment or use of a compression hip screw and plate with ancillary compression screw augmentation (Fig. 3). In a recent report of 12 patients treated with a ventral compression plate placed through an anterior approach, union occurred in 83%. The favored position of arthrodesis is 20° to 30° of hip flexion, neutral abduction-adduction (or up to 5° of adduction), and neutral internal-external rotation (or slight external rotation). Insufficient flexion makes sitting

difficult, too much flexion causes excessive lumbar lordosis when standing. Abduction or internal rotation of the hip should be avoided. Because hip position is so critical, an intraoperative radiograph confirming position is advisable. Long-term results of arthrodesis have shown a high rate of patient satisfaction, pain relief, and surprisingly good function for 20 years or more in most patients. Over decades, many patients develop back pain (60% at 30 years in one series) and ipsilateral knee pain. Conversion of the surgically fused hip to a total hip arthroplasty is more difficult than routine primary total hip arthroplasty. Relief of back pain after conversion is more predictable than relief from ipsilateral knee pain.

Osteotomy

Osteotomies around the hip continue to have a central role in the treatment of younger patients with a number of hip diseases including developmental hip dysplasia, ON of the femoral head, and femoral neck nonunions, as well as the sequelae of childhood hip disease, including Perthes disease and slipped capital femoral epiphysis. Osteotomies about the hip include reconstructive and salvage pelvic osteotomies, as well as varus, valgus, flexion, and extension intertrochanteric femoral osteotomies and greater trochanteric osteotomy.

Pelvic Osteotomy Reconstructive pelvic osteotomies have broadened the surgical options available to manage acetabular dysplasia in young adults. Several reconstructive pelvic osteotomies have been described, but all are designed to allow rotation of the acetabulum to a more favorable position,

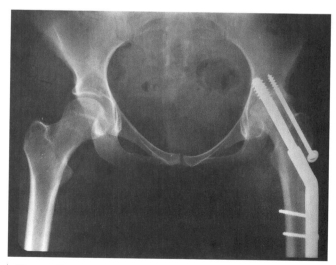

Figure 3

Hip arthrodesis using a sliding hip screw and plate with ancillary screw fixation.

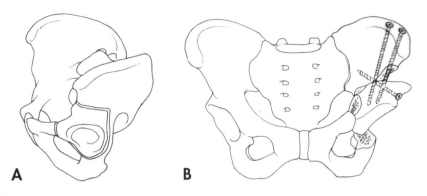

Figure 4

A, Pelvic model demonstrating the osteotomies used to create a mobile acetabular fragment during the Bernese periacetabular osteotomy. B, Pelvic model showing typical position and fixation of the osteotomy fragment after correction. (Reproduced with permission from the Mayo Foundation, Rochester, MN.)

thereby providing better femoral head coverage with acetabular articular cartilage. Presurgical radiographic evaluation of a young adult with hip dysplasia should include routine plain radiographs of the hip and a false profile view of the hip to determine the severity of anterior acetabular deficiency. Reconstructive pelvic osteotomies include triple osteotomy, spherical osteotomies, and the Bernese periacetabular osteotomy. Triple osteotomy has the disadvantage of necessitating bone cuts at a distance from the acetabulum. The large acetabular fragment thus created allows limited rotational correction, and when rotated creates a large pelvic deformity. Spherical osteotomies about the hip are technically difficult, require special spherical osteotomes, and do not allow medial translation of the acetabular fragment but have been reported to provide good results.

In the last 5 years, the Bernese periacetabular osteotomy has become the most popular reconstructive pelvic osteotomy because it allows large rotational corrections, does not cause significant pelvic deformity, allows medial translation of the acetabular fragment, and does not devascularize the fragment. The technique involves partial osteotomy of the ischium, complete osteotomy of the pubis, and biplanar osteotomy of the ilium. The posterior column is left intact (Fig. 4). The fragment can then be rotated (in most cases of acetabular dysplasia anteriorly and laterally), then fixed with screws in an appropriate position. Overcorrection is possible because of the mobility of the fragment after osteotomy. A high rate of bony union has been reported, and favorable early to midterm results have been reported (Fig. 5). A recent study found that when the procedure was performed for patients with dysplasia and associated arthritis the results correlated with the severity of arthritis: 32 of 33 hips with

minimal or moderate arthritis had good results but only 1 of 9 with severe arthritis had a good result at 5 or more years after surgery.

The primary candidate for reconstructive pelvic osteotomy is a young patient with hip pain associated with acetabular dysplasia in the absence of advanced degenerative arthritis. In patients with severe coxa valga and marked acetabular dysplasia, pelvic osteotomy can be combined with varus intertrochanteric osteotomy. Pelvic osteotomies are technically challenging procedures even when performed by experienced hip surgeons. Reported complications include neurovascular injuries, intra-articular osteotomies, delayed osteotomy union, prolonged abductor gait, and heterotopic ossification. The potential morbidity of the surgery has led most surgeons not to recommend surgery for asymptomatic hips with acetabular dysplasia.

Chiari osteotomy medializes the hip center of rotation (biomechanically advantageous) and provides some lateral femoral head coverage with hip joint capsule and bone. Unlike reconstructive pelvic osteotomies, Chiari osteotomy does not cover the femoral head with articular cartilage. Therefore, Chiari osteotomy is considered in patients who have unsatisfactory acetabular anatomy or articular cartilage for reconstructive osteotomy and are not candidates for joint replacement surgery.

Femoral Osteotomy Femoral osteotomies include intertrochanteric and greater trochanteric osteotomies. Intertrochanteric osteotomies are named according to the direction of rotation through the osteotomy site: in a varus intertrochanteric osteotomy, the proximal femur is rotated to a varus position; in an extension osteotomy, the femoral head is directed posteriorly; and in a flexion osteotomy, it is directed anteriorly. A prerequisite for intertrochanteric osteotomy is adequate hip motion in the planned plane of correction to allow the hip to return to a functional position after osteotomy. Indications for femoral osteotomies have decreased as pelvic osteotomies have improved, because most young patients who are osteotomy candidates have acetabular dysplasia. Because most of the bony deformity usually is on the acetabular side in these patients, pelvic osteotomies have the advantage of correcting the problem at the site of the anatomic deformity (on the pelvic side of the joint). However, varus intertrochanteric osteotomy is still indicated

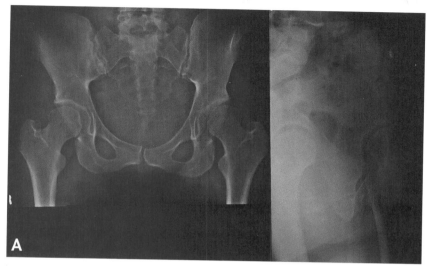

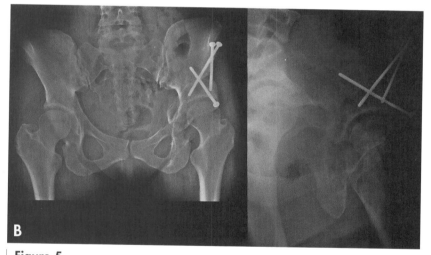

Figure 5

A, Preoperative anteroposterior and false profile radiograph of young female with acetabular dysplasia. B, Radiograph 2 years after Bernese periacetabular osteotomy demonstrates osteotomy healing and improved anterior and lateral femoral head coverage.

for symptomatic patients with minimal acetabular dysplasia but significant coxa valga and a relatively spherical femoral head. Varus osteotomies shorten the limb, and techniques that do not remove a large wedge of bone from the osteotomy site are preferred.

Valgus intertrochanteric osteotomy is reserved for the few patients with femoral head deformities that become more congruent with the hip in an adducted position or for patients with a mushroom-shaped femoral head in which a large medial osteophyte ("capital drop") is present. In such patients, valgus osteotomy may allow loading of the medial osteophyte, and thus medialization of the center of hip joint

rotation and reduction of joint reactive forces. Valgus osteotomy also is used to treat femoral neck nonunions with a vertically oriented nonunion site: a valgus intertrochanteric osteotomy places the femoral neck nonunion perpendicular to the joint reactive force, and thus under compression, thereby stimulating healing.

Varus and valgus osteotomies are most commonly performed in the intertrochanteric region and fixed with blade plates. During osteotomy, extension through the osteotomy site can improve anterior femoral head coverage while flexion through the osteotomy site can deliver the anterior femoral head from the acetabulum. Extension often is added during varus intertrochanteric osteotomy in the patient with coxa valga and mild anterior acetabular dysplasia. Flexion intertrochanteric osteotomy is most commonly done for ON of the femoral head to remove an anterior femoral head lesion from the weightbearing zone of the acetabulum. Intertrochanteric osteotomies should be done with future total hip arthroplasty in mind: efforts should be made to minimize translation of the proximal fragment relative to the femoral shaft. Results of intertrochanteric femoral osteotomy vary according to the indication and patient cohort, but in almost all series less arthritis correlates with better results.

Femoral Osteotomy for the Dysplastic Hip
Two recent papers have reported good results of intertrochanteric osteotomy in dysplastic hips when the femoral head was round and there was little arthritis. Both also showed poorer results when the procedure was used in patients with advanced arthritis. In a separate recent series of 31 valgus-extension osteotomies for severe osteoarthritis secondary to acetabular dysplasia, 15 patients had good pain relief and a satisfactory result 12 to 18 years after surgery.

Femoral Osteotomy for Osteonecrosis of the Femoral Head
Intertrochanteric osteotomy continues to play a limited but valuable role in treatment of ON of the femoral head. Many different osteotomies have been described, but the goal of most is to rotate the osteonecrotic portion of the femoral

head to a position in which it is either delivered from the weightbearing zone of the hip or rotated to position in which it is completely contained within the acetabulum. Results of osteotomy for this diagnosis have varied widely, probably in part due to differences in patient selection criteria. One recent series in which strict selection criteria were used to choose 45 hips with Ficat stage III ON for valgus-flexion intertrochanteric osteotomy had an 87% 5-year survivorship free of revision to total hip arthroplasty. Osteotomy appears to have the highest chance of success in patients with a relatively small amount of femoral head involvement, and the best results have been reported when the sum of the arcs of involved femoral head on AP and lateral views of the femoral head is less than 200°.

Rotational osteotomy through the base of the femoral neck theoretically allows large amounts of rotation of the femoral head. Excellent results of the procedure have been reported from Japan, even for large osteonecrotic lesions, but reports of smaller series from Europe and North America have been less favorable.

Femoral Osteotomy for Degenerative Arthritis Long-term follow-up studies of large series of intertrochanteric osteotomies done for osteoarthritis have demonstrated that for a significant number of patients quality of pain relief deteriorates with time. Therefore, as a general rule, older patients with more advanced arthritis are more likely to be candidates for total hip arthroplasty, whereas younger patients with less arthritis are considered more strongly for osteotomy. Patients with symmetric joint space loss and relatively normal proximal femoral anatomy may be less likely to benefit from osteotomy than patients with anatomic abnormalities that can be corrected by osteotomy or patients with areas of well-preserved cartilage that can be rotated to a weightbearing position of the hip while maintaining or improving joint congruence.

Greater Trochanteric Osteotomy The indications for greater trochanteric advancement are limited. The procedure can effectively relieve pain when trochanteric overgrowth or a foreshortened femoral neck leaves the tip of the trochanter (and therefore the insertion of the abductor muscles) in a biomechanically disadvantageous position. Such patients may have discomfort as a result of abductor muscle fatigue that can be relieved by trochanteric advancement to a more distal and lateral position.

Resection Arthroplasty

Resection arthroplasty may relieve pain from advanced hip disease, but for most patients the procedure provides poorer function than total hip arthroplasty, osteotomy, or arthrode-

sis. Shortening of the limb is expected, and most patients require external support for ambulation. Oxygen consumption has been reported to be more than 200% higher than for patients with normal hips. This procedure is most commonly used to treat infected or unreconstructable hip arthroplasty. As a primary procedure, resection arthroplasty is typically reserved for patients with severe hip pain and advanced hip disease, who by virtue of underlying diagnosis or functional or medical status are not candidates for a reconstructive hip procedure.

Osteonecrosis

ON, also referred to as avascular necrosis, aseptic necrosis, and ischemic necrosis, is a poorly understood condition in which circulation to a specific area of bone is impaired, leading to death of marrow and bone cells and eventually to collapse of the necrotic segment. Displaced femoral neck fractures are the most common cause of ON, but this section focuses primarily on nontraumatic ON in adults, where the diagnosis and management are much more difficult than in posttraumatic ON.

This condition most commonly affects adults between 20 and 50 years of age. The femoral head is most often involved. The condition is bilateral in over 60% of patients, and in approximately 15% other bones are affected, most frequently the humeral head, knee, talus, and small bones of the hands and feet. ON is being diagnosed with increasing frequency because of both an increased incidence and a greater awareness. It has been estimated that approximately 10,000 to 20,000 new cases of ON are diagnosed annually in the United States and that 10% of primary total hip replacements are done for ON.

Etiology

ON develops after approximately 10% of undisplaced femoral neck fractures, 15% to 30% of displaced fractures, and 10% of hip dislocations. In displaced fractures, it is caused by tearing of the vessels supplying the femoral head. In dislocation, mechanical compression of vessels also occurs; therefore, prompt reduction of a dislocated hip is essential, preferably within 6 hours of injury, to decrease the incidence of ON.

Several mechanisms have been implicated in nontraumatic ON. These include external compression of vessels, venous thrombosis, arterial embolization, and primary diseases of or injury to regional vessels. A number of conditions and factors have been associated with ON, although the mechanism of action is not always clear. Excess alcohol intake and prolonged high doses of corticosteroids have been implicated in approximately 70% of patients and may act by increasing or altering circulating lipids and coagulation mechanisms. In the past, 15% to 20% of cases have been labeled "idiopathic," but with increasing knowledge about etiologic factors, this number is steadily decreasing. The relationship to sickle cell anemia, dysbarism, and Gaucher's disease is well established, but the number of patients who fall into these categories is relatively small in the North American population. A number of medical conditions have been associated with ON, such as systemic lupus erythematosus (SLE), gastrointestinal disorders, allergic conditions, and organ transplantation. Although vascular pathology may occur in some, the most likely common denominator is corticosteroid administration. A certain minimal dose and duration of steroid is required to induce ON; however, the exact amount has not been conclusively determined, and there is a marked difference in the sensitivity of patients to this and other insults. It is presumed that certain patients have an underlying proclivity for the development of ON; however, it is not always clear just what factors may be involved. Recently it has been noted that up to 75% of patients with ON have subtle coagulation defects not diagnosed by routine testing. These include thrombophilia, an increased tendency to form blood clots, and hypofibrinolysis, a relative inability to dissolve clots that have already formed. Studies have also shown increased or abnormal circulating lipids in many patients with ON. Other factors may be identified in the future. A recent study of corticosteroid-induced ON in an animal model demonstrated efficacy of prophylaxis with a lipid clearing agent.

Pathogenesis

Within 6 to 12 hours after the vascular insult, death of marrow elements occurs. Death of bone, diagnosed by absent osteocytes, may not become apparent for several days. Bone and not articular cartilage is affected initially, because cartilage receives its nourishment from synovial fluid and not the intraosseous circulation. Increased intraosseous pressure has been measured in the femoral head and neck and may contribute to the development of necrosis. An attempt at repair takes place. Necrotic material is removed and new bone is formed directly on old dead trabeculae. Usually there is more bone removal than formation, which leads to mechanical weakness of the necrotic segment. If this is small and not near a weightbearing surface, spontaneous healing often occurs. If the area of necrosis is large and is in a region of high stress, spontaneous healing is unlikely and collapse of the articular surface usually occurs within 6 to 12 months of the insult. This occurs in approximately 80% of patients with clinically diagnosed ON

and, in turn, leads to increased pain and disability, damage to articular cartilage, acetabular involvement, and eventually to secondary arthritis of the hip. Approximately 70% of untreated patients eventually require some form of arthroplasty.

Diagnosis

Although there is no completely satisfactory method of treating ON, results are considerably better if treatment is started well before the femoral head has begun to collapse. Early diagnosis is therefore essential. The most important factor in making a diagnosis is to have a high index of suspicion and to be aware of the predisposing factors that are associated with ON in over 80% of patients.

The clinical picture of ON is nonspecific. Early after a vascular insult the joint is asymptomatic and may remain so if the lesion is small. Pain usually develops gradually and may be related to increased intraosseous pressure. A sudden increase in pain often is associated with collapse of the articular surface. Eventually the patient may develop a limp and decreased range of motion.

Most routine laboratory studies are negative, although the diagnosis of sickle cell anemia and SLE can be made by appropriate tests. Patients should be evaluated for abnormal amounts of circulating lipids and special testing for coagulopathies may be indicated. These include screening for decreased levels of proteins C and S and antithrombin III, as well as increased levels of plasminogen activator inhibitor-1. At present these tests may not be available at all centers.

Routine, good quality AP and lateral radiographs of both hips and any other suspected joints are essential. Often these are diagnostic of ON. Radiographic changes do not generally appear until at least 3 months after the insult. The earliest findings may include subtle osteopenia, but more frequently there is a mottled appearance of the anterosuperior aspect of the femoral head, consisting of patchy areas of sclerosis and lucency. These are related to regions of bone formation and resorption. Later a sclerotic rim may form around the necrotic segment. In some patients, collapse of trabeculae beneath the subchondral plate produces a radiolucent crescent sign. Still later, the articular surface becomes flattened. Secondary degenerative changes follow, with joint space narrowing and eventually sclerosis and "cyst" formation in the acetabulum associated with marginal osteophytes (Fig. 6). If bilateral hip involvement is noted on plain radiographs, further studies rarely are required. If ON is suspected, but is not seen on radiographs, or if ON is seen in only 1 hip, an MRI of both hips should be obtained. The sensitivity and specificity of this study is over 95% and MRI is the single best test for the early diagnosis of ON. Limited coronal sections with T1-weighted

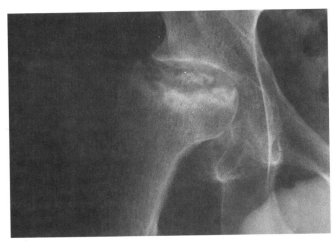

Figure 6

Radiograph showing extensive collapse of femoral head with early joint line narrowing, stage VB.

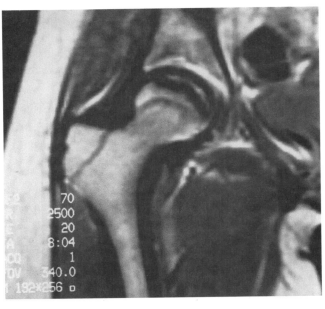

Figure 7

Magnetic resonance imaging scan of patient with stage IA osteonecrosis of the right hip. Plain films were normal.

imaging usually are sufficient to make the diagnosis, and a full sequence rarely is needed (Fig. 7). Other conditions that affect the femoral head, such as transient osteoporosis of the hip (also referred to as bone marrow edema syndrome), usually can be ruled out.

Staging

Once ON has been diagnosed it is important to determine the type and extent of involvement by means of an effective system of staging. This enables the orthopaedist to establish a prognosis, determine the best method of treatment, follow the progression or resolution of the condition, and evaluate and compare the effectiveness of various methods of treatment. A number of different staging systems have been described. The one most commonly used at present was described initially in the 1960s by Arlet and Ficat and modified twice since then. The latest version, published in 1985, is shown in Table 1. Bone biopsies, pressure measurements, and angiography were used to determine preradiographic ON. MRI was not specifically included. No attempt was made to quantitate lesion size. By 1982 a quantitative system of staging had been developed at the University of Pennsylvania, which included MRI, did not incorporate invasive diagnostic techniques or symptomatology, and enabled quantitative measurement of the size of the lesion in both early and late stages (Table 2). This system provides several advantages and in particular has documented the importance of lesion size in determining prognosis and treatment. It has long been recognized that the use of a standardized international system of staging would provide several advantages, including the ability to compare the effectiveness of various methods of treatment. To this end, the University of Pennsylvania System was endorsed in 1991 by the Association Research Circulation Osseous (ARCO) and subsequently modified in 1992 and 1993.

Treatment: Early

Prevention is, of course, the best treatment and risk factors, such as steroids, should be avoided or minimized. Medical treatment may be indicated for patients with coagulopathies and lipid abnormalities.

In approximately 80% of clinically diagnosed cases, the natural course of untreated ON is one of steady progression. The goal is, therefore, to make an early diagnosis and to treat the condition so as to retard progression and preserve the femoral head.

Symptomatic Treatment and Restricted Weightbearing
"Conservative" treatment relying on restricted weightbearing is generally ineffective. However, very small asymptomatic lesions and those located in the medial aspect of the femoral head have a much better prognosis and may heal spontaneously without specific treatment. Restricted weightbearing using a cane or crutches is indicated primarily as a symptomatic treatment for patients in whom definitive prophylactic surgery is not indicated and who are not yet ready for hip

Table 1
Ficat stages of necrosis

Stage	Clinical Features	Radiographic Signs	Bone Scan	Abnormal Hemodynamics	Diagnosis Without Core Biopsy
Early					
0, Preclinical	0	0	Decreased uptake?	+	Impossible
I, Preradiographic	0 or +	0	Increased uptake	++	Impossible
II, Before flattening of head or sequestrum	+	Diffuse porosis, sclerosis or cysts	+	++	Probable
Transition		Flattening crescent sign			
Late					
III,Collapse	++	Broken contour of head Sequestrum Normal joint space	+	+ or normal	Certain
IV, Osteoarthritis	+++	Collapse of head Decreased joint space	+	+	Arthritis

(Reproduced with permission from Ficat RP: Idiopathic bone necrosis of the femoral head. *J Bone Joint Surg* 1985;67B:3—9.)

reconstruction. This includes patients with advanced stages of ON as well as those with earlier stages whose prognosis and life expectancy is such that a total hip replacement (THR) will most likely be the definitive procedure required.

Electrical Stimulation Different types of electrical signals have been used to treat ON, either alone or as an adjunct to decompression and grafting. Direct current and capacitive coupling have not demonstrated a clear benefit, whereas a small number of investigators have noted a beneficial effect with pulsing electromagnetic fields applied externally without adjunctive surgery. Different signals are available and it should be noted that these results were achieved with a specific signal designed to treat ON. Further study of this investigational method is needed to determine its efficacy.

Decompression Because increased intraosseous pressure has been found in conjunction with ON, a variety of procedures

have been designed to decompress the femoral head. "Core decompression" was first described in 1964 by Arlet and Ficat and involves removal of an 8- to 10-mm core of bone from the femoral head and neck. In addition to providing decompression, this also establishes a pathway for vascular ingrowth and stimulates new bone formation. This is perhaps the most commonly used procedure for the treatment of ON, although it remains somewhat controversial. It often provides prompt relief of pain, even in hips in which ON progresses. It can be supplemented by the addition of bone graft and by various agents used to stimulate bone formation, such as bone morphogenetic protein and demineralized bone matrix. It is a simple and safe procedure, although reports on its effectiveness vary considerably. A recent extensive review of the literature compared 1,206 hips treated by core decompression to 819 treated nonsurgically. Satisfactory clinical results were achieved in 64% of those treated with core decompression versus only 23% treated nonsurgically. In

Table 2
University of Pennsylvania system for staging osteonecrosis

Stage	Criteria	
0	Normal or nondiagnostic radiograph, bone scan, and MRI	
I	Normal radiograph; abnormal bone scan and/or MRI	
	A-Mild	(< 15% of head affected)
	B-Moderate	(15% to 30%)
	C-Severe	(> 30%)
II	Lucent and sclerotic changes in femoral head	
	A-Mild	(< 15%)
	B-Moderate	(15% to 30%)
	C-Severe	(> 30%)
III	Subchondral collapse (crescent sign) without flattening	
	A-Mild	(< 15% of articular surface)
	B-Moderate	(15% to 30%)
	C-Severe	(> 30%)
IV	Flattening of femoral head	
	A-Mild	(< 15% of surface or < 2 mm depression)
	B-Moderate	(15% to 30% of surface or 2 to 4 mm depression)
	C-Severe	(> 30% of surface or > 4 mm depression)
V	Joint narrowing and/or acetabular changes	
	A-Mild	(Average of femoral head
	B-Moderate	involvement as determined
	C-Severe	in Stage IV, and estimated acetabular involvement)
VI	Advanced degenerative changes	

MRI, magnetic resonance imaging (Reproduced with permission from Urbaniak JR, Jones JP (eds): *Osteonecrosis: Etiology, Diagnosis and Treatment.* Rosemont, IL, American Academy of Orthopaedic Surgeons, 1997, p 279.)

hips treated before femoral head collapse, satisfactory results were found in 71% and 35%, respectively. In other more recent studies, these findings were confirmed and a distinct relationship was noted between outcome and lesion size as well as stage. In 1 study, in stages I and II, good results were achieved in 80% of hips with less than 15% head involvement

compared to 60% satisfactory results in hips with more than 15% head involvement.

Bone Grafting A large number of grafting procedures have been described. Generally a portion of necrotic bone is removed and replaced with cancellous or cortical graft. This can be done by going directly through the articular surface of the femoral head, the "trap door" procedure; through the neck; or through the lateral cortex of the proximal femur. These procedures combine the advantages of core decompression with those of bone grafting, which helps stimulate vascular ingrowth and new bone formation. When cortical struts are used, they also provide mechanical support to prevent femoral head collapse. Recently there has been considerable interest in the use of a vascularized fibular graft. At 1 institution, this procedure has been performed over 1,000 times and has given satisfactory clinical results in 80% of the patients treated before femoral head collapse and in 70% of those treated even after collapse. This procedure is difficult and time consuming and requires special equipment and experience. Complications may occur in 13% to 20% of patients. It appears to hold promise for certain patients with ON but it should not be undertaken lightly because the specific indications for this procedure have yet to be defined.

Osteotomy Different types of osteotomies have been used to treat ON with variable and often temporary results. These results were discussed earlier.

Treatment: Late
If a patient is first encountered after significant femoral head collapse has occurred, stage IV-B or beyond, especially if accompanied by pain, a limp, and a decreased range of motion, the hip may well be beyond the point where the prophylactic measures just described are likely to be of benefit. These patients usually are treated symptomatically until such time as reconstructive surgery is required.

Femoral Endoprostheses Because ON affects primarily the femoral head and not the acetabulum, it is tempting to consider replacing only the femoral head with either a unipolar or bipolar endoprosthesis rather than a THR. This approach is still used by many experienced surgeons. However, even a normal acetabulum is not designed to accept a metal bearing surface and in virtually all hips that require arthroplasty, the acetabular cartilage is no longer normal. Studies comparing results with endoprostheses to THR clearly favor the latter.

Cup or Surface Replacement Arthroplasty (SRA) Standard cup arthroplasty or SRA is a procedure previously used as an alternative to THR. Results were inferior and this procedure was for the most part abandoned. Recently there has been a renewed interest in a hemisurface replacement in which the femoral head alone is resurfaced with a metal or ceramic cup, with or without a small stem. The acetabulum is left intact. With improved techniques and components, recognizing the importance of fitting the acetabulum as closely as possible, the preliminary results with this approach have been gratifying. More cases with longer follow-up will be required to determine whether this is to become a standard approach for patients with ON.

Total Hip Replacement Older reports on THR in patients with ON were disappointing and indicated a significantly higher failure rate than in patients with other disorders. However, more recent reports in which new techniques and devices were used indicate a better outcome in ON and less difference between these patients and age-matched controls with other diagnoses. Results with THR are significantly better than with femoral endoprostheses. Despite the concerns about performing THR in younger patients with ON, it usually is the procedure of choice when reconstructive surgery is needed. With improvements in components and techniques, the durability of a THR should increase steadily, making surgeons less reluctant to perform THR in younger patients who have ON.

Miscellaneous Procedures Rarely, a patient with an advanced stage of ON requires hip reconstruction but is not a candidate for THR. Two procedures that might be considered in selected situations are resection arthroplasty and arthrodesis. Indications and contraindications for these procedures must be kept clearly in mind.

Total Hip Arthroplasty

Total hip arthroplasty (THA) is one of the most successful surgical procedures. More than 120,000 primary THAs are performed in the United States each year at an estimated cost of over 2.5 billion dollars. Because most hip replacements are done in patients older than 65 years of age, the number of procedures is expected to increase as the population ages. The utility of THA has been well documented in a variety of outcome studies that have documented marked improvements in pain, sleep, range of motion, and physical ability after THA. Overall, the data have documented that there is a significant improvement in functional status and quality of life. However, there is some disagreement as to how these patients fare compared to their "healthy" counterparts of similar age. Data from 1 study suggested that after surgery, patients were less healthy than the

general population of the same age. In contrast, in another study the life expectancy of patients with THA was actually greater than that of their counterparts, with 78% of patients surviving an additional 10 years after age 65.

Measuring Outcome

Recently, much attention has been placed on outcome measures. Historically, the surgeon or another medical professional evaluated outcomes, but more recently emphasis has been placed on the importance of the patient evaluating his or her own outcome as much as possible. This is based on the fact that there is perceived or real bias when physicians are the evaluators. A recent study showed that patient and physician evaluations of outcome after THA were similar when the patients had little or no pain and were satisfied with their results. However, as the level of the patients' overall satisfaction decreased, the disparity increased between the patients' rating of pain and the physicians' rating.

Several possible explanations for the differences between patients' and physicians' evaluations have been suggested. First, and perhaps most important, is the difference between their expectations for the procedure. The physician and patient may have different definitions of what constitutes a good outcome. In addition, the patients may not state their problems clearly for fear of disappointing their physicians. There may be a comprehension problem between a patient's statement of his or her problem and the physician's understanding of that problem. Finally, the quality of the physician/patient relationship may influence the patient's level of satisfaction significantly. Currently, most researchers are using a combination of patient self-administered questionnaires and physician-generated assessment to provide a more complete evaluation of outcome.

Another problem in measuring outcomes is the difference in definitions used to define failure. The failure rate reported depends on how failure is defined, and several criteria have been used, including revision surgery, clinical failure (a painful arthroplasty), and radiographic failure. Assessment of these variables is not uniform among authors. The need for revision surgery depends on the operating surgeon's indications for revision, for example, severe pain, moderate pain, or bone loss in the absence of pain. Clinical function may depend on who is doing the evaluation and what scoring system is used. Historically, these have not included the patient's assessment of failure or success. Radiographic failure depends on the criteria used for definition of a loose implant.

Cost

In terms of the cost-benefit analysis, THA is one of the most beneficial surgical procedures currently performed. A study demonstrated that the actual cost of THA rose 46.5% between 1981 and 1990. However, when this was adjusted for inflation, it represented a real increase of only 1.9%. During that same time period, costs associated with the implant grew 212%, for a real increase after inflation of 117%. Implant costs in 1990 represented 24% of the total cost associated with the procedure versus 11% in 1981. These data show the important role the surgeon has played in decreasing nonimplant-related costs, mainly through shorter hospital stays and more judicious use of ancillary services.

Third party payers, including the government, have a keen interest in cost and variables that relate to cost. Several studies have looked at the relationships between the volume of THRs performed by providers and mortality, morbidity, and hospital charges, which have some relationship to actual cost. One study used a comprehensive hospital abstract reporting system that is a computerized data set of the Washington State Department of Health to examine the relationship between volume of hip replacements performed by surgeons and hospitals and the postoperative rate of complications. The rate of surgical complications was modeled as the function of the volume of procedures performed by the surgeon or hospital with adjustment for age of the patient, gender, comorbidity, and surgical diagnosis. There was a significant difference in case mix of the low volume providers compared to that of the high volume providers. Surgeons and hospitals with a volume below the fortieth percentile had a more adverse risk profile in terms of age and comorbidity. However, after adjusting for this, surgeons who averaged fewer than 2 hip replacements annually had a worse outcome. They tended to have higher mortality rates, more infections, higher rates of revision operations, and more serious complications.

In another study in which similar data were examined, the hospitals and doctors were arbitrarily divided into 3 case volume groups (low, medium, and high). Surgeons with a low volume of primary cases (fewer than 10) had a significantly higher mortality rate, higher average charges, and increased length of stay. The results were similar with revision cases.

These studies suggest that the outcome of a surgical procedure such as THA is related to the surgeon's experience as well as the experience of the hospital. However, these data were not collected for purposes of scientific evaluations. The data collection process used by these agencies focuses on economic aspects of medicine. In addition, the accuracy of the coding has not been validated. In many centers, for example, a revision surgery automatically has a complication code associated with that surgery. On the other hand, posthospital complications such as dislocation or pulmonary embolus cannot be tracked. Current algorithms consider only medical factors

and neglect orthopaedic aspects of the case, such as the technical difficulty of the arthroplasty. A patient with a significant femoral deformity requiring osteotomy would have the same severity of illness score as a patient with normal anatomy provided their medical condition was similar.

Cemented Acetabular Components: Metal-Backed Versus All Polyethylene

Metal-backed acetabular components were initially designed so that the polyethylene would be exchangeable. Finite element studies supported the concept of metal backing in that it more evenly distributed forces throughout the cement mantle. In vitro laboratory testing using strain gauge analysis has subsequently supported this hypothesis. However, clinical studies have not demonstrated superior outcomes with metal backing of the acetabular component compared with cemented all polyethylene components. In a study of THAs with cemented titanium stems and cemented acetabular components, one patient group had metal-backed components and another group had all-polyethylene cups. Wear, loosening, and revision rates were compared between these 2 groups. In the metal-backed group, both the linear wear and volumetric wear were greater. In addition, the metal-backed components showed increased rates of radiolucency, loosening, and revision. There were some unique features to the design of this cemented component. The surface finish of the metal-backed component was relatively smooth. Some of these implants failed at the metal-cement interface and not at the bone-cement interface. This raises questions about the strength of the metal-cement interface and supports the suggestion that the surface finish may play a role in the failure of this particular component. Despite that, no series has documented superior results with metal-backed cemented components.

Other aspects of acetabular component design may be important variables, although autopsy studies demonstrated that the mechanism of failure of cemented acetabular components is primarily a biologic event rather than a mechanical event. Therefore, improving the stress distribution of the cement may not be as important on the acetabular side as it is in the femoral side. Flanged acetabular components have been reported to have a decreased radiolucency when compared to standard components. This supports the hypothesis that particle-induced bone resorption at the cement-bone interface is a likely mechanism of failure for cemented components, because the flanged components may actually reduce access to the interface.

Although metal backing has an influence on the load transfer and stress distribution through the cement mantle, it likely does not impact the mechanism of failure of these implants. Autopsy studies have demonstrated that cemented components fail primarily at the cement-bone interface. Bone resorption begins circumferentially at the outer edge of the component and progresses toward the dome of the acetabulum. The bone resorption at the cement-bone interface appears to be the result of the biologic response to polyethylene wear debris. There is essentially an extension of the pseudocapsule that resorbs bone along this interface. Although changes in cementing technique have produced no clear improvement in the long-term results of cemented components, 1 study showed that the state of the cement-bone interface on the early postoperative radiograph was predictive of longevity. Only 2.2% of components graded as well-fixed on early postoperative radiographs were loose at final follow-up. In contrast, the rate of aseptic loosening for those components graded as not well-fixed on early radiographs was 14.4%.Patient-related factors that tend to be associated with higher failure rates of cemented acetabular components include heavy weight, young age, and diagnosis of posttraumatic arthritis or ON.

Cement Fixation: The Femoral Side

The results of cemented THA, especially on the femoral side, have been related to surgical cementing technique. It is less clear that changes in cementing technique have had any effect on the long-term results of cemented acetabular replacement. Better results have been documented with improved femoral cementing techniques, such as plugging the distal canal and injecting the cement retrograde with a cement delivery system. Of 90 patients (102 hips) who were alive 14 or more years after surgery, 1 had had both hips revised (2%) because of bilateral aseptic loosening of the femoral component. An additional 7 femoral components (7%) were loose radiographically but were not revised.

In another study, patients younger than 51 years at the time of surgery did as well as the group as a whole. Only 1 patient in this group of 51 consecutive THAs in a group of patients aged 50 or younger required revision for femoral loosening. Two additional components were loose radiographically. Again, the rate of aseptic loosening on the acetabular side was much higher in this group.

In a follow-up of Charnley THAs using so-called second generation cementing technique, revision of the femoral component for aseptic loosening was required in 4 (1%) of the entire series of 356 hips and

in 3 (2%) of the 142 hips in 130 patients who survived at least 15 years. Failure of the femoral component, defined as aseptic loosening leading to revision or definite or probable radiographic loosening, occurred in 10 of 356 hips (3%)and in 6 of 116 hips (5%) of which radiographs were made at least 15 years after surgery. Acetabular component revision for aseptic loosening was required in 17 (5%) of the entire series and in 14 (10%) of the 142 hips in patients who survived at least 15 years. In addition, aseptic loosening of the acetabular component occurred in 41 of the 356 hips (12%)and in 26 of the 116 hips (22%)for which radiographs were made available at 15 years. These findings support the concept that long-term durability of the femoral component can be achieved with cementing, but cement fixation on the acetabular side is less reliable even when the surgeon is experienced and improved techniques of cementing are used.

Recent attempts have been made to grade the cement mantle and to look at the effect of cement mantle thickness on long-term results. In one commonly used grading system the cement mantles are graded on a scale of A through D (Table 3). A 15-year study demonstrated that femoral implants graded C2 had a statistically significantly higher aseptic loosening than the combined group of implants graded A, B, and C1. Despite the widespread use of this grading system, the relationship of cement grade with implant survivorship has not been established. Moreover grading of a cement mantle depends on the quality of the radiographs and the number of views obtained.

Because newer generation cementing techniques (porosity

Table 3
Grading of the cement mantle in total hip arthroplasty

Grade	Radiographic Appearance
A	Complete filling of proximal portion of medullary canal of diaphysis; no distinction between cortical bone and bone cement ("white-out")
B	Complete distribution, but cortical bone and cement can be distinguished in some areas
C1	Extensive radiolucent line of more than 50% of cement-bone interface or voids in cement
C2	Thin (< 1 mm) mantle; mantle defect in which metal is in direct contact with cortical bone
D	Gross deficiencies of mantle, such as no cement distal to tip of stem, major defects in mantle, or multiple large voids

reduction, bond-enhancing surface finishes) are relatively new, there are few long-term follow up reports in the literature. In 3 studies of a hybrid hip replacement with a cemented femoral component and a cementless acetabular component, mechanical failure rates ranged from 1% to 5% with no clear reasons for the different rates.

Technical factors, such as varus positioning of the implant, mantle defects, and lack of cement distal to the tip of the implant, have been implicated as causes of premature loosening. To assure an adequate cement mantle it is important to know the relationship of the rasp and stem for the system being used because this will determine the appropriate thickness of the cement mantle. Reaming of the femoral canal is not advised with the use of a cemented femoral component because reaming transforms a rough, irregular endosteal surface into a smooth surface, which decreases the shear strength at the cement-bone interface.

Although cementing technique is important in the long-term outcome of cemented femoral components, it is likely that there is a complex interaction between cementing technique and stem design, including such variables as the cross-sectional geometry, length, offset, and surface finish of the stem. There is no consensus on the optimal surface finish for cemented femoral components. In general, 3 different surface finishes have been used for cemented femoral components: polished, matte finish, and grit blasted. The surface roughness (RA) can be measured in microinches, with a polished stem typically less than 10 RA, a matte finish stem approximately 30 RA, and a grit blasted stem 80 RA or greater. In a clinical report, the authors noted a higher failure rate in Iowa femoral components with a matte surface than had been reported for components with a smooth surface. They postulated that the geometry, a cylindric distal shape, and the surface finish were responsible for the progressive pattern of loosening seen in this series. The most recent follow-up report on this group of patients noted a mechanical failure rate of 6.9% on the femoral side at 8 to 9 years after surgery.

Cementless Fixation

Cementless implants were developed in hopes of eliminating periprosthetic bone resorption ("cement disease"), but the use of cementless components did not eliminate the problem of periprosthetic bone resorption or osteolysis. In addition, first generation cementless designs were associated with thigh pain, rapid polyethylene wear, and stress shielding.

Second generation designs and improvements in surgical technique have corrected many problems. The importance of obtaining both axial and rotational stability is now well understood. Implant design and instrumentation have evolved to ensure that the implant is inserted in a stable fashion in most patients. This has resulted in a much higher percentage of bone ingrowth as determined by radiographic evaluation and autopsy studies.

Porous Coated Acetabular Components

In general, the results of porous coated acetabular components have been encouraging. At 5 to 10 years, the revision rates for aseptic loosening have been low. The main problem associated with porous coated acetabular components has been accelerated polyethylene wear in some patients. This is a multifactorial problem that includes issues related to design, femoral head size, patient variables, and surgical technique. If excessive polyethylene wear can be avoided, these devices will offer more durable fixation than offered by cemented components.

Autopsy studies have demonstrated that reliable bone ingrowth can be obtained with these implants. Unlike early studies in which the percent of bone ingrowth into the pore space of porous coated components was examined in failed THAs, more recent autopsy studies evaluated the remodeling that occurs at the interface between bone and metal in clinically successful THAs. These studies routinely demonstrated that a high percentage of porous coating is in direct apposition with periprosthetic bone. In addition, they also demonstrate a higher percentage of ingrowth of bone into the pore space than did the early studies.

Several reports of the Harris-Galante type I acetabular component (Zimmer, Warsaw, IN) inserted without cement have been published. In a series of 204 consecutive primary hip arthroplasties performed using this acetabular component, 173 hips were available for clinical review at a mean of 104 months after surgery. Two patients had an exchange of an excessively worn polyethylene liner and 1 had debridement and grafting of a osteolytic lesion. None of the cups required revision for aseptic loosening.

In another series, 136 consecutive primary THAs were reviewed at a mean of 7 years after surgery. The acetabular components had been revised for loosening and none were radiographically loose. There were no complications related to the use of screws, and no screw had bent or broken. The mean rate of polyethylene wear in this group of patients was 0.1 mm/year. Finally, there were no dissociations of the acetabular liner in this series. Two patients did have asymptomatic osteolysis of the ischium and adjacent rim of the acetabulum, which was treated with exchange of the acetabular liner and grafting of the lesions.

The results of the porous coated anatomic (PCA) component (Howmedica, Rutherford, NJ) have been more variable. This component is a metal backed 1-piece chrome cobalt acetabular component with polyethylene and metal preassembled at the factory. It has beads sintered to the metal backing and 2 pegs to supplement initial fixation. Many of the components were mated to 32-mm femoral heads. In one study, 6 of 100 of the acetabular components had migrated, but only 2 had been revised between 5 and 7 years after surgery. In contrast, failure was reported of 23 (12%) of 199 PCA acetabular components because of either migration or severe osteolysis. Osteolysis was correlated with duration of implantation and was significantly greater with acetabular components that had an outer diameter of 55 mm or less (polyethylene thickness of less than 8.5 mm). Thirteen of the hips were revised at a mean of 69.5 months after the initial operation. Examination of retrieved acetabular components revealed extensive polyethylene damage on the articular and back surfaces of the liner.

In another study, revision for aseptic loosening of uncemented cups was used as an end point in analysis of 4,352 primary THAs done with the 11 porous-coated acetabular components most commonly used in that country. The overall cumulative revision rates of acetabular components were 3.2% after 5 years and 7.1% after 6 years. With hydroxyapatite (HA) coated cups and hemispheric porous coated cups the failure rate was less than 0.1%. Of the 626 unthreaded hemispheric porous coated cups (Harris-Galante, Zimmer, Warsaw, IN and Gemini, DePuy, Warsaw, IN) none had been revised and of the 1,943 HA coated cups, (Atoll and Tropic, Landes, Chaumont, France) only 1 had been revised. In contrast, there was great variation in the performance of threaded uncoated metal-backed components. The PM (Aesculap, Tuttlingen, Germany) had no revisions compared with a 21% revision rate at 6 years for the Ti-Fit (Richards, Memphis, TN) components. An all polyethylene uncemented component had a cumulative revision rate of 14%.

Surgical technique for implantation of hemispheric porous coated acetabular components has evolved over the past decade. At first, most components were implanted using a line-to line surgical reaming technique, in which the acetabulum was reamed to the same size as the component. This technique required some form of supplemental fixation, such as pegs, spikes, or screws, for initial implant stability. Currently most porous coated acetabular components are implanted with a "press fit" technique, in which the component is larger than the last reamer used. The "press fit" provides implant stability and often, no supplemental fixation is used. Good results have been reported with both techniques at 5 years after implantation of the Harris-Galante I (Zimmer, Warsaw, IN) components. Further follow-up is necessary to ensure that both techniques provide reliable bony ingrowth.

The role of screws and screw holes in the etiology of osteol-

ysis remains controversial. Retrieval studies have documented small granulomas in the screw holes, and wear debris can potentially gain access to the pelvis through screw holes. However, a study of multiple factors, including cup design and the presence of screws and screw holes, and their association with pelvic osteolysis did not show a detrimental effect of screws or screw holes in the acetabular components. The first priority at the time of implantation is to obtain a stable construct. The implant must be rigidly fixed to sustain physiologic loads and not allow motion at the interface if bone ingrowth is to occur. Screws are one way to improve the chances of ingrowth occurring.

Threaded Acetabular Components

The reported results of threaded acetabular components in North America have been disappointing. One study showed an 85% cup survivorship at 4 years after primary surgery and only 52% survivorship after revision. Another review of a different titanium cup revealed 31% of primary cups had been revised or were pending revision at 5 to 9 years. Based on these reports, threaded acetabular components have not gained popularity in North America.

In Europe, however, some threaded acetabular components are quite popular, but results vary greatly depending on the cup used and the center implanting them. An independent report evaluated 300 uncoated cementless PM (Aesculap, Tuttlingen, Germany) prostheses and found survivorship rates of 93% at 4 to 7 years and 84% at 7 to 8 years.

The Zweymuller (Allo Pro AG, Baar, Switzerland) truncated self-tapered threaded ring is made of pure titanium with a 3 to 5 µm grit blasted surface roughness. Of 167 consecutive primary THAs done with these threaded components, 2 failed to achieve initial stability, with 1 requiring almost immediate revision. In 126 hips followed for a minimum of 5 years, the average Harris hip score at 7 years was 91 points. At 9 to 10 years, the implant survivorship with definite loosening as the end point was 98.7%.

In a report on the Integral (Biomet, Warsaw, IN) porous femoral component, 179 patients were reviewed. Thirty-two percent of the hips were implanted with a threaded titanium plasma sprayed hemispherical cup. In this subset, the failure rate of the socket was 22% (32 hips). The authors believed that the use of 28- and 32-mm titanium femoral heads as well as thin polyethylene liners, with first generation components (nonconforming shell liner contact and inadequate locking mechanism) contributed significantly to these failures.

Extensively Porous Coated Stems

The longest follow-up of extensively porous coated stems in North America has been with the anatomic medullary locking (AML, DePuy, Warsaw, IN) prosthesis, a cobalt-chrome stem with a cobalt-chrome beaded fixation surface. In a recent report of 167 patients (174 hips), who were followed for a minimum of 10 years, there were 20 reoperations involving a component. At 12 years after surgery, the rate of survival was 0.97 ± 0.02 (mean ± standard error) for the stem and 0.92 ± 0.03 for the cup . There was a statistically significant increase in the rate of osteolysis in younger patients, who also had a statistically significant higher reoperation rate. The most frequent cause of reoperation in this group was severe polyethylene wear of the acetabular component.

Of the 147 patients (154 hips) who did not have an exchange of a component, 87% reported no pain or mild pain that did not limit activity, 10% had pain that occasionally limited activity, and 3% had pain that always limited activity. Fifty-three percent of the patients stated that they had no limitations with relation to the hip, and an additional 31% said that they had only slight limitations. Of the 117 surviving femoral components, 90% had bone ingrowth, and an additional 8% had a stable fibrous interface; only 2% were definitely loose. With the addition of the 3 revised femoral components there was a total of 5 loose stems in this study.

Analysis of autopsy specimens with this implant in place indicated that a mean of 35% of the surface had bone ingrowth. In areas where bone was present, 67% of the pore space was occupied by bone on the extensively coated stems. The most bone ingrowth was at the level where the porous coating ended. This corresponds to the so-called "spot weld" seen on radiographic evaluation. These studies clearly show the potential of cobalt-chrome implants to become osseointegrated.

Proximally Porous Coated Stems

First generation proximally porous coated stems, in general, have not performed as well as first generation extensively porous coated stems. Often these stems had patched porous coating or limited areas of ingrowth surface, increasing rates of loosening or failure to become osseointegrated. In addition, the prevalence of diaphyseal osteolysis has been associated with patch porous coating. It is hypothesized that the patched porous coating allows ingress of joint fluid and wear debris into the endosteal canal and therefore contributes to the process.

The Harris-Galante (Zimmer, Warsaw, IN) porous coated femoral component is a titanium alloy implant with patched porous coating on the anterior, posterior, and medial aspects of the implant. In a report of 100 consecutive THAs with these components 4.8 years after surgery, 2 femoral components were revised for aseptic loosening, and 6% of patients had moderate thigh pain. Ingrowth was classified as bony in 89%, stable fibrous in 8%, and unstable in 3%. However, a pedestal formed

in 18%, measurable subsidence occurred in 22%, and endosteal erosion occurred in 12%. Up to 50% of these implants have demonstrated endosteal erosion in some studies.

The anatomic porous replacement (APR-I) hip system (Intermedics Orthopaedics, Austin, TX) was also a titanium implant. It was designed for metaphyseal bone attachment and had proximal patch porous coating. The results of 100 consecutive primary THAs were reported by 1 group at an average of 6.7 years after surgery. Selection for these implants was limited to patients in whom a satisfactory interoperative fit could be obtained. In contrast to the Harris-Galante and Multi-Lock (Zimmer, Warsaw, IN) stems, which are straight stems, the APR-I is a curved "anatomic" stem. Revision rate in this group of patients was 16%, with a mechanical failure rate of 11%. Seventy percent of the hips had progressive loss of fixation. Loss of fixation on the femoral side correlated with young patient age, higher patient activity level, and metaphyseal fill of less than 90%. The authors concluded that the APR-I stem failure rate was unacceptably high.

The PCA total hip prosthesis was another first generation cementless proximally porous coated implant in which the stem was made of chrome cobalt alloy. In a group of 100 primary PCA THAs followed for 5 to 7 years, the average Harris hip ratings were between 92 and 93 points. Ninety-four percent of femoral components were graded as ingrown by radiographic evaluation using the criteria of Engh and associates. Five percent of the femoral components had subsided and 1 femoral revision was pending.

In another group of 116 PCA implants, the average Harris hip score was 91 at a minimum of 6 years after surgery. Seven hips had confirmed loosening of the femoral component, with subsidence ranging from 13 to 20 mm; all of these required revision. Unlike previous groups, these authors correlated implant stability with good fit on the AP and lateral radiographs.

Cementless Tapered Stems

Tapered stems are designed to be wedged into the femoral canal to obtain implant stability. Early reports have been encouraging. A retrospective review of 314 Mallory-Head titanium femoral components at a mean follow-up of 3.7 years reported no femoral revisions for instability of the stem, pain, or femoral osteolysis. Of the stems, 11% had initial subsidence; however, it nearly always stabilized within 6 months and did not affect eventual stem stability. In a matched paired analysis, another group reported the effect of HA coating on the Taperloc stem. At a mean follow-up of 2.2 years, all stems in both groups were stable. The authors concluded there was no advantage to HA coating over the time period of the study. A study on bone remodeling compared a cobalt-chrome stem to a titanium alloy Trilock (DePuy, Warsaw, IN) stem. Both were radiographically stable at 3 to 4 years after surgery, and the difference in the modulus of elasticity between the 2 types of stems had little effect on the loss of bone mineral density in most of the proximal part of the femur.

Cementless Press Fit Stems: Nonporous

Several nonporous femoral components designed for insertion without cement are popular in Europe but have limited clinical use in North America. A review of 2,907 arthroplasties with uncemented femoral components indicated that, in the 8 designs used, the estimated probability of revision for aseptic loosening of 2 press-fit stems was more than 3 times that of the other 6 stems.

Hydroxyapatite-Coated Acetabular and Femoral Components

HA and tricalcium phosphate (TCP) are potentially resorbable compounds that may bond to bone directly. The osteoconductive properties of these substances have been well documented. Several methods are available for the application of HA coating to metal substrates, and the coating method affects the chemical, mechanical, and biologic properties of the coating. Techniques used for coating include dip coating, electrophoretic deposition, immersion coating, hot isostatic pressing, solution deposition, sputter coating, and flame spraying. Only the last 3 methods are used for application to orthopaedic implants.

Europeans have had a large experience with the use of HA-coated components. One of the more commonly used implants is a titanium femoral stem (Omnifit, Osteonics, Allentown, NJ) that has a 50µm thickness of plasma sprayed HA coating over the proximal third of the surface of the stem. In one report, the rate of survivorship for HA-coated prostheses at 6 years was 100% for the femoral component and 99% for the threaded acetabular component.

In a randomized prospective study, titanium alloy straight stems were implanted with either cement, HA coating, or porous coating. The HA applied to the proximal third of the surface was 200 µm thick. At 2 years, the clinical results did not differ with respect to Harris hip scores, but the HA coated components demonstrated less subsidence.

In a large North American clinical trial, 436 hip arthroplasties were done with grit blasted, straight, collarless titanium implants with a 50-µm thick air-plasma sprayed HA coating on the proximal third. The acetabular components were either porous-coated or HA coated and of 3 different designs. The investigators reported good results at 2, 3, and 5 years. At 5 years, the failure rate for mechanical loosening of the femoral component was only 0.46%. Two stems had been

revised for aseptic loosening and none were radiographically loose. Endosteal osteolysis was present in only one patient (0.8%).

Similar clinical and radiographic results with HA-coated stems and stems without HA coating have been reported in several other studies. Similarly, no clear benefit of HA coating has been demonstrated for acetabular components.

In a multicenter study, the failure rate of nonthreaded hemispheric HA-coated hemispheric components was 19%, while that of HA-coated threaded components was 3% and of non-HA porous coated components, 6%.

Remodeling around HA-coated implants has been studied radiographically and in retrieved implants. Proximally coated HA femoral components have a characteristic remodeling pattern, with frequent radiolucent lines around the distal uncoated portion of the stem and a few radiolucent lines around the HA-coated portion. Cancellous condensation at the distal extent of the coating resembles a "spot weld" around beaded chrome cobalt noncemented stems. In 2 prospective studies of proximally coated HA stems, dual energy X-ray absorptiometry demonstrated 8% to 12% decrease in bone mineral density in the proximal part of the femur between 18 and 24 months after surgery.

The results of analysis of retrieved HA coated components depends on the type of implant and on whether the implant is retrieved at revision surgery or at autopsy. One report of 14 implants retrieved for failure noted that HA particulate material was seen in the periprosthetic tissues and embedded in the surfaces of the polyethylene liner. This finding raised some concerns about the role of HA particles in accelerated polyethylene wear, which has not been demonstrated to be a problem in clinical studies. In general, data from autopsy studies have indicated that bone is in direct apposition to the implants. Resorption of HA coating has been identified, but delamination has not been demonstrated to be a major problem. Some studies of failed implants, however, have revealed delamination of the coating as well as HA debris. Some of these stems may have failed because of the failure of the HA coating, but stem failure may have been related to other factors, such as infection, malposition, or excessive wear of the polyethylene, which damaged the HA coating.

Total Hip Arthroplasty Complications

Pain

Although THA is one of the most successful procedures in orthopaedic surgery, a small percentage of patients have pain after surgery. A systematic approach to the evaluation of this pain, with careful attention to the patient's history, physical examination, and laboratory and radiographic studies, is necessary to reach a correct diagnosis. The time of onset of hip pain is important. Pain that occurs early after surgery and is out of proportion to the usual postoperative pain may indicate a postoperative infection or an unstable implant. Some patients form heterotopic ossification, which may be painful. Late pain may result from component loosening, but late hematogenous infection and soft-tissue problems, such as tendinitis or bursitis, are other possible causes. Osteolysis usually is painless unless it is associated with spontaneous fracture of the greater or lesser trochanter or acute synovitis of the hip joint.

The location of the pain is important in identifying its source. Groin pain usually is caused by acetabular component loosening, which can also cause buttock pain. Femoral component loosening usually causes thigh or knee pain. Thigh pain, especially with prolonged activity, can be associated with a stable uncemented femoral component and is usually localized to a specific region of the thigh near the tip of the stem. Pain caused by local tissue inflammation usually is felt in the anatomic location of the inflammation. The most common site, over the trochanter, is related to trochanteric bursitis or gluteal tendinitis. Nonunion of the greater trochanter usually is painless, but can occasionally cause pain that is localized over the lateral aspects of the hip. Iliopsoas inflammation is more common with collared implants in small patients in whom the collar overhangs the medial calcar. Iliopsoas irritation also can be caused by impingement on cementless sockets that are prominent anteriorly or inferiorly, causing groin pain.

It is important to determine whether the patient has pain with activity, pain at rest, or both. Pain caused by component instability usually is activity related. Clinically, a history of "start-up" pain may indicate a loose component. The patient may report that after 5 or 10 steps there is less pain in the groin. Pain with a loose component often is triphasic in that the first few steps cause acute sharp pain, the pain lessens with more walking, and then with a moderate amount of walking, pain again increases. With loose components, the pain is either in the groin or thigh, with occasional buttock pain caused by a loose socket. A pain caused by subluxation usually occurs when the patient is arising from the seated position. This is a sharp pain, and the patient usually corrects the position before dislocation occurs. Pain that occurs at night should suggest the possibility of infection, a neoplastic process, or spinal stenosis. It also is important to determine the presence of peripheral vascular disease because activity related pain can also result from vascular claudication.

Prosthetic Loosening

Serial radiographs are the mainstay for evaluation of the status of prosthetic fixation. For cemented acetabular components, an implant that has migrated or has a complete cement-bone radiolucency usually is considered loose. Loosening of a cemented femoral component has been historically graded as definite, probable, or possible. A definitely loose cemented femoral component is denoted by a change in implant position (subsidence, varus or valgus tilt, and/or rotation), a new metal-cement radiolucency, a new cement fracture, or a broken implant. Probable loosening has been defined as a complete radiolucency at the cement-bone interface. Possible loosening is defined as a cement-bone radiolucency occupying between 50% and 99% of the surface area. Autopsy studies have made the diagnosis of possible and probable loosening somewhat less clear, because bone remodeling at the cement-bone interface can lead to the appearance of a radiolucency on plain radiographs. This apparent radiolucency results from formation of a so-called second medullary canal between the inner cortex, which is in intimate contact with the bone cement, and the outer cortex.

Definite migration or change in implant position are accepted criteria for loosening of cementless acetabular components. The significance of a complete radiolucent line at the prosthesis-bone interface is not known but may suggest failure of bone ingrowth. Porous surface shedding and screw breakage also suggest loosening of uncemented components. A change in component position or subsidence, and/or a complete radiolucent line at the prosthesis-bone interface encompassing the areas of the porous coating are considered criteria for loosening of femoral components. Divergent sclerotic lines about the prosthesis suggest a change in implant position and loosening. A pedestal across the endosteal canal at the tip of the stem and sclerosis of the calcar region of the femur often are visible on radiographs. In contrast, proximal femoral osteopenia, streaming trabeculae from the porous surface finish to the endosteum, and densification of bone at the distal level of the porous coating are all radiographic signs denoting bone ingrowth.

Osteolysis

Osteolysis is a common complication of cementless total joint replacement. Marked periprosthetic bone resorption can occur without clinical symptoms, emphasizing the need for periodic radiographic evaluation after THA. Three primary etiologies have been suggested: generation of particulate debris, access of debris to the implant-bone interface and periprosthetic bone, and the biologic reaction to the wear particles. Osteolysis appears to be caused by particle-induced bone resorption. Data from autopsy studies and in vivo experiments have shown that bulk materials used in orthopaedic implants are well tolerated biologically, and no signs of toxicity were found in cemented femoral replacements harvested at autopsy up to 17 years after surgery. In these well-functioning implants, little fibrous tissue was present at the cement-bone interface. Findings from histologic analysis and scanning electron microscopy of the cement-bone interface were compatible with osseointegration. An autopsy study of cementless chrome-cobalt and titanium components also found that the metal-bone interface was free of fibrous tissue.

The most common source of small particulate wear debris is the articulation. Wear at the articulation is inevitable with current prostheses, with average wear rates in cemented THAs of 0.1 mm/year reported. Polyethylene wear is related to several factors, including head size, implant design, counterface abrasions, and 3-body wear. Modularity has introduced another potential source of particulate debris: corrosion of the modular connections between the femoral head and neck. Burnishing has been found at other modular connections, including the distal and proximal sleeves. Wear also has been found on the back side of modular acetabular components. Other potential sources of wear particles include the metal-cement interface in debonded cemented components and the metal-bone interface in uncemented components. In addition to the potential biologic consequences of metallic debris, it may enter the articulation and lead to 3-body wear. The effective joint space is defined as not only the articulation, but the entire periprosthetic space that is accessible to joint fluid and thus wear particles. Most wear particles (> 90%) are less than 1 μm in size. Routine histologic analysis is not adequate to study this small wear debris.

To have an adverse effect on bone, particulate debris must gain access to the bone. Osteolysis appears at this time to be a biologic response to wear particles locally. There is no evidence that a response at one site can induce osteolysis at another site. The location of osteolysis can, in part, be predicted based on implant design. For example, patch porous coated implants provide channels for debris to gain access to the endosteal canal, even in the presence of excellent bone ingrowth. This has been demonstrated in an animal study, in which bone ingrowth into a porous surface served as a barrier to migration of polyethylene particles. However, polyethylene debris migrated along the smooth, nonporous portion of the implant. This phenomenon also has been seen clinically. The original Harris-Galante (Zimmer, Warsaw, IN) femoral component was a patch porous coated implant with the coating limited to the proximal aspect of the implant. Because the incomplete porous coating provided channels for debris to

access the endosteal canal, diaphyseal osteolysis with this implant was common. Similar findings were noted with the APR-I femoral component (Intermedics Orthopedics, Austin, TX), which also had an incomplete porous coating. In contrast, osteolysis in association with circumferentially porous coated femoral components almost always appears in the greater and lesser trochanteric regions. These findings have obvious implications for implant design.

Information on the biocompatibility of wear debris comes from several sources including in vitro and in vivo studies, autopsy material, revision material, and clinical follow-up studies. Many studies based on findings at revision surgery have described the histology of the membrane that forms at the implant-bone interface in association with aseptic loosening and osteolysis. Typically, there are abundant macrophages and giant cells consistent with a foreign body granuloma. Cell cultures of the retrieved membranes indicate that this tissue has the capacity to produce a variety of substances, such as prostaglandin E^2, collagenase, interleukin-1, and tumor necrosis factor. All of these substances have been implicated in bone resorption, and it is postulated that these substances may be responsible for osteolysis.

Stress Shielding

After THA, there is a marked change in the transfer of load from the hip joint to the proximal femur. Load normally carried by the bone alone is now shared by the implant and bone. This change results in remodeling of the proximal femur, which is characterized by decreased density and thinning of the cortex, especially in the calcar region. This phenomenon is commonly referred to as stress shielding. Although useful for providing information on gross architectural changes, clinical radiographs are not a sensitive method to quantitate bone loss. Differences in radiographic technique with respect to target distance, exposure setting, and field variability make it impossible to accurately measure density change. Dual energy X-ray absorptiometry has been used to evaluate change in bone mineral content after THA, but does not permit determination of the remodeling processes that account for the change in density. Direct examination of autopsy specimens has been used to more critically evaluate the change in bone architecture after THA.

Clinically, the most severe stress shielding occurs with extensively porous coated, chrome-cobalt stems. An average 45% decrease in bone mineral content was reported after THA with this stem design. However, in a group of patients characterized as having severe stress shielding based on plain radiographs, no adverse effects were noted in terms of hip scores, the presence of osteolysis, or the need for revision surgery in this group of patients.

The factors that can influence the extent of the remodeling process after THA include age, gender, weight, activity level, disease state, medications, duration of implantation, stem stiffness, and the quality (density) of bone. Analysis of autopsy specimens from patients with unilateral THAs using either cemented or extensively porous coated femoral components demonstrated a strong correlation between the bone mineral density of the control femur and the percentage decrease in bone mineral density of the remodeled femur. These findings suggest that the less dense the bone is before hip replacement surgery, the greater the extent of bone loss after THA regardless of whether the stems were cemented or had extensive porous coating. Studies also have shown that the posterior cortex is more prone to bone loss after hip replacement than was previously appreciated.

Dislocation

Dislocation occurs after 1% to 10% of THAs, and further surgery is often required for correction of the problem. The posterior approach to the hip has been associated with a higher dislocation rate than other approaches, and posterior dislocation is the most common direction of instability reported after THA. In 3,199 Charnley THAs, the incidence of dislocation in the first year was 2.3% for the transtrochanteric approach and 2.7% for the posterior approach. At 2 years, the incidence was 2.8% in each group. Arthroplasty performed by less experienced surgeons through the posterior approach resulted in especially frequent dislocations. Regardless of the approach, there was a higher risk of dislocation in patients with rheumatoid arthritis and nonhealed hip fractures than in patients with osteoarthritis. Half of the male patients with dislocations (10 of 20) had histories of alcohol abuse.

Size of the femoral prosthesis head also has been cited as a factor in hip stability. Historically, it has been thought that 32-mm heads, for example, had fewer dislocations than 22-mm heads. The relation of head size to hip stability, however, is a complex one that depends on the femoral neck geometry. This, in turn, relates to the risk of impingement of the neck on the acetabular component. In 4,230 primary THAs, the rate of dislocation was 3.7% with 22-mm heads and only 1.1% with 32-mm heads.

Most (40% to 70%) dislocations occur in the first month after surgery. The chance of recurrent dislocation is related to the time of first dislocation. An initial dislocation in the first month after surgery is less likely to recur than is an initial dislocation 3 months or more after surgery. Late dislocation is uncommon. Fewer than 1% of patients first dislocate their hip 5 years after their index procedures. Recurrent dislocation almost always requires surgical intervention. Important factors in the evaluation of recurrent dislocation include component position, restoration of the normal offset after hip replacement and its relationship to abductor muscle tension, leg length, implant design, and patient-related factors such as compliance. The chance of successful surgical management of a recurrent dislocation is related to the ability to identify its cause, but the success rate is only about 70% when a cause can be identified. If no obvious cause can be identified, a trochanteric advancement has been advocated. Simple trochanteric advancement is successful in about 75% of patients.

Elevated rim liners have been used to improve hip stability after THA, and most manufacturers now provide an elevated rim liner as an option. A concern has been that the use of elevated rim liners may improve stability in 1 direction, but also lead to increased risk of impingement and subsequent polyethylene wear. In a large study, there was no increase in rates of loosening with use of elevated rim liners. Laboratory studies confirmed that elevated rim liners can improve stability in 1 direction, but decrease overall arc of motion. In a study of 2,469 acetabular components with elevated rim liners and 2,698 with standard liners, the probability of dislocation at 2 years was 2.19% for the hips with elevated rim liners and 3.85% for those with standard liners. A similar trend was seen at 5 years.

Constrained sockets can be used to correct recurrent dislocation or intraoperative instability. In a study of 21 constrained acetabular components placed to remedy either preoperative or intraoperative instability, 15 patients had no further dislocations or subluxations at a minimum follow-up of 2 years. However, 8 dislocations occurred in the remaining 6 patients. An increased acetabular inclination angle was the only predictive factor in the hips that dislocated. This increase was presumably caused by impingement of the femoral stem on the rim of the insert.

Periprosthetic Fractures

Periprosthetic fractures are becoming increasingly frequent. Before the advent of press fit porous coated implants, intraoperative femoral fractures occurred during fewer than 1% of THAs. The use of press fit implants has increased this number, but most of the fractures have no clinical significance because they are small cracks around the proximal opening of the femur. Revision surgery is associated with a higher incidence of intraoperative femoral fractures. The incidence of postoperative fractures reported in the literature varies from 0.1% after primary THA to 4.2% after revision surgery.

Periprosthetic fractures can be classified according to the American Academy of Orthopaedic Surgeons (AAOS) Committee on the Hip classification system, which takes into account fracture location and pattern. Another classification is based on fracture location, fixation of the stem, and quality of the bone. Complications associated with periprosthetic fractures include malunion, nonunion, and loosening of the femoral component. In general, displaced fractures distal to the tip of the femoral component usually require surgical management. When the fracture is associated with a loose femoral component, revision is recommended. The choice of the most appropriate type of fixation depends on the factors discussed above, as well as the age of the patient and the experience of the surgeon. If the fracture and the prostheses are stable, the fracture can be treated nonsurgically.

If the fracture is unstable, treatment depends on the stability of the prostheses. If the prostheses is loose and the bone stock is adequate, revision with a long-stem implant can be performed. If the bone stock is inadequate as a result of extensive osteolysis or severe comminution, the proximal femur may require replacement with either an implant or proximal femoral allograft, depending on the age of the patient and the degree of bone loss. If the prostheseis is not loose, open reduction and internal fixation is the preferred treatment for displaced fractures that are unstable. Plate fixation is preferred unless the fixation violates the cement mantle of the femoral stem. Cable plates are now available that allow plate fixation without the use of screws in the area of the femoral component. Bicortical structural allografts are useful when bone quality is poor.

The stability of various constructs in repairing periprosthetic fractures has been evaluated in laboratory studies. In an experimental study comparing several different methods of fracture fixation, good strength and stability were achieved by supplementing the long-stem conversion component with allograft struts and cable cerclage. Good stability also was obtained by lateral compression plating.

In a clinical study of periprosthetic fractures of the acetabulum after THA, the authors concluded that, while periprosthetic acetabular fractures were associated with a poor prognosis regarding the survival of the original acetabular component, some minimally displaced fractures heal with nonsurgical treatment without compromising the function of the component. When the component fails after a fracture, either because of nonunion or because of loosening, salvage is possible by acetabular revision in a high percentage of patients. If possible, periacetabular fractures should be allowed to unite before revising the acetabular component.

Heterotopic Ossification

Heterotopic ossification (HO) is atypical bone formation in the muscle and connective tissue after THA. The reported prevalence of HO after hip procedures ranges from 2% to 3% up to 90%. Most HOs are asymptomatic and do not lead to functional limitation. Risk factors for HO differ from study to study, but most authors believe that patients with ankylosing spondylitis are at increased risk. It appears that men with bilateral hypertrophic osteoarthritis also are at risk. In addition, those patients who have HO in 1 hip after THA will often have HO after THA in the contralateral hip. If HO is resected, it will almost always recur if prophylactic measures are not used.

Both nonsteroidal anti-inflammatory medications and external beam radiation therapy have been shown to be effective prophylactic agents. Indomethacin, ibuprofen, diclofenac, and aspirin have all been shown to inhibit HO formation in both animals and humans. The effectiveness of a 6-week postoperative course of indomethacin was evaluated in 100 patients. Although 22% of the patients had some side effects from the anti-inflammatory, most completed at least 4 weeks of treatment. There was a statistically significant reduction in HO in the treatment group. In another study, the effectiveness of a 10 day course of indomethacin in high risk patients was evaluated. Of 109 patients (123 hips), 106 (119 hips) successfully completed the 10 day course, and no significant (Brooker class 3 or 4) HO formation occurred in any of these patients. Of 45 patients with HO after THA on the contralateral side, only 2 formed new heterotopic bone.

A 1-week course of naproxen was reported to prevent HO in 24 (89%) of 27 patients; 12 of 23 patients (52%) in the control group had HO. In other studies, tenoxicam and ketorolac have been shown to be effective for HO prophylaxis. Nonsteroidal anti-inflammatory drugs must be used cautiously in those patients who are being anticoagulated postoperatively for deep venous thrombosis prophylaxis.

In initial studies of external beam radiation, 20 Gy in 2 Gy fraction doses over a 10 dose course was used. The radiation dose has been substantially reduced, and in recent studies lower doses have been found to be as effective. In one report, a single dose of 5.50 Gy was compared to a single dose of 7 Gy. Twelve of 19 hips (63%) that were treated with 5.5 Gy developed HO compared with only 9 of 88 (10%) that were treated with 7 Gy. The authors concluded that a single dose consisting of 5.5 Gy was inadequate for HO prophylaxis in high risk patients. Another prospective, randomized study of 86 compared radiation therapy (8 Gy) given 4 hours before THA to radiation therapy given 72 hours postoperatively. No difference was noted between the 2 groups in terms of the prevalence of grade 3 or 4 HO. The authors concluded that preoperative radiation was as effective as postoperative radiation and that it eliminated the discomfort and morbidity associated with conventional postoperative treatment. When using external beam radiation after THA, it is important to shield bone ingrowth components and trochanteric osteotomies to avoid retardation of bone ingrowth and nonunion.

Infection

Infection after total joint arthroplasty may lack the classic symptoms of fever and chills, and physical examination of the patient also may not find signs of warmth, redness, or sinus track formation with drainage. The erythrocyte sedimentation rate (ESR) and C-reactive protein (CRP) are both acute-phase reactants that when elevated are not specific for the infectious process but are clearly helpful. The sensitivity for the ESR and CRP ranges from 61% to 96%, while the specificity ranges from 85% to 100%. Aspiration of the hip is indicated for patients with a history suggesting infection or whose radiographs show focal osteolysis, aggressive non-focal osteolysis, or periostitis. The polymerase chain reaction (PCR) is a newer diagnostic test enabling production of large specific sequences of DNA from very small quantities of material. Further clinical evaluation of the PCR is necessary before it can be widely applied.

Nuclear Scans Technetium Tc 99m bone scans and gallium 67 citrate scans are nonspecific and do not differentiate between aseptic and septic loosening. The scan most commonly used is leukocyte scintigraphy, which has 80% to 90% percent sensitivity and 85% to 100% specificity. Immunoscintography is a newer technique that labels immunoglobulins. Indium In 111-labeled human nonspecific immunoglobulin G (^{111}In IgG) is a type of immunoscintigraphy that has been studied clinically for the evaluation of infection and inflammation. The success of the scans have varied between 67% and 100% for specificity and 88% and 100% for sensitivity.

Frozen Section Analysis During revision arthroplasty, frozen section analysis is an important step to determine whether the component has become loose because of a septic or aseptic process. Tissue specimens are obtained from those tissues that are most grossly inflamed and adjacent to the prosthesis. Specimens also are obtained from the bone-prosthesis interfaces on the femur and acetabulum. Tissues are analyzed on high magnification, and the number of polymorphonuclear cells is quantified. A frozen section analysis of at least 1 polymorphonuclear cell per high-powered field (average of 1 per 10 high-powered fields) lowers the threshold and increases the sensitivity but does reduce the specificity to diagnose infection. Counting 10 polymorphonuclear cells per high powered field lowers the sensitivity, but is more specific and has a higher positive predictive value. At this time 5 polymorphonuclear cells per high powered field is the accepted standard.

Table 4
Success of treatment for periprosthetic infection

Treatment	Hip (% success)	Knee (% success)
Antibiotic suppression	—	18
Debridement with antibiotics	25 to 35	25 to 35
One-stage exchange without antibiotics—polymethylmethacrylate (PMMA)	55 to 60	55 to 60
One-stage exchange with antibiotics—PMMA	80 to 85	70 to 80
Two-stage exchange without antibiotics—PMMA	80 to 85	85 to 90
Two-stage exchange with antibiotics—PMMA	88 to 93	90 to 95

Outline 1
Patients at potenial increased risk of hematogenous total joint infection

Immunocompromised/Immunosuppressed patients

Inflammatory arthropathies: rheumatoid arthritis, systemic lupus erythematosus

Disease, drug, or radiation-induced immunosuppression

Other Patients

Insulin-dependent (type 1) diabetes

First 2 years following joint placement

Previous prosthetic joint infections

Malnourishment

Hemophilia

Outline 2
Incidence stratification of bacteremic dental procedures

Higher Incidence*
Dental extractions

Periodontal procedures including surgery, subgingival placement of antibiotic fibers/strips, scaling and root planing, probing, recall maintenance

Dental implant placement and reimplantation of avulsed teeth

Endodontic (root canal) instrumentation or surgery only beyond the apex

Initial placement of orthodontic bands but not brackets

Intraligamentary local anesthetic injections

Prophylactic cleaning of teeth or implants where bleeding is anticipated

Lower Incidence†

Restorative dentistry§ (operative and prosthodontic) with/without retraction cord

Local anesthetic injections (nonintraligamentary)

Intracanal endodontic treatment; postplacement and buildup

Placement of rubber dam

Postoperative suture removal

Placement of removable prosthodontic/orthodontic appliances

Taking of oral impressions

Fluoride treatments

Taking of oral radiographs

Orthodontic appliance adjustment

---

*Prophylaxis should be considered for patients with total joint replacement that meet the criteria in Table 1. No other patients with orthopaedic implants should be considered for antibiotic prophylaxis prior to dental treatment/procedures

†Prophylaxis not indicated

§This includes restoration of carious (decayed) or missing teeth

Clinical judgement may indicate antibiotic use in selected circumstances that may create significant bleeding

(Adapted from: *Prevention of Bacterial Endocarditis; Recommendations by the American Heart Association,* from the Committee on Rheumatic Fever, Endocarditis, and Kawasaki Disease. Council on Cardiovascular Disease in the Young. Reproduced with permission from the *Journal of the American Medical Association.*)

Outline 3
Suggested antibiotic prophylaxis regimens*

Patients not allergic to penicillin: cephalexin, cephradine or amoxicillin: 2 grams orally 1 hour prior to dental procedure

Patients not allergic to penicillin but unable to take oral medications: cefazolin 1 gram or ampicillin 2 grams IM/IV 1 hour prior to the procedure

Patients allergic to penicillin: clindamycin 600 mg orally 1 hour prior to the dental procedure

Patients allergic to penicillin and unable to take oral medications: clindamycin 600 mg IM/IV 1 hour prior to the procedure

---

*No second doses are recommended for any of these dosing regimens

It is critical that grossly inflamed granulation tissue be selected because taking tissue from less inflamed areas not in contact with the joint can result in false-negative sampling. In contrast, false positives rarely occur but can be associated with acutely inflamed tissue near a fracture, such as a trochanteric avulsion. It is imperative that the orthopaedist and pathologist have a working relationship and the pathologist be experienced in the analysis and interpretation of frozen sections for patients with prosthetic infection.

Treatment Once the diagnosis has been established, the treatment of periprosthetic infections of the hip or knee arthroplasty relies on the basic principles for treatment of infection elsewhere in the body. The infected site must be surgically debrided to remove infected and necrotic tissue and foreign material, and the surgical site must be thoroughly irrigated. Once this is completed, final cultures of the debrided tissues are obtained and parenteral antibiotic therapy is initiated to treat any microscopically retained bacteria. If any of these steps in treatment are not successfully performed, the infection has a greater chance of persisting or recurring. Debridement with retention of the components may be possible in the early postoperative infections (less than 3 months), if symptoms have been present for a short time (less than 1 to 2 weeks), or if the infection is hematologic and the components are well fixed. Even if these strict criteria are met, the failure rate approaches 50% when the components are retained.

The standard treatment for an infected implant, removal of the components, may be done in 1 stage, with the components replaced at the time of the surgical debridement, or in 2 stages, with an interval from 6 weeks to 1 year between surgical debridement and reimplantation. Results of these treatment methods are summarized in Table 4. Rarely, surgical debridement is followed by reconstruction with bone graft at a second surgery and a final prosthetic placement at a third surgery. Local antibiotic delivery systems have been developed for use at the time of debridement. One such system incorporates an implant and is known as the prosthesis of antibiotic-loaded acrylic cement or PROSTALAC. The combination of 2.4 to 2.6 grams of tobramycin and 1 to 1.5 grams of vancomycin per package of bone cement can be used. The local antibiotic delivery systems are removed at the time of joint reimplantation.

Antimicrobial Prophylaxis The routine use of antibiotic prophylaxis for dental patients with total joint replacements has been scrutinized more recently because of the lack of scientific evidence supporting its use, the risk of emerging antibiotic resistant bacteria, the risk of anaphylactic reaction associated with antibiotics, and the cost of continued routine usage of antibiotics. It is recommended that patients have

good dental health before undergoing joint arthroplasty and, when necessary, seek professional care. Patients who already have a total joint in place also should maintain this good oral health. The patients most at risk for hematogenous total joint infection are those who are immunocompromised, immunosuppressed, have had their implant placed within the last 2 years, or have other problems making them more at risk (Outlines 1 and 2). Particular oral and dental procedures may have higher incidences of bacteremia and thus are more likely to cause prosthetic infection. If the dentist, who is ultimately responsible for making treatment recommendations to these patients, determines antibiotic prophylaxis is necessary, antibiotics should be given before the procedure. The antibiotic selected (Outline 3) should be specific for bacteria of the oral cavity.

Acetabular Component Revision Arthroplasty

Bone Defects

The AAOS published a classification system for acetabular deficiencies (Table 5) in which defect types are divided into 2 main categories: segmental and cavitary deficiencies. This classification system allows accurate intraoperative classification of acetabular defect configuration and severity (except when otherwise noted, defects will be classified according to this system throughout this section). Another acetabular defect classification system is based on the presence or absence of an intact acetabular rim, the stability of the acetabular dome and walls, the integrity of the acetabular columns, and the amount of coverage that can be obtained for cementless acetabular fixation. Defects are classified by type (I to III), indicating the extent to which the remaining acetabular bone can support an acetabular component (Table 6). This system helps predict the method of acetabular reconstruction and the acetabular component type that will be required. In Type I defects, a press-fit acetabular ingrowth implant (regular or oversized) can be used with or without particulate graft and bone screws. Type II defects still have adequate support for the acetabular component so that structural allograft is not necessary and generally oversized components and graft with supplemental screw fixation are recommended. Acetabular component placement in the high hip center also can be useful if adequate superior column support can be obtained. Cemented cups with morcellized graft also may be appropriate when an adequate rim remains. Type III defects usually require bulk allograft reconstruction of the acetabulum to support a cemented acetabular implant. Antiprotrusio cages also may be used. Additionally, the sur-

Table 5
The American Academy of Orthopaedic Surgeons classification system for acetabular deficiencies in total hip arthroplasty

Type	Description
Type I	Segmental deficiencies
	Peripheral
	Superior
	Anterior
	Posterior
	Central (medial wall absent)
Type II	Cavitary deficiencies
	Peripheral
	Superior
	Anterior
	Posterior
	Central (medial wall intact)
Type III	Combined deficiencies
Type IV	Pelvic deficiencies
Type V	Arthrodesis

Table 6
Acetabular defect types and characteristics (Paprosky) classification system for acetabular deficiencies in total hip arthroplasty

Type	Rim	Walls/Domes	Columns	Bone Bed
Type I	Intact	Intact	Intact and supportive	> 50%: cancellous
Type II	Distorted	Distorted	Intact and supportive	< 50%; cancellous
Type III	Missing	Severely compromised	Nonsupportive	Membranous/ sclerotic

nique. Proximal placement of the acetabulum decreases leg length, requiring correction on the femoral side with implants that have neck extensions.

Fixation of a cementless acetabular component in the high hip center requires the use of small components. A press-fit should be augmented by screw fixation. The small number of screw holes must be carefully aligned to access the remaining bone of the ilium and posterior column. The zones for safe screw placement are significantly narrowed as the cup is positioned proximal to the anatomic hip center, requiring the placement of fixation screws in the outer half of the posterior quadrants.

geon should be prepared to fix bulk allograft to the pelvis or reconstruct pelvic discontinuities by plating the anterior or posterior columns.

Avoiding severe bone deficiencies may be the most important consideration in acetabular revision. In a recent report of 54 revisions of failing cementless implants, it was suggested that early intervention for polyethylene wear and pelvic osteolysis is beneficial even in asymptomatic patients.

Joint Restoration

The goals of revision acetabular arthroplasty are a stable construct, restoration of bone stock, and restoration of the hip center to its anatomic location whenever possible. In principle, restoration of the hip center to its normal anatomic location will optimize biomechanical hip function. When acetabular bone loss is moderate, this is most frequently accomplished by expanding the acetabulum at the anatomic center and using an oversized component fixed with transacetabular screws. Even in some of the most difficult cases of bone loss the hip center can be restored by using bulk allograft reconstruction or augmentation devices.

However, because stability of the construct is the most important goal of revision arthroplasty, it is not prudent to restore the center of hip rotation if this results in tenuous acetabular component fixation. Placing a small cup into the high hip center is another option if adequate superior bone is available for implant fixation. Lateral cup placement should be avoided because it alters hip biomechanics and increases acetabular and femoral component loosening. The superior-only hip center relocation does not significantly affect the total joint force magnitudes or directions, probably accounting for the good long-term results reported with this tech-

Methods of Reconstruction

Porous Fixed Component Although cementless revision acetabular arthroplasty usually requires some further loss of bone during fashioning of the acetabulum, this method is popular because it is a relatively simple and reproducible way to correct all types of acetabular deficiencies. In a study of 61 consecutive so-called hybrid revision THAs, no cementless acetabular components required re-revision, and only 1 cup demonstrated radiographic evidence of loosening. Compared to a group of 74 hips that had revision THA using contemporary cementing techniques, survival of the cementless acetabular components was significantly better ($p = 0.001$). Surgery was performed by the same surgeon and followed up for a comparable time interval. In another study of 115 hips followed for 7 to 11 years, no re-revisions of cementless acetabular components were required. Complete radiolucencies were present in 4%, an additional 3% had progressive radiolucencies, radiolucencies about screws were seen in 2%, and acetabular osteolysis was seen in 4%. The authors concluded that revision with a cementless porous-coated hemispherical fiber-metal component provided superior results to cemented acetabular revision.

Even large type III acetabular defects can be treated with large spherical cementless acetabular components without bulk allograft. Success of this technique relies on the cup being placed in a stable position against host bone and using multiple transacetabular screws to augment fixation. In a study of 19 patients with an average follow-up of 46 months, only 3 (11%) required re-operation. In another study of 32 hips with type II and type IV defects, only 3 (9%) components required re-revision for aseptic loosening at an average of 64 month postoperatively. The results of both these studies compare favorably with results obtained using bulk allograft reconstruction methods.

Cemented Acetabular Component The results of cemented acetabular revision are most influenced by the generally poor quality of the remaining deficient sclerotic bone. The importance of bone stock is illustrated in a study of 82 young patients with cemented acetabular revision implants. Loosening of the component occurred in 51% of patients who had poor bone stock (massive or global collapse of the acetabulum and defects involving at least 2 columns) compared to only 14% in those with small local defects. The relationship between bone stock and loosening was highly significant ($p = 0.0002$). Others also have reported less than favorable rates of acetabular component loosening, even when improved cementing techniques were used. In a study of 76 patients (81 hips), 13 hips (16%) required re-revision for aseptic loosening of the cemented acetabular component, whereas only 5.4% of the cemented femoral stems required re-revision. These results confirm that cemented femoral revision is a durable option when improved cementing techniques are used, but that cemented acetabular revision performs poorly.

Cemented acetabular revision with the use of compressed morcellized graft may be indicated when contained bone deficiencies are present and reconstitution of bone stock is desired. In a series of 88 hips reconstructed with impacted graft and a cemented acetabular component, 4 clinical and 6 radiographic failures had occurred at an average follow-up of 70 months. In another study of 102 patients, there was a 3% rate of aseptic cup loosening at 5 years and an 18% rate at 10 years. Both studies found that graft incorporation was successful and facilitated subsequent revision surgery. Postmortem retrieval analysis also has demonstrated that graft incorporation does occur, and that impacted morcellized graft is useful in restoring bone deficiency within contained acetabular defects.

Bipolar Reconstruction Bipolar reconstruction has been used largely for massive bone loss or instability. In a study of 81 patients who had hip reconstruction with bone graft and bipolar endoprostheses for severe acetabular deficiency, the Harris hip score was improved from 49.9 preoperatively to 70.8 at the most recent follow-up (3 to 8 years postoperatively). However, although the overall probability of implant survival was 96% at 1 year, it deteriorated to only 47% at 6.5 years. Recent evidence also suggests that the use of bipolar implants is associated with osteolysis. In a membrane retrieval study, the amount of polyethylene debris in the

interface tissues surrounding bipolar endoprostheses was found to be greater than around THA. Because of its high failure rate and potential for osteolysis, bipolar reconstruction has a limited role in revision hip reconstruction.

Threaded Socket Threaded acetabular components have fallen out of favor because of mounting evidence of poor performance. A meta-analysis of the orthopaedic literature evaluated the performance of threaded acetabular components. A review of 95 articles yielded 1,269 in the threaded group, 1,979 in the porous control group, and 10,230 in the cemented control group. The threaded cup group had a significantly higher rate of revision than the control groups. The use of this implant has largely been abandoned.

Constrained Socket These components are useful when only acetabular revision is required in conjunction with a well-fixed nonmodular stem (particularly when proximal location of the hip center is required). Because length and offset are not adjustable, a constrained component may be needed to prevent instability. These components will be subjected to high stresses, because forces cannot be dissipated normally at the articulation; therefore, supplemental screw fixation is warranted to optimize construct stability.

Structural Allograft The massive defects associated with failed acetabular components can require structural allografts to provide component stability and restore the hip center. Although initial reports of acetabular reconstruction using structural allografts were not encouraging, they helped define the variables responsible for failure. A refinement of techniques has led to improved success. In a recent study of 61 cemented acetabular revisions using bulk structural allograft and followed for an average of 16.5 years, these constructs were highly successful at an average of 5 years postoperatively but much less so by 11.8 years. These patients had a small average cup size of 40 mm (range, 34 to 50 mm). The authors found that 78% of the acetabular components that remained rigidly fixed were supported by graft over less than 50% of the contact area, while only 36% of those components requiring revision were so supported ($p < 0.05$). The need for the acetabular component to be supported by predominantly host bone was corroborated by results of another study of 29 patients who had shelf structural allografts, done in conjunction with cemented and cementless acetabular revision. After an average follow-up of 7.1 years, 86% of revisions were successful both clinically and radiographically. The authors believed their success was a result of their technique of ensuring that at least 50% of the cup was supported by host bone.

Cementless acetabular reconstruction in combination with

bulk allograft is usually feasible because not enough host bone can be apposed to the ingrowth surface. However, several recent studies conclude that success with a cementless cup is possible if the graft supports less than 50% of the cup. In a series of 16 revisions treated with cementless cups and structural allografts, only 1 failure occurred after a minimum follow-up of 5 years. In a postmortem retrieval analysis of 2 successful cementless bulk allograft constructs, both demonstrated > 50% of the cup apposed to viable host bone, with ingrowth noted only in these regions. The allograft was found to be united to the host bone, but it did not revascularize or remodel, or grow into the porous coating.

Augmentation Devices When acetabular defects are severe (type III and IV), metal supporting rings or an antiprotrusio cage are a means of optimally using the remaining acetabular bone for revision arthroplasty. Even in the most severe acetabular bone deficiency, ischial and pubic bone stock usually is preserved. Supporting rings with iliac and ischial or pubic extensions can accommodate screws in these regions, allowing the acetabular bone defect to be bridged. Bone graft must be packed behind the device, and an all polyethylene acetabular component is then cemented into this construct. This technique may allow reconstruction of the hip at its original location in situations where reliance on host bone stock alone would have made this impossible.

In a study of 72 revision surgeries using the Müller acetabular reinforcement ring examined after a mean of 6.4 years, only 2 patients required re-revision surgery. However, the authors found that progressive radiolucencies and loosening were associated with proximal and lateral position of the ring. Stable hips were associated with restoration of the anatomic hip center and adequate bone coverage for the acetabular component. Cages that allow fixation into both the ilium and ischium seem to provide even better long-term results. In a study of 42 failed acetabular arthroplasties treated with a Burch-Schneider antiprotrusio cage, 32 hips (76%) showed no evidence of acetabular component failure or loosening at a mean 5 years after revision. In another study using roof reinforcement rings with structural allografts, 7 of 8 revisions were successful at an average of 7.5 years.

Femoral Component Revision Arthroplasty

Removal of the Failed Femoral Component

The indications for femoral component revision include aseptic loosening, infection, polyethylene wear, component malposition, osteolysis, and component failure. Good quality preoperative radiographs including anteroposterior (AP) and lateral hip views and an AP pelvis view are essential in planning the surgical technique for exposure, implant removal, and reconstruction. The mode of implant failure may affect the quality of the remaining bone, thus influencing the type of reconstruction used.

It is important to correctly identify the component system to be revised and to make sure that compatible replacement femoral heads and liners are available. Some early designs did not incorporate modular acetabular components and, therefore, are not compatible with a simple liner exchange. During an acetabular revision with a well-fixed nonmodular femoral component, inability to achieve stability is an indication for femoral revision. The type of implant to be revised may affect the surgical approach used and which components are revised.

Revision arthroplasty surgery requires more extensive surgical exposure, which can be achieved through a variety of approaches. The standard trochanteric osteotomy may provide the additional exposure necessary for difficult acetabular or femoral component removal or reconstruction. The trochanteric slide differs from the standard trochanteric osteotomy in that the attachment of the vastus lateralis is left intact, providing additional insurance against proximal migration of the trochanteric fragment. In the revision setting, proximal femoral bone stock is compromised and provides only a limited surface area for healing of the trochanteric fragment. Both techniques are associated with a delayed or nonunion rate of about 10%.

The more recently described extended proximal femoral osteotomy has supplanted the trochanteric osteotomy in femoral revision arthroplasty for a number of reasons (Fig. 8). The proximal femoral osteotomy consists of the trochanter and the lateral third of the femur. The length is determined during preoperative planning to optimize ease of component removal and femoral reconstruction. Soft-tissue stripping is kept to a minimum and the distal soft-tissue attachment is preserved. An oscillating saw and high-speed pencil tip burr are used to cut the femur. The extended osteotomy provides a greater exposure than the standard osteotomy, allowing easier removal of the well-fixed implant, greater access to the distal bone-cement interface, decreased inadvertent cortical perforations during cement removal, enhanced exposure of the acetabulum, proper tensioning of the abductors with distal ad-vancement, decreased time in surgery, and predictable healing of the osteotomized fragment. When used with an extensively porous coated revision stem, the osteotomy allows a more neutral reaming of the femoral canal and direct inspection of the distal press fit and decreases the incidence of complications, such as eccentric reaming, femoral perforations, and fractures. Varus remodeling seen in as many as 30%

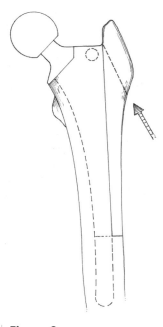

Figure 8

Extended proximal femoral osteotomy. Arrow points to standard trochanteric osteotomy.

of femurs to be revised complicates femoral preparation and reconstruction. Although somewhat more difficult, a technique for using the extended osteotomy with cement reconstruction has been described.

Many stems can be extracted before performing the extended osteotomy. However, well-fixed fully coated cementless stems and highly textured or pre-coated cemented stems are much more difficult to remove. In these cases, the osteotomy must frequently be performed with the prosthesis in situ.

In fully coated stem removal, this osteotomy exposes the lateral aspect of the stem; a Gigli saw is then passed around the medial aspect of the stem and is directed distally to the level where the stem profile becomes cylindrical. Using a metal cutting burr, the stem is sectioned at this point. Trephines are then used over the cylindrical portion to complete stem removal.

In well-fixed cemented stem removal, access to the lateral cement column is provided by the extended osteotomy. This simplifies the removal of the well-fixed component. Although rarely necessary, a stubborn cemented stem also can be sectioned at a point where it becomes cylindrical and the distal aspect trephined for removal.

Bone Loss

A simplified classification system based on the location and extent of femoral bone loss has been developed, which replaced the American Academy of Orthopaedic Surgeons' Committee on the Hip classification of femoral defects. There are 4 categories of bone loss: types I–IV (Fig. 9). This new classification allows planning of the revision procedure and prediction of the probability of bone ingrowth based on the femoral deficit present and the amount of canal fill during reconstruction.

Femoral Reconstruction Allograft bone is an effective means of restoring bone stock in the revision setting where host bone is compromised because of osteolysis, stress shielding, aseptic loosening, or damage caused by removal of well-fixed components or cement.

Cancellous Bone Graft Cavitary defects can be filled effectively with cancellous graft. Radiographic incorporation is frequently observed. Cancellous bone cannot be relied on to provide stability with an uncemented implant. The impaction grafting technique uses cancellous bone and cement to create a stable femoral construct in the presence of ballooned cortices found in some type IIIB and all type IV femoral defects.

Cortical Strut Allograft Cortical strut allograft is useful in the revision setting when proximal cortical bone is deficient. Cortical struts should not be relied on to provide structural support. In type II and III femoral defects, 309 freeze-dried cortical strut allografts were secured with cerclage wire and allograft/autograft slurry along with an uncemented calcar replacement stem. In 99% of patients, the strut grafts incorporated with a solid union at 8.6 months, and the graft maturation took between 3 and 5 years. Allograft structural support of the prosthesis was associated with poor results.

Allograft Prosthetic Composite For massive defects (type IV) not amenable to other reconstructive methods, such as a tumor prosthesis, an allograft prosthetic composite (APC) can be used to reconstruct the hip. An APC consists of the proximal portion of a modular prosthesis, which is cemented to a proximal femoral allograft, and the distal stem, which is fixed to the host femoral diaphysis using cementless or cement fixation. When cementless fixation is achieved with good rotational control, a butt joint can be used at the allograft host junction. If the cementless fixation has less than ideal rotational control, a step cut can be used at the allograft host junction to provide additional rotational stability. In elderly osteopenic patients, cement can be used for distal fixation. At a minimum of 2 years' follow-up, 85% of 130 APCs were considered successful, 10% were revised, and 5% were considered to have radiographic nonunions at the host allograft junction.

Cemented Femoral Fixation for Revision

Revision surgery is complicated by damage to the proximal femoral bone stock that compromises the quality of cemented femoral fixation. Data from studies in human cadavers and canine models have demonstrated a marked reduction in pull-out strength in revised cemented femurs compared to primary femurs. A further reduction in strength was also seen with each subsequent revision. The main mode of failure in

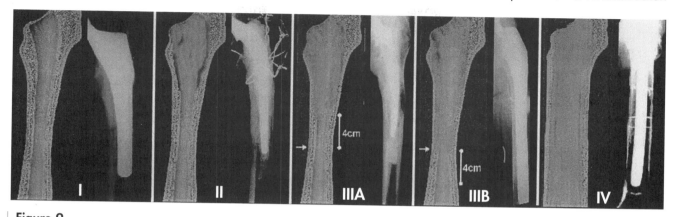

Figure 9

Femoral defect classification. Type I has minimal metaphyseal involvement and adequate cancellous bone. Type II has metaphyseal damage with a minimally involved diaphysis. Type IIIA has metadiaphyseal damage with 4 cm of reliable cortex proximal to the isthmus and type IIIB has metadiaphyseal damage with 4 cm of reliable cortex distal to the isthmus. Type IV has extensive metadiaphyseal and thin ballooned cortices with widened canals precluding reliable fixation.

cemented revisions is loosening at the cement-bone interface, further demonstrating the difficulties associated with cementing into a sclerotic bony bed.

First-generation cement methods used in femoral revision had a repeat revision rate of 3% to 60%. With longer follow-up, ongoing deterioration of results has been observed both radiographically and by clinical criteria. Forty-four percent of 166 femoral revisions were considered radiographically loose, 21% were considered clinically loose, and 5% were re-revised at 4.5 years postoperatively according to an early report from 1 institution. In a more recent multicenter evaluation of 204 cemented revision hips, 27% were radiographically loose and 10% were re-revised at a mean of 6 years after the operation.

Contemporary cementing methods have led to some improvement in both clinical and radiographic results. However, a combined failure rate of 0.5% to 3% per year over the first decade has been reported with second-generation cemented methods on the femoral side. Other studies have failed to indicate an improved revision survival rate with "modern" cement techniques. When the bony bed precludes significant cement interdigitation, it is reasonable to expect a reduction in fixation durability over time. The relative value in revision surgery of more recent so-called third-generation cement methods, including the use of spacers and stem centralizers, cement porosity reduction, and stem surface enhancements, remains to be seen.

Age at time of revision and the length of the cemented revision stem both appear to have a strong correlation with its survival. A younger age at time of revision and a shorter revision stem are associated with less than ideal results after cemented revision. In low demand octogenarians, cement fixation in the revision setting has had good results. Cemented femoral revision components that extend at least 2 femoral diameters beyond the area of cancellous defect minimize the stresses associated with loosening of the cemented revision. The addition of antibiotics to cement may improve the outcome of those patients revised for infection.

Cementless Femoral Revision

Proximally Porous Coated Implants Proximally porous coated revision implants rely on the proximal femoral bone stock that is frequently deficient. Therefore, proximal cementless fixation is more reliable in type I and II femoral defects. Sixty-six revisions using the Anatomic Porous Replacement Revision Hip System (Intermedics, Austin, TX) in 65 patients with predominantly type I and II femoral defects were followed for a mean of 4.7 years. Ninety-four percent of stems were deemed stable, and 6% of the stems were re-revised for loosening.

Modular design in a proximally fixed implant provides more options. Rotational stability is essential to the design of a proximally fixed device. The incorporation of distal flutes in the S-ROM (Joint Medical Products Corp, Stamford, CT) device has demonstrated relatively good results in femoral revision. In a series of 52 complex revisions using this component with a mean of 3 years follow-up the overall femoral mechanical loosening rate was 10%, and complications included intraoperative fractures in 28%.

Intraoperative fractures compromise the initial stability of the proximally coated implant, and in stems without supplemental distal fixation the results have been quite poor. At 5 years follow-up of 69 revisions with proximally tapered long stem designs to maximize fill of the proximal femur, 82% of the entire series were free of revision or moderate pain, compared to only 58% of those with an intraoperative femoral fracture during implant insertion.

A recent report of 375 consecutive revisions using 6 different proximally porous-coated implant designs (both long and short stem) indicated that during the first 5 years postrevision the re-revision rate for the overall series was 20%. Twenty-four percent of patients had moderate to severe pain and 29% had mild pain. Of the devices, 40% were radiographically loose and an additional 17% were possibly loose. Increased subsidence and decreased survivorship were noted when more severe bone loss was present.

Extensively Porous Coated Stem Difficulty in obtaining initial stability leading to poor intermediate-term results has tempered the initial enthusiasm for proximally coated implants. The extensively porous coated cementless stems bypass the often deficient proximal bone; they obtain initial diaphyseal fit and stability in the relatively normal distal bone, allowing for reliable biologic fixation with bony ingrowth. Extensively porous coated implants are proving dependable in intermediate and long-term follow up.

Long-term success of cementless femoral revisions depends on achieving initial axial and torsional stability by maximizing canal fill at time of implantation. Bone ingrowth correlates with the ability to fill the femoral canal. In one study, with greater than 90% canal fill, subsidence of the stem was less than 2 mm, and there were no unstable stems. When the average canal fill was 75%, subsidence was greater than 2 mm (average, 7 mm), and all of the stems were unstable. Increased initial axial and torsional prosthetic stability decreases micromotion and allows for long-term biologic fixation. A minimum interference fit of 4 cm is necessary for stability, with 6 cm of intimate contact preferred. Maximizing canal fill not only provides prosthetic stability, but also provides a circumferential biologic seal after bone ingrowth to prevent wear debris from migrating distally and creating osteolysis. Maximal canal fill also is associated with decreased complaints of thigh pain. Thigh pain is less common in stems achieving fixation with bone ingrowth (4.2 %) than in stems that have stable fibrous fixation (18.5%).

Since 1988, a second generation of extensively porous coated implants has been available; these are made of cobalt chromium with bullet-shaped distal tips and a larger selection of diameters and lengths and are available with standard, modified medial, and calcar replacement proximal geometries. They are also available in straight or an anterior bowed

stem. This bow is made to resemble the normal femoral curvature. These modifications were made to improve canal fill and decrease cortical impingement.

These second-generation extensively porous coated implants were used in 83 patients for 87 femoral revisions; 67 patients with 71 revisions (average follow-up, 5.8 years) were reviewed. Aseptic loosening was the primary indication for revision. At a minimum of 5 years' follow-up, 96% of the femoral components remained in place, 54 (79%) achieved fixation with bone ingrowth, and 14 (21%) had stable fibrous fixation. No re-revisions were performed for loosening and no femoral components exhibited radiographic instability. Three patients who underwent resection arthroplasty for infection had stable fixation of the femoral component at time of surgery. Two of the stems were bone ingrown and the other was fibrous stable. There was a strong correlation between canal fill and bony ingrowth. As a result, the reviewers proposed that the ability to obtain fixation with bone ingrowth better correlates with obtaining canal fill than with the type of femoral defect present.

Distal fixation provides a number of advantages over proximal fixation. The relatively cylindrical femoral diaphysis enables the surgeon to dictate component placement to maximize hip stability without compromising component stability. Both femoral version and length can be adjusted without adversely affecting cortical contact. On the other hand, the anatomy of the proximal femur determines optimal component positioning with a proximally fixed device. The position of the proximally fixed device cannot be altered without adversely affecting cortical contact and/or risking fracture of the comparatively thin metaphyseal cortical bone.

Impaction Allograft Technique An alternative approach to the challenge of bone loss in the revision setting is the impaction allograft technique. For large tubulous canals devoid of cancellous bone, allograft cancellous bone is tightly packed within the canal of the host femur, and a smooth polished stem is cemented within the grafted endosteal surface. In a cadaver model, the stability of the allograft/cemented reconstruction was found to be intermediate between those of conventional cemented and cementless stems. This stability is essential for healing of the graft to occur. Evaluations of biopsy specimens have demonstrated that remodeling occurs and there is at least some restoration of bone stock using this technique.

Clinical evaluations seem optimistic in these otherwise unreconstructable patients. Early results of 56 of 67 patients treated with impaction grafting included 2 septic failures and no evidence of femoral component loosening; 79% of the patients were pain free. In a second short-term review of 34 impaction grafting revisions there were 2 major concerns with the technique: fractures and subsidence. Femoral integrity was compromised in 8 of 34 (2 perforations, 4 intraoperative fractures, 2 postoperative fractures). Subsidence of the construct occurred in 40% of the patients, and these stems subsided an average of 10.1 mm.

Annotated Bibliography

Hip Arthroscopy

Edwards DJ, Lomas D, Villar RN: Diagnosis of the painful hip by magnetic resonance imaging and arthroscopy. *J Bone Joint Surg* 1995;77B:374–376.

Small chondral defects, osteochondral loose bodies, and labral tears not diagnosed by MRI were identified and treated with hip arthroscopy.

McCarthy JC, Busconi B: The role of hip arthroscopy in the diagnosis and treatment of hip disease. *Can J Surg* 1995;38(suppl 1):S13–S17.

At arthroscopy, positive correlations ($p < 0.05$) were identified between preoperative clicking or giving way and locking symptoms and labral tears and loose bodies. Arthroscopy allowed treatment of these problems.

Hip Arthrodesis

Duncan CP, Spangehl M, Beauchamp C, McGraw R: Hip arthrodesis: An important option for advanced disease in the young adult. *Can J Surg* 1995;38(suppl 1):S39–S45.

The authors review principles and techniques of hip arthrodesis.

Matta JM, Siebenrock KA, Gautier E, Mehne D, Ganz R: Hip fusion through an anterior approach with the use of a ventral plate. *Clin Orthop* 1997;337:129–139.

A new method of hip arthrodesis with a ventral compression plate placed through a Smith-Peterson approach is described. Union was achieved in 10 of 12 patients.

Osteotomy

Gotoh E, Inao S, Okamoto T, Ando M: Valgus-extension osteotomy for advanced osteoarthritis in dysplastic hips: Results at 12 to 18 years. *J Bone Joint Surg* 1997;79B:609–615.

For 31 hips with advanced osteoarthritis in patients with hip dysplasia, the 15-year survivorship of valgus extension osteotomy was 51%.

Iwase T, Hasegawa Y, Kawamoto K, Iwasada S, Yamada K, Iwata H: Twenty years' followup of intertrochanteric osteotomy for treatment of the dysplastic hip. *Clin Orthop* 1996;331:245–255.

Fifteen-year survivorship was 87% for varus intertrochanteric osteotomies (for dysplasia with early or no degenerative disease) and 38% for valgus osteotomy (for dysplasia with advanced degenerative disease).

Millis MB, Murphy SB, Poss R: Osteotomies about the hip for the prevention and treatment of osteoarthrosis. *J Bone Joint Surg* 1995;77A:626–647.

This is a comprehensive discussion of the present status of hip osteotomy with an extensive reference list.

Wedge JH: Osteotomy of the pelvis for the management of hip disease in young adults. *Can J Surg* 1995;38(suppl 1):S25–S32.

The author reviews the available procedures, indications, and results of pelvic osteotomy in young adults.

Osteonecrosis

Fairbank AC, Bhatia D, Jinnah RH, Hungerford DS: Long-term results of core decompression for ischaemic necrosis of the femoral head. *J Bone Joint Surg* 1995;77B:42–49.

This authoritative review of the long-term results of a large number of cases of ON treated by core decompression, gives an objective evaluation of the indications, contraindications, and results of this technique.

Glueck CJ, Freiberg R, Tracy T, Stroop D, Wang P: Thrombophilia and hypofibrinolysis: Pathophysiologies of osteonecrosis. *Clin Orthop* 1997;334:43–56.

The authors discuss the role that certain subtle coagulopathies may play in the pathogenesis of ON.

Mont MA, Carbone JJ, Fairbank AC: Core decompression versus nonoperative management for osteonecrosis of the hip. *Clin Orthop* 1996;324:169–178.

This comprehensive review of 42 reports of hips treated either by core decompression or nonsurgical management shows significantly better outcomes in hips treated surgically than in those treated nonsurgically.

Mont MA, Hungerford DS: Non-traumatic avascular necrosis of the femoral head. *J Bone Joint Surg* 1995;77A:459–474.

This excellent and comprehensive review of ON of the femoral head includes a description of etiology, staging, diagnosis, and treatment.

Steinberg ME, Hayken GD, Steinberg DR: A quantitative system for staging avascular necrosis. *J Bone Joint Surg* 1995;77B:34–41.

This in-depth discussion of a quantitative system for staging avascular necrosis, referred to in the text, shows the advantages of this system over older, nonquantitative methods of staging.

Urbaniak JR, Coogan PG, Gunneson EB, Nunley JA: Treatment of osteonecrosis of the femoral head with free vascularized fibular grafting: A long-term follow-up study of one hundred and three hips. *J Bone Joint Surg* 1995;77A:681–694.

This is a review of a large series of patients with long-term follow-up treated by a single surgeon with resection of the necrotic segment and grafting with both cancellous graft and a vascularized fibula. Results were excellent even in patients with some degree of femoral head collapse.

Urbaniak JR, Jones JP Jr (eds): *Osteonecrosis: Etiology, Diagnosis, and Treatment.* Rosemont, IL, American Academy of Orthopaedic Surgeons, 1997.

This is the published proceedings of an international symposium on ON, which includes participants from several countries and the latest information concerning etiology, pathogenesis, and treatment. It is perhaps the most comprehensive compendium on this topic currently available.

Cost Effectiveness/Outcome Assessment

Espehaug B, Havelin LI, Engesaester LB, Langeland N, Vollset SE: Patient-related risk factors for early revision of total hip replacements: A population register-based case-control study of 674 revised hips. *Acta Orthp Scand* 1997;68:207–215.

The authors identify a set of patient-related factors associated with poor THR prognosis. Increasing weight was a risk factor among men older than 67 years and taller than 1.77 m. Smoking had no overall effect, but former heavy smokers had risk of 2.6 compared to non-smokers. Alcohol intake was associated with an increased risk of dislocation. Revision due to infection was more common among patients taking antidiabetic drugs than among patients taking no medication. An increased overall revision risk was found among patients using systemic steroids or local pulmonary steroids.

Lavernia CJ, Guzman JF: Relationship of surgical volume to short-term morality, morbidity, and hospital charges in arthroplasty. *J Arthroplasty* 1995;10:133–140.

The authors detail the effects of surgical volume on short-term outcome as measured by mortality, morbidity, length of stay, and hospital charges for primary and revision arthroplasty as a function of the surgeon and the hospital.

Lieberman JR, Dorey F, Shekelle P, et al: Differences between patients' and physicians' evaluations of outcome after total hip arthroplasty. *J Bone Joint Surg* 1996;78A:835–838.

The authors report a comparison study of the patients' and physicians' ratings of pain and function.

Cement Fixation

Madey SM, Callaghan JJ, Olejniczak JP, Goetz DD, Johnston RC: Charnley total hip arthroplasty with use of improved techniques of cementing: The results after a minimum of fifteen years of follow-up. *J Bone Joint Surg* 1997;79A:53–64.

A 15-year follow-up of 356 THAs by 1 surgeon is reported. The authors demonstrate long-term durability of fixation of the femoral component but less reliable fixation of the acetabular component, even when the surgeon is experienced and improved techniques of cementing are used.

Mohler CG, Callaghan JJ, Collis DK, Johnston RC: Early loosening of the femoral component at the cement-prosthesis interface after total hip replacement. *J Bone Joint Surg* 1995;77A: 1315–1322.

This is a report on 1,941 THAs performed by 2 surgeons on patients 41 to 77 years of age at arthroplasty. Of these patients, 27 had early loosening of the femoral component 2 to 10 years postoperatively. The authors believe that both the geometry (cylindrical shape distal to the proximal cobra shape) and the surface finish of the Iowa femoral component were responsible for the pattern of progressive loosening.

Mohler CG, Kull LR, Martell JM, Rosenberg AG, Galante JO: Total hip replacement with insertion of an acetabular component without cement and a femoral component with cement: Four to seven-year results. *J Bone Joint Surg* 1995;77A:86–96.

This is a report on 120 hybrid THAs performed by 4 surgeons on 117 patients (average age, 67 years) at arthroplasty. Follow-up averaged 62 months (range, 48 to 85). Two percent of cups and 2% of stems were definitely radiographically loose. The authors believe that this procedure is an excellent alternative for older patients who have a painful hip caused by osteoarthrosis.

Mulroy WF, Estok DM, Harris WH: Total hip arthroplasty with use of so-called second-generation cementing techniques: A fifteen-year-average follow-up study. *J Bone Joint Surg* 1995;77A: 1845–1852.

The 14- to 17-year results of a single surgeon series of 102 hips reveals a revision rate for aseptic loosening of 2% for femoral components and 10% for acetabular components. An additional 42% of cups were definitely radiographically loose. Femoral components implanted with the use of second-generation cementing techniques appear to have fared much better than acetabular components.

Mulroy WF, Harris WH: Acetabular and femoral fixation 15 years after cemented total hip surgery. *Clin Orthop* 1997;337: 118–128.

The 15-year results of a single surgeon series of 47 hips reveals a revision rate for aseptic loosening of 1 femoral component and 10 acetabular components. Overall, 8% of stems and 64% of cups were definitely radiographically loose.

Woolson ST, Haber DF: Primary total hip replacement with insertion of an acetabular component without cement and a femoral component with cement: Follow-up study at an average of six years. *J Bone Joint Surg* 1996;78A:698–705.

In a 6-year follow-up study of 121 Hybrid THAs, there was a stem revision rate of 5% and cup loosening rate of 0%. The clinical results in the 104 patients (115 hips) for whom clinical and radiographic data were available were excellent at the time of intermediate follow-up.

Uncemented Total Hip Arthroplasty

Astion DJ, Saluan P, Stulberg BN, Rimnac CM, Li S: The porous-coated anatomic total hip prosthesis: Failure of the metal-backed acetabular component. *J Bone Joint Surg* 1996;78A:755–766.

This is review of 199 THAs performed with a PCA, at 19 to 94 months (mean 58 ± 18 months) postsurgery. The results of this study suggest that factors related to both the design and the material contributed to the failure of these porous-coated anatomic acetabular components.

Bleobaum RD, Mihalopoulus NL, Jensen JW, Dorr LD: Postmortem analysis of bone growth into porous-coated acetabular components. *J Bone Joint Surg* 1997;79A:1013–1022.

The authors report a retrieval study of 7 porous-coated acetabular components, at 10 to 64 months (mean 38 ± 21 months) postimplantation. Microradiographic analysis of all 7 components showed that an average of 84% ± 9% of the porous coating was in direct apposition to the periprosthetic bone. The authors believe that consistent bone growth into anatomic porous replacement acetabular components can be achieved.

Engh CA Jr, Culpepper WJ III, Engh CA: Long-term results of use of the anatomic medullary locking prosthesis in total hip arthroplasty. *J Bone Joint Surg* 1997;79A:177–184.

The authors report an 11-year follow-up (range, 10 to 13 years) of 174 AML THAs. There were 20 reoperations involving a component.

Engh CA, Hooten JP Jr, Zettl-Schaffer KF, Ghaffarpour M, McGovern TF, Bobyn JD: Evaluation of bone ingrowth in proximally and extensively porous-coated anatomic medullary locking prostheses retrieved at autopsy. *J Bone Joint Surg* 1995;77A:903–910.

The authors report a retrieval study of 8 AML femoral components (3 proximally and 5 extensively) at 17 to 84 months postimplantation (mean, 63 months). All 8 components had some bone ingrowth into the porous surface. A mean of 35% of the implant surface had bone ingrowth. In the areas where bone was present, 67% of the available porous surface on the extensively coated stems and 74% on the proximally coated stems contained bone.

Geesink RT, Hoefnagels NH: Six-year results of hydroxyapatite-coated total hip replacement. *J Bone Joint Surg* 1995;77B:534–547.

This is a 5.6- to 7.6-year follow-up study of 118 Omnifit THAs, all in patients younger than 66 years of age at arthroplasty. The survival rate at a mean of 6 years was 100% for the HA-coated stems and 99% for the HA-threaded cups. The authors believe that HA coatings can provide early pain relief and durable implant fixation.

Latimer HA, Lachiewicz PF: Porous-coated acetabular components with screw fixation: Five to ten-year results. *J Bone Joint Surg* 1996;78A:975–981.

In this 5- to 10-year follow-up study of 136 Harris-Galante 1 porous coated acetabular components, none required revision for acetabular component loosening. The low prevalence of polyethylene wear and pelvis osteolysis is a notable improvement compared with the results of arthroplasty with other porous-coated acetabular components.

Complications of Total Hip Arthroplasty

Osteolysis and Wear

Jacobs JJ, Urban RM, Gilbert JL, et al: Local and distant products from modularity. *Clin Orthop* 1995;319:94–105.

The local and distant distribution of solid and soluble products of corrosion from the head and neck junction of modular femoral total hip prosthetic components were characterized. The authors believe that it is premature to eliminate femoral implants with head and neck modularity from the surgeon's armamentarium; improvements in fretting corrosion resistance are required to ensure the durability and safety of these devices.

Jasty M, Goetz DD, Bragdon CR, et al: Wear of polyethylene acetabular components in total hip arthroplasty: An analysis of one hundred and twenty-eight components retrieved at autopsy or revision operations. *J Bone Joint Surg* 1997;79A;349–358.

The authors report a retrieval study of 128 cemented hips analyzed for polyethylene wear. The rate of volumetric wear was higher in 32-mm femoral heads than in 22-mm heads.

Mckellop HA, Campbell P, Park SH, et al: The origin of submicron polyethylene wear debris in total hip arthroplasty. *Clin Orthop* 1995;311:3–20.

The microscopic morphology of the surfaces of polyethylene acetabular cups tested in a hip joint stimulator was compared to that of cups retrieved from patients. The authors believe that future modifications of the bearing materials should be directed toward maximizing the resistance of the materials to the wear mechanisms producing the submicron wear particles.

Stress-Shielding

Bugbee WD, Culpepper WJ II, Engh CA Jr, Engh CA Sr: Long-term clinical consequences of stress-shielding after total hip arthroplasty without cement. *J Bone Joint Surg* 1997;79A:1007–1012.

The authors report 207 hips followed up for at least 2 years, with a 23% incidence of stress-shielding (pronounced femoral bone remodeling).

Maloney WJ, Sychterz C, Bragdon C, et al: Skeletal response to well fixed femoral components inserted with and without cement. *Clin Orthop* 1996;333:15–26.

The authors report a study of 48 anatomic specimen femora from 24 patients with unilateral cemented and cementless hip replacements retrieved 13 months to 16 years postimplantation. The maximum cortical bone loss by level was at the middle section for the cemented femurs and at the midproximal and middle sections for the cementless femurs. A strong correlation was noted between the bone mineral density of the control femur and percentage decrease of bone mineral density in the remodeled femur.

Dislocation

Cobb TK, Morrey BF, Ilstrup DM: The elevated-rim acetabular liner in total hip arthroplasty: Relationship to postoperative dislocation. *J Bone Joint Surg* 1996;78A:80–86.

Authors compare data on 2,469 acetabular components with an elevated-rim liner (10° of elevation) and 2,698 with a standard liner. Dislocation rates were higher in the standard liner group than in the elevated-rim liner group. The authors do not advocate the routine insertion of an acetabular component with an elevated-rim liner at this time.

Hedlundh U, Ahnfelt L, Hybbinette CH, Weckstrom J, Fredin H: Surgical experience related to dislocations after total hip arthroplasty. *J Bone Joint Surg* 1996;78B:206–209.

The authors document the effect of surgical experience on the dislocation rate after 4,230 primary THAs at 3 orthopaedic centers. There were 129 postoperative dislocations (3%). Twice the number of dislocations were registered for inexperienced surgeons as for their more experienced colleagues.

Periprosthetic Fractures

Peterson CA, Lewallen DG: Periprosthetic fracture of the acetabulum after total hip arthroplasty. *J Bone Joint Surg* 1996;78A:1206–1213.

The authors believe that periprosthetic acetabular fractures are associated with a poor prognosis with regard to the survival of acetabular component but that it is possible to achieve union and to salvage a functional prosthesis in patients who have sustained such a fracture.

Heterotopic Ossification

Amstutz HC, Fowble VA, Schmalzried TP, Dorey FJ: Short-course indomethacin prevents heterotopic ossification in a high-risk population following total hip arthroplasty. *J Arthroplasty* 1997;12:126–132.

This study was performed on 109 patients to prevent HO after THA. A 10-day course of indomethacin prevents the more significant grades of HO and is effective at reducing the incidence of HO following THA.

Knelles D, Barthel T, Karrer A, Kraus U, Eulert J, Kolbl O: Prevention of heterotopic ossification after total hip replacement: A prospective, randomized study using acetylsalicylic acid, indomethacin and fractional or single-dose irradiation. *J Bone Joint Surg* 1997;79B:596–602.

The authors report a prospective randomized controlled study using acetylsalicylic acid, indomethacin for 7 and 14 days, 1 fractional irradiation, and 2 different single doses of irradiation after surgery. A single irradiation of 7 Gy is recommended for patients who have developed HO after previous operations or to whom administration of indomethacin is contraindicated.

Pellegrini VD Jr, Gregoritch SJ: Preoperative irradiation for prevention of heterotopic ossification following total hip arthroplasty. *J Bone Joint Surg* 1996;78A:870–881.

The authors compare efficacy of preoperative and postoperative irradiation at minimum 6-months' follow-up. The authors suggest that preoperative irradiation is effective for the prevention of HO following THA and that it eliminates the discomfort and morbidity associated with conventional postoperative treatment.

Infection

Becker W, Palestro CJ, Winship J, et al: Rapid imaging of infections with a monoclonal antibody fragment (LeukoScan). *Clin Orthop* 1996;329:263–272.

The diagnostic accuracy for imaging infection with a technetium Tc 99m-labeled antigranulocyte Fab' fragment (LeukoScan) was prospectively examined in a multicenter study in 53 patients. Sensitivity, specificity, and diagnostic accuracy of LeukoScan were 90.0%, 84.6%, and 87.9%, respectively; and with autologous leukocyte scintigraphy were 93.9%, 76.5%, and 81.3%, respectively.

Fitzgerald RH, Jacobson JJ, Luck JV Jr, et al: Antibiotic prophylaxis for dental patients with total joint replacements. *AAOS Bulletin* 1997;45:9–11.

Representatives from the AAOS and American Dental Association (ADA) met and developed guidelines for the use of antimicrobial prophylaxis for dental patients with total joint replacements. The group was able to stratify dental procedures by the risk of bacteremia and patients by their susceptibility to infection. Recommendations on antibiotics to be used are also provided.

Garvin KL, Evans BG, Salvati EA, Brause BD: Palacos gentamicin for the treatment of deep periprosthetic hip infections. *Clin Orthop* 1994;298:97–105.

Between 1983 and 1986, 40 hip arthroplasties in 40 patients with documented deep infection were reimplanted using Palacos gentamicin. At an average follow-up of 5 years (range, 2 to 10), 2 hips (5%) developed recurrent infection.

Garvin KL, Hanssen AD: Infection after total hip arthroplasty: Past, present, and future. *J Bone Joint Surg* 1995;77A: 1576–1588.

The authors review diagnostic and treatment standards for patients with infection after THA. Two-stage reimplantation with local antibiotic delivery was successful in 285 of 423 patients (91%) reviewed. Future methods using polymerase chain reaction to assist in diagnosis, and methods to amplify cell-mediated immune response are described.

Hanssen AD, Osmon DR, Nelson CL: Prevention of deep periprosthetic joint infection. *J Bone Joint Surg* 1996;78A: 458–471.

The authors provide strategies to help prevent infection after total joint arthroplasty.

Lachiewicz PF, Rogers GD, Thomason HC: Aspiration of the hip joint before revision total hip arthroplasty: Clinical and laboratory factors influencing attainment of a positive culture. *J Bone Joint Surg* 1996;78A:749–754.

The authors review the results of hip aspiration performed on 142 hips. Twenty-one hips (15%) were infected; however, the intraoperative culture for 2 hips was considered to be false-positive and excluded. Preoperative aspiration had a sensitivity of 92%, a specificity of 97%, and an accuracy of 96%.

Lonner JH, Desai P, Dicesare PE, Steiner G, Zuckerman JD: The reliability of analysis of intraoperative frozen sections for identifying active infection during revision hip or knee arthroplasty. *J Bone Joint Surg* 1996;78A:1553–1558.

The authors performed a prospective study to determine the reliability of analysis of intraoperative frozen sections for the identification of infection during 175 consecutive revision total joint arthroplasties (142 hip and 33 knee). Twenty-three patients had at least 5 polymorphonuclear leukocytes per high-power field on analysis of the frozen sections and were considered to have an infection. The authors suggest that it is valuable to obtain tissue for intraoperative frozen sections during revision hip and knee arthroplasty.

Masteron EL, Masri BA, Duncan CP: Treatment of infection at the site of total hip replacement. *J Bone Joint Surg* 1997;79A: 1740–1749.

The authors review the treatment of patients who develop infection at the site of THA. Using the PROSTALAC technique the authors successfully healed 44 of 48 patients (94%) at a minimum 2-year follow-up.

Nijhof MW, Oyen WJ, van Kampen A, Claessens RA, van der Meer JW, Corstens FH: Evaluation of infections of the locomotor system with indium-111-labeled human IgG scintigraphy. *J Nucl Med* 1997;38:1300–1305.

Indium In 111 labeled human nonspecific immunoglobin G (^{111}InIgG) was used to evaluate 226 patients with 232 possible foci of infection or inflammation. The authors concluded that careful interpretation is necessary in cementless THA up to 1 year after insertion and in recent fractures and pseudarthrosis, in which uptake may be caused by sterile inflammation and not by infection.

Tsukayama DT, Estrada R, Gustilo RB: Infection after total hip arthroplasty: A study of the treatment of one hundred and six infections. *J Bone Joint Surg* 1996;78A:512–523.

Ninety-seven patients (106 infections in 98 hips) were studied. A good result was noted after the initial treatment of 28 (90%) of the 31 infections diagnosed on the basis of positive intraoperative cultures at the time of revision, 25 (71%) of the 35 early postoperative infections, 29 (85%) of the 34 late chronic infections, and 3 of the 6 acute hematogenous infections. The factors associated with recurrent infection were retained bone cement, the number of previous operations, potential immunocompromise, and early postoperative infection after arthroplasty without cement.

Acetabular Revision

Anderson MJ, Murray WR, Skinner HB: Constrained acetabular components. *J Arthroplasty* 1994;9:17–23.

Sixteen of 21 constrained acetabular components were successful in preventing further dislocations. An increased cup abduction angle averaging 70° was the only predictive factor of the failure of the constrained cup ($p = 0.05$).

Garbuz D, Morsi E, Gross AE: Revision of the acetabular component of a total hip arthroplasty with a massive structural allograft: Study with a minimum five-year follow-up. *J Bone Joint Surg* 1996;78A:693–697.

The authors examined their results with massive structural acetabular allografts in 33 hips followed up for a minimum of 5 years. The only factor that was found to be clinically important with respect to outcome was the method of reconstruction.

Kelley SS: High hip center in revision arthroplasty. *J Arthroplasty* 1994;9:503–510.

In this study of 23 hips reviewed at an average follow-up of 35 months, only 1 acetabular implant was radiographically loose while 2 cemented femoral implants were radiographically loose. Superior cup placement an average 24.7 mm did not result in concomitant lateralization.

Lee BP, Cabanela ME, Wallrichs SL, Ilstrup DM: Bone-graft augmentation for acetabular deficiencies in total hip arthroplasty: Results of long-term follow-up evaluation. *J Arthroplasty* 1997;12:503–510.

The authors evaluate their results of 102 acetabular arthroplasties using bone graft augmentation. Although their early results were encouraging, acetabular failure increased to 18% at 10 years. They conclude that graft incorporation was successful and facilitated subsequent revision surgery.

Morsi E, Garbuz D, Gross AE: Total hip arthroplasty with shelf grafts using uncemented cups: A long-term follow-up study. *J Arthroplasty* 1996;11:81–85.

The authors review results of their series of 33 hips treated with cementless cups and structural graft at a minimum follow-up of 5 years. The 16 revisions with allograft improved patients' hip score from 44.4 preoperatively to an average score of 82 at the most recent review.

Papagelopoulos PJ, Lewallen DG, Cabanela ME, McFarland EG, Wallrichs SL: Acetabular reconstruction using bipolar endoprosthesis and bone grafting in patients with severe bone deficiency. *Clin Orthop* 1995;314:170–184.

Eighty-one patients who had hip reconstruction with bone grafting and bipolar endoprosthesis for severe acetabular deficiency were reviewed retrospectively at 3 to 8 years postoperatively. Thirty-five procedures were considered unsuccessful at the most recent follow-up with only 54.7% of patients considering themselves improved.

490 Lower Extremity

Paprosky WG, Perona PG, Lawrence JM: Acetabular defect classification and surgical reconstruction in revision arthroplasty: A 6-year follow-up evaluation. *J Arthroplasty* 1994;9:33–44.

The authors discuss their experience reconstructing acetabular defects around 147 failed cemented acetabular components. They develop a defect classification system based on the ability of remaining bone to support acetabular reconstruction.

Slooff TH, Buma P, Schreurs BW, Schimmel JW, Huiskes R, Gardeniers J: Acetabular and femoral reconstruction with impacted graft and cement. *Clin Orthop* 1996;323:108–115.

The authors conducted a clinical and radiographic evaluation of 88 patients whose acetabular defects were reconstructed with impacted morcellized allograft and a cemented cup. After a mean follow-up of 70 months, clinical and 6 radiographic failures had occurred. These results encourage the authors to continue the use of this technique.

Sutherland CJ: Treatment of type III acetabular deficiencies in revision total hip arthroplasty without structural bone-graft. *J Arthroplasty* 1996;11:91–98.

This is a prospective randomized study of 19 hips, reviewed at an average follow-up of 46 months. The Harris hip score improved from 46 to 75. Although 26% of hips demonstrated some evidence of loosening, only 11% required revision.

Stockl B, Beerkotte J, Krismer M, Fischer M, Bauer R: Results of the Muller acetabular reinforcement ring in revision arthroplasty. *Arch Orthop Trauma Surg* 1997;116:55–59.

The use of reinforcement rings to reconstruct the acetabulum were successful if the craniolateral position was avoided and the hip center was positioned more closely to the anatomic hip center.

Woolson ST, Adamson GJ: Acetabular revision using a bone-ingrowth total hip component in patients who have acetabular bone stock deficiency. *J Arthroplasty* 1996;11:661–667.

The authors conclude that cementless acetabular revision with supplemental screw fixation and bone-graft appeared to be successful in restoring moderate or severe bone loss and providing a stable, painless reconstruction.

Femoral Revision

Aribindi R, Barba M, Solomon M, Paprosky WG: Bypass fixation. *Orthop Clin North Am* 1998;29:319–329.

This article reviews femoral fixation in revision arthroplasty and presents 5-year data on a second generation of extensively porous coated stems used in 87 revisions in 83 patients. No femoral components were revised for loosening. Three patients were revised for infection. Eighty percent were bone ingrown and 20% were fibrous stable.

Buoncristiani AM, Dorr LD, Johnson C, Wan Z: Cementless revision of total hip arthroplasty using the anatomic porous replacement revision prosthesis. *J Arthroplasty* 1997;12:403–415.

Sixty-six hips in 65 patients (average age, 56) received an APR revision stem and were followed up for a mean of 4.7 years. Only 6% of the stems were revised and 94% of the stems were considered stable. The hydroxyapatite coating used in 31 stems was associated with an improved Harris hip score.

Chandler HP, Ayres DK, Tan RC, Anderson LC, Varma AK: Revision total hip replacement using the S-ROM femoral component. *Clin Orthop* 1995;319:130–140.

Fifty-two femoral revisions using the S-ROM femoral component were performed in 48 patients (average age, 60 years). At an average of 3 years' follow-up 5 (10%) stems were loose.

Elting JJ, Mikhail WE, Zicat BA, Hubbell JC, Lane LE, House B: Preliminary report of impaction grafting for exchange femoral arthroplasty. *Clin Orthop* 1995;319:159–167.

Fifty-six patients were followed up 2 to 5 years after impaction grafting femoral revision. There were 2 septic failures, no loose femoral components, and 79% were pain free.

Gross AE, Hutchison CR, Alexeeff M, Mahomed N, Leitch K, Morsi E: Proximal femoral allografts for reconstruction of bone stock in revision arthroplasty of the hip. *Clin Orthop* 1995;319:151–158.

The authors followed up 168 proximal femoral allografts used in femoral revisions for 4.8 years and they found 85% of the femoral reconstructions were successful and 10.1% required revisions.

Katz RP, Callaghan JJ, Sullivan PM, Johnston RC: Long-term results of revision total hip arthroplasty with improved cementing technique. *J Bone Joint Surg* 1997;79B:322–326.

Eighty-one hips in 76 patients (average age, 64 years) were followed up for a mean of 11.9 years following a femoral component revision using second generation techniques. Thirteen (16%) were revised due to aseptic loosening and 10 (24%) were felt to be radiographically loose.

Krishnamurthy A, MacDonald S, Paprosky WG: Five to 13-year follow-up study on cementless femoral components in revision surgery. *J Arthroplasty* 1997;12:839–847.

This review of 297 cementless revision arthroplasties using extensively coated components includes a basic classification of femoral defects.

Mann KA, Ayers DC, Damron TA: Effects of stem length on mechanics of the femoral hip component after cemented revision. *J Orthop Res* 1997;15:62–68.

In a 3-dimensional finite element model of cemented revision stems of 5 different lengths, relative motion at the cement bone interface was reduced using stem lengths that extended greater than 2 femoral diameters beyond the original defect.

McGrory BJ, Bal BS, Harris WH: Trochanteric osteotomy for total hip arthroplasty: Six variations and indications for their use. *J Am Acad Orthop Surg* 1996;4:258–267.

This is a review of 6 trochanteric osteotomy techniques, indications for use, and results in the literature. Also described is the technique for using the extended trochanteric osteotomy with a cemented component.

McLaughlin JR, Harris WH: Revision of the femoral component of a total hip arthroplasty with the calcar-replacement femoral component: Results after a mean of 10.8 years postoperatively. *J Bone Joint Surg* 1996;78A:331–339.

Thirty-eight cemented revision hips using second generation cement techniques and a calcar replacement stem in patients with a mean age of 55 years were followed up a mean of 10.8 years. Thirty-two percent were felt to be loose and 18% had been revised.

Meding JB, Ritter MA, Keating EM, Faris PM: Impaction bone-grafting before insertion of a femoral stem with cement in revision total hip arthroplasty: A minimum two-year follow-up study. *J Bone Joint Surg* 1997;79A:1834–1841.

In a study of 34 revisions performed with impaction grafting and cement, femoral integrity was compromised in 8 and subsidence occurred in 7.

Mulroy W, Harris WH: Revision total hip arthroplasty with use of so-called second-generation cement techniques for aseptic loosening of the femoral component: A fifteen-year average follow-up study. *J Bone Joint Surg* 1996;78A:325–330.

Forty-three femoral revisions in 41 patients with an average age of 51 years were followed up an average of 15 years. Seven (20%) were revised due to aseptic loosening; 9 (26%) were considered radiographically loose.

Younger TI, Bradford MS, Magnus RE, Paprosky W: Extended proximal femoral osteotomy: A new technique for femoral revision arthroplasty. *J Arthroplasty* 1995;10:329–338.

The authors provide detailed surgical technique on the extended proximal femoral osteotomy as well as their clinical results. No nonunions or delayed unions were seen in 20 patients who underwent this osteotomy in the revision setting.

Classic Bibliography

Barrack RL, Harris WH: The value of aspiration of the hip joint before revision total hip arthroplasty. *J Bone Joint Surg* 1993;75A:66–76.

Berry DJ, Muller MM: Revision arthroplasty using an anti-protrusio cage for massive acetabular bone deficiency. *J Bone Joint Surg* 1992;74B:711–715.

Callaghan JJ, Brand RA, Pedersen DR: Hip arthrodesis: A long-term follow-up. *J Bone Joint Surg* 1985;67A:1328–1335.

D'Antonio JA, Capello WN, Borden LS, et al: Classification and management of acetabular abnormalities in total hip arthroplasty. *Clin Orthop* 1989;243:126–137.

Ficat RP: Idiopathic bone necrosis of the femoral head: Early diagnosis and treatment. *J Bone Joint Surg* 1985:67B:3–9.

Ganz R, Klaue K, Vinh TS, Mast JW: A new periacetabular osteotomy for the treatment of hip dysplasias: Technique and preliminary results. *Clin Orthop* 1988;232:26–36.

Glick JM: Hip arthroscopy using the lateral approach, in Bassett FH III (ed): *Instructional Course Lectures XXXVII.* Park Ridge, IL, American Academy of Orthopaedic Surgeons, 1988, pp 223–231.

Havelin LI, Vollset SE, Engesaeter LB: Revision for aseptic loosening of uncemented cups in 4,352 primary total hip prostheses: A report from the Norwegian Arthroplasty Register. *Acta Orthop Scand* 1995;66:494–500.

Hooten JP Jr, Engh CA, Heekin RD, Vinh TN: Structural bulk allografts in acetabular reconstruction: Analysis of two grafts retrieved at post-mortem. *J Bone Joint Surg* 1996;78B:270–275.

Marti RK, Schuller HM, Raaymakers EL: Intertrochanteric osteotomy for non-union of the femoral neck. *J Bone Joint Surg* 1989;71B:782–787.

Paprosky WG, Magnus RE: Principles of bone grafting in revision total hip arthroplasty: Acetabular technique. *Clin Orthop* 1994;298:147–155.

Raut VV, Siney PD, Wroblewski BM: Revision of the acetabular component of a total hip arthroplasty with cement in young patients without rheumatoid arthritis. *J Bone Joint Surg* 1996;78A:1853–1856.

Schutzer SF, Harris WH: High placement of porous-coated acetabular components in complex total hip arthroplasty. *J Arthroplasty* 1994;9:359–367.

Shinar AA, Harris WH: Bulk structural autogenous grafts and allografts for reconstruction of the acetabulum in total hip arthroplasty: Sixteen-year average follow-up. *J Bone Joint Surg* 1997;79A:159–168.

Silverton CD, Rosenberg AG, Sheinkop MB, Kull LR, Galante JO: Revision total hip arthroplasty using a cementless acetabular component: Technique and results. *Clin Orthop* 1995;319:201–208.

Sponseller PD, McBeath AA, Perpich M: Hip arthrodesis in young patients: A long-term follow-up study. *J Bone Joint Surg* 1984;66A:853–859.

492   Lower Extremity

Steel HH: Triple osteotomy of the innominate bone. *J Bone Joint Surg* 1973;55A:343–350.

Steinberg ME: Osteonecrosis of the hip. *Semin Arthroplasty* 1991;2:159–249.

Stromberg CN, Herberts P, Palmertz B: Cemented revision hip arthroplasty: A multicenter 5-9 year study of 204 first revisions for loosening. *Acta Orthop Scand* 1992;63:111–119.

Tanzer M, Drucker D, Jasty M, McDonald M, Harris WH: Revision of the acetabular component with an uncemented Harris-Galante porous-coated prothesis. *J Bone Joint Surg* 1992;74:987–994.

Trousdale RT, Ekkernkamp A, Ganz R, Wallrichs SL: Periacetabular and intertrochanteric osteotomy for the treatment of osteoarthrosis in dysplastic hips. *J Bone Joint Surg* 1995;77A:73–85.

Weber KL, Callaghan JJ, Goetz DD, Johnston RC: Revision of a failed cemented total hip prosthesis with insertion of an acetabular component without cement and a femoral component with cement: A five to eight-year follow-up study. *J Bone Joint Surg* 1996;78A:982–994.

Chapter 39
Femur: Trauma

Femoral Shaft Fractures

Classification

Femoral shaft fractures are classified by their bony configuration as well as the degree of injury to the surrounding soft tissues. Fracture location, fracture pattern, and the amount of comminution are the important determinants in the commonly used classification developed by Winquist, Hansen, and Clawson (Fig. 1). This classification system was developed to assess the degree of bony stability and its relationship to

standard and interlocked intramedullary nailing techniques. Fractures with comminution involving 50% or less of the bony circumference (types I and II) and located in the middle third of the femoral diaphysis are axially and rotationally stable after standard reamed intramedullary nailing. Fractures with a proximal or distal location are rotationally and, in some cases, axially unstable, requiring interlocking intramedullary nailing. Spiral fractures and those with comminution involving more than 50% of the bony circumference (types III, IV, and V) are axially and rotationally unstable (Fig. 1).

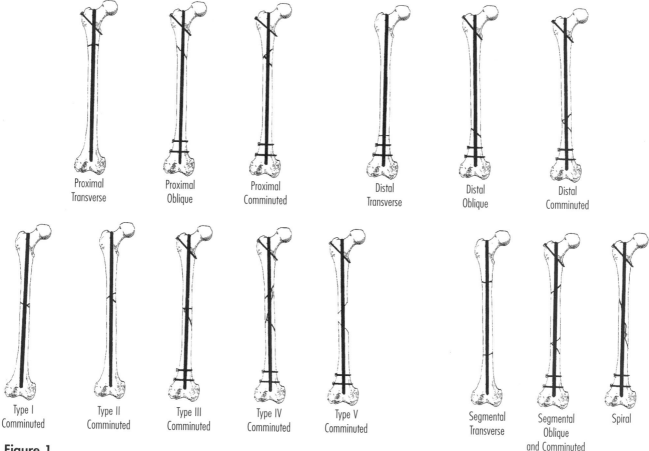

Proximal Transverse | Proximal Oblique | Proximal Comminuted | Distal Transverse | Distal Oblique | Distal Comminuted

Type I Comminuted | Type II Comminuted | Type III Comminuted | Type IV Comminuted | Type V Comminuted | Segmental Transverse | Segmental Oblique and Comminuted | Spiral

Figure 1

Winquist classification of femoral shaft fractures and recommended method of nail fixation. (Reproduced with permission from Kasser JR (ed): *Orthopaedic Knowledge Update 5*. Rosemont, IL, American Academy of Orthopaedic Surgeons, 1996, pp 427–436.)

Table 1
Gustilo classification of open fractures

Type	Description
I	A wound less than 1 cm long with little soft-tissue damage; fracture pattern is simple with little comminution
II	A wound more than 1 cm long without extensive soft-tissue damage, flaps, or avulsion; contamination and fracture comminution are moderate
III	Extensive soft-tissue damage, contamination, and fracture comminution
	A. Soft-tissue coverage is adequate; comminuted and segmental high-energy fractures are included regardless of wound size
	B. Extensive soft-tissue injury with massive contamination and severe fracture comminution requiring local or free flap coverage
	C. Arterial injury requiring repair

As part of their Comprehensive Classification of Fractures of Long Bones, the AO/ASIF group has developed a classification scheme for femoral shaft fractures that has been adopted by the Orthopaedic Trauma Association. With 27 different categories, the complete system is too complex and cumbersome. Even when reduced to 9 categories for clinical application, it seems ill-suited to the femoral diaphysis in which a simple description of fracture location and the degree of axial stability will suffice. The additional information may be helpful for research purposes. However, it currently does not appear to offer any additional therapeutic or prognostic advantage.

For open fractures, the method of Gustilo and Anderson, later modified by Gustilo and associates, is commonly used for clarification (Table 1). The accepted supposition is that these subdivisions correlate with the level of wound contamination and/or impaired vascularity, allowing them to serve as a basis for decision-making and prognosis. Unfortunately, because of the subjective nature of this method, determining the "type" for each individual injury is subject to a high degree of interobserver variability and is not consistently reproducible. Nonetheless, this system continues in general use pending development of a superior grading system.

Patient Evaluation

Overview In most cases, patients with a femoral shaft fracture have sustained high-energy trauma. Associated occult injuries are not uncommon. A small but significant (3.5%) relationship with fractures of the thoracic and lumbar spine has been reported, with more than half being initially unrecognized. Therefore, examination of the injured extremity, even in those with an apparent isolated injury, should be just one part of a well-organized overall evaluation of the entire musculoskeletal system.

Examination of the injured extremity is carried out during the secondary survey of the patient except in cases of obvious exsanguinating hemorrhage in accordance with the Advanced Trauma Life Support evaluation sequence (Chapter 13). A closed fracture of the femoral shaft, occurring alone or in combination with other extremity fractures, should not be considered the cause of hypotensive shock. An alternative source of hemorrhage should always be sought.

Multiple System Injury Patients with multiple injuries in association with a femoral shaft fracture are best treated by fracture stabilization within 24 hours of injury. Surgical intervention should proceed as soon as possible after completion of the initial resuscitation and the disposition of any head, chest, or abdominal injuries. Despite the controversy regarding presence of severe head injury (Glasgow Coma Score ≤ 8), early fracture stabilization does not predispose to central nervous system complications as long as hypotension and hypoxia are avoided. This approach allows early mobilization of the multiply injured patient and is instrumental in preventing pulmonary complications.

Open Fractures An open fracture should be irrigated and debrided and appropriate intravenous antibiotics instituted on an emergent basis. Initially, the traumatic wounds are left open. Subsequent treatment depends on the delay from injury to surgical intervention, the magnitude of the soft-tissue injury, the degree of wound contamination, and the presence of any additional injuries.

Patients with multiple injuries and open fractures require early fracture stabilization. Intramedullary nailing is preferred for fixation of type I, II, and IIIA open fractures. For type IIIB and IIIC injuries, treatment must be individualized. External fixation, plating, and intramedullary nailing all have a place in the treatment.

In patients with an isolated open femoral fracture, an accepted (but not ideal) treatment method is the traditional sequence of tibial pin traction for temporary fracture stabilization, delayed primary wound closure 5 to 7 days after the initial debridement, followed by closed intramedullary nail fixation 5 to 7 days later. However, type I, II, and IIIA open fractures preferably are treated by emergent debridement and intramedullary nailing. Type IIIB and IIIC open fractures require careful individual assessment, but emergent fracture fixation is preferable for type IIIB and required for type IIIC injuries.

For type IIIB and IIIC open fractures, the external fixator should be considered as an interim device for patients with isolated or multiple injuries. Conversion to an intramedullary nail is performed as soon as allowed by the status of the local soft tissues and the patient's general condition. In the majority of cases, especially within 2 weeks of injury, the external fixator can be replaced by the intramedullary nail as a 1-stage procedure. Alternatively, pin site colonization may necessitate an interval of skeletal traction or use of the external fixator as definitive fracture treatment.

Open fractures caused by gunshots present a special situation. Low-velocity gunshot fractures do not require formal fracture site debridement but should otherwise be handled as type I injuries. High-energy injuries, such as close-range shotgun blasts and high-velocity gunshots, should be managed as type IIIB injuries.

Vascular Injury Although concomitant vascular injury is uncommon (< 2%), it can occur with any of the fracture types. It is most commonly associated with fractures caused by penetrating trauma. In general, evidence of vascular injury can be divided into "hard and soft signs." The specific hard signs include distal ischemia or pulse deficit, presence of a bruit, an expanding or pulsatile hematoma, and obvious arterial bleeding. The less specific soft signs include a small stable hematoma, adjacent nerve injury, unexplained hypotension, and proximity of a penetrating or displaced fracture, such as a fracture at the level of the adductor hiatus. Although the finding of any hard signs reliably indicates the presence of arterial injury, their absence does not exclude injury. Furthermore, the detection of a Doppler signal may be helpful in assessing limb viability and limb patency, but it does not exclude a proximal arterial injury.

Arteriography is indicated in patients with overt signs of arterial injury only when needed to further define or localize the lesion prior to surgical intervention, such as in patients who have preexisting peripheral arterial disease and those sustaining blunt trauma with multiple level ipsilateral bony or ligamentous injury who are at risk for a segmental arterial injury. The Doppler-derived arterial pressure index is a valuable screening test for occult arterial injury, especially when swelling caused by hemorrhage or edema interferes with pulse palpation. An ankle-brachial systolic pressure ratio (ankle-brachial index or ABI) < 0.9 or a 20 mm Hg pressure difference between limbs is abnormal, necessitating further evaluation by angiography.

The treatment of an arterial injury depends on a number of factors, including blood loss amount, limb perfusion quality, and duration of ischemia. Ideally, distal limb ischemia time should be limited to less than 6 hours; this requires a team approach. Temporary vascular shunts can be helpful in limiting ischemia time. The femoral shaft fracture can then be stabilized without the risk of disrupting the vessel repair. Plate fixation, external fixation, and, to a lesser extent, intramedullary nailing are fracture treatment options. Fracture fixation is followed by the definitive vascular repair. Fasciotomy is indicated if there has been a period of limb ischemia exceeding 8 hours or subsequent elevation in compartment pressures.

Nerve Injury Peripheral nerve injury is not commonly associated with femoral shaft fractures caused by blunt trauma. The incidence is higher with penetrating injury and can result in an incomplete lesion and a patchy neurologic deficit. A detailed examination is needed to define these injuries. Functional recovery is variable, depending on the type and severity of the nerve lesion. Iatrogenic nerve palsy can result from both direct pressure and stretch injury, depending on the treatment modality. The prognosis for recovery is good in these cases.

Compartment Syndrome Although uncommon, compartment syndrome of the thigh must always be considered when evaluating a patient with a femoral shaft fracture. Predisposing factors include multiple injuries, systemic hypotension, vascular injury, coagulopathy, a history of external limb compression, and the use of military antishock trousers. Open fractures are also at risk because of high-energy injury. An associated high incidence of infection and neurologic deficit make early diagnosis mandatory in order to provide the best chance for recovery. A high index of suspicion and judicious use of compartment pressure monitoring and fasciotomy are essential.

Ipsilateral Knee Ligament and Meniscal Injury Ipsilateral knee ligament injury should be suspected in any patient with a femoral shaft fracture. The incidence is quite high, up to almost 50% in some reported series. The presence of a femoral shaft fracture makes evaluation of the ipsilateral knee very difficult. Before any traction is applied, the knee should be clinically examined and appropriate radiographs taken. Knee ligament injury with instability precludes use of a tibial traction pin. After fracture fixation, the knee should

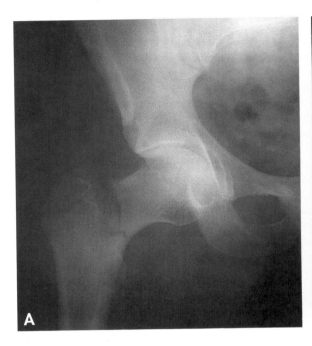 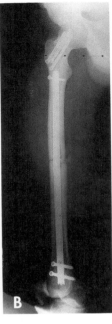 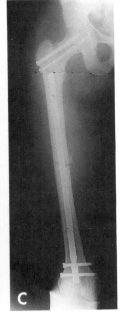

Figure 2

A, Ipsilateral femoral neck fracture showing typical vertical fracture line. The femoral neck fracture was provisionally stabilized with Kirschner wires prior to retrograde nailing (B), followed next by definitive femoral neck fracture reduction and cannulated screw fixation (C).

be reexamined and any identified ligamentous injury should be treated. Meniscal injury also is not uncommon (> 30% in one series). All patients with a femoral fracture and concomitant knee effusion and/or ligament laxity should be considered at risk for intra-articular injury. However, there may be no acute clinical evidence of meniscal injury or cruciate ligament injury. Therefore, knee symptoms that occur later should be viewed with a high index of suspicion for intra-articular pathology.

Associated Extremity Fractures Patients with multiple fractures warrant the same aggressive approach as that required for the treatment of patients with multiple system injury. Bilateral fractures of the femoral shaft are usually associated with additional musculoskeletal or systemic injuries. Closed intramedullary nailing is the treatment of choice. The floating knee syndrome, ipsilateral fracture of the femoral and tibial shafts, is a serious high-energy injury. Open fractures of one or both bones are common. Associated injuries are also common with a reported mortality rate ranging from 5% to 15%. The best results are achieved when both fractures are stabilized, allowing the early restoration of knee motion.

Ipsilateral fractures of the femoral neck and shaft (2.5% to 6% of all femoral shaft fractures) usually occur in association with other injuries and from high-energy trauma. The femoral neck fracture may be minimally or nondisplaced, presenting as an almost vertical fracture line, and it is often either missed or not clinically evident at the time of initial patient evaluation. Radiographs of the hip (preferably in 15° of internal rotation) should be obtained in all patients with a fracture of the femoral shaft on initial presentation, after fracture fixation, including image intensifier views during and after surgery, and, again, in the early (2 to 4 week) postinjury period. Furthermore, any patient complaining of groin or hip pain should have additional studies. Potential for a poor outcome is related to the complications from the neck fracture. Therefore, although simultaneous fixation of both the hip and shaft fractures is desirable, optimal management of the femoral neck fracture cannot be compromised. Reduction and stabilization of the femoral neck fracture is the main priority. Screw fixation of the femoral neck in combination with either compression plating or retrograde nailing of the femoral shaft (Fig. 2) has been shown to provide excellent results in a few small series. One commonly used and recommended technique, antegrade intramedullary femoral nailing with screw fixation of the femoral neck fracture, has not been uniformly successful. Although good results have been reported with a second-generation (reconstruction) locked intramedullary nail, its use remains controversial. The technique is demanding and is best reserved for experienced surgeons treating fractures with a nondisplaced femoral neck component.

Ipsilateral intertrochanteric and diaphyseal fractures of the femur are to be differentiated from femoral neck/shaft fractures. Although technically demanding, this fracture combination does not present the same potential for complications

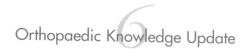

as that associated with a femoral neck fracture. Second-generation locked intramedullary nails allow stabilization of this ipsilateral hip/shaft fracture pattern. Care must be taken to avoid varus malposition or medial displacement of the intertrochanteric fracture component. A promising and relatively new implant, the full-length intramedullary hip screw, awaits further study. The compression hip screw and plate implant combination remains a viable alternative treatment option.

Thromboembolic Disease Deep-vein thrombosis (DVT) and pulmonary embolism are now well-recognized problems associated with high-energy trauma in general, and specifically with fractures of the femoral shaft. In one series, DVT was found in 80% of femoral fracture patients in whom prophylaxis against thromboembolism was not used. DVT is usually clinically occult. Proximal DVT are at high risk for embolization. Approximately 30% of calf vein DVT extend proximally with the attendant embolization risk. Therefore, prophylactic therapy and/or screening for the development of DVT should be considered for these patients with identified high risk factors: older age, blood transfusions, surgery, and spinal cord injury.

Treatment Methods

Nonsurgical Care Traction is used mainly for the temporary stabilization of a femoral shaft fracture if definitive surgical fixation must be delayed. Traction can be applied through a pin placed through either the proximal tibia or distal femur. A distal femoral pin is required in the presence of ipsilateral knee ligament injury, but should be avoided if delayed intramedullary nailing is planned. Indications for traction as part of a definitive nonsurgical fracture treatment plan are few. These include the lack of equipment or expertise to perform surgical fixation, systemic contraindications to anesthesia, or a local contraindication, such as infection at the surgery site. In these cases, a variable period of traction, usually 6 weeks, is followed by hip spica cast or cast-brace application. Although this treatment method has a high fracture union rate, its long list of problems, such as prolonged recumbency and hospital stay, knee stiffness, and fracture malunion, preclude its general use.

External Fixation External fixation is not indicated for the routine treatment of fractures of the femoral shaft. Its main indication is in the management of open fractures with severe soft-tissue injury (types IIIB and IIIC). An external fixator also should be considered in patients with severe burns, closed fractures with associated vascular injury, and infected

fractures previously treated by internal fixation. Because the surgical procedure is quick and generally has a low complication rate, external fixation can be of use for the patient, multiply injured or otherwise, who cannot tolerate prolonged anesthesia. External fixators can be applied for temporary fracture stabilization, allowing healing of the soft tissues prior to delayed internal fixation, or as the definitive method of fracture management. Although early mobilization of the patient is facilitated, external fixation as a definitive treatment is associated with significant late complications, including knee stiffness, malunion, nonunion, pin-site infection, and osteomyelitis. Delayed conversion to internal fixation carries with it an additional increased risk of subsequent infection.

Plating Accurate reduction and stable fixation that will allow early mobilization of the patient and the limb can be achieved using plating techniques. The relative disadvantages of these techniques are infection, hardware failure, delayed union, and residual muscle weakness. Over the past few years, concern regarding an increased potential for pulmonary injury associated with reamed intramedullary nailing in the multiply injured patient with concomitant chest injury created renewed interest in plate fixation. However, a recent study comparing plate fixation to reamed intramedullary nailing in this patient group failed to support this concern. Therefore, current indications for plate fixation continue to be diaphyseal fractures associated with an ipsilateral femoral neck fracture or a vascular injury requiring repair.

The surgical procedure involves the application of a single broad plate to the lateral aspect of the femur. An "indirect reduction," using an intraoperative distraction device or precontouring of the plate, is instrumental in limiting periosteal stripping and medial dissection. Comminuted fragments are not directly dissected free and anatomically reduced, but are bridged by the plating, theoretically eliminating the need for bone graft and decreasing the rate of complications.

Intramedullary Nailing Intramedullary nailing is the treatment of choice for the majority of fractures of the femoral shaft. Closed antegrade locked nailing with reaming is the preferred method. Open nailing, using a small incision at the fracture site to allow fracture reduction and passage of the guide wire, may provide results similar to those of closed nailing. A formal open procedure, exposing the bone ends for nailing or supplemental wire fixation, is to be avoided because of higher rates of infection and impaired fracture healing. The usual surgical technique requires a fracture table with the patient in a supine or lateral position. An alternative method, in which a femoral distractor or manual traction is used for fracture reduction with the patient placed on a radiolucent operating room table, has been shown to be effective, especially in patients with multiple injuries.

Antegrade Locked Intramedullary Nailing With Reaming
This method remains the treatment of choice for closed and type I, II, and IIIA open fractures. With the advent of interlocking, direct manipulation of the fracture site for cerclage wiring or any other supplemental fixation is no longer necessary. Static interlocking (insertion of cross-locking screws in both the proximal and distal fracture fragments), as dictated by the fracture configuration (Fig. 1), was once thought to require dynamization (removal of either the proximal or distal screws) to optimize fracture healing. Many reports now indicate that static interlocking does not clinically affect fracture union. Errors in the initial radiographic assessment and subsequent locking screw decision-making can result in loss of fracture reduction. Therefore, initial static interlocking is recommended in all cases. For proximal and midshaft fractures, only 1 distal locking screw is required in the interlocking nail construct. In distal third fractures, 2 screws should be used to prevent angulatory deformity. Dynamization is reserved for those fractures that radiographically demonstrate minimal callus formation 16 to 20 weeks after nailing.

The reported results of reamed intramedullary nailing are superior to those of other treatment methods for closed and open type I, II, and IIIA fractures. Almost complete return of hip and knee motion and a union rate of over 95% can be expected. Infection rates are also extremely low (< 1%). The reported numbers are small and the situation is not so clear-cut for type IIIB and IIIC open fractures, however. In type IIIB injuries, improved fracture alignment and joint motion are obtained in exchange for an increased risk of infection. Intramedullary nailing for type IIIC fractures places the vascular repair or shunt at risk. This risk, however, should be decreased by using a femoral distractor, rather than the fracture table, to bring the femur to length prior to vessel repair.

Although results of antegrade intramedullary nailing are reported to be excellent in terms of fracture union, return of joint motion, and a low overall complication rate, there is little information regarding the functional outcome from the patients' perspective. One such study indicates that this outcome is not as good as expected. Thirty-nine percent had limited walking, standing, and stair-climbing ability, and 37% had residual discomfort. Recent studies have also revealed a high rate (41% in one series) of residual proximal thigh pain (relieved in two thirds by nail removal) and hip abductor weakness. Further study is needed to define the actual functional outcome.

Antegrade Locked Intramedullary Nailing Without Reaming
Unreamed intramedullary nailing became popular as a result of reports indicating increased pulmonary complications and mortality rate in the multiply injured patient treated with reamed intramedullary nailing. Subsequent studies, including one in which outcomes in patients with severe chest trauma and a femoral fracture were compared to outcomes in those without fracture, have failed to support these claims of increased risk with reaming. Furthermore, it appears that fracture healing may be impaired with unreamed nailing. At the present time, intramedullary nailing of the femur without reaming offers no clear-cut advantage.

Complications of Antegrade Nailing Significant complications of reamed antegrade locked intramedullary nailing are infrequent. Infection (< 1%, closed fractures) requires thorough debridement at the fracture site. If the nail is providing fracture stability, it may be left in place. Otherwise, the nail should be removed, the medullary canal reamed, and a larger nail inserted. This approach is usually successful, assuming an early diagnosis, an intact soft-tissue envelope, and the absence of extensive necrotic bone and purulence. Staged sequential reconstructive methods incorporating the use of temporary external fixation may otherwise be required.

Although low in incidence, malunion continues to occur even with static interlocking. One series reported malrotation (> 15°) in almost 20% of patients and a leg-length discrepancy (> 10 mm) in 9%. Fracture malalignment, especially malrotation, should be evaluated in the immediate postoperative period at which time it can usually be corrected by revision of the position of the locking screws. Aseptic nonunion can be addressed by exchange to a larger-diameter reamed nail, with an expected union rate of approximately 95%.

Difficulty in placing the nail entry portal accurately in the piriformis fossa is associated with many problems, including iatrogenic fracture of the femoral neck or trochanter and fracture malunion. This technical difficulty is most apparent in nailings of morbidly obese patients.

Heterotopic ossification about the hip is common after reamed antegrade nailing but infrequently (< 5%) has any effect on hip motion. If necessary, delayed excision is usually successful in regaining functional joint motion. Of more concern is a recent study in which 88% of those with heterotopic ossification had significant proximal thigh pain. However, the cause and effect of this relationship remains to be determined.

Other complications of antegrade nailing can be directly attributed to the use of the fracture table for the maintenance of fracture reduction. Iatrogenic nerve palsy, which can involve 1 or both divisions of the sciatic nerve or, more commonly, the pudendal nerve, has been directly related to the fracture table-related problems of poor patient positioning, excessive traction, and prolonged surgical times. Prognosis for spontaneous recovery is good. Compartment syndrome in the uninjured leg has also been reported in association with the fracture table; it is caused by the combination of the hemilithotomy position and prolonged surgical time. In patients with bilateral femoral shaft fractures, this combination of the hemilithotomy position on the fracture table and prolonged surgical time has also resulted in peroneal nerve palsy and compartment syndrome involving both the thigh and leg in the limb initially placed in the well-leg holder. Excessive traction and prolonged surgical time, especially in the hemilithotomy position, should be avoided. As noted previously, satisfactory alternatives to the fracture table exist.

Retrograde Reamed Nailing Retrograde intramedullary nailing of fractures of the femoral shaft using a distal extra-articular entry portal via the medial femoral condyle was initially advocated for the treatment of patients with ipsilateral fracture of the femoral neck and shaft. Its indications were later expanded to include those with multiple injuries to facilitate the performance of simultaneous or sequential procedures. In this application, the patient was placed supine on a radiolucent operating room table. However, technical difficulties and an increased potential for femoral malunion limited its use. These problems were mainly related to the entry portal, which is not in line with the intramedullary canal, a situation exacerbated by the unavailability of purpose-specific implants or instrumentation. Modification of this technique, using an intercondylar entry portal and a nail having proximal locking holes with an anteroposterior orientation and inserted without reaming, has been shown to be successful in treating a small group of multiply injured patients. Indications include multiple system injury, multiple fractures, ipsilateral vascular injury, periprosthetic fractures, and ipsilateral proximal femoral fracture (Fig. 2). Before this method is applied for the routine treatment of isolated femoral shaft fractures, further study is required to delineate the adverse effect, if any, on knee joint function and to evaluate the initial higher observed rate of nonunion and malunion as compared to antegrade reamed nailing.

Supracondylar Fractures of the Femur

Introduction
Supracondylar fractures of the femur occur in a bimodal age distribution. In the younger, predominantly male patient group, the fractures result from high-energy trauma with a greater incidence of intra-articular damage and associated systemic or skeletal injuries. Fractures in the elderly, predominantly female group are low-energy injuries, often preceded by radiographic evidence of generalized osteopenia or other "age-related fractures" of the hip, spine, or pelvis. Knee stiffness and osteoarthrosis are common sequelae of this injury. Fracture management depends on many factors, including the fracture type, bone quantity, and the patient's overall medical condition. Although treatments vary, both patient groups will benefit from restoration of joint congruity and the institution of early knee motion.

Classification
Ideal prerequisites for a classification system require that it be simple enough to remember and understand, allow description of all the fracture variations, assist in formulating a treatment plan, and provide prognostic information. The AO/ASIF classification of supracondylar fractures (Fig. 3), which divides fractures into extra-articular (A), unicondylar (B), or bicondylar intra-articular (C) fracture types, appears to satisfy most of these criteria.

Treatment Methods

Nonsurgical Care Skeletal traction is not appropriate for the majority of supracondylar fractures of the femur because better results can be obtained with internal fixation. Patients with displaced fractures who present with contraindications to surgical intervention are the main candidates for this treatment method. It must be understood that these fractures are difficult to manage in traction and require constant vigilance to minimize the significant risks of malunion and knee stiffness as well as the potential complications of recumbency. A variable period of traction is usually followed by mobilization using a cast brace. Low-energy impacted fractures or those with minimal displacement can be managed with a cast or knee brace. Frequent follow-up is required to guard against fracture displacement and soft-tissue compromise.

Antegrade Locked Intramedullary Nailing With Reaming This method has been successfully used to stabilize type A and selected type C_1 and C_2 fractures occurring both alone and in combination with ipsilateral femoral shaft fractures. Careful presurgical evaluation is required to ensure that type C_3 injuries with coronal plane fracture lines are not inadvertently treated using this technique. Many modifications to the standard nailing procedure are required, including supplemental lag screw fixation of the intra-articular component in the C-type fractures and removing the distal 15 mm of the nail to allow satisfactory purchase of the distal locking screws.

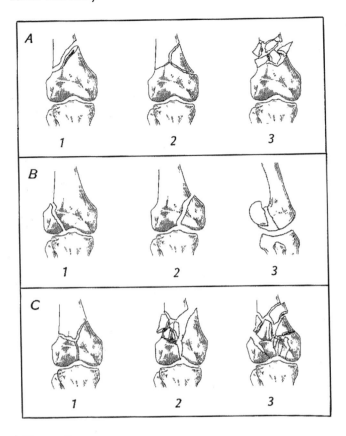

Figure 3

Current AO/ASIF classification of supracondylar fractures. Fractures are A, extra-articular fracture; A_1, simple; A_2, metaphyseal wedge; A_3, metaphyseal complex; B, partial articular fracture; B_1, lateral condyle, sagittal; B_2, medial condyle, sagittal; B_3, frontal; C, complete articular fracture; C_1, articular simple, metaphyseal simple; C_2, articular simple, metaphyseal multifragmentary; C_3, multifragmentary. (Adapted with permission from Müller ME, Allgöwer M, Schneider R, et al (eds): *Manual of Internal Fixation*. Berlin, Germany, Springer-Verlag, 1991, pp 140–141.)

The procedure is performed with the patient supine to avoid a valgus reduction. Displaced intercondylar fracture lines that cannot be anatomically reduced by closed means require either an arthrotomy for visualization and manipulation of the intra-articular component or selection of an alternative method of fixation. Overall, results are best for the type A fractures. Caution must be advised, because an increased risk of fatigue failure in stainless steel nails has been reported when the fracture line is within 5 cm of the most proximal of the distal locking screw holes. This risk is minimized by using large-diameter nails and avoiding early weightbearing.

Retrograde Interlocking Intramedullary Nailing With Reaming A relatively new device, a supracondylar intramedullary nail, allows closed locked retrograde fixation of all type A fractures and has the potential for limited opening for reduction and fixation of the intra-articular component in type C fractures. For the surgical technique, the patient is supine with the limb draped free. A split patellar tendon approach is used unless open reduction of the condyles is required. In this case a formal medial parapatellar tendon arthrotomy is performed. Preliminary reports have been cautiously optimistic. Initial problems with fatigue failure through empty locking holes in stainless steel nails, especially evident when treating nonunions, have necessitated implant redesign. Good results have been reported for subsequent small series. However, concerns continue as to the potential for septic arthritis related to the intra-articular entry portal and for fracture proximal to the implant. The ongoing evolution in the design of the implants indicates that this promising technique is still under development. This device may find its best application in the stabilization of type A fractures above a total knee arthroplasty.

Plate Fixation Plating techniques provide stable anatomic fracture fixation, which allows early limb mobilization. A recent biomechanical study has demonstrated the superiority of plate fixation when compared to antegrade and retrograde nailing in a cadaver model. It is currently the standard to which all other treatment methods must be compared. The standard surgical approach uses a midlateral incision directed toward the midpoint of the lateral femoral condyle, extending, as needed, toward a point just distal to the tibial tubercle to address intra-articular fracture lines. Type C_3 fractures may require additional medial exposure, which can be obtained by osteotomizing the tibial tubercle or performing a Z-plasty of the patellar tendon. An "indirect reduction" technique, limiting medial dissection and periosteal stripping, is desirable because it has been shown to limit the need for bone grafting. Therefore, using a second, medial counter-incision should be avoided, if possible.

A blade plate or condylar compression screw can be used for type A, C_1, most C_2, and selected C_3 fractures. With these devices, good to excellent results are reported in over 70% of patients. The surgical technique is demanding, however. Careful preoperative planning and strict adherence to the described surgical details are necessary to approximate the reported results. Complications are often the result of avoidable technical errors.

The condylar buttress plate should be used when the fracture pattern does not allow insertion of the blade plate or condylar screw (type C_3 and severely comminuted C_2 fractures). This plate is not very strong and does not control varus-valgus alignment very well. A deficient medial cortical buttress, evident after buttress plate application, is an indication for supplemental medial fixation using either a 2-pin external fixator (indirect technique) or a plate.

External Fixation As in the case of femoral shaft fractures, external fixation is most often used as an interim fracture stabilization measure for severe injuries and can be applied spanning the knee joint so that the pin sites do not compromise the area planned for later definitive fracture fixation. A retrospective review of 13 cases treated using monolateral external fixation until fracture union has reported good results, and this method appears to be a viable option in selected patients with multiple injuries, open fractures, or vascular injury.

Special Considerations

Bone Grafting Autogenous cancellous iliac crest bone should be used whenever there is metaphyseal comminution, medial stability cannot be obtained, and the indirect reduction method cannot be applied. This currently applies to all type A_3, C_2, and C_3 fractures in which the surgical approach has resulted in excessive soft-tissue stripping and in type IIIB and IIIC open fractures that present with significant bony and soft-tissue injury requiring staged reconstruction.

Type B Fractures Adequate fixation of displaced unicondylar fractures can be obtained using cancellous lag screws. Occasionally, type B_1 and B_2 fractures require supplemental buttress plating, especially in osteoporotic bone. Excellent long-term results have been reported in over 80% of patients.

Fractures in the Elderly Stable internal fixation with plates and screws is difficult to achieve in osteoporotic bone. In this situation, screw purchase can be greatly improved by the use of methylmethacrylate. This technique may be applicable for selected type A and C fractures. Alternatively, type A fractures with minimal comminution can be adequately stabilized using flexible intramedullary devices, such as the Zickel supracondylar nail, or standard locked nailing as described above. Type B_1 and B_2 fractures usually require a supplemental buttress plate. Other options, nonsurgical treatment and primary total knee arthroplasty, should always be carefully considered in all of these patients. However, a prospective, randomized study has demonstrated the clear benefits of adequately performed internal fixation as compared with nonsurgical treatment.

Fracture Following Total Joint Arthroplasty Nondisplaced fractures can be managed by closed means. Displaced fractures are best treated with surgical treatment (Chapter 43).

Closed treatment for displaced fractures carries a high risk of malunion and knee stiffness.

Annotated Bibliography

Femur Fractures

Multiple System Injury

Bone LB, Babikian G, Stegemann PM: Femoral canal reaming in the polytrauma patient with chest injury: A clinical perspective. *Clin Orthop* 1995;318:91–94.

Three groups of patients (97 total)—femoral fracture treated using a reamed nail, femoral fracture fixed with a plate, and no femoral fracture—with Injury Severity Scores (ISS) of ≥ 18 and a severe chest injury were retrospectively studied. ISS was similar for all groups. Mortality and adult respiratory rates were lowest in the nailing group. Mortality was highest in the no fracture group. Chest injury, not the method of fracture fixation, was the significant risk factor.

Bosse MJ, MacKenzie EJ, Riemer BL, et al: Adult respiratory distress syndrome, pneumonia, and mortality following thoracic injury and a femoral fracture treated either with intramedullary nailing with reaming or with a plate: A comparative study. *J Bone Joint Surg* 1997;79A:799–809.

Three groups of patients—acute femur fracture and thoracic injury, femur fracture without thoracic injury, and thoracic injury without femur fracture—with ISS ≥ 17 from 2 centers were retrospectively studied. In all, 707 patients were studied. Those with femur fractures were treated with either intramedullary nailing with reaming (235) or plating (218). No significant differences were found. Nailing with reaming did not increase the risk of pulmonary complications, multiple organ failure, or death.

Starr AJ, Hunt JL, Chason DP, Reinert CM, Walker J: Treatment of femur fracture with associated head injury. *J Orthop Trauma* 1998;12:38–45.

Thirty-two patients with a femur fracture and head injury were retrospectively studied. There were three groups: immediate (within 24 hours) stabilization (14), delayed stabilization (14), and no fracture fixation (4). Patients were divided into severe (Glasgow Coma Scale [GCS] ≤ 8) and mild (GCS > 8) head injury groups. Early fracture stabilization did not increase central nervous system complications and delay in fracture stabilization appeared to increase risk of pulmonary complications.

Open Fractures

Grosse A, Christie J, Taglang G, Court-Brown C, McQueen M: Open adult femoral shaft fracture treated by early intramedullary nailing. *J Bone Joint Surg* 1993;75B:562–565.

Between 1984 and 1990, 115 consecutive open femur fractures (36 type I, 42 type II, 20 type IIIA, 12 type IIIB, 5 type IIIC) were treated by debridement of the wound and early nailing. The procedure was performed in 106 on the day of injury. Union was delayed in 4, requiring bone grafting in 3. Infection occurred in 3. Early intramedullary nailing was a safe and efficient treatment method.

Van den Bossche MR, Broos PL, Rommens PM: Open fractures of the femoral shaft, treated with osteosynthesis or temporary external fixation. *Injury* 1995;26:323–325.

Of 54 patients, 20 were treated with initial external fixation because of the severity of the systemic or soft-tissue injury. In the 18 survivors, 16 fractures were treated with locked intramedullary nailing and 2 with plating. There were no deep infections or pin site infections. The fixator was converted to internal fixation, on average, at 21 days after injury.

Vascular Injury

Bandyk DF: Vascular injury associated with extremity trauma. *Clin Orthop* 1995;318:117–124.

A general review of the recent literature and a diagnostic algorithm is presented including the use of the Doppler-derived ankle-brachial systolic pressure index.

Ipsilateral Knee Ligament and Meniscal Injury

Vangsness CT Jr, DeCampos J, Merritt PO, Wiss DA: Meniscal injury associated with femoral shaft fractures: An arthroscopic evaluation of incidence. *J Bone Joint Surg* 1993;75B:207–209.

In 47 patients with closed, displaced, diaphyseal fractures of the femur caused by blunt trauma there were 12 medial meniscal injuries (5 tears) and 13 injuries of the lateral meniscus (8 tears). Two patients had tears of both menisci. Examination under anesthesia revealed ligamentous laxity in 23 patients (49%), but meniscal injuries had a similar incidence in knees with and without ligament injury.

Associated Extremity Fractures

Kang S, McAndrew MP, Johnson KD: The reconstruction locked nail for complex fractures of the proximal femur. *J Orthop Trauma* 1995;9:453–463.

The authors experienced a 75% complication rate in 4 patients with ipsilateral femoral neck and shaft fractures.

Wolinsky PR, Johnson KD: Ipsilateral femoral neck and shaft fractures. *Clin Orthop* 1995;318:81–90.

A review of the epidemiology, diagnosis, treatment, and complications is presented as well as a discussion detailing the problems with the reconstruction nail.

Thromboembolic Disease

Geerts WH, Code KI, Jay RM, Chen E, Szalai JP: A prospective study of venous thromboembolism after major trauma. *New Engl J Med* 1994;331:1601–1606.

Serial impedance plethysmography and lower extremity contrast venography were performed to detect DVT in 716 patients. DVT prophylaxis was not used. DVT was found in 201 of 349 patients (58%) with adequate venographic studies; 18% had proximal DVT. Of 74 patients with femur fractures, 59 (80%) had DVT. One third of DVT were proximal in patients with lower extremity fractures. Only 2% had clinical signs suggestive of DVT. Five independent risk factors were identified: older age, blood transfusion, surgery, fracture of the femur or tibia, and spinal cord injury.

Intramedullary Nailing

Bain GI, Zacest AC, Paterson DC, Middleton J, Pohl AP: Abduction strength following intramedullary nailing of the femur. *J Orthop Trauma* 1997;11:93–97.

As part of a larger study including nailing for closed femoral shortening, 32 patients with an acute isolated fracture of the femoral shaft were evaluated at a minimum of 24 months after injury. Findings included residual trochanteric pain (40%), thigh pain (10%), and limp (13%). Abductor strength was diminished as compared to the normal, contralateral hip ($p < 0.01$). Abductor weakness correlated with the incidence of complaints.

Benirschke SK, Melder I, Henley MB, et al: Closed interlocking nailing of femoral shaft fractures: assessment of technical complications and functional outcomes by comparison of a prospective database with retrospective review. *J Orthop Trauma* 1993;7:118–122.

An abbreviated functional assessment was performed in 56 patients at a minimum of 12 months postinjury. Thirty-seven percent of the patients had pain; 39% had some limitation in ability to ambulate or stand; 9% had to obtain new employment or seek job modifications. A significant portion of patients with femoral shaft fractures treated with interlocking nails will have permanent functional loss.

Braten M, Terjesen T, Rossvoll I: Femoral shaft fractures treated by intramedullary nailing: A follow-up study focusing on problems related to the method. *Injury* 1995;26:379–383.

Of 116 patients evaluated, 23 had a true torsional deformity $\geq 15°$; 11 had shortening ≥ 10 mm. Hip pain was present in 26% and knee pain in 20% of patients with a retained nail versus 4% and 2%, respectively, of patients who had the nail removed.

Dodenhoff RM, Dainton JN, Hutchins PM: Proximal thigh pain after femoral nailing: Causes and treatment. *J Bone Joint Surg* 1997;79B:738–741.

Eighty patients treated with reamed antegrade nailing for an acute femoral fracture were retrospectively evaluated for thigh pain. At an average 21 months of follow-up, 33 (41%) had residual pain that interfered with routine activities. Seventeen patients had the nails removed but pain persisted in 6. The presence of heterotopic bone was found to be related to the presence of pain ($p < 0.001$).

Karpos PA, McFerran MA, Johnson KD: Intramedullary nailing of acute femoral shaft fractures using manual traction without a fracture table. *J Orthop Trauma* 1995;9:57–62.

The technique and advantages of using manual intraoperative traction was evaluated in 32 fractures. Surgical time was significantly decreased (95 minutes average). The authors concluded that the method was of added benefit, especially in polytrauma patients.

Moed BR, Watson JT: Retrograde intramedullary nailing, without reaming, of fractures of the femoral shaft in multiply injured patients. *J Bone Joint Surg* 1995;77A:1520–1527.

Twenty consecutive multiply injured patients with 22 femoral shaft fractures were treated using retrograde nailing without reaming and an intercondylar entry portal. Surgical time averaged 75 minutes. There were no infections, 1 rotational malunion, no hardware failures, and all but 1 patient regained normal knee motion. However, there were 3 nonunions (86%) and time to union was prolonged.

Tornetta P III, Tiburzi D: The treatment of femoral shaft fractures using intramedullary interlocked nails with and without intramedullary reaming: A preliminary report. *J Orthop Trauma* 1997;11:89–92.

Eighty-one consecutive patients were treated using locked nails randomized to either reamed or unreamed groups. There were more intraoperative technical complications in the unreamed group. Time to union was similar for both groups except for distal fractures, which healed faster with reaming. No advantage to unreamed nailing was noted.

Supracondylar Fractures

Bolhofner BR, Carmen B, Clifford P: The results of open reduction and internal fixation of distal femur fractures using a biologic (indirect) reduction technique. *J Orthop Trauma* 1996;10: 372–377.

Fifty-seven type A or C fractures were treated by plating using indirect reduction techniques. No bone grafting or dual plating was used. All fractures healed. There was 1 malunion and 1 deep infection. Results were good to excellent in 84%.

Butt MS, Krikler SJ, Ali MS: Displaced fractures of the distal femur in elderly patients: Operative versus non-operative treatment. *J Bone Joint Surg* 1996;78B:110–114.

Forty-two fractures were evaluated in a prospective randomized trial comparing surgical (95° dynamic condylar screw) to closed treatment (traction followed by cast-brace application at 6 weeks). Excellent or good results were obtained in 53% of the surgery cases versus 31% in the traction group.

Iannacone WM, Bennett FS, DeLong WG Jr, Born CT, Dalsey RM: Initial experience with the treatment of supracondylar femoral fractures using the supracondylar intramedullary nail: a preliminary report. *J Orthop Trauma* 1994;8:322–327.

A retrograde supracondylar intramedullary nail was used to treat 38 patients with 41 supracondylar femur fractures (3 A_2, 16 A_3, 6 C_1, 6 C_2, and 10 C_3). Nineteen fractures were closed and 23 were open. Complications included 4 nonunions and 5 delayed unions, 7 of which required revision surgery. Four patients developed fatigue failure of the nail, which was subsequently redesigned. Further clinical trials and additional biomechanical testing are needed prior to general use of this implant.

Koval KJ, Kummer FJ, Bharam S, Chen D, Halder S: Distal femoral fixation: A laboratory comparison of the 95 degrees plate, antegrade and retrograde inserted reamed intramedullary nails. *J Orthop Trauma* 1996;10:378–382.

In this cadaver study, the 95° plate was significantly stiffer than either the antegrade Russell-Taylor nail or the supracondylar (GSH) nail. The antegrade nail was the least rigid and the supracondylar nail had significantly lower loads to failure.

Koval KJ, Seligson D, Rosen H, Fee K: Distal femoral nonunion: Treatment with a retrograde inserted locked intramedullary nail. *J Orthop Trauma* 1995;9:285–291.

Sixteen distal femoral nonunions were treated using a stainless steel supracondylar nail. Four united with a single surgery; 1 united after nail dynamization and later nail failure; 2 more healed after exchange of a broken nail. Additional surgery was required in 6 of the remaining 9 patients; none of these 9 fractures had healed at the last follow up. In all, 9 nails broke with failure occurring through a screw hole near the nonunion. It was concluded that this device should not be used in treating distal femoral nonunions.

Marsh JL, Jansen H, Yoong HK, Found EM Jr: Supracondylar fractures of the femur treated by external fixation. *J Orthop Trauma* 1997;11:405–410.

Thirteen patients with supracondylar fractures (2 A_2, 1 A_3, 7 C_2, 3 C_3) were definitively treated using a monolateral fixator. The main indications for patient selection were multiple system injury, soft-tissue compromise, and vascular injury requiring repair. Twelve fractures healed. There was one infected nonunion. Nine patients had pin site infections, but all resolved. Knee range of motion averaged 111° but was less than 90° in 2 patients; 4 had shortening or malunion. It was concluded that this is a satisfactory treatment in highly selected patients.

Moran MC, Brick GW, Sledge CB, Dysart SH, Chien EP: Supracondylar femoral fracture following total knee arthroplasty. *Clin Orthop* 1996;324:196–209.

Twenty-nine fractures above total knee arthroplasty implants were retrospectively studied. Five nondisplaced fractures treated nonsurgically had satisfactory results; 9 displaced fractures treated closed had poor results. Fifteen displaced fractures were treated with plate fixation; there were 10 satisfactory results with 2 malunions and 3 requiring revision surgery due to nonunion. It was concluded that despite the high complication rate displaced fractures are best treated by early fixation.

Classic Bibliography

Bone LB, Johnson KD, Weigelt J, Scheinberg R: Early versus delayed stabilization of femoral fractures: A prospective randomized study. *J Bone Joint Surg* 1989;71A:336–340.

Brumback RJ, Ellison PS Jr, Poka A, Lakatos R, Bathon GH, Burgess AR: Intramedullary nailing of open fractures of the femoral shaft. *J Bone Joint Surg* 1989;71A:1324–1331.

Brumback RJ, Ellison TS, Poka A, Bathon GH, Burgess AR: Intramedullary nailing of femoral shaft fractures: Part III. Long-term effects of static interlocking fixation. *J Bone Joint Surg* 1992;74A:106–112.

Brumback RJ, Reilly JP, Poka A, Lakatos RP, Bathon GH, Burgess AR: Intramedullary nailing of femoral shaft fractures: Part I. Decision-making errors with interlocking fixation. *J Bone Joint Surg* 1988;70A:1441–1452.

Brumback RJ, Uwagie-Ero S, Lakatos RP, Poka A, Bathon GH, Burgess AR: Intramedullary nailing of femoral shaft fractures: Part II. Fracture-healing with static interlocking fixation. *J Bone Joint Surg* 1988;70A:1453–1462.

Bucholz RW, Ross SE, Lawrence KL: Fatigue fracture of the interlocking nail in the treatment of fractures of the distal part of the femoral shaft. *J Bone Joint Surg* 1987;69A:1391–1399.

Butler MS, Brumback RJ, Ellison TS, Poka A, Bathon GH, Burgess AR: Interlocking intramedullary nailing for ipsilateral fractures of the femoral shaft and distal part of the femur. *J Bone Joint Surg* 1991;73A:1492–1502.

Carr CR, Wingo CH: Fractures of the femoral diaphysis: A retrospective study of the results and costs of treatment by intramedullary nailing and by traction and a spica cast. *J Bone Joint Surg* 1973;55A:690–700.

Connolly JF, Whittaker D, Williams E: Femoral and tibial fractures combined with injuries to the femoral or popliteal artery: A review of the literature and analysis of fourteen cases. *J Bone Joint Surg* 1971;53A:56–68.

Feliciano DV, Herskowitz K, O'Gorman RB, et al: Management of vascular injuries in the lower extremities. *J Trauma* 1988;28: 319–328.

Giles JB, DeLee JC, Heckman JD, Keever JE: Supracondylar-intercondylar fractures of the femur treated with a supracondylar plate and lag screw. *J Bone Joint Surg* 1982;64A:864–870.

Johnson KD, Cadambi A, Seibert GB: Incidence of adult respiratory distress syndrome in patients with multiple musculoskeletal injuries: Effect of early operative stabilization of fractures. *J Trauma* 1985;25:375–384.

Kang S, McAndrew MP, Johnston KD: The reconstruction locked nail for complex fractures of the proximal femur. *J Orthop Trauma* 1995;9:453–463.

Kempf I, Grosse A, Beck G: Closed locked intramedullary nailing: Its application to comminuted fractures of the femur. *J Bone Joint Surg* 1985;67A:709–720.

Mize RD, Bucholz RW, Grogan DP: Surgical treatment of displaced, comminuted fractures of the distal end of the femur. *J Bone Joint Surg* 1982;64A:871–879.

Neer CS II, Grantham SA, Shelton ML: Supracondylar fracture of the adult femur: A study of one hundred and ten cases. *J Bone Joint Surg* 1967;49A:591–613.

Olerud S: Operative treatment of supracondylar-condylar fractures of the femur: Technique and results in fifteen cases. *J Bone Joint Surg* 1972;54A:1015–1032.

Schatzker J, Home G, Waddell J: The Toronto experience with the supracondylar fracture of the femur, 1966–72. *Injury* 1974;6:113–128.

Schwartz JT Jr, Brumback RJ, Lakatos R, Poka A, Bathon GH, Burgess AR: Acute compartment syndrome of the thigh: A spectrum of injury. *J Bone Joint Surg* 1989;71A:392–400.

Stewart MJ, Sisk TD, Wallace SL Jr: Fractures of the distal third of the femur: A comparison of methods of treatment. *J Bone Joint Surg* 1966;48A:784–807.

Swiontkowski MF, Hansen ST Jr, Kellam J: Ipsilateral fractures of the femoral neck and shaft: A treatment protocol. *J Bone Joint Surg* 1984;66A:260–268.

Webb LX, Winquist RA, Hansen ST: Intramedullary nailing and reaming for delayed union and nonunion of the femoral shaft: A report of 105 consecutive cases. *Clin Orthop* 1986;212: 133–141.

Winquist RA, Hansen ST Jr, Clawson DK: Closed intramedullary nailing of femoral fractures: A report of five hundred and twenty cases. *J Bone Joint Surg* 1984;66A:529–539.

Wiss DA, Fleming CH, Matta JM, Clark D, et al: Comminuted and rotationally unstable fractures of the femur treated with an interlocking nail. *Clin Orthop* 1986;212:35–47.

Chapter 40
Knee and Leg: Pediatric Aspects

Pediatric Lower Extremity Deformities

Fibular Deficiency

Fibular deficiency is one of the most common congenital anomalies of the lower extremity. This longitudinal deficiency may be complete or partial, involving either end of the fibula. It should be considered a deficiency of the entire lower extremity with associated anomalies in the femur, tibia, foot, and ankle. Femoral valgus, knee instability, tibial bowing and shortening, malalignment of the ankle, tarsal coalitions, and lateral foot ray aplasia are all common (Fig. 1).

Choice of treatment depends on the global lower extremity involvement of this condition. Syme's amputation with prosthetic fitting is the mainstay of treatment for severely involved lower limbs with significant shortening and ankle and foot involvement. These patients, treated at a young age, have fewer surgical procedures, hospital admissions, and psychological consequences of treatment than those in whom

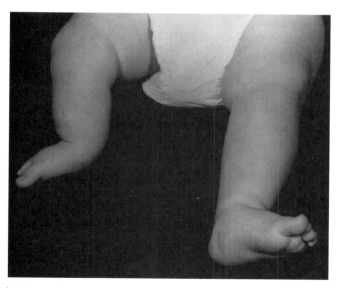

Figure 1

Fibular deficiency. This demonstrates the global lower extremity involvement with this condition. There is femoral shortening, knee valgus, tibial shortening with bowing, and foot and ankle deformities.

definitive treatment is delayed. There is a high level of prosthetic function in children fitted with a prosthesis after amputation. Procedures to salvage the limb are available for those with a lesser constellation of anomalies or in cases in which the parents refuse amputation. The cartilaginous fibular anlage may be resected distally, attempting to stabilize the ankle. It is difficult to align the foot directly under the tibia, and this may require a significant soft-tissue release and tibial osteotomy with long-term bracing. The foot may also need surgical realignment in order to render it plantigrade and functional. Significant foot anomalies may preclude such an approach. The potential retardation of tibial growth needs to be considered in the overall management of these patients.

If tibial growth is inhibited less than 25% to 30%, lengthening procedures offer an alternative to amputation, and the foot and ankle can be salvaged. These methods allow angular correction and lengthening with foot and ankle stabilization. For larger discrepancies, the lengthenings may have to be staged. There is a tendency to redevelop knee or ankle valgus and tibial bowing. Ankle arthrodesis is often needed after lengthening. This approach can yield a functional extremity, but requires multiple hospitalizations and surgical procedures with a high complication rate and the risk of long-term emotional and psychological trauma. Careful preoperative screening of the patients and families should be undertaken to decrease the incidence of complications and to decide between amputation or reconstruction.

Tibial Hemimelia

Tibial hemimelia is a less common longitudinal deficiency, with an estimated incidence of 1 in 1 million live births. This may be an inherited anomaly associated with other limb deficiencies, such as cleft hand. Developmental dysplasia of the hip and bilateral deficiencies are common. Tibial hemimelia is characterized as partial or complete and terminal or intercalary (grades I to III). There may be a proximal tibial anlage that affords some knee stability. The primary clinical features of this condition are shortening and angulation of the leg, severe rigid foot deformities, and knee instability with quadriceps aplasia or weakness (Fig. 2). Knee flexion contractures may develop, complicating the condition.

Treatment options vary according to the severity of involvement. Severe deformities with shortening, knee instability, no

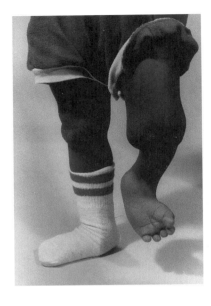

Figure 2

Tibial hemimelia. Foot and ankle deformities are common in this condition along with severe shortening and bowing of the tibia. This patient underwent amputation and prosthetic fitting.

quadriceps function, and significant foot deformities are best treated with a primary amputation and prosthetic fitting. A knee disarticulation for complete absence of the tibia is very functional in the young child, allowing active end bearing. A Syme's amputation may be performed if there is an acceptable residual limb and no significant flexion contracture. Tibia-fibula synostosis is an option when the proximal tibia is present with a functional knee. The Brown procedure (centralization of the fibula under the femur) creates a one-bone leg; reported results are mixed and indications for this procedure are very limited. The fibula has been noted to hypertrophy after centralization. There must be strong quadriceps function and a minimal knee flexion contracture for this procedure to succeed. Many patients develop postoperative flexion contractures and have mediolateral instability. Some revision procedure, such as femoral or fibular osteotomy, is usually required, and a frequent end result is amputation. Therefore, early amputation and prosthetic fitting have been the primary methods of treatment of severe tibial hemimelia. The centralized fibula can be lengthened in the limb with milder involvement, if there is a stable knee and functional foot. As with fibular deficiency, the patient must be carefully screened preoperatively, complications expected, and staged lengthenings considered in selected cases.

Discoid Meniscus

Discoid menisci are a rare cause of lateral knee pain in children. Various etiologies have been proposed, including failure of normal central absorption of the developing meniscus, abnormal posterior motion, and hereditary transmission. The classic symptoms are pain, clicking, and locking with loss

of extension. The Watanabe classification grades a discoid meniscus as complete, incomplete, and Wrisberg ligament type (no posterior capsular attachments). There is a high incidence of bilaterality, with symptoms generally presenting in childhood; discovery of a discoid meniscus has been made in infants as young as 6 months. Plain radiographs are frequently unremarkable; magnetic resonance imaging (MRI) is the diagnostic tool of choice. The usual image is a thickened, flat meniscus with an increased intrameniscal signal (Fig. 3).

Treatment should be reserved for symptomatic knees. Arthroscopic partial excision or trimming of the meniscus to a more normal shape yields excellent results in the complete or partial discoid meniscus with posterior stability. Complete meniscectomy is recommended only if the posterior attachments are deficient (Wrisberg type), although there are some reports of successful posterior reattachments. Long-term follow-up has not demonstrated degenerative changes in cases treated surgically using these methods but complete meniscectomy should be avoided, if possible.

Osteochondritis Dissecans

Osteochondritis dissecans (OCD) is a condition in which there is fragmentation or separation of a portion of the articular surface of the knee. The classic location is in the lateral portion of the medial femoral condyle. There is a male predominance (2:1) with up to 33% bilaterality reported. The average age of presentation is between 5 and 15 years. Possible etiologic factors include direct external trauma, indirect trauma from the tibial spine, osteonecrosis, genetic predisposition, or defects in ossification such as seen in epiphyseal dysplasia. The typical symptoms can be vague pain,

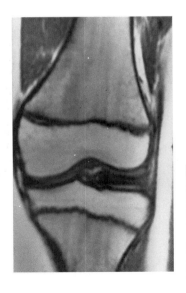

Figure 3

Discoid meniscus. Magnetic resonance imaging of a discoid lateral meniscus showing flattening and thickening of the meniscus with increased intrameniscal signal and femoral condyle adaptive changes.

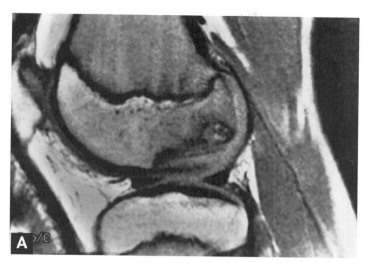

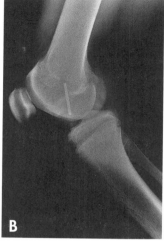

Figure 4

Osteochondritis dissecans (OCD). A, Magnetic resonance image of an OCD lesion illustrating fragmentation and sclerosis. B, The fragment may be reattached and held with screws.

clicking, popping, or effusion. OCD may present with mechanical symptoms related to a loose body. Tenderness to palpation may be present over the area of the lesion. Initial radiographic evaluation includes anteroposterior, lateral, and tunnel radiographs. MRI and bone scan can be supplemental examinations. Radiographic studies generally demonstrate a well-circumscribed area of sclerosis in the subchondral bone, whereas bone scans may be used to document increased uptake, indicative of healing potential. The MRI scan is of value not only to outline the extent of the lesion and articular cartilage involvement, but also to detect loose bodies and to determine if the OCD is surrounded by synovial fluid (Fig. 4).

Initial treatment in children is nonsurgical (limitation of activity and/or knee immobilization) unless the lesion is unstable or a loose body is present. Failure of nonsurgical measures after 3 to 6 months warrants surgical intervention. Small lesions may be arthroscopically excised and drilled, whereas large defects may require open curettage, reduction, and fixation. Absorbable implants have been used in recent years, with only preliminary results available. The patients should maintain limited weightbearing until healing occurs. Osteochondral allografts may be used for the largest defects, with osseous bridging being reported as early as 12 weeks.

Congenital Dislocation of the Knee

Congenital dislocation of the knee is a rare condition, frequently bilateral, and more prevalent in females. It commonly is asso-

ciated with neuromuscular conditions, such as arthrogryposis and myelomeningocele, and includes other anomalies such as developmental dysplasia of the hip, foot deformities, and elbow dislocation. There is an association with ligamentous laxity and with Down, Larsen's, and Turner's syndromes. The classic types (I–III) include hyperextension, subluxation, and complete dislocation. With complete dislocation, there is an irreducible hyperextended separation of the femur and tibia (Fig. 5). This condition should not be confused with positional hyperextension, which is reducible and responsive to nonsurgical treatment, usually passive stretching and a Pavlik harness in the first few months.

Initial treatment should be serial stretching of the soft tissues during the newborn period, which may be supplemented with a Pavlik harness or a cast in types I and II. The complete dislocation requires an open reduction consisting of

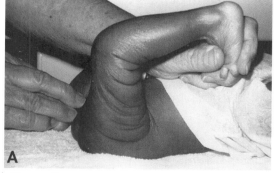

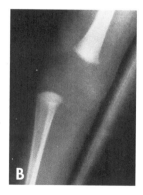

Figure 5

Congenital dislocation of the knee. The knee is locked in hyperextension, and is frequently associated with neuromuscular conditions. Clinical (A) and radiographic (B) appearances demonstrate the irreducible nature of this dislocation and anterior dislocation of the tibia from the femur.

anterior incision; quadriceps V-Y plasty, and release of the rectus femoris, vastus intermedius, and capsule. The hamstrings and iliotibial band may need lengthening or realignment. The knee should flex to 90° intraoperatively and be casted at 45° postoperatively. A knee-ankle-foot orthosis is used to allow stabilized weightbearing and encourage flexion. There are preliminary reports of early percutaneous lengthening of the quadriceps, but no long-term outcomes.

Quadriceps Contracture

Isolated quadriceps contracture is a rare condition that develops after repeated injections into the newborn's quadriceps muscle. Intramuscular antibiotics have a local sclerosing effect leading to fibrosis, scarring, and contracture. The knee is typically extended with a significant loss of flexion (Fig. 6). The condition is also seen in arthrogryposis and myelomeningocele as an isolated problem. There may be an associated patellar dislocation if the vastus lateralis and iliotibial band are involved. Rectus femoris contractures may affect both hip and knee motion. More than 1 muscle is usually involved, including the deep muscles such as the vastus intermedius.

Treatment is generally surgical, with release of any fibrosis and V-Y plasty of the quadriceps giving the best results. At least 90° of flexion should be obtained intraoperatively and maintained postoperatively with casting, bracing, and rehabilitation.

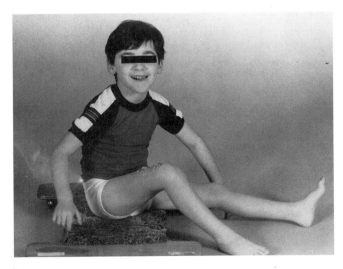

Figure 6

Quadriceps contracture. Bilateral quadriceps contracture secondary to repeated intramuscular injections. The left knee is hyperextended, and the right has been treated by fibrosis release and quadriceps lengthening.

Angular Deformities

Congenital Posteromedial Bowing of the Tibia

Posteromedial bowing of the tibia is a congenital anomaly characterized by apex posterior and medial bowing of the middle or distal portion of the tibia and fibula. The foot is typically in a marked calcaneovalgus position, giving the appearance at birth of being folded up into the tibial deformity created by the bowing. There is apparent limitation of ankle plantarflexion. The diagnosis can usually be made on the basis of physical examination and radiographs.

The calcaneovalgus foot position will resolve, and may be replaced by a mild equinus contracture. The bowing also usually spontaneously resolves, so that a decision to perform corrective osteotomy should be deferred at least 2 years from birth. Corrective tibial osteotomy should be carried out only for the rarely inadequate spontaneous correction. Unlike anterolateral bowing of the tibia, union can be expected if osteotomy is performed.

The tibial shortening does not correct spontaneously. Slight growth velocity retardation compared to the opposite side results in progressive limb-length inequality. Shortening may vary from mild, requiring no treatment, to a severity (> 4 to 5 cm) at which contralateral epiphysiodesis or limb lengthening of the involved extremity may be considered. Once the tibial bowing has resolved, the growth inhibition remains constant, so that the ultimate discrepancy can be determined from serial radiographic assessments.

Congenital Pseudarthrosis of the Tibia

Congenital pseudarthrosis of the tibia varies from simple anterolateral bowing of an intact tibia to frank pseudarthrosis present prior to walking age. In contradistinction to posteromedial bowing, the tibia with anterolateral bowing is a variant of congenital pseudarthrosis of the tibia and has a strong propensity to progress to further deformity, fracture, and nonunion. Approximately 50% of patients have neurofibromatosis (type I). The family history or other stigmata of neurofibromatosis must be carefully assessed in order to detect other manifestations.

Treatment of congenital pseudarthrosis of the tibia often is difficult. If the tibia is intact, deformity correction is rarely warranted because of the high risk of nonunion after osteotomy. Protective bracing, particularly if the medullary canal is narrow or the diaphyseal cortex seems tenuous, is indicated in childhood. Surgical intervention will almost always be required after fracture occurs; rarely can union be achieved by simple external immobilization. The basic surgical requirements are resection of the pseudarthrosis, bone grafting, and stable fixation. The role of adjunctive therapy, such as electromagnetic stimulation, is not clearly established. The technique of Williams intramedullary rodding of the tibia and fibula has met with relatively good success (80%)(Fig.7). With this procedure, a retrograde intramedullary rod is introduced into the tibia through the calcaneus and talus. The tibial rod is left across the ankle and subtalar joint if the distal fragment is short or osteopenic, and the leg is immobilized in a protective brace at least until the rod has migrated proximal to the ankle mortise with growth.

A circular external fixator may also be used to stabilize and compress a persistent nonunion. The most successful application of this method has been in patients older than 5 years, and in whom stabilization of the nonunion site was combined with proximal tibial corticotomy to stimulate blood flow to the affected leg and perform simultaneous lengthening as required. Refracture rate after union can be as high as 25%.

An alternative treatment is vascularized fibular transposition into the defect of the resected pseudarthrosis with fixation to the proximal and distal tibial segments. The contralateral healthy leg is the typical donor site. Union with this treatment has been reported to be 90%. However, problems with distal or proximal bony union, persistent deformity, refracture, and donor site morbidity, especially ankle valgus, can occur. Some authors use vascularized fibulae only in case of failed intramedullary rodding or may use it primarily in severe cases.

Patients must be apprised of the risk of refracture at any time, and protective bracing implemented when warranted by the fragility of the leg. The patient should not undergo excessive or prolonged treatment. The final salvage procedure for a congenital pseudarthrosis of the tibia remains amputation. Although amputation may be proximal or through the nonunion site, Syme's amputation is also a consideration. Although the residual limb will not be end bearing, preservation of the tibial articular surface will prevent the young child from facing diaphyseal overgrowth, requiring subsequent revisions with growth.

Delayed Pseudarthrosis

A delayed type of congenital pseudarthrosis presents at age 3 to 5 years or older, with a transverse fracture secondary to mild trauma with delayed union or subsequent nonunion. There may or may not be antecedent history of mild limb atrophy or subtle anterolateral bow of the affected tibia. Although surgery will often be required to effect union, the prognosis for union is somewhat better than for the more typical congenital types.

Finally, a rare resolving type of anterolateral bow has been described. This relatively rare condition may be recognized

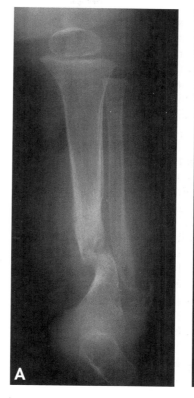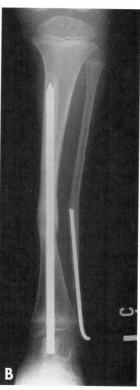

Figure 7

Congenital pseudarthrosis of the tibia treated with Williams intramedullary rod and bone grafting. Preoperative anteroposterior (A) radiograph of an infant with congenital pseudarthrosis of the tibia. Note the established nonunion of the tibia. B, Postoperative radiographic appearance after intramedullary fixation of the tibia with a Williams rod, intramedullary fixation of the fibula with a Kirschner wire, and bone grafting.

clinically at birth as anterolateral bowing of the tibia, but with distinct radiographic features. The tibial medullary canal is intact, the fibula is relatively unaffected, and there is evidence of new bone formation and cortical hypertrophy within the concavity of the tibial deformity, suggesting early favorable spontaneous remodeling. Reminiscent of posteromedial bowing of the tibia, such unusual cases will spontaneously correct the angular deformity without propensity to fracture, but may have limb-length inequality that requires treatment.

Physiologic Varus and Valgus

The standing femoral-tibial angle varies during the first half of childhood. The typical child has a varus femoral-tibial angle at birth averaging 10°, which gradually corrects to a neutral relationship between the ages of 18 to 24 months.

Persistent varus after this stage in an otherwise healthy infant should raise suspicion for the presence of infantile tibia vara. Children pass through this neutral phase to one of femoral-tibial valgus, usually maximal at age 3.5 years, and averaging approximately 15°. Subsequently, the femoral-tibial angle returns to the normal adult relationship of 5° to 7° of valgus, usually by the age of 6 to 7 years, although severe valgus deformity may persist for a longer period.

Provided that the child has the appearance of being healthy and the femoral-tibial relationship falls within these normal parameters, radiographs are not necessary, and no treatment is required. If, however, the deformity is extreme, asymmetric, or occurring at an inappropriate phase of development, radiographs are warranted. Varus or valgus malalignment may also result from epiphyseal dysplasias, unrecognized metabolic bone disease, such as renal osteodystrophy or true nutritional rickets, remote physeal trauma or other injury, tibia vara, focal fibrocartilaginous dysplasia, or a host of other uncommon conditions. Unresolving physiologic varus is uncommon; it usually evolves to an obvious infantile tibia vara if it persists. When genu valgum does not resolve by the age of 6 to 10 years, medial distal femoral and/or proximal tibial extraperiosteal stapling or hemiepiphysiodesis may be indicated at the appropriate age (usually early adolescence).

Infantile Tibia Vara (Blount Disease)

Infantile tibia vara is characterized by a combination of proximal tibial varus deformity and distinctive radiographic appearance as described by Langenskiöld. The disorder presents as a persistent or progressive varus deformity after walking age, typically presenting between the ages of 1 and 3 years. There is a distinct predilection for the condition in African-Americans, blacks of Caribbean origin, and people of Mediterranean origin. In addition, early weightbearing, particularly in large and overweight children, may represent an etiologic factor.

The clinical and radiographic distinction between persistent physiologic varus and early (Langenskiöld stage I) infantile tibia vara can be difficult prior to 24 to 36 months of age. In the absence of clear radiographic evidence of infantile tibia vara, the determination of the radiographic metaphyseal-diaphyseal angle has been reported to be helpful. When this angle is < 11°, the diagnosis is usually physiologic varus, and progressive varus rarely occurs. When it is > 15°, progressive varus with worsening radiographic findings must be carefully evaluated.

The role of daytime, valgus-producing braces in preventing progressive deformity and effecting correction is uncertain. A bracing trial may be warranted in patients younger than 3 years old with Langenskiöld stage III or less involvement; close monitoring for compliance and progression of the disorder is necessary, and results from bracing are variable.

Patients with Langenskiöld stage IV radiographic deformity, who are older than 3 years, or who have progressive clinical and radiographic deformity despite bracing, are candidates for proximal tibial osteotomy. Recurrent deformity in spite of osteotomy can occur in children older than 4 to 5 years, and early correction of the varus deformity may be advisable. Once complete medial physeal arrest has occurred (Langenskiöld stage VI), recurrence after high tibial osteotomy is inevitable. In such cases, transphyseal osteotomy with epiphysiodesis, physeal bar resection with osteotomy, or elevation of a severely depressed medial tibial plateau are surgical options that have mixed results. Unilateral cases must be monitored for the presence and extent of limb-length inequality in addition to recurrence, because the length inequality itself may require treatment.

Late-Onset Tibia Vara

Late-onset tibia vara can be classified as juvenile and adolescent types. Adolescent tibia vara is characterized by progressive varus deformity, with radiographic widening of the medial proximal tibial physis during adolescence. This radiographic widening represents fibrosis and disruption of normal physeal architecture, occurring in response to excessive compressive stresses in the presence of mild persistent physiologic varus and obesity.

The natural history of adolescent tibia vara has not been determined, yet in one study it was suggested that at least some cases resolve spontaneously. The majority present because of progressive deformity or mild knee symptoms. Significant intra-articular symptoms may be evaluated independently by MRI or arthroscopy as clinically indicated. Bracing is not indicated in adolescent tibia vara.

Proximal tibial osteotomy is effective in correcting the deformity in adolescents near skeletal maturity. This can be performed either transphyseally or distal to the physis. After correction, if the physis has been preserved, physeal healing often occurs with subsequent normal growth. Thus, overcorrection of the deformity is not indicated. Internal fixation with accurate correction after osteotomy is challenging because of a combination of obesity, joint laxity, and subtle deformity in the distal femur or distal tibia. The presence of varus or valgus deformity in the distal femur or distal tibia should be determined by the treating surgeon, and a decision made as to the need for combined tibial and femoral osteotomy. Achieving accurate correction of the deformity as viewed in the weightbearing position is not easy when the osteotomy is performed in a supine patient with joint laxity. External fixation with either acute or gradual correction is an attractive alternative that allows for postoperative adjustment of alignment, if necessary, and correction of the mild limb-length inequality often present in unilateral cases.

An alternative, less invasive surgical procedure is lateral hemiepiphysiodesis, with medial completion of the epiphysiodesis if and when full correction occurs (Fig. 8). This procedure has been reported to correct this deformity in 50% of cases, and it avoids the potential complications associated with osteotomy and either internal or external fixation. However, it does not address any rotational deformity, and in some patients, the medial tibial physis does not grow normally to allow correction. Attention must be paid to limb-length inequality in unilateral cases, and it should be treated as clinically indicated.

An intermediate form of tibia vara, "juvenile" tibia vara, occurs in patients between the ages of 6 and 10 years. Radiographically, the entire proximal tibia appears to be disrupted with severe bowing, but there is less epiphyseal distortion than in the later stages of infantile tibia vara. Treatment is similar to adolescent tibia vara, but the risk for recurrence is increased, and the amount of growth remaining must be taken into account before recommending epiphysiodesis.

Limb-Length Inequality

Etiology

Limb-length inequality arises from many causes; most can be determined by careful history and physical examination and by radiographs, when a clinically significant discrepancy or deformity exists. The physician should specifically look for soft-tissue hypertrophy or atrophy, mild reductions characteristic of fibular hemimelia, such as valgus knee and hypoplastic lateral foot rays, café-au-lait spots associated with neurofibromatosis or fibrous dysplasia, or vascular anomalies of the affected extremity. Radiographs of the lower extremity may detect unrecognized bone lesions, such as enchondroma affecting the physis, fibrous dysplasia, mild fibular hemimelia, and other possible causes. Orthoroentgenograms or scanograms should be taken to document the magnitude of discrepancy if it exceeds 1.5 to 2 cm, or if the etiology is expected to result in progressive deformity. If no specific etiology can be found, idiopathic hemihypertrophy or hemiatrophy may be the etiology. Many patients have no explanation for a mild (< 1.5 cm) discrepancy; they remain static and often have a family history with similar body habitus in a parent. The physician, however, should use serial examinations to be sure that a mild discrepancy in a skeletally immature child remains static.

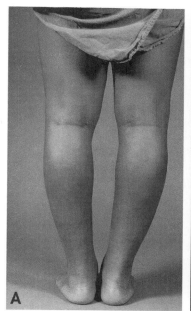 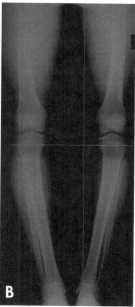 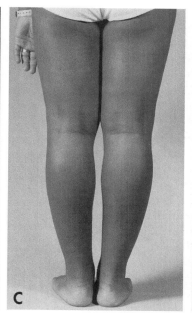 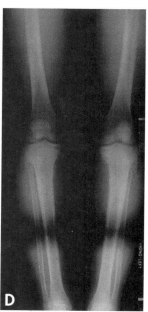

Figure 8

Treatment of adolescent tibia vara by lateral hemiepiphysiodesis. Preoperative clinical appearance (A) and standing anteroposterior radiograph (B) of a patient with adolescent tibia vara. Postoperative clinical appearance (C) and standing radiograph (D) of the same patient after treatment with lateral proximal tibial hemiepiphysiodesis.

Serial examinations and radiographs should be performed to determine the dynamics of the limb-length inequality when it is not obvious (such as known complete physeal arrest after trauma). The Moseley straight line graph can predict with reasonable accuracy the ultimate limb-length discrepancy at maturity when the percentage of growth inhibition of the shorter limb remains constant. This is usually the case in congenital deficiencies and physeal injuries, but it may be less constant in discrepancies associated with inflammatory arthritis, vascular anomalies, nonphyseal trauma, or Legg-Perthes disease. In the latter circumstance, more careful and frequent assessment may be necessary. Radiographs are rarely warranted more frequently than every 6 months.

Treatment

Treatment plans are based on the projected discrepancy at skeletal maturity and any associated functional limb deficits. Surgical options are appropriately timed epiphysiodesis or stapling, lengthening, or acute shortening. Gait abnormalities and compensatory strategies can be detected by gait analysis when leg length discrepancies exceed 2 cm; thus a discrepancy > 2 cm remains the threshold beyond which intervention is usually recommended. Complaints of pain or functional disability related to anything other than extreme inequality are unusual in the pediatric population; however, if significant symptoms exist, they should be assessed independently. Generally accepted guidelines are epiphysiodesis for discrepancies of 2 to 5 cm and limb lengthening for 5 to 15 cm.

Epiphysiodesis remains the simplest, safest, and least complicated method of surgically correcting limb-length inequality. The timing of surgery is determined from Green-Anderson growth remaining charts or the Moseley straight line graph method. A recent evaluation of the accuracy of these methods, however, has shown that the Menelaus chronologic age-growth remaining method is as reliable as the others. Several clinical series have confirmed the efficacy and safety of percutaneous epiphysiodesis using fluoroscopically guided drills and curettes.

Significant advances in limb-lengthening have occurred in the last 10 years, with the introduction of circular external fixators and the technique of gradual callus distraction (callotasis) fostering greater interest in this more complex approach to limb-length inequality. The callotasis technique, used with a circular ring fixator and wires, monolateral devices and half-pins, or combinations of these, results in more certain new bone formation and rarely requires internal fixation or bone grafting. Furthermore, the newly formed bone may be subsequently lengthened again, so that staged, repeated lengthenings can be planned, permitting recon-

struction for more severe shortening than previously suggested. Clinical and experimental studies show that bone and soft-tissue complications, although fewer than with the Wagner technique, are frequent. Furthermore, permanent muscle and articular cartilage damage have been documented with lengthening, particularly with larger percentage lengthenings. Careful patient selection and education are still required.

Acute shortening of the femur may be performed in the skeletally mature patient as an alternative to lengthening. Closed femoral shortening of 5 to 7 cm with intramedullary fixation can provide good results. Prolonged rehabilitation to regain muscle strength in the shortened segment may be required, and some studies suggest that full recovery may not occur with more extensive shortening.

Traumatic Disorders of the Knee and Leg

Distal Femoral Physeal Fractures

Most distal femoral physeal fractures are Salter-Harris type I or II injuries (Fig. 9). The distal femoral physis has a central undulation directed into the metaphysis that increases its shear strength. It also increases the risk of a physeal arrest following Salter-Harris type I and II fractures. Displaced type I injuries are reduced closed, and stabilized with retrograde, smooth Steinmann pins. The pins should cross centrally in the femur proximal to the physis. Salter-Harris type II fractures with a small metaphyseal fragment are treated in a similar manner. Injuries with a large metaphyseal fragment can be stabilized after a closed reduction with cannulated screws directed parallel to the physis. Salter-Harris type III and IV injuries often require an open reduction to verify physeal and articular reduction. Cannulated screws through the epiphysis parallel to the physis normally suffice for both injuries.

Evaluation of Knee Ligament and Meniscal Injuries in Children/Adolescents

Knee ligament and meniscal injuries are rare in young children. Disruptions of the anterior cruciate ligament (ACL) normally occur in preadolescent and adolescent patients. MRI is useful in diagnosis with a sensitivity of 85% for medial meniscal injuries, 87% for lateral meniscal injuries, and 64% for ACL injuries in children with acute knee trauma. Its specificity is 95% for meniscal injuries and 94% for ACL disruptions. An MRI study should be obtained in children and adolescents when clinical examination suggests a ligament injury. Diagnostic arthroscopy may be required.

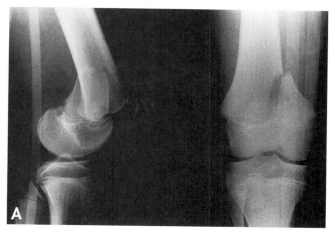 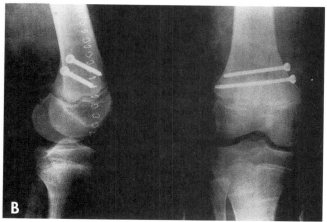

Figure 9

A, Anteroposterior and lateral radiograph of the knee in a 12-year-old with a Salter-Harris type II distal femoral physeal fracture. B, This injury was treated with reduction and internal fixation parallel to the physis utilizing the large metaphyseal fragment.

Anterior Cruciate Ligament Injuries Recent data suggest that skeletally immature patients with an ACL disruption treated nonsurgically (physical therapy, bracing) have persistent instability, generating interest in ACL reconstruction. They are subject to recurrent meniscal injuries and may not return to their preinjury level of activity. Good results recently were reported for ACL reconstruction in this older adolescent age group. A 7-mm hole was placed centrally through the tibial physis. The graft was then placed "over the top" in the femur. Reconstruction with hamstring tendons placed in a groove over the front of the tibia and in a groove over the top of the femur, avoiding violation of the growth plates, is also acceptable. Children with 2 cm or more of growth remaining in the knee and an ACL disruption should be treated nonsurgically with rehabilitation and bracing. ACL reconstruction can be performed when they near skeletal maturity, if symptomatic.

Meniscal Injuries Traumatic meniscal injuries in children and skeletally immature adolescents are rare but have been recognized more frequently in recent years. The majority of meniscal tears in young children are associated with a discoid meniscus. Most traumatic injuries to nondiscoid menisci in skeletally immature patients are in the peripheral portion. These injuries should be repaired surgically. A tear in the nonvascular zone of the meniscus will necessitate debridement as in the adult.

Osteochondral Fractures

Osteochondral fractures in the knee are typically associated with patellar dislocations. Half of these injuries are capsular avulsions of the medial patellar margin in which the bony

fragment remains attached to the capsule. Free intra-articular fragments usually originate from the lateral femoral condyle or the central ridge of the patella. Chondral lesions without an osseous component occur in approximately one third of the patients with a chondral disruption. Small loose fragments should be removed arthroscopically. Lesions ≥ 1 cm with a larger osseous component should be reduced and stabilized.

Patellar Fractures/Overuse Injuries

Patellar fractures are uncommon in skeletally immature patients. Direct trauma can produce a fracture of the body of the patella. These are managed by open reduction and internal fixation as is a comparable patellar injury in an adult. The most common patellar fracture in older children and adolescents is a "sleeve fracture" separating the distal patellar "sleeve" from the bony nucleus of the patella. Recognition requires a careful examination because the osseous component may be small and difficult to detect by radiograph. The patellar tendon extensor mechanism can become abnormally elongated if the injury is severe, unrecognized, and unrepaired. Malunion reduces extension force of the knee and may compromise gait.

Overuse injuries and development-related malalignment problems involving the patella are common in adolescents. Patellar tendinitis presents with pain and tenderness to palpation in the substance of the patellar tendon. This is associated with an increase in activity and normally occurs during periods of growth acceleration. If untreated, this condition can progress to Sinding-Larsen-Johansson syndrome. These patients have tenderness to palpation at the inferior pole of the patella, limited knee flexion secondary to pain, and radio-

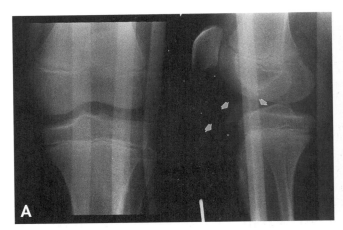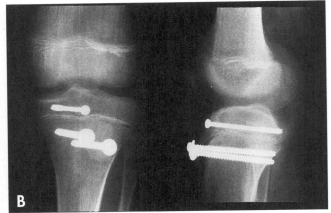

Figure 10

A, Anteroposterior and lateral radiograph of the knee in a 13-year-old boy who sustained a type III tibial tubercle fracture (arrows). B, This patient was treated with open reduction and screw fixation to reconstruct the extensor mechanism of the knee and to maintain an anatomic reduction of the articular surface of the proximal tibia.

graphic evidence of distal pole fragmentation. The treatment for these overuse conditions is activity modification, anti-inflammatory agents, ice, and stretching. The patient may resume normal activities once the symptoms resolve. Patellar tendon strapping can be effective in reducing the risk of recurrence.

Tibial Intercondylar Eminence Fractures

Meyers and McKeever (1959) classified tibial intercondylar eminence fractures into 3 types. A type I injury is nondisplaced or has only "slight elevation" of the anterior margin with excellent bony apposition of the avulsed fragment. The anterior third to half of the avulsed fragment is displaced from its bed in a type II injury. The posterior aspect of the fragment remains intact. There is complete displacement of the tibial intercondylar eminence in a type III injury.

Type I injuries should be treated with cast immobilization in approximately 10° of flexion and early frequent follow-up to make sure the fragment does not displace. The treatment of type II injuries is controversial. Some authors suggest that closed treatment with cast immobilization in full extension or slight flexion is the treatment of choice. They cite recent reports of less than optimal results in patients treated surgically. Other authors believe that an anatomic reduction of the fractured fragment reduces the risk of late instability and loss of extension.

Arthroscopically assisted or formal open reduction with internal fixation should be used for all displaced type III fractures, especially if there is a loss of extension in the knee before surgical repair or suspected entrapment of the medial meniscus. There have been several recent reports on arthroscopic techniques to reduce and stabilize these injuries. A

technique of arthroscopic reduction and stabilization of tibial eminence fractures using a cannulated screw in the epiphysis has been reported, as well as the use of an ACL tibial drill guide to assist in the passage of an absorbable suture around the fractured fragment. This suture may then be tied, reducing the fragment into its bed.

Approximately 50% of children with a tibial intercondylar eminence fracture may have clinical evidence of ACL laxity, even when the fracture unites in an anatomic position, possibly caused by a concomitant interstitial injury of the ACL itself.

Proximal Tibial Physeal/Apophyseal Fractures

Fractures of the proximal tibial physis are rare, accounting for only 0.5% to 2% of all physeal injuries. The most common fracture pattern is a Salter-Harris type II with a posterior metaphyseal fragment. This occurs because the posterior physis closes earlier than the anterior physis. The posterior metaphyseal fragment can be used to assist in closed reduction of the fracture. Many injuries are stable following closed manipulation and cast application. The extremity is casted in extension if the injury is stable. Unstable injuries can be treated with crossed-pin fixation after a reduction is achieved. In some cases, a child with a proximal tibial physeal fracture will have lower extremity ischemia secondary to a disruption of flow in the popliteal artery near the trifurcation. This ischemia resolves in the majority of patients following closed reduction. An urgent evaluation and treatment of the popliteal artery injury should be performed in any patient in whom ischemia does not quickly resolve after closed reduction.

Apophyseal injuries of the proximal tibial tubercle have been classified into 3 types by Watson-Jones. A small fragment of the distal, anterior, tibial apophysis is displaced in a superior direction in a type I injury. Type II fractures have a larger fragment involving the majority of the secondary ossification center. The fracture line passes through the apophyseal growth plate and the proximal tibial epiphysis into the joint in a type III injury (Fig. 10). Type I fractures are treated with cast immobilization. Displaced type II and III fractures normally require an open reduction and screw fixation. The majority of these injuries occur in adolescents near skeletal maturity so growth disturbances are uncommon. If this injury occurs in a younger child, smooth pins may be used to maintain the reduction and to help prevent premature closure of the anterior apophysis, which may result in a genu recurvatum deformity.

Proximal Tibia Metaphyseal Fractures

Fractures of the proximal tibial metaphysis are uncommon, with a reported prevalence of 6 fractures per 100,000 children per year. These rare injuries should be treated aggressively to achieve an anatomic reduction. Progressive valgus deformity following proximal tibial metaphyseal fractures has been reported, and may result from inadequate reduction. Documentation and maintenance of adequate reduction are difficult when a flexed knee cast is used. Occasionally, periosteum and the insertion of the pes anserine can be trapped in the fracture site, preventing a complete reduction. This soft tissue may need to be removed surgically if a near anatomic reduction cannot be obtained closed. The second, more widely held theory on the development of postfracture tibia valgus is overgrowth of the proximal medial tibia. This overgrowth may be secondary to fibular tethering or a differential blood flow between the medial and the lateral side of the proximal tibial physis. Postfracture bracing does not prevent the development of the tibia valgus, which peaks 12 to 18 months after injury.

Children who develop postfracture tibia valgus (age at injury: 3 to 8 years) should be treated by observation. Osteotomy of the proximal tibia should be performed rarely in adolescents and only for significant deformity that does not correct after observation (greater than 20°). Postfracture tibia valgus greater than 15° in the adolescent may be treated with selective proximal tibial medial hemiepiphysiodesis. Evaluation of the patient's leg length is performed at the same time.

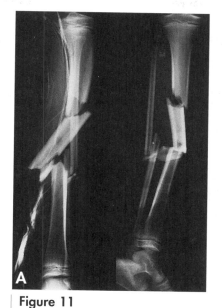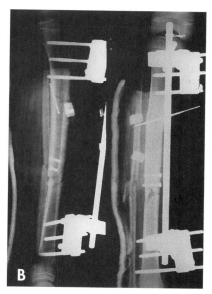

Figure 11

A, Comminuted middle third fracture of the tibia and fibula in a 6-year-old who was involved in a pedestrian motor vehicle accident. B, This grade IIIB injury was treated with irrigation and debridement, limited internal fixation, and the placement of an external fixator.

Tibial Diaphyseal Fractures

Diaphyseal fractures of the tibia in children usually occur as a result of indirect forces. Axial loading with lower extremity rotation is the most common indirect force producing this fracture. These injuries are normally oblique. Fractures resulting from direct trauma may be transverse or comminuted. Child abuse is considered the most common etiology in a child younger than 1 year of age. Displaced tibial fractures without an associated fibular fracture may angulate into varus. Complete fractures of the tibia and fibula have a tendency to displace into valgus angulation. Valgus angulation should be avoided because of the association of postfracture tibia valgus in skeletally immature patients. Varus angulation up to 10° is acceptable in the child younger than 8 years of age.

Indications for surgical treatment of a tibial shaft fracture in a skeletally immature patient include multiple system injuries, an open fracture, a floating knee, or a fracture that cannot be adequately reduced. Options for fixation include an external fixator, elastic/flexible intramedullary nails, or a compression plate as indicated.

Open tibial fractures and fractures associated with a compartment syndrome should be treated in the same way as comparable injuries in adults. External fixation is the method of choice to stabilize the injury in both cases (Fig. 11). This provides access to the soft-tissue wounds and maintains fracture alignment.

Distal Tibia Metaphyseal Fractures

Fractures of the distal tibial metaphysis may be complete or incomplete. The anterior cortex may become impacted, producing recurvatum at the fracture site. Casting may produce recurvatum if the foot is placed in dorsiflexion. The foot should, therefore, be kept in mild equinus until the fracture is stable. A long leg cast is usually applied for 3 to 4 weeks, followed by a short leg walking cast with the ankle in neutral dorsiflexion until union has occurred.

Annotated Bibliography

Fibular Hemimelia

Gibbons PJ, Bradish CF: Fibular hemimelia: A preliminary report on management of the severe abnormality. *J Pediatr Orthop* 1996;5B:20–26.

Results of limb lengthening in 8 cases of fibular hemimelia are presented. There was an average length gain of 10.5 cm with adequate length achieved in all patients. There is a high complication rate with this procedure, which is, however, a viable alternative to amputation.

Grogan DP, Holt GR, Ogden JA: Talocalcaneal coalition in patients who have fibular hemimelia or proximal femoral focal deficiency: A comparison of the radiographic and pathological findings. *J Bone Joint Surg* 1994;76A:1363–1370.

Amputation specimens of patients with fibular hemimelia underwent both pathologic and radiographic evaluation. Six of 8 patients exhibited talocalcaneal coalition, an important consideration if foot salvage is contemplated.

Naudie D, Hamdy RC, Fassier F, Morin B; Duhaime M: Management of fibular hemimelia: Amputation or limb lengthening. *J Bone Joint Surg* 1997;79B:58–65.

The authors compared patients with hemimelia who had a Syme's amputation and those with Ilizarov lengthening. The Syme group had excellent function. The lengthening group had more complications, surgery, hospitalization, and school absence.

Tibial Hemimelia

Herring JA, Birch JG (eds): *The Child With a Limb Deficiency*. Rosemont, IL, American Academy of Orthopaedic Surgeons, 1998.

This book provides detailed discussion of fibular and tibial deficiencies in children.

Simmons ED Jr, Ginsburg GM, Hall JE: Brown's procedure for congenital absence of the tibia revisited. *J Pediatr Orthop* 1996;16: 85–89.

The authors present their experience using the Brown centralization procedure for tibial hemimelia with a Syme's amputation of the foot. They report good results in long-term follow-up. Quadriceps function of at least grade 3 is needed for this procedure to be successful.

Turker R, Mendelson S, Ackman J, Lubicky JP: Anatomic considerations of the foot and leg in tibial hemimelia. *J Pediatr Orthop* 1996;16:445–449.

The authors describe multiple foot and ankle anomalies in this condition including coalitions, tendon anomalies, and ankle articulations. This is similar to fibular hemimelia and anomalies should be evaluated if foot salvage is contemplated.

Discoid Meniscus

Washington ER III, Root L, Liener UC: Discoid lateral meniscus in children: Long-term follow-up after excision. *J Bone Joint Surg* 1995;77A:1357–1361.

This long-term follow-up study (average 17 years) revealed excellent or good results with no evidence of degenerative knee changes in the majority of patients who underwent arthroscopic meniscectomy for symptomatic discoid menisci.

Osteochondritis Dissecans

Garrett JC: Fresh osteochondral allografts for treatment of articular defects in osteochondritis dissecans of the lateral femoral condyle in adults. *Clin Orthop* 1994;303:33–37.

The use of allografts for large OCD defects is presented. This extensive procedure had overall good results and should be reserved for the lesion not amenable to drilling and reimplanting.

Schenck RC Jr, Goodnight JM: Osteochondritis dissecans. *J Bone Joint Surg* 1996;78A:439–456.

This extensive review of the etiology, presentation, diagnosis, and treatment of OCD provides a thorough discussion of this topic.

Congenital Dislocation of the Knee

Haga N, Nakamura S, Sakaguchi R, Yanagisako Y, Taniguchi K, Iwaya T: Congenital dislocation of the knee reduced spontaneously or with minimal treatment. *J Pediatr Orthop* 1997;17: 59–62.

The authors present their positive experience using a Pavlik harness when no other anomalies or syndromes are present. Ninety percent of the postural deformities resolved with this method and they recommend waiting until the infant is at least 1 month of age prior to intervening surgically.

Angular Deformity

General

Mielke CH, Stevens PM: Hemiepiphyseal stapling for knee deformities in children younger than 10 years: A preliminary report. *J Pediatr Orthop* 1996;16:423–429.

Hemiepiphyseal stapling was used for correction of angular deformity from a variety of causes in 25 children younger than age 10 (mean, 6 years, 4 months). Minimal complications were encountered, although 7 patients required restapling for recurrent deformity. No physeal arrests occurred.

Pinkowski JL, Weiner DS: Complications in proximal tibial osteotomies in children with presentation of technique. *J Pediatr Orthop* 1995;15:307–312.

The authors describe only 3 superficial wound infections and 1 delayed union after 37 osteotomies using a technique of distal fibulectomy and prophylactic anterior compartment fasciotomy.

Scheffer MM, Peterson HA: Opening-wedge osteotomy for angular deformities of long bones in children. *J Bone Joint Surg* 1994;76A:325–334.

The surgical technique of opening wedge osteotomy with bone graft and minimal or no internal fixation is described with results of 31 osteotomies. The authors recommend the technique for angular deformity less than 25°, and projected limb-length inequality of < 25 mm.

Congenital Pseudarthrosis of the Tibia

Boero S, Catagni M, Donzelli O, Facchini R, Frediani PV: Congenital pseudarthrosis of the tibia associated with neurofibromatosis-1: Treatment with Ilizarov's device. *J Pediatr Orthop* 1997;17:675–684.

The authors assessed 21 patients with congenital pseudarthrosis of the tibia 2 years or more after removal of an Ilizarov apparatus. At follow-up, 9 were consolidated without residual deformity, 5 healed but had residual deformity, and 7 had not united. Resection of the pseudarthrosis and patient older than 5 years were favorable prognostic factors.

Gilbert A, Brockman R: Congenital pseudarthrosis of the tibia: Long-term followup of 29 cases treated by microvascular bone transfer. *Clin Orthop* 1995;314:37–44.

In a review of 29 skeletally mature patients treated by vascularized fibular transfer, 75% had neurofibromatosis. The average age at surgery was 6 years, and at follow-up, 17.5. Twenty-eight patients had a healed tibia; 17 patients required only 1 operation, but 12 required between 2 and 4 secondary procedures.

Grill F: Treatment of congenital pseudarthrosis of tibia with the circular frame technique. *J Pediatr Orthop* 1996;5B:6–16.

Nine patients with congenital pseudarthrosis of the tibia were treated by simultaneous resection of the pseudarthrosis and proximal tibial lengthening using a circular external fixator. At average follow-up of 4 years, all tibiae united, although proximal tibial valgus, distal tibial valgus, and limb-length inequality were present in some.

Guidera KJ, Raney EM, Ganey T, Albani W, Pugh L, Ogden JA: Ilizarov treatment of congenital pseudarthroses of the tibia. *J Pediatr Orthop* 1997;17:668–674.

Nine of 11 children were successfully treated using the Ilizarov apparatus. The 2 who failed to unite required amputation.

Tuncay IC, Johnston CE II, Birch JG: Spontaneous resolution of congenital anterolateral bowing of the tibia. *J Pediatr Orthop* 1994;14:599–602.

Five patients with anterolateral bowing resolved spontaneously. These patients were characterized by early spontaneous subperiosteal new bone formation in the concavity of the tibial deformity, and no fibular involvement.

Physiologic Varus and Valgus

Fraser RK, Dickens DR, Cole WG: Medial physeal stapling for primary and secondary genu valgum in late childhood and adolescence. *J Bone Joint Surg* 1995;77B:733–735.

Forty-three patients with primary or secondary genu valgum were treated by medial tibial and/or femoral stapling. All patients with primary, and 85% of patients with secondary deformity had good or excellent results. At least 1 year of growth remaining was a prerequisite. Rebound phenomenon was minimal but unpredictable.

Infantile Tibia Vara

Doyle BS, Volk AG, Smith CF: Infantile Blount disease: Long-term follow-up of surgically treated patients at skeletal maturity. *J Pediatr Orthop* 1996;16:469–476.

Seventeen patients with infantile tibia vara were evaluated at an average of 15 years after initial surgery. Patients undergoing initial osteotomy later than age 4 or with Langenskiöld stage III or greater disease had significantly more pain and intra-articular abnormalities than those operated on earlier.

Price CT, Scott DS, Greenberg DA: Dynamic axial external fixation in the surgical treatment of tibia vara. *J Pediatr Orthop* 1995;15:236–243.

Percutaneous osteotomy of the proximal tibia with acute correction and dynamic axial external fixation is described for 31 tibiae with infantile, juvenile, or adolescent tibia vara. Two patients had transient neurapraxias, but no other significant complications occurred.

Stricker SJ, Edwards PM, Tidwell MA: Langenskiöld classification of tibia vara: An assessment of interobserver variability. *J Pediatr Orthop* 1994;14:152–155.

Twelve orthopaedic surgeons and residents classified 60 radiographs according to the 6-stage Langenskiöld classification. Exact agreement overall was only 50%. Agreement was greatest for stages I and VI, but poor for stages II through IV.

Adolescent Tibia Vara

Coogan PG, Fox JA, Fitch RD: Treatment of adolescent Blount disease with the circular external fixation device and distraction osteogenesis. *J Pediatr Orthop* 1996;16:450–454.

Twelve tibiae in 8 patients with adolescent Blount's disease were treated using a circular fixator and gradual deformity correction. One patient required reoperation for premature consolidation. Distal tibial valgus was corrected as well in 4 patients.

de Pablos J, Azcarate J, Barrios C: Progressive opening-wedge osteotomy for angular long-bone deformities in adolescents. *J Bone Joint Surg* 1995;77B:387–391.

Seventeen patients with 27 angular deformities, including 20 with adolescent Blount's disease were treated by percutaneous osteotomy and progressive lengthening using a modified Wagner apparatus applied for an average of 12 weeks. No major complications were encountered.

Ingvarsson T, Hägglund G, Ramgren B, Jonsson K, Zayer M: Long-term results after adolescent Blount's disease. *J Pediatr Orthop* 1997;6B:153–156.

Twenty-three patients with 27 limbs affected by adolescent tibia vara were assessed for knee problems at an average age of 47. Nine had no treatment, 11 had hemiepiphysiodesis, and 7 had osteotomy. At follow-up, most had little or no pain; 9 had arthrosis.

Limb-Length Inequality

Aaron AD, Eilert RE: Results of the Wagner and Ilizarov methods of limb-lengthening. *J Bone Joint Surg* 1996;78A:20–29.

In this comparison of the Wagner and Ilizarov lengthening methods (not fixators) in 20 and 21 patients, respectively, consolidation averaged 44 days per cm with the Wagner method and 26 days with the Ilizarov method. There were 30 major complications in the Wagner-treated limbs and only 13 in the Ilizarov-treated limbs.

Aronson J: Limb-lengthening, skeletal reconstruction, and bone transport with the Ilizarov method. *J Bone Joint Surg* 1997;79A: 1243–1258.

This is an excellent review of the history, basic science, indications, and summary of results of the Ilizarov apparatus in limb lengthening, nonunion, angular deformity, and bone transport.

Ghoneem HF, Wright JG, Cole WG, Rang M: The Ilizarov method for correction of complex deformities: Psychological and functional outcomes. *J Bone Joint Surg* 1996;78A:1480–1485.

This is a retrospective functional and psychological evaluation of 45 children between the ages of 3 and 18 (average, 12 years) treated with the Ilizarov apparatus for lower extremity shortening and/or deformity. All had a normal psychological profile, 42 of 45 had no limitation of activities of daily living, and 37 were satisfied with the results of treatment.

Holm I, Nordsletten L, Steen H, Folleras G, Bjerkreim I: Muscle function after mid-shaft femoral shortening: A prospective study with a two-year follow up. *J Bone Joint Surg* 1994;76B: 143–146.

Isokinetic testing of knee function was performed in 12 limbs before and serially for 2 years after femoral shortening of between 27 and 70 mm. Two years afer surgery, significant quadriceps and hamstring function reduction was still present; recovery was greater in the hamstrings.

Hope PG, Crawfurd EJ, Catterall A: Bone growth following lengthening for congenital shortening of the lower limb. *J Pediatr Orthop* 1994;14:339–342.

Lower limb growth velocity before and after Wagner lengthening was evaluated in 20 patients with congenital limb deficiency. No significant alterations in limb growth velocity were noted at follow-up.

Horton GA, Olney BW: Epiphysiodesis of the lower extremity: Results of the percutaneous technique. *J Pediatr Orthop* 1996; 16:180–182.

Twenty-six patients underwent 42 percutaneous epiphysiodeses using drill bits and curette under image intensifier control. All achieved physeal arrest. No angular deformities, fractures, or neurovascular complications occurred.

Kaufman KR, Miller LS, Sutherland DH: Gait asymmetry in patients with limb-length inequality. *J Pediatr Orthop* 1996;16: 144–150.

A gait analysis of 20 subjects with documented limb-length inequality revealed that asymmetry of gait was detectable for discrepancies greater than 2 cm and increased with increasingly greater discrepancy.

Little DG, Nigo L, Aiona MD: Deficiencies of current methods for the timing of epiphysiodesis. *J Pediatr Orthop* 1996;16: 173–179.

Prediction of the results of epiphysiodesis in 71 patients using Anderson and Green, Moseley, and Menelaus methods were compared. No method proved superior; the authors recommend the Menelaus method because it is the simplest and based on chronologic age.

Paley D, Herzenberg JE, Paremain G, Bhave A: Femoral lengthening over an intramedullary nail: A matched-case comparison with Ilizarov femoral lengthening. *J Bone Joint Surg* 1997;79A: 1464–1480.

In this comparison of 32 femoral lengthenings over an intramedullary nail with 32 traditional Ilizarov femoral lengthenings, lengthening over nail patients were in the external fixator half as long as those treated traditionally, incurred no regenerate fractures (6 in the traditional group), recovered knee motion more quickly, and had a lower major complication rate.

Synder M, Harcke HT, Bowen JR, Caro PA: Evaluation of physeal behavior in response to epiphyseodesis with the use of serial magnetic resonance imaging. *J Bone Joint Surg* 1994;76A: 224–229.

Evaluation of growth recovery lines on sequential MRI scans of 14 patients after percutaneous epiphysiodesis led the authors to conclude that the effect of surgery on longitudinal growth was immediate, and that no discernible effect was noted in the physes that were not operated on.

Stanitski DF, Shahcheraghi H, Nicker DA, Armstrong PF: Results of tibial lengthening with the Ilizarov technique. *J Pediatr Orthop* 1996;16:168–172.

The results of 62 tibial lengthenings in 52 patients using the Ilizarov apparatus are reviewed. Lengthening averaged 7.5 cm (32% of original length). Unplanned reoperations were required 28 times.

Traumatic Disorders of the Knee and Leg

Andrews M, Noyes FR, Barber-Westin SD: Anterior cruciate ligament allograft reconstruction in the skeletally immature athlete. *Am J Sports Med* 1994;22:48–54.

Allograft fascia lata or Achilles tendon ACL reconstruction (7-mm tunnel centrally placed through the tibial physis and placed "over-the-top" in femur) can be effective in select skeletally immature athletes who do not want to modify activities or who have an associated meniscal injury.

Beaty JH, Kumar A: Fractures about the knee in children. *J Bone Joint Surg* 1994;76A:1870–1880.

This is an excellent review of fractures around the knee in children.

Berg EE: Pediatric tibial eminence fractures: Arthroscopic cannulated screw fixation. *Arthroscopy* 1995;11:328–331.

An arthroscopic reduction and stabilization technique is described in which cannulated screws are used for tibial eminence fractures in children.

Buess-Watson E, Exner GU, Illi OE: Fractures about the knee: Growth disturbances and problems of stability at long-term follow-up. *Eur J Pediatr Surg* 1994;4:218–224.

The authors present clinical and radiographic data on complications (leg length discrepancy, axis deviation, instability) resulting from fractures about the knee in childhood. Growth disturbances making secondary procedures necessary occurred in 5 of 14 distal femoral physeal fractures. Complex instability was observed in 3 of 7 proximal tibial physeal fractures.

Matelic TM, Aronsson DD, Boyd DW Jr, LaMont RL: Acute hemarthrosis of the knee in children. *Am J Sports Med* 1995; 23:668–671.

Children with an acute traumatic knee hemarthrosis often have an intra-articular injury (67% osteochondral fractures, 10% ACL injury). Preoperative radiographs failed to identify the osteochondral fractures in 36% of the patients. Arthroscopic evaluation may be valuable in identifying the etiology of an acute hemarthrosis of the knee in a child or adolescent.

Matsusue Y, Nakamura T, Suzuki S, Iwasaki R: Biodegradable pin fixation of osteochondral fragments of the knee. *Clin Orthop* 1996;322:166–173.

Biodegradeable ultra-high strength poly L-lactide pins are effective in stabilizing fractures and osteochondritis of the knee. Bone union was obtained in all cases without a single inflammatory reaction.

Medler RG, Jansson KA: Arthroscopic treatment of fractures of the tibial spine. *Arthroscopy* 1994;10:292–295.

The authors report use of an ACL tibial drill guide to assist in the passage of suture for the reduction and stabilization of tibial immature fractures in children.

Nietosvaara Y, Aalto K, Kallio PE: Acute patellar dislocation in children: Incidence and associated osteochondral fractures. *J Pediatr Orthop* 1994;14:513–515.

The authors report a prospective study of acute patellar dislocation in children. Incidence of dislocation was 43/100,000.

Parker AW, Drez D Jr, Cooper JL: Anterior cruciate ligament injuries in patients with open physes. *Am J Sports Med* 1994;22: 44–47.

Six children with ACL and meniscal injuries were treated surgically. One patient also had a grade III medial collateral ligament injury and a lateral patellar dislocation. The hamstring tendons were placed in a groove over the front of the tibia and a groove over the top of the femur.

Thomson JD, Stricker SJ, Williams MM: Fractures of the distal femoral epiphyseal plate. *J Pediatr Orthop* 1995;15:474–478.

Best results were obtained with anatomic reduction and pin fixation. Forty-three percent of fractures treated without pin fixation lost reduction during casting. Operating room reductions were more likely to be anatomic than reductions done in the emergency room.

Williams JS Jr, Abate JA, Fadale PD, Tung GA: Meniscal and nonosseous ACL injuries in children and adolescents. *Am J Knee Surg* 1996;9:22–26.

This is a retrospective review of 24 children and adolescents with suspected meniscal or ACL injuries. Nonosseous ACL injuries were identified arthroscopically in 18 patients (75%), 10 of whom had a coexistent meniscal lesion. Four of the 5 patients with a lateral meniscal injury, both patients with an ACL injury, and all 3 patients with a medial meniscal tear were identified by MRI.

Zobel MS, Borrello JA, Siegel MJ, Stewart NR: Pediatric knee MR imaging: Pattern of injuries in the immature skeleton. *Radiology* 1994;190:397–401.

Medial meniscal injuries were identified by MRI studies in 29 of the 104 knees (posterior horn: 93%, body: 52%). Lateral meniscal abnormalities were found in 18% of the patients; the ACL was abnormal in 15 knees. One posterior cruciate disruption, 7 medial collateral ligament injuries, and 1 lateral collateral type injury were also identified.

Classic Bibliography

Aichroth PM, Patel DV, Marx CL: Congenital discoid lateral meniscus in children: A follow-up study and evaluation of management. *J Bone Joint Surg* 1991;73B:932–936.

Aitken GT: The child amputee: An overview. *Orthop Clin North Am* 1972;3:447–472.

Buckley SL, Smith G, Sponseller PD, Thompson JD, Griffin PP: Open fractures of the tibia in children. *J Bone Joint Surg* 1990; 72A:1462–1469.

Cramer KE, Limbird TJ, Green NE: Open fractures of the diaphysis of the lower extremity in children: Treatment, results and complications. *J Bone Joint Surg* 1992;74A:218–232.

Drennan JC: Congenital dislocation of the knee and patella, in Heckman JD (ed): *Instructional Course Lectures 42*. Rosemont, IL, American Academy of Orthopaedic Surgeons, 1993, pp 517–524.

Gabriel KR, Crawford AH, Roy DR, True MS, Sauntry S: Percutaneous epiphyseodesis. *J Pediatr Orthop* 1994;14: 358–362.

Hughston JC, Hergenroeder PT, Courtenay BG: Osteochondritis dissecans of the femoral condyles. *J Bone Joint Surg* 1984; 66A:1340–1348.

Lloyd-Roberts GC, Thomas TG: The etiology of quadriceps contracture in children. *J Bone Joint Surg* 1964;46B:498–502.

Loder RT, Herring JA: Fibular transfer for congenital absence of the tibia: A reassessment. *J Pediatr Orthop* 1987;7:8–13.

Macnicol MF, Gupta MS: Epiphysiodesis using a cannulated tubesaw. *J Bone Joint Surg* 1997;79B:307–309.

Maguire JK, Canale ST: Fractures of the patella in children and adolescents. *J Pediatr Orthop* 1993;13:567–571.

Meyers MH, McKeever FM: Fracture of the intercondylar eminence of the tibia. *J Bone Joint Surg* 1959;41A:209–222.

Schoenecker PL, Capelli AM, Millar EA, et al: Congenital longitudinal deficiency of the tibia. *J Bone Joint Surg* 1989;71A: 278–287.

Sharma M, MacKenzie WG, Bowen JR: Severe tibial growth retardation in total fibular hemimelia after limb lengthening. *J Pediatr Orthop* 1996;16:438–444.

Simpson AH, Williams PE, Kyberd P, Goldspink G, Kenwright J: The response of muscle to leg lengthening. *J Bone Joint Surg* 1995;77B:630–636.

Stanitski CL, Harvell JC, Fu F: Observations on acute knee hemarthrosis in children and adolescents. *J Pediatr Orthop* 1993;13:506–510.

Stanitski DF, Rossman K, Torosian M: The effect of femoral lengthening on knee articular cartilage: The role of apparatus extension across the joint. *J Pediatr Orthop* 1996;16:151–154.

Suzuki S, Kasahara Y, Seto Y, Futami T, Furukawa K, Nishino Y: Dislocation and subluxation during femoral lengthening. *J Pediatr Orthop* 1994;14:343–346.

Willis RB, Blokker C, Stoll TM, Paterson DC, Galpin RD: Long-term follow-up of anterior tibial eminence fractures. *J Pediatr Orthop* 1993;13:361–364.

Chapter 41
Knee and Leg: Bone Trauma

Patellar Fractures

The most common mechanism of injury resulting in a patellar fracture is a direct blow to the anterior aspect of the knee. In motor vehicle accidents, this most often occurs when the knee strikes the dashboard; common associated injuries include ipsilateral femoral shaft fracture, hip fracture-dislocation, and posterior cruciate ligament rupture. An eccentric contraction of the quadriceps mechanism may result in a tension fracture of the patella.

Diagnosis

A direct blow to the patella generates compressive forces that can cause longitudinal, stellate, or comminuted fractures. These injuries usually are not widely displaced because the retinaculum is intact. However, tension force failure of the patella can result in wide displacement secondary to associated tearing of the quadriceps expansion.

History and physical examination are usually diagnostic. Pain, swelling, reduced ability or inability to extend the leg against gravity, and a palpable defect between the patellar fragments and extensor retinaculum all occur with displaced fractures. Minimally displaced fractures may cause only pain and swelling.

Patellar fractures can be classified by the mechanism of injury, the amount of displacement, or the configuration of the major fracture lines (transverse, vertical, osteochondral, or comminuted). Important to this classification scheme is the amount of displacement. Displaced fractures are defined as those with a step-off of more than 2 mm or a fracture gap of more than 3 mm.

Radiographic evaluation should include anteroposterior (AP), and lateral views. Tangential views of the patella with the knee in varying degrees of flexion are helpful to identify osteochondral or nondisplaced longitudinal fractures. Additional imaging studies, such as computed tomography (CT) or magnetic resonance imaging (MRI) scans, are rarely required but may be helpful to further define osteochondral fractures after patellar dislocations or sleeve fractures in children.

Treatment

Minimally Displaced Fractures Patients with minimally displaced patellar fractures that have less than 1 mm of step-off and slight separation are usually able to extend the leg fully against gravity and thus demonstrate an intact retinaculum. These patients can be managed with cylinder casting or a knee immobilizer for 4 to 6 weeks. Weightbearing with the knee in full extension is allowed. Follow-up within the first 4 weeks should ensure that the position is maintained, because even slight degrees of knee flexion can cause distraction at the fracture site.

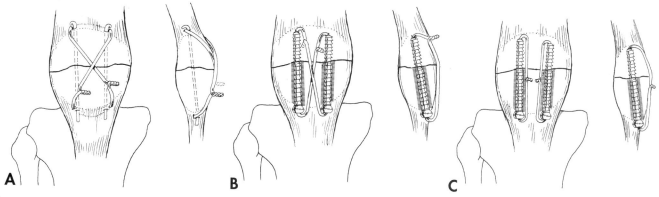

Figure 1

Patellar fixation. A, Modification of the modified tension-band technique with use of an 18-gauge wire crossed anteriorly. B, Cannulated screws with tension band crossed anteriorly. C, Cannulated screws with separate tension bands. Wire twists should not protrude anteriorly; they are rotated laterally or medially to prevent soft-tissue irritation. (Reproduced with permission from Cramer KE, Moed BR: Patellar fractures: Contemporary approach to treatment. *J Am Acad Orthop Surg* 1997;5:323-331.)

Displaced Fractures For displaced or comminuted fractures, efforts should be directed to restore and preserve the articular surface as well as the knee extensor mechanism. A vertical midline incision is used to provide surgical exposure. In general, transverse incisions should be avoided. However, transverse lacerations often occur in concert with open patellar fractures, and these should be incorporated into a longitudinal extensile incision to facilitate secondary reconstructive procedures.

Reduction should be confirmed by direct palpation of the articular surface, which can be felt through the torn retinaculum. If the retinaculum is intact, a small longitudinal retinacular incision should be made to confirm articular congruency. An intraoperative lateral radiograph is useful to confirm reduction as well as accurate hardware placement.

Fixation varies with the fracture pattern involved. Displaced transverse fractures are commonly stabilized with a tension-band wiring technique in which either interfragmentary Kirschner wire (K-wire) fixation is combined with a tension-band wire or interfragmentary cannulated lag-screw fixation is combined with a tension band threaded through the cannulated screws and then crossed over the anterior patella in the typical figure-of-8 configuration (Fig. 1).

As the degree of fracture comminution increases, as much articular surface as possible should be preserved. Lag screws can be used for large fragments with smaller fragments stabilized with multiple interfragmentary K-wires. This fixation is supplemented with a tension-band wire. If the inferior patellar fragment is too small or significant comminution precludes lag-screw or K-wire fixation, the fragment should be excised and the patellar tendon advanced. The tendon is attached through multiple drill holes spaced along the fractured surface near the articular surface to prevent tilting of the patella and minimizes step-off between the articular surface and the tendon. Care should be taken to avoid patella baja during the reattachment. Patellectomy is reserved for severely comminuted fractures that cannot be reasonably reconstructed.

With secure fixation, gentle active flexion with passive extension can be instituted within 2 weeks after surgery. Immediate weightbearing in extension is allowed. Extensive comminution, advancement of the patellar tendon, and noncompliance may preclude early range of motion. In these cases, the knee should be immobilized in extension for 4 to 6 weeks before the initiation of range-of-motion exercises. Resistive exercises should be avoided until adequate healing is evident. Common complications related to surgical fixation include decreased range of motion, loss of reduction (0% to 2%), infection (3% to 10%), and hardware irritation that necessitates surgical removal (15%).

Tibial Plateau Fractures

Injuries to the tibial plateau result from a medially or laterally directed force or an axial compressive load. The resulting fracture pattern is a reflection of the forces involved. When a plateau fracture is suspected, the physical examination should thoroughly document the neurovascular status, especially in suspected cases of fracture-dislocation. Plateau fractures associated with fracture extension into the tibial diaphysis may also be associated with acute compartment syndrome secondary to hemorrhage and edema of the involved compartments. Severe contusion and internal degloving occur particularly in high-energy injuries. Even in the absence of open fractures, the contused soft tissues may be in jeopardy because of fracture instability or associated severe swelling. Physical examination should focus on the continuity of the soft tissues and the presence of blisters or superficial abrasions; these areas must be avoided during any subsequent surgical approach. In some cases, surgery should be delayed or temporized until the soft-tissue envelope has recovered sufficiently to allow for surgical intervention.

Routine radiographic evaluation consists of AP and lateral views supplemented with 2 oblique projections and a "plateau view." CT scans provide additional information regarding the cross-sectional anatomy of the fracture, which aids in the preoperative planning, especially for high-energy fracture patterns. The use of magnetic resonance imaging (MRI) has been shown to be superior in assessing associated soft-tissue injury, such as meniscal and ligamentous disruptions, but is not routinely used on an emergent basis. Arteriography should be considered for those high-energy fracture patterns in which an intimal tear is suspected by clinical presentation.

The Schatzker classification scheme (Fig. 2) is used to group fractures that are similar in their mechanisms of injury and fracture pattern, require a similar approach in their treatment, and have a similar prognosis. Schatzker types I, II, and III are typically the result of a lower energy mechanism of injury, as opposed to the more complex Schatzker types IV, V, and VI fractures, which result from a high-energy mechanism of injury.

Nonsurgical Management

Nonsurgical treatment is indicated following a low-energy injury with an incomplete or nondisplaced fracture and in select instances of tibial plateau fractures in the elderly in whom future total knee replacement is anticipated. Relative indications for nonsurgical management include severe medical disabilities, such as pulmonary or cardiovascular compromise or severe systemic metabolic disease (eg, peripheral

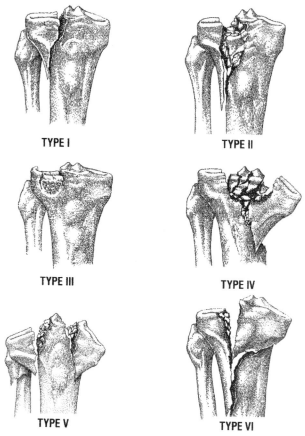

Figure 2

Schatzker classification of tibial plateau fractures. Type I is a pure split of the lateral plateau; type II is a split depression fracture of the lateral plateau; type III is a pure depression of the lateral plateau; type IV is a fracture of the medial tibial plateau; type V is a bicondylar fracture; and type VI includes extensive soft-tissue injury in association with a bicondylar fracture and diametaphyseal disassociation.

vascular occlusive disease, diabetes). Severe soft-tissue compromise in which the risk of skin slough and associated postoperative wound infection is high is also an indication for nonsurgical treatment.

Immobilization and nonweightbearing are maintained for 4 weeks, followed by conversion to a hinged fracture brace with gradual range of motion. Avoiding knee stiffness is a priority. Weightbearing is delayed until radiographic evidence of healing is noted.

Traction, or a spanning external fixator, is indicated for injuries with excessive comminution or fracture displacement, advanced osteoporosis, or soft-tissue compromise in which early casting is contraindicated. A supramalleolar traction pin is used with balanced suspension, and use of a Thomas splint and Pearson knee attachment is helpful to ini-

tiate early range of motion. At 4 to 6 weeks, radiographs obtained out of traction are used to assess healing. If no further displacement has occurred, the patient is placed in a hinged knee brace, and progressive range of motion and advancement of weightbearing are initiated.

Surgical Management

The primary indications for surgical management include significant articular depression and displacement of condylar fragments. No universal agreement exists on the amount of articular depression that can be accepted; from 4 to 10 mm has been described. If joint instability (excessive varus or valgus angulation with the knee in full extension) is caused by articular depression or axial displacement of a tibial condyle, then surgery is indicated. Other absolute indications for surgery include open tibial plateau fractures and those associated with an acute compartment syndrome, an acute vascular lesion, or an ipsilateral femoral shaft fracture (floating knee).

The overall condition of the soft tissues will determine the extent of any surgical approach. As the soft-tissue damage increases, a less invasive approach combining closed reduction with percutaneous fixation and external stabilization would be favored over extensile approaches and associated hardware implantation. Fractures with large condylar fragments and without excessive comminution or extensive articular impaction are also amenable to this less invasive approach.

Closed or Limited Open Reduction Preoperative manual traction radiographs may indicate which fragments will be reduced with ligamentotaxis alone and identify those fracture components that will require a direct surgical approach (limited surgical exposure). If traction radiographs do not demonstrate a reasonable reduction, then a more formal open reduction should be considered.

Intraoperative traction delivered by a femoral distractor or external fixator is used to reduce the tibial condyles. Further condylar manipulation with large percutaneous reduction clamps as well as percutaneous wires (joysticks) is often necessary. Articular reduction is evaluated with either fluoroscopy or arthroscopy. Residual articular depression is elevated percutaneously through a metaphyseal window. Percutaneous articular reduction has been most successful for Schatzker type I fractures and has not been satisfactory for the split depression or more complex fracture patterns. If the tibial condyles are incompletely reduced, a limited incision is directed to this area to elevate the joint and/or to remove a section of an entrapped meniscal fragment. Fixation is completed with cannulated screws. If no condylar comminution exists and an anatomic reduction has been

achieved, the leg can be casted or placed in a fracture brace. If neutralization of the fracture is required, then a monolateral or circular hybrid external fixator can be applied. Good results have been reported with this method provided the mechanical axis of the leg is maintained. Complications have been reported primarily as a result of tensioned wires or fixation half pins in close proximity to the knee joint (Fig. 3).

Open Reduction With Internal Fixation As comminution and displacement of the condylar fragments increase with increasing degrees of joint impaction, the ability to achieve a satisfactory indirect reduction decreases. Increased comminution requires more stability than can generally be obtained by percutaneous screws alone and, therefore, direct plating of these injuries is necessary to avoid loss of fixation.

A straight midline or a medial or lateral parapatellar incision is used to achieve adequate exposure for acute fracture fixation and to facilitate later reconstruction as needed. Menisci must be preserved if possible. Submeniscal arthrotomy or release of the anterior horn of the meniscus is used to expose the articular surface. Articular reduction may be achieved directly by hinging open the condylar wedge fracture or indirectly through a metaphyseal window. The depressed fragment is reduced and bone graft applied. Condylar reduction is achieved using femoral distractors and large reduction forceps. The medial or lateral condyles are fixed using buttress or antiglide plates. When comminution exists at the diaphyseal/metaphyseal junction, a stronger compression plate should be used as a bridge plate to span this area.

For posteromedial condylar pathology, an additional posteromedial exposure can be used. Direct fixation using an extraperiosteal antiglide or buttress plate may be needed for these fracture patterns.

With severe fractures, the paramount concern is to preserve the integrity of the soft-tissue envelope. By limiting the use of large plates to one side of the fracture and using an extraperiosteal plate or external fixator to buttress the opposite condyle, good results can be achieved in patients with high-energy fracture patterns.

Open Plateau Fractures

For severe open injuries or injuries with significant soft-tissue compromise, staged reconstruction can be used. Articular fixation is achieved in a percutaneous or limited fashion, and the knee is bridged using a spanning external fixator placed at the time of the initial surgery. Buttress plating and bone grafting can be carried out 3 to 4 weeks after injury (following recovery of the soft tissues).

Tibial Shaft Fractures

The tibia is the most commonly fractured long bone; frequently, these injuries are caused by high-energy trauma. The tibia is subcutaneous throughout its length, with a relatively poor blood supply. This factor combined with a high-energy mechanism of injury predicts major complications and a poor functional outcome, especially in patients with open fractures.

Fractures are classified by anatomic location, described as

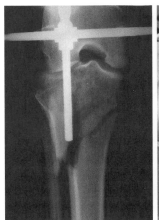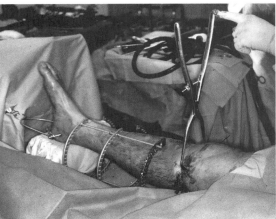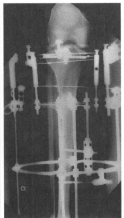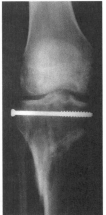

Figure 3

Schatzker type VI plateau fracture. Large condylar fragments and minimal comminution at the joint and major fracture lines make this fracture amenable to a less-invasive surgical approach. Distraction techniques in combination with percutaneous fixation and hybrid external fixation can obtain excellent results.

either proximal, mid or distal third (distal third fractures have demonstrated a higher incidence of delayed union, malunion, and nonunion). Fracture configurations are classified as simple, butterfly, and comminuted. Further subclassification describes the presence and extent of comminution, which correlates with absorbed energy as an indication of severity. This classification has been adopted by the AO/ASIF and the Orthopaedic Trauma Association. From their results, it is evident that simple fractures requiring surgery have the best prognosis. Comminuted or crush injuries have a significantly worse prognosis.

The extent of soft-tissue injury is a predictor of outcome. As the severity of the soft-tissue injury increases so does the incidence of nonunion, malunion, infection, and the likelihood of a limited functional outcome.

Open fractures should be graded after the first debridement. Preoperative classification of open fractures often underestimates the degree of bone and soft-tissue compromise. The modified Gustilo-Anderson classification divides open fractures into 5 groups (Table 1). Type I have an open wound < 1 cm in length; type II have an open wound > 1 cm, but < 10 cm in length without contamination and can be closed without flap coverage. Type IIIA have an open wound > 10 cm that can be closed by delayed primary techniques; periosteal stripping and contamination are absent. Type IIIB fractures have soft-tissue loss requiring rotational or free-flap coverage; periosteal stripping with bone loss and contamination is frequently present. Type IIIC fractures are any open fracture with an associated vascular injury requiring repair.

Early aggressive debridement and soft-tissue coverage with regional flaps or free tissue transfer minimizes infection and optimizes healing. The zone and extent of soft-tissue injury must be appreciated even when the tibial fracture is closed. Soft-tissue injury in closed fractures has been classified:

Table 1
Open fracture classification

	Description of Wound	Condition of Soft Tissues	Fracture Pattern	Fracture Contamination
Type I	1cm or less	Minimal muscle contusion	Simple transverse or short oblique	None
Type II	>1cm, without extensive flaps or avulsion	Moderate muscle crushing	Simple transverse or short oblique with minimal communition	None
Type IIIA	Extensive laceration or flaps; adequate soft-tissue coverage of fracture site or high-energy trauma regardless of the size of the wound	Extensive soft-tissue damage including skin and muscle with crushing component	Segmental fractures; gunshot injuries	May be present
Type IIIB	Extensive soft-tissue loss requiring secondary coverage procedures	Periosteal stripping and exposed bone	Extensive communition	Usually extensive
Type IIIC	Open fracture with arterial injury requiring repair			

type 0, indirect injury with minimal soft-tissue damage (low-energy fracture); type I, low-to-moderate energy fracture with superficial abrasions and contusions; type II, moderate-energy injury with muscle contusion and deep abrasions; type III, high-energy fracture with an internal degloving injury with deep contusion, skin blisters, and full-thickness abrasions. Compartment syndrome and associated neurovascular injury may be present.

The most practical classification determines treatment (surgical versus nonsurgical management). In general, unstable fractures tend to preclude nonsurgical management. Severe soft-tissue injury, involvement of an articular surface, 100% initial displacement of the fracture, comminution greater than 50% of the bone circumference, and transverse fracture orientation are all hallmarks of an unstable fracture pattern. Presence of a fibular fracture in association with a tibial fracture at the same level often indicates an unstable fracture. Predictably, high-energy injuries are more severe with a much higher prevalence of delayed union and are less likely to be treated successfully in a nonsurgical fashion.

Treatment Options for Fractures of the Tibial Shaft

It is generally accepted that the treatment standard for stable closed tibial shaft fractures is closed reduction with the application of a long leg cast followed by functional bracing with early weightbearing. Following closed reduction, alignment should be maintained such that there is < 1 cm of shortening with angulation < 5° and rotational deformity limited to 5° or less.

One group advises that functional closed treatment be limited to closed injuries that have no more than 15 mm of initial shortening or are axially stable reduced transverse fractures. In their series of 1,000 closed tibial fractures treated initially with closed reduction and long leg casting, weightbearing as tolerated in the cast was permitted. If length and alignment were acceptable and pain and swelling had subsided, the cast was replaced with a fracture brace at an average of 3.7 weeks. In 95% of the fractures, the final shortening was < 12 mm (average, 4.28 mm). Final angulatory deformity was ≤ 6° in 90% of patients. In this series, the rate of nonunion was 1.1%. The presence of an intact fibula was a relative contraindication to functional bracing, because significant varus deformity (> 5°) was more likely to develop. Time to union was increased for comminuted fractures.

Prospective studies comparing intramedullary (IM) nailing versus closed treatment revealed longer healing times, increased residual angular deformity and fracture shortening, and increased disability with closed treatment methods. Hindfoot stiffness occurred in 15% of the patients treated

with casts. Twenty-two percent of the patients in the closed treatment group eventually underwent surgical intervention for failure to maintain adequate reduction. Although closed treatment with functional bracing is appropriate for some fractures, recognition of fractures for which this approach will ultimately fail is key.

Plate Osteosynthesis Plate fixation after severe soft-tissue injury should be cautiously considered because of possible complications, such as tissue loss and infection. Relative indications for plate fixation include those tibial shaft fractures that have fracture extension into the ankle or knee joint, select open fractures with little soft-tissue stripping, and arterial injury requiring rapid stabilization.

Closed Intramedullary Nailing The development of interlocked IM nails has expanded the indications for closed nailing of the tibia. Treatment with an interlocked nail results in a high union rate with a low incidence of malunion and infection. By interlocking the nail, length and alignment can be restored, even in comminuted fractures. IM nails are primarily indicated to stabilize diaphyseal fractures, and they usually restore axis alignment for fractures in the mid and distal diaphysis to within 4 cm of the ankle joint. Nailing of proximal third tibial metaphyseal fractures has been shown to be fraught with potential complications, primarily valgus malunion. In one series, 84% of these proximal fractures had residual angulation of 5° or more. Technical errors included use of a medialized nail entry portal and a posteriorly and laterally directed nail trajectory. Suggested techniques for the successful nailing of proximal shaft fractures include use of an adjunctive antiglide plate located at the level of the fracture apex or use of the semiextended position of the knee. These techniques all help prevent the development of apex anterior angulation (Fig. 4). However, in general, alternative methods for proximal third fractures should be thoroughly investigated prior to IM nailing.

If a reamed nail is chosen, sequential reaming of the canal is undertaken and performed without tourniquet control to avoid cortical necrosis. Compartment syndrome following reamed IM nailing has been reported to be related to the duration and force of traction in combination with the reaming, which causes extravasation of the reamed bone through the site of the fracture as well as contributing additional hemorrhage into a traumatized compartment. However, the cause of compartment syndrome in this situation is probably multifactorial.

Small diameter interlocking nails were designed to be inserted without reaming, and it was hoped that the benefits of unreamed nailing (low infection rate, high rate of union) would be realized, especially in open fractures or in fractures with compromised soft tissue where reaming was to be avoided. A recent randomized prospective study of closed tibial shaft fractures compared 73 fractures treated with reamed nails and 63 fractures treated with unreamed nails. The surgical time, fluoroscopic duration, and blood loss were identical for the 2 groups. The union rate was not significantly different for either group: 96% union for reamed nailing and 89% for unreamed nailing. The rate of malunion and infection was not significantly different for either group. The authors concluded that there were no major advantages to IM nailing without reaming as compared to nailing with reaming for the treatment of closed tibial shaft fractures. There was a higher incidence of delayed union and device failure (breakage of interlocking screws and nail fracture) in the group treated without reaming.

If union is not achieved when using unreamed nails, fatigue failure of the nail or the interlocking screw with subsequent nonunion may occur. Numerous secondary procedures have been advocated to promote union and avoid hardware failure. Nail dynamization, exchange reamed nailing, open bone grafting, and fibular osteotomy have all been used alone or in combination to promote union.

For unstable closed tibial fractures without soft-tissue compromise or significant swelling, reamed IM nailing appears to be the treatment of choice. In those fractures, with significant swelling, impending compartment syndrome, compromised soft tissues, or in the treatment of a polytraumatized patient, unreamed nailing is believed to be a satisfactory alternative.

Knee pain is a common sequela following tibial nailing; it occurs in approximately 60% of patients. A recent study correlated insertion of the nail through the patellar tendon with a high incidence of anterior knee pain. There was no correlation between nail protrusion and knee pain. Of those patients with knee pain, 77% had the nail inserted via a patellar tendon splitting approach, compared to 50% of those with a paratendon insertion site. Eighty percent experienced partial or total relief of pain following nail removal.

External Fixation External fixation minimizes additional disruption of the soft-tissue envelope or the vascularity of the fracture fragments and other osseous structures. Among fix-

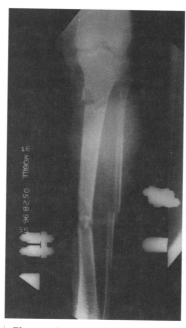
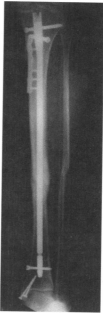
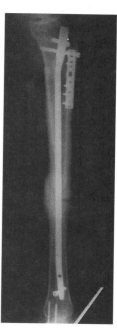

Figure 4

A segmental tibial fracture with proximal one third fracture extension. A subcutaneous anti-glide plate was placed across the proximal fracture following reduction. The plate was used to facilitate nailing and prevent translation of the proximal fragment. A reamed nail was used.

ation devices, external fixation is the least traumatic to apply. Indications for external fixation in closed tibial fractures include periarticular fractures with compromised soft tissues in which extensile incisions necessary for plate application are contraindicated. External fixation is also indicated in open tibial fractures, providing stabilization and adjunctive wound care without foreign-body implantation. Relative indications include the use of external fixation in polytrauma patients in whom urgent stabilization is necessary to facilitate the care of multiple injuries and to avoid the harmful effects of prolonged traction and recumbency.

Complications are primarily pin related and delayed union or nonunion. Patient compliance has a direct correlation to the longevity of the pin. Weightbearing is inconsistent in the external fixation frames. Postframe immobilization (cast or orthotic management) is often necessary.

Treatment of Open Fractures
Open tibial shaft fractures are a surgical emergency. Care begins in the emergency department with a thorough description of the wound and neurovascular status. A sterile saline dressing is placed over the wound and the fracture is splinted. Wound manipulation prior to surgery should be minimized. Immediate debridement of all devitalized soft tis-

sue and bone is performed in the operating room in concert with skeletal stabilization. Debridement is repeated every 48 to 72 hours until a healthy wound is produced. Soft-tissue coverage over exposed bone should be achieved within 5 to 7 days. Prophylactic antibiotics are given routinely for 24 hours postdebridement and repeated for every succeeding surgical intervention.

The primary goal in treating open tibial fractures should be to obtain a biologically sound wound as well as a stable fracture with the use of whichever fixation device is preferred by the surgeon. Controversy over IM nailing for severe tibial shaft fractures has developed because of the osseous devascularization that occurs through the inner two thirds of the tibial cortex and the entire cortex at the fracture region following IM reaming. Animal studies have shown that nailing without reaming causes cortical vascular changes similar to those caused by reaming; however, the phenomenon was limited to tight-fitting nails with extensive cortical contact. Cortical circulation was spared to a much greater degree with the use of a loose-fitting nail without reaming, compared to insertion of a nail after reaming. These studies suggest that small-diameter unreamed nails may spare medullary blood supply and cortical vascularity, which are important in the management of open fractures. Relative and theoretical biologic benefits of unreamed nails have been balanced by the biomechanical limitations of these devices. Unlike large-diameter reamed nails, the small-diameter nails may cause a large discrepancy between the canal and the nail, accentuating motion at the interlocking bolts. By necessity, both the nail and the locking bolts are of a smaller diameter, producing another potential site of implant failure. Because open fractures heal more slowly than closed injuries, fatigue failure of these components is a possibility that may be especially problematic when using small-diameter solid core nails without a cannulation. These nails may be very difficult to remove should the distal segment of the nail fracture.

The use of reamed IM nails for closed and type I fractures has a very low rate of infection, less than 3% in several recent studies. However, the rate of infection for reamed nailing of severe open fractures (type IIIB) has been reported as high as 23%. The rate of infection with external fixation for type III injuries has ranged from 4% to 7%. This relatively low and comparable rate of infection has been offset by the increased rate of malunion that has been reported when treating open tibial shaft fractures to completion with an external fixator.

Recent studies in which open tibial fractures were stabilized with unreamed interlocking nails have reported rates of union greater than 96% with minimal rates of malunion and rates of infection in the range of 4% to 8% for type IIIB frac-

tures. Numerous randomized prospective studies have compared the results of unreamed interlocking nails with those of external fixation for the treatment of open fractures. All of the studies demonstrate the superiority of nailing without reaming. Similar rates of infection and nonunion were present for both treatment modalities, but there was a significantly higher prevalence of malunion with external fixation. Unreamed nailing facilitates other procedures, such as soft-tissue procedures and delayed bone grafting for the overall management of open fractures without the hindrance of an external frame.

External fixation is still the choice for stability in the highly contaminated open fracture or in those fractures that experience a long delay prior to surgical treatment. Because unreamed nails may require secondary procedures to achieve union and hardware failure is seen more frequently, their routine use is being reevaluated.

A recent prospective randomized study evaluated 50 open fractures treated with nailing after reaming and 44 fractures treated with nailing without reaming. The groups were similar with respect to the number of fractures and fracture types treated. No clinically significant differences were noted with regard to the technical aspects of nailing or in the rate of early postoperative complications. No difference in average time to union was seen (29 weeks for unreamed nails and 30 weeks for reamed nails). Nine percent of reamed and 12% of unreamed fractures went on to nonunion (not significant). The rates of infection were similar with 2 reamed and 1 unreamed fractures developing an infection. There was a significant increase in the number of broken screws (29% in the unreamed group) compared to the reamed group (9%). The functional outcome between the groups was similar. The authors concluded that the clinical and radiographic results of nailing after reaming were similar to those without reaming for fixation of open fractures; however, the unreamed nails had a higher rate of hardware failure.

Regardless of the method of open fracture stabilization, all these studies demonstrate the principles of intensive debridement and the ability to achieve a biologically sound wound prior to skeletal reconstruction. Rates of infection have been low for both reamed and unreamed nails used for type I, II, and IIIA fractures. Controversy still exists as to the efficacy of reamed versus unreamed nailing for the treatment of severe IIIB injuries.

Antibiotic Therapy
Second-generation cephalosporins are administered for closed grade I, II, and IIIA fractures. With extensive comminution, periosteal stripping, and contamination, an amino

glycoside is added (types IIIB and IIIC). Secondary to possible anaerobic contamination, penicillin is added for farm injuries.

Use of an antibiotic bead pouch technique to provide local antibiotic administration and temporary dead space management for open fracture treatment has been described. Following thorough debridement and skeletal stabilization, the soft-tissue and bony defect is filled with a chain of polymethylmethacrylate/antibiotic beads laden with gentamicin. The wound is sealed by direct closure or with an impermeable plastic drape.

In a study of 81 open tibial shaft fractures treated with a reamed IM nail and delayed wound closure, 26 had prophylactic antibiotics only. The other 55 were managed identically except that an antibiotic bead pouch was used following the initial debridement. There was a 16% incidence of infection in those fractures treated without a bead pouch, compared to a 4% infection rate with a bead pouch. The authors recommended the addition of the bead pouch to the overall wound management protocol.

Limb Salvage

The Mangled Extremity Severity Score (MESS) is a retrospective effort to relate the severity of the injury, limb ischemia, shock, and patient age to predict which limbs can be successfully reconstructed. This and other rating scales have been shown to have many pitfalls and should not be used as the sole determining factor for instituting limb salvage. They also do not address the long-term function and general well-being of the patient. Clinical studies have highlighted the tremendous expense to society for limb salvage of type IIIB and IIIC open tibial fractures and have demonstrated that successful limb salvage does not always equal a successful functional outcome.

Complications

Complications of tibial shaft fractures include nonunion, malunion, and infection. Nonunion refers to the nonhealing or arrest of the bony repair process with formation of intervening fibrous or cartilaginous tissue. The usual time frame is 6 to 8 months minimum to classify a fracture as having a nonunion. Tibial nonunions are differentiated into 2 major categories: the vital or hypertrophic nonunion versus an atrophic (avascular) nonunion. Infected nonunions may be either atrophic or hypertrophic. Hypertrophic nonunions require mechanical stability to unite. The surgical approach should be biologic in that the hypertrophic callus should not be disturbed or taken down. Closed reamed IM nailing has the advantages of indirect reduction and stable fixation but limited deformity correction. Tension-band plating rigidly

stabilizes the nonunion and has a greater potential to restore significant malalignment. Limiting the surgical exposure by indirect reduction using a femoral distractor, application of a tension band plate, and the use of a tensioning device with interfragmental compression lag screws allow excellent deformity correction and consolidation of hypertrophic nonunions. External fixation techniques, particularly closed distraction of hypertrophic nonunions, have been successful to restore leg-length discrepancy and correct malalignment.

Atrophic nonunions require rigid mechanical stabilization as well as a biologic stimulus for healing. The preferred treatment for atrophic nonunion is autogenous cancellous bone graft placed in a posterolateral location. For defects greater than 3 to 4 cm, numerous graft attempts may be necessary. In addition, these patients require prolonged periods of cast or brace protection in order to avoid fatigue fracture and late deformation across the graft region. For this reason, defects greater than 4 cm have been treated with bone transport techniques using either monolateral or circular small-wire external fixators with excellent results. A significant disadvantage to these techniques is the prolonged period of time the patient must remain in the external fixator and the risk of nonunion at the docking site. Recent studies have shown that routine bone grafting of the bone transport docking site can significantly reduce the overall time in the external fixator.

Malunion is defined as 5° of varus, valgus, or rotational malalignment, 5° of apex, anterior, or posterior angulation, and more than 1 cm of shortening. Malunion alters the mechanical axis of the leg and may accelerate the onset of arthritis in the knee and ankle. Symptomatic nonunions should be osteotomized, realigned, and stabilized using either a nail or plate. Gradual distraction osteogenesis has been shown to correct multiple deformities simultaneously as well as restore overall limb length.

The etiology of posttraumatic osteomyelitis is related to the magnitude of the initial trauma. Treatment of infected fractures uses a staged reconstruction protocol. In an infected nonunion, implants are left in place if they are providing stability. If the implants provide no stability at the time of debridement, all fracture hardware should be removed. In addition, all necrotic bone should be excised at debridement. Stabilization is necessary and is usually provided by external fixation. Debridements are necessary to obtain a biologically sound wound. Dead-space management involves use of antibiotic beads or open wound packing. Eventual soft-tissue closure may be achieved using free-flap coverage. Deep, culture-specific antibiotics are administered for 4 to 6 weeks. Following resolution of the infection and healing of the soft tissues, delayed skeletal reconstruction is performed.

Compartment Syndrome

The diagnosis of compartment syndrome is based on clinical signs and measurements of the intracompartmental pressure. The physical signs of compartment syndrome are severe pain, resistance to analgesics, and pain that is out of proportion to what is expected from the primary problem. Pain is not relieved by immobilization, ice, elevation, or narcotics. Circumferential casts or dressing may actually aggravate the discomfort by decreasing the relative volume of the compartment. Most patients will exhibit a tense, firm, swollen muscle running the length of the anatomic compartment involved. The firmness is not localized to the site of a fracture or area of contusion. Early clinical signs, such as pain on passive stretch and regional hypesthesia, are variable, yet may herald an evolving compartment syndrome. Most compartments have sensory nerves that travel through the bulk of the muscular compartment. The first sign of nerve ischemia is altered sensation. This ischemia can progress to frank anesthesia if untreated. The appearance of paresthesia in the distribution of the deep peroneal nerve has been documented with pressures > 30 mm Hg. However, the physician must be aware of the possibility of superimposed traumatic peripheral nerve deficit. Paresis caused by compartment syndrome is a late finding that warrants emergent treatment and is of little help in the diagnosis of early compartment syndrome.

The universal factor that must be present for compartment syndrome to exist is increased tissue pressure. Measurement of this pressure is the most effective means of diagnosis, especially in patients in whom the signs and symptoms are not clear-cut or in patients who are comatose or unresponsive. Pressures are measured by inserting a needle or catheter, which is connected to a manometer, into the compartment. A small amount of fluid is injected into the compartment. The pressure at which the fluid enters the compartment is the intracompartmental pressure. Single measurements are made with a side-port catheter or simple needles. Catheters can be left in place for long-term monitoring and are useful in the diagnosis of exercise-induced compartment syndrome. New hand-held pressure monitors with an interchangeable side-port catheter attached to a syringe plunger mechanism are universally available. This technique imitates that of needle injection in which the side-port catheter or needle is placed in the compartment in question. The advantage of these devices is that they are totally self-contained, extremely portable, and very simple to use. Comparisons of these units to the infusion method have shown that they are as reliable in determining compartment pressures. However, values obtained with simple needles were less consistent and indicated

pressure 15 to 20 mm greater than those obtained with a wick catheter and side-port needles.

Needle location in relation to the fracture is important. When pressures were measured at varying distances from the fracture, the highest pressures were found adjacent to the fracture in the anterior and deep posterior compartments. The controversy in establishing a maximum tolerable compartment pressure is no doubt related to the large degree of individual variation and tolerance to elevated pressures. There are 2 basic definitions of critical pressure: (1) an absolute value (> 30 mm Hg) or (2) a derived value (Δp = diastolic blood pressure-compartment pressure [< 30 mm Hg]).

Progressive elevation of compartment pressure may be a more reliable sign of an evolving compartment syndrome than any absolute level of increased pressure. Serial determinations of compartment pressure, however, have the disadvantage of requiring either the presence of an indwelling catheter or multiple catheter insertions into an already potentially ischemic and compromised compartment. In a prospective study, 116 patients with diaphyseal fractures had continuous monitoring of anterior compartment pressure for 24 hours. Three patients had acute compartment syndrome (2.6%). In the first 12 hours of monitoring, 53 patients had absolute pressures > 30 mm Hg and 30 had pressures > 40 mm Hg with 4 > 50 mm Hg. Only one patient had a Δp = diastolic pressure - compartment pressure of < 30 mm Hg. In the second 12-hour period, 28 patients had absolute pressures > 30 mm Hg and 7 > 40 mm Hg. Only 2 had Δp of < 30 mm Hg and required fasciotomies. None of the 116 patients had any sequela of compartment syndrome at least 6 months after injury. The authors found the use of a Δp of 30 mm Hg as a threshold for a fasciotomy led to no missed cases of acute compartment syndrome, and the authors recommend that decompression should be performed if the Δp drops to < 30 mm Hg. In spite of this study, a prolonged absolute value of > 30 mm Hg should be considered an indication for presence of a compartment syndrome.

Management of compartment syndrome is surgical decompression. This is usually accomplished through medial and lateral incisions. The lateral incision allows access to the anterior and lateral compartments and the medial incision allows decompression of the superficial and deep posterior compartments. The dual incision method is less risky, primarily because the fascial incisions are all superficial and avoid deep neuromuscular structures. Alternatively, all 4 compartments can be decompressed through a single lateral incision. The benefit of a single incision is balanced by the risk of incomplete decompression. The importance of long skin incisions is illustrated by a study in which 8 patients with compartment syndrome underwent surgical decompression while their intracompartmental pressures were being monitored. Initial decompression was through a skin incision 8 cm in length. The pressure remained > 30 mm Hg in 9 compartments of the 8 patients and it dropped < 30 mm Hg only after the length of the skin incision was increased to 16 cm.

Following surgical decompression, the leg is elevated until swelling decreases. After 5 to 7 days of elevation, the swelling decreases substantially in many cases. Techniques to prevent skin contracture (retention with elastic bands) will improve the likelihood of delayed primary closure. Occasionally, a split-thickness skin graft is required.

Complications of compartment syndrome include scarring, contractures, and decreased nerve function. Decompression of nerves and excision of contracted scarred muscle can be partially effective in the management of these complications.

Annotated Bibliography

Patellar Fractures

Smith ST, Cramer KE, Karges DE, Watson JT, Moed BR: Early complications in the operative treatment of patellar fractures. *J Orthop Trauma* 1997;11:183–187.

Consecutive series of 87 patellar fractures were reviewed to identify and review the early complications in the surgical treatment using a modified tension-band wire fixation. Twenty-two percent of fractures treated with tension-band wiring and early motion displaced > 2 mm within the early postoperative period. Technical errors or patient noncompliance were identified as factors.

Tibial Plateau Fractures

Duwelius PJ, Rangitsch MR, Colville MR, Woll TS: Treatment of tibial plateau fractures by limited internal fixation. *Clin Orthop* 1997;339:47–57.

Seventy-six plateau fractures were treated according to a prospective protocol using instability in extension as the principal indication for surgical fixation. Closed manipulative reduction under fluoroscopy with elevation of joint depression and fixation using cannulated screws or buttress plates was used. Of patients, 87% had a successful outcome using Rasmussen's criteria. Significant articular comminution or metaphyseal diaphyseal extension may not be suitable for this technique.

Marsh JL, Smith ST, Do TT: External fixation and limited internal fixation for complex fractures of the tibial plateau. *J Bone Joint Surg* 1995;77A:661–673.

Twenty-one complex fractures of the tibial plateau in 20 patients were treated with closed reduction interfragmentary screw fixation of the articular fragment and application of a unilateral half-pin external fixator. Most patients had function close to that of age-matched controls. Complications were attributable primarily to the proximal half-pins of the external fixator.

Weiner LS, Kelley M, Yang E, et al: The use of combination internal fixation and hybrid external fixation in severe proximal tibia fractures. *J Orthop Trauma* 1995;9:244–250.

Fifty severe fractures of the proximal tibia were treated using limited internal fixation combined with circular external fixation. All fractures healed in an average 12 weeks with 2 nonunions requiring bone graft. This treatment method is associated with a high percentage of good and excellent results, combines the advantages of anatomic stable fixation with less soft-tissue dissection, and eliminates the need for large implants.

Tibial Shaft Fractures

Blachut PA, O'Brien PJ, Meek RN, Broekhuyse HM: Interlocking intramedullary nailing with and without reaming for the treatment of closed fractures of the tibial shaft: A prospective, randomized study. *J Bone Joint Surg* 1997;79A:640–646.

Seventy-three closed tibial shaft fractures were managed with reamed IM nailing, and 63 fractures were managed with unreamed nails.

Duwelius PJ, Schmidt AH, Rubinstein RA, Green JM: Nonreamed interlocked intramedullary tibial nailing: One community's experience. *Clin Orthop* 1995;315:104–113.

Forty-nine acute displaced tibial fractures were treated with a standard surgical protocol using a femoral distractor without a fracture table and an unreamed interlocking tibial nail. Ninety-four percent of the fractures healed; however, 57% required at least 1 additional operation to obtain union. Unreamed tibial nails provide adequate stabilization and can be used in the management of most open or closed tibial fractures; however, early dynamization or exchange nailing and bone grafting should be considered to hasten union and avoid hardware failure.

Keating JF, Orfaly R, O'Brien PJ: Knee pain after tibial nailing. *J Orthop Trauma* 1997;11:10–13.

This retrospective analysis of patients treated by tibial nailing evaluates a consecutive series of patients analyzed to determine the incidence of knee pain, time of onset, and relationship of nail position. Results indicate a parapatellar tendon incision for nail insertion and nail removal for those patients with a painful knee. The causes of knee pain after tibial nailing are multifactorial.

Konrath G, Moed BR, Watson JT, Kaneshiro S, Karges DE, Cramer KE: Intramedullary nailing of unstable diaphyseal fractures of the tibia with distal intraarticular involvement. *J Orthop Trauma* 1997;11:200–205.

Twenty diaphyseal fractures with distal intra-articular involvement were stabilized with lag screw fixation with or without supplemental plating of the intra-articular extensor ankle fracture followed by IM nailing of the diaphyseal fracture. Two fractures had excellent alignment after healing with no subsequent displacement of the articular fracture. Indications for IM nailing of unstable diaphyseal tibial fractures may be extended to include fractures with distal extension into the ankle joint as well as fractures occurring in combination with noncontiguous ipsilateral ankle fractures.

532   Lower Extremity

Lang GJ, Cohen BE, Bosse J, Kellam JF: Proximal third tibial shaft fractures: Should they be nailed? *Clin Orthop* 1995;315:64–74.

Thirty-two extra-articular fractures of the proximal third of the tibia were treated with locked intramedullary nails. Eighty-four percent had angulation of 5° or greater in the frontal or sagittal plane with 59% having displacement at the fracture site. Twenty-five percent incurred loss of fixation associated with the placement of a single proximal locking screw. The authors would limit the use of intramedullary nailing for proximal third tibial shaft fractures and would consider alternate forms of fixation.

Sarmiento A, Sharpe FE, Ebramzadeh E, Normand P, Shankwiler J: Factors influencing the outcome of closed tibial fractures treated with functional bracing. *Clin Orthop* 1995;315: 8–24.

One thousand consecutive closed diaphyseal tibial fractures were treated with prefabricated functional below knee braces. The high union rate and low morbidity associated with functional bracing of closed tibial fractures confirms that the final shortening does not increase beyond the initial shortening. Presence of an intact fibula is a relative contraindication for functional fracture bracing because angular deformity is more likely to develop.

Compartment Syndrome

McQueen MM, Court-Brown CM: Compartment monitoring in tibial fractures: The pressure threshold for decompression. *J Bone Joint Surg* 1996;78B:99–104.

In a prospective study, 116 patients with tibial shaft fractures were evaluated for compartment syndrome using Δp = diastolic pressure - compartment pressure. No cases of missed acute compartment syndrome occurred if the Δp of 30 mm Hg or higher was measured.

Classic Bibliography

Alho A, Benterud JG, Hogevold HE, Ekeland A, Stromsoe K: Comparison of functional bracing and locked intramedullary nailing in the treatment of displaced tibial shaft fractures. *Clin Orthop* 1992;277:243–250.

Bone LB, Johnson KD: Treatment of tibial fractures by reaming and intramedullary nailing. *J Bone Joint Surg* 1986;68A: 877–887.

Carpenter JE, Kasman R, Matthews LS: Fractures of the patella. *J Bone Joint Surg* 1993;75A:1550–1561.

Court-Brown CM, Christie J, McQueen MM: Closed intramedullary tibial nailing: Its use in closed and Type I open fractures. *J Bone Joint Surg* 1990;72B:605–611.

Cramer KE, Moed BR: Patellar fractures: Contemporary approach to treatment. *J Amer Acad Orthop Surg* 1997;5: 323–331.

Gustilo RB, Gruninger RP, Davis T: Classification of type III (severe) open fractures relative to treatment and results. *Orthopedics* 1987;10:1781–1788.

Helfet DL, Jupiter JB, Gasser S: Indirect reduction and tension-band plating of tibial nonunion with deformity. *J Bone Joint Surg* 1992;74A:1286–1297.

Johner R, Wruhs O: Classification of tibial shaft fractures and correlation with results after rigid internal fixation. *Clin Orthop* 1983;178:7–25.

Lottes JO: Medullary nailing of the tibia with the triflange nail. *Clin Orthop* 1974;105:53–66.

Marsh JL, Nepola JV, Wuest TK, Osteen D, Cox K, Oppenheim W: Unilateral external fixation until healing with the dynamic axial fixator for severe open tibial fractures. *J Orthop Trauma* 1991;5:341–348.

Moore TM, Patzakis MJ, Harvey JP: Tibial plateau fractures: Definition, demographics, treatment rationale, and long-term results of closed traction management or operative reduction. *J Orthop Trauma* 1987;1:97–119.

Mubarak SJ, Owen CA, Hargens AR, Garetto LP, Akeson WH: Acute compartment syndromes: Diagnosis and treatment with the aid of the wick catheter. *J Bone Joint Surg* 1978;60A: 1091–1095.

Oestern HJ, Tscherne H: Pathophysiology and classification of soft tissue injuries associated with fractures, in Tscherne H, Gotzen L (eds): *Fractures With Soft Tissue Injuries*. Berlin, Germany, Springer-Verlag, 1984, pp 1–9.

Paley D, Catagni MA, Argnani F, Villa A, Benedetti GB, Cattaneo R: Ilizarov treatment of tibial nonunions with bone loss. *Clin Orthop* 1989;241:146–165.

Rasmussen PS: Tibial condylar fractures: Impairment of knee joint stability as an indication for surgical treatment. *J Bone Joint Surg* 1973;55A:1331–1350.

Schatzker J, McBroom R, Bruce D: The tibial plateau fracture: The Toronto experience 1968-1975. *Clin Orthop* 1979;138: 94–104.

Weber MJ, Janecki CJ, McLeod P, Nelson CL, Thompson JA: Efficacy of various forms of fixation of transverse fractures of the patellar. *J Bone Joint Surg* 1980;62A:215–220.

Whittle AP, Russell TA, Taylor JC, Lavelle DG: Treatment of open fractures of the tibial shaft with the use of interlocking nailing without reaming. *J Bone Joint Surg* 1992;74A:1162–1171.

Wiss DA, Johnson DL, Miao M: Compression plating for nonunion after failed external fixation of open tibial fractures. *J Bone Joint Surg* 1992;74A:1279–1285.

Chapter 42
Knee and Leg: Soft-Tissue Trauma

Knee Ligament Injuries

Background

The incidence of knee ligament injuries in the United States has increased over the last 2 decades, possibly because of increased activity levels in the middle-aged population as well as increased participation at all levels in a variety of sports. Injuries to the anterior cruciate ligament (ACL) continue to generate major interest because of their frequency and the extent of the resulting disability. More than 200,000 new ACL injuries occur in the United States annually. Women have a higher risk of injury with similar exposure rates in basketball, soccer, and rugby. Although ACL injury can be caused by contact, it is more common in noncontact sports, with the plant-and-pivot or stop-and-jump mechanisms predominating.

Approximately 50% of patients with ACL tears also have meniscal tears. The lateral meniscus is torn more frequently than the medial meniscus in acute ACL injuries, but in chronic ACL tears the medial meniscus is more commonly involved. Several recent studies suggest that the classically described "unhappy triad" of torn ACL, torn medial collateral ligament (MCL), and torn medial meniscus is actually less common than the association of torn ACL, torn MCL, and torn lateral meniscus.

Because most ACL injuries occur in noncontact situations, some authors have suggested that the shoe-surface interface may contribute to the frequency of ACL tears. In a prospective study, ACL tears were approximately 3 times more frequent in high school football players who wore edge cleat designs than in athletes wearing the classic screw-in variety or soccer-style cleats.

MCL injury remains the most common isolated knee ligament injury, and it also is the injury most commonly associated with ACL injury. Fortunately, it does not require surgical treatment in most patients.

The posterior cruciate ligament (PCL) is a vertically oriented ligament that is approximately 1.5 times as strong as the ACL. It is the primary restraint to posterior translation of the knee and the secondary restraint to posterolateral rotation,

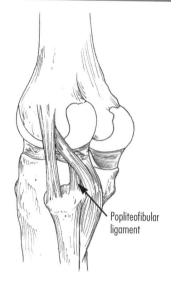

Popliteofibular ligament

Figure 1

Schematic of the posterolateral corner of the knee demonstrating the popliteofibular ligament arising from the fibular head and joining the popliteus tendon.

assists in the screw home mechanism, and is important in knee proprioception. Approximately 5% of all knee ligament injuries in a general population involve the PCL, but as many as 60% of knee ligament injuries treated in emergency rooms involve the PCL.

The posterolateral corner is a combination of structures that includes the iliotibial band (ITB), biceps femoris (long and short heads), fibular collateral ligament, popliteus complex (tendon, tibial attachment, popliteofibular ligament, lateral meniscal attachments), arcuate complex, fabellofibular ligament, middle third of the capsular ligament, and joint capsule. The popliteofibular ligament (Fig. 1) has been identified as an important contributor to posterolateral stability both in anatomic dissections and in resection studies. Injuries to the posterolateral structures most commonly occur with PCL injuries (approximately 60%), occasionally with ACL injuries, and rarely as isolated injuries.

History and Physical Examination

The history remains a key factor in diagnosing knee ligament injuries through identification of the mechanism involved. Most ACL injuries are associated with a hemarthrosis that

Table 1
Tests for specific knee ligament injuries

Injured Ligament*	Key Test	Secondary Test
ACL	Lachman	Pivot shift
MCL	Valgus laxity at 30°	
PCL	Posterior drawer at 90°	Posterior sag at 90°
LCL	Varus laxity at 30°	
Posterolateral corner	Posterolateral drawer at 30°	Posterolateral drawer at 90°

*ACL, anterior cruciate ligament; MCL, medial collateral ligament; PCL, posterior cruciate ligament; LCL, lateral collateral ligament

maximum manual side-to-side difference of 3 mm or more is diagnostic of an ACL tear. Table 1 shows the tests that are indicative of specific ligament injuries. Laxity is graded by the increased translation compared to the uninjured knee: grade 1, 1 to 5 mm; grade 2, 6 to 10 mm; grade 3, 10 to 15 mm; grade 4, > 15 mm.

The pivot shift phenomenon is diagnostic of ACL insufficiency and reflects the instability that results from ACL injury. There are a number of ways to elicit the pivot shift, which is an anterior subluxation of the tibia in extension with reduction in flexion. The position of the thigh and leg alters the degree of the pivot shift: adduction of the thigh or internal rotation of the leg tends to reduce the translation elicited. Although the anterior drawer test is of little value in the diagnosis of acute ACL injury, it is of more value in a chronic ACL-deficient knee. Performing the test with the leg in internal or external rotation gives additional information about the secondary stabilizers at the posterolateral or posteromedial corners. As with the Lachman test, the examiner must determine if increased anterior translation represents reduction of a posterior subluxated tibia. A proximal anterior tibial abrasion suggests PCL injury, as does asymmetric knee hyperextension. The resting position of the anterior tibial plateau relative to the femoral condyles during the drawer test indicates whether there is ACL or PCL laxity. A decrease of the normal anterior resting position of the tibial plateaus (posterior tibial sag) suggests that any increased sagittal plane laxity is from PCL injury.

Although partial tears of the ACL have been extensively described in the literature, their detection by physical examination is problematic. Several authors have suggested that a partial tear is present if the Lachman is 2+ or less with a firm end point and the pivot shift is no more than a glide. A recent cadaver study demonstrated an inability to identify by clinical examination the partially transected (anteromedial bundle) ACL.

The collateral ligaments are evaluated by determining varus and valgus laxity at 0 and 30° of flexion. Laxity in full extension implies complete collateral ligament tear, with injury to the secondary restraints, such as the ACL, PCL, and posteromedial or posterolateral corners. The evaluation of posterolateral laxity includes identification of asymmetric thigh-foot angles in external rotation, greater at 30° of flexion than at 90°, as well as the reverse pivot shift and external rotation recurvatum tests.

occurs within the first few hours after injury. An audible pop is noted by approximately half of the patients sustaining an ACL injury.

Mechanisms of PCL injury include a fall onto the ground with the foot plantarflexed (striking the tibial tubercle), a direct posterior blow to a flexed knee (such as a dashboard injury), hyperflexion, hyperextension, severe varus or valgus loads after failure of the collaterals, or knee dislocations. Injuries may be complicated by concurrent injuries of the MCL, ACL, or posterolateral complex. In some series, isolated PCL injuries account for only 3.5% of all PCL injuries, although this is probably low because an isolated PCL injury may go unrecognized. Whether the injury mechanism was low energy or high energy also affects the long-term prognosis and treatment recommendations. Hemarthrosis or popliteal ecchymosis may be apparent in an isolated PCL injury. Popping or tearing sensations are infrequently noted. PCL tears often are associated with femoral fractures from motor vehicle trauma (10% to 40% in various series of femoral fractures). Posterolateral complex injuries can result from a blow on the anteromedial tibia or an external rotation injury to the extended knee and usually occur in conjunction with partial or complete PCL tears.

The examination of the knee with acute ligament injury often is difficult within the first several hours, because swelling and pain cause guarding by the patient. Early examination is advantageous, and comparison to the uninjured knee is mandatory. In a patient with an acute hemarthrosis, the Lachman and varus-valgus tests often are the only tests that can be reliably performed. In an acute injury, any difference in translation or the feeling of a soft end point may indicate a ligament tear. Instrumented arthrometry testing can be a helpful adjunct in the diagnosis of an acute knee injury; a

Imaging

Routine radiographs are indicated in all patients with a traumatic hemarthrosis or chronic ligamentous deficiency. These should include as a minimum anteroposterior (AP) and lateral views to identify a tibial spine fracture or Segond fracture, an avulsion fracture from the lateral tibial margin, which is diagnostic of ACL injury. An avulsion fracture of the PCL tibial insertion may be noted on the lateral radiograph, and if this fragment is displaced more than 5 mm, primary repair and fixation are indicated. Posterior tibial subluxation may occur with PCL injury. Tunnel and sunrise views will help to identify osteochondral injuries and the patellofemoral compartment degeneration that develops in 5% to 8% of patients with chronic PCL injuries. In long-standing ligamentous insufficiency, posteroanterior (PA) weightbearing views in 45° of flexion are indicated to identify the joint space narrowing of posttraumatic arthrosis. Standing views from hip to ankle on a long cassette are recommended in patients suspected of having an abnormal alignment. Patients with chronic PCL injuries and posterolateral corner injuries may have a varus thrust and alignment should be further quantitated with a long cassette radiograph.

Magnetic resonance imaging (MRI) can be helpful when the clinical examination is limited because of pain and swelling and to identify associated injuries to the menisci and articular cartilage. Although the sensitivity of MRI in identifying ACL injury may be high (90% to 98%), its specificity, particularly in differentiating partial from complete tears, is low (less than 50% in some series). The overall accuracy of MRI in determining acute ACL injury (< 24 hours) is approximately 90%, below that of clinical examination. MRI can, however, identify bone bruising, which occurs in more than 90% of acute ACL tears and may predict deterioration of the articular surfaces and a possible risk of delamination of the cartilage from underlying bone. Although MRI is extremely sensitive for determining PCL injury, the diagnosis should be established by history and physical examination. In one study, 77% of complete PCL ruptures appeared on MRI to be in continuity at 4 months after injury, but increased posterior laxity was found by clinical examination.

Anterior Cruciate Ligament Injuries

The treatment of ACL injuries should be tailored to the individual patient. Factors to be considered in determining treatment include activity level, amount of time involved with high demand activities, willingness of the patient to modify these activities, laxity of the joint, and presence of associated ligament, articular cartilage, or meniscal injuries. Activity levels should be classified according to the International Knee Documentation Committee evaluation form, which has 4 levels: level I, jumping, pivoting, or hard cutting (eg, football, soccer); level II, heavy manual work or side-to-side sports (eg, skiing, tennis); level III, light manual work or noncutting sports (eg, jogging, running); and level IV, sedentary activity without sports.

The natural history of the ACL-deficient knee often includes repetitive buckling episodes with level I or II activities, although some patients with significant laxity do not have functional instability. Patients who frequently participate in level I or II activities and have concomitant ligament or meniscal pathology fare less well. The status of the menisci is a key determinant of long-term function in the ACL-injured knee. Meniscectomy, even partial, leads to decreased function with increased risk of degenerative changes. Because meniscal injury with ACL deficiency is in large part related to buckling episodes, treatment is directed toward eliminating functional instability.

Nonsurgical Treatment Nonsurgical treatment generally is recommended for patients limited to level III and IV activities, and may be considered for patients with limited participation in level I or II activities who are willing to modify their activities. Although some patients with significant ACL laxity are able to participate in level I activities without instability, there is at present no reliable means to identify these patients. The risk of meniscal injury from instability does not justify a trial of nonsurgical treatment or a delay in surgery until the end of a season in a high-demand athlete.

Initial nonsurgical treatment is directed at regaining range of motion and decreasing posttraumatic capsular swelling and effusion. Regaining strength and proprioceptive skills follows. Scarring of the tibial stump to the lateral wall or roof of the intercondylar notch may reduce long-term laxity. To this end, early open chain quadriceps exercises should be avoided, with reliance on closed kinetic chain strengthening, which is less likely to stretch any scar. Although some studies have suggested that preferentially strengthening the hamstrings reduces symptoms of instability, quadriceps strengthening should not be ignored. Gastrocnemius strength also is important in maintaining a more normal gait pattern after ACL injury.

The use of functional braces often is part of a nonsurgical program for ACL insufficiency; approximately two thirds of patients feel more stable, but a substantial number of knees buckle in the brace. In carefully controlled studies, functional braces helped to limit anterior translation of the tibia in ACL-deficient knees at low loads (far below loads placed on the knee in sport). Unfortunately, most braces slow voluntary reaction times of the hamstring muscles, which are important dynamic stabilizers of the joint.

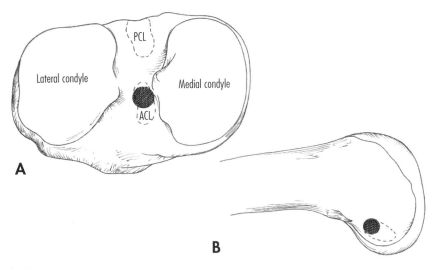

Figure 2

Schematic of tibial (A) and femoral (B) drill hole positions (shaded areas) in relation to the anterior cruciate ligament footprints (dashed lines). Note that the tunnels are still made within the anatomic insertions.

After an ACL injury, loss of nerve endings in the remaining stumps diminishes proprioception. Proprioceptive reeducation using balance boards or similar devices may be of benefit in a nonsurgical program.

Surgical Treatment With steady advances in arthroscopically assisted ACL reconstruction techniques and rehabilitation protocols, outcomes of ACL reconstruction have improved substantially since the 1980s. Current minimally invasive techniques of reconstruction emphasize the anatomic placement of high-strength ligament grafts using rigid fixation techniques. Delaying reconstruction until full extension has been achieved reduces the risk of arthrofibrosis and hastens the recovery of function after surgery.

Many systems are available for the accurate placement of guide pins in the tibia and femur. Identification of possible notch impingement with placement of a graft in the anterior half of the ACL tibial footprint, accentuated in a knee with hyperextension, has lead many to recommend tibial graft placement in the posterior two thirds of the tibial footprint (Fig. 2, *A*). There is consensus that the femoral drill hole should be placed in the 11 o'clock position in right knees and the 1 o'clock position in left knees. Placement of the femoral guide pin in a suitably posterior position (Fig. 2, *B*) is easier with the use of a drill guide that keys off the over-the-top position. Although the concept of isometry was popular in the 1980s, it has largely been supplanted by anatomic positioning. The use of an isometer demonstrating 3 mm or less of translation through a full range of motion can be helpful

for less experienced surgeons; however, its routine use by experienced ACL surgeons is not necessary. If the arthroscopic placement of the guide wire on the tibia or femur is uncertain, an intraoperative lateral radiograph should be obtained to confirm the pin placement before drilling. The use of acorn type drills to make the tibial hole may result in an entry site into the joint that is more anterior than guide pin placement. This is caused by an asymmetric breakthrough into the joint and can be avoided by using a uniform diameter fluted drill for the tibial hole.

Endoscopic techniques (femoral drill hole reamed transarticularly) have proven to produce stability equal to 2-incision techniques while reducing short-term morbidity of ACL reconstruction. As with any technically demanding procedure, there is a learning curve associated with the switch to the endoscopic techniques. The use of a tourniquet is not necessary for ACL reconstruction; surgical times and final stability results are the same with or without a tourniquet. The preoperative intra-articular injection of dilute epinephrine solution (1:100,000 to 1:200,000) or the use of a pump reduces the need for routine tourniquet use. If used, the tourniquet should be deflated after 2 hours.

Graft Selection Bone-patellar tendon-bone (B-PT-B) graft, with the most long-term results because of its popularity in the 1980s and early 1990s, is the benchmark to which other graft materials are compared. Quadrupled hamstring tendon (4-HT) is another graft with wide popularity and an increasing body of literature supporting its use. The 4-HT technique is quite different from the double hamstring techniques that were used in the 1980s with unacceptably high failure rates.

A 10-mm wide graft from the central third of the patellar tendon has an initial strength more than 150% that of the ACL. If the graft is to be rigidly fixed at both ends with a technique that allows rotation of the graft (eg, interference screws), rotation of the graft 90° or more increases its strength approximately 20%. Although there is debate as to the more appropriate direction of rotation of the graft, external rotation seems to best reproduce the normal anatomy of the ACL.

Interference screw fixation with titanium screws is the most popular technique for fixation of B-PT-B grafts. Divergence of the screw (particularly on the femoral side) from the direction of the tunnel reduces the strength of fixation. The strength of the initial graft fixation depends on the size of the gaps between the bone blocks and the tunnels, as well as the diameter of screw used. When the gap between the bone plug and the tunnel is 2 mm or less, fixation is just as good with a 7- or 9-mm screw, and the smaller screw should be used because it reduces the chance of splitting the block. As the gap size increases to 4 mm, 9-mm screws are used; laboratory testing found 60% better holding power with the larger screw when the gap was 4 mm. Biodegradable screws made from polylactide (PLA) have been suggested as an alternative to metal screws and have the same initial fixation strength as metal screws. Animal studies indicate that the screw is not replaced by bone, but rather by fibrous tissue. Intra-articular use of PLA may lead to sporadic aseptic synovitis, probably mediated by activation of the complement system.

Pretensioning the graft before implantation, or cycling under tension before fixation of the tibial end, increases the initial tension in the graft and decreases laxity of the joint. The tensioning technique probably is the least well understood facet of ACL reconstruction. Applying large initial tension to the graft and then fixing it with the knee extended to 0° has reliably obtained stable knees with little loss of motion.

The use of 4-HT grafts, most commonly double-looped semitendinosus and gracilis tendons, is increasing in popularity because studies have shown that stability with this technique is similar to that of B-PT-B grafts and significantly better than that of double thickness hamstring grafts. The 4-HT grafts have been reported to be 1.5 to 2 times as strong as the ACL. Several techniques give strong initial fixation; these include looped polyester tape with button, blunt threaded interference screw, and double screw and washer. Keeping fixation points closer to the joint decreases the overall graft length and potential for creep and may improve the long-term laxity with 4-HT grafts. Several authors have cautioned against using interference screws without additional fixation for the tibial side in 4-HT grafts. Postoperative expansion of the tibial drill hole has been reported with all graft materials, but appears to be more common with hamstring techniques.

Because of the variety of fixation techniques, the recommended forces applied while tensioning the 4-HT graft vary widely. In 1 study, mean laxity at 2-year follow-up was significantly reduced by increased initial graft tension at 30° (mean laxity = 0.6 ± 1.7 mm at 80 N versus mean laxity = 2.2 ± 2.4 mm at 20 N). Overtensioning can be prevented by assuring that full passive extension is possible after fixing the graft.

Postoperative Treatment Delaying surgery until full knee extension is possible and obtaining full extension after surgery with early range of motion have reduced the frequency of stiffness after ACL reconstruction to less than 3%.

Several studies revealed no benefit from the use of continuous passive motion after reconstruction. Cryotherapy devices do not have lasting effects, but do reduce early swelling and pain, as well as having high patient acceptance. Most uncomplicated ACL reconstructions can be done on an outpatient or short-stay (< 24 hour) basis.

Early rehabilitation programs should protect the graft from excessive strain because of transient weakness before revascularization and healing. Weightbearing with protection (drop lock brace and/or crutches) for the first 3 to 4 weeks after surgery often is recommended. Fixation is the weak link for the first 2 weeks with patellar tendon grafts and for up to 8 weeks with hamstring grafts. Therefore, during the initial rehabilitation, most surgeons recommend a more cautious and less aggressive therapy program. Closed kinetic chain strengthening exercises decrease strain on the graft from joint compression and simultaneous hamstring contraction, when compared to open chain quadriceps exercises. A randomized, controlled study showed decreased laxity, decreased anterior knee pain, and a more rapid return to function when closed kinetic chain exercises were used. Several studies have confirmed that early return to athletics (often by 4 to 6 months) can occur with no increased risk of failure, if return is based on recovery of quadriceps muscle strength (> 50% for jogging, > 65% for sports-specific agility training, > 80% for full athletics). Self-directed rehabilitation programs with limited physical therapy visits are successful and cost-effective for most patients with ACL reconstructions, but patients who need a more rapid recovery or have a complication may require more frequent visits over a longer time. Functional braces may decrease the strain on the graft, but inhibit the protective effect of hamstring contraction.

Proprioceptive reeducation and sports-specific training should be the final phase of rehabilitation. The mature ACL graft is enervated with mechanoreceptors. Animal studies have shown reenervation of ACL grafts by 6 months. The timing of reenervation probably is similar to the limited revascularization of the grafts.

Results of ACL Surgery Results should be quantitated not only by measurable laxity (pivot-shift, Lachman, and instrumented laxity testing) but also by functional status and activity level. Objectively stable knees often are defined as those with a pivot-shift ≤ 1+ and instrumented laxity ≤ 3 mm. Stable knees are reported in 88% to 95% of patients with ACL reconstructions at midterm (3- to 5-year) follow-up. There is a slow but steady increase in failures with time. Subjective success, defined as full return to preinjury activity levels without significant symptoms, is reported to occur 80% to 92% at midterm follow-up. Function is adversely affected by meniscal resection or articular surface damage. Because of increased healing rates of meniscal repairs performed with ACL reconstruction, the zone of meniscal preservation/repair should be extended.

Objectively stable knees can be obtained in 90% to 95% knee reconstructions with B-PT-B autografts, and approximately 85% of patients return to previous levels of activity with this graft. However, 10% to 40% of patients report long-standing anterior knee pain of varying degrees. Permanent quadriceps strength deficits of nearly 10% are usual after B-PT-B grafting, and kneeling may be uncomfortable. Patellar fractures have been reported to occur in approximately 2% of patients with this graft, but patellar tendon rupture is rare.

Donor site morbidity is less with 4-HT grafts than with B-PT-B grafts. Hamstring strength deficits usually are 10% or less, and anterior knee pain is substantially reduced (from 30% to 6% in 1 study). Anterior knee pain after reconstruction with 4-HT grafts probably is caused by fat pad scarring.

Although several randomized, controlled studies have compared 4-HT to B-PT-B grafts, all have been too small to reveal significant differences in most measures of outcome, with the exception that females have greater postoperative laxity with 4-HT grafts than with B-PT-B grafts. Combining data from different studies (meta-analysis) reveals that B-PT-B techniques yield a significantly higher percentage of stable knees with a higher rate of return to preinjury sports, while 4-HT grafts lead to a faster recovery with significantly less long-term anterior knee pain.

Alternative Graft Sources Synthetic materials (Dacron, Gortex, carbon fiber) were used briefly as ACL prostheses during the 1980s and early 1990s. Their use has been abandoned because of high time-related failure rates (> 40% at 4- to 6-year follow-up). A polypropylene ligament augmentation device (LAD) remains available. Although it can improve the success rate of the biomechanically inferior quadriceps-patella tendon graft to almost equal that of B-PT-B grafts, several studies comparing the use of the LAD with high strength grafts have shown no significant benefit in its use.

A number of allograft tissues (including B-PT-B, Achilles tendon, fascia lata, and hamstring tendons) are available. They can be processed in a number of ways, including fresh freezing, irradiation, and freeze drying. Irradiation at doses > 1 Mrad causes biomechanical alterations of the tissue, but doses > 3 Mrad are needed to eliminate viruses from the tissue. The current risk of transmission of the human immunodeficiency virus (HIV) by ligament allograft tissues screened by all available techniques, including polymerized

chain reaction (PCR), is estimated to be less than 1 in 1,000,000. Transmission of any of the hepatitis viruses is also possible, and donor tissue is routinely screened for hepatitis B and C. Freeze dried grafts have been demonstrated to have limited shelf life, with increasing risk of failure as the duration between harvest and implantation increases. Deep freezing of allograft tissues reduces their antigenicity by altering the major histocompatibility antigens. Fewer than 50% of patients implanted with deep frozen grafts have any signs of immune recognition of the graft.

Results of ACL reconstruction with allograft tissues are similar to those with autografts. Currently most surgeons use allografts for revision ACL surgery, for ACL reconstruction in older patients (particularly those with significant degenerative changes) and those with potentially weakened autografts (eg, chronic patellar tendinitis or partial or complete patellar tendon ruptures), and for multiple ligament injuries.

Alternative autograft donor sites have been used, and there is significant current interest in the central quadriceps tendon with patellar bone. It has been suggested as an alternative graft source for revision and primary ACL reconstruction because of its low donor site morbidity. Graft harvest is technically demanding, and no long-term prospective studies have evaluated outcomes with this technique. Table 2 summarizes the advantages and disadvantages of the more commonly used grafts.

Failed ACL Reconstruction Failure can be divided into 3 categories: arthrofibrosis or loss of motion, pain that limits function and is caused by arthrosis or extensor mechanism dysfunction, and recurrent patholaxity. The common causes of failure of ACL surgery are: (1) surgical technique, with malpositioned tunnels, misplaced fixation devices, or inadequate notchplasty; (2) lack of graft incorporation because of avascularity, rejection, or stress shielding; and (3) trauma from reinjury or overaggressive rehabilitation. Failure also can be caused by lack of appropriate treatment of associated laxities or inappropriate graft choice. The most common cause of graft failure is malpositioning of the drill holes, more commonly the femoral drill hole. Anterior placement of the femoral drill hole (more than 40% forward on Blumensaat's line on the lateral radiograph) leads to a significantly greater risk of failure. Anterior placement of the tibial drill hole also increases the risk of failure because of notch impingement. Malposition of either drill hole can cause arthrofibrosis or graft rupture.

Arthrofibrosis is more difficult to treat than graft rupture, because of secondary contracture of other structures in the joint and potential articular surface damage to the patello-

Table 2
Various graft sources

Tissue Source	Major Advantages	Major Disadvantages
Autologous B-PT-B*		
Ipsilateral	High strength	Anterior knee pain
	Rigid fixation	Patellar fracture
	Long track record	
	More aggressive initial rehabilitation	
Contralateral	Available for revisions	Injury to other knee
Quadrupled hamstring tendons (4-HT)	High strength	Lower static stability
	Low donor site morbidity	Slower initial rehabilitation
	Reduced anterior pain	Shorter follow-up
Central quadriceps tendon (CQT)	Potentially less pain	No long-term data
	Available for revisions	Difficult harvest
Allograft tendons	No donor site morbidity	Delayed incorporation
	Suitable for multiple ligaments	Slightly lower success
		Infectious disease transmission

*Bone-patellar tendon-bone

femoral joint. Although the cause of arthrofibrosis often is technical, abnormal expression of multiple growth factors may ensue, increasing scarring.

Revision surgery for recurrent laxity requires careful technical planning in several areas: placement of skin incisions, removal of fixation devices, notchplasty revision, location and size of previous tunnels, graft selection, graft fixation, and rehabilitation. A 2-stage procedure may be necessary to bone graft expanded tunnels before revision ACL reconstruction.

Medial Collateral Ligament Injuries

Nonsurgical treatment of all degrees of isolated MCL injury is well established. Grade 1 injuries (1 to 5 mm opening in 30° of flexion) can be treated symptomatically, often requiring only crutches for a week or 2. Patients with grade 2 MCL injuries (6 to 10 mm opening) are best treated with crutches and a hinged brace for 2 to 3 weeks. Grade 3 injuries (11 to 15 mm opening) are treated with a hinged brace for 3 to 4 weeks. Early quadriceps and hamstring strengthening should be encouraged, and return to athletics should be delayed until strength and endurance have been recovered. Functional braces were shown to support the injured MCL in laboratory studies, but there are no clinical studies to support their use. A protracted period of weakness may accompany healing of the MCL, because animal data indicate it takes 6 weeks for an MCL with a partial tear to return to full strength. A functional brace may be necessary in an athlete with an MCL injury who returns early to competition.

For MCL tears with associated posterior capsule injuries, both surgical and nonsurgical treatment has been recommended. Surgical treatment for proximal injuries to the MCL carries a higher risk of stiffness, and nonsurgical treatment is recommended for these injuries.

Posterior Cruciate Ligament Injuries

Instability is a less frequent complaint after isolated PCL injuries than after isolated ACL injuries; isolated PCL injuries are more frequently associated with pain than with instability. Over time (10 to 20 years) medial and patellofemoral compartment arthritis occurs in patients with PCL-deficient knees. In addition, cadaver studies have shown that isolated tears of the PCL resulted in increased contact pressures in the medial and patellofemoral compartments.

The nonsurgical treatment of PCL injuries should focus on quadriceps rehabilitation. There is no evidence to support the use of functional bracing for isolated PCL laxity. Several authors have reported little functional disability and low risk of degeneration with nonsurgical treatment despite static laxity. In 1 study of arthroscopically confirmed PCL injuries, 14 of 15 patients treated without surgery continued to function at a high level without pain 4 years after injury. Other studies have noted higher degrees of disability with nonsurgical treatment. Serial technetium bone scanning has been recommended in nonsurgically treated patients to identify early articular surface degeneration as a possible indication for reconstruction.

True isolated PCL injuries generally do not require surgery, because there usually is only a partial tear of the PCL with no associated injury to any other structure, especially the posterolateral corner. Combined injuries, however, may result in residual instability and disability after nonsurgical treatment. Most knee surgeons recommend reconstruction or repair of the PCL and associated ligament injuries, preferably within the first 2 weeks. The most common injury associated with a PCL injury is to the posterolateral corner (60% of patients with PCL injuries have posterolateral corner injuries). A patient with these injuries will have a 3+ posterior drawer test (> 10 mm posterior subluxation) and a positive increase in external tibial rotation at 30° and 90° of flexion. Because a 1+ posterior drawer often persists after reconstruction, and it is unusual to restore the posterior drawer test to normal, surgical treatment usually is considered only for higher-grade lesions (grade III). Twenty percent of athletes with PCL-deficient knees eventually require reconstruction.

For surgical reconstruction of the PCL, there is increasing consensus regarding graft placement, the position of the knee when securing the graft, and the methods of fixation. Recent studies have shown that the PCL consists of 2 distinct components that are not isometric. The larger and biomechanically stronger anterolateral component is taut in flexion and should be the focus of PCL reconstructive procedures (Fig. 3). Graft selection includes all of the grafts used for ACL reconstruction. Achilles tendon allograft offers the advantage of a large soft-tissue graft with excellent biomechanical properties that can be easily passed through the bony tunnels. The patellar tendon autograft has the problems of added morbidity due to the harvest and a more difficult graft passage. In addition, it does not provide as much collagen tissue as the Achilles tendon. Quadriceps tendon autograft is attractive but currently is not used by most surgeons in the United States. There is an increasing interest in using a 2-bundle technique for reconstruction of the PCL, but there have been very few basic science studies and only a few surgeons are currently using this technique. Postoperative rehabilitation protocols after PCL reconstruction are much less aggressive than those after ACL reconstruction. This difference results from the concomitant surgery to other structures (especially the posterolateral corner) and the need to protect the PCL graft from posterior tibial subluxation until biologic healing occurs (approximately 6 to 8 weeks).

Posterolateral Complex Injuries

Injuries to the posterolateral complex can involve all or various combinations of the popliteus tendon and its attachments, the arcuate ligament, and the lateral collateral ligament (LCL). These infrequent injuries are associated most commonly with PCL injuries and knee dislocations (ACL and PCL), and rarely with ACL injuries. Patients with posterolateral injury may complain of knee instability, especially when descending inclines. Injury to the peroneal nerve occurs in 10% or more of posterolateral corner disruptions. Biomechanical studies show that cutting of the posterolateral structures leads to increased external tibial rotation, increased varus rotation, and increased posterior tibial translation. Biomechanically, loss of lateral and posterolateral soft-tissue restraints results in increased tensile forces on the lateral side of the knee and increased compressive forces on the medial side. Data from gait analysis studies indicate that patients with posterolateral complex injuries in association with varus aligned knees and ACL deficiencies have increased adduction movements within the medial compartment. These movements may result in accelerated wear of the medial compartment or increased articular surface injury to the lateral compartment because of the excessive spin.

Direct primary repair is recommended for acute posterolateral complex injuries. In addition, any bony avulsion, such as of

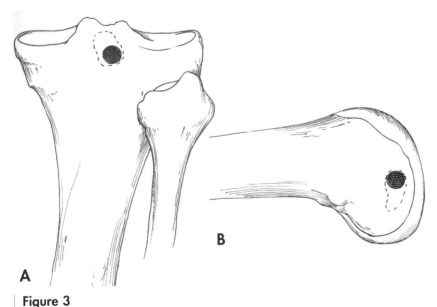

Figure 3

Schematic of tibial (A) and femoral (B) drill hole positions (shaded areas) in relation to the posterior cruciate ligament (PCL) footprints (dashed lines) that most accurately reproduce the insertion of the anterolateral component of the PCL.

the fibular head, should be repaired. Because of the complex anatomy of this area, primary repair can be done only within a few weeks of injury. Careful exposure and repair of all injured structures through a lateral approach is recommended. The surgeon should be prepared for reconstruction if primary repairs are not possible. Reconstructive surgery is required for chronic injuries. Traditional procedures, such as biceps tenodesis and arcuate ligament advancement, have mixed results. More anatomic procedures, such as popliteal ligament reconstruction with or without LCL reconstruction with autograft or allograft, are being done, but results of these procedures are still pending. For a chronic posterolateral complex injury with varus malalignment (varus thrust), a high tibial osteotomy (HTO) is indicated before posterolateral corner surgery. Often the HTO alone eliminates the need for reconstruction of the posterolateral structures.

Few reports are available on the results of posterolateral repairs or reconstructions. One recent study reports a 64% success rate for restoration of posterolateral stability with arcuate complex bony recession, whereas another study by the same author reports a 78% success rate using Achilles tendon allograft for a loop reconstruction of the LCL.

Combined Injuries

MCL tears in conjunction with ACL tears are common. Partial tears of the MCL can be ignored if ACL reconstruction is performed after full knee motion is regained. With complete tears of both ligaments, surgery usually is indicated to maintain functional stability. Opinions about the treatment remain divided. Most authors favor ACL reconstruction after a period of protection in a hinged brace to promote healing of the MCL and regain motion. However, in some patients with both ACL and MCL injuries, the MCL does not completely heal and residual laxity persists. Therefore, for grade III tears of the MCL with opening in full extension, some experienced surgeons recommend early repair of the MCL combined with ACL reconstruction. Because this increases the risk of postoperative stiffness, special precautions (early range of motion and keeping the brace locked in full extension) must be taken.

Grade III MCL tears associated with complete PCL disruptions are likely to result in a grossly unstable knee with little chance for healing of the MCL; therefore, most surgeons favor early repair (within the first 2 weeks) of the MCL in conjunction with PCL reconstruction. Brace treatment for 4 to 6 weeks, followed by arthroscopic PCL reconstruction, may yield similar results if the tibia remains reduced in the brace.

Knee Dislocations

Dislocation of the tibiofemoral joint often causes extensive disruption of the ligamentous structures and may injure tendon and neurovascular structures. Dislocations are classified by the position of the tibia: anterior, posterior, medial, lateral, or rotatory. The pattern of ligamentous injury with knee dislocations is variable and cannot be accurately predicted from the direction of dislocation.

Vascular injury is a potential catastrophic complication of knee dislocation, and careful assessment of distal perfusion before and after reduction of the joint is mandatory. The risk of vascular injury appears to be less when the dislocation is relatively low energy (except with hyperextension), as might be encountered on the athletic field (5% to 50% in various series), than with high-energy trauma (20% to 50%). Arteriography is mandatory if there is any diminution of distal perfusion before or after reduction and should be considered in all high-energy dislocations, because of the potential for subintimal tears that may later occlude the vessel. Early revascularization is crucial, because delay of more than 6 hours increases the risk of compartment syndrome and amputation. Four-compartment fasciotomies should be done to minimize the consequences of reperfusion edema in all patients who undergo vascular repair. Major ligamentous repair or reconstruction probably should not be done at the time of vascular repair, although minimal stabilization or temporary external fixation may be necessary to protect the vascular repair in grossly unstable joints. Any patient who has complete tears of the ACL and PCL should be presumed to have sustained a dislocation with spontaneous reduction and with a high risk of vascular injury.

Peroneal nerve injury is the most common major neurologic problem associated with knee dislocation, and some degree of dysfunction (from sensory deficit to complete disruption) occurs in up to 50% of patients. Complete injury is associated with a poor prognosis for recovery. With joints that are grossly unstable on the lateral side, peroneal nerve injury may result from manipulation required to treat vascular injuries or associated fractures. In one series, 25% of patients with knee dislocations had peroneal nerve injuries that occurred during repair of other structures.

Ligament injuries resulting from knee dislocation are more commonly avulsions from bone or with a bone fragment than occur with lesser trauma. In a recent series, one third of all disrupted ligaments had been avulsed and only two thirds had midsubstance tears. Tendon avulsions also are common, including avulsions of the biceps, patellar, popliteus, and pes anserinus tendons.

Current indications for immediate surgery include vascular injury and irreducible or open dislocations. Entrapment of the MCL within the joint may prevent reduction or block motion after reduction. Dimpling of the overlying skin suggests MCL entrapment.

There is no consensus on the treatment of knee dislocations because of their low frequency and the wide spectrum of associated ligament and other soft-tissue injuries. Most authors believe that non-surgical treatment should be reserved for older or inactive patients, because of the high rates of residual laxity. Early surgery with repair of the collateral and capsular ligaments and reconstruction of the cruciates has been advocated, but even with early motion postoperatively, up to two thirds of patients have difficulty regaining full motion. If the ACL or PCL is avulsed, the ligament should be repaired and augmented. Surgical treatment can be delayed without compromising stability if appropriate care is given for injuries to the MCL (brace for 6 weeks, then combined ACL and PCL reconstruction) or posterolateral structures (brace for 2 weeks, then combined ACL and PCL reconstruction with posterolateral repair and augmentation).

Various tissues (autograft and allograft) have been used successfully for these combined reconstructions. Because of the number of grafts required and the frequency of associated injuries, reconstruction with allograft tissues is an attractive alternative.

Meniscal Injuries

Meniscal injuries are among the most commonly reported knee problems. The mechanism usually involves a twisting maneuver on a weightbearing knee. Patients frequently complain of joint line pain, swelling, and occasionally of "clicking" or even locking of the knee. The diagnosis can be made through a careful history and physical examination in 90% of patients. PA 45° flexion (weightbearing), lateral, and Merchant radiographs should be obtained. When questions remain, MRI of the knee has been shown to be an accurate method of confirming the diagnosis. Medial meniscal tears are more common in stable knees; however, when associated with an acute ACL tear, lateral tears are more prevalent. The incidence of medial meniscal tears in ACL-deficient knees increases with time.

History has shown that total meniscectomy results in an increased risk of progressive gonarthrosis. Recent treatment of meniscal tears has emphasized preserving as much of the normal meniscus as possible. Treatment options include meniscal repair and partial meniscectomy; in some tears, no treatment is required.

Certain meniscal tears are appropriate for repair. Tears repaired concurrently with ACL reconstruction heal more predictably than those in unstable knees. Vertical longitudinal tears within 3 mm of the peripheral edge of the meniscus are likely to heal, whereas tears longer than 4 cm have a higher chance of failure. Patient age, age of tear, patient gender, and medial versus lateral location are not good predictors of healing potential.

Meniscal repairs can be done with arthroscopic or open technique. Open repairs are limited to tears at the meniscocapsular junction. Techniques for arthroscopic repair include inside-out, outside-in, and all-inside. Vertically oriented sutures have significantly higher strength to failure than those placed in a horizontal plane (Fig. 4). In addition, it appears that tears repaired with permanent rather than absorbable sutures heal better. A fibrin clot sutured into the repair site also has been reported to improve healing. Newer implants, such as T-shaped soft-tissue suture anchors and

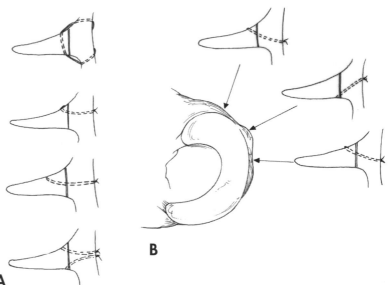

Figure 4

A, Diagram demonstrating suture placement patterns for meniscal repair. Note that the vertical and centrally placed horizontal sutures will reapproximate the tear surfaces, whereas a suture placed off-center superiorly or inferiorly may inadequately close the tear. B, Diagram illustrating "stacking" or horizontal mattress sutures on the superior and inferior surfaces of the meniscus. (Reproduced with permission from Cooper DE: Arthroscopic meniscal repair: "Outside-in" technique. *Oper Tech Sports Med* 1994;2:190–200.)

absorbable meniscal darts or arrows, make the all-inside technique easier. Although initial holding strength appears to equal that obtained by horizontal suturing techniques, no long-term outcome studies have been reported, and implant breakage, failure, and migration are potential complications unique to these devices. Other reported complications after meniscal repair include entrapment or damage to the peroneal nerve with lateral meniscal repairs, and entrapment of the saphenous nerve with medial repairs. If a nerve injury is suspected after repair and no recovery occurs within 24 hours, surgical exploration should be strongly considered.

The use of meniscal allograft tissue to reconstruct the meniscus has elicited a great deal of interest within the last several years. Indications for meniscal allograft transplantation are currently being defined, but the best surgical candidate appears to be a young symptomatic individual, who has had previous arthroscopic meniscectomy, articular cartilage changes of grade II or less, and normal physiologic lower extremity alignment on long (hip to ankle) standing radiographs. The lack of uniformity in patient selection, surgical technique, and follow-up criteria have made the clinical results of allograft meniscal transplantation difficult to interpret. Only frozen allograft or cryopreserved allograft tissues have shown promising results at early follow-up. It appears that soft-tissue techniques for anchoring the meniscal horns do not adequately secure the graft during weightbearing, and results are inferior to those achieved with bone plug or bone bridge attachment of the meniscal horns.

Basic science animal studies and clinical studies have contributed to the identification of several concerns relating to meniscal allograft transplantation. Although it is clear that the meniscal allograft heals to peripheral tissue, biopsy specimens have revealed persistent changes within the cellular make-up, cellular content, and collagen architecture, thereby raising questions about the long-term viability and the predisposition for further injury in these menisci. Currently, there are only 2 objective ways of evaluating clinical results of meniscal transplantation: MRI and arthroscopy. Both have been shown to be accurate for determining the anatomic location of the meniscus, but neither technique can evaluate the effectiveness of the transplanted meniscus as a load-bearing structure.

For those tears judged to be unreparable, partial meniscectomy reliably reduces or eliminates symptoms, but still results in an increased risk of late arthrosis. This is especially true when the lateral meniscus is removed, articular surface damage is already present, or malalignment results in overload of the involved compartment. It is important to remove only the offending portion of the structure, preserving as much of the meniscus as possible. An attempt should be made to achieve a smooth transition between the torn remnant and the normal portions of the meniscal body. Some meniscal tears can be treated without repair or excision. If found arthroscopically, surgical adjuncts such as trephination or synovial abrasion may encourage the healing of stable tears.

Rehabilitation after meniscal repair is controversial. Good results have been reported with aggressive rehabilitation in patients who have simultaneous ACL reconstruction and meniscal repair. Recent studies suggest that accelerated rehabilitation, including full weightbearing, early motion, and return to sports within 2 to 3 months, has no negative effect on healing rates.

Second look arthroscopy in short-term follow-up studies has shown that many patients who have clinically healed menisci may actually have only partially healed menisci. The re-tear rate and long-term function of such incompletely healed menisci remains to be determined.

A recent study compared radiographic findings in matched groups of patients who had arthroscopic partial meniscectomy or open meniscal repair. At 7 years, significantly more arthrosis was seen in the meniscectomy group. However, when the same patients were reexamined at 13 years there was no significant difference in the radiographic changes between the 2 groups. This finding suggests that further investigation into the treatment of meniscal injuries is indicated.

Knee Braces

Background
The use of braces for the knee is controversial. Although they usually are well accepted by patients, there is little biomechanical evidence that supports their use. Braces can be classified as functional, rehabilitative, or prophylactic.

Functional Braces
Functional braces are designed to improve function in an abnormal knee. This group can be subclassified into derotational, patellofemoral, and unloading types of braces. Derotational braces are used in cruciate deficient knees to reduce recurrent giving way episodes. Current literature suggests that they may increase stability under low-loading conditions, and most subjective studies indicate that patients feel a marked improvement in knee stability. Braces appear to be ineffective in resisting higher loads and may have detrimental effects on neuromuscular performance.

Patellofemoral braces can be used to decrease symptoms in individuals with patellofemoral pain or in an attempt to eliminate patellar subluxation. Biomechanical studies show no effect on knee function, but patients again report a significant perception of increased patellar stability. Several recent studies have questioned the value of bracing in the treatment of patellofemoral pain.

Unloading braces are used to decrease arthritic pain in patients with unicompartmental degenerative arthritis of the knee. One study reported improvement in pain and function in patients with moderate to severe medial compartment osteoarthritis.

Rehabilitative Braces

Rehabilitative braces are used in the immediate postinjury or postoperative period to allow protected range of motion. Many surgeons use a range of motion type of brace initially and then change to a functional brace during rehabilitation of patients with ACL reconstructions. Braces also are frequently used after meniscal repair and to protect healing collateral ligament injuries. There is no clinical or biomechanical proof of efficacy for brace use in the injured or surgically repaired knee.

Prophylactic Braces

Conflicting results have been reported in the use of prophylactic braces for prevention of injury during contact sports. Biomechanical studies demonstrated that a brace cannot prevent transmission of heavy translational or torsional loads to the ACL, but these studies were done on cadaver knees or on intact knees at rest. A more recent article suggested that in a weightbearing knee with an intact ACL, braces may offer more protection to the ligaments. Although 1 clinical trial found that players wearing prophylactic single upright braces had an increased incidence of knee injury, others showed that there is a trend toward protection against all knee injuries and a statistically significant reduction in MCL injuries, especially in defensive football players. It is unknown whether a double upright brace might offer even more protection. Prophylactic patellar bracing may decrease the incidence of patellofemoral pain in active individuals. The literature is unclear as to the effect of brace wear on athletic performance.

Articular Cartilage Injuries

Injuries to the articular cartilage can be classified as chondral and osteochondral. Acute osteochondral injuries are in many ways the easiest to repair. Large osteochondral fragments resulting from acute trauma should be replaced and internally fixed whenever possible. The same is true for large osteochondral fragments resulting from osteochondritis dissecans. Chronic defects involving cartilage and underlying bone may require the use of osteochondral allografts. Chondral injuries are more challenging because of the limited healing potential of articular cartilage. Two common grading systems for articular cartilage damage are shown in Outline 1. Large areas of severe articular surface damage, especially involving opposing joint surfaces, are unlikely to respond to current repair techniques. Most of these techniques depend on a shoulder of normal cartilage around the lesion to protect the transplanted cells or tissue. However, for focal full-thickness lesions involving a single surface, most commonly the femoral condyle, a number of treatment options exist. The various articular cartilage repair strategies can be classified as techniques for subchondral bone penetration, osteochondral grafting, and cell and tissue engineering.

Subchondral Bone Penetration

Partial-thickness articular surface injuries generate little if any healing response, whereas injuries that reach the subchondral bone result in a repair attempt by marrow-derived cells. Drilling, abrasion, and microfracture of the subchondral bone have all been suggested as techniques to stimulate this type of healing response. Although many patients show clinical improvement after such treatment, it is clear that the resulting repair fibrocartilage is histologically and biomechanically different from normal hyaline cartilage.

Outline 1
Grading systems for osteochondral damage

Outerbridge System

Grade I:	Softening and swelling of cartilage
Grade II:	Fragmentation and fissuring, less than 0.5-in diameter
Grade III:	Fragmentation and fissuring, greater than 0.5-in diameter
Grade IV:	Erosion of cartilage down to exposed subchondral bone

Noyes System

Grade 1:	Cartilage surface intact (1A = some remaining resilience; 1B = deformation)
Grade 2A:	Cartilage surface damaged (cracks, fibrillation, fissuring, or fragmentation); with less than half of cartilage thickness involved
Grade 2B:	Depth of involvement greater than half of cartilage thickness but without exposed bone
Grade 3:	Bone exposed (3A = surface intact; 3B = surface cavitation)

Osteochondral Grafts

Although the use of osteochondral autografts to treat focal cartilage defects is not new, arthroscopic techniques for transferring these grafts of cartilage and bone only date to 1993. In the existing systems, tubular cutters are used to harvest 4.5- to 10-mm cylindrical osteochondral grafts from the articular margins of the intercondylar notch or from the far lateral aspect of the anterior lateral femoral condyle. Identically sized holes are then made in the defect and 1 or more grafts are transplanted. The efficacy of these procedures remains to be determined. Past experience with cartilage repair raises questions regarding the ability of the donor cartilage to heal to the adjacent recipient cartilage. Defect size and depth restrictions for these techniques are also unclear. Most of the experience to date is with small lesions that can be treated with 1 large or several small cylindrical grafts. Lesions larger than 2.5 cm^2 may not be appropriate for this technique and, in fact, may create significant problems because of the large area of donor site harvest.

Autologous Cell and Tissue Engineering

The transplantation of autologous cells, natural and synthetic matrices, and bioactive factors into articular cartilage defects is currently being investigated. Tissues such as rib cartilage, perichondrium, periosteum, and even fracture callus have been used to fill defects, and chondrocytes or osteochondral progenitor cells have been isolated for culture and transplantation. Collagen and other materials are being studied as matrices for cultured cells with or without the addition of growth factors.

To date, the largest clinical experience has been with autologous chondrocyte transplantation. In this procedure, articular cartilage is harvested from a nonweightbearing area of the knee and sent to a laboratory for chondrocyte isolation, culture, and propagation. In a second procedure, a periosteal flap is sutured over the lesion and the resuspended cells are injected into the defect. In the first published series, good to excellent results at 2 years were reported in 14 of 16 patients with femoral condylar lesions, but in only 2 of 7 patients with patellar defects. In a recent canine study in which the same technique and chondrocytes processed by the same laboratory were used, 4-mm defects in the trochlear groove treated with cultured chondrocytes under a periosteal flap were compared with defects treated with a periosteal flap alone and with untreated defects. The authors detected no difference among the groups with regard to any of the parameters used to evaluate the quality of the repair. These results contrast sharply with those of a similar study in rabbits, in which the addition of chondrocytes significantly improved the quality of the repair tissue. These conflicting reports highlight the need for both large controlled clinical studies and animal research to validate new techniques for cartilage repair.

Plica Syndrome

A synovial plica is an inward fold or ridge of the synovial lining. In the knee, incomplete reabsorption of the mesenchymal tissue that occupied the space between the femur and tibia in the embryo leaves these synovial folds in the joint. Arthroscopically they appear as bands or ridges extending into the intra-articular space. Synovial plicae should be differentiated from bands of dense scar tissue that can be present after trauma or surgery. Suprapatellar and infrapatellar plicae have been reported to be present in nearly 90% of knees examined arthroscopically, with a variety of patterns and locations. The medial patellar plica, present in approximately 75% of knees, is more clinically significant; the lateral patellar plica is rare (1%). In general, the medial patellar plica runs from the medial aspect of the suprapatellar space obliquely down in a nearly coronal plane to attach to the superior portion of the infrapatellar fat pad. It is most commonly seen as a complete fold with a sharp free margin commonly called a shelf, but occasionally has other configurations, such as a fenestrated band or several small folds. As the medial plica courses distally it lies immediately anterior to the medial femoral condyle near the inferior medial region of the patella. It is believed that in this position it can be a source of pain as it contacts the medial femoral condyle.

Clinically, patients have pain and tenderness along the medial patellar retinaculum directly over the medial femoral condyle. On examination, this location is above the medial joint line, but not anterior enough to cause patellofemoral joint pain. In most patients, a palpable thickening or band is present. The most common causes of a symptomatic medial plica are direct trauma and repetitive overuse activities, such as running, biking, or stair stepping, as well as kneeling. Other possible sources of pain should be ruled out by history and examination because this is primarily a diagnosis of exclusion. Computed tomography (CT) arthrogram of the knee can display these synovial folds and may help determine whether a fold is thin or thick. A medial plica is routinely seen on MRI scans of the knee. Plica thickness on CT or MRI scan has not been correlated with symptoms. Local injection can be helpful to confirm the diagnosis of symptomatic medial plica, but does not seem to have a significant role in treatment because very few patients have long-lasting relief.

The most effective treatment of a symptomatic medial synovial plica remains arthroscopic resection. A number of recent studies have demonstrated the effectiveness of resection in selected patients, and resection has been demonstrated to be superior to diagnostic arthroscopy alone. A complete arthroscopic examination of the knee should always be done, with special attention to possible medial meniscal tears or patellofemoral articular lesions. In properly selected patients, results of arthroscopic plica resection are good or excellent in 90%, with low morbidity and rapid recovery. The most common complication is postoperative hemarthrosis. Because of this risk, asymptomatic plicae generally should not be resected.

Arthroscopy of the Knee

Arthroscopy of the knee continues to be one of the most common and successful orthopaedic procedures. It generally is done in a hospital outpatient surgery department or at a free-standing surgery center. Recently, there has been an increase in the use of arthroscopy in the physician's office setting, but this has not gained widespread acceptance. It has, however, rekindled interest in using local anesthetic, usually with intravenous sedation, for arthroscopic procedures. In properly selected patients, local anesthesia has been shown to be safe and effective for diagnostic and therapeutic arthroscopies. Patient satisfaction has been high, and cost savings have been approximately $400 per procedure. However, some procedures are too painful for the use of local anesthesia, and if conversion to general anesthesia is required, this cannot be done in the office, and the procedure will have to be aborted. This may result in incomplete treatment and the need for a second procedure with general anesthesia.

The increased interest in office arthroscopy has stimulated the development of a number of new arthroscopic optical catheter systems designed to be less invasive while providing acceptable images. These devices are smaller in diameter and less expensive than standard arthroscopes. They are similar to older needle arthroscopic tools, but have improved characteristics and video output. Several studies comparing optical catheter systems to conventional arthroscopy in similar situations found that the newer systems tended to underestimate the number of intra-articular injuries. The sensitivity for meniscal and chondral injuries has been reported to be 25% to 67%. It has been suggested that these devices may compromise visual acuity, resulting in missed and incorrect diagnoses. Improvements in equipment and technique may make these devices more attractive in the future.

There is an ever increasing variety of arthroscopic fluid pump systems available. These systems have gained increasing acceptance and have become simpler and more reliable for operating room personnel. The simplest ones provide a constant inflow pressure with the ability to maintain high flow volumes. Some systems monitor direct intra-articular fluid pressure, while others rely on pressure measurements at the pump source. Finally, some designs control flow rate as well as pressure by controlling the fluid outflow. There have been concerns that the use of arthroscopic pumps unnecessarily increases the volume of fluid used during arthroscopic procedures, thereby increasing costs and stressing operating room personnel. This can be avoided through judicious use of pump pressures and attention to control of fluid outflow. Another concern has been the increased risk of fluid extravasation, either into the thigh or calf, which at high pressures generated by arthroscopic pumps could lead to a situation resembling a compartment syndrome. There have been several reports of this type of complication. However, because the fluid used is a physiologic saline and there is no associated muscle injury or other trauma within the compartments, the extravasated fluid dissipates relatively quickly with no residual effects. Should this situation arise, the procedure should be finished as quickly as possible at low pump pressures and the patient should be observed in the recovery room for dissipation of the fluid. Only if compartment swelling and measured intracompartmental pressures do not resolve should a formal fasciotomy be considered.

The use of arthroscopic electrocautery has become increasingly common over the past several years. Although not as common as in shoulder arthroscopy, electrocautery in knee arthroscopy can be very helpful. It is used most commonly in arthroscopic lateral release to decrease the risk of significant postoperative hemarthrosis, a common complication. In addition, it is helpful when a tourniquet is not recommended, such as in patients with significant peripheral vascular disease or a previous vascular reconstruction, and for surgeons who prefer to perform knee arthroscopy without a tourniquet. The development of electrocautery tips that are insulated to near the very end allows the use of these tips in conductive fluid, such as normal saline. It is no longer necessary to use nonconductive fluids, such as water or glycerol.

Lasers continue to be used in a small number of arthroscopic knee procedures. They work by creating heat in the tissue as it absorbs the intense laser light. Lasers have been described as effective in smoothing frayed or degenerative tissues, and because they can coagulate tissue, they reduce the amount of bleeding during synovial resection. In addition, it has been reported that lasers can weld or fuse tissue clefts, such as small meniscal splits. However, these effects are likely more visual than structural or functional. There has been increasing interest in the reported ability of lasers to shrink or contract tissue by heating of the collagen protein. Clinically, lasers are being used in the shoulder to shrink or reduce the joint capsule; the procedure is called a laser capsulorrhaphy. There has been interest in treating patellar instability with laser tissue shrinking of the lax medial patellar retinaculum to reduce patellar subluxation or dislocation, but this use of lasers remains investigational. There continue to be a number of drawbacks to the use of lasers in knee arthroscopy. They have not been shown to be any more effective than standard mechanical debridement and meniscectomy. In addition, they are expensive, and the cost is prohibitive for most operating room settings at this time. They are not as effective for removing large quantities of tissue, and there are significant issues with regard to safety and training of operating room personnel. Recently, osteonecrosis in the femoral condyles of several patients has been associated with arthroscopic surgery augmented with the use of lasers. This seems to be more than a coincidence, although the mechanisms are not well understood.

More recently, electrothermal devices have been developed that, like lasers, are designed to deliver thermal energy to the tissues using a specially designed probe. These devices could effect the same tissue shrinking as a laser, but the amount of tissue heating may be easier to control and the cost is significantly less. Again, these devices are generating widespread interest in shoulder arthroscopy and may have some future role in knee arthroscopy.

Local anesthetics have long been used for reducing immediate postoperative pain after knee arthroscopy, and long-acting anesthetics such as bupivacaine generally are used in the arthroscopic portals and/or intra-articularly. More recently, the use of intra-articular morphine after knee arthroscopy has been recommended. Doses have ranged from 1 to 5 mg. A large number of studies have compared the effects of these various treatments on postoperative pain. Although some reported a reduction in pain with the additional use of morphine, others have found no such effect. Studies in which higher doses, such as 3 to 5 mg, were used were more likely to report significant reduction of pain. Whether pain relief from the use of intra-articular morphine is based on a local anesthetic or a systemic effect is not clear.

Reflex Sympathetic Dystrophy

In recent years there has been an evolution in the terminology used to describe the condition commonly known as reflex sympathetic dystrophy (RSD). The terminology used more recently is sympathetically maintained pain (SMP). SMP is pain that results from sympathetic nervous system dysfunction. In general, SMP is not present alone, but is part of a pain dysfunction syndrome. One component of this syndrome is sympathetically independent pain, which includes the primary components of a local painful organic condition such as an injury, psychological factors such as personality disorder or secondary gain factors, and systemic factors such as peripheral neuropathy or systemic disease. In most patients with RSD several sources of pain coexist, including a component that is sympathetically independent as well as a component that is sympathetically maintained. It is this secondary component, or the SMP that is relieved by sympathetic blockade. This terminology helps surgeons understand that pain present from sympathetic nervous system dysfunction complicates and coexists with pain from other sources. SMP generally is initiated by some noxious triggering event and does not occur de novo. This event may be a significant pathologic condition, such as a meniscus tear or patellofemoral dysfunction, or a trivial injury that would be expected to resolve spontaneously.

The hallmark for identification of SMP is the presence of pain out of proportion to that expected for the degree of injury. SMP often extends well beyond the involved area in a nonanatomic distribution. Frequently the pain is described as a burning sensation with extreme sensitivity to light touch, such as clothing or bed linens. A frequently present early and suggestive sign is intolerance to cold, such as from ice used after an injury or surgery. In addition, there can be abnormal color changes, commonly a blue or dusky change as well as an increase in sweating. As a result of the pain, there is limitation of knee joint range of motion and inhibition of muscle contraction causing weakness. These symptoms should alert the clinician to consider the possibility of SMP. Later in the course of an ongoing RSD there are trophic changes, such as hair loss, smooth shiny skin, osteopenia, joint contractures, and atrophy.

The cornerstones of the management of SMP are early recognition and intervention (Fig. 5). Treatment of SMP includes sympathetic blockade, oral medication, and physical therapy. Sympathetic blockade generally is achieved through the use of intrathecal injection of a low dose of local anesthetic. Because the sympathetic fibers are less myelinated than the motor and sensory nerve fibers, they are more susceptible to the effects of the local anesthetic. Thus the use of a low concentration of anesthetic can achieve a relatively selective block of these sympathetic fibers. This blockade should be associated with a temperature increase in the involved extremity as a result of vasodilatation. The SMP should be relieved by the block, while the sympathetically independent pain may persist. Therefore, there may not be complete pain relief, but a substantial amount should be relieved, or the diagnosis of SMP is probably incorrect. More prolonged treatment can be achieved using an indwelling epidural catheter in an inpatient setting. Direct block of the sympathetic chain through a paravertebral block also is effective, but more difficult to perform. Finally, a surgical sympathectomy can be considered but is rarely indicated.

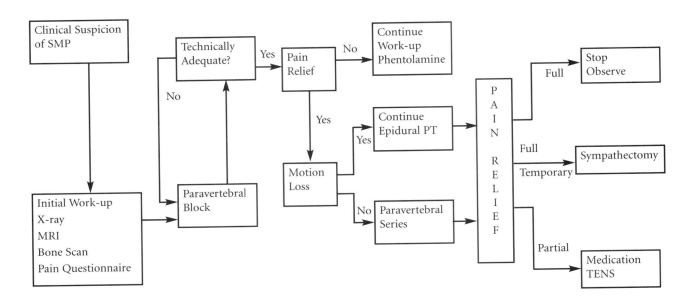

Figure 5

A flowchart for the management of sympathetically maintained pain (SMP) in the lower extremity. MRI, magnetic resonance imaging; TENS, transcutaneous electrical stimulation. (Reproduced with permission from Lindenfeld TN, Bach BR Jr, Wojtys EM: Reflex sympathetic dystrophy and pain dysfunction in the lower extremity, in Springfield DS (ed): *Instructional Course Lectures 46*. Rosemont, IL, American Academy of Orthopaedic Surgeons, 1997, pp 261–268.)

Pharmacologic treatment of SMP has a less predictable response than sympathetic blockade. Drugs that have been used for treatment of SMP include anticonvulsants, especially carbamazepine, antidepressants, especially amitriptyline, and alpha receptor blockers. In general, orthopaedists have little experience prescribing these medications, and because the medications all have a number of side effects, they are probably best left for use by other health care providers.

Finally, physical therapy is an important aspect of treatment of SMP. It is essential for the therapy provider to develop a constructive, supportive relationship with involved patients because this is a difficult condition to recover from. Generally, active assisted range of motion exercises are preferable to passive range of motion. Avoidance of noxious stimuli such as ice is important. Gentle soft-tissue massage can be effective in reducing sensitivity and improving function. Emphasis should be on slow but steady progress and on returning to functional activities without excessive protection; avoidance of the involved extremity should be encouraged.

Patellofemoral Disorders

Pain and disability from disorders of the patellofemoral joint are among the most common knee conditions requiring treatment. Most of these problems can be treated nonsurgically, although occasionally surgery is indicated. Differential diagnoses include patellofemoral arthritis, patellar instability, lateral facet overload, patellofemoral pain resulting from patellar and/or trochlear chondral defects, patellar tendinitis, medial plica syndrome, symptomatic bipartite patella, and meniscal tears. A careful history and physical examination generally can identify the source of pathology. However, some patients do not have clearly identifiable sources of anterior knee pain. Clinical assessment should include structural findings, such as tibial-femoral alignment, Q angle, hip rotation, quadriceps function and atrophy, patellar mobility and tilt, patellofemoral crepitus, and standard knee evaluation. Functional testing should include gait assessment, active knee extension against resistance, and provocative tests, such as patellar apprehension and patellar grind.

Plain radiography views should include a tangential view of the patella, such as a Merchant view. Comparison of these views to a contralateral asymptomatic knee may be helpful. In recent years, CT scanning has been recommended to evaluate patellar tilt and/or subluxation. This is typically done with the knee flexed to 30°, and abnormalities may be accentuated by active quadriceps contraction during the scanning process. Although MRI can better identify articular cartilage lesions, it generally is not indicated in patellofemoral disorders unless needed to rule out other joint pathology such as meniscal tears.

Treatment should be focused on the identified source of pain. In most patients a directed exercise program is successful in reducing symptoms. This program should include initial activity modification and should emphasize closed chain resistance exercises, as well as improving quadriceps and hamstring flexibility. Open chain, active knee extension exercises, although effective in strengthening the quadriceps muscle, frequently aggravate patellofemoral symptoms. Emphasis should be on pain-free, functional exercises. Patellar taping and/or patellar bracing can be effective as an adjuvant therapy. Most patients have relief with this program, although they may not have not complete resolution of their symptoms. Clinical studies assessing results of treatment have suffered from a lack of a standard means of evaluating outcomes, as well as a lack of long-term follow-up.

Surgical treatment for patellofemoral pain is best reserved for those with identifiable and correctable lesions, including patellar malalignment, a tight lateral retinaculum, and patellofemoral articular cartilage disorders. Usually the articular surfaces are examined arthroscopically and the lateral retinaculum is released, either arthroscopically or through a limited open approach. This release should be done relatively close to the patella to reduce the risk of bleeding and not extend into the tendon of the vastus lateralis. Isolated or concomitant debridement of the patellofemoral joint articular surface generally is not recommended. However, clearly loose fragmented portions of articular cartilage that may get caught with knee flexion and extension should be removed. Debridement of softening or fissuring of the articular surface should be avoided. In properly selected patients, arthroscopic lateral release relieves symptoms in approximately 80%; however, this procedure is indicated in only a small number.

Patellar instability, including both subluxation and dislocation, also is generally effectively treated with a structured exercise program. Acute dislocations usually require a short period of immobilization in extension and occasionally require aspiration of a hemarthrosis. However, prolonged immobilization increases the risk for joint contractures and worsens muscle atrophy. In a series of 100 patients with acute first time dislocations, the recurrence rate was 44% after an average of 13 years. Recent MRI evaluation of acute dislocations demonstrated acute injuries to the medial patellofemoral ligament near its femoral insertion (Fig. 6). This finding has important implications in the surgical management of these patients. Surgical treatment of acute dislocations generally has not been indicated unless an associated osteochondral fragment requires removal. However, acute ligament repair might be indicated for an athlete with a high risk for recurrence who cannot afford an in-season injury. The criteria for recommending acute ligament repair are not clear at this time.

Recurrent patellar subluxation or dislocation that persists despite appropriate nonsurgical treatment should be treated surgically. The 3 options in surgical treatment are lateral retinacular release or lengthening, medial soft-tissue repair or reconstruction, and repositioning of the patellar tendon, usually through tibial tubercle transfer. In general, lateral release alone is insufficient for treatment of recurrent instability. There is no clear consensus on whether proximal soft-tissue realignment procedures in which medial tissues are tightened or reconstructed and lateral tissues are released or lengthened, or distal realignment procedures, such as medial tibial tubercle transfer (usually done along with a lateral release), are preferable.

Medial soft-tissue repair or reconstruction, advocated by some surgeons to correct the injured structures directly, is simpler, less invasive, and has better cosmetic results. Open proximal soft-tissue realignment procedures recommended include distal and lateral advancement of the vastus medialis obliquus, imbrication of the medial capsule and ligaments, direct repair of the patellofemoral ligament (Fig. 7), and reconstruction using soft-tissue grafts such as the semitendi-

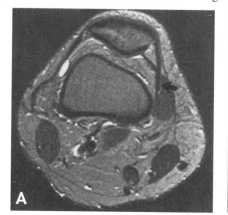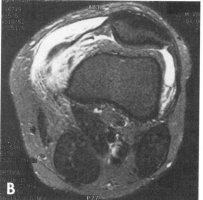

Figure 6

Axial magnetic resonance imaging views of a normal knee (A) and the contralateral knee (B) following acute lateral patellar dislocation. Note the disruption of the medial patellofemoral ligament off of the medial femoral epicondyle compared to the normal ligament (shown by the dark arrow). (Reproduced with permission from Boden BP, Pearsall AW, Garrett WE Jr, Feagin JA Jr: Patellofemoral instability: Evaluation and management. *J Am Acad Orthop Surg* 1997; 5:47–57.)

nosus tendon. These procedures are done along with a lateral release. Several authors have reported good results with arthroscopically-assisted proximal realignment.

Distal realignment is believed by some to correct a biomechanical malalignment that led to the dislocation in the first place. The Elmslie-Trillat procedure or a modification is the most commonly recommended of the distal realignment procedures. In this procedure the tibial tubercle is osteotomized and transferred medially, leaving the most distal portion of the osteotomy hinged to improve stability. The degree of transfer depends on the individual patient, and the stability of the transferred patella should be assessed intraoperatively to determine adequate, but not excessive, displacement. The transferred tubercle generally is stabilized with screw fixation, which allows early postoperative motion. With this transfer, the insertion of the patellar tendon is moved only medially, not anteriorly or posteriorly. Any procedure, such as the Hauser procedure, that results in a posterior displacement of the tibial tubercle is not recommended because this can increase patellofemoral forces. Clinical series generally show that good results can be obtained with either approach, with a success rate above 90% in preventing recurrent dislocation; however, some patients have persistent pain and are not be able to return to their preinjury levels of activity.

When a reduction in patellofemoral forces is desired, such as in patients with significant patellofemoral joint articular cartilage abnormalities, anterior displacement of the tubercle may be done to reduce patellofemoral forces. This can be achieved through an anteromedial tibial tubercle transfer. In this procedure, the osteotomy of the tubercle is angled from anteromedial to posterolateral depending on the degree of anterior displacement desired (Fig. 8). Then, as the tubercle is displaced medially, it is also displaced anteriorly. If additional anterior displacement is desired, a bone graft can be placed in the osteotomy gap before it is stabilized. Results with this technique have been quite good in patients with patellofemoral malalignment plus lateral facet chondral changes, although many patients continue to have some degree of discomfort. Direct anterior displacement of the tibial tubercle, such as the Maquet procedure, can be used in patients with patellofemoral arthrosis without malalignment; however, the results are less satisfactory. Wound healing problems over an anteriorly displaced tibial tubercle are an occasional complication with the Maquet procedure, but do not seem to be a significant problem with the anteromedial transfer. Other complications of tibial tubercle transfer include postoperative stiffness, persistent anterior knee pain, and fracture of the proximal tibia.

In rare circumstances, a patellectomy may be considered for salvage of a patellofemoral joint disorder. However, this

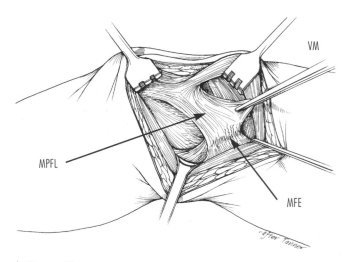

Figure 7

Surgical exposure of the medial patellofemoral ligament (MPFL) at its attachment to the medial epicondyle of the femur (MFE). The vastus medialis (VM) has been retracted anteriorly. (Reproduced with permission from Boden BP, Pearsall AW, Garrett WE Jr, Feagin JA Jr: Patellofemoral instability: Evaluation and management. *J Am Acad Orthop Surg* 1997;5:47–57.)

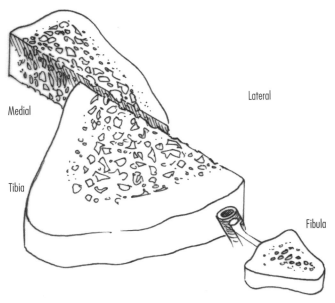

Figure 8

Schematic of a cross-section through the tibia at the level of the tubercle demonstrates how an oblique osteotomy results in anterior as well as medial transfer of the tibial tubercle. This has the effect of realigning the extensor mechanism as well as decreasing the patellofemoral contact forces. (Reproduced with permission from Fulkerson JP, Becker GJ, Meaney JA, Miranda M, Folcik MA: Anteromedial tibial tubercle transfer without bone graft. *Am J Sports Med* 1990;18:490.)

should be done for clear, objective, otherwise untreatable joint disease, and not for pain in the absence of significant pathology. When considering patellectomy, the patient needs to be well informed that pain and crepitus may persist and that significant knee extension weakness will ensue. If a patellectomy is done, preservation and repair of the extensor mechanism is essential, along with ensuring centralization and stability of the residual extensor tendon.

Extensor Mechanism Disruption

The extensor mechanism consists of the quadriceps muscle, quadriceps tendon, patella, and patellar tendon. Any disruption in this chain of structures can result in weakness and/or the inability to actively extend the knee. Clearly, proper function is essential for normal daily activities. Patellar tendinitis, or "jumper's knee" probably is a partial tear of the patellar tendon at its attachment to the distal pole of the patella. Repetitive use and recurrent injuries of this tendon prevent adequate healing and result in persistent pain. Patellar tendinitis is characterized by tenderness at the distal pole of the patella, occasionally with localized swelling or enlargement, and pain with strenuous quadriceps activities such as jumping or squatting. In general, treatment with activity modification, stretching, and strengthening, especially with eccentric exercises, is successful. Some individuals feel more secure with a strap placed around the knee at the level of the patellar tendon. Steroid injections into the painful area are not recommended because they can increase the risk of complete patellar tendon rupture. MRI typically demonstrates an area of abnormal tendon at the deep surface adjacent to the patellar attachment (Fig. 9). Patients not responsive to nonsurgical treatment and who cannot participate at the desired level of activity generally can be treated successfully with surgical resection of the diseased tendon and reattachment of the normal tendon to the patella, combined with continued postoperative rehabilitation.

Complete disruption of the patellar tendon is an uncommon injury. It generally occurs in younger patients as an isolated injury, but can be associated with other injuries in patients with knee dislocation. It generally is a result of a vigorous eccentric quadriceps contraction, such as in a fall or landing. A number of these injuries are misdiagnosed initially. Anatomically, the tears are at the patellar attachment or midsubstance and frequently extend medially and laterally beyond the tendon into the anterior portions of the joint capsule. Even when diagnosis is delayed, direct surgical repair and/or reconstruction should be performed. Usually, a primary repair can be achieved and can be augmented with a hamstring tendon autograft (gracilis or semitendinosus) placed through drill holes in the patella and tibia. Although such augmentation may not be necessary for all acute repairs, it should be used in repairs of chronic tears.

Some surgeons choose to support or protect the repaired tendon by placing a loop of wire or heavy suture from the tibia to the patella, shielding the repair (Fig. 10). This procedure may allow early and more aggressive range of motion,

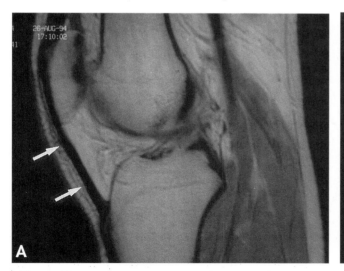
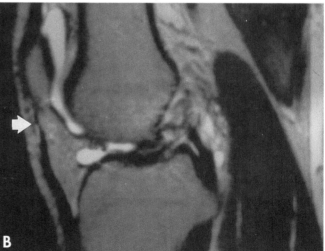

Figure 9

Magnetic resonance images through the patellar tendon of a normal tendon (A) and a tendon with a subacute tear (B). Such studies are most helpful in cases of partial tears. (Reproduced with permission from Matava MJ: Patellar tendon ruptures. *J Am Acad Orthop Surg* 1996;4:287–296.)

but if a wire is used it generally requires removal and frequently the wire breaks. Care should be taken to avoid creation of an iatrogenic patella baja. Comparison to the uninjured knee by intraoperative examination or radiographs can help determine the correct length of the patellar tendon. Postoperative management generally includes weightbearing in extension, progressively increasing protected range of motion with patellar mobilization, and electrical stimulation or straight leg raising to maintain quadriceps muscle function.

Quadriceps tendon rupture generally occurs in older patients and is more commonly associated with systemic diseases such as systemic lupus erethematosus, diabetes, and gout. Delay in diagnosis is even more common with quadriceps tendon tears than with patellar tendon tears because there are no radiographic abnormalities. In addition, a degree of active extension usually is preserved, although it is significantly weak. This weakness, along with a palpable tenderness or defect in the tendon proximal to the patella and an index of suspicion can make the diagnosis. If necessary, confirmation can be obtained from ultrasonography or MRI. Early primary repair is indicated when the diagnosis is made. Postoperatively, immobilization and protection from overloading of the tendon are continued for somewhat longer than after repair of the patellar tendon, because the risk for knee contracture is less and the healing in these typically elderly patients with systemic diseases is slower.

For chronic quadriceps or patellar tendon tears, surgical repair should be considered if functional limitations are significant. Mobilization of the torn tendon edges, as well as a more proximal quadriceps lengthening, may help bring the tendon ends together. Typically, reinforcement with autogenous graft, such as the semitendinosus, or a quadriceps turndown should be done followed by more extended immobilization and slower rehabilitation than after repair of an acute tear. Education of emergency room and primary care physicians about extensor mechanism disruptions may help reduce the number of misdiagnosed tears of the extensor mechanism.

Annotated Bibliography

Background

Arendt E, Dick R: Knee injury patterns among men and women in collegiate basketball and soccer: NCAA data and review of literature. *Am J Sports Med* 1995;23:694–701.

This is an epidemiologic study over 5 years from the National Collegiate Athletic Association (NCAA) Injury Surveillance System. It shows the increased risk of all knee injuries in women compared to men, particularly ACL tears, which occur 2.4 times more often in soccer and 4.1 times more often in basketball.

Lambson RB, Barnhill BS, Higgins RW: Football cleat design and its effect on anterior cruciate ligament injuries: A three-year prospective study. *Am J Sports Med* 1996;24:155–159.

Football shoes with longer irregular cleats placed on the outer rim of the sole have greater traction (torsional resistance) on both grass and artificial surfaces. This design lead to a significantly greater risk of ACL injury.

History and Physical Examination

Lintner DM, Kamaric E, Moseley JB, Noble PC: Partial tears of the anterior cruciate ligament: Are they clinically detectable? *Am J Sports Med* 1995;23:111–118.

In a cadaver study, in which experienced examiners were blinded as to ligament status, they were able to recognize 100% of intact ligaments and 77% of complete transections, but only 13% of partial transections (anteromedial band). The authors suggest that any partial ACL tear identified by increased laxity on physical examination is a complete tear.

Imaging

Adalberth T, Roos H, Laurén M, et al: Magnetic resonance imaging, scintigraphy, and arthroscopic evaluation of traumatic hemarthrosis of the knee. *Am J Sports Med* 1997;25:231–237.

This is a prospective study of 40 patients with acute hemarthrosis evaluated as noted. When compared with arthroscopy for ACL tears, MRI had a sensitivity of 97%, specificity of 50%, and accuracy of 50%. MRI findings of partial rupture of the ACL were wrong almost all the time, and tears should be regarded as complete if the Lachman is at all positive.

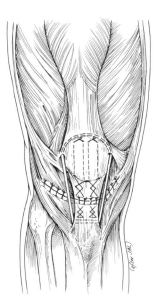

Figure 10

Acute repair of a ruptured patellar tendon using Bunnell type suturing to the patella and a reinforcing suture placed from the quadriceps tendon to the tibial tubercle. The repair extends medially and laterally well beyond the patellar tendon. (Reproduced with permission from Matava MJ: Patellar tendon ruptures. *J Am Acad Orthop Surg* 1996;4: 287–296.)

Treatment Options

Anterior Cruciate Ligament

Beynnon BD, Fleming BC, Johnson RJ, Nichols CE, Renstrom PA, Pope MH: Anterior cruciate ligament strain behavior during rehabilitation exercises in vivo. *Am J Sports Med* 1995;-23:24–34.

In vivo instrumentation data from patients with intact ACLs are presented. Ranges of motion where isometric quadriceps contraction and simultaneous quadriceps-hamstring contraction strain the intact ACL are identified, assisting in the design of postsurgical rehabilitation protocols.

Bynum EB, Barrack RL, Alexander AH: Open versus closed chain kinetic exercises after anterior cruciate ligament reconstruction: A prospective randomized study. *Am J Sports Med* 1995;23:401–406.

In a prospective randomized study using B-PT-B, closed versus open kinetic chain exercise rehabilitation protocols were compared. At 1-year follow-up, anterior laxity at maximum manual (1.6 mm versus 3.3 mm) and anterior knee pain great enough to restrict activities (15% versus 38%) were both significantly less in the closed chain group.

Fulkerson JP, Langeland R: An alternative cruciate reconstruction graft: The central quadriceps tendon. *Arthroscopy* 1995;11:252–254.

The central quadriceps tendon is described as an alternative graft for ACL reconstruction, primary and revision. The technique is described, but no results are presented.

Howard ME, Cawley PW, Losse GM, Johnston RB III: Bone-patellar tendon-bone grafts for anterior cruciate ligament reconstruction: The effects of graft pretensioning. *Arthroscopy* 1996;12:287–292.

Pretensioning patellar tendon grafts at 89 N for 4 minutes or more resulted in a 10% to 14% increase in length prior to implantation. Without pretensioning, it is likely postimplantation creep will occur leading to increased knee laxity.

Khalfayan EE, Sharkey PF, Alexander AH, Bruckner JD, Bynum EB: The relationship between tunnel placement and clinical results after anterior cruciate ligament reconstruction. *Am J Sports Med* 1996;24:335–341.

In a prospective study, clinical function and knee laxity correlated with tibial and femoral tunnel placement. Placement of the femoral tunnel 60% or more posteriorly on Blumensaat's line and tibial placement 20% to 40% posteriorly on the tibial plateau on the lateral radiograph were good predictors of function and laxity.

O'Neill DB: Arthroscopically assisted reconstruction of the anterior cruciate ligament: A prospective randomized analysis of three techniques. *J Bone Joint Surg* 1996;78A:803–813.

This is one of the few prospective randomized studies comparing the results of B-PT-B reconstructions of the ACL with those of 4-HT. Due to small sample sizes, few results reached statistical significance, although there was a trend for less laxity (measured with KT-2000) and greater return to preinjury athletics in the endoscopic B-PT-B group.

Shelbourne KD, Foulk DA: Timing of surgery in acute anterior cruciate ligament tears on the return of quadriceps muscle strength after reconstruction using an autogenous patellar tendon graft. *Am J Sports Med* 1995;23:686–689.

Delaying ACL surgery following injury until full range of motion is obtained resulted in a quicker return of quadriceps strength and athletic participation. In the delayed group, 73% had 80% quadriceps strength by 6 months, whereas this was only 47% in the early group.

Shelton WR, Barrett GR, Dukes A: Early season anterior cruciate ligament tears: A treatment dilemma. *Am J Sports Med* 1997;25:656–658.

In a prospective study of athletes sustaining an early season ACL tear without meniscal damage (MRI documented), 70% were able to return to athletics an average of 6 weeks postinjury. Two thirds of the patients required ACL reconstruction due to instability an average of 7 months postinjury, with 59% of these knees having sustained meniscal injury.

Snyder-Mackler L, Fitzgerald GK, Bartolozzi AR III, Ciccotti MG: The relationship between passive joint laxity and functional outcome after anterior cruciate ligament injury. *Am J Sports Med* 1997;25:191–195.

The authors describe a group of patients who were able to continue to participate at a very high level after complete ACL tear with significant laxity (approximately 7 mm at max man). Unfortunately, there are no reliable means to identify this population early on after injury.

Wojtys EM, Kothari SU, Huston LJ: Anterior cruciate ligament functional brace use in sports. *Am J Sports Med* 1996;24:539–546.

In an in vivo study on ACL-deficient patients at low loads, various functional braces reduced anterior translation 29% to 39% with muscles relaxed. This increased to 70% to 85% with muscle activation. This was at a cost of significant slowing of hamstring muscle reaction times, an important dynamic stabilizer.

Yasuda K, Tsujino J, Tanabe Y, Kaneda K: Effects of initial graft tension on clinical outcome after anterior cruciate ligament reconstruction: Autogenous doubled hamstring tendons connected in series with polyester tapes. *Am J Sports Med* 1997;25:99–106.

In a prospective randomized study with quadrupled hamstring grafts tensioned at 30° of flexion, increasing tension from 20 N to 80 N significantly reduced laxity at 2 years from 2.2 mm to 0.6 mm.

Posterior Cruciate Injuries

Harner CD, Höher J: Evaluation and treatment of posterior cruciate ligament injuries. *Am J Sports Med* 1998;26:471–482.

This article provides a review of relevant basic science and current nonsurgical and surgical treatment of combined and isolated PCL injuries.

Miller MD, Harner CD: The anatomic and surgical considerations for posterior cruciate ligament reconstruction, in Jackson DW (ed): *Instructional Course Lectures 44*. Rosemont, IL, American Academy of Orthopaedic Surgeons, 1995, pp 431–440.

Macro- and microanatomy, insertion sites, and biomechanics are discussed. Current surgical techniques are described, including graft placement, portal placement, and graft fixation.

Shino K, Horibe S, Nakata K, Maeda A, Hamada M, Nakamura N: Conservative treatment of isolated injuries to the posterior cruciate ligament in athletes. *J Bone Joint Surg* 1995;77B: 895–900.

Twenty-two athletes with acute isolated PCL injuries were examined arthroscopically. Four were removed from sports because of severe medial articular cartilage damage, 3 had PCL reconstructions because of reparable meniscal tears, and 15 were treated conservatively. At an average 51-month follow-up, only 1 of the 15 had developed arthritic symptoms despite continued athletic activity.

Posterolateral Complex Injuries

Fanelli GC, Giannotti BF, Edson CJ: Arthroscopically assisted combined posterior cruciate ligament/posterior lateral complex reconstruction. *Arthroscopy* 1996;12:521–530.

This is a retrospective series of 21 PCL/posterolateral arthroscopically assisted reconstructions. Various autologous and allograft tissues were used for the PCL, while the posterolateral biceps tenodesis of Clancy was used. Excellent functional and static stability results are reported.

Noyes FR, Barber-Westin SD: Treatment of complex injuries involving the posterior cruciate and posterolateral ligaments of the knee. *Am J Knee Surg* 1996;9:200–214.

This article reviews multiple studies on treatments for PCL and posterolateral injuries of the knee, biomechanical studies of isometry and graft placement, gait analysis, surgical techniques, and rehabilitation principles.

Terry GC, LaPrade RF: The posterolateral aspect of the knee: Anatomy and surgical approach. *Am J Sports Med* 1996;24: 732–739.

Surgical anatomy of the posterolateral corner is meticulously described. A new, anatomically based, surgical approach is proposed. The article contains photographs of posterolateral knee anatomy.

Combined Injuries

Hillard-Sembell D, Daniel DM, Stone ML, Dobson BE, Fithian DC: Combined injuries of the anterior cruciate and medial collateral ligaments of the knee: Effect of treatment on stability and function of the joint. *J Bone Joint Surg* 1996;78A:169–176.

In a retrospective review of combined complete ACL tears with grade II or III MCL tears treated in various ways, the authors note no increased valgus laxity if the MCL was not repaired. The authors recommend ACL reconstruction only for these combined injuries.

Hughston JC: The importance of the posterior oblique ligament in repairs of acute tears of the medial ligaments in knees with and without an associated rupture of the anterior cruciate ligament: Results of long-term follow-up. *J Bone Joint Surg* 1994;76A: 1328–1344.

With an average follow-up of 22 years in 41 patients following repair of complete MCL and posterior corner tears, the authors obtained excellent results with primary repair and augmentation of the MCL and posterior oblique ligament. More than half of the patients had an ACL tear as well, and the 17 patients with untreated ACL tears had little or no laxity or degenerative changes.

Knee Dislocations

Fanelli GC, Giannotti BF, Edson CJ: Arthroscopically assisted combined anterior and posterior cruciate ligament reconstruction. *Arthroscopy* 1996;12:5–14.

Arthroscopically assisted combined ACL/PCL reconstruction with posterolateral biceps tenodesis, for those patients with laxity, yielded good stability and excellent function. MCL tears were braced to promote healing prior to reconstruction.

Shapiro MS, Freedman EL: Allograft reconstruction of the anterior and posterior cruciate ligaments after traumatic knee dislocation. *Am J Sports Med* 1995;23:580–587.

Early repairs and reconstruction following knee dislocations (average 10 days postinjury) in a small series (7 patients) led to good stability (mean increased sagittal laxity 3.3 mm) with 6 of 7 being clinically good to excellent. Arthrofibrosis requiring manipulation (4 of 7) was a common problem.

Wascher DC, Dvirnak PC, DeCoster TA: Knee dislocation: Initial assessment and implications for treatment. *J Orthop Trauma* 1997;11:525–529.

This retrospective review shows that bicruciate ligament injuries are similar to knee dislocations in mechanism of injury, ligamentous injury, and major vascular injury.

Meniscus

Albrecht-Olsen P, Lind T, Kristensen G, Falkenberg B: Failure strength of a new meniscus arrow repair technique: Biomechanical comparison with horizontal suture. *Arthroscopy* 1997;13:183–187.

The authors describe a new repair technique using the Biofix meniscal arrow. There was no difference in pullout strengths when comparing a single horizontal suture to a single arrow or to a single arrow that had been incubated in isotonic saline after repair and prior to testing.

Asahina S, Muneta T, Yamamoto H: Arthroscopic meniscal repair in conjunction with anterior cruciate ligament reconstruction: Factors affecting the healing rate. *Arthroscopy* 1996;12: 541–545.

Results of 98 second-look arthroscopies in 121 patients who underwent meniscal repair and ACL reconstruction were reviewed. Age, sex, location (medial or lateral), or residual laxity were not predictors of outcome. Repairs of peripheral third tears did significantly better than central third (87% compared to 59% healing). History of locking had a significantly negative effect on results (63% healed in contrast to 84% with no locking).

DeHaven KE, Lohrer WA, Lovelock JE: Long-term results of open meniscal repair. *Am J Sports Med* 1995;23:524–530.

Thirty-three consecutive open meniscal repairs followed for an average of 10 years, had a retear rate of 21% (7/33). All retears occurred in knees with a compromised ACL. Standing radiographs revealed degenerative changes in 15% (4/26) of knees with successful repairs while 57% (4/7) of knees with repeat tears showed degenerative joint disease, p = 0.04.

Eggli S, Wegmuller H, Kosina J, Huckell C, Jakob RP: Long-term results of arthroscopic meniscal repair: An analysis of isolated tears. *Am J Sports Med* 1995;23:715–720.

The authors report the long-term follow-up (average, 7.5 years) of 52 repairs of isolated meniscal tears, examining the failure rate in relationship to patient age, acuity of tear, distance of tear from the periphery, location of tear, and type of suture used in the repair. There was no significant difference in acuity of tear, location of tear, or length of tear. Tears within 3 mm of peripheral rim repaired with permanent suture fared significantly better. Age < 30 years approached statistical significance. MRI results did not correlate with healing.

Horibe S, Shino K, Maeda A, Nakamura N, Matsumoto N, Ochi T: Results of isolated meniscal repair evaluated by second-look arthroscopy. *Arthroscopy* 1996;12:150–155.

Short-term follow-up (2 to 10 months) by second-look arthroscopy in 35 patients is reported. Medial repairs (82% excellent) appeared to heal better than lateral (50% excellent). Age of patient and age of tear had no influence on outcome.

Knee Brace

BenGal S, Lowe J, Mann G, Finsterbush A, Matan Y: The role of the knee brace in the prevention of anterior knee pain syndrome. *Am J Sports Med* 1997;25:118–122.

A prospective study in athletes participating in an 8-week program of progressive strenuous physical exercise is reported. One group wore a silicone ring knee brace during physical activity. The second group remained unbraced. At the end of 8 weeks there was a significant subjective reduction in the incidence of anterior knee pain in braced male participants. No difference was seen in female participants.

Beynnon BD, Johnson RJ, Fleming BC, et al: The effect of functional knee bracing on the anterior cruciate ligament in the weightbearing and nonweightbearing knee. *Am J Sports Med* 1997;25:353–359.

Intraoperative strain measurements were performed in normal ACLs in braced and unbraced knees while "injury mechanism" loads were applied externally. Bracing produced a protective effect on the ligament by significantly reducing the strain values for anterior directed loading of the tibia up to 140 n in both weightbearing and nonweightbearing knees.

Greenwald AE, Bagley AM, France EP, Paulos LE, Greenwald RM: A biomechanical and clinical evaluation of a patellofemoral knee brace. *Clin Orthop* 1996;324:187–195.

A biomechanical study of a patellofemoral knee brace showed that although the brace had essentially no effect on knee mechanics, patients noted a significant improvement in pain and a decreased sense of instability.

Howell SM, Taylor MA: Brace-free rehabilitation, with early return to activity, for knees reconstructed with a double-looped semitendinosus and gracilis graft. *J Bone Joint Surg* 1996;78A:814–825.

Forty-one patients were followed up for 2 years after ACL reconstruction during which they were treated with an intensive, brace-free rehabilitation; 88% had less than 3 mm side-to-side difference when tested at maximum manual force with the KT-1000 device.

Wojtys EM, Kothari SU, Huston LJ: Anterior cruciate ligament functional brace use in sports. *Am J Sports Med* 1996;24: 539–546.

Five patients with chronically unstable knees due to ACL disruption were tested for amount of tibial translation using a specifically designed device. Six different braces were used and each knee was tested in the braced and unbraced state. A significant decrease in anterior tibial translation was seen at low levels of force in knees with and without the stabilizing contractions of the hamstring, quadriceps, and gastrocnemius muscle groups.

Articular Cartilage Injuries

Breinan H, Minas T, Hsu HP, Nehrer S, Sledge CB, Spector M: Effect of cultured autologous chondrocytes on repair of chondral defects in a canine model. *J Bone Joint Surg* 1997;79A: 1439–1451.

Forty-four 4-mm cartilage defects were created in the trochlear groove of dogs and treated by cultured autologous chondrocytes under a periosteal flap, a periosteal flap alone, or no treatment. At 12 and 18 months, no significant differences among the groups were identified with regard to any of the parameters used to assess the quality of the repair.

Brittberg M, Lindahl A, Nilsson A, Ohlsson C, Isaksson O, Peterson L: Treatment of deep cartilage defects in the knee with autologous chondrocyte transplantation. *N Engl J Med* 1994; 331:889–895.

The authors review the results of autologous chondrocyte transplantation in 23 people with deep cartilage defects in the knee. At 2 years, 14 of 16 patients with femoral condylar transplants had good to excellent results, compared to only 2 of 7 patients with patellar transplants.

Buckwalter JA, Mankin HJ: Articular cartilage: Degeneration and osteoarthritis, repair, regeneration, and transplantation, in Cannon WD (ed): *Instructional Course Lectures 47*. Rosemont, IL, American Academy of Orthopaedic Surgeons, 1998, pp 487–504.

The authors provide an excellent review of articular cartilage degeneration and osteoarthrosis, including repair, regeneration, and transplantation techniques.

Caplan AI, Elyaderani M, Mochizuki Y, Wakitani S, Goldberg VM: Principles of cartilage repair and regeneration. *Clin Orthop* 1997;342:254–269.

The authors summarize their rationale for the use of mesenchymal stem cells for articular cartilage regeneration.

Hangody L, Kish G, Karpati Z, Udvarhelyi I, Sgigeti I, Bely M: Mosaicplasty for the treatment of articular cartilage defects: Application in clinical practice. *Orthopedics* 1998;21:751–756.

The authors describe their technique of mosaicplasty and present a preliminary report on 57 patients with a minimum 3-year follow-up. Ninety-one percent had good or excellent results according to the modified Hospital for Special Surgery knee score.

Plica Syndrome

Flanagan JP, Trakru S, Meyer M, Mullaji AB, Krappel F: Arthroscopic excision of symptomatic medial plica: A study of 118 knees with 1–4 year follow-up. *Acta Orthop Scand* 1994; 65:408–411.

In this review of a large series of patients treated arthroscopically for plica resection, 92% had little to no pain postoperatively.

Arthroscopy

Garino JP, Lotke PA, Sapega AA, Reilly PJ, Esterhai JL Jr: Osteonecrosis of the knee following laser-assisted arthroscopic surgery: A report of six cases. *Arthroscopy* 1995;11:467–474.

This is 1 of several reports on the association of osteonecrosis of the femoral condyle found following use of the laser during arthroscopy. A mechanism for injury is lacking.

Lintner S, Shawen S, Lohnes J, Levy A, Garrett W: Local anesthesia in outpatient knee arthroscopy: A comparison of efficacy and cost. *Arthroscopy* 1996;12:482–488.

In a series of selected patients, arthroscopy was performed under local anesthesia with sedation with good success. An average savings of $400 per case over standard techniques was achieved.

Meister K, Harris NL, Indelicato PA, Miller G: Comparison of an optical catheter office arthroscope with a standard rigid rod-lens arthroscope in the evaluation of the knee. *Am J Sports Med* 1996;24:819–823.

This prospective randomized study compares an optical catheter fiberoptic system to a standard arthroscope in the same patient in the operating room setting. In 47 patients the optical catheter system was significantly worse in visualizing pathologic changes.

Small NC, Glogau AI, Berezin MA, Farless BL: Office operative arthroscopy of the knee: Technical considerations and a preliminary analysis of the first 100 patients. *Arthroscopy* 1994;10: 534–539.

The report suggests that arthroscopy in an office setting under local anesthesia with light intravenous sedation can be successful in properly selected patients.

Reflex Sympathetic Dystrophy

Lindenfeld TN, Bach BR Jr, Wojtys EM: Reflex sympathetic dystrophy and pain dysfunction in the lower extremity, in Springfield DS (ed): *Instructional Course Lectures 46*. Rosemont, IL, American Academy of Orthopaedic Surgeons, 1997, pp 261–268.

This is an up-to-date review of RSD, its terminology, pathogenesis, and treatment.

O'Brien SJ, Ngeow J, Gibney MA, Warren RF, Fealy S: Reflex sympathetic dystrophy of the knee: Causes, diagnosis, and treatment. *Am J Sports Med* 1995;23:655–659.

In this retrospective study of 60 patients with RSD, 92% had relief with a sympathetic block. Patients with no or correctable lesions had a good prognosis while those with uncorrectable lesions did not.

Patellofemoral Disorders

Bellemans J, Cauwenberghs F, Witvrouw E, Brys P, Victor J: Anteromedial tibial tubercle transfer in patients with chronic anterior knee pain and a subluxation-type patellar malalignment. *Am J Sports Med* 1997;25:375–381.

The authors report a series of selected patients treated with a Fulkerson type of tibial tubercle transfer for patellar instability/malalignment and pain. A dramatic improvement was achieved in 28 of 29 patients.

Bellemans, J, Cauwenberghs F, Brys P, Victor J, Fabry G: Fracture of the proximal tibia after Fulkerson anteromedial tibial tubercle transfer: A report of four cases. *Am J Sports Med* 1998; 26:300–302.

The authors report on 4 patients with fractures 4 to 8 weeks after Fulkerson tibial tubercle osteotomy. All fractures occurred at the distal end of the osteotomy. The authors concluded that the osteotomy is not fully healed at 4 weeks and patients should be protected for 8 weeks after surgery.

Maenpaa H, Lehto MU: Patellar dislocation: The long-term results of nonoperative management in 100 patients. *Am J Sports Med* 1997;25:213–217.

This is 1 of the few reports on the natural history following first time patellar dislocation. Overall there was a high (44%) recurrence rate.

Naramja RJ Jr, Reilly PJ, Kuhlman JR, Haut E, Torg JS: Long-term evaluation of the Elmslie-Trillat-Maquet procedure for patellofemoral dysfunction. *Am J Sports Med* 1996;24:779–784.

Of 55 knees evaluated 1 to 16 years (average, 6 years) after the Elmslie-Trillat-Maquet procedure, 19 knees (35%) had excellent results, 10 (18%) had good results, and 11 (20%) had fair results. The best results were in patients with instability as a primary symptom.

Sallay PI, Poggi J, Speer KP, Garrett WE: Acute dislocation of the patella: A correlative pathoanatomic study. *Am J Sports Med* 1996;24:52–60.

MRI evaluation of 23 patients with acute patellar dislocations demonstrated medial patellofemoral ligament tears at the femoral insertion in 87%. Open exploration confirmed these tears in 15 of 16 patients. Only 58% of results were good and excellent.

Classic Bibliography

Boden BP, Pearsall AW, Garrett WE Jr, Feagin JA Jr: Patellofemoral instability: Evaluation and management. *J Am Acad Orthop Surg* 1997;5:47–57.

Clancy WG Jr, Shelbourne KD, Zoellner GB, Keene JS, Reider B, Rosenberg TD: Treatment of knee joint instability secondary to rupture of the posterior cruciate ligament: Report of a new procedure. *J Bone Joint Surg* 1983;65A:310–322.

Cooper DE, DeLee JC: Reflex sympathetic dystrophy of the knee. *J Am Acad Orthop Surg* 1994;2:79–86.

Cooper DE, DeLee JC, Ramamurthy S: Reflex sympathetic dystrophy of the knee: Treatment using continuous epidural anesthesia. *J Bone Joint Surg* 1989;71A:365–369.

Daniel DM, Stone ML, Dobson BE, Fithian DC, Rossman DJ, Kaufman KR: Fate of the ACL-injured patient: A prospective outcome study. *Am J Sports Med* 1994;22:632–644.

Dupont JY: Synovial plicae of the knee: Controversies and review. Clin Sports Med 1997;16:87–122.

Fulkerson JP, Kalenak A, Rosenberg TD, Cox JS: Patellofemoral pain, in Eilert RE (ed): *Instructional Course Lectures XLI*. Park Ridge, IL, American Academy of Orthopaedic Surgeons, 1992, pp 57–71.

Harner CD (ed): Symposium: Failed anterior cruciate ligament surgery. *Clin Orthop* 1996;325:1–139.

Harner CD, Xerogeanes JW, Livesay GA, et al: The human posterior cruciate ligament complex: An interdisciplinary study: Ligament morphology and biochemical evaluation. *Am J Sports Med* 1995;23:736–745.

Johnson DP, Eastwood DM, Witherow PJ: Symptomatic synovial plicae of the knee. *J Bone Joint Surg* 1993;75A:1485–1496.

Karlsson J, Kalebo P, Goksor LA, Thomee R, Sward L: Partial rupture of the patellar ligament. *Am J Sports Med* 1992;20:390–395.

McConville OR, Kipnis JM, Richmond JC, Rockett SE, Michaud MJ: The effect of meniscal status on knee stability and function after anterior cruciate ligament reconstruction. *Arthroscopy* 1993;9:431–439.

Parolie JM, Bergfeld JA: Long-term results of nonoperative treatment of isolated posterior cruciate ligament injuries in the athlete. *Am J Sports Med* 1986;14:35–38.

Post WR, Fulkerson JP: Distal realignment of the patellofemoral joint: Indications, effects, results, and recommendations. *Orthop Clin North Am* 1992;23:631–643.

Rasul AT Jr, Fischer DA: Primary repair of quadriceps tendon ruptures: Results of treatment. *Clin Orthop* 1993;289:205–207.

Rougraff BT, Reeck CC, Essenmacher J: Complete quadriceps tendon ruptures. *Orthopedics* 1996;19:509–514.

Shea KP, Fulkerson JP: Preoperative computed tomography scanning and arthroscopy in predicting outcome after lateral retinacular release. *Arthroscopy* 1992;8:327–334.

Shelbourne KD, Nitz P: Accelerated rehabilitation after anterior cruciate ligament reconstruction. *Am J Sports Med* 1990;18:292–299.

Small NC, Glogau AI, Berezin MA: Arthroscopically assisted proximal extensor mechanism realignment of the knee. *Arthroscopy* 1993;9:63–67.

Steiner ME, Hecker AT, Brown CH Jr, Hayes WC: Anterior cruciate ligament graft fixation: Comparison of hamstring and patellar tendon grafts. *Am J Sports Med* 1994;22:240–246.

Veltri DM, Warren RF: Posterolateral instability of the knee. *J Bone Joint Surg* 1994;76A:460–472.

Chapter 43
Knee: Reconstruction

Nonarthroplasty Considerations

Patients with degenerative joint disease of the knee may have a variety of symptoms and disabilities; however, the overwhelming complaint usually is pain, the severity, duration, and location of which should be recorded. These patients also may have mechanical symptoms such as locking episodes. The functional assessment of any given patient is closely related to that patient's pain and may prove important to the choice of treatment option. Many patients with degenerative joint disease of the knee are elderly, and general medical or neurologic problems should be evaluated. The lumbosacral spine and hips should be examined as well as the knee(s). Careful assessment of the neurovascular status of the involved extremity is critical. Radiographs are extremely important; routine radiographic views should include standing anteroposterior (AP), lateral, and patellar axial views. A 45° posteroanterior (PA) flexion weightbearing radiograph of the knee may help to further assess suspected arthritic changes (Fig. 1). Bone scans of the knee may be useful in assessing sus-

pected osteonecrosis or early degenerative changes. Similarly, magnetic resonance imaging (MRI) may be used for diagnosis of suspected meniscal tears. Although MRI is a useful adjunct in evaluating painful knees, it is often overused. Advanced degenerative knee disease can usually be diagnosed with plain radiographs, and cost-efficient criteria for MRI use should be followed. One important area in which MRI can be helpful is in the diagnosis of osteonecrosis (Fig. 2).

Initial treatment of degenerative joint disease of the knee is typically nonsurgical, including patient-directed strengthening of the lower extremity, use of acetaminophen or nonsteroidal anti-inflammatory medications, and occasional corticosteroid injections. Recently, interest has emerged in hyaluronic acid injection and the use of oral agents, glucosamine and chondroitin sulfate. Heel wedges, sorbithane inserts, and functional braces designed to "unload" the knee joint and remove painful symptoms may be considered for specific patients. Surgical treatment options may be considered when nonsurgical measures fail.

The role of arthroscopic debridement in the treatment of the arthritic knee remains controversial. Although the efficacy of the procedure in degenerative joint disease is not well defined, limited morbidity and swift recovery have been reported. The most optimistic results indicate that clinical success occurs in approximately 60% to 70% of patients at 5-year follow-up. Recent longer-term evaluations have had less satisfactory results when more advanced degenerative changes were found in older patients undergoing partial meniscectomy with existing articular cartilage degeneration.

Surgical arthroscopy may allow more accurate definition of existing degenerative disease or synovitis. Arthroscopic debridement with copious joint lavage and removal of unstable meniscal fragments and loose bodies with minimal chondral shaving appear to offer maximum benefit with minimal morbidity. Although the precise etiology of pain relief is not clear, joint lavage alone appears to provide some

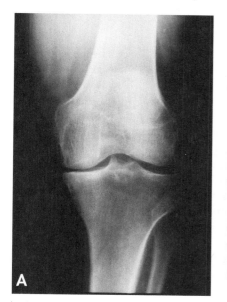 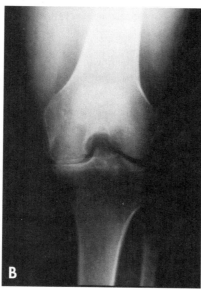

Figure 1

A, Standing anteroposterior radiograph of left knee. B, 45° posteroanterior view of the left knee demonstrataing increased narrowing of the medial joint space.

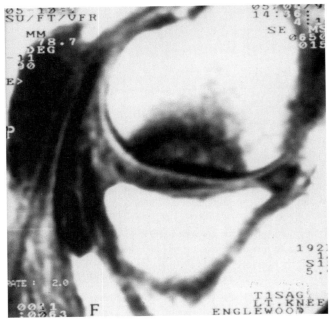

Figure 2

Magnetic resonance imaging (MRI) scan showing osteonecrosis of the medial femoral condyle. MRI may be useful if radiographs are negative.

relief of symptoms. Data from a recent preliminary pilot study suggest that the benefits may result from a placebo effect.

Arthroscopic debridement is well suited for older patients with mild to moderate degenerative joint disease. The 45° PA standing radiograph or bone scan may be helpful in identifying more subtle degenerative changes. Inferior results can be expected in patients with loss of joint space, significant angular deformity, patellofemoral arthrosis, chondrocalcinosis, and rest pain. Patients with short-term mechanical symptoms are more favorable candidates.

Multiple techniques have been attempted to stimulate repair or reformation of the articular surfaces of the knee. Subchondral drilling and abrasion arthroplasty are designed to penetrate the subchondral bone. These procedures do not appear to offer any additional benefit in the treatment of osteoarthritis of the knee with both tibial and femoral involvement. Early results of a microfracture technique using a surgical awl to create multiple "microfractures" in exposed bone combined with limited weightbearing and continuous passive motion have been optimistic. However, longer-term follow-up is required to more accurately define the role of this procedure.

Recently, there has been great interest in regenerating articular cartilage. Published techniques include the use of peri-

chondral grafts, periosteal grafts with and without autologous chondrocytes, carbon fiber scaffolds, articular matrices and growth factors, mesenchymal cell based repairs, osteochondral autografts and allografts, and articular cartilage autografts. Although preliminary studies have been promising, these techniques at the present time appear to be focused more on isolated chondral lesions and not advanced degenerative joint disease.

Synovectomy

Synovectomy may be used to treat a number of synovial proliferative disorders. Particularly good results have been reported in patients with rheumatoid arthritis, pigmented villonodular synovitis, and synovial chondromatosis. Less satisfactory results have been reported in patients with nonspecific synovitis, seronegative arthritis, and posttraumatic arthritis. Indications for synovectomy are persistent synovitis for at least 6 months despite adequate medical management that may include anti-inflammatory agents, corticosteroid injections into the knee, physiotherapy, rehabilitation, and use of drugs such as gold or methotrexate. The results of synovectomy are superior when it is performed early in the disease process and range of motion (ROM) is well preserved. More advanced joint destruction is not well suited for this procedure.

Synovectomy in hemophilia is indicated in patients with recurrent hemarthroses and subacute or chronic synovitis. Again the best results are obtained in patients with minimal degenerative changes on standing radiographs.

Surgical synovectomy of the knee may be performed using either open or arthroscopic techniques. In arthroscopic synovectomy, multiple surgical portals are used. Careful posterior portal placement is mandatory, because complications associated with the posteromedial portal, including residual pain or numbness from neuroma formations have been reported. Large diameter motorized synovial resectors are used to remove the superficial layer of synovium down to the plane between the synovium and subsynovial tissues. Smaller diameter shavers may be helpful in managing the submeniscal, posterior compartment, and intercondylar synovial tissues. Early range of motion, with or without the use of continuous passive motion, is recommended. Clinical results are similar using open or arthroscopic synovectomy techniques. However, arthroscopic techniques more rapidly restore motion and function and have less postoperative morbidity. Study results indicate that a number of synovectomized knees may ultimately require total knee arthroplasty (TKA). A single anterior midline incision is recommended with open synovectomy to lessen future wound or exposure problems at the time of arthroplasty.

Initial reports of radioisotope synovectomy techniques have indicated 80% clinical success. Investigation of radiation synovectomy continues with the use of yttrium and other agents. Results of these nonsurgical techniques must be compared with the present results of arthroscopic synovectomy.

Proximal Tibial Osteotomy

Degenerative joint disease of the knee may be associated with limb malalignment, which accentuates the stress on damaged articular cartilage, causing further degenerative changes and angular deformity. The redistribution of these forces to the less involved compartment after an osteotomy facilitates reparative healing and potentially increases the life span of the knee joint. Thus, the goals of osteotomy include relief of pain, improved function, and providing individuals with heavy functional demands the opportunity to continue activities that may be precluded by TKA. The successful long-term clinical results of TKA have redefined the role of osteotomies.

In a normal knee, approximately 60% of the weightbearing forces are transmitted through the medial compartment. In a knee with unicompartmental arthritis, the altered limb alignment redistributes more load to the affected compartment. The associated increase in angular deformity may affect ligamentous support of the knee. This vicious cycle of progressive angular deformity and loss of articular cartilage may progress with time.

A straight line drawn from the center of the femoral head through the center of the knee to the center of the ankle mortise defines the mechanical axis of the limb. A normal mechanical axis is a straight line and defined as 0°. The tibiofemoral angle of the knee is defined by the angle created by a line drawn down the longitudinal axis of the femur and a line drawn down the longitudinal axis of the tibia. A normal tibiofemoral alignment is approximately 5° to 7° of valgus (Fig. 3). These angles may be determined from full-length, 3-joint weightbearing radiographs and are used to determine the degree of existing angular deformity, which is critical to the goals of corrective surgical osteotomy.

Valgus Osteotomy

In medial tibiofemoral osteoarthrosis with a varus deformity, an upper tibial valgus osteotomy may be performed. Patient selection for this procedure has undergone reevaluation over the past decade. Despite 5-year success rates of 80% to 90%, clinical results with tibial osteotomy appear to deteriorate with time. For 2 large series, 61% good results were reported at an average follow-up of 10 years, and 63% good results for 95 knees at an average follow-up of 8.5 years. These results must be compared with favorable long-term clinical results after TKA in similar series. A tibial osteotomy is preferred for

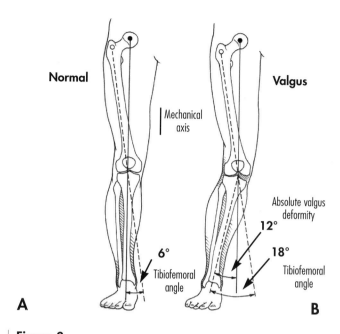

Figure 3

A, Normal alignment with a tibiofemoral angle of 6° of valgus. The tibial shaft axis and the mechanical axis are colinear. B, Valgus deformity of 12° and tibiofemoral angle, 18° of valgus. The tibial shaft axis deviates 18° from the mechanical axis. (Reproduced with permission from Healy WL, Anglen JO, Wasilewski SA, Krackow KA: Distal femoral varus osteotomy. *J Bone Joint Surg* 1988;70A:102–109.)

young active patients because of its potential to allow unlimited strenuous activity. However, in a recent retrospective study no improvement was revealed in the level of patient activity after tibial osteotomy; the best predictor of postoperative activity was the preoperative level of activity.

Given the available information, it is difficult to precisely identify the indication for upper tibial valgus osteotomy. In 1 study, patients older than 60 years had less satisfactory results after osteotomy. Candidates for this procedure appear to be younger (< 60 years), heavier patients with mild to moderate medial compartment osteoarthritis and a varus deformity and patients involved in heavy labor or aggressive athletic activities. Adequate motion (flexion greater than 90° and flexion contracture less than 15°) and a competent medial collateral ligament are prerequisites.

Relative Contraindications Patients suffering from inflammatory arthritis should not be considered for tibial osteotomy. Similarly, patients with limited ROMs are not good candidates because osteotomy is unlikely to improve motion. Advanced patellofemoral arthritis and anatomic varus deformity > 10° are relative contraindications. Varus deformities greater than 15° are frequently associated with lateral tibial subluxation and ligamentous laxity or increased loss of bone in the medial tibial plateau, both of which are associated with inferior clinical results.

Obesity has been associated with early clinical failures after tibial osteotomy. However, in young, active, overweight patients with osteoarthritis, upper tibial osteotomy may still be preferred to a prosthetic replacement. Finally, acceptance of the cosmetic appearance of the lower extremity after valgus tibial osteotomy is an important selection criterion.

Preoperative Assessment Preoperative physical examination should document adequate ROM, ligament stability, angular deformity, and normal ipsilateral hip function. Careful evaluation of the patellofemoral compartment and suspected meniscal pathology should be performed. A standard knee radiographic series including standing AP and axial views of the patella will allow evaluation of existing degenerative joint disease. A 3-joint weightbearing radiograph to determine the existing tibiofemoral anatomic axis and mechanical axis is mandatory to calculate the desired correction and to assess deformities of the tibia or femur that exist above or below the knee. Although no consensus exists on the ideal postoperative alignment, most would favor correcting the mechanical axis into 2° to 5° of valgus alignment.

Gait analysis has demonstrated a relationship between preoperative gait patterns and clinical outcome. Patients with a low adduction moment during gait had better clinical results than those with high adduction moment gait patterns. This relationship has been further substantiated with longer-term follow-up (5.9 years). The adaptive mechanisms used to lower the adduction moment during gait included shortening the stride and toeing out. Patients with low adduction moments (79%) maintained valgus alignment of the knee compared with those who had high adduction moments (29%). Although gait analysis may allow a more sensitive approach to patient selection, the lack of availability has limited its usefulness.

A relationship between clinical improvement after osteotomy and postoperative alignment has been noted. A preoperative method for calculating the desired correction results in a mechanical axis passing through 30% to 40% of the width of the lateral tibial plateau. Ligamentous laxity may alter these determinations. A number of methods to calculate the desired osteotomy correction have been reported, including recent use of computer-generated systems to determine the precise correction. Clearly, careful preoperative planning is critical to the ultimate success of this operation. Arthroscopic assessment of the knee before osteotomy to confirm the indications does not appear to be of prognostic value.

Surgical Technique The surgeon may choose between a wedge (opening or closing) or dome osteotomy technique. Typically, both of these techniques are performed through the cancellous bone of the upper tibia proximal to the tibial tubercle. A lateral closing wedge tibial osteotomy is most frequently performed for genu varum, and dome osteotomy is used for larger degrees of angular correction. Some surgeons prefer a medially based opening wedge osteotomy with bone grafting or distraction osteogenesis techniques using external fixation.

Multiple fixation techniques have been reported. Present trends include stable internal fixation to allow early motion and weightbearing. External fixation risks pin tract infection and historically has been associated with an increased rate of postoperative complications.

The fibula may exert a tethering effect on osteotomy closure. Satisfactory solutions include fibular shaft osteotomy, disruption of the proximal tibiofibular syndesmosis, or fibular head excision with lateral soft-tissue repair.

Complications The most significant complications of high tibial osteotomy include peroneal nerve paralysis, undercorrection, excessive overcorrection, intra-articular fracture, nonunion, and early loss of surgical correction. Compartment syndrome may occur after tibial osteotomy. Fortunately, vascular injuries are uncommon. Deep venous thrombosis varies between 1.2% and 13.5% with a low incidence of pulmonary embolism.

High tibial osteotomy has proven to relieve pain in the treatment of varus gonarthrosis. The association of undercorrection of deformity with decreased survivorship and early deterioration of good results emphasizes the importance of accurate surgical technique. The surgical technique for subsequent knee replacement often is affected by the previous osteotomy. Surgical exposure and patellofemoral mechanics may be more problematic, and careful preoperative planning is required. A large proportion of patients who have a tibial osteotomy will eventually require TKA, and selection of skin incisions for tibial osteotomy should reflect this.

Varus Osteotomy

Primary involvement of the lateral compartment associated with a valgus deformity is less commonly encountered. Although upper tibial varus osteotomy has been used for minor deformities (12° to 15°), more exaggerated angular correction may result in excessive tibial obliquity and predispose the knee to mediolateral laxity. The preferred osteotomy is in the distal femur, which will allow correction of the superolateral tilt of the joint line.

Indications for distal femoral osteotomy are similar to those for tibial osteotomy and must be considered relative to TKA. Relative contraindications include inflammatory arthritis, severe patellofemoral arthritis, and significant joint instability with a medial thrust on gait. A flexion contracture < 20° and flexion > 90° is preferred. Again, the osteotomy appears indicated in younger, active patients with valgus deformity and moderate lateral compartment degenerative joint disease. Additionally, patients should be able to tolerate the more rigorous postoperative recovery with extended period of limited weightbearing (4 to 12 weeks). Preoperative assessment should include careful evaluation of the ipsilateral hip.

A variety of surgical techniques have been described for distal femoral osteotomy. Typically, a closing wedge osteotomy is used. Future considerations of possible TKA should dictate the surgeon's preference for skin incision. Early ROM and limited weightbearing are recommended. Stable internal fixation and correct alignment (the transcondylar axis should be perpendicular to the tibiofemoral axis in neutral [0°] or slight varus) are critical to success.

Short-term clinical success (4 years) has been reported after distal femoral osteotomy. A recent longer-term study noted probability of survival (without need for further arthroplasty) after distal femoral osteotomy was 64%. Early failures were attributed to poor patient selection and fixation failure. Late failures were associated with painful advanced degenerative joint disease. These authors noted little technical difficulty in revising these knees to TKA, although they preferred a staged procedure, removing the blade plate 6 months before the anticipated arthroplasty. Occasional use of a stemmed femoral component was needed. With proper patient selection, adequate angular correction, and stable fixation, distal femoral osteotomy appears to be an effective procedure.

Unicompartmental Replacement

Unicompartmental knee arthoplasty, a replacement of either the medial or lateral portion of the tibiofemoral joint, is an alternative to tibial osteotomy or tricompartmental replacement. Unicompartmental replacement preserves both cruciate ligaments, theoretically yielding a knee with more normal kinematics.

Indications for unicompartmental knee replacement are varied. Some would argue that TKA, rather than unicompartmental knee replacement, should be done for older patients because the results from the TKA are very predictable. Others believe that older patients do very well with unicompartmental replacement and are ideal candidates for this cost-effective approach, noting that these patients have quicker rehabilitation and excellent long-term results. The ideal candidate for unicompartmental replacement is a patient with a physiologic age older than 60, a relatively sedentary lifestyle, and a diagnosis of osteoarthritis. Ideally, patients should have > 90° of flexion and a flexion contracture of less than 15°. When reviewing patients for possible unicompartment replacement, 1 group reported that only 6% of patients were good candidates.

Although most surgeons use these criteria for unicompartmental selection, some have advocated unicompartmental replacement for patients who are young but do not meet the indications for proximal tibial osteotomy. For most patients, the ultimate decision as to whether or not to perform unicompartmental replacement must be made at the time of surgery. If the anterior cruciate ligament is not in good condition, unicompartmental replacement should not be performed because subluxation will lead to early arthritic change in the opposite compartment. The patellofemoral joint and the other femorotibial compartment must be thoroughly evaluated for arthritis. Mild areas of chondromalacia may be acceptable, but significant arthritis in one of the other compartments is certainly a contraindication to unicompartmental replacement as are synovial proliferation and chondrocalcinosis. Surgical details include proper component sizing, ligamentous balancing, and preservation of the coronary ligament of the anterior meniscal horn of the opposite compartment.

Review of large groups of patients with unicompartmental replacement indicated greater than 85% survival at 10 years. Early failures have been secondary to poor surgical technique and poor design features, including thin polyethylene, metal-backed tibial components, uncemented designs, excessive tibial resection, and femoral components that were too narrow.

Revision TKA after unicompartmental replacement may be quite challenging. Initial studies suggest significant bone loss from the unicompartmental replacement and subsequent need for bone augmentation with either allograft or metallic wedges. Newer prostheses are more resurfacing in nature and have decreased the need for augmentation at the time of revision. Early results of revision arthroplasty after failure of a more modern unicompartmental replacement are promising.

Total Knee Arthroplasty

The rate of TKA procedures continues to increase annually for a variety of reasons, including increased longevity in the general population, the outstanding success associated with TKA, and the gradual expansion of TKA indications to include younger patients. Recent literature has focused primarily on assessment of new surgical techniques and prosthetic designs to optimize patellofemoral function and minimize polyethylene wear. The controversies regarding the proper role of the posterior cruciate ligament in TKA and whether the patella should be resurfaced during TKA are under investigation. The increase in prospective, randomized trials evaluating the various aspects of TKA is laudable.

Patient Selection and Outcomes

The primary indications for TKA include pain, functional impairment, and radiographic evidence of intra-articular disease in a relatively sedentary individual. The excellent patient satisfaction and clinical function achieved with TKA make knee replacement one of the most successful surgical procedures currently available. In many clinical series, > 95% survival rates of tibial and femoral fixation have been reported at 10 to 15 years' follow-up. Because of the long-term durabilty and excellent clinical results of TKA, the indications have slowly expanded to include younger and more active patients. In 114 patients with osteoarthritis who had cemented posterior stabilized TKA at an average age of 51 years (range, 21 to 55 years), 94% of femoral and tibial components survived for 18 years. This survival rate was 90% when patellar revisions were included.

Contraindications to TKA include active infection, severe neurologic compromise of the extremity, prior knee arthrodesis, extensor mechanism disruption, and severe recurvatum deformity of the knee. Although some investigators have performed TKA for selected patients with a knee arthrodesis, an extensor mechanism disruption, or severe recurvatum deformity, caution is advised because there are many special considerations regarding surgical technique and prosthetic design when performing TKA for these patients. It is important to emphasize that specific indications for TKA cannot be considered in an isolated manner. Rather, all variables, such as age, medical comorbidities, psychological components, and technical considerations, must be integrated when recommending surgical intervention.

Despite the excellent results of TKA in most patients, emerging data from outcome studies suggest that it may be possible to identify patients at risk for a less favorable outcome. Medical conditions such as Parkinson's disease or rheumatoid arthritis may cause reduction of function reflected in overall knee scores; however, pain relief and implant survival are comparable to those of the typical primary TKA. Patients with diabetes mellitus have more early complications, fewer good and excellent knee scores, and worse long-term outcomes than control patients.

Reports of TKA after failed proximal tibial valgus osteotomy continue to suggest a more complicated surgery with inferior clinical results when compared to typical primary TKA. These observations contrast with those for supracondylar varus femoral osteotomies, which do not appear to affect the clinical outcome of subsequent TKA. Preoperative assessment of patients older than 75 years reveals that poorer mental health scores, decreased physical function, and increased bodily pain scores are associated with poorer outcomes; appraisal of baseline psychological status and social functioning may help identify patient subsets at risk for a poor functional outcome.

Surgical Approaches

The medial parapatellar approach is used most often for TKA; however, alternative surgical approaches are being investigated and have shown favorable results in patellofemoral function and stability. The midvastus approach, which separates the vastus medialis muscle in the direction of its fibers beginning at the superior pole of the patella, was shown to be an efficacious alternative to the medial parapatellar approach in 118 randomized TKAs; in a retrospective comparison, 50% of the TKAs done through a parapatellar approach required a lateral retinacular release compared with only 3% of TKAs using a midvastus approach. The subvastus approach, which leaves the entire vastus medialis obliquus intact, required lateral retinacular release in 27.5% compared with 51% for the parapatellar approach.

Surgical approaches for the difficult primary TKA exposure include the use of a quadriceps snip, a V-Y turndown quadricepsplasty, or an extended tibial tubercle osteotomy. The quadriceps snip does not induce additional weakness when compared with the contralateral TKA and requires no special postoperative precautions or special rehabilitation. An extended tibial tubercle and tibial crest osteotomy can be useful, and fixation usually is obtained with multiple screws or wires. Nonunion, displacement, and tibial shaft fracture have been reported complications following osteotomy.

Soft-Tissue Balancing

The collateral ligaments should be balanced throughout the motion arc although the presence of slight varus-valgus laxity in the midflexion range is expected. There is no consensus on the proper sequence of soft-tissue releases; however, the valgus knee often has been associated with postoperative instability after extensive lateral soft-tissue release. A new method of intra-articular release for the valgus knee, which usually spares the lateral collateral ligament and lengthens rather than transects the iliotibial tract, can significantly improve postoperative stability.

Limb Alignment

The entry point for proper femoral intramedullary (IM) alignment is medial to the notch center. Preoperative templating of the anatomic axis helps to determine when to use a medial entry point, because central entry in these knees will cause excessive valgus malalignment. Medial femoral bowing or a capacious femoral canal also can lead to inconsistent cuts when using IM systems. IM goniometers may facilitate more accurate distal femoral preparation than standard instruments. IM tibial cutting guides are as accurate as conventional extramedullary guides; however, tibias with coronal plane bowing deformity lead to a less than ideal cut with IM systems.

Femoral Component Rotation

There is considerable interest in establishing the proper femoral rotation to optimize knee kinematics, improve patellar tracking, and facilitate soft-tissue balancing. The 3 basic anatomic landmarks used to determine femoral rotation include: (1) the posterior condylar (PC) axis, (2) the transepicondylar (TE) axis, and (3) the AP axis (Fig. 4). In general, the AP axis is perpendicular to the TE axis, which is externally rotated an average of 3° in relationship to the PC axis. There is variation of up to 10° in this relationship because use of the PC axis in the valgus knee with severe posterior bone loss induces internal femoral component rotation, whereas in the varus knee the PC axis often correlates with the other axes. It is probably best to be familiar with the use of all 3 axes when assessing femoral component rotation because localization of the medial epicondylar sulcus often may be indistinct when defining the TE axis, and severe

trochlear wear or trochlear dysplasia obscures discernment of the AP axis.

An analogous method of determining the femoral rotational axis is to base the posterior femoral bone resection on a line perpendicular to the tibial shaft axis. The tibial shaft axis method usually correlates with the TE axis. Clinically, these femoral rotational landmarks appear to be helpful by decreasing the need for lateral retinacular release (LRR), increasing the total flexion arc, decreasing the incidence of medial tibial pain, and decreasing the incidence of patellar fracture. Some instrumentation systems and prosthetic designs account for an additional 3° of external femoral rotation; however, this averaging approach does not account for the large individual variation of these rotational axes between knees and may result in significant component malrotation.

Patellar Preparation

The decision of whether or not to resurface the patella during TKA has been evaluated in several randomized clinical trials. In 100 TKAs, significantly less pain and better knee flexor torques were observed in the group that did not have patellar resurfacing, while knee function scores, stair climbing, and knee extensor torques were similar. In a bilateral comparison study, no differences were noted in subjective performance, ascending or descending stairs, or the incidence of anterior knee pain. Anterior knee pain requiring reoperation for patellar resurfacing was noted in 2 separate studies. Currently, the use of an appropriate prosthetic design with careful surgical technique in selected patients permits the surgeon to decide whether or not to perform patellar resurfacing during TKA.

LRR for intraoperative correction of patellar maltracking should be performed if deemed necessary; however, postoperative problems associated with LRR include pain, wound healing complications, longer rehabilitation, and patellar fracture. Preservation of the superior geniculate artery during a lateral release does not appear to have any effect on patellar loosening or fracture. In addition, proper rotation of the femoral and tibial components and accurate reproduction of original patellar height can help minimize the need for LRR (Fig. 5). In 121 TKAs with a slightly reduced postoperative patellar composite height (average, 1.58 mm), the LRR rate was reduced to 12.4% compared with 55% in 100 control TKAs. Careful attention to patellar thickness and use of the TE axis further reduced the need for LRR to less than 2%.

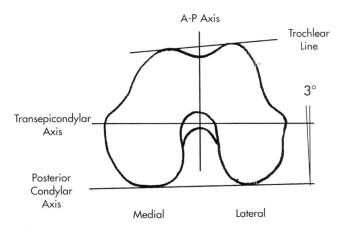

Figure 4

Femoral rotation landmarks.

Prosthesis Design

In general, the long-term results of TKA have been extremely favorable with total condylar knee designs. Historically,

Femoral Component Rotation

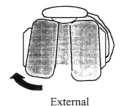
External

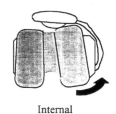
Internal

Patellar Component Translation

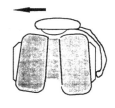
Medialized

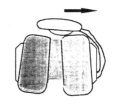
Lateralized

Patellar Thickness

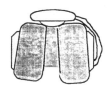
Anatomic

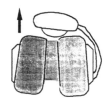
Increased

Figure 5

Component positioning in relation to patellar tracking.

posterior cruciate ligament (PCL) substituting designs have been associated with more patellofemoral problems, whereas PCL-retaining designs have been associated with more osteolysis and polyethylene wear problems related to flat-on-flat articular designs. Changes to improve patellofemoral tracking and increase the tibiofemoral conformity are key elements in current prosthetic designs aimed at improved long-term outcomes. The concept of careful balancing of the PCL to allow more favorable femoral component kinematics is important in the relationship between prosthetic design and surgical technique.

Femoral components associated with a higher incidence of patellar maltracking and more frequent revision patellofemoral surgery tend to have features that include a short and narrow anterior flange, a shallow trochlea, an abrupt anteri-

or to distal transition of the patellar groove, and a larger radius of curvature. Many new prosthetic designs emphasize improvement of patellofemoral function by closely replicating the position and orientation of the anatomic femoral trochlea. This improvement has required deepening the trochlear groove and aligning the trochlea in a valgus anatomic position in most designs. In a gait analysis of 2 prosthetic designs differing only in the shape and depth of the trochlear notch, significant functional differences during the late stance phase of stair climbing were observed in the patients with a nonanatomic trochlear design. In a biomechanical patellofemoral tracking study, in which 3 prostheses with recent design changes to the patellofemoral articulation were compared, there were no significant patellar tracking differences.

Controversy regarding the role of the PCL continues, and results of several clinical studies suggest strong consideration of a PCL-substituting TKA for a varus contracture of at least 15°, knees with prior patellectomy, and patients with rheumatoid arthritis. Studies that deal with the theoretical advantages of cruciate-substituting versus cruciate-retaining TKA have revealed the following: (1) preservation of the PCL does not appear to improve proprioception after TKA; (2) the ability to reproduce normal PCL strains after cruciate-retaining TKA occurs in less than 37% of patients (in 1 study); (3) normal femoral rollback has been more reproducible in cruciate-substituting than in cruciate-retaining TKA or cruciate sacrificed TKA; (4) paradoxical anterior femoral translation and lateral liftoff often are observed with cruciate-retaining TKA, and cruciate-substituting TKA more closely reproduces normal joint kinematics; (5) new stair climbing gait analysis revealed that cruciate substituting and retaining TKA are equivalent and both are superior to cruciate sacrificing TKA; and (6) in a prospective study, the ROM was significantly better in cruciate-substituting than in cruciate-retaining TKA.

The long-term studies of cemented TKA have set the standard that other fixation methods must achieve, although durable results have been reported with some cementless designs. The 14-year survivorship of 106 consecutive cemented total condylar TKAs was 95.6%. Similarly, the survival of cemented cruciate-substituting TKAs at 11 years was 96.4%. Ten-year survival of the cemented cruciate-retaining TKA has been more variable because of different design issues, such as flat-on-flat articular surfaces; however, 10- to 12-year survival rates of 96% to 98% are being reported. The overall 10-year survival rate of 163 cementless TKAs was 94%, and when only loosening or revision of the tibial or femoral components was the criterion for failure, the 10-year survival rate was 96.7%.

The incidence of osteolysis associated with the use of screws and cemented tibial fixation with a press-fit femoral component was 30%, with a press-fit femoral component and cemented tibial component without screws it was 10%, and with a cemented femoral component with a cemented tibia and no screws it was 0. The configuration of porous coating on the undersurface of the tibial component appears to contribute to the extent of osteolysis. Tibial trays with patches of porous coating connected by smooth metal tracks had more osteolysis than components with uninterrupted porous coating, suggesting that the smooth tracks conduct polyethylene debris. A tibial component, designed for cement fixation of the tray and biologic fixation of porous coated stems and pegs, has been reported to have good clinical results at short-term follow-up.

Polyethylene Wear

Ultra-high molecular weight polyethylene (UHMWPE) wear is multifactorial, including the manufacturing process, articular geometry, limb alignment, type of material used for the femoral component, thickness of the polyethylene, and modularity of tibial inserts. Male gender, younger age, increased patient weight, and the underlying diagnosis of osteoarthritis are statistically significant patient factors. The amount of UHMWPE wear correlates with the number of loose beads.

Oxidation resulting from gamma sterilization in air significantly decreases the resistance of UHMWPE to fatigue and wear, and this effect is potentiated by prolonging the length of shelf life prior to implantation. Ethylene oxide sterilization resulted in less UHMWPE wear than sterilization with gamma radiation in air in 1 study. In a finite element analysis of 8 different contemporary knee designs, the advantage of designs with more conforming articulating surfaces and thicker UHMWPE components was validated. An in vitro model of UHMWPE cold extrusion suggests that a minimum thickness of 12 mm is required to eliminate cold extrusion. A high revision rate (21.5%) of the femoral-tibial articulation in 186 knee replacements with a flat articular surface at an average follow-up of 6.1 years was attributed to polyethylene wear in 57.5% of knees. Comparison of polyethylene wear in 2 groups of patients with the same prosthetic design but different materials and processing methods for the polyethylene tibial inserts suggests that improved quality control can improve the wear characteristics of UHMWPE.

Perioperative Considerations

Cost containment issues have modified current thinking regarding many perioperative aspects of TKA, and many studies have been performed to specifically address these issues. Several studies have compared TKA outcomes with and without the use of a tourniquet during the operation. In a randomized study of 80 patients, there was no significant difference in the total operating time or overall blood loss; however, in the patients without tourniquet use there was less postoperative pain, earlier knee flexion and straight-leg raising, and fewer superficial wound infections and deep venous thromboses. In another randomized study, the effects were compared of timing of tourniquet release after wound closure and bandaging or tourniquet release before quadriceps closure to achieve hemostasis. Operating times and postoperative blood loss were similar, yet less postoperative pain and fewer wound complications were observed in patients with efforts at hemostasis. In another study, 3 patient groups included no tourniquet, a tourniquet for cementing only, and a tourniquet for the entire operation. The incidence of deep venous thrombosis was not related to tourniquet use, but blood loss was significantly increased without the use of a tourniquet.

Postoperative Pain In a randomized, double-blind trial of 82 patients, the patients who received an intra-articular injection of 0.5% bupivacaine and 1:200,000 epinephrine after wound closure used less morphine in the first 24 hours after the operation and experienced better knee flexion at discharge. In another similar trial of 105 TKAs, no difference in the use of postoperative morphine was noted with the use of postoperative intra-articular bupivacaine or morphine. In 90 TKAs, no correlation was seen between the use of cryotherapy and use of postoperative morphine.

Range of Motion Several studies of the use of continuous passive motion (CPM) machines reveal no significant differences in time of hospital discharge or final ROM. A maximal early flexion routine of 70° to 100° with CPM appears to reduce the length of the hospital stay and increase motion at 1 year. In a prospective study of 103 TKAs, knee scores and ROM did not differ at 2 years, but more manipulations were necessary in the non-CPM group. Cost analysis suggests that CPM may be a cost-effective method to increase short-term flexion and decrease the need for knee manipulation. Knees closed at 90° of flexion and rehabilitated with early passive flexion (drop and dangle) and no CPM had less drainage, earlier hospital discharge, and better extension than knees with CPM. In a study of 108 patients, knees closed in 90° to 110° of flexion required less home physical therapy and had significantly better flexion measurements at all time intervals than knees closed in extension. In a randomized prospective study of 75 TKAs, there was no effect on early rehabilitation of the degree of knee flexion at the time of capsular closure. Final ROM appears to correlate best with preoperative ROM.

Complications Associated With Total Knee Arthroplasty

Although the majority of TKAs are extremely successful, this procedure has potential complications. The issues of infection and thromboembolic disease associated with TKA are discussed elsewhere.

Fat Embolism

Embolic showers seen by transesophageal echocardiography can be reduced with the use of extramedullary guide systems. Newer extramedullary systems are being developed to match the accuracy of intramedullary systems. However, in 1 study, no difference in the incidence of venous emboli was noted with the use of extramedullary or intramedullary guide systems. These investigators believe that venous emboli arise from the thrombogenic effect of the tourniquet rather than intramedullary instrumentation. Although fat embolism is a multifactorial problem, simultaneous bilateral TKA procedures appear to be associated with a higher prevalence of this condition.

Neurovascular

The cumulative prevalence of peroneal palsy after TKA has been reported to be 0.58%. In 32 TKAs with associated peroneal nerve palsies, epidural anesthesia for postoperative pain, previous lumbar laminectomy, and preoperative valgus deformity (especially when combined with a flexion contracture) were statistically significant predisposing factors. Diagnosis usually is made in the first few days after surgery, and initial treatment should include loosening of any constricting dressings and flexion of the knee between 20° and 30°. Intraoperative exploration of the peroneal nerve in high-risk patients and early postoperative exploration remain controversial. There are no data supporting early postoperative exploration of the nerve, except when there is clear evidence of a compressive hematoma. For patients with no recovery of peroneal nerve function after 2 months of nonsurgical treatment, surgical decompression of perineural fibrosis may be worthwhile.

The prevalence of arterial complication with TKA is 0.03% to 0.2%. Absent pedal pulses and arterial calcification on preop-

erative radiographs are predisposing factors. Direct injury to vascular structures can be minimized when thorough knowledge of the arterial anatomy about the knee joint is combined with careful surgical technique. Rapid diagnosis and treatment are essential to optimize the outcome.

Periprosthetic Fractures

Fractures associated with TKA can occur in the femur, tibia, or patella, and the treatment approach is clarified by categorizing them into intraoperative and postoperative fractures. Most intraoperative fractures are nondisplaced or minimally displaced fractures that occur during component insertion or with component removal during a revision procedure. Intraoperative, intercondylar distal femoral fracture is a complication of posterior stabilized TKA that can be avoided with careful resection technique and size verification with an intercondylar sizing guide.

Postoperative supracondylar femoral fractures can be classified as type I, undisplaced fractures associated with a stable or well-functioning prosthesis; type II, displaced fractures that have resulted in unacceptable alignment of the extremity or the prosthetic components; and type III, either nondis-

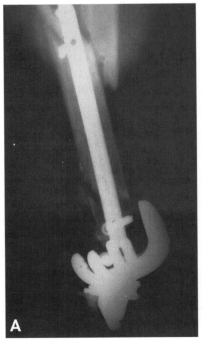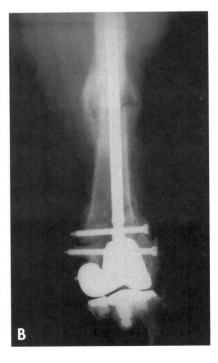

Figure 6

Treatment of supracondylar fracture with intramedullary nail with interlocking screws. A, Femoral fracture in the early postoperative period at the proximal end of a supracondylar nail used for fixation of a supracondylar fracture above a total knee implant. B, Salvage was obtained with a full-length, locked retrograde nail.

placed or displaced supracondylar fractures adjacent to a failing implant. Closed treatment for type I fractures generally is recommended; type II fractures are managed best with surgical fixation such as plate and screw fixation. The use of supracondylar intramedullary nails for these fractures has gained popularity (Fig. 6). Type III fractures can be treated in 1 of 2 ways: by initially treating only the fracture and then revising the implant at a later date or by incorporating the fracture treatment into the implant revision procedure.

Periprosthetic tibial fractures associated with TKA can be classified into 4 anatomic fracture types (Fig. 7). Type I fractures involve the tibial metaphysis and adjacent tibial baseplate, type II fractures occur in the metaphyseal-diaphyseal region adjacent to the tibial stem, type III generally are diaphyseal fractures that occur below the tibial stem tip, and type IV fractures involve the tibial tubercle. Fractures can be further subclassified as postoperative A (a well-fixed prosthesis) or postoperative B (a radiographically loose prosthesis), and intraoperative C. A fracture associated with a loose prosthesis is managed best with revision surgery, and fractures associated with well-fixed prostheses can be managed with the usual principles of tibial fracture management.

In general, patellar fractures in which the quadriceps mechanism remains intact can be treated nonsurgically, and those with quadriceps disruption require surgery.

Extensor Mechanism Problems

A variation of the patellar clunk syndrome, the "patellar catch syndrome," has been described in a cruciate-retaining knee design that has a wide intercondylar space and a shorter posterior extension of the intercondylar notch. This phenomenon was observed in 11 of 192 (5.7%) TKAs, all with this spe-

cific prosthetic design and unresurfaced patellae. The mechanism includes entrapment of the superior pole of the patella in the intercondylar notch at 60° to 90° of flexion, and the problem often can be treated by shaving off the superior pole of the patella or by resurfacing the patella. Higher rates of complications occurred with metal-backed components, a diagnosis of osteoarthritis, or obesity.

Heterotopic Ossification

The largest areas of heterotopic ossification usually are located on the anterior aspect of the distal femur after TKA. Marked hypertrophic arthrosis and excessive periosteal damage to the anterior femur are associated with the development of postoperative heterotopic ossification. This is correlated with restriction of postoperative motion and an increased lumbar bone density index.

Hemarthrosis

Recurrent hemarthrosis after TKA is most commonly caused by entrapment of synovial tissue or the fat pad between the prosthetic surfaces; however, in most patients the etiology remains unknown. Treatment includes aspiration, rest, ice, and discontinuation of medications that alter hemostasis. Recurrent symptoms often require open synovectomy with tibial insert exchange to allow access to the posterior compartment.

Arthroscopy of Total Knee Arthroplasty

The overall success rate for arthroscopic treatment of 40 TKAs was 73%. Specific surgical diagnoses included patellar clunks in 82%, other soft-tissue impingement syndromes in 60%, and arthrofibrosis in 63%. In another study of 29 TKAs, arthroscopic resection of fibrous plicae apparently resolved symptoms in 25; in another study of 48 knees, arthroscopic treatment of peripatellar fibrosis was unpredictable. The latter authors recommended that specific limited goals be established before surgery.

The popliteus tendon may cause a painful snap as it rolls over the overhanging edge of the metallic posterior femoral condyle or a retained lateral femoral osteophyte. If this phenomenon is identified during the operation, removal of all osteophytes and, if necessary, surgical release of the femoral insertion are beneficial. After arthroplasty, arthroscopic release of the painful popliteus tendon has been described for this condition.

A symptomatic pseudomeniscus after TKA can be treated with arthroscopic debridement. Arthroscopic release of the PCL for a stiff TKA, at a mean interval of 29 months after TKA, was deemed successful in 8 of 9 patients. ROM increased from 74° of flexion before arthroscopy to 112° at final

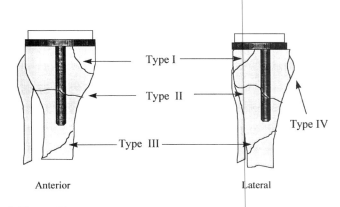

Type I

Type II

Type III

Type IV

Anterior

Lateral

Figure 7
Periprosthetic tibial fracture classification.

follow-up. Because of the increased risk of infection associated with arthroscopy of TKA, perioperative antibiotics are recommended for these procedures.

Skin and Wound

Lateral skin flap numbness with a midline incision typically involves an area of more than 40 cm² and does not improve with time in most patients. A 20% incidence of suture reaction with subcuticular wound closure using polydioxanone suture compared with no suture reactions using polyglycolic acid suture suggests that subcuticular polydioxanone be avoided in TKA. Aggressive wound management of superficial wound healing problems and early soft-tissue coverage of full-thickness skin slough are essential.

Evaluation of the Painful Knee

TKA is among the most reliable, predictable procedures in orthopaedic surgery for relieving pain and restoring knee function. Nevertheless, some patients will have significant persistent symptoms or will develop symptoms postoperatively. A thorough history and physical examination are crucial in making an accurate diagnosis. This requires a greater time investment on the part of the orthopaedic surgeon than evaluating a straightforward symptomatic knee with severe degenerative arthritis prior to a primary TKA. Examining the patient on more than 1 occasion is helpful to ensure that findings are consistent and to allow the surgeon to develop a rapport with the patient to better interpret the findings. Combining selective use of diagnostic tests with history and physical examination should allow for an accurate diagnosis in most symptomatic total knees.

History

It is helpful to determine the history of the primary surgical procedure. Persistent swelling or drainage after the original arthroplasty is associated with a higher risk of subsequent infection. It is important to determine whether primary wound healing occurred and whether good pain relief was obtained from the primary arthroplasty. It is useful to determine specifically if the current symptoms are different from the original symptoms for which the patient underwent the primary arthroplasty. If the current symptoms are exactly like those that existed prior to the original operation, the question arises as to whether the original diagnosis was in error.

At the outset, the exact nature of the patient's complaint must be established. Although pain is frequently given as a reason for seeking consultation, more specific questioning may elicit an actual problem of giving way, weakness, or swelling. Weakness may be a manifestation of spinal stenosis, and giving way may be caused by muscle atrophy or by quadriceps weakness or inhibition. Once it is established as the primary problem, pain should be localized as precisely as possible. Radicular pain points to a possible lumbar spine origin, medial thigh pain occasionally is referred from the hip, and pain in the thigh or calf may be of vascular origin. If the pain is localized to a very small area and can be consistently located with a single finger, a neuroma or localized bursitis may be the cause. Pain that is well localized in the anterior portion of the knee frequently is of patellofemoral origin. Pain in the posterior, popliteal region is less common and points to the possibility of a popliteal cyst, pseudaneurysm, or deep vein thrombosis. Most often, the pain is more diffuse in nature, but is localized in the immediate vicinity of the knee joint.

Start-up pain that is worse with the first few steps is most typical of loosening and could represent inadequate ingrowth in a cementless knee or early loosening in a cemented component. Inadequate ingrowth in a cementless knee typically occurs in the first or second year, whereas loosening of a cemented knee usually occurs much later. Pain that occurs at night or that is constant and unrelated to activity may indicate infection. Popping and clicking associated with the pain may indicate the presence of meniscal remnants, loose bodies, or a patellar clunk syndrome.

A patient's social history may also be relevant. Patients receiving workers' compensation have been shown to have less predictable results after TKA. The physician also needs to be aware if there is pending litigation or legal action regarding the knee. If a patient is taking antidepressants or is being treated for a psychiatric condition, it may affect the way he or she interprets symptoms originating in the knee. In such patients, it is advisable to make sure that the underlying psychiatric condition is being optimally treated before making any definitive decisions on elective reoperation.

Physical Examination

It is useful to first focus on extrinsic causes of pain. Careful examination of the lumbar spine is warranted if there is any radicular component to the pain. Examination of the hip should be routine. If hip rotation is limited or if ROM of the hip reproduces pain in the knee, radiographs should be obtained. In some cases injecting the hip with local anesthetic is useful to determine if the knee symptoms are alleviated. The feet should be examined for peripheral neuropathy and neurovascular status. Absent pulses may indicate peripheral vascular disease, which may cause symptoms and warrants vascular evaluation. After careful evaluation for extrinsic causes of knee pain, the knee joint should be examined. It is helpful to watch patients walk with and without assistive devices and with the knee joint clearly visible. Collapse of the knee into varus or valgus with weightbearing may indicate ligamentous instability or component loosening and subsidence (Fig. 8). Patients that go into hyperextension or back knee deformity with weightbearing may have developed posterior cruciate insufficiency or excessive posterior wear.

The knee should be observed for swelling or effusion, which may indicate the presence of infection or particulate wear debris. Shiny skin that is hypersensitive raises the suspicion of reflex sympathetic dystrophy. The leg and foot should be observed for vascular changes, such as discoloration or abnormal hair distribution, that may indicate the presence of vascular insufficiency. Careful palpation about the knee also yields helpful information. Point tenderness of the proximal medial tibia, for instance, may represent pes anserine bursitis. Point tenderness and crepitus at the joint line may indicate a symptomatic remnant of soft tissue or impingement of an underlying prominence, such as an osteophyte, cementophyte, or overhanging implant. Point tenderness away from the joint line may be from a neuroma. Presence of a Tinel's sign and elimination of the point tenderness by a local injection support a diagnosis of neuroma. Authors of a recent study have recommended neuroma excision in this clinical situation.

ROM, both active and passive, as well as the presence of crepitation with active motion should be recorded. Grinding may be associated with a metal-backed patella that has dissociated. Patellar clunk also is associated with distinctive audible popping as the knee goes from flexion into extension. Extension lag is most often caused by laxity in the extensor mechanism. The degree of maximum active flexion also is important to record because decreased postoperative flexion is most closely correlated with lack of flexion preoperatively.

Stability should be tested after ROM is measured. Opening to varus and valgus stress should be recorded in extension as well as 30° and 90° of flexion. It should be noted whether there is a firm end point on stress testing. Laxity to stress testing is typically recorded as 1+, 2+, and 3+ as with a knee ligament examination. Sagittal plane laxity should also be tested.

Finally, the patellofemoral joint should be the specific focus of careful physical examination. Patellofemoral problems are

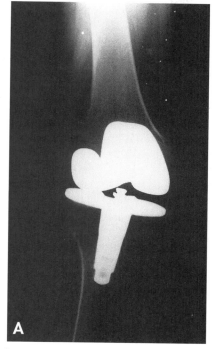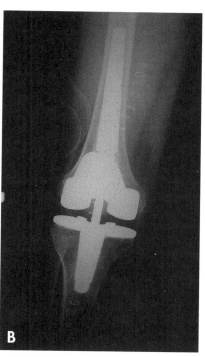

Figure 8

Weightbearing radiograph demonstrates ligamentous imbalance with medial opening and valgus deformity (A). Release of the lateral ligaments from the femur along with revision to a posterior stabilized type femoral component with a thicker insert corrected the symptomatic giving way with weightbearing (B).

the most common single cause of reoperation after primary TKA and thus deserve special attention. Patellar tracking should be watched during active and passive flexion and extension of the knee and compared to that of the contralateral side, particularly if the other side is normal and asymptomatic. The presence of tilting, crepitus, or clunking often indicates a problem with patellar tracking. The patella should be palpated and ballotted to determine if pain can be reproduced with these maneuvers, and patellar mobility should be checked with the knee slightly flexed. Lack of mobility may indicate excessive scarring or patella baja, which is often associated with loss of motion. Hypermobility and apprehension from laterally directed pressure is suggestive of lateral subluxation of the patella, particularly if this reproduces the patient's symptoms.

Radiographic Evaluation

The next step in arriving at a diagnosis of a symptomatic knee after TKA is careful review of sequential plain radiographs. Initial postoperative radiographs should be reviewed for radiolucent lines at the bone-cement interface or the implant-bone interface. Extensive radiolucencies that have developed over a short period of time have an entirely different meaning than those that may have been present on the immediate postoperative radiographs and have not progressed. Radiolucent lines at the bone-cement interface are a common finding after cemented TKA. Incomplete radiolucencies over a minority of the interface do not correlate with the presence of loosening. A complete radiolucent line that is progressive and 1 to 2 mm in thickness is consistent with loosening. Component subsidence or change in position is the most specific finding indicative of component loosening. Because the implant-bone interface is more difficult to assess with cementless components, fluoroscopic examination is helpful. The tibial component is best assessed using AP fluoroscopy, while the implant-bone interface of the femoral component is best assessed on a lateral view.

A current full-length film including the hip, knee, and ankle is useful for determining component alignment. Ideally, the femoral component should be aligned at 90° to the mechanical axis, and the tibial component should be oriented at 90° to the axis of the tibial shaft. On the lateral view, the anterior flange of the femoral component should be parallel with the anterior cortex of the femur. The orientation of the tibial component on the lateral view depends somewhat on the type of component. Cruciate-retaining implants are generally positioned in 7° of posterior slope while cruciate-substituting designs are frequently implanted at 0° to 3° of posterior slope.

The lateral view is useful in assessing the thickness of the patellar cut. Underresection of the patella, leaving a thick bone fragment, may be associated with a lack of motion or patellofemoral symptoms. A lateral view also is useful in measuring the AP dimension of the femoral component, which can be compared to the AP dimension of the contralateral normal knee. An increase in the AP dimension can be associated with lack of motion, while a decrease can be associated with instability, particularly in flexion. Patella baja can be assessed on the lateral view, and can cause restricted flexion. Elevation of the joint is a common cause. Excessive rollback of the femoral component in a cruciate-retaining knee can also be seen on the lateral view. This problem may be indicative of excessive tightness in the PCL that can cause pain and lack of flexion.

Although these measurements give useful information as to the static alignment of

the components, plain radiographs may be used to determine dynamic alignment as well. Weightbearing radiographs give information on ligament balance as well as component alignment (Figs. 8 and 9). If the patient is unable to bear weight to assess ligamentous balance, stress views can be obtained. The sunrise view or other tangential views are useful in assessing the patellofemoral joint. Although small degrees of tilt may not be clinically significant, gross subluxation or dislocation may be apparent on a tangential view. In addition, direct contact of a metal-backed patella with the femoral component may be apparent on a tangential view, indicating polyethylene wear-through or dissociation.

Radionuclide Evaluation

In a small percentage of cases, the fixation status of total knee components remains in doubt after careful review of plain radiographs. In these problematic cases, nuclear medicine scans are used to try to diagnose loosening and infection as well as to differentiate loosening from infection. Studies of asymptomatic knees, however, have shown that increased uptake is present in many components that persists for several years, particularly with cementless knee replacements. Therefore, a single scan is not nearly as helpful as a comparison with previous scans. Using indium In 111, an accuracy of 84%, sensitivity of 83%, and specificity of 85% have been obtained in the diagnosis of infection. False positives have

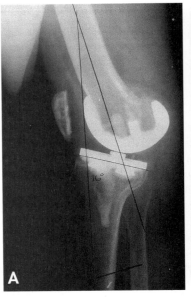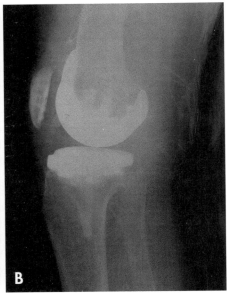

Figure 9

A standing lateral view demonstrates hyperextension of the knee on weightbearing, which was painful (A). Insertion of a more constrained, thicker insert blocked the hyperextension and alleviated the symptoms (B).

been observed in patients with rheumatoid arthritis or osteolysis. An accuracy as high as 95% has been reported for diagnosing infection using a combination of indium In 111 and technetium Tc 99 diphosphonate scanning. Unfortunately, the scans seem to be less helpful in patients with chronic indolent infection. Nuclear medicine scans are most helpful when the knee is entirely normal, in which case it is unlikely that the knee is either infected or loose. Continued observation, further diagnostic investigations, and possibly referral for a second opinion are most appropriate in such cases.

Laboratory Analysis

Although blood cell count, erythrocyte sedimentation rate, and C-reactive protein are often obtained as screening tests for infection, the white blood cell count is the least useful and is only elevated in a minority of cases that prove to be infected. The sedimentation rate has a sensitivity of 60% to 80% when 30 mm per hour is used as the cutoff for diagnosing the infection. The C-reactive protein returns to normal sooner than the erythrocyte sedimentation rate and is therefore more useful in evaluating knees that are within 3 months of the surgical procedure.

The most useful laboratory test by far in evaluating the painful knee is analysis of aspirated fluid. It is important to ascertain whether a patient is on antibiotics at the time of the aspiration or has been on antibiotics in the immediate past because antibiotic use is a major contributor to false negative aspirations. When antibiotics have been used in the recent past, it is prudent to delay aspiration for 4 to 6 weeks. A small percentage of patients may develop an acute exacerbation of infection requiring intervention prior to the desired delay. In patients who have not been on antibiotics, aspirations have been found to be 75% sensitive in detecting infection. If there is a high index of suspicion for infection, performance of repeat aspiration can increase the sensitivity to 85%. A differential blood cell count and analysis of aspirated fluid also are helpful. A white blood cell count of greater than 25,000/mm^3 or greater than 90% polymorphonuclear leukocytes is strongly indicative of infection. Gram stain of aspirated fluid has been found not to be particularly helpful in diagnosing infection. In 1 series, the Gram stain was negative in 32 consecutive cases of infected total joints. In another series looking specifically at total knees, the Gram stain was positive in only 10% of infected total knees. A negative Gram stain is, therefore, not indicative of the absence of infection.

Recently, molecular genetic testing has been described as a useful method of analyzing fluid from painful total knees. A technique has been developed that allows the application of the polymerase chain reaction on aspirated fluid to detect the presence of bacterial DNA. Initial tests reported an accuracy of 100%. Application of this technology to a larger sample size has resulted in an accuracy of approximately 92%. One major advantage of this type of testing is that it is not affected by the presence of antibiotics in the joint fluid. This technique may well prove to be a significant advance in the diagnosis of the infected total knee.

Revision Total Knee Replacement

Whereas the principles of revision TKA are similar to those of primary arthroplasty, numerous additional difficulties are encountered, including soft-tissue scarring, bone loss, flexion-extension imbalance, ligamentous instability, and disturbance of the anatomic joint line. Thorough preoperative planning and meticulous surgical technique are necessary to obtain optimal results.

Preoperative Planning

Evaluation begins with clinical assessment of alignment, ROM, ligamentous stability, status of the extensor mechanism (ie, instability, lag), and signs of infection. Careful evaluation of the skin and soft tissues is paramount, particularly in the location of previous surgical incisions. Radiographs are evaluated to assess bone stock, the presence of osteolysis, the level of the joint line, and the type and status of prosthetic fixation. Laboratory workup, including complete blood count, acute phase reactants, and preoperative aspiration of the knee for cultures is required to rule out infection.

Additional planning should include review of the previous surgical report to determine the size and type of the present prosthetic implant, the method of fixation used, and the extent of previous soft-tissue releases. Preoperative preparation is completed by ordering bone graft in cases of substantial bone loss and appropriate equipment, including extraction devices and revision prosthetic components. Modular TKA systems, which provide modular metal augmentations, various options of prosthetic constraint, and diaphyseal engaging stems, are helpful in managing the problems of bone loss, instability, joint line restoration, and prosthetic fixation.

Surgical Technique

Use of the previous surgical incision is recommended whenever possible. If long parallel incisions exist, choice of the lateralmost skin incision is favorable to avoid a large lateral skin flap that has been compromised at the time of the initial lateral skin incision. Transcutaneous oxygen measurements, both before and after skin incisions about the knee, have demonstrated reduced oxygenation of the lateral skin region. In complex situations, such as knees with multiple skin incisions or previously burned or irradiated skin, obtaining a plastic surgery consultation may be necessary, both for the design of the upcoming skin incision and for consideration of preoperative muscle flap procedures if the risk of skin necrosis is substantial. Soft-tissue expansion techniques also have been shown to be beneficial in reducing skin necrosis in complex cases.

Because of intra-articular scarring from previous surgical procedures, exposure, particularly eversion of the extensor mechanism, can be demanding. Techniques to assist exposure include performing a longer capsulotomy, release of intra-articular adhesions, extensive release of the deep medial collateral ligament to allow increased external rotation of the tibia (relieving tension on the extensor mechanism), and early lateral retinacular release to assist patellar eversion. If exposure difficulties remain after these maneuvers, extensile exposure options, such as a quadriceps snip, modified V-Y quadricepsplasty, or extended tibial tubercle osteotomy, are required (Fig. 10). Use of the quadriceps snip has gained in popularity because of favorable exposure, minimal postoperative morbidity (such as extensor lag or tendinous disruption) and the ability to proceed with customary postoperative rehabilitation programs.

Prosthetic components must be removed with patience to decrease bone loss. Numerous devices are available including thin osteotomes, a Gigli saw (best for cementless devices), and universal or prosthesis-specific extractors. When removing cemented prostheses, it is best to initially disrupt the prosthesis-cement rather than the cement-bone interface. This sequencing is better to preserve bone because the cement can be secondarily removed under direct vision with less bone loss after the prosthetic components are initially removed.

After component removal, bone and soft-tissue deficits, the level of the joint line, flexion-extension balance, and symmetry are assessed. The remaining sequence of surgical events varies, but typically initially involves reconstruction of the tibial plateau because this affects dimensions of both the flexion and extension spaces. The flexion gap is then reconstructed followed by balancing of the extension gap to the flexion gap through additional femoral resection or bone or metal augmentation of the distal femur. Last, the joint line is adjusted, the patellofemoral joint reconstructed, and the wound meticulously closed.

Additional bone resection must be minimized. A general principle is to remove only 1 to 2 mm of bone from the most prominent femoral or tibial condyle to provide a platform onto which cutting guides can be placed. Contralateral condylar defects are later treated with bone graft or metal prosthetic augmentation. The scientific data are unclear regarding whether it is better to use bone graft or prosthetic augmentations to reconstruct bone deficits. Both options appear to work well if prosthetic components are well fixed in a knee with good alignment and stability. If metal prosthetic augmentations are chosen, biomechanical studies favor rectangular over angular augmentations because of reduction in shear stress at the fixation interface, although both designs have performed equally well clinically.

Prosthetic components are selected based on intraoperative findings. Prosthetic constraint should be minimized to enhance the durability of fixation. In many patients, however, PCL deficiency is common and the choice of a posterior cruciate-substituting device is wise. In most revisions, either large bony defects or weak remaining condylar bone is encountered, necessitating the use of either press-fit or cemented diaphyseal engaging stems for additional support and load distribution (Fig. 11). These methods of stem fixation have had equivalent results. Press-fit stems provide the advantage of easier removal and improved remaining bone stock should additional revision arthroplasty become necessary. Cemented stems are favored in cases with anatomic osseous distortion or when adequate fixation is not obtained with press-fit designs.

Prosthetic components must be posi-

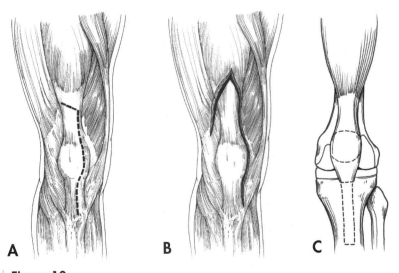

Figure 10

Schematic diagram demonstrating extensile exposure options available in cases of complex revision total knee arthroplasty. Options include quadriceps snip (A), V-Y turndown (B), and tibial tubercle osteotomy (C).

tioned to restore the mechanical axis. Data from recent studies have shown the importance of restoring rotational component alignment to enhance both symmetry and balance of the flexion and extension spaces as well as patellofemoral tracking. These reports suggest placement of the femoral component externally rotated 3° to 4° relative to the posterior condylar line is optimal (Fig. 4). This is best accomplished by placement of the femoral component parallel to the transepicondylar axis, which usually remains as an anatomic landmark, even in cases of substantial distal femoral bone loss.

Previous analyses have shown restoration of the joint line to within 8 mm of its normal anatomic level enhances TKA performance and durability. Determination of the anatomic joint line can be obtained from review of radiographs of the contralateral knee, if it is normal, or assessment of the original radiograph before the index TKA was performed. Additional guidelines include placement of the joint line approximately 1 finger width below the inferior pole of the patella, 1 finger width above the fibular head, level with the old meniscal scar, 2.53 cm distal to the lateral epicondyle, or 3.08 cm distal to the medial epicondyle.

Reconstruction of the patellofemoral joint requires restoration of the joint line to assure proper patellar height, accurate placement of all 3 prosthetic components for proper tracking, and soft-tissue balancing of the extensor mechanism via

lateral retinacular release and medial soft-tissue imbrication if necessary. The surgeon must avoid either medial shift or internal rotation of the femoral or tibial components, or lateral positioning of the patellar component on the patella to avoid patellar malalignment. Patellar resurfacing is not possible in all patients because of loss of patellar bone stock. In patients with remaining patellar thickness of less than 12 mm, the surgeon should consider performing a patellar arthroplasty by simply smoothing the remaining patellar articular surface and assuring central tracking. Wound closure must be performed with precision, avoiding excessive wound tension.

Results

Results of revision TKA have been inferior to those of primary TKA. Literature review of results of the 1970s and 1980s reveals numerous reports with clinical success rates of less than 70%. Improvement in results is evident in more recent studies because of improvements in surgical technique and prosthetic design (Table 1). A recent review of treatment of major bone defects with structural allografts in 30 patients revealed 87% satisfactory results. The best results were obtained with use of cement fixation of the implant to allograft along with use of stemmed components, which reduced stress on the allograft, host bone, and fixation inter-

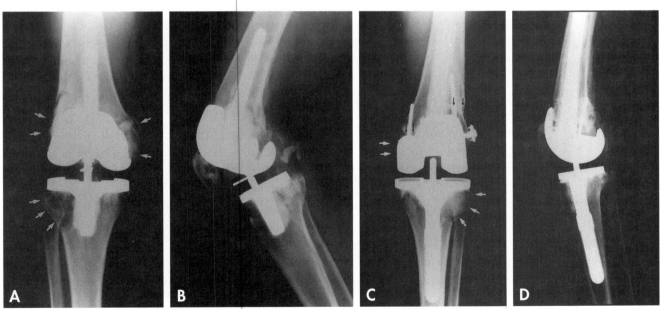

Figure 11

Preoperative anteroposterior (A) and lateral (B) radiographs of a failed revision total knee arthroplasty (TKA) due to femoral component loosening and elevation of the joint line. C, Postoperative anteroposterior and D, lateral radiographs of the repeat revision TKA using structural allografting of the distal femur and proximal tibia (arrows) and diaphyseal-engaging femoral and tibial stems with restoration of an acceptable joint line.

Table 1
Results of revision total knee arthroplasty: The 1990s

Author*	Publication Date	Cases (No.)	Follow Up (yrs)	Satisfactory Results (%)	Complications (%)
Friedman et al	1990	137	5.2	62	6
Mnaymneh et al	1990	10	3.3	58	50
Wilde et al	1990	12	2.7	75	42
Chotivichit et al	1991	18	4.3	78	NA
Rand	1991	21	4.0	50	33
Elia et al	1991	40	3.4	75	30
Hohl et al	1991	29	6.1	72	NA
Rosenberg et al	1991	36	4.0	69	47
Stockley et al	1992	18	4.2	83	28
Mow et al	1994	15	5.6	80	20
Whiteside	1994	163	9.0-11.0	94	10
Murray et al	1994	40	4.8	NA	5
Takahashi et al	1994	39	2.0	NA	21
Tsahakis et al	1994	15	2.1	100	0
Harris et al	1995	14	3.6	93	29
Vince et al	1995	44	2.0-6.0	86	7
Haas et al	1995	76	3.5	84	13
Gustilo et al	1996	56	8.3	73	4
Ghazavi et al	1997	30	4.2	77	23
Engh et al	1997	30	4.2	87	23

*See following "Bibliography" with full references
NA = Data not available

face. Another review of 76 revision TKAs performed with use of modular components with press-fit diaphyseal engaging stems demonstrated 84% good to excellent results at a follow-up of 2 to 9 years.

Knee Fusion and Resection Arthroplasty

Although rarely required, the end-stage procedure for a failed TKA may be fusion or resection arthroplasty. IM rods or external fixation devices have been used for fusion. Resection arthroplasty is usually reserved for the low demand patient and the patient with extensive bone loss.

Annotated Bibliography

Nonarthroplasty Considerations

Akizuki S, Yasukawa Y, Takizawa T: Does arthroscopic abrasion arthroplasty promote cartilage regeneration in osteoarthritic knees with eburnation? A prospective study of high tibial osteotomy with abrasion arthroplasty versus high tibial osteotomy alone. *Arthroscopy* 1997;13:9–17.

In this prospective study, 51 knees treated by osteotomy with abrasion arthroplasty were compared to 37 knees treated only with high tibial osteotomy. Articular cartilage was evaluated by arthroscopy at surgery and 1 year postoperatively; improvement was more common in the abrasion arthroplasty group.

Brittberg M, Lindahl A, Nilsson A, Ohlsson C, Isaksson O, Peterson L: Treatment of deep cartilage defects in the knee with autologous chondrocyte transplantation. *N Engl J Med* 1994; 331:889–895.

Cultured autologous chondrocytes were used to repair full-thickness cartilage defects of the knee in 23 patients. Two years after transplantation, 14 of the 16 patients with femoral condyle transplants had good to excellent results. At 36 months, 5 of 7 patients with patellar transplants had inferior results.

Cartier P, Sanouiller JL, Grelsamer RP: Unicompartmental knee arthroplasty surgery: 10-year minimum follow-up period. *J Arthroplasty* 1996;11:782–788.

Excellent long-term results (93% at 10 to 12 years) are reported for unicompartmental replacements. Slight undercorrection of varus alignment and adequate polyethylene thickness are important for long-term successful outcome.

Finkelstein JA, Gross AE, Davis A: Varus osteotomy of the distal part of the femur: A survivorship analysis. *J Bone Joint Surg* 1996;78A:1348–1352.

In this long-term evaluation of 21 patients after corrective varus osteotomy of the distal femur for lateral compartment osteoarthrosis associated with a valgus deformity, probability of survival at 10 years was 64%, representing a continued deterioration over time compared to an earlier report of survival of 83%.

Gill T, Schemitsch EH, Brick GW, Thornhill TS: Revision total knee arthroplasty after failed unicompartmental knee arthroplasty or high tibial osteotomy. *Clin Orthop* 1995;321:10–18.

A retrospective matched pair comparative analysis was performed after TKA in 30 patients after failed high tibial osteotomy and 30 patients after failed unicompartmental arthroplasty. Average follow-up was 3.8 years with a minimum of 2 years. Results in the osteotomy group were superior to those in the unicompartmental arthroplasty group.

Grelsamer RP: Unicompartmental osteoarthrosis of the knee. *J Bone Joint Surg* 1995;77A:278–292.

This excellent current concepts review discusses the rationale for treatment of unicompartmental arthritis using basic science principles as guidelines.

Levine WN, Ozuna RM, Scott RD, Thornhill TS: Conversion of failed modern unicompartmental arthroplasty to total knee arthroplasty. *J Arthroplasty* 1996;11:797–801.

Revision of modern unicompartmental replacement to TKA was accomplished without the need for structural allografts. Early results are similar to those for primary TKA.

Matsusue Y, Thomson NL: Arthroscopic partial medial meniscectomy in patients over 40 years old: A 5- to 11-year follow-up study. *Arthroscopy* 1996;12:39–44.

The authors report a retrospective study of 68 knees from 65 patients older than 40 years who had a partial medial meniscectomy. The mean follow-up period was 7.8 years (5 to 11 years). Patients with grade III or IV cartilage damage at the time of arthroscopic partial medial meniscectomy had significantly worse results than patients without any significant articular cartilage degeneration at the time of surgery.

Mont MA, Antonaides S, Krackow KA, Hungerford DS: Total knee arthroplasty after failed high tibial osteotomy: A comparison with a matched group. *Clin Orthop* 1994;299:125–130.

The authors reviewed 73 TKAs in 67 patients after a high tibial osteotomy (HTO) at an average follow-up of 73 months (24 to 132). Factors associated with a worse outcome in the HTO patients included (*p* < 0.01): (1) workers' compensation patient, (2) history of reflex sympathetic dystrophy after HTO, (3) less than 1 year or no pain relief after HTO, (4) multiple surgeries before HTO, and (5) occupation as a laborer.

Moseley JB Jr, Wray NP, Kuykendall D, Willis K, Landon G: Arthroscopic treatment of osteoarthritis of the knee: A prospective, randomized, placebo-controlled trial. Results of a pilot study. *Am J SportsMed* 1996;24:28–34.

This pilot study was designed to evaluate the placebo effect of arthroscopic debridement. A placebo group was compared to a group with arthroscopic joint lavage and arthroscopic debridement. All 3 treatment groups appeared to have improvement in pain up to 6 months, suggesting a possible placebo effect of the surgery.

Nagel A, Insall JN, Scuderi GR: Proximal tibial osteotomy: A subjective outcome study. *J Bone Joint Surg* 1996;78A:1353–1358.

This is a retrospective study of the level of participation in work and sport activities of 34 men following proximal tibial osteotomy. The average age of patients at the time of surgery was 49 years; average follow-up was 8 years. The best predictor of postoperative activity was preoperative activity, and the level of activity tended to decrease with time.

Ogilvie-Harris DJ, Weisleder L: Arthroscopic synovectomy of the knee: Is it helpful? *Arthroscopy* 1995;11:91–95.

The authors reviewed 211 arthroscopic synovectomies utilizing a standard 6-portal technique with a minimum 2-year follow-up were reviewed. Good results were noted in patients with rheumatoid arthritis, pigmented villonodular synovitis, and synovial chondromatosis, with 90% experiencing elimination of synovitis and relief of pain. Patients with nonspecific synovitis, seronegative arthritis, and posttraumatic arthritis did not respond as well.

Total Knee Arthroplasty

Barrack RL, Wolfe MW, Waldman DA, Milicic M, Bertot AJ, Myers L: Resurfacing of the patella in total knee arthroplasty: A prospective, randomized, double-blind study. *J Bone Joint Surg* 1997;79A:1121–1131.

In 118 TKAs, at average follow-up of 30 months (range, 24 to 44 months), there were no differences in the overall knee scores, patient satisfaction, or patellar fractures in patients with resurfaced or retained patellae. Of the 60 TKAs without resurfacing, 8 knees (13%) had anterior knee pain and 6 patients (10%) deemed the pain to be severe enough to warrant additional surgery for patellar resurfacing.

Colizza WA, Insall JN, Scuderi GR: The posterior stabilized total knee prosthesis: Assessment of polyethylene damage and osteolysis after a 10-year-minimum follow-up. *J Bone Joint Surg* 1995;77A:1713–1720.

Of 101 TKAs with metal-backed tibial components followed up an average 10 years and 8 months, there were no loose tibial components and minor nonprogressive tibial radiolucencies in only 11%. The preoperative ROM arc of 94° improved to a final ROM arc averaging 110°. Polyethylene wear and osteolysis were not observable problems.

Dennis DA, Komistek RD, Hoff WA, Gabriel SM: In vivo knee kinematics derived using an inverse perspective technique. *Clin Orthop* 1996;331:107–117.

Fluoroscopic video studies of 64 knees demonstrated an anterior position of the average initial contact point (ICP) during full extension in normal knees and posterior stabilized TKAs. The average ICP in posterior cruciate-retaining (CR) TKA and anterior cruciate ligament (ACL) deficient knees was located posterior to the tibial midpoint.

Feinstein WK, Noble PC, Kamaric E, Tullos HS: Anatomic alignment of the patellar groove. *Clin Orthop* 1996;331:64–73.

Electronic digitization and 3-dimensional reconstruction of 15 anatomic specimens revealed large variability of the patellar groove in relationship to the anatomic and mechanical femoral axes, the transepicondylar axis, and transcondylar axis. In relationship to these axes, there was a range variation of 11° to 16° of the patellar groove in the coronal and transverse planes. None of the axes were deemed reliable as a reference guide.

Hirsch HS, Lotke PA, Morrison LD: The posterior cruciate ligament in total knee surgery: Save, sacrifice, or substitute? *Clin Orthop* 1994;309:64–68.

Three groups of patients were studied in 242 consecutive TKAs: In group I the PCL was sacrificed at the tibial attachment, in group II the PCL was retained, and a posterior cruciate-substituting TKA was performed in group III. At 2 years, no differences were found between the 3 groups regarding knee scores and radiographic evaluation.

Jordan LR, Olivo JL, Voorhorst PE: Survivorship analysis of cementless meniscal bearing total knee arthroplasty. *Clin Orthop* 1997;338:119–123.

Of 473 consecutive cementless TKAs followed up an average of 5 years, 17 (3.6%) required a change of components as a result of mechanical failure for polyethylene fracture, dislocation, or ligamentous instability. Using the endpoint of revision surgery for any reason, the 8-year survival rate was 94.6%.

Laskin RS: Total knee replacement with posterior cruciate ligament retention in patients with a fixed varus deformity. *Clin Orthop* 1996;331:29–34.

The 10-year outcome of posterior cruciate-retaining TKA with a preoperative contracture of at least 15° varus was compared with posterior cruciate-substituting TKA with similar preoperative contracture, and cruciate-retaining TKA with no contracture. For patients with a preoperative varus contracture of at least 15°, the PCL should be released and a cruciate- substituting TKA used.

Laskin RS, O'Flynn H: Total knee replacement with posterior cruciate ligament retention rheumatoid arthritis: Problems and complications. *Clin Orthop* 1997;345:24–28.

A comparison of 116 posterior cruciate-retaining TKAs in rheumatoid arthritis (RA) patients with 674 in osteoarthritis (OA) patients at average 8.2 years follow-up revealed posterior instability in 40% of RA patients and 2% of OA patients.

Malkani AL, Rand JA, Bryan RS, Wallrichs SL: Total knee arthroscopy with the kinematic condylar prosthesis: A ten-year follow-up study. *J Bone Joint Surg* 1995;77A:423–431.

In 118 cemented posterior cruciate-retaining TKAs followed for 10 ± 0.7 years, the 10-year survival for the end point of revision surgery was 96%. When revision surgery, complete radiolucent lines, and a poor knee score were combined as end points, the 10-year survival was only 76%.

Miyasaka KC, Ranawat CS, Mullaji A: 10- to 20-year followup of total knee arthroplasty for valgus deformities. *Clin Orthop* 1997;345:29–37.

In a group of 160 knees with an average preoperative valgus deformity of 17.6° (range, 10° to 45°), the classic method of lateral soft-tissue release was compared with a new method that involves intra-articular release of the posterolateral capsule and arcuate complex, lengthening rather than transection of the iliotibial band, and occasional release of the popliteus tendon. The new technique resulted in varus-valgus stability in 94% of knees compared with 79% using the older method.

Paletta GA Jr, Laskin RS: Total knee arthroplasty after a previous patellectomy. *J Bone Joint Surg* 1995;77A:1708–1712.

In a retrospective study, 9 posterior stabilized TKAs and 13 posterior cruciate-retaining TKAs in 22 patients with a prior patellectomy and subsequent TKA were compared with 2 posterior stabilized and cruciate-retaining TKAs in patients with no prior patellectomy. Cruciate-retaining TKA provides less predictable results for knees with a prior patellectomy.

Poilvache PL, Insall JN, Scuderi GR, Font-Rodriguez DE: Rotational landmarks and sizing of the distal femur in total knee arthroplasty. *Clin Orthop* 1996;331:35–46.

Measurements of multiple angles and anatomic landmarks, including the transepicondylar axis, the AP axis, the posterior condylar line, and the mechanical axis, were assessed in 100 TKAs. The AP axis was difficult to define in knees with trochlear wear or intercondylar osteophytes. The transepicondylar axis was determined to be a more reliable landmark than the AP axis for proper femoral component rotation.

Ritter MA, Herbst SA, Keating EM, Faris PM, Meding JB: Long-term survival analysis of a posterior cruciate-retaining total condylar total knee arthroplasty. *Clin Orthop* 1994;309:136–145.

For 394 cemented total condylar TKAs followed up at a mean of 8 years (range, 1 to 18 years), the Kaplan-Meier survival rate at 12 years was 96.8%. Nine patients with an infection were excluded from the survival analysis.

Scott RD, Thornhill TS: Posterior cruciate supplementing total knee replacement using conforming inserts and cruciate recession: Effect on range of motion and radiolucent lines. *Clin Orthop* 1994;309:146–149.

A consecutive case study of the same posterior cruciate-retaining TKA design in 50 knees with flatter tibial inserts compared with 50 knees using curved inserts with careful attention to posterior cruciate balancing revealed no difference in the ROM and incidence of tibial radiolucencies between the 2 groups.

Stiehl JB, Cherveny PM: Femoral rotational alignment using the tibial shaft axis in total knee arthroplasty. *Clin Orthop* 1996;331:47–55.

Comparison of 2 different techniques of posterior femoral condyle resection in 100 TKA using the posterior condylar axis or the tibial shaft axis revealed a lower incidence of lateral retinacular release (72% versus 28%) and postoperative patellar fracture (7% versus 0%) when using the tibial shaft axis resection method.

Whiteside LA: Cementless total knee replacement: Nine- to 11-year results and 10-year survivorship analysis. *Clin Orthop* 1994;309:185–192.

In 163 cementless TKAs with 9- to 11-year follow-up, the 10-year survival rate was 96.7% when considering loosening and revision as the survival end points. When considering patellar revision and tibial polyethylene wear, the overall 10-year survival rate was 94%.

Complications Associated With Total Knee Arthroplasty

Ayers DC, Dennis DA, Johanson NA, Pellegrini VD Jr: Common complications of total knee arthroplasty. *J Bone Joint Surg* 1997; 79A:278–311.

This comprehensive review describes the prevention and treatment of specific problems related to wound healing, neurovascular injury, infection, thromboembolic disease, extensor mechanism problems, stiffness, and periprosthetic fractures associated with TKA.

Dellon AL, Mont MA, Krackow KA, Hungerford DS: Partial denervation for persistent neuroma pain after total knee arthroplasty. *Clin Orthop* 1995;316:145–150.

Fifteen patients with persistent knee pain after TKA were diagnosed as having a neuroma based on well-localized pain with an area of cutaneous hypesthesia or dysesthesia. Other criteria included the presence of a positive Tinel's sign and response to a local anesthetic block.

Engh GA, Ammeen DJ: Periprosthetic fractures adjacent to total knee implants: Treatment and clinical results. *J Bone Joint Surg* 1997;79A:1100–1113.

This article provides an extensive review of periprosthetic fractures associated with TKA includes diagnosis, classification, management options, and the clinical results of intraoperative and postoperative fractures of the distal femur, proximal tibia, and patella. It includes an excellent discussion of the management of periprosthetic patellar fractures and use of extensor mechanism allografts for disruption of the extensor mechanism.

Felix NA, Stuart MJ, Hanssen AD: Periprosthetic fractures of the tibia associated with total knee arthroplasty. *Clin Orthop* 1997; 345:113–124.

A 4-part anatomic classification system and treatment algorithm is proposed based on a retrospective review of 102 fractures. Fractures associated with a loose prosthesis are managed best with revision surgery, and fractures associated with well-fixed prostheses can be managed with the usual principles of tibial fracture management.

Levine MJ, Mariani BA, Tuan RS, Booth Jr RE: The use of PCR molecular genetic techniques in revisional knee arthroplasty: The first 200 cases. *Clin Orthop*, in press.

The use of molecular genetic techniques in 200 consecutive patients undergoing TKA were studied with preoperative aspiration, Gram stain, and culture in a polymerase chain reaction analysis. The accuracy rate in diagnosing the infection was 92% compared to 100% accuracy reported in an earlier study. This test has the advantage of not being affected by the presence of antibiotics.

Lynch NM, Trousdale RT, Ilstrup DM: Complications after concomitant bilateral total knee arthroplasty in elderly patients. *Mayo Clin Proc* 1997;72:799–805.

There were significant differences in the incidence of postoperative cardiovascular and neurologic complications in patients 80 years of age or older who undergo concomitant bilateral TKA in comparison with matched patients who undergo unilateral TKA. Episodes of congestive heart failure and acute delirium were significantly increased, and a trend toward increased mortality was also observed in the bilateral TKA group.

Markel DC, Luessenhop CP, Windsor RE, Sculco TA: Arthroscopic treatment of peripatellar fibrosis after total knee arthroplasty. *J Arthroplasty* 1996;11:293–297.

A description of the arthroscopic management of the entity of symptomatic peripatellar fibrosis following TKA in 48 knees revealed good results in 20 knees (42%) and poor results in 19 knees (40%).

Mont MA, Dellon AL, Chen F, Hungerford MW, Krackow KA, Hungerford DS: The operative treatment of peroneal nerve palsy. *J Bone Joint Surg* 1996;78A:863–869.

This retrospective review of 31 cases of surgical decompression of the peroneal nerve to release bands of fibrous tissue and epineural fibrosis suggests that peroneal palsy does not always resolve with nonsurgical measures and if improvement is not observed after 2 months surgical decompression of the nerve may be indicated.

Rand JA: The patellofemoral joint in total knee arthroplasty. *J Bone Joint Surg* 1994;76A:612–620.

This is an excellent review of the anatomy and biomechanics of the patellofemoral joint in TKA including patellar resurfacing techniques, patellar maltracking, patellar component wear and failure mechanisms, management of patellar fractures, soft-tissue impingement syndromes, patellar ligament rupture, and revision of the patellar component.

Evaluation of the Painful Knee

Barrack RL, Jennings RW, Wolfe MW, Bertot AJ: The value of preoperative aspiration before total knee revision. *Clin Orthop* 1997;345:8–16.

Routine aspiration of the symptomatic total knee prior to reoperation was performed in a consecutive series of 69 knees in 67 patients. The sensitivity of aspiration was only 42% in patients who had been on antibiotics compared to 75% in patients who had never been on antibiotics.

Beight JL, Yao B, Hozack WJ, Hearn SL, Booth RE Jr: The patellar "clunk" syndrome after posterior stabilized total knee arthroplasty. *Clin Orthop* 1994;299:139–142.

Out of a group of 1,484 posterior stabilized total knees, 20 patellar clunks in 19 patients were identified. Eleven arthroscopic debridements and 3 patellar component revisions were performed in 12 patients, all of whom demonstrated suprapatellar fibrous nodule that lodged in the intercondylar notch during flexion and dislodged during extension.

580   Lower Extremity

Chimento GF, Finger S, Barrack RL: Gram stain detection of infection during revision arthroplasty. *J Bone Joint Surg* 1996; 78B:838–839.

Intraoperative Gram stain was performed in 169 revision total joints of which 32 were found to be infected (11 hips and 21 knees). The intraoperative Gram stain was negative in all cases (sensitivity = 0%) indicating that the absence of a positive Gram stain is not indicative of the absence of infection.

Fehring TK, McAvoy G: Fluoroscopic evaluation of the painful total knee arthroplasty. *Clin Orthop* 1996;331:226–233.

Twenty postoperative total knee patients evaluated for pain and instability had normal-appearing plain radiographs. Diagnosis of aseptic loosening was made with fluoroscopically guided radiographs in 14 of the 20 patients. Fluoroscopic analysis predicted fixation status of the components at revision surgery in all cases.

Fehring TK, Valadie AL: Knee instability after total knee arthroplasty. *Clin Orthop* 1994;299:157–162.

Twenty-five cases of total knees revised for tibiofemoral instability were examined out of a group of 126 total knee revisions. Preoperative aspiration consistently showed a predominance of red blood cells. Physical examination and dynamic radiographs were helpful in confirming the diagnosis of instability.

Revision Total Knee Replacement

Chen F, Krackow KA: Management of tibial defects in total knee arthroplasty: A biomechanical study. *Clin Orthop* 1994;305: 249–257.

An in vitro biomechanical study was performed to evaluate the effects of modifying the shape of tibial bone defects on the subsequent stability of defect repair. Conversion of oblique angular defects into a stepped (rectangular) pattern resulted in improved rigidity of the system when either cement or metal augmentations were used to reconstruct the defect.

Dennis DA: Wound complications in total knee arthroplasty, in Springfield DS (ed): *Instructional Course Lectures 46*. Rosemont, IL American Academy of Orthopaedic Surgeons, 1997, pp 165–169.

This chapter thoroughly reviews the risk factors and preventative measures, including choice of skin incision, to reduce wound complications following TKA. Treatment options for management of prolonged serous drainage and superficial or full-thickness soft-tissue necrosis are outlined.

Duff GP, Lachiewicz PF, Kelley SS: Aspiration of the knee joint before revision arthroplasty. *Clin Orthop* 1996;331:132–139.

Sixty-four revision TKAs were evaluated to assess the value of preoperative aspiration of the knee joint. Preoperative aspiration of the prosthetic knee was found to have a sensitivity, specificity, and accuracy. Preoperative aspiration proved to be the most helpful study for diagnosis or exclusion of infection in a prosthetic knee joint.

Engh GA, Herzwurm PJ, Parks NL: Treatment of major defects of bone with bulk allografts and stemmed components during total knee arthroplasty. *J Bone Joint Surg* 1997;79A:1030–1039.

The results of 35 structural allografts performed in 30 patients undergoing primary or revision TKA were reviewed at an average of 50 months. Results were good or excellent in 87% and no additional revisions were necessary.

Garvin KL, Scuderi G, Insall JN: Evolution of the quadriceps snip. *Clin Orthop* 1995;321:131–137.

Sixteen patients underwent revision TKA in which the quadriceps snip was used to gain surgical exposure. This technique proved to be safe and simple, and did not require alteration of the patient's postoperative physiotherapy regimen. Clinical quadriceps strength was weaker than that of the contralateral normal leg, but similar to that of the opposite knee, which had had TKA.

Ghazavi MT, Stockley I, Yee G, Davis A, Gross AE: Reconstruction of massive bone defects with allograft in revision total knee arthroplasty. *J Bone Joint Surg* 1997;79A:17–25.

Allograft bone was used to reconstruct major defects in the proximal tibia or distal femur in 30 knees of 28 patients undergoing revision TKA. At an average of 50 months' follow-up, success was obtained in 77%.

Gold DA, Scott SC, Scott WN: Soft tissue expansion prior to arthroplasty in the multiply- operated knee: A new method of preventing catastrophic skin problems. *J Arthroplasty* 1996; 11:512–521.

Ten knees with multiple prior surgical procedures around the knee underwent soft-tissue expansion before major knee surgery. The resultant multiple skin incisions were believed to potentially jeopardize normal wound healing. Following soft-tissue expansion, the major surgical procedures were accomplished without wound complications in all cases.

Stiehl JB, Abbott BD: Morphology of the transepicondylar axis and its application in primary and revision total knee arthroplasty. *J Arthroplasty* 1995;10:785–789.

A morphologic anatomic study of 13 cadaveric lower extremities was performed. The mean distance of the transepicondylar axis (TEA) to the joint line was 3.08 cm medial and 2.53 cm lateral. The TEA is an important landmark that is virtually perpendicular to the mechanical axis of the lower extremity and parallels the knee flexion axis.

Whiteside LA: Surgical exposure in revision total knee arthroplasty, in Springfield DS (ed): *Instructional Course Lectures 46*. Rosemont, IL, American Academy of Orthopaedic Surgeons, 1997, pp 221–225.

This chapter reviews the various extensile exposures used in revision TKA, including the quadriceps turndown, quadriceps snip, and extended tibial tubercle osteotomy. The surgical technique as well as the advantages and disadvantages of each exposure are outlined.

Classic Bibliography

Barrett WP, Scott RD: Revision of failed unicondylar unicompartmental knee arthroplasty. *J Bone Joint Surg* 1987;69A: 1328–1335.

Chotivichit AL, Cracchiolo A III, Chow GH, Dorey F: Total knee arthroplasty using the total condylar III knee prosthesis. *J Arthroplasty* 1991;6:341–350.

Coventry MB, Ilstrup DM, Wallrichs SL: Proximal tibial osteotomy: A critical long-term study of eighty-seven cases. *J Bone Joint Surg* 1993;75A:196–201.

Elia EA, Lotke PA: Results of revision total knee arthroplasty associated with significant bone loss. *Clin Orthop* 1991;271: 114–121.

Friedman RJ, Hirst P, Poss R, Kelley K, Sledge CB: Results of revision total knee arthroplasty performed for aseptic loosening. *Clin Orthop* 1990;255:235–241.

Gustilo T, Comadoll JL, Gustilo RB: Long-term results of 56 revision total knee replacements. *Orthopedics* 1996;19:99–103.

Haas SB, Insall JN, Montgomery W III, Windsor RE: Revision TKA with use of modular components with stems inserted without cement. *J Bone Joint Surg* 1995;77A:1700–1707.

Harris AI, Poddar S, Gitelis S, Sheinkop MB, Rosenberg AG: Arthroplasty with a composite of an allograft and a prosthesis for knees with severe deficiency of bone. *J Bone Joint Surg* 1995; 77A:373–386.

Healy WL, Anglen JO, Wasilewski SA, Krackow KA: Distal femoral varus osteotomy. *J Bone JointSurg* 1988;70A:102–109.

Heck DA, Marmor L, Gibson A, Rougraff BT: Unicompartmental knee arthroplasty: A multicenter investigation with long-term follow-up evaluation. *Clin Orthop* 1993;286:154–159.

Hofmann AA, Wyatt RW, Beck SW: High tibial osteotomy: Use of an osteotomy jig, rigid fixation, and early motion versus conventional surgical technique and cast immobilization. *Clin Orthop* 1991;271:212–217.

Hohl WM, Crawfurd E, Zelicof SB, Ewald FC: The total condylar III prosthesis in complex knee reconstruction. *Clin Orthop* 1991; 273:91–97.

Insall JN, Joseph DM, Msika C: High tibial osteotomy for varus gonarthrosis: A long-term follow-up study. *J Bone Joint Surg* 1984;66A:1040–1048.

Katz MM, Hungerford DS, Krackow KA, Lennox DW: Results of total knee arthroplastyafter failed proximal tibial osteotomy for osteoarthritis. *J Bone Joint Surg* 1987;69A:225–233.

Kozinn SC, Scott R: Unicondylar knee arthroplasty. *J Bone Joint Surg* 1989;71A:145–150.

Lai CH, Rand JA: Revision of failed unicompartmental total knee arthroplasty. *Clin Orthop* 1993;287:193–201.

Matthews LS, Goldstein SA, Malvitz TA, Katz BP, Kaufer H: Proximal tibial osteotomy: Factors that influence the duration of satisfactory function. *Clin Orthop* 1988;229:193–200.

Mnaymneh W, Emerson RH, Borja F, Head WC, Malinin TI: Massive allografts in salvage revisions of failed total knee arthroplasties. *Clin Orthop* 1990;260:144–153.

Mow CS, Wiedel JD: Noncemented revision total knee arthroplasty. *Clin Orthop* 1994;309:110–115.

Murray PB, Rand JA, Hanssen AD: Cemented long-stem revision total knee arthroplasty. *ClinOrthop* 1994;309:116–123.

Odenbring S, Lindstrand A, Egund N, Larsson J, Heddson B: Prognosis for patients with medial gonarthrosis: A 16-year follow-up study of 189 knees. *Clin Orthop* 1991;266:152–155.

Ogilvie-Harris DJ, Fitsialos DP: Arthroscopic management of the degenerative knee. *Arthroscopy* 1991;7:151–157.

Ogilvie-Harris DJ, McLean J, Zarnett ME: Pigmented villonodular synovitis of the knee: The results of total arthroscopic synovectomy, partial arthroscopic synovectomy, and arthroscopic local excision. *J Bone Joint Surg* 1992;74A:119–123.

Rand JA: Role of arthroscopy in osteoarthritis of the knee. *Arthroscopy* 1991;7:358–363.

Rand JA: Revision total knee arthroplasty using the total condylar III prosthesis. *J Arthroplasty* 1991;6:279–284.

Rosenberg AG, Verner JJ, Galante JO: Clinical results of total knee revision using the total condylar III prosthesis. *Clin Orthop* 1991;273:83–90.

Scott RD, Cobb AG, McQueary FG, Thornhill TS: Unicompartmental knee arthroplasty: Eight- to 12- year follow-up evaluation with survivorship analysis. *Clin Orthop* 1991; 271:96–100.

Smiley P, Wasilewski SA: Arthroscopic synovectomy. *Arthroscopy* 1990;6:18–23.

Stockley I, McAuley JP, Gross AE: Allograft reconstruction in total knee arthroplasty. *J Bone Joint Surg* 1992;74B:393–397.

582   Lower Extremity

Takahashi Y, Gustilo RB: Nonconstrained implants in revision total knee arthroplasty. *ClinOrthop* 1994;309:156–162.

Tsahakis PJ, Beaver WB, Brick GW: Technique and results of allograft reconstruction in revision total knee arthroplasty. *Clin Orthop* 1994;303:86–94.

Vince KG, Long W: Revision knee arthroplasty: The limits of press fit medullary fixation. *Clin Orthop* 1995;317:172–177.

Wang JW, Kuo KN, Andriacchi TP, Galante JO: The influence of walking mechanics and time on the results of proximal tibial osteotomy. *J Bone Joint Surg* 1990;72A:905–909.

Wilde AH, Schickendantz MS, Stulberg BN, Go RT: The incorporation of tibial allografts in total knee arthroplasty. *J Bone Joint Surg* 1990;72A:815–824.

Chapter 44
Ankle and Foot: Pediatric Aspects

Congenital and Acquired Deformities

Metatarsus Adductus

Metatarsus adductus is the term used most commonly to describe a foot shape characterized by medial deviation of the forefoot on the midfoot with neutral or slight valgus alignment of the hindfoot. Metatarsus varus refers to a similar but more severe and rigid deformity in which the forefoot is also supinated. A skewfoot combines adduction and plantarflexion of the forefoot on the midfoot, with moderate to severe valgus deformity of the hindfoot. There are no strict clinical or radiographic criteria for defining these entities. A developmental abnormality resulting in a trapezoid shape of the medial cuneiform with medial and dorsal alignment of the first cuneiometatarsal joint may be an important pathogenic factor.

Spontaneous correction of metatarsus adductus occurs in approximately 95% of patients. Serial casting occasionally can be used for rigid feet in children between 6 and 12 months of age. A holding device, such as reverse or straight last shoes, can be used at night for several months thereafter to prevent recurrence of deformity. Good results can be expected at long-term follow-up without a need for surgery, even when there is mild to moderate residual deformity. Severe deformity in an older, untreated child may cause pain, callus formation, and shoe fitting problems that may require surgery.

The techniques of tarsometatarsal capsulotomies and osteotomies at the base of the metatarsals are associated with complications. An opening wedge osteotomy of the trapezoid-shaped medial cuneiform treats the deformity at the site of deformity and is associated with few risks or complications. Concurrent osteotomies at the base of the lesser metatarsals or a closing wedge osteotomy of the cuboid may be necessary.

Clubfoot (Talipes Equinovarus)

Idiopathic clubfoot occurs in approximately 1 of every 1,000 live births, affects males twice as often as females, and is bilat-

eral in approximately 50% of cases. Clubfoot also is associated with other conditions, such as myelomeningocele, arthrogryposis, and amniotic band syndrome. Recent genetic research supports the hypothesis of a multifactorial pattern of inheritance.

In a clubfoot, the talus is smaller than normal, and the talar neck is deviated in a plantarmedial direction. The axes of the anterior and middle facets of the calcaneus create a more acute angle than in the normal foot, with the anterior facet oriented inward. There is often a corresponding varus deformity of the distal end of the calcaneus, resulting in a medial orientation of the calcaneocuboid joint with varying degrees of subluxation at that joint.

The goal of treatment for patients who have a clubfoot is a plantigrade foot with good joint mobility that is functional, painless, stable over time, and free of calluses. Most clubfeet can be only partially corrected with manipulation and serial casting. Complete deformity correction, however, usually is achieved by one of the many described surgical procedures, which can range from minimal surgery as in the Ponseti technique to complete posteromedial and posterolateral release.

The best age for surgery is between 6 and 12 months. General anesthesia with supplemental caudal epidural anesthesia has been shown to decrease the postoperative narcotic requirement and provide good pain control for several hours after surgery. The Cincinnati incision is an extensile posteromedial and lateral approach to the clubfoot deformity that leaves a reasonably cosmetic scar. In a severe clubfoot, it may not be possible to immediately approximate the incision with the foot in the fully corrected position without compromising the circulation of the skin. A pin may be inserted across the talonavicular joint, the cast can be applied with the foot in plantarflexion, and the foot can be manipulated safely into further dorsiflexion during a cast change under anesthesia 2 weeks later.

The most difficult aspect of clubfoot is management of residual or uncorrected deformity (Fig. 1), which may require repeat soft-tissue release combined with osteotomies and, occasionally, tendon transfers.

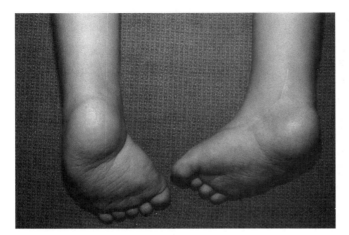

Figure 1

Residual deformity in a 3-year-old child after posteromedial release, without comprehensive lateral release.

Cavus Foot

Cavus foot deformity is defined as fixed plantarflexion of the forefoot on the hindfoot, resulting in an abnormally high arch (Fig. 2). A careful neurologic examination is vital because, in over two thirds of patients, the etiology of the cavus foot deformity is a neuromuscular disorder, such as Charcot-Marie-Tooth disease, poliomyelitis, lipomeningocele, tethered cord, or spinal cord tumor. Radiographs and magnetic resonance imaging (MRI) of the spine and electrodiagnostic studies of the extremity may be indicated, especially with unilateral deformity.

Cavovarus, with or without equinus, is the most common type of cavus foot deformity. It can be caused by several different patterns of muscle imbalance. Calcaneocavus is much less common and is seen in conditions such as myelomeningocele and poliomyelitis in which there is paralysis of the triceps surae with preservation of strength in the muscles that plantarflex the forefoot on the hindfoot. Initially, all components of the cavovarus deformity are flexible. The first metatarsal becomes rigidly plantarflexed. The effect is one of fixed pronation of the forefoot on the hindfoot, which in turn leads to inversion of the subtalar joint. The Coleman block test helps to identify when the flexible hindfoot varus becomes rigid.

With rare exception, cavus foot deformities progressively increase in severity and rigidity. Management of the deformity must be individualized because it is based on the severity and the etiology of the deformity. There are few indications for prolonged nonsurgical management. Indications for surgery include instability of the foot and ankle and painful calluses under the first metatarsal head and the base of the fifth metatarsal. Reconstruction involves concurrent correction of the deformities and balancing of the muscle forces. The deformities should be corrected using (1) soft-tissue releases to align the joints and (2) osteotomies to correct the secondary bone deformities (Fig. 3). Tendon transfers are chosen based on the existing and anticipated patterns of muscle imbalance. The best chance for long-term success rests with an approach based on early correction of deformity, maintenance of joint mobility, appropriate muscle balancing, and the performance of additional nonarthrodesing procedures and tendon transfers as indicated for recurrent deformities during the remainder of the child's growth. This frequently requires plantar medial release and medial cuneiform or first metatarsal osteotomy to correct forefoot cavus, and calcaneal osteotomy to correct hindfoot varus. Arthrodeses are reserved as salvage procedures for older adolescents and adults. Triple arthrodesis, which for many years was considered to be the treatment of choice for the cavovarus foot, has been shown to lead frequently to the development of long-term degenerative arthritis in the ankle and midtarsal joints as a result of stress transfer.

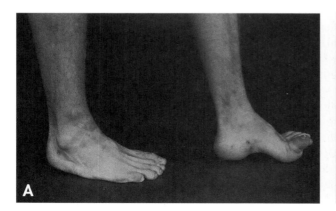

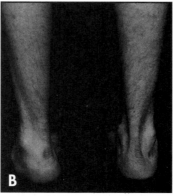

Figure 2

Cavovarus foot deformity in a 16-year-old boy with Charcot-Marie-Tooth disease.

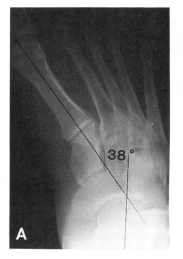

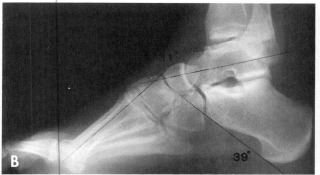

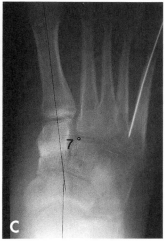

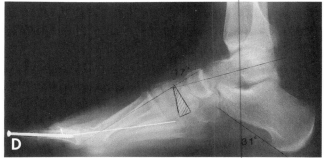

Figure 3

Cavovarus foot in a boy with Charcot-Marie-Tooth disease. A and B, Moderately severe deformity with rigid forefoot and stiff hindfoot. On the lateral radiograph, the axes of the talus and first metatarsal cross in the body of the medial cuneiform, the apex of the deformity. C and D, Following 2-stage reconstruction of the forefoot and midfoot. Stage 1, plantarmedial soft-tissue release. Stage 2 (3 weeks later), medial cuneiform plantar opening-wedge osteotomy, tibialis posterior transfer to middle cuneiform, Jones transfer, Hibbs transfer, fusion of interphalangeal joint of hallux.

Calcaneovalgus Foot

Calcaneovalgus is a benign, positional foot deformity with a reported incidence of 1 in every 1,000 live births (Fig. 4). The ankle joint is dorsiflexed and there is limitation of passive plantarflexion. The subtalar joint is everted, but flexible. The forefoot can be plantarflexed on the hindfoot to create a longitudinal arch. Spontaneous and stimulated active plantarflexion and inversion efforts can be observed. It is important to distinguish calcaneovalgus from congenital vertical talus, congenital posteromedial bowing of the tibia, and weakness of plantarflexion related to a neurologic disorder, such as spinal dysraphism.

Most calcaneovalgus feet correct spontaneously. Passive stretching exercises may be helpful, but are not scientifically proven. Serial casting into plantarflexion is indicated only for the rare calcaneovalgus foot that is more rigid than usual and slow to correct spontaneously.

Idiopathic (Flexible) Flatfoot

Idiopathic flexible flatfoot is a normal variation of the shape of the foot that rarely causes disability or requires treatment. There is no agreement on strict clinical or radiographic crite-

ria for defining a flatfoot, so incidence figures are only approximations. Nevertheless, it is believed that the majority of infants and at least 20% of adults have flexible flatfeet. A flatfoot is considered flexible if the subtalar joint is mobile and can be inverted from valgus to varus. At least 10° of dorsiflexion of the ankle is possible in individuals with the common, benign flexible flatfoot. The physician must be certain that the subtalar joint is in neutral alignment and that the knee is fully extended when testing for contracture of the Achilles tendon.

It has been established by both clinical and radiographic studies that the average arch height is lower in the child than in the adult, the height of the longitudinal arch generally increases spontaneously during the first decade of life in most children, there is a wide range of normal arch heights at all ages (particularly in young children), and there is no benefit from shoe modifications and inserts over spontaneous natural improvement in the development of the longitudinal arch. Over-the-counter and custom-molded shoe inserts have limited use but have been shown to increase the useful life of shoes and to relieve activity-related, nonlocalized aching pain in the legs and feet of some children with symptomatic flexi-

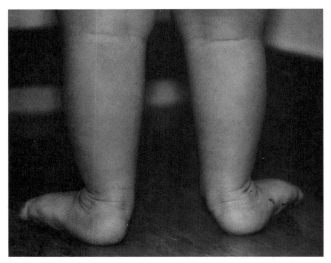

Figure 4
Severe bilateral calcaneovalgus deformity in a 2-year-old child.

ble flatfeet. Surgery for flexible flatfoot is rarely indicated.

A child with a flexible flatfoot and a short Achilles tendon may experience pain and callus formation under the rigidly plantarflexed head of the talus. An orthosis, particularly a rigid type, may exacerbate the symptoms. These individuals should perform Achilles tendon stretching exercises daily. If significant symptoms persist and deformity is mild, a simple Achilles tendon lengthening may be adequate treatment. For severe deformity, lengthening of the Achilles tendon should be combined with a calcaneal lengthening osteotomy. The calcaneal lengthening osteotomy has been shown to correct all components of the deformity, restore function to the subtalar complex, and relieve symptoms. Many other procedures have been proposed, most involving arthrodesis of one or more joints. Long-term studies have demonstrated that arthrodesis of even the small joints of the child's foot should be avoided if possible because of the significant risk of developing degenerative arthritis at the adjacent joints.

Accessory Navicular

An accessory navicular is a congenital structural abnormality of the tarsal navicular that is frequently bilateral and occurs in 5% to 15% of the population. Type I is a rarely symptomatic, small pea-shaped sesamoid bone located in the center of the most distal portion of the tibialis posterior tendon. Type II, the most frequently symptomatic, is a bullet-shaped ossicle joined to the tuberosity of the navicular by a syndesmosis or synchondrosis. Type III is a large, horn-shaped navicular that probably results from fusion of a type II with

the body of the navicular. The association between an accessory navicular and flexible flatfoot remains controversial.

The typical patient is an active adolescent girl with a history of minor trauma who presents with pain, callus formation, tenderness, and, occasionally, swelling over the bony prominence on the plantarmedial aspect of the navicular. Radiographs will demonstrate the pathology. For pain caused by tibialis posterior tendinitis or a fracture through the synchondrosis of the accessory navicular, immobilization in a below-the-knee cast is recommended for 4 to 6 weeks. An orthosis and a change in shoe style may help to maintain comfort. Surgery is indicated when symptoms persist after prolonged attempts at nonsurgical management. Very good and reliable pain relief can be expected from simple excision of the accessory navicular with shaving of the medial prominence of the main body of the navicular. Advancement of the tibialis posterior tendon does not improve the results and is not necessary.

Congenital Vertical Talus

A congenital vertical talus is a dorsolateral dislocation of the talonavicular joint associated with extreme plantarflexion of the talus. The foot has a rocker-bottom appearance, and the head of the talus is prominent and palpable on the plantar surface. A longitudinal arch cannot be created by passive manipulation of the foot. It is reported that the deformity occurs in association with syndromes, such as arthrogryposis, myelomeningocele, and sacral agenesis, in over 50% of cases. The deformity is bilateral in 50% of affected children. The etiology is most likely muscle imbalance or intrauterine contracture from lack of movement.

A lateral radiograph of the foot in maximum dorsiflexion demonstrates fixed equinus of the talus. A stress lateral radiograph in maximum plantarflexion demonstrates an irreducible dislocation of the talonavicular joint and confirms the diagnosis. A congenital oblique talus is a less well-defined deformity that seems to exist on the continuum between a congenital vertical talus and a flexible flatfoot with a short Achilles tendon. On initial evaluation, the oblique talus can be dorsiflexed slightly from its severe equinus position, and the alignment at the talonavicular joint can be improved with plantarflexion of the forefoot. The oblique talus may correct completely with casting or may require a limited surgical reconstruction.

For congenital vertical talus, the forefoot is serially casted or stretched into plantarflexion to stretch the dorsal tendons, skin, and neurovascular structures of the foot. Reduction of the talonavicular joint dislocation is desired, but is not expected. Surgical reconstruction by a single-stage circumferential release through a Cincinnati incision is indicated between 6 and 18 months of age in almost all feet. Naviculectomy, by shortening the elongated medial column of the foot, is an effective operation for correcting recurrent or untreated vertical talus deformity in the older child. This procedure preserves some motion in the resultant pseudosubtalar joint complex. Subtalar and triple arthrodeses have also been recommended in this age group, but it is technically challenging to correct severe valgus deformity of the hindfoot with either procedure, and these operations lead to stress transfer to adjacent joints. Subtalar arthrodesis has also been associated with progressive overcorrection of the deformity in some feet.

Tarsal Coalition

Tarsal coalition is a fibrous, cartilaginous, or bony connection between two or more tarsal bones that results from a congenital failure of differentiation and segmentation of primitive mesenchyme. It is most commonly seen as an autosomal dominant condition (with nearly full penetrance) that may affect up to 1% of the general population. Talocalcaneal and calcaneonavicular coalitions occur with about equal frequency, are usually bilateral, and together account for nearly all coalitions. There may be more than one coalition in the same foot. Tarsal coalition may also be seen in association with other congenital disorders, such as fibular and tibial hemimelia and Apert's syndrome. The coalitions in the latter group are often more extensive than the idiopathic variety and are rarely, if ever, symptomatic.

Maturation of the coalition coincides with the development of progressive valgus deformity of the hindfoot, flattening of the longitudinal arch, and restriction of subtalar motion, all of which are more severe in feet with talocalcaneal coalitions. For the individuals with tarsal coalition who develop pain, the onset of symptoms may coincide with bony transformation of a previously cartilaginous coalition. This generally occurs between 8 and 12 years of age for those children with calcaneonavicular coalitions, and between 12 and 16 years of age for those with talocalcaneal conditions. The onset of vague, aching, activity-related pain in the sinus tarsi area or along the medial aspect of the hindfoot is often insidious. The peroneal tendons may appear to be in spasm and can develop a late contracture. The exact etiology and location of the pain and spasm are debated. The foot examination reveals stiffness or rigidity of an everted subtalar joint. The hindfoot remains in valgus alignment even with toe standing. Calcaneonavicular conditions are best seen on the oblique radiograph. Talocalcaneal coalitions are best seen on computed tomography (CT) images in the coronal plane. MRI is helpful in identifying coalitions that are still in the fibrous

stage and not visualized on radiographs or CT scan, but it should not be a first-line study. A bone scan can be helpful in evaluating a rigid flatfoot with an atypical presentation of pain to look for other etiologies (ie, osteoid osteoma, infection, fracture).

Treatment is indicated only for the tarsal coalitions that are symptomatic. Pain should be almost completely relieved on application of a below-the-knee walking cast. A soft orthosis can be placed in the shoe when the cast is removed 4 to 6 weeks later. Lasting pain relief has been reported as variable in patients with tarsal coalitions who were treated by nonsurgical means. Surgical management is indicated if pain recurs or nonsurgical treatment fails. A good long-term result can be expected following resection of calcaneonavicular coalitions with interposition of the extensor digitorum brevis. The short-term results of resection and soft-tissue interposition for talocalcaneal coalitions have been good, but the results deteriorate with time and long-term studies are not available. Unsatisfactory results from resection have been reported in feet in which the ratio of the surface area of the coalition to the surface area of the posterior facet was greater than 50% (as determined by CT scan) and in which there was even greater valgus deformity of the hindfoot. The independent influence of the size of the coalition was not determined in that or any other study. Some authors recommend initial resection of a symptomatic talocalcaneal coalition regardless of size if the foot is not fixed in valgus. The presence of a talar beak does not necessarily indicate the presence of degenerative arthrosis and is not, by itself, a contraindication for resection. Documented degenerative arthrosis and persistence or recurrence of pain following coalition resection are indications for triple arthrodesis. Severe, symptomatic valgus deformity of the hindfoot associated with a talocalcaneal coalition can be corrected with a calcaneal lengthening osteotomy with or without resection of the coalition.

Cerebral Palsy

Spastic muscle imbalance creates deformities of the foot and ankle in children with cerebral palsy. Dynamic equinus in young children with cerebral palsy may be managed by an ankle foot orthosis (AFO). Serial casts can be used in children under the age of 4 years to stretch a mildly contracted Achilles tendon. Surgery is appropriate for older children with fixed deformities. The gastrocnemius alone can be lengthened if the soleus is not contracted. Open or percutaneous lengthening of the Achilles tendon is a safe and effective procedure as long as the tendon is not overlengthened and as long as contractures of the hamstrings and iliopsoas are lengthened concurrently.

Equinovalgus, caused by overactivity of the triceps surae and the peroneus brevis, is common in children with diplegia and quadriplegia. Severe contractures can result in pain and callus formation under the rigidly plantarflexed head of the talus. Subtalar and triple arthrodeses have been the most commonly used procedures to manage this deformity; however, long-term follow-up studies have consistently reported high rates of complications including the frequent development of degenerative arthrosis in the ankle and adjacent joints of the foot. A medial displacement osteotomy of the posterior aspect of the calcaneus can improve the clinical appearance of the valgus deformity of the hindfoot, but it does not correct the external rotation deformity in the subtalar complex or align the talonavicular joint. A calcaneal lengthening osteotomy has been shown to correct all components of the deformity, restore function to the subtalar complex, and relieve symptoms. The Achilles and peroneus brevis tendons must be lengthened and it is often necessary to correct the supination deformity of the forefoot.

Equinovarus, resulting from overactivity of the Achilles tendon and the tibialis anterior or posterior muscles or both, is often seen in children with hemiplegia. The treatment options are a split tibialis anterior or split tibialis posterior tendon transfer combined with an Achilles tendon lengthening. Some authors believe that split transfer of the tibialis anterior is the more physiologic of the 2 in that it preserves free motion of the subtalar joint; others recommend split transfer of the tibialis posterior tendon if it is the primary deforming force. Long-standing, rigid equinocavovarus deformity may require tendon lengthenings and transfers along with plantar fasciotomy, capsulotomies, and osteotomies as for any cavovarus foot deformity.

Myelomeningocele

The incidence of foot deformities in children with myelomeningocele ranges from 60% to 90%. Proposed etiologies include muscle imbalance, intrauterine positioning, and subclinical spasticity. Children with myelomeningocele require reasonably plantigrade and supple feet that can be braced and accept shoe wear. Correction of deformities with preservation of joint motion is extremely important. Insensate skin and joints along with osteopenia put these children at risk for the development of neurotrophic ulceration, Charcot arthropathy, and pathologic fracture.

Clubfoot accounts for approximately 50% of the deformities. It should be treated with circumferential release between 12 and 18 months of age, similar to the treatment protocol for idiopathic clubfoot. Tendons should be divided rather than lengthened. There is a higher risk of recurrence than for the idiopathic deformity. Repeat circumferential release or talectomy may be used for revision surgery or the rigid foot.

Calcaneus deformity arises because of unopposed activity of the tibialis anterior muscle and is commonly seen in children who are high functioning, low lumbar level ambulators. The deformity can cause callus formation and ulceration of the heel pad and a progressive crouched gait disturbance. It remains unclear whether transfer of the tibialis anterior through the interosseous membrane to the calcaneus provides any benefit over simple tenotomy. Spasticity and weakness of the tibialis anterior are contraindications to transfer. Achilles tendon tenodesis may be an option in the child prior to skeletal maturity.

Valgus deformity of the ankle joint, accompanied by external tibial torsion, is commonly seen in children with myelomeningocele. Valgus deformity can lead to pressure concentration under the medial malleolus with skin breakdown. The external tibial rotation will contribute to valgus stress at the knee and gradual worsening of gait. Supramalleolar varus derotational osteotomy can correct both deformities of the tibia simultaneously, but loss of fixation, malunion, and nonunion have been reported in up to 10% of cases in most series. An attractive alternative is the gradual correction of the ankle valgus using a transphyseal medial malleolar screw and acute correction of tibial torsion by means of a pure rotational osteotomy. Children with myelomeningocele may also have valgus deformity of the subtalar joint associated with a flatfoot or skewfoot deformity. They will exhibit callus formation and, occasionally, ulceration under the head of the talus. The Achilles tendon may not be contracted. A calcaneal lengthening osteotomy has been shown to correct even severe valgus deformity of the subtalar joint in these children. It can be carried out under the same anesthetic as the tibial osteotomy. Rigid supination, abduction, or adduction of the forefoot may be present and must be corrected with an osteotomy of the medial column of the foot. Arthrodesis of the subtalar joint should be avoided, particularly in children who ambulate. Stress transfer in these children may lead to degenerative arthritis in adjacent joints or to the even more serious condition of Charcot arthropathy.

Juvenile Hallux Valgus

Juvenile hallux valgus is defined as greater than 14° of lateral deviation of the hallux on the first metatarsal that develops in children and adolescents. There is maternal inheritance in over 70% of cases. Metatarsus primus varus, defined as angulation between the first and second metatarsals of greater than 8°, and medial deviation of the cuneiform-first metatarsal joint are often present. Controversy surrounds the associations of juvenile hallux valgus with pes planus, metatarsus adductus, a long first metatarsal, ligamentous laxity, and shoe wear. The defining characteristic of juvenile hallux valgus may be an increased distal metatarsal articular angle (DMAA) (Fig. 5). Approximately 50% of children have an increased DMAA, and the percentage is highest in those with a long first metatarsal, those younger than 10 years, and those with a positive family history of hallux valgus. Congruency of the metatarsophalangeal joint is greater with higher DMAA values in adolescents. In juvenile hallux valgus, the first metatarsophalangeal joint is often well-aligned on a first metatarsal bone in which there is a valgus deformity at its distal end. In adults, the DMAA is more often normal and joint congruity is poor. The physician must, however, be circumspect with data based on the DMAA because reported interobserver reliability for this measurement is low, even though intraobserver reliability is high.

Most adolescents with hallux valgus are asymptomatic and have learned to choose their shoe wear so as to avoid pressure and pain. Shoe modifications should be prescribed to accommodate the deformity. Foot orthoses have no proven efficacy in correcting the deformity. Surgical correction of the deformity should be reserved for those adolescents in whom shoe modifications have been unsuccessful in relieving pain that regularly interferes with normal activities. Perhaps the most important preoperative considerations are a clear understanding by the patient of the goals and risks, and a clear understanding by the surgeon of the patient's expectations. Poor results with high complication rates from surgery have been consistently reported in 30% to 60% of cases of juvenile hallux valgus. Many of the poor results can be attributed to poor patient selection or procedure selection, especially in

light of the recent understanding of the DMAA and joint congruity. The typical adolescent with metatarsus primus varus, an increased DMAA, and a congruent joint should undergo a 2-level proximal valgus and distal varus osteotomy of the first metatarsal without release of the lateral capsule of the metatarsophalangeal joint. The risk of osteonecrosis of the first metatarsal head is increased when distal osteotomy is combined with lateral capsular release. An alternative to the proximal metatarsal osteotomy is an opening wedge osteotomy of the medial cuneiform, which simultaneously avoids damage to the physis of the first metatarsal and corrects the malalignment of the cuneiform-first metatarsal joint.

Traumatic Disorders

Fractures of Distal Tibial and Fibular Physes

These common fractures account for 25% of all physeal fractures and occur most frequently between the ages of 8 and 15 years. When the fracture is nondisplaced, the radiographic findings may be subtle. The goals of treatment are to restore joint congruity for those fractures extending into the joint, to restore mechanical alignment, and to minimize the potential for growth abnormalities resulting from physeal injury.

Nondisplaced Salter-Harris types I and II distal tibial fractures are immobilized for 3 to 6 weeks in a long leg cast with no weightbearing, followed by 3 to 4 weeks in a short leg walking cast. When displaced, these fractures should undergo gentle closed reduction. Approximately 10° of valgus and anterior angulation can be accepted. Varus should be avoided. If 1 or 2 attempts at closed reduction do not produce adequate fracture alignment, open reduction is indicated to correct any soft-tissue interposition.

Salter-Harris types III and IV distal tibial fractures can result in articular incongruity and are associated with a significant (approximately 20%) risk of growth problems even when treated optimally. It is important to ascertain that apparently nondisplaced fractures remain nondisplaced and to follow fractures not requiring internal fixation closely to detect any late displacement. Displacement of these fractures, even when minimal (1 to 2 mm), should not be accepted and usually requires open reduction. The surgeon should try to avoid crossing the physis with pins and screws used for internal fixation. Current use of cannulated 4.0-mm screws inserted in a transepiphyseal manner is accepted (Fig. 6).

Prolonged follow-up after these fractures heal is advisable because even Salter-Harris type II fractures have a substantial risk (approximately 16%) of growth abnormalities. Small posttraumatic physeal bars of the distal tibia are frequently amenable to surgical removal. Larger bars may require surgi-

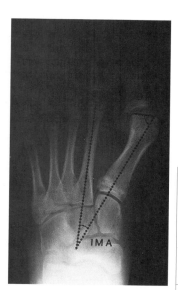

Figure 5

The distal metatarsal articular angle (DMAA), the angle created by the intersection of a line across the articular surface of the first metatarsal with the axis line of the first metatarsal shaft, is an important determinant in the management of juvenile hallux valgus.

cal closure of the remainder of the physis to avoid the need for osteotomy for angular deformity. Contralateral epiphysiodesis or, occasionally, limb lengthening may be required for leg length discrepancy.

Physeal fractures involving the distal fibula, when isolated, are usually minimally displaced and can be treated with immobilization. When widely displaced, they are usually

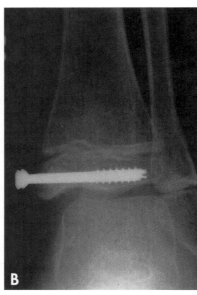

Figure 6

A, Salter-Harris type IV fracture of the distal tibia. B, After open reduction and internal fixation with transepiphyseal screws.

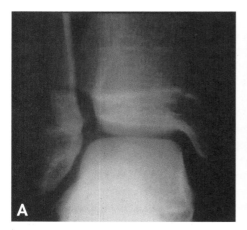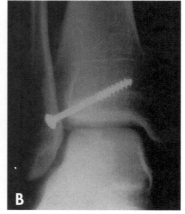

Figure 7

A, Juvenile Tillaux fracture. B, After open reduction and internal fixation.

associated with a displaced distal tibial fracture and can be reduced and if necessary stabilized at surgery.

Juvenile Tillaux and Triplane Fractures

The distal tibial physis closes centrally first, then medially, and finally laterally over 18 months of time. Injury to the ankle occurring during this period produces fracture patterns in late adolescence not typically seen in younger children.

When only the anterolateral part of the physis remains open at the time of injury, external rotation injury results in avulsion of the anterolateral part of the epiphysis by the anterior tibiofibular ligament, the juvenile Tillaux fracture (Fig. 7). Because patients with this injury have little growth remaining, growth abnormality is not generally a problem. Significant (> 2 mm) displacement of the fragment has been associated with posttraumatic arthritis and, therefore, should not be accepted. Closed reduction, percutaneous reduction and fixation, or if necessary, open reduction and internal fixation (ORIF) of displaced fractures is required.

In slightly younger adolescents, external rotation injury produces triplane fractures. They usually appear as a Salter-Harris type III fracture on the anteroposterior (AP) and mortise views, and a Salter-Harris type II fracture on the lateral view. Such fractures may consist of 2 or more fragments. CT scanning may delineate the number and the amount of displacement of the fragments. As with the juvenile Tillaux fracture, > 2 mm of intraarticular displacement has been associated with posttraumatic arthritis and requires closed reduction or, if necessary, ORIF. Current technique favors closed manipulation and percutaneous fixation or limited ORIF of displaced intra-articular fracture fragments.

Fractures of the Talus

Fractures of the talus in children are rare. Most occur in teenagers. The mechanism of injury is generally forced dorsiflexion. Most of these fractures involve the neck of the talus. They are often nondisplaced or minimally displaced. Findings on physical examination may be subtle and only consist of mild swelling or pain on palpation, especially when the fracture is nondisplaced. Nondisplaced fractures can be treated with cast immobilization. A long leg cast, with the knee flexed to prevent weightbearing, is recommended initially. Displaced fractures require reduction. This is first attempted by closed manipulation consisting of plantarflexion, longitudinal traction, and either inversion or eversion as necessary. Five millimeters of displacement and 5° of malalignment are acceptable on the AP radiograph. When reduction is successful and the fracture stable, long leg cast immobilization with close follow-up to detect late displacement may be sufficient. Unstable fractures may be internally stabilized using the newer technique of cannulated screws inserted from posterior to anterior just lateral to the Achilles tendon. Fractures not satisfactorily reduced by closed means require open reduction. An anteromedial approach medial to the extensor hallucis longus is recommended. Dissection around the talar neck should be kept to the minimum necessary for adequate reduction. Osteonecrosis of the talus has been reported in up to 25% of fractures in this age group. Revascularization of the talus may occur more rapidly in children than adults, a possibility that makes prolonged nonweightbearing using a patellar tendon bearing orthosis desirable when this complication is detected. The large cartilaginous component of the subchondral bone of the talus may make the Hawkin's sign unreliable for the detection of osteonecrosis in this age group. MRI is probably the best test to establish the diagnosis when in doubt.

Fractures of the Calcaneus

Calcaneal fractures, similar to fractures of the talus, are less common in children than adults. Extra-articular calcaneal fractures can be occult in young children. These occult fractures, often detected by bone scan, have been called a nontibial type of "toddler fracture." Older children with nondisplaced, extra-articular calcaneal fractures are casted in a long leg cast and made nonweightbearing. Children with displaced beak fractures and apophyseal avulsion fractures require ORIF. Fractures involving the anterior process of the calcaneus can occasionally result in painful nonunion. All other extra-articular calcaneal fractures seem to have a favorable outcome. Intra-articular fractures, even those with significant joint depression, have been reported to do well with nonsurgical treatment in very young children. Joint depression can be documented at follow-up, but the talus seems to remodel to accommodate the deformity and symptoms seem to be uncommon. ORIF is indicated for older adolescents with significant joint depression, similar to the adult injury.

Lisfranc Fractures

Lisfranc fracture-dislocations are rare in children. In the largest series reported in the literature confined to patients younger than 16 years, only 4 of 18 patients were younger than 10 years old. Displaced fracture-dislocations require closed reduction and pin fixation or ORIF when satisfactory closed reduction is not possible.

Metatarsal Fractures

Metatarsal fractures are common in the pediatric age group. Most involve the metatarsal shaft and can be treated nonsurgically with 3 to 4 weeks of immobilization and early weightbearing. Surgical treatment is generally reserved for open fractures. Fractures at the proximal diaphyseal/metaphyseal junction of the fifth metatarsal that do not unite, displaced intra-articular metatarsal head fractures, and completely displaced metatarsal neck fractures may be other indications for ORIF.

Annotated Bibliography

Metatarsus Adductus

Farsetti P, Weinstein SL, Ponseti IV: The long-term functional and radiographic outcomes of untreated and non-operatively treated metatarsus adductus. *J Bone Joint Surg* 1994;76A:257–265.

Passively correctable deformities resolved spontaneously. Good results were obtained in 90% of the partly flexible and rigid deformities with serial casts. There were no long-term functional disabilities in patients with mild or moderate residual deformity. No patient had surgical correction.

Morcuende JA, Ponseti IV: Congenital metatarsus adductus in early human fetal development: A histologic study. *Clin Orthop* 1996;333:261–266.

The shape of the medial cuneiform was altered in a trapezoid shape, and the first cuneometatarsal joint tilted toward the medial and dorsal directions.

Clubfoot (Talipes Equinovarus)

Cooper DM, Dietz FR: Treatment of idiopathic clubfoot: A thirty-year follow-up note. *J Bone Joint Surg* 1995;77A:1477–1489.

With the use of pain and functional limitation as the outcome criteria, 78% of 45 patients treated by the "nonoperative" method of Ponsetti had an excellent or good outcome compared with 85% of 97 individuals who did not have congenital deformity of the foot at an average age of 34 years. This may be the gold standard long-term outcome study on clubfeet.

Epeldegui T, Delgado E: Acetabulum pedis: Part II. Talocalcaneonavicular joint socket in clubfoot. *J Pediatr Orthop* 1995;4B:11–16.

Pathoanatomic observations of the socket, or acetabulum pedis, of the talocalcaneonavicular joint in clubfoot revealed that the axes of the anterior and middle facets of the calcaneus create a more acute angle than in the normal foot. The anterior facet is oriented inward.

Ferlic RJ, Breed AL, Mann DC, Cherney JJ: Partial wound closure after surgical correction of equinovarus foot deformity. *J Pediatr Orthop* 1997;17:486–489.

The Cincinnati incision was left open to heal by secondary intent if primary closure led to compromise to the circulation of the skin or loss of the corrected position. One or 2 additional anesthetics were required for wound care.

Foulk DA, Boakes J, Rab GT, Schulman S: The use of caudal epidural anesthesia in clubfoot surgery. *J Pediatr Orthop* 1995;15:604–607.

General anesthesia with supplemental caudal epidural anesthesia provided excellent postoperative pain relief for over 8 hours, almost routinely allowed safe discharge on the same day as surgery, and resulted in a statistically significant decrease in intraoperative narcotic requirement. Parent satisfaction was high, but cost savings were low.

Rebbeck TR, Dietz FR, Murray JC, Buetow KH: A single-gene explanation for the probability of having idiopathic talipes equinovarus. *Am J Hum Genet* 1993;53:1051–1063.

The probability of having clubfoot is explained by the Mendelian segregation of a single gene with 2 alleles plus the effects of some unmeasured factor(s).

Tolat V, Boothroyd A, Carty H, Klenerman L: Ultrasound: A helpful guide in the treatment of congenital talipes equinovarus. *J Pediatr Orthop* 1995;4B:65–70.

Ultrasound may be used to distinguish the unossified cartilage and the ossification centers of the tarsal bones. The technique does not take much time, is easily tolerated by the child, and may be repeated frequently to assess the response to treatment.

Cavus Foot

Holmes JR, Hansen ST Jr: Foot and ankle manifestations of Charcot-Marie-Tooth disease. *Foot Ankle* 1993;14:476–486.

This is an overview of the problem from the perspective of a single individual with decades of experience.

Idiopathic (Flexible) Flatfoot

Mosca VS: Calcaneal lengthening for valgus deformity of the hindfoot: Results in children who had severe, symptomatic flatfoot and skewfoot. *J Bone Joint Surg* 1995;77A:500–512.

The calcaneal lengthening osteotomy was shown to effectively correct severe, intractably symptomatic valgus hindfoot deformity and eliminate the signs and symptoms associated with the deformity while avoiding arthrodesis. Most of the deformities were in children with myelomeningocele and cerebral palsy. Lengthening of the Achilles tendon and peroneus brevis were required along with plication of the talonavicular joint and tibialis posterior tendon. Osteotomy of the medial cuneiform was sometimes necessary to correct rigid deformity of the forefoot.

Theologis TN, Gordon C, Benson MK: Heel seats and shoe wear. *J Pediatr Orthop* 1994;14:760–762.

Helfet heel seats improved shoe wear and pain in children with excessive heel valgus, but did not influence the natural history of arch development.

Accessory Navicular

Prichasuk S, Sinphurmsukskul O: Kidner procedure for symptomatic accessory navicular and its relation to pes planus. *Foot Ankle Int* 1995;16:500–503.

An association of pes planus and symptomatic accessory navicular was shown. Simple excision, without advancement of the tibialis posterior, is recommended for the management of this condition.

Congenital Vertical Talus

Napiontek M: Congenital vertical talus: A retrospective and critical review of 32 feet operated on by peritalar reduction. *J Pediatr Orthop* 1995;4B:179–187.

Thirty-two feet were treated for congenital vertical talus by peritalar reduction. The Green-Grice procedure combined with the peritalar reduction method led to overcorrection in 7 of 16 feet.

Tarsal Coalition

Kitaoka HB, Wikenheiser MA, Shaughnessy WJ, An KN: Gait abnormalities following resection of talocalcaneal coalition. *J Bone Joint Surg* 1997;79A:369–374.

There were 5 excellent, 4 good, 3 fair, and 2 poor clinical results at a mean duration of 6 years after resection. Good results deteriorate over time, and most patients have a residual functional deficit with decreased motion of the hindfoot and the ankle.

McCormack TJ, Olney B, Asher M: Talocalcaneal coalition resection: A 10-year follow-up. *J Pediatr Orthop* 1997;17:13–15.

Satisfactory results persisted for 10 years or more after surgery in 8 of 9 cases. There was no deterioration of symptom relief, loss of motion, or development of degenerative joint changes. These are the best reported intermediate-term results.

Moyes ST, Crawfurd EJ, Aichroth PM: The interposition of extensor digitorum brevis in the resection of calcaneonavicular bars. *J Pediatr Orthop* 1994;14:387–388.

Nine of 10 feet that underwent resection with interposition of the extensor digitorum brevis became asymptomatic and mobile and showed no evidence of recurrence. Three of 7 feet in which the resection was not accompanied by extensor digitorum brevis interposition developed recurrence of the bar along with pain and stiffness.

Wechsler RJ, Schweitzer ME, Deely DM, Horn BD, Pizzutillo PD: Tarsal coalition: Depiction and characterization with CT and MR imaging. *Radiology* 1994;193:447–452.

MRI depicts all tarsal coalitions but may not be able to help differentiate synovitis from fibrous coalitions. CT has limitations in the depiction of fibrous coalitions.

Wilde PH, Torode IP, Dickens DR, Cole WG: Resection for symptomatic talocalcaneal coalition. *J Bone Joint Surg* 1994;76B:797–801.

Indications for successful resection of a symptomatic talocalcaneal coalition are: the area of the coalition measures 50% or less of the area of the posterior facet of the calcaneus on the preoperative coronal CT, there are less than 16° of heel valgus, and there are no radiographic signs of arthritis of the posterior talocalcaneal joint. Talar beaking does not impair the clinical result.

Cerebral Palsy

Horton GA, Olney BW: Triple arthrodesis with lateral column lengthening for treatment of severe planovalgus deformity. *Foot Ankle Int* 1995;16:395–400.

Triple arthrodesis with lateral column lengthening through the calcaneocuboid joint provides for reliable arthrodesis and allows correction of severe planovalgus deformity while maintaining foot length. Mild deformities can be corrected with lateral column lengthening alone.

Myelomeningocele

Abraham E, Lubicky JP, Songer MN, Millar EA: Supramalleolar osteotomy for ankle valgus in myelomeningocele. *J Pediatr Orthop* 1996;16:774–781.

Fifty-five supramalleolar osteotomies were performed in 35 patients. Loss of correction or nonunion occurred in 5 (9%).

Broughton NS, Graham G, Menelaus MB: The high incidence of foot deformity in patients with high-level spina bifida. *J Bone Joint Surg* 1994;76B:548–550.

Deformities were found in 89% of the feet. Spasticity of the muscles controlling the foot was detected in 36 (51%) of the 70 calcaneus feet and in 22 (17%) of the 126 equinus feet.

Davids JR, Valadie AL, Ferguson RL, Bray EW III, Allen BL Jr: Surgical management of ankle valgus in children: Use of a transphyseal medial malleolar screw. *J Pediatr Orthop* 1997;17:3–8.

This is a minimally invasive, minimally morbid, technically simple method of reversible partial epiphysiodesis at the ankle. Resumption of physeal growth and recurrence of deformity was seen when the screws were removed before skeletal maturity.

de Carvalho Neto J, Dias LS, Gabrieli AP: Congenital talipes equinovarus in spina bifida: Treatment and results. *J Pediatr Orthop* 1996;16:782–785.

Good and fair results were achieved in 77% of clubfeet in children with spina bifida treated by radical posteromedial-lateral release. In the children with thoracic/high lumbar level, only 50% had a good or fair result.

Stevens PM, Belle RM: Screw epiphysiodesis for ankle valgus. *J Pediatr Orthop* 1997;17:9–12.

Retarding medial malleolar growth by means of a vertical screw is a safe, predictable, and effective technique. Neither recurrence nor permanent physeal closure occurred following screw removal before skeletal maturation.

Stott NS, Zionts LE, Gronley JK, Perry J: Tibialis anterior transfer for calcaneal deformity: A postoperative gait analysis. *J Pediatr Orthop* 1996;16:792–798.

Transfer of the tibialis anterior muscle to the calcaneus arrests progression of the calcaneal deformity, but cannot prevent excessive dorsiflexion of the ankle during stance. Continued bracing is necessary to provide a more normal-appearing, energy-efficient gait.

Hallux Valgus

Coughlin MJ: Juvenile hallux valgus: Etiology and treatment. *Foot Ankle Int* 1995;16:682–697.

This excellent summary of the state of knowledge on juvenile hallux valgus includes a clear discussion of DMAA and congruency.

Jones KJ, Feiwell LA, Freedman EL, Cracchiolo A III: The effect of chevron osteotomy with lateral capsular release on the blood supply to the first metatarsal head. *J Bone Joint Surg* 1995;77A:197–204.

Latex injection was used in cadaveric specimens. Technical errors in the performance of the chevron osteotomy, alone or in conjunction with extensive capsular stripping, can result in damage to the vessels that supply the metatarsal head.

Vittetoe DA, Saltzman CL, Krieg JC, Brown TD: Validity and reliability of the first distal metatarsal articular angle. *Foot Ankle Int* 1994;15:541–547.

This cadaver radiograph study showed that although intraobserver reliability for DMAA measurement was high, interobserver reliability for the clinical technique of measurement was poor.

Traumatic Disorders

Cole RJ, Brown HP, Stein RE, Pearce RG: Avulsion fracture of the tuberosity of the calcaneus in children: A report of four cases and review of the literature. *J Bone Joint Surg* 1995;77A: 1568–1571.

Four patients with displaced calcaneal tuberosity fractures that required ORIF are reported.

Jensen I, Wester JU, Rasmussen F, Lindequist S, Schantz K: Prognosis of fracture of the talus in children: 21 (7-34)-year follow-up of 14 cases. *Acta Orthop Scand* 1994;65:398–400.

Fourteen children who had talar fractures were reviewed at follow-up from 7 to 34 years. All patients with displaced fractures had exercise-induced pain at follow-up.

Schindler A, Mason DE, Allington NJ: Occult fracture of the calcaneus in toddlers. *J Pediatr Orthop* 1996;16:201–205.

Five children younger than 36 months of age presented with refusal to walk after trauma and were treated with long leg casts. Radiographs were normal at presentation but showed occult calcaneus fracture at follow-up.

Shin AY, Moran ME, Wenger DR: Intramalleolar triplane fractures of the distal tibial epiphysis. *J Pediatr Orthop* 1997; 17:352–355.

Three types of intramalleolar triplane fractures were identified by CT scans on 5 patients.

Classic Bibliography

Berman A, Gartland JJ: Metatarsal osteotomy for the correction of adduction of the fore part of the foot in children. *J Bone Joint Surg* 1971;53A:498–506.

Bleck E: Metatarsus adductus: Classification and relationship to outcomes of treatment. *J Pediatr Orthop* 1983;3:2–9.

Crawford AH, Marxen JL, Osterfield DL: The Cincinnati incision: A comprehensive approach for surgical procedures of the foot and ankle in childhood. *J Bone Joint Surg* 1982;64A: 1355–1358.

Cowell HR, Elener V: Rigid painful flatfoot secondary to tarsal coalition. *Clin Orthop* 1983;177:54–60.

Cummings RJ, Lovell WW: Current concepts review: Operative treatment of congenital idiopathic club foot. *J Bone Joint Surg* 1988;70A:1108–1112.

Dennyson WG, Fulford GE: Subtalar arthrodesis by cancellous grafts and metallic internal fixation. *J Bone Joint Surg* 1976;58B: 507–510.

Ertl JP, Barrack RL, Alexander AH, vanBuecken K: Triplane fracture of the distal tibial epiphysis: Long-term follow-up. *J Bone Joint Surg* 1988;70A:967–976.

Goldner J, Gaines R: Adult and juvenile hallux valgus: Analysis and treatment. *Orthop Clin North Am* 1976;7:863–887.

Jayakumar S, Cowell HR: Rigid flatfoot. *Clin Orthop* 1977;122: 77–84.

Johnson GF: Pediatric Lisfranc injury: "Bunk bed" fracture. *Am J Roentgenol* 1981;137:1041–1044.

Kling TF, Bright RW, Hensinger RN: Distal tibial physeal fractures in children that may require open reduction. *J Bone Joint Surg* 1984;66A:647–657.

Kumar SJ, Cowell HR, Ramsey PL: Foot problems in children: Part I. Vertical and oblique talus, in Frankel VH (ed): American Academy of Orthopaedic Surgeons *Instructional Course Lectures XXXI*. St. Louis, MO, CV Mosby, 1982, pp 235–251.

Kumar SJ, Guille JT, Lee MS, Coute JC: Osseous and non-osseous coalition of the middle facet of the talocalcaneal joint. *J Bone Joint Surg* 1992;74A:529–535.

McKay DW: New concept of and approach to clubfoot treatment: Section I. Principles and morbid anataomy. *J Pediatr Orthop* 1982;2:347–356.

McKay DW: New concept of and approach to clubfoot treatment: Section II. Correction of clubfoot. *J Pediatr Orthop* 1983;3:10–21.

McKay DW: New concept of and approach to clubfoot treatment: Section III. Evaluation and results. *J Pediatr Orthop* 1983;3:141–148.

Peterson HA, Newman SR: Adolescent bunion deformity treated with double osteotomy and longitudinal pin fixation of the first ray. *J Pediatr Orthop* 1993;13:80–84.

Scranton PE, Zuckerman JD: Bunion surgery in adolescents: Results of surgical treatment. *J Pediatr Orthop* 1984;4:39–43.

Simons GW: Complete subtalar release in club feet: Part I. A preliminary report. *J Bone Joint Surg* 1985;67A:1044–1055.

Simons GW: Complete subtalar release in club feet: Part II. Comparison with less extensive procedures. *J Bone Joint Surg* 1985;67A:1056–1065.

Stark JG, Johanson JE, Winter RB: The Heyman-Herndon tarsometatarsal capsulotomy for metatarsus adductus: Results in 48 feet. *J Pediatr Orthop* 1987;7:305–310.

Swiontkowski ME, Scranton PE, Hansen S: Tarsal coalitions: Long-term results of surgical treatment. *J Pediatr Orthop* 1983;3:287–292.

Turco VJ: Surgical correction of the resistant club foot: One-stage posteromedial release with internal fixation. A preliminary report. *J Bone Joint Surg* 1971;53A:477–497.

Wiley JJ: Tarso-metatarsal joint injuries in children. *J Pediatr Orthop* 1981;1:255–260.

Chapter 45
Ankle and Foot: Trauma

Ankle Fractures

Introduction

The frequency and severity of ankle fractures have been increasing over the last 3 decades because of an active older population. Generally, women are at higher risk than men of the same race, and whites have a higher risk than do blacks of the same gender. Before the age of 50 years, ankle fractures are most frequent in men; after this age, they are more common in women. In fact, ankle and foot fractures are among the most common fractures sustained by elderly women. One recent epidemiologic study identified the highest age-specific incidence of ankle fractures in women between 75 and 84 years of age. People who are overweight or obese are more predisposed to ankle fractures than are those of normal weight, and reduction of displaced malleolar fractures is lost more often in overweight patients. Data from motor vehicle collisions indicate that seat belts are ineffective in preventing ankle or tarsal injuries and that the incidence of these injuries is increased among shorter drivers.

Ankle fractures are only weakly related to bone density. Increased dietary calcium most likely does not reduce the risk of ankle fracture, and the benefits of vitamin D are unclear. Patients with healed ankle fractures have a twofold increased incidence of new fractures of all kinds, but without any predilection for the side of the injured ankle. The reasons for the increased number of additional fractures in these patients are unknown.

Pilon Fractures

Pilon fractures, which cause severe disruption of the tibial plafond, are rare, constituting 7% to 10% of tibial injuries (Fig. 1). This scarcity limits the experience that the average orthopaedic surgeon has in treating this injury.

High-energy axial loading is responsible for most pilon fractures, but some are caused by low-energy rotational forces. The classification scheme of Rüedi and Allgöwer takes into account the complex axial loading injuries of the tibial plafond and has been shown to accurately predict outcome. A type I fracture is a cleavage fracture of the distal tibia without major disruption of the articular surface. In a type II fracture, the articular fragments are displaced, and in a type III fracture articular fragments are displaced, comminuted, and impacted. Final functional outcome correlates with both the magnitude of the injury and the accuracy of the articular reduction, but anatomic reduction of severe injuries reduces the risk of late arthrosis and pain.

Two methods of treatment are used: traditional open reduction and internal fixation (ORIF) with plates and screws and hybrid using limited open reduction combined with external fixation. Excellent or good results can be expected in approximately 86% of patients treated with traditional ORIF of types I and II low-energy fractures because damage to the soft tissues is not severe and fracture displacement and comminution are minimal. Infection is infrequent, but nonunions occur in 7% of such fractures, malunions in 3%, and wound dehiscence in about 17%.

Complications are more frequent after ORIF of high-energy types II and III fractures and multiple additional procedures often are required. Wound problems and deep infection are reported to occur in as many as 37%, malunion in 23%, and nonunion in 27%. Complications are fewer after external fixation of high-energy pilon fractures than after plate fixation.

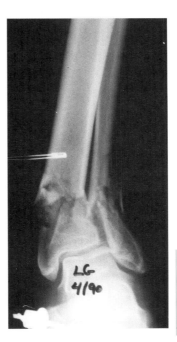

Figure 1

Type II pilon fracture with minimal articular surface displacement but comminution of the tibial diaphysis. (Courtesy of Kenneth J. Koval, MD)

Traditional half-pin fixators, articulated half-pin fixators, ring fixators, and hybrid combinations have been used, often with limited internal fixation of the articular surface, with or without plate fixation of the fibula. For fractures with severe soft-tissue injuries or articular comminution, half-pin fixators provide stability to aid bone-graft incorporation and soft-tissue healing. The obvious disadvantage of a rigid, joint-spanning fixator is that early ankle motion is not possible. Articulated fixators allow early range of motion of the ankle, although motion is somewhat restricted and abnormal. Malalignment of the fixator can allow motion through the fracture site and displacement of fracture fragments, leading to pin loosening and pin track infection.

The articulated fixator is applied with pins inserted into the medial neck of the talus, parallel to the talar dome, and into the tuberosity of the calcaneus so that the hinge of the fixator is roughly aligned horizontally along the axis of the ankle. Because this is not the true axis of the ankle, motion is not normal. The proximal pins are placed through a template into the medial border of the tibia. Distraction is applied, and the fracture is reduced by ligamentotaxis. Articular fragments that remain displaced can be reduced by open or percutaneous manipulation. The fibula is fixed as the surgeon chooses. Bone grafting improves fracture stability and helps prevent delayed union.

Hybrid external fixators consist of tensioned wires in the tibial epiphyseal fragment connected to half-pins in the diaphysis. This leaves the subtalar and tibiotalar joints free for early motion. However, the thin wires may not adequately stabilize a fracture with extensive articular comminution.

The frequency of early complications, such as infection, wound problems, and tibial osteomyelitis, has been decreased with the use of external fixation of high-energy pilon fractures. Although unusual, loss of reduction can occur, but usually can be corrected by adjustment of the fixator. Pin track infections occur in approximately 21% of patients, but most can be treated successfully with aggressive wound care and oral antibiotics.

External fixation of high-energy injuries also reduces some late complications: reported rates of nonunion and malunion are less than 8%. Unfortunately, most patients with these severe injuries develop posttraumatic arthritis, and 3% to 9% eventually required ankle arthrodesis for pain control.

Ankle Fractures

Ankle trauma accounts for between 3% and 12% of all emergency room visits. Although most patients with ankle injuries have radiographic examinations, fractures are diagnosed in only 7% to 36%. In an effort to curb excessive use of radiologic procedures and to reduce waiting time and radiation exposure of patients, the Ottawa clinical decision rule was developed to guide physicians in their use of radiographs for evaluation of acute ankle injuries. This rule states that an ankle radiograph is needed only if the patient has pain near the malleoli and one or more of these findings: (1) age 55 years or older, (2) inability to bear weight immediately after the injury and for 4 steps in the emergency department, or (3) bony tenderness at the posterior edge or tip of either malleolus. The rule does not apply in the presence of deformity with a clinically obvious fracture, and it may be unreliable in patients with altered mental status, intoxicated patients, or those with language difficulties.

The original researchers reported the Ottawa rule to be 100% sensitive and 40% specific for detecting malleolar fractures. Waiting times, medical charges, and the use of radiography were reduced significantly. However, independent studies in different environments showed the Ottawa rule to have a sensitivity ranging from 93% to 94.6% and a specificity ranging from 11% to 15.5% in the detection of ankle fractures. Missed fractures included those of the calcaneus, navicular, and malleoli. Overall the Ottawa rule is more sensitive than clinical impression and can assist in decision-making, but it cannot replace the judgment and common sense of physicians.

Lateral and mortise views are sufficient for the diagnosis and classification of almost all ankle fractures, and additional views generally do not add any useful information. Occasionally, a nondisplaced or avulsion fracture may not be visible. Approximately 1% of fractures of the posterior tibial plafond, lateral and medial malleoli, talar dome and neck, and calcaneus are not detected by plain radiography.

Undiagnosed ankle fractures can lead to prolonged disability and pain. A marked ankle joint effusion on plain radiographs is an indication of an occult fracture (Fig. 2). The size of the ankle effusion is determined by measuring the total capsular distension (anterior plus posterior distention of the capsule) on the lateral radiograph. A total joint capsule distention of 15 mm has a positive predictive value for occult ankle fracture of 83% and a specificity of 86%. Plain or computed tomography (CT) should then be used to identify the fracture.

Isolated Lateral Malleolar Fractures

Published reports support nonsurgical treatment of isolated distal fibular fractures that have no clinical or radiographic evidence of injury to the medial side of the joint. Successful results have been reported in approximately 96% of such fractures treated with casts, ankle braces, or ankle strapping. Immediate weightbearing and early ankle motion result in a shorter rehabilitation period and a notable improvement in

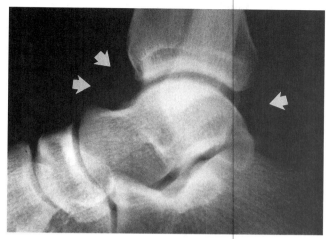

Figure 2

The appearance of an ankle joint effusion on a lateral ankle radiograph. Arrows highlight convex soft-tissue lines that reflect distention of the ankle joint capsule anteriorly and posteriorly.

the range of motion in the first 2 months compared to treatment by immobilization for 4 weeks in a plaster walking cast. Patients treated with early motion also have fewer ankle-related symptoms in the first 3 months after injury.

CT studies of such injuries demonstrate an undisturbed ankle mortise, although approximately a third of ankles with isolated lateral malleolar fractures have a slight widening of the lateral joint space, the clinical significance of which is unknown. In cadaver studies, a simulated fracture of the lateral malleolus alone did not result in abnormal ankle motion, but when accompanied by a tear of the deltoid ligament, the fracture was unstable. After the initial radiograph, further displacement of the talus or fibula is uncommon after isolated lateral malleolar fracture. Because of the inherent stability of this fracture pattern, frequent radiographic monitoring probably is not justified.

Bimalleolar or Trimalleolar Fractures and Equivalent Injuries

Fracture of the lateral malleolus with a tear of the deltoid ligament is caused by the same mechanism that produces bimalleolar fractures: supination and external rotation. Instead of the medial malleolus being fractured, the deltoid ligament is torn, allowing the talus to displace laterally. Deltoid ligament tear should be suspected when a lateral malleolar fracture is accompanied by tenderness, swelling, and hematoma on the medial side of the ankle.

Stress radiographs can be used to evaluate stability when a lateral malleolar fracture is present with medial tenderness but without a definite talar shift. The radiograph is taken with the leg stabilized in slight internal rotation while external rotation is applied to the foot. An increase of more than 2.5 to 3.0 mm in the width of the medial clear space is indicative of a deltoid ligament tear.

A lateral malleolar fracture with major injury to the deltoid ligament generally requires ORIF of the fibula, with or without repair of the ligament. Usually the deltoid ligament is avulsed from the medial aspect of the talus and can be reattached with sutures through holes drilled in the talar body and neck. The fibular fracture can be stabilized with a one-third tubular plate and cortical screws (most commonly used), lag screws alone, Kirschner wires (K-wires) and tension band fixation, or a small, interlocked intramedullary nail. Lateral or posterolateral plate fixation remains the gold standard because of its rigidity and ability to control rotation and length.

Stable, nondisplaced bimalleolar and trimalleolar fractures can be treated with cast immobilization. Weekly radiographs are necessary for at least 4 weeks to detect loss of reduction in the cast. Weightbearing depends on the surgeon's judgment, but usually can begin at 4 to 6 weeks.

Displaced fractures of both the medial and lateral malleoli are best treated with open repair to reestablish a congruent joint surface. Plates, screws (metallic or absorbable), staples, and tension bands have all been used successfully. Fixation of a posterior malleolar fragment is controversial, but most surgeons recommend surgical stabilization of posterior malleolar fragments that involve 25% to 33% or more of the articular surface, or if there is instability or incongruity after fixation of the fibula and medial malleolus.

Reports of anatomic reduction and internal fixation of unstable bimalleolar and trimalleolar fractures indicate good to excellent results in 71% to 95% of patients. Complications are infrequent. Marginal wound necrosis and superficial infection occur in approximately 5% of patients, and deep infection, nonunion, and failure of fixation are uncommon in young, healthy patients. Complications, especially infection, are more frequent in diabetic patients, in whom wound infections occur in 13% to 40%. Superficial wound infections usually can be treated successfully with oral antibiotics. Deep infections require antibiotic therapy, hardware removal, and, occasionally, ankle fusion. Uncontrolled osteomyelitis can lead to loss of limb. Significant risk factors in diabetic patients include peripheral vascular disease with absent pedal pulses and preexisting neuropathy.

Ankle Fractures With Diastasis

Recent clinical and biomechanical studies have clarified the indications for repair of syndesmotic injuries. In cadaver ankle fracture models, when the deltoid ligament was intact, widening of the ankle mortise did not significantly affect joint contact areas nor was ankle motion altered significantly by fibular osteotomy with syndesmotic disruption. Once the deltoid ligament, especially its deep portion, was divided, however, dramatic aberrations in motion occurred. Repair of the lateral and syndesmotic structures did not result in normal motion, but did prevent tibiotalar dislocation, suggesting that syndesmotic stabilization is needed only if rigid bimalleolar fixation cannot be obtained.

Most clinical studies also indicate that, even if the deltoid ligament is ruptured, the syndesmosis often is not stabilized if rigid bimalleolar fixation is obtained or if the fibular fracture is within 4.5 cm of the ankle joint. An absolute indication for syndesmosis stabilization is intraoperative instability of the distal tibiofibular joint after rigid fixation of the medial and lateral malleoli; screws (3.5 or 4.5 mm) can be used. For syndesmosis fixation, a screw should be placed 2 cm proximal and parallel to the ankle joint and directed 30° anteriorly. A nonparallel screw may shorten or lengthen the fibula. Lag technique should be avoided. The screw should be left in until the syndesmosis is completely healed, at least 3 months. Late widening of the syndesmosis has been reported after early screw removal.

Good to excellent results have been reported in from 63% to 72% of patients with syndesmosis injuries. Ankle dislocation, postoperative deep infection, and early screw removal are associated with poorer results.

Traumatic Injury to the Foot

General Principles

In its simplest form the foot represents a 3-legged stool. The talar dome is the seat and the calcaneus and the first and fifth metatarsal heads represent the 3 legs. The stool is stable when the seat is located within the triangle formed by the 3 legs. The stability of these weightbearing points depends on the position and interaction of the individual bones of the foot. The medial column consists of the talus, navicular, and cuneiforms, along with their respective metatarsals. The lateral column includes the calcaneus, cuboid, and fourth and fifth metatarsals. The relative interaction between these 2 columns determines foot position and the weightbearing line of the foot. When trauma shortens the medial column, a relative cavus foot is created. When the lateral column is shortened, an abductoplanus deformity occurs.

Two types of joints are present in the foot: those that function as traditional diarthrodial joints with significant motion and those that are relatively immobile and provide structure and a small amount of shock absorption. The joints in which motion

is important are the tibiotalar, fibulotalar, talonavicular, talocalcaneal, and fourth and fifth tarsometatarsal. The metatarsophalangeal joints also are mobile but do not have as much effect on the stability of the foot when injured. Motion in other joints is limited and can be sacrificed for structure or stability.

Functionally, the foot is divided into 3 sections, the hindfoot, midfoot, and forefoot. The competing issues of mobility and stability must be considered carefully when treating injuries in each section. The hindfoot comprises the talus and calcaneus and is the section responsible for most of the motion in the foot. Midfoot function is clearly related to its gross anatomic shape and is responsible for medial and lateral columnar stability. The forefoot consists of 5 metatarsal bones constituting the 6 weightbearing contacts for the forefoot (the 2 sesamoids under the first metatarsal are the actual contact with the ground).

Talar Fractures

The talus is composed of 7 articular surfaces covering 60% of the bony surface. Vascular access to the bone is limited to nonarticular areas. The talus defines ankle and subtalar motion and anchors the medial column of the foot. Fractures of the talus are classified depending on their primary area of involvement: body, neck, head, posterior or lateral process. Imaging includes an anteroposterior (AP) view of the ankle, and AP, lateral, and modified AP (Canale) views of the foot to show all articular surfaces. CT scans may be helpful in comminuted fractures to delineate articular involvement and fracture pattern. In lateral and posterior process fractures, a CT scan is necessary to determine the true amount of subtalar articular involvement.

Uncorrected articular incongruity or misalignment along any talar fracture pattern results in significant impairment of foot function. Displaced intra-articular fractures should be treated by open reduction and rigid internal fixation (Fig. 3). Bone graft should be used where it is needed to restore structural integrity, and fragments too small for fixation or stabilization should be excised to minimize the formation of intra-articular debris leading to arthrosis.

Surgical approaches to the talar neck vary with the fracture pattern and should be planned to maximize fracture and joint surface exposure and minimize soft-tissue stripping and vascular compromise. Medial or lateral malleolar osteotomies can be used for access to body fractures. Medial and anterolateral incisions are recommended for talar neck fractures, but a posterior approach also is acceptable. Posterior to anterior screws provide the most rigid fixation, but fracture reduction is difficult without a medial or lateral surgical approach. Postoperatively, patients should be treated in a nonweightbearing cast for 6 to 8 weeks before beginning

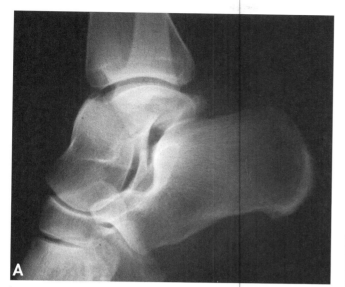 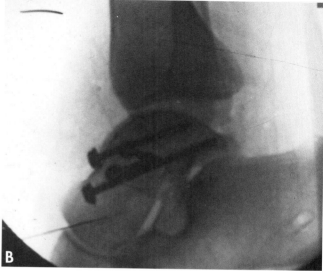

Figure 3

A, Displaced fracture of the talar body with disruption of the subtalar joint. B, After open reduction and screw fixation. (Courtesy of Kenneth J. Koval, MD)

range-of-motion exercises. The ankle should be placed in at least a plantigrade position. Nonweightbearing should continue for a full 3 months.

Approximately 20% of talar fractures are open injuries. Infection has been reported in as many as 38% of open talar fractures. Acute arthrodesis or excision of involved joint surfaces has not been shown to produce better results than restoration of bone stock. The likelihood of talar body osteonecrosis increases with the severity of the injury. The diagnosis of osteonecrosis is routinely made radiographically by the absence of a Hawkins sign; this lucency deep to the subchondral surface of the talar dome on an AP radiograph of the ankle obtained 6 to 8 weeks after injury is an indication of revascularization. Talar osteonecrosis does not always lead to collapse. Accepted practice is to allow weightbearing when the fracture has healed, but patients with radiographic evidence of osteonecrosis should be cautioned about the possibility of collapse and followed periodically. The role of magnetic resonance imaging (MRI) in determining treatment is not yet established, but it may be helpful to determine the extent of blood flow.

Peritalar Dislocations

Dislocations of the subtalar complex involve disruption of both the tibiocalcaneal and talonavicular articulations. Medial dislocation occurs with forceful inversion of the foot with the sustentaculum acting as a lever arm against the talar head. Forceful eversion positions the anterior process of the

calcaneus as the lever arm against the talar head, resulting in lateral displacement of the foot. Significant trauma causes most of these injuries, but a surprising number come from athletic activities. Between 10% and 40% of peritalar dislocations are open and have a significant risk of subsequent infection. The clinical deformity usually is apparent, but an AP view of the foot is helpful to show the position of the talonavicular joint and evidence of impaction before attempted reduction.

In closed dislocations, timely reduction is important to minimize vascular compromise to the overlying soft tissues. Patient sedation, knee flexion, and firm longitudinal traction are needed for a successful closed reduction. Usually the joint is stable after reduction. A CT scan is recommended to ensure that no occult articular fractures are overlooked, because long-term results deteriorate when articular fractures are present. Closed reduction may be unsuccessful because of articular fracture, talonavicular impaction, or soft-tissue interposition.

Regardless of the type of peritalar dislocation, early range of motion is essential to prevent ankle stiffness, but the time to weightbearing varies. After a closed, congruent reduction of a dislocation without fracture, early weightbearing is allowed. After closed reduction of a dislocation with a nondisplaced fracture, weightbearing should be delayed for 4 to 6 weeks; weightbearing may be delayed even longer after ORIF.

Calcaneal Fractures

Fractures of the calcaneus are disabling. The need for surgical treatment of calcaneal fractures continues to be controversial. Recently, in small prospective studies, outcomes in comfort and activity level have been improved with ORIF of intra-articular calcaneal fractures. Open reduction generally is recommended for fractures with substantial displacement of the tuberosity, reversal of the Böhler angle, or displacement of the articular surfaces. AP, lateral, and axial radiographs define the position of the tuberosity. CT scans should be used for planning treatment or to supplement radiographs if the need for intervention is unclear. Scans used to be done in the coronal and transverse planes. With improved software, scans can be done in any plane and reformatted in transverse, coronal, and sagittal planes as needed.

Treatment falls into 3 categories: closed treatment without reduction, manipulative reduction with or without fixation, and ORIF. The treatment should be based on the fracture pattern; the patient's needs, health, and activity; and the knowledge and skill of available medical personnel. Reduction parameters include narrowing of the talar body, elevation of the posterior facet, and reduction of the 4 joint surfaces of the calcaneus. Restoration of the normal relationship of all these components is important to restore any of the normal calcaneal function. Arthritic changes and subtalar stiffness are common. Early motion is an important part of open treatment, but weightbearing should be avoided for 2 to 3 months, based on the pattern and healing. Patients with stable fractures should begin range-of-motion exercises as soon as the surgical wound is healed.

Treatment of highly comminuted fractures is controversial. There are advocates for closed treatment, traditional ORIF, and primary subtalar arthrodesis. No controlled data exist to guide this decision. If primary arthrodesis is chosen, the anatomy should be restored at the time of treatment.

The use of bone graft or bone graft substitutes is controversial. In the absence of data, good surgical principles should be used to determine whether a graft is needed.

Anterior process fractures occur either as avulsion or through compression forces. The anterior process may provide an important bony support to the talus on weightbearing and should be maintained in its anatomic position. Sustentacular fractures rarely are isolated but can cause significant morbidity if missed. The sustentaculum provides bony support for the talar head and is the attachment site of the spring ligament. A CT scan is best at defining the extent of damage. Nondisplaced sustentacular fractures can be treated in a nonweightbearing cast for 4 weeks. Any displacement should be reduced and rigidly fixed to allow early motion. Weightbearing should be avoided for 3 months. Symptomatic nonunions or malunions should be excised.

Lesser Tarsal Bones

The midfoot joints are relatively immobile. With the exception of the talonavicular and fourth and fifth tarsometatarsal joints, motion need not be preserved for satisfactory outcome of midfoot fractures. Isolated fracture to any of the bones in this region is uncommon, and great care should be taken to rule out instability of the remaining bones if an injury to 1 is found. Navicular fractures are important if they involve disruption of the talonavicular articular surface or tibialis posterior insertion. Joint surface disruption is caused by axial loading with a medially or laterally directed shear component. Tuberosity avulsion is caused by significant forefoot abduction forces in relation to the hindfoot with tibialis posterior resistance or by a direct blow. A cuboid fracture is the result of an axial load along the lateral column; it rarely occurs alone. Dislocation or subluxation of the cuboid is caused by ligamentous disruption and can occur with or without a fracture. Cuneiform injuries usually involve some degree of both fracture and dislocation and may be part of a severe destabilizing injury to the whole foot or may occur from a direct blow. Many cuneiform injuries are associated with Lisfranc disruptions.

Radiographic evaluation includes normal AP, lateral, and oblique radiographs of the foot. These are best done with simulated weightbearing if possible to accentuate any ligamentous instability. Stress films also are helpful. CT scans may be helpful for assessment of midfoot fracture-dislocations. Treatment of tarsal injuries should emphasize restoration of stability to the midfoot as a whole, with preservation of the relative length of the medial and lateral column and the motion of essential joints, if possible. If nondisplaced, midfoot fractures can be treated in a nonweightbearing short leg cast for 6 weeks, followed by protected weightbearing until symptoms resolve. Displaced fractures or unstable joints should be surgically reduced, with length restored, and rigidly fixed. Restoration and preservation of the talonavicular, fourth and fifth tarsometatarsal, and to a lesser extent calcaneocuboid joints should be considered a priority. There are times when severe comminution makes reduction impossible. Under these circumstances, treatment should focus on restoration of the length and shape of the foot without regard for the individual tarsal bones. Fusion to adjacent midfoot bones can be used to preserve structural integrity. All voids created by the reduction should be filled with bone graft.

Lisfranc Injuries

Lisfranc injury is the term used to describe injuries that involve tarsometatarsal joints, including both joint dislocation and fracture (Fig. 4). Functionally, the weightbearing position of the forefoot depends on the proper alignment of this joint complex. The second and third joints are stiff to provide structural support to the medial column and arch of the foot. Laterally, the fourth and fifth joints exhibit up to 3 times the available movement of the medial joints. Identifying these injuries requires good radiographs focusing on the alignments of the second and fourth tarsometatarsal joints. Nondisplaced fractures without ligament instability should be treated in a nonweightbearing cast for 6 weeks. If there is demonstrable instability, treatment should include open anatomic reduction and rigid fixation. Any residual instability within the lateral column is treated with K-wire fixation to minimize stiffening of the joint. With severe comminution, the tarsometatarsal joints within the medial column can be fused acutely to provide lasting stability. Injuries that are initially unrecognized can be treated by arthrodesis.

Metatarsal Injuries

Weightbearing studies show that weight distribution is relatively equal among the 6 points of contact in the forefoot. This translates to the first metatarsal (the 2 sesamoids) assuming a third of the weightbearing load, with the second, third, fourth, and fifth metatarsals each assuming a sixth of the forefoot load during stance. The soft-tissue support for forefoot alignment consists mainly of multiple dense ligaments between the lesser metatarsals. There are no significant ligamentous attachments between the first and second metatarsals.

Treatment should preserve the symmetry of the weight dis-

tribution of the forefoot. If displacement results in disruption of the weightbearing surface, reduction may be indicated. Fractures of the first metatarsal should be treated to preserve the position of the first metatarsal head as a major weightbearing point. Anatomically nondisplaced fractures of the first metatarsal head can be treated in a nonweightbearing cast for 6 weeks; otherwise, ORIF is used to restore position. Isolated fractures of the lesser metatarsals usually do well in a hard sole shoe with progressive weightbearing as tolerated. Any significant displacement can be treated with closed reduction and casting for 3 weeks. Multiple metatarsal fractures usually require stabilization with K-wires or ORIF with plates. The pins should remain in place for 6 weeks. In open injuries involving bone loss, it is important to try and maintain metatarsal head position using transfixation pins and bone grafting the defect after wound stabilization.

Athletic Injuries

Ankle Sprains

Inversion sprains to the lateral ankle ligaments are the most common injuries in sports, accounting for 40% of all athletic injuries. The anterior talofibular ligament (ATFL) and calcaneofibular ligament (CFL) are injured sequentially during inversion of the plantarflexed foot. The posterior talofibular ligament rarely is injured except in complete dislocation of the ankle, and the distal tibiofibular ligaments are almost never injured during inversion sprains. Subtalar joint sprains can be isolated or associated with lateral ankle ligament sprains and frequently are overlooked in patients who have inversion ankle injuries. Other conditions that may be associated with lateral ankle ligament sprains include osteochondral fractures of the talus, peroneal tendon injuries, and injury to branches of the superficial peroneal nerve.

On examination, swelling and tenderness are noted over the ATFL and CFL areas. Tenderness posterior to the fibula may be indicative of peroneal tendon injury. Patients who are unable to bear weight should be suspected of having a fracture or an injury to the distal tibiofibular syndesmosis. Anterior drawer testing to assess the status of the ATFL is done with the knee flexed and the ankle in slight plantarflexion. Talar tilt is tested with the ankle in neutral dorsiplantarflexion, and is increased in injuries to both the ATFL and CFL. Grade I sprains are partial tears of the ATFL and are stable to stress testing. Grade II sprains are characterized by moderately increased anterior drawer with no increase in talar tilt. Grade III sprains are unstable to both anterior drawer and talar tilt stress, indicating complete tear of the ATFL and at least partial tear of the CFL.

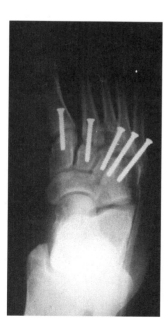

Figure 4

Severe Lisfranc injury that required screw stabilization of all tarsometatarsal joints. (Courtesy of Kenneth J. Koval, MD)

Treatment of grade I and II sprains starts with rest, ice, compression, and elevation (RICE). Hyperbaric oxygen therapy, while recently popular in the treatment of ankle sprains in professional athletes, has been shown to have no measurable effect when compared to controls. Surgical treatment of grade III sprains is rarely, if ever indicated. One to 3 weeks of cast immobilization may be appropriate in patients with grade III sprains accompanied by severe pain and swelling, but most patients are best treated with RICE and functional bracing. Early weightbearing is encouraged, and range-of-motion exercises avoiding inversion are begun as soon as pain and swelling permit. Stage II of rehabilitation begins with isometric, progressive resistive, and proprioceptive exercises. Athletes can return to sports when they are able to run and pivot without pain while the ankle is braced. Functional bracing or taping for sports has been shown to improve peroneal muscle reaction time and proprioception and to provide a mild increase in resistance to inversion stress. Bracing or taping for sports is continued for 6 months after injury.

Up to 20% of patients develop functional instability (giving way, recurrent sprains) after an acute inversion injury. Electromyographic studies have demonstrated prolonged peroneal muscle reaction times in patients with chronic ankle instability, and most of these patients will be improved by strengthening and proprioceptive exercises. Patients with persistent functional instability and demonstrated mechanical laxity are candidates for lateral ligament reconstruction.

Stress radiographs are used to determine mechanical laxity in patients with chronic lateral instability. Although normal values for lateral ankle laxity vary widely, it is generally agreed that anterior translation of the talus of more than 9 mm, or 5 mm more than the uninvolved ankle, is indicative of deficiency of the ATFL. Talar tilt of more than 10° or 5° more than the opposite side is indicative of excessive laxity in both the ATFL and CFL.

Surgical reconstruction is directed at restoring the anatomy and function of the ATFL and CFL. The Gould modification of the Broström procedure (Fig. 5) remains the most widely used reconstruction. In addition to repair of the ATFL and CFL, the lateral talocalcaneal ligament and extensor retinaculum are reefed to control excessive subtalar joint motion, which is frequently associated with lateral ankle instability. A longitudinal incision can be used to inspect the peroneal tendons in patients with pain posterior to the fibula. Patients with long-standing severe instability, failed previous anatomic repair, or generalized ligamentous laxity may require a reconstruction augmented with tendon graft. In addition, patients with severe subtalar joint laxity, varus hindfoot, or weakness of the peroneal musculature may require a nonanatomic, augmented reconstruction that limits subtalar joint motion. A varus hindfoot may contribute to instability as well as contribute to a failed reconstruction. A lateralizing calcaneal osteotomy may be a helpful adjunct to soft-tissue reconstruction.

Subtalar Joint Instability

Subtalar joint instability may be isolated or associated with lateral ankle instability, and is frequently overlooked. Because the CFL is a primary stabilizer of the subtalar joint, ankle sprains involving this ligament also affect the stability of the subtalar joint. After acute inversion injury, patients with injury to the bifurcate ligament have tenderness over the anterior calcaneal process, which is palpated half way between the lateral malleolus and the fifth metatarsal base. Nonunions of fractures of the anterior calcaneal process are not uncommon and may require excision with repair of the bifurcate ligament. Diagnosis of chronic subtalar joint laxity can be made clinically by determining total inversion of the foot and ankle, then subtracting talar tilt measured on stress radiographs, and comparing with the uninvolved side. Subtalar stress radiographs are obtained with the ankle in dorsiflexion and 30° internal rotation. The tube is angled in a 40° caudocephalad direction. Medial displacement of the calcaneus on the talus of more than 5 mm is indicative of excessive subtalar joint laxity. The clinical and radiographic diagnosis of subtalar joint instability often is difficult, and the clinician must be alert to the possibility of subtalar instability when evaluating patients with recurrent inversion injuries.

Direct repair of the subtalar joint ligaments alone may not achieve sufficient stability because of weak and attenuated tissues. Nonanatomic reconstruction augmented with tendon graft usually is required to reliably stabilize the subtalar joint. Subtalar joint instability is usually associated with ankle instability, and both joints can be successfully stabilized by procedures such as the Watson-Jones, Evans, or Chrisman-Snook reconstructions, which use a portion of the peroneus brevis tendon as a tenodesis that limits subtalar joint motion.

Syndesmosis Sprains

Approximately 1% of ankle sprains result in injury to the ankle syndesmosis. These injuries occur secondary to external rotation or hyperdorsiflexion of the ankle and usually are associated with injury to the deltoid ligament. Patients have pain and swelling over the deltoid ligament and the distal tibiofibular ligaments and complain of pain with weightbearing. Pain also may be elicited with forced external rotation or dorsiflexion of the ankle. The "squeeze test" is performed by compressing the fibula to the tibia above midcalf level; it is

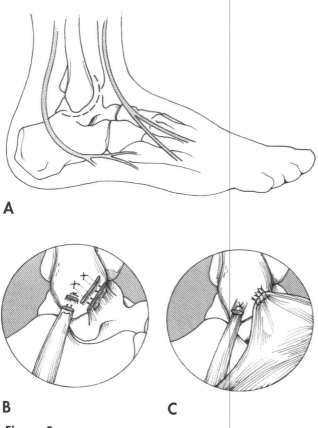

A

B   **C**

Figure 5

The modified Broström procedure (Broström-Gould). A, Curved anterolateral incision. A longitudinal incision may be used, allowing conversion to an augmented reconstruction, and inspection of the peroneal tendons. B, The anterior talofibular and calcaneofibular ligaments are divided 3 mm distal to their origin. The ligaments are sutured to the fibula through drill holes and the proximal stumps are repaired over the ligament in a pants over vest fashion. C, The lateral extensor retinaculum and the lateral talocalcaneal ligament are sutured to the fibula to control subtalar motion. (Reproduced with permission from McCluskey LC, Black K: Ankle injuries in sports, in Gould JS (ed): *Operative Foot Surgery*. Philadelphia, PA, WB Saunders, 1994, pp 901–936.)

positive when squeezing results in pain at the distal syndesmosis. Radiographs are required to rule out diastasis of the tibiofibular joint. Acute frank diastasis of as little as 1 mm may require internal fixation using a tibiofibular screw placed just proximal to the syndesmosis, along with repair of the ATFL. Patients who do not have diastasis are treated with a brief period of immobilization until pain and swelling are controlled, followed by mobilization in a functional brace. Weightbearing is delayed until the patient is pain free. Early weightbearing and accelerated return to sports activities may delay recovery and adversely affect outcome. Recovery time after syndesmosis sprain is prolonged, approximately double

that after grade III inversion ankle sprains. In patients with chronic pain after syndesmosis sprain, eversion stress radiographs or bone scan may be required to diagnose late subtle instability of the syndesmosis. Heterotopic ossification or frank synostosis may cause chronic pain after syndesmosis injury, requiring late resection.

Peroneal Tendon Injuries

Acute peroneal tendon dislocations frequently are misdiagnosed as ankle sprains because of associated lateral pain and swelling and a history of a twisting injury to the ankle. In peroneal tendon dislocations, however, the ankle is swollen and tender over the peroneal retinaculum, posterior to the fibula. On examination, the tendons may dislocate with active eversion of the ankle against resistance. Although cast immobilization may result in successful healing of the torn retinaculum in some patients, acute surgical repair is the most reliable method to achieve a satisfactory outcome. For chronic recurrent dislocation, deepening of the posterior fibular groove with repair of the superior retinaculum to the lateral fibula is a highly successful method of surgical treatment. Longitudinal tears in the peroneal tendons frequently are seen at the time of surgery and usually are treated by repair or excision of the damaged portion of the tendon.

Achilles Tendinitis/Tendinosis

The term "tendinosis" has become popular to differentiate inflammation of the tendon (tendinitis) from more chronic conditions that cause degeneration of the tendon substance. Peritendinitis is inflammation of the peritenon, and is characterized by inflammation and thickening of the peritenon. It is most common in middle-aged male runners as an overuse injury. Examination may reveal crepitus about the tendon with active motion. Mechanical causes also may be present and include excessive tibial varus, calcaneal valgus, and decreased elasticity of the gastrocnemius-soleus complex. Initial treatment consists of rest, nonsteroidal anti-inflammatory medication, heel wedges, and a stretching program. Neutral position orthotics and Achilles tendon taping may be successful in patients with mechanical malalignment.

Achilles peritendinitis with tendinosis is inflammation of the peritenon combined with alteration of the Achilles tendon. The tendon becomes thickened and may contain degenerative areas within its substance. Vascular studies have shown a decreased blood supply to the Achilles tendon 4 to 6 cm proximal to the calcaneal insertion, with this area being the most common site of tendinosis and rupture. Ultrasound and MRI are both sensitive tests for diagnosing and staging tendinosis. Patients with combined peritendinitis and tendinosis are treated similarly to those with isolated tendinitis.

Up to 25% of patients require surgery after failing to improve with at least 6 months of conservative management.

Surgical treatment consists of excision of the inflamed peritenon and exploration of the Achilles tendon with excision of degenerative tissue. In patients with insertional pain, the calcaneal tuberosity and retrocalcaneal bursa also are excised. Immediate motion is begun postoperatively. Despite aggressive rehabilitation, decreased calf muscle strength persists for over 6 months after surgery. Patients with intractable pain and significant degeneration may benefit from tendon augmentation. The flexor hallucis longus (FHL) is anatomically suited for this transfer, which adds both the tendon function and increased blood supply because the muscle belly may be approximated to the underside of the Achilles tendon and the tendon passed through a drill hole in the calcaneus. The distal part of the FHL is attached to the flexor digitorum longus but remains somewhat weak.

Achilles tendinosis leading to rupture is characterized by mucinoid degeneration and fatty infiltration of the tendon. Approximately 85% of patients have no history of pain before acute rupture, and in these patients mechanical factors such as eccentric overloading may be the primary etiologic factor, rather than degeneration of the tendon. Acute rupture is characterized by a palpable defect 6 to 8 cm proximal to the calcaneal insertion and failure of the foot to passively plantarflex when the calf is squeezed (Thompson test). Because the diagnosis is missed in up to 25% of patients, careful attention to the status of the Achilles tendon is required when examining patients with acute ankle injuries. In spite of the frequency of the injury, the need for surgical treatment remains unclear. Most physicians treating elite athletes recommend surgical treatment. Acute repair followed by early protected motion is recommended in active individuals. Repair is accomplished with heavy nonabsorbable sutures and can be reinforced with a tendon graft. Full return to sports usually is possible at 6 months, with minimal strength deficits. MRI studies of repaired tendons show complete continuity at 6 months. A recent prospective randomized study from Europe compared open and closed treatment of those without a gap in the tendon and found no difference in outcome or rerupture rate. Patients were excluded from the randomization if, with the foot plantarflexed by gravity, the gap between the proximal and distal ends of the ruptured tendon was > 1 cm. Nonsurgical treatment may be suitable in inactive patients; however, it is associated with a 25% rerupture rate and significant residual calf muscle weakness.

Stress Fractures

Stress fractures of the foot and ankle account for up to half of all stress fractures in athletes. Diagnosis may be delayed because of poor localization on physical examination and failure of standard radiographs to show the fracture. Technetium Tc 99m bone scanning frequently shows multiple areas of increased uptake in the feet of running athletes and, therefore, is not always definitive in diagnosing or localizing stress fractures in this area.

Medial Malleolus Although the tibia is the most common site for stress fractures in track athletes, medial malleolar stress fractures are rare. Medial malleolar stress fractures are associated with jumping sports and are characterized by a vertical fracture line extending from the medial articular surface of the tibial plafond. Although nonsurgical immobilization is adequate for incomplete fractures, complete fractures require ORIF. After fixation, early motion is allowed with protected weightbearing until radiographs show complete healing.

Fibula Fibular stress fractures occur 6 to 8 cm proximal to the tip of the lateral malleolus. Full weightbearing in a below knee cast is the initial treatment followed by gradual return to sports in a pneumatic protective splint once the pain and swelling permit (4 to 6 weeks). Healing is usually complete at 8 to 12 weeks after fracture. Valgus hindfoot alignment may be causative and should be corrected in severe or recalcitrant cases.

Tarsal Navicular Navicular stress fractures are the most common stress fractures in the athlete's foot, accounting for 15% of all stress fractures in track athletes. The fracture propagates in the sagittal plane secondary to repetitive impact from the head of the talus, and it may be more common in athletes with a cavus foot. Microangiographic studies demonstrate a relative avascularity of the central third of the bone. Pain is poorly localized, and standard radiographs frequently fail to show the fracture, making delayed and missed diagnosis of this fracture common. Although technetium Tc 99m bone scan is the most sensitive test for stress fracture, high impact athletes frequently have multiple areas of increased uptake in the foot, making the test less valuable in these individuals. MRI may more reliably locate an early stress fracture in the tarsal bones. CT scanning reliably shows an established fracture (Fig. 6). Treatment consists of nonweightbearing and immobilization for 8 weeks. CT scanning should be repeated to document healing before return to sports, and orthotics frequently are used to reduce stress and refracture. Weightbearing has been associated with a high nonunion rate, leading to severe midfoot degenerative arthritis and loss of function. Delayed union or nonunion is treated by excision of the sclerotic fracture margins and bone grafting, with or without internal fixation. Because the blood supply enters by radial penetrating arteries originating in a circumferential vessel, the dissection should be limited. When internal fixation is needed, it can be inserted percutaneously under fluoroscopic guidance.

Tarsal Stress Fractures Other Than the Navicular Stress fractures of the calcaneus, cuboid, and cuneiform bones are less common and can be treated with relative rest, weightbearing as pain permits in a rigid orthosis, and gradual advancement of activities. Custom orthotics may prevent recurrence after healing.

Metatarsal Stress Fractures Metatarsal stress fractures are more frequently associated with military recruits undergoing physical conditioning than with athletes; however, these fractures are common in athletes. The distal diaphysis of the second or third metatarsal is the most common site. Standard radiographs usually are negative for the first 2 to 3 weeks, followed by the appearance of bone callus at the fracture site. Patients are placed in a rigid orthosis and can resume athletic training when pain permits. Fracture at the second metatarsal base is less common and is associated with prolonged morbidity resulting from delayed union. The fracture should be immobilized, with the patient nonweightbearing for 8 weeks or until radiographic evidence of healing is seen. The use of an orthosis is recommended with the resumption of sports. An anatomic cause should be sought for stress fractures of the neck of the second or third metatarsal. Possible problems—excessive tightness of the heel cord, a long second or short first metatarsal, or an excessively mobile first metatarsal or ray—are amenable to surgical correction.

Stress fractures of the base of the fifth metatarsal distal to the tuberosity, or "Jones fractures," are common athletic injuries and are more likely to occur in the cavus foot as a result of increased ground reaction force over the fifth metatarsal. Acute fractures often heal with strict nonweightbearing in a below knee cast for 8 weeks. Stress fractures are characterized by widening of the fracture site with sclerosis of the fracture margins and are less likely to heal with nonsurgical treatment. Because of the high incidence of delayed unions, nonunions, and refractures in athletes and other young active persons sustaining this injury, intramedullary fixation with a screw is the treatment of choice in this group of patients. Intramedullary screw fixation allows early protected weightbearing and return to sports in 6 to 8 weeks if radiographs show evidence of healing.

Annotated Bibliography

Epidemiology

Baron JA, Karagas M, Barrett J, et al: Basic epidemiology of fractures of the upper and lower limb among Americans over 65 years of age. *Epidemiology* 1996;7:612–618.

Ankle fracture rates for women are higher than those for men, and whites have higher rates than do blacks of the same gender. Ankle fracture rates do not increase with age.

Seeley DG, Kelsey J, Jergas M, Nevitt MC: Predictors of ankle and foot fractures in older women: The study of Osteoporotic Fractures Research Group. *J Bone Miner Res* 1996;11:1347–1355.

Data from 9,704 women over 65 years of age were analyzed. Ankle fractures are only weakly related to bone density and are not age-related in older women.

Tibial Pilon

Aktuglu K, Ozsoy MH, Yensel U: Treatment of displaced pylon fractures with circular external fixators of Ilizarov. *Foot Ankle Int* 1998;19:208–216.

Twenty cases of pylon fractures were treated with Ilizarov external fixators. Results were good to excellent in 75% of patients. Pin tract infections occurred in 55%.

Babis GC, Vayanos ED, Papaioannou N, Pantazopoulos T: Results of surgical treatment of tibial plafond fractures. *Clin Orthop* 1997;341:99–105.

Three parameters significantly influenced the outcome of tibial plafond fractures: (1) the clinical type of fracture, (2) the quality of reduction attained at surgery, and (3) the specific surgical procedure used to manage the fracture.

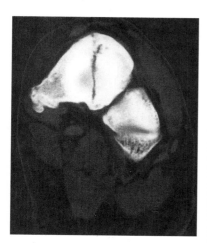

Figure 6

Stress fractures of the tarsal navicular are often not detected on standard radiographs. Computed tomography scan is the most accurate method for visualizing the sagittally oriented fracture.

Marsh JL, Bonar S, Nepola JV, Decoster TA, Hurwitz SR: Use of an articulated external fixator for fractures of the tibial plafond. *J Bone Joint Surg* 1995;77A:1498–1509.

In a prospective study, 49 displaced tibial plafond fractures were treated with an articulated external fixator combined (in most cases) with limited internal fixation of the joint. No deep infections were recorded; 18 patients considered their results excellent or satisfactory.

Martin JS, Marsh JL, Bonar SK, DeCoster TA, Found EM, Brandser EA: Assessment of the AO/ASIF fracture classification for the distal tibia. *J Orthop Trauma* 1997;7:477–483.

Good observer agreement was achieved among the examiners for the type of pilon fracture, but poor agreement was observed when grouping the fractures. Using CT scans did not improve examiner agreement on classification.

Teeny SM, Wiss DA: Open reduction and internal fixation of tibial plafond fractures: Variables contributing to poor results and complications. *Clin Orthop* 1993;292:108–117.

ORIF was used in 60 tibial plafond fractures. Outcomes correlated well with the magnitude of the injury and the ability to obtain a stable anatomic reduction. Thirty-seven percent of the severe fractures became infected.

Williams TM, Marsh JL, Nepola JV, DeCoster TA, Hurwitz SR, Bonar SB: External fixation of tibial plafond fractures: Is routine plating of the fibula necessary? *J Orthop Trauma* 1998; 12:16–20.

ORIF of the fibula fracture in tibial plafond fractures treated with external fixation was associated with a significant rate of wound complications. Good clinical results may be obtained without fixing the fibula.

Ankle

Auleley GR, Kerboull L, Durieux P, Cosquer M, Courpied JP, Ravaud P: Validation of the Ottawa ankle rules in France: A study in the surgical emergency department of a teaching hospital. *Ann Emerg Med* 1998;32:14–18.

Use of the Ottawa ankle rules by French emergency physicians resulted in 99% sensitivity in detecting ankle fractures and had the potential of reducing radiography requests by 33%. The rules failed to predict 1 avulsion fracture.

Brage ME, Rockett M, Vraney R, Anderson R, Toledano A: Ankle fracture classification: A comparison of reliability of three X-ray views versus two. *Foot Ankle Int* 1998;19:555–562.

Four different observers independently classified 99 sets of ankle radiographs using both the Lauge-Hansen and Danis-Weber systems. Good to excellent agreement was demonstrated overall among the examiners when using the Danis-Weber system with either 3 or 2 views, and there was good agreement using the Lauge-Hansen system with either 2 or 3 views.

Clark TW, Janzen DL, Logan PM, Ho K, Connell DG: Improving the detection of radiographically occult ankle fractures: Positive predictive value of an ankle joint effusion. *Clin Radiol* 1996; 51:632–636.

The presence of a large ankle effusion on radiographs after acute ankle trauma suggests an underlying fracture. The positive predictive value of an effusion 15 mm or greater on the initial lateral ankle radiograph was 83%.

Jensen SL, Andresen BK, Mencke S, Nielsen PT: Epidemiology of ankle fractures: A prospective population-based study of 212 cases in Aalborg, Denmark. *Acta Orthop Scand* 1998;69: 48–50.

Below the age of 50, ankle fractures were commonest in men. After this age, ankle fractures in women became predominant. Alcohol and slippery surfaces were each involved in nearly a third of ankle fractures. Nine tenths of ankle fractures are the result of indirect trauma.

Kelly AM, Richards D, Kerr L, et al: Failed validation of a clinical decision rule for the use of radiography in acute ankle injury. *NZ Med J* 1994;107:294–295.

In a multicenter trial, the Ottawa rule had a sensitivity of 93% for ankle fracture detection, with a specificity of 11%. Fractures that were missed included an unstable ankle fracture, a calcaneus fracture, and a talus fracture.

Konrath G, Karges D, Watson JT, Moed BR, Cramer K: Early versus delayed treatment of severe ankle fractures: A comparison of results. *J Orthop Trauma* 1995;9:377–380.

A retrospective review of 202 closed Weber B bimalleolar ankle fractures showed no significant differences in the results or complications of those fractures treated early versus those treated with delay.

Low CK, Tan SK: Infection in diabetic patients with ankle fractures. *Ann Acad Med Singapore* 1995;24:353–355.

Ten patients with diabetes underwent ORIF for displaced ankle fractures. Infection occurred in 50%, 4 had wound infections, and the last patient developed an infected pressure sore from the cast. Two patients required below-knee amputations. With treatment, the infection in the other 3 patients resolved.

McBryde A, Chiasson B, Wihelm A, Donovan F, Ray T, Bacilla P: Syndesmotic screw placement: A biomechanical analysis. *Foot Ankle Int* 1997;18:262–266.

In a cadaver study, syndesmotic fixation with the screw placed 2.0 cm above the ankle joint provided the strongest fixation when compared to the screw placed 3.5 cm above the joint.

Michelson JD, Ahn U, Magid D: Economic analysis of roentgenogram use in the closed treatment of stable ankle fractures. *J Trauma* 1995;39:1119–1122.

Review of serial radiographs in 82 patients with stable ankle fractures showed that secondary displacement of the talus or fibula is rare. Frequent radiographs for evaluation of stable ankle fractures may not be needed.

Musgrave DJ, Fankhauser RA: Intraoperative radiographic assessment of ankle fractures. *Clin Orthop* 1998;351:186–190.

To determine whether 3 or 2 radiographic ankle views are necessary to properly evaluate the reduction of low energy, rotational ankle fractures during surgery, 4 surgeons independently reviewed 2 sets of 93 ankle fractures treated with ORIF. The authors concluded that fracture reduction and fixation can be assessed adequately with only the lateral and mortise views.

Omeroglu H, Gunel U, Bicimoglu A, Tabak AY, Ucaner A, Guney O: The relationship between the use of tourniquet and the intensity of postoperative pain in surgically treated malleolar fractures. *Foot Ankle Int* 1997;18:798–802.

Postoperative pain with tourniquet use was harder to control in males and patients older than 30 years of age.

Pelto-Vasenius K, Hirvensalo E, Vasenius J, Partio EK, Bostman O, Rokkanen P: Redisplacement after ankle osteosynthesis with absorbable implants. *Arch Orthop Trauma Surg* 1998;117: 159–162.

Redisplacement of the ankle fracture following fixation occurred in 2.5% of patients and was more common in more severe ankle fractures. Absorbable implants may not be suitable for comminuted, unstable ankle fractures.

Stiell I, Wells G, Laupacis A, et al: Multicentre trial to introduce the Ottawa ankle rules for use of radiography in acute ankle injuries: Multicentre Ankle Rule Study Group. *BMJ* 1995; 311:594–597.

The Ottawa ankle rule was used by more than 200 physicians evaluating more than 12,000 adults with acute ankle injuries. There were significant reductions in the use of ankle radiography and in waiting times for patients. The sensitivity of the rule in detecting ankle fractures approached 100%.

Yamaguchi K, Martin CH, Boden SD, Labropoulos PA: Operative treatment of syndesmotic disruptions without use of a syndesmotic screw: A prospective clinical study. *Foot Ankle Int* 1994; 15:407–414.

Transyndesmotic fixation was not used if rigid bimalleolar fixation was obtained or if lateral without medial fixation was achieved when the fibular fracture was within 4.5 cm of the joint line. With these guidelines, only 3 of the 21 patients in the study need stabilization of the syndesmosis.

Traumatic Foot Injuries

Bohay DR, Manoli A II: Occult fractures following subtalar joint injuries. *Foot Ankle Int* 1996;17:164–169.

The authors discuss the late findings of 4 cases of subtalar joint disruption and the effect of occult fractures on the joint long term. The problem of subsequent arthritis is enough to warrant a CT scan of subtalar joint disruptions to identify articular fractures.

Burdeaux BD Jr: Fractures of the calcaneus: Open reduction and internal fixation from the medial side. A 21-year prospective study. *Foot Ankle Int* 1997;18:685–692.

Sixty-one calcaneal fractures were treated by a medially directed open reduction; 80% were considered successful, and a mean American Orthopaedic Foot and Ankle Society score of 94.7 was obtained.

Freeman BJ, Duff S, Allen PE, Nicholson HD, Atkins RM: The extended lateral approach to the hindfoot: Anatomical basis and surgical implications. *J Bone Joint Surg* 1998;80B:139–142.

This article provides an extensive review of the anatomy for the lateral approach to the calcaneus and includes tips to minimize surgical wound complications.

Inokuchi S, Ogawa K, Usami N, Hashimoto T: Long-term follow up of talus fractures. *Orthopedics* 1996;19:477–481.

This article covers a 10-year follow-up of 86 talar fractures. Poor outcome was caused by the onset of osteoarthritis secondary to osteonecrosis and joint surface incongruity. Early nonweightbearing is recommended for best results.

Miric A, Patterson BM: Pathoanatomy of intra-articular fractures of the calcaneus. *J Bone Joint Surg* 1998;80A:207–212.

Two hundred twenty calcaneal fractures are reviewed radiographically and the fracture anatomy defined. CT scans are critical for determining the true fracture anatomy. Usually there were associated joint injuries in addition to the posterior facet.

Myerson MS: Primary subtalar arthrodesis for the treatment of comminuted fractures of the calcaneus. *Orthop Clin North Am* 1995;26:215–227.

The article discusses the selection and technique for primary fusion, which is indicated for a badly comminuted posterior facet. Good results can be obtained with attention to anatomic reduction of the fracture.

Quill GE Jr: Fractures of the proximal fifth metatarsal. *Orthop Clin North Am* 1995;26:353–361.

In depth review of the injuries to the base of the fifth metatarsal and accepted treatments are discussed.

Ruiz Valdivieso T, de Miguel Vielba JA, Hernandez Garcia C, Castrillo AV, Alvarez Posadas JI, Sanchez Martin MM: Subtalar dislocation: A study of nineteen cases. *Int Orthop* 1996;20:83–86.

Nineteen cases of subtalar dislocation were reviewed approximately 8 years after injury and reduction. Poor results were due to open injuries, associated bone lesions, and prolonged immobilization.

Sanchez Alepuz E, Vicent Carsi V, Alcantara P, Llabres AJ: Fractures of the central metatarsal. *Foot Ankle Int* 1996; 17:200–203.

Fifty-seven patients with central metatarsal fractures were reviewed. Treatments were mixed. Poor outcomes as judged by metatarsalgia were seen with comminution, sagittal plane displacement, open fracture, or severe soft-tissue injury.

Thordarson DB, Krieger LE: Operative vs. nonoperative treatment of intra-articular fractures of the calcaneus: A prospective randomized trial. *Foot Ankle Int* 1996;17:2–9.

Thirty interarticular calcaneal fractures were prospectively randomized to standardized surgical or nonsurgical care. Functional outcome studies at 2 years showed better outcome with surgical care (86.7) than with nonsurgical care (55.0).

Athletic Injuries

Lateral Ankle Sprains

Borromeo CN, Ryan JL, Marchetto PA, Peterson R, Bove AA: Hyperbaric oxygen therapy for acute ankle sprains. *Am J Sports Med* 1997;25:619–625.

This randomized, double-blind study found no difference between patients treated with hyperbaric oxygen versus controls.

Burks RT, Morgan J: Anatomy of the lateral ankle ligaments. *Am J Sports Med* 1994;22:72–77.

Location and orientation of the lateral ankle ligaments is precisely defined, enabling the surgeon to perform an anatomically correct reconstruction.

Louwerens JW, Ginai AZ, van Linge B, Snijders CJ: Stress radiography of the talocrural and subtalar joints. *Foot Ankle Int* 1995;16:148–155.

Diagnostic techniques for talocrural and subtalar stress radiography are reviewed, and clinical significance is discussed.

Mascaro TB, Swanson LE: Rehabilitation of the foot and ankle. *Orthop Clin North Am* 1994;25:147–160.

An in-depth, step by step review of functional rehabilitation of the injured ankle is presented.

Thermann H, Zwipp H, Tscherne H: Treatment algorithm of chronic ankle and subtalar instability. *Foot Ankle Int* 1997;18:163–169.

A rationale for anatomic versus nonanatomic reconstruction is presented based on the presence of combined talocrural and subtalar instability.

Syndesmosis Sprains

Miller CD, Shelton WR, Barrett GR, Savoie FH, Dukes AD: Deltoid and syndesmosis ligament injury of the ankle without fracture. *Am J Sports Med* 1995;23:746–750.

The authors advocate the use of stress radiographs to detect subtle instability of the syndesmosis, and internal fixation of diastasis of 1 mm or more.

Achilles Tendinitis and Tendinosis

Karjalainen PT, Aronen HJ, Pihlajamaki HK, Soila K, Paavonen T, Bostman OM: Magnetic resonance imaging during healing of surgically repaired Achilles tendon ruptures. *Am J Sports Med* 1997;25:164–171.

MRI is an accurate method for determining rate of healing following repair of Achilles tendon ruptures.

Mandelbaum BR, Myerson MS, Forster R: Achilles tendon ruptures: A new method of repair, early range of motion, and functional rehabilitation. *Am J Sports Med* 1995;23:392–395.

Early motion and full weightbearing after repair resulted in no reruptures and no isokinetic strength deficit at 12 months postoperatively.

Scioli MW: Achilles tendinitis. *Orthop Clin North Am* 1994;25:177–182.

This is a review of the pathogenesis, diagnosis, and treatment of Achilles tendinitis.

Peroneal Tendon Injuries

Kollias SL, Ferkel RD: Fibular grooving for recurrent peroneal tendon subluxation. *Am J Sports Med* 1997;25:329–335.

The authors describe the fibular grooving procedure for recurrent peroneal tendon dislocation. All 11 patients were rated excellent at follow-up with no recurrent dislocations.

Stress Fractures

Bennell KL, Malcolm SA, Thomas SA, Wark JD, Brukner PD: The incidence and distribution of stress fractures in competitive track and field athletes: A twelve-month prospective study. *Am J Sports Med* 1996;24:211–217.

The authors report a prospective study, documenting the incidence and distribution of stress fractures in track and field athletes.

Classic Bibliography

Ankle Fractures

Bauer M, Jonsson K, Nilsson B: Thirty-year follow-up of ankle fractures. *Acta Orthop Scand* 1985;56:103–106.

Boden SD, Labropoulos PA, McCowin P, Lestini WF, Hurwitz SR: Mechnical considerations for the syndesmosis screw: A cadaver study. *J Bone Joint Surg* 1989;71A:1548–1555.

Bourne RB, Rorabeck CH, Macnab J: Intra-articular fractures of the distal tibia: The pilon fracture. *J Trauma* 1983;23:591–596

Eisele SA, Sammarco GJ: Fatigue fractures of the foot and ankle in the athlete, in Heckman JD (ed): *Instructional Course Lectures 42*. Rosemont, IL, American Academy of Orthopaedic Surgeons, 1993, pp 175–183.

Finsen V, Saetermo R, Kibsgaard L, et al: Early postoperative weight-bearing and muscle activity in patients who have a fracture of the ankle. *J Bone Joint Surg* 1989;71A:23–27.

Franklin JL, Johnson KD, Hansen ST Jr: Immediate internal fixation of open ankle fractures: Report of thirty-eight cases treated with a standard protocol. *J Bone Joint Surg* 1984;66A: 1349–1356.

Gould N, Seligson D, Gassman J: Early and late repair of lateral ligaments of the ankle. *Foot Ankle* 1980;1:84–89.

Hopkinson WJ, St. Pierre P, Ryan JB, Wheeler JH: Syndesmosis sprains of the ankle. *Foot Ankle* 1990;10:325–330.

Kannus P, Renstrom P: Treatment for acute tears of the lateral ligaments of the ankle: Operation, cast, or early controlled mobilization. *J Bone Joint Surg* 1991;73A:305–312.

Kellam JF, Waddell JP: Fractures of the distal tibial metaphysis with intra-articular extension: The distal tibial explosion factor. *J Trauma* 1979;19:593–601.

Kristensen KD, Hansen T: Closed treatment of ankle fractures: Stage II supination-eversion fractures followed for 20 years. *Acta Orthop Scand* 1985;56:107–109.

Lauge-Hansen N: Fractures of the ankle. II: Combined experimental-surgical and experimental-roentgenologic investigations. *Arch Surg* 1950;60:957–985.

Lindsjö U: Operative treatment of ankle fracture-dislocations: A follow-up study of 306/321 consecutive cases. *Clin Orthop* 1985;199:28–38.

Lundberg A, Svensson OK, Nemeth G, Selvik G: The axis of rotation of the ankle joint. *J Bone Joint Surg* 1989;71B:94–99.

Pankovich AM: Fractures of the fibula proximal to the distal tibiofibular syndesmosis. *J Bone Joint Surg* 1978;60A:221–229.

Schaffer JJ, Manoli A II: The antiglide plate for distal fibular fixation: A biomechanical comparison with fixation with a lateral plate. *J Bone Joint Surg* 1987;69A:596–604.

Torg JS, Balduini FC, Zelko RR, Pavlov H, Peff TC, Das M: Fractures of the base of the fifth metatarsal distal to the tuberosity: Classification and guidelines for non-surgical and surgical management. *J Bone Joint Surg* 1984;66A:209–214.

Torg JS, Pavlov H, Cooley LH, et al: Stress fractures of the tarsal navicular: A retrospective review of twenty-one cases. *J Bone*

Joint Surg 1982;64A:700–712.

Weber BG, Simpson LA: Corrective lengthening osteotomy of the fibula. *Clin Orthop* 1985;199:61–67.

Wilson FC Jr, Skilbred LA: Long-term results in the treatment of displaced bimalleolar fractures. *J Bone Joint Surg* 1966;48A: 1065–1078.

Yablon IG, Heller FG, Shouse L: The key role of the lateral malleolus in displaced fractures of the ankle. *J Bone Joint Surg* 1977; 59A:169–173.

Yde J, Kristensen KD: Ankle fractures: Supination-eversion fractures stage II. Primary and late results of operative and non-operative treatment. *Acta Orthop Scand* 1980;51:695–702.

Zeegers AV, van der Werken C: Rupture of the deltoid ligament in ankle fractures: Should it be repaired? *Injury* 1989;20:39–41.

Traumatic Injuries to the Foot

Arntz CT, Veith RG, Hansen ST Jr: Fractures and fracture-dislocations of the tarsometatarsal joint. *J Bone Joint Surg* 1988; 70A:173–181.

Benirschke SK, Sangeorzan BJ: Extensive intraarticular fractures of the foot: Surgical management of calcaneal fractures. *Clin Orthop* 1993;292:128–134.

Böhler L: Diagnosis, pathology, and treatment of fractures of the os calcis. *J Bone Joint Surg* 1931;13:75–89.

Buckley RE, Meek RN: Comparison of open versus closed reduction of intraarticular calcaneal fractures: A matched cohort in workmen. *J Orthop Trauma* 1992;6:216–222.

Canale ST, Kelly FB Jr: Fractures of the neck of the talus: Long-term evaluation of seventy-one cases. *J Bone Joint Surg* 1978; 60A:143–156.

Carr JB, Hansen ST, Benirschke SK: Subtalar distraction bone block fusion for late complications of os calcis fractures. *Foot Ankle* 1988;9:81–86.

Essex-Lopresti P: The mechanism, reduction technique, and results in fractures of the os calcis. *Br J Surg* 1952;39:395–419.

Foster SC, Foster RR: Lisfrancís tarsometatarsal fracture-dislocation. *Radiology* 1976;120:79–83.

Gallie WE: Subastragalar arthrodesis in fractures of the os calcis. *J Bone Joint Surg* 1943;25:731–736.

Hawkins LG: Fractures of the neck of the talus. *J Bone Joint Surg* 1970;52A:991–1002.

612   Lower Extremity

Kalamchi A, Evans JG: Posterior subtalar fusion: A preliminary report on a modified Gallie's procedure. *J Bone Joint Surg* 1977;59B:287–289.

Lindsay WRN, Dewar FP: Fractures of the os calcis. *Am J Surg* 1958;95:555–576.

Sanders R, Fortin P, DiPasquale T, Walling A: Operative treatment in 120 displaced intra-articular calcaneal fractures: Results using a prognostic computed tomography scan classification. *Clin Orthop* 1993;290:87–95.

Sangeorzan BJ, Benirschke SK, Carr JB: Surgical management of fractures of the os calcis, in Jackson DW (ed): *Instructional Course Lectures 44.* Rosemont, IL, American Academy of Orthopaedic Surgeons, 1995, pp 359–370.

Sangeorzan BJ, Mayo KA, Hansen ST: Intraarticular fractures of the foot: Talus and lesser tarsals. *Clin Orthop* 1993;292: 135–141.

Sangeorzan BJ, Benirschke SK, Mosca V, Mayo KA, Hansen ST Jr: Displaced intra-articular fractures of the tarsal navicular. *J Bone Joint Surg* 1989;71A:1504–1510.

Sangeorzan BJ, Swiontkowski MF: Displaced fractures of the cuboid. *J Bone Joint Surg* 1990;72B:376–378.

Stephenson JR: Treatment of displaced intra-articular fractures of the calcaneus using medial and lateral approaches, internal fixation, and early motion. *J Bone Joint Surg* 1987;69A:115–130.

Swanson TV, Bray TJ, Holmes GB Jr: Fractures of the talar neck: A mechanical study of fixation. *J Bone Joint Surg* 1992;74A: 544–551.

Chapter 46
Ankle and Foot Reconstruction

Hindfoot and Ankle Reconstruction

Introduction

The biomechanics of the subtalar and talonavicular joints determine the function of the foot. The subtalar joint is the major contributor to inversion (heel varus) and eversion (heel valgus), but it does not move in a strictly coronal plane. When the hindfoot is inverted, as happens in midstance to toe-off, the foot becomes rigid, allowing for propulsion. When the hindfoot is everted, the foot is supple, allowing shock absorption at heel strike and accommodation to uneven ground while walking. Loss of these important functions leads to a rigid foot and ultimately places more stress across the midfoot and ankle. Over an extended time this may lead to degenerative joint disease in adjacent joints. The subtalar and transverse tarsal joints also contribute to dorsiflexion and plantarflexion, primarily at the limits of the arc of motion.

Because of longer life expectancy, the frequency of surgical arthrodesis of major joints is declining. Selective arthrodesis of the talonavicular or talocalcaneal joints substantially reduces hindfoot motion. Selective arthrodesis of the calcaneocuboid joint in neutral position, however, does not cause significant loss of functional motion of the subtalar joint. Arthrodesis in malposition, however, leads to significant loss of subtalar motion, which initiates the degenerative cascade. As in other weightbearing joints, valgus is better tolerated than varus. Inversion and eversion, while primarily attributed to the subtalar joint, are to a small extent cumulative, because the ankle joint is capable of coronal plane motion in the extremes of the arc.

Pes Planus

Pes planus is characterized by flattening of the medial longitudinal arch, with or without forefoot abduction, hindfoot valgus, or a tight heel cord. The deformity is classified as flexible or rigid. A rigid deformity in a child or adolescent is indicative of peroneal spastic flatfoot, which is rare in adults. A diminished medial longitudinal arch is present in 10% to 20% of the population; however, if the heel cord is not tight and the hindfoot is flexible, this is not abnormal. Recent evidence suggests that some patients with asymptomatic flexible flatfoot may progress to a symptomatic deformity, because patients with symptomatic flatfoot often have a painless flexible deformity on the contralateral side. Most adult flatfoot deformities develop when a normal foot loses its arch after rupture of the posterior tibial tendon (Fig. 1).

Treatment of pes planus is indicated if the foot becomes painful or the deformity progresses and makes shoe wear difficult. The goal of nonsurgical treatment is to prevent progression of the deformity while achieving permanent correction. This typically involves the use of an arch support. If the hindfoot is flexible and in a neutral position, a simple accommodative insert can be used. Significant hindfoot valgus may require a University of California, Berkeley (UCB) L-type orthosis with medial posting. If the posterior tibial tendon is ruptured, a brace above the ankle usually is required to relieve pain.

Surgical treatment is indicated for painful pes planus if conservative treatment fails or if significant deformities cannot be corrected nonsurgically. Such deformities include forefoot abduction, hindfoot valgus, talonavicular or navicular cuneiform or tarsal-metatarsal sag, and significant heel-cord contracture. Surgical treatment includes soft-tissue balancing, usually by lengthening of the Achilles tendon and augmentation with the flexor digitorum longus (FDL), and correction of bony alignment by osteotomy or arthrodesis. Because the deformity includes attrition of the stabilizing ligaments, correction of bony alignment often is needed. Medial

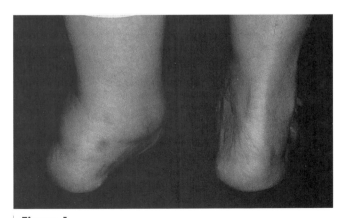

Figure 1

Flatfoot deformity in an adult secondary to posterior tibial tendon rupture.

column stabilization at the level of the naviculocuneiform or cuneiform metatarsal joints may correct the longitudinal arch. When significant hindfoot valgus accompanies the loss of arch, a medializing calcaneal osteotomy may be used. When forefoot abduction is present as well, lateral column lengthening can complete the correction. Soft-tissue reconstruction should not be done without bony stabilization, because without structural stability, the soft tissues will eventually stretch. Major arthrodesis should probably be reserved for elderly patients and patients with uncorrectable deformity or degenerative joint changes, because normal motion and function are sacrificed. Early surgical intervention in a foot with a supple subtalar joint may help to maintain normal function.

Posterior Tibial Tendon Incompetence

Etiology Several factors are thought to contribute to dysfunction of the posterior tibial tendon, including mechanical wear, Achilles tendon tightness, increased extratendinous pressure from a bony or soft-tissue injury, accessory navicular, preexisting flexible flatfoot deformity, and steroid injection.

The posterior tibial tendon makes a sharp turn at the medial malleolus, which may contribute to the mechanical wear. A tight Achilles tendon complex or equinus contracture also overloads the foot, causing the heel to come off the ground early in the gait cycle. The downward force of body weight must be counteracted by the upward pull of the posterior tibial tendon, which stresses the tendon further and leads to hypermobility of the medial column. Instability of the medial column of the weightbearing tripod of the foot may contribute to tendon overload and failure.

A nondisplaced fracture or soft-tissue injury in the area of the posterior tibial tendon that does not disrupt the soft-tissue envelope may, theoretically, cause local bleeding thereby increasing extratendinous pressure. Because this area is hypovascular, the end arteriole pressure may not be sufficient to overcome this increase.

Rupture of the posterior tibial tendon has been reported to occur after surgical sectioning of the plantar fascia for plantar fasciitis or heel pain. Loss of the plantar fascia, which serves as part of the static arch support and helps to evenly distribute forces on the plantar surface of the foot, can hasten arch collapse and development of posterior tibial tendon incompetence. Steroid injections also have been implicated in these tendon ruptures.

Patients who are obese, have hypertension, diabetes, or rheumatoid arthritis are susceptible to posterior tibial tendon rupture. Although diabetes is believed to be a contributing factor in some patients, it is unclear whether the tendon incompetence is the result of the disease process, neuropathic sequelae, or a combination of multiple factors. Patients with rheumatoid arthritis may develop posterior tibial tendon rupture as a result of direct invasion of the tendon or secondary strain from a valgus hindfoot.

Anatomy The posterior tibial tendon arises in the deep posterior compartment of the leg from the posterior surface of the tibia, interosseous membrane, and fibula and passes behind the medial malleolus to insert onto the medial navicular. Fibers from the posterior tibial tendon that pass under the medial arch extend to the cuneiforms and cuboid, as well as to the bases of the second, third, and fourth metatarsals, dynamically supporting the arch. The plantar interosseous ligaments are extremely strong and form a static support sling. If the posterior tibial tendon becomes incompetent, the static support soon stretches. Both traumatic and attritional ruptures of the spring ligament have been linked to adult flatfoot.

Clinical Presentation Symptoms of posterior tibial tendon rupture may start after a seemingly minor injury. Pain usually is located medially at first, but after the tendon ruptures, discomfort is more diffuse in the arch. As the foot begins to sag and abduct, pain can move laterally into the area of the sinus tarsi or beneath the fibula where bony impingement occurs (Fig. 2). On clinical examination, the foot has a diminished arch and may have hindfoot valgus or forefoot abduction. When viewed from behind, the hindfoot valgus can allow more than the fifth toe to be visible (the "too-many-toes" sign).

Radiographs should include weightbearing anteroposterior (AP) and lateral views and a hindfoot alignment (Harris) view. Uncovering of the talar head medially is a sign of fore-

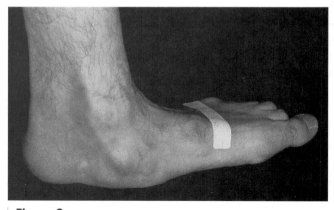

Figure 2

Flatfoot deformity with collapse of the medial arch in a foot with an intact but insufficient posterior tibial tendon.

foot abduction. The lateral weightbearing view may show an altered talo-first metatarsal axis. Degenerative changes at the talonavicular and talocalcaneal joints, with spurring and dorsal talar bossing, also may be present. The hindfoot alignment view is a reliable method of measuring coronal plane alignment. Patients stand on a radiolucent platform with equal weight on both feet. The X-ray tube is oriented 20° from the horizontal so it is perpendicular to the plane of the film, and the beam is centered at the level of the ankle.

Treatment Nonsurgical treatment may be appropriate in an elderly or sedentary patient with a normal arch on the other foot. A custom-molded ankle-foot orthosis (AFO) with medial posting to invert the valgus hindfoot or shoe modifications with wedging can be used.

When symptoms are related entirely to synovitis of the posterior tibial tendon, as in patients with rheumatoid arthritis, synovectomy alone may be appropriate (Fig. 3). When the tendon has completely ruptured, soft-tissue balancing combined with osteotomy or arthrodesis usually is necessary, often with augmentation of the posterior tibial tendon by transfer of the FDL into the navicular or cuneiform. Most patients also require lengthening of the Achilles or gastrocnemius tendon because of equinus contracture.

For patients without significant forefoot abduction deformity and with a mobile subtalar joint, medial displacement calcaneal osteotomy may be a helpful adjunct to soft-tissue augmentation. Lateral column lengthening can be effective in patients with combined deformities that include forefoot abduction, hindfoot valgus, and a low calcaneal pitch angle. This technique involves lengthening the calcaneus with osteotomy and bone grafting or lengthening the lateral column through the calcaneocuboid joint with arthrodesis and bone grafting. For patients without severe hindfoot valgus deformity, the medial column can be stabilized by arthrodesis of the naviculocuneiform or tarsometatarsal joint (Fig. 4), or both (Miller procedure). Calcaneal osteotomy can be added to the procedure for more correction.

In long-standing ruptures of the posterior tibial tendon, the deformity is more rigid. If the subtalar joint is still supple, the goal of treatment is to correct the deformity without sacrificing functional motion of the subtalar joint. Double, triple, and isolated talonavicular or calcaneocuboid arthrodeses have all demonstrated some efficacy. Triple arthrodesis corrects the deformity, but subtalar function is lost and flattening may occur distal to the arthrodesis if the soft tissues are not supported. A medializing osteotomy of the calcaneus can restore the shape of the arch if the deformity is not severe.

If the subtalar joint is rigidly fixed in valgus, a motion sparing procedure cannot be used, and arthrodesis is necessary as

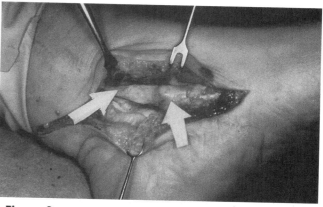

Figure 3

Partial rupture of posterior tibial tendon required debridement and synovectomy because of continued pain and swelling.

a salvage procedure. Often several procedures are combined to treat the deformity and dysfunction. In the presence of an equinus contracture, a lengthening procedure of the gastrocnemius-soleus complex is required to decrease the abnormal forces.

Accessory Navicular

Anatomy The accessory navicular is a secondary ossification center along the medial midfoot that has been found in 9% to 15% of autopsy dissections. Often this anomaly is asymptomatic. Accessory navicular is classified into 3 types: (1) a completely separate ossicle just proximal to the navicular within the posterior tibial tendon or an extension of the medial navicular, (2) a contiguous extension of the navicular, or (3) an incomplete fibrous union with a cleavage plane between the 2 bones. The presence of the ossicle indicates a decrease in the plantar supportive "sling" extension to the remainder of the midfoot by the posterior tibial tendon, which weakens the dynamic support of the medial arch.

Clinical Presentation Usually a patient has pain along the medial arch. The prominence may be tender from shoe or boot pressure. If the fibrous type of separate ossicle is stressed as in a twisting injury, symptoms may occur. At times, an associated deformity with arch collapse is present (Fig. 5). Problems may arise from the prominence of the medial bone or weakening associated with posterior tibial tendon symptoms.

The reverse or medial oblique view is especially helpful to clearly delineate the navicular. A bone scan may be used to evaluate an acute injury or to determine if the source of pain is in fact the accessory navicular in patients with chronic symptoms.

Treatment If symptoms are caused by direct pressure on the accessory navicular, a stress-relieving soft orthosis may be helpful. If symptoms are caused by insufficient function of the posterior tibial tendon due to its weakened attachment, cast immobilization and physical therapy can be tried. If nonsurgical methods are not successful, surgical treatment should be considered. Procedures used for flatfoot deformities may be appropriate. A type 2 accessory navicular can be attached by excavating the primary navicular and arthrodesing the accessory navicular to the primary navicular. The posterior tibial tendon is advanced and reattached to the navicular by leaving a cortical shell attached to the tendon. However, many believe that simple excision with reefing of the soft tissue and reconnecting the tendon to the medial navicular is sufficient. Removal of the medial buttress from the navicular is necessary to provide a cancellous surface for the repair and to decrease the medial prominence. In patients with posterior tibial tendon weakness without deformity, an augmented Kidner procedure reinforces the posterior tibialis by transferring the FDL tendon into the underside of the navicular and medial cuneiform.

Cavus Foot

Clinical Presentation Cavus foot is characterized by elevation of the medial arch, medial forefoot plantarflexion and adduction, and hindfoot varus (Fig. 6). The hindfoot and forefoot deformities may be fixed or dynamic and may be accompanied by hyperextenion of the metatarsophalangeal joints, with the lesser toes positioned dorsally. Symptoms can be diffuse because of the abnormal position of the foot or specific to a particular deformity, such as pain beneath the base of the fifth metatarsal or recurrent hindfoot inversion caused by displacement of the foot relative to the weightbearing axis of the limb.

Cavus foot deformity can result from many conditions, including residual clubfoot deformity or other childhood foot problems; arthrogryposis; neuromuscular diseases, such as Charcot-Marie-Tooth, stroke, or polio; and trauma with

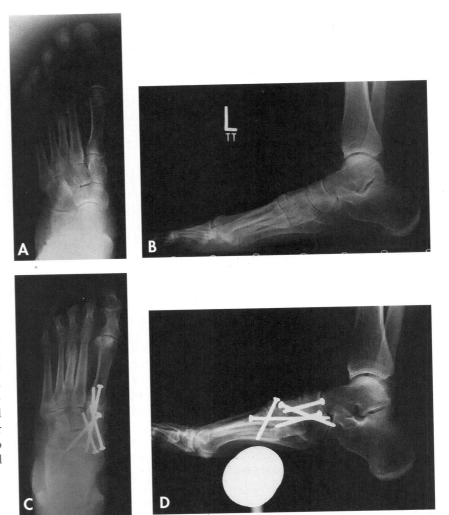

Figure 4

A and B, Foot of a 52-year-old woman who had a flat, valgus, abducted foot with midfoot aching. Note the stress shielding of the first ray and relative thickening of the second ray. C and D, The same foot after stabilization of the naviculocuneiform, cuneiform-metatarsal, and intercuneiform joints.

untreated deep posterior compartment syndrome.

The Coleman block test can be used to determine whether the hindfoot deformity is fixed or supple. A block is placed under the lateral forefoot such that the first metatarsal is not supported along the medial edge of the block. If the foot rotates and the hindfoot varus corrects, the deformity is caused by forefoot plantarflexion, not by a fixed varus hindfoot.

Any patient with a cavus foot should have a neurologic evaluation, including examination of the spine and testing of motor strength and deep tendon reflexes. Examination should include each of the muscles in the leg. This will help in the treatment decision-making process.

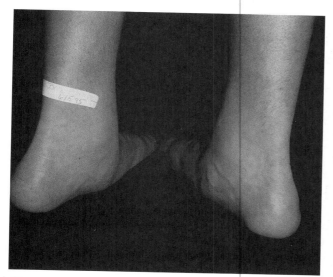

Figure 5

Accessory navicular and flatfoot deformity in a 15-year-old boy.

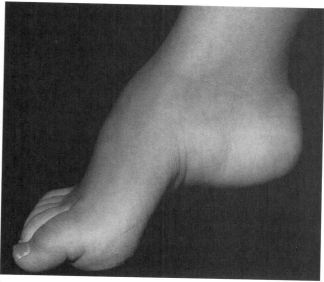

Figure 6

Cavus foot deformity in a patient with Charcot-Marie-Tooth disease.

Treatment The goal of treatment is a balanced, stable, plantigrade foot that resists ankle inversion and can fit into a shoe. Nonsurgical treatment of the cavus foot includes supportive shoe wear, a solid ankle cushioned heel (SACH), or a cushioned accommodative insert with lateral posting. Varus alignment of the hindfoot causes rigidity and makes bracing more difficult. The shoes can be modified to include more cushioning and a lateral heel wedge. For patients with weakness, additional support is achieved by use of an AFO or double-upright hinged posts with a patellar-tendon-bearing (PTB) attachment.

Reconstruction for cavus foot is among the most challenging orthopaedic endeavors. To fully correct the deformity and balance the foot, multiple procedures are required. If surgery is elected, osteotomy, arthrodesis, and tendon transfers are used to restore the bony alignment and motor balance of the foot. In general, anterior or posterior tibial tendons with excessive pull on the medial side of the foot are moved or split to create balance with pull on the lateral side of the foot. Excessive pull of the peroneus longus should be neutralized by transferring it to the peroneus brevis. Dorsiflexion of the foot can be improved by transferring the extensor digitorum longus (EDL) to the midfoot and lengthening the Achilles tendon. Release of the plantar fascia and spring ligament contributes to the correction as well.

Excessive plantarflexion of the first ray also can be treated by a proximal dorsiflexion osteotomy or arthrodesis at the first metatarcal cuneiform joint. The calcaneus can be moved into more valgus with a midfoot osteotomy to correct the high arch and change the pitch angle. Although every attempt is made to maintain subtalar motion, it is sometimes necessary to perform a triple arthrodesis. Derotation of the subtalar joint is important to correct hindfoot alignment.

Hammertoes frequently accompany the more complex hindfoot and midfoot deformities. The lesser toes are treated by flexor-to-extensor tendon transfers. Resection arthroplasty of the proximal interphalangeal joint can be used to correct fixed deformities. The Jones transfer, which transfers the EHL to the first metatarsal and the flexor hallucis longus (FHL) to the base of the proximal phalanx, also is effective in correcting deforming forces in the first ray.

Hindfoot and Ankle Arthritis

The most common cause of arthritis is posttraumatic degenerative joint disease. Fixation of fractures about the foot and ankle requires meticulous attention to detail with respect to the joint surfaces. A step-off of as little as 2 mm in the subtalar joint greatly increases stress. Although much of the injury to the articular cartilage occurs at the time of the initial trauma, continued displacement of the weightbearing surface leads to further degeneration. Fracture of the talus can involve the ankle or talocalcaneal (subtalar) joints directly, and if not properly reduced, can cause abnormal mechanical stresses on the more distal talonavicular joint. As in the shoulder, joint laxity with multiple episodes of subluxation or dislocation can damage the articular cartilage, resulting in degenerative joint disease.

Inflammatory arthropathies, such as rheumatoid arthritis or gout, can affect the foot and ankle. Arthritis can develop in one or more joints. If the inflammatory process involves tendinopathy as well, rupture can occur leading to foot deformity. Hemarthrosis, either from hemophilia or intra-articular bleeding from anticoagulation, can affect the ankle. Often this occurs from a seemingly trivial injury. Idiopathic arthropathy can present as synovitis, with localized pain and mild swelling. Finally, infectious sources must be ruled out.

Clinical Presentation Patients complain of pain and swelling. Deformity of the involved joints also may be present, and motion may be limited by pain or blocking osteophytes. Long-standing deformity may cause secondary tendon contracture. The pain may be relieved by rest and exacerbated by standing or walking.

Weightbearing radiographs, including oblique, Broden, and Harris views, can be used to evaluate alignment, osteophyte formation, and joint space loss. A computed tomography (CT) scan is helpful, especially in postfracture evaluation of the subtalar joint. A CT is done in 2 planes, perpendicular to the subtalar joint (semicoronal) and parallel to the plantar surface of the foot.

Treatment Early arthritis can be treated symptomatically with nonsteroidal anti-inflammatory drugs and increased cushioning in shoes. Medical conditions should be aggressively treated if possible. Physical therapy is helpful to maintain strength and motion as well as general conditioning. A period of immobilization with a cast or an AFO often decreases the pain and inflammation. Prolonged immobilization, however, can lead to permanent loss of motion. The AFO can be removed for motion exercises. Judicious limited use of intra-articular injection also may decrease symptoms.

Surgical treatment of early arthritis aims to relieve pain and maintain function. Synovectomy, removal of loose bodies, and removal of degenerative osteophytes can prolong the functional life of the joint. Arthrodesis is the primary surgical treatment for the small joints of the foot and ankle. Success of hindfoot or ankle arthrodesis is dependent on final position. Although many techniques are used, including external and internal fixation and arthroscopically-assisted arthrodesis with limited arthrotomy, the position of the arthrodesis is more important than the technique used.

Ankle arthrodesis should be done with the ankle in neutral position or slight plantarflexion, neutral to slight valgus, and a small amount of external rotation relative to the contralateral limb. Placement of the ankle in slight plantarflexion (in women), however, has been reported to lead to abnormal stresses about the ankle and higher failure rates with subsequent arthritis in the adjacent joints. Currently, internal fixation is used more often than external fixation for ankle arthrodesis.

The talus should be shifted posterior under the tibia to shorten the lever arm acting on the remainder of the foot. Leaving the talus too far anterior leads to accelerated degenerative changes in the remainder of the foot and backward thrust at the knee. Neutral to slight external rotation (10° maximum) of the talus also prevents stress on the subtalar joint. Neutral to slight valgus keeps the medial part of the foot in weightbearing alignment. The talo-first metatarsal angle should be restored in 2 planes. Triple, or subtalar, arthrodesis should derotate any deformity from within the subtalar, talonavicular, or calcaneocuboid joint. If substantial deformity is present, bone grafting may be required.

Arthrodesis of the ankle remains the standard for surgical treatment of ankle arthritis in older adults. However, it is less than ideal under some circumstances. New techniques using small pin fixator distraction devices or osteocartilaginous autografts have shown some early promise, although long-term results are not available. The latter technique is suited for a localized defect in the talus. Small dowels of bone and cartilage are grafted to the dome of the talus.

Recent advances in ankle arthroplasty have been more encouraging. In general, ankle arthroplasty is not considered as successful as shoulder, elbow, hip, or knee arthroplasty. Complications of ankle arthroplasty have included loss of implant position, loosening, extrusion, and deformity. Recently, use of tibia or fibular arthrodesis combined with newer implant arthroplasty has shown a relatively high rate of patient satisfaction (Fig. 7). At an average follow-up of 4.5 years, 92% of patients reported that they were satisfied with the result, 80% of ankles were slightly painful or painless, and only 6% required revision. Although the incidence of component migration at this intermediate follow-up is worrisome, patient satisfaction was relatively high and revision rate was relatively low. Until long-term results are available, ankle arthroplasty occasionally should be considered an option for select middle-aged patients (20 to 30 years of age) who have had triple or subtalar arthrodesis for severe ankle arthritis, or in patients who have bilateral ankle disease and need some type of propulsion.

Forefoot Problems

Hallux Valgus

An estimated 200,000 surgeries for hallux valgus are performed each year in the United States. Despite this high incidence, there is little consensus on optimal surgical treatment.

Both intrinsic and extrinsic factors have been implicated in the development of hallux valgus. Intrinsic factors include neuromuscular disorders, collagen disorders, first metatarsocuneiform hypermobility, pes planus, and a laterally-directed distal first metatarsal articular surface. The principal external factor is the mechanical effect of constriction from wearing shoes. Inappropriate footwear initially forces the hallux into valgus leading to a cascade of events that includes (1) attenuation of the medial joint capsule and ligaments, (2) plantar and lateral migration of the abductor hallux tendon, (3) sesamoid subluxation, (4) lateral deviation of the flexor and extensor tendons with resultant eccentric loading of the first metatarsal head, and (5) metatarsus primus varus. Mechanical and in vivo tests have shown that these events result in the loss of strength at push-off of the first ray and transfer of load primarily to the central and lateral metatarsal heads.

Clinical Presentation The primary symptom of hallux valgus is pain over the medial eminence. This is typically related to pressure from footwear and can be associated with bursal inflammation, skin irritation, and ulceration. Metatarsosesamoid joint pain also is common and appears to be related to focally elevated stress between the medial sesamoid and the ridge separating the sesamoid sulci and the intersesamoid crista. In some patients, hallux valgus deformity causes profound weakness of great toe push-off strength, resulting in transfer of load to a symptomatic second metatarsophalangeal (MTP) joint.

Physical examination for hallux valgus should include evaluation for benign joint hypermobility syndrome. The area of tenderness should be localized. Tenderness in the metatarsosesamoid region indicates that this articulation may have arthritis or subluxation. Tenderness along the medial eminence implies that successful treatment will need to unload this focal pressure area. MTP and tarsometatarsal (TMT) joint range of motion should be determined. The foot should be inspected for calluses indicating focal overload, especially under the second

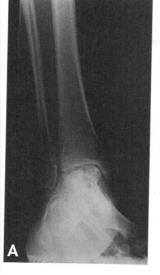
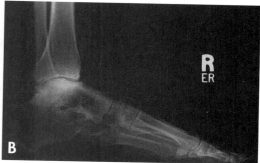
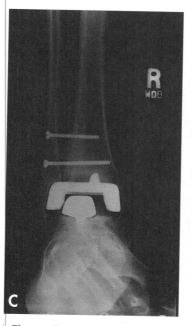
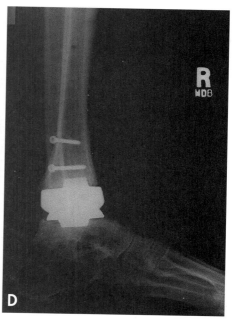

Figure 7

A and B, Arthritis of the tibiotalar joint with avascular collapse of the talus. Note previous triple arthrodesis. C and D, Six months after ankle arthroplasty, the patient is pain-free and pleased with the result despite radiographic signs of screw loosening and lucency around the lateral side of the implant.

metatarsal head. The longitudinal arch should be inspected for collapse, and posterior tibial tendon function should be evaluated.

AP, lateral, and axial (tangential) standing radiographs should be obtained. On the AP view, the first MTP joint is evaluated for evidence of degenerative arthritis, congruence, and lateral deviation of the distal metatarsal articular surface. Both the MTP angle and the first-to-second intermetatarsal angle are measured to quantify the relative degree of axial plane deformity. The AP view also demonstrates signs of arch collapse (talocalcaneal divergence, talonavicular subluxation, or midfoot pronation), relative shortening of the first metatarsal, and valgus deviation of the first interphalangeal joint (hallux valgus interphalangeus). On the lateral view, degenerative arthritis of the first MTP and TMT joints can be identified as well as instability of the first TMT joint with plantar widening. The standing axial radiograph helps to understand the fundamental biomechanical imbalance in hallux valgus. Hallucal and metatarsal rotation can be determined on the basis of these radiographs, and the degree of metatarsal sesamoid subluxation can be accurately defined.

Treatment Nonsurgical and surgical treatment modalities are used to treat hallux valgus. Patients with mild deformity and a congruent joint are best treated conservatively. The principal nonsurgical treatment option is avoidance of ill-fitting shoes. Physical therapy, exercises, and splints have all been advocated as adjuncts to decrease the amount of valgus deviation of the great toe; however, there are limited published data to support these approaches. The occasional use of arch supports can be helpful if pes planus is present; however, they are not indicated in most patients with a primary diagnosis of hallux valgus. Patients with heel cord tightness may benefit from heel cord stretching exercises.

Surgical treatment is indicated after all conservative treatment modalities have been exhausted and the patient remains symptomatic. Before surgical intervention, the patient must be counseled regarding postoperative expectations, the uncertainty of long-term results, the probable need for life-long footwear change, and the possibility of complications. Common problems after surgery include decreased MTP joint motion, recurrence, sensory nerve dysfunction, localized infection, hallux varus, and, rarely, osteonecrosis of the metatarsal head.

Over 150 operations have been described for treating hallux valgus deformity, confirming the complexity of the condition and the lack of concensus and a complete understanding of the problem and its treatment. Important factors in decision making include congruency of the MTP and metatarso-sesamoid joints, severity of deformity, presence of midfoot or hindfoot deformity, presence of arthritis, and intrinsic joint stability. Congruency is assessed by the relationship of the articular surface of the proximal phalanx to the metatarsal head on the AP view and the metatarsosesamoid articulation on the axial view. Incongruent joints require that a soft-tissue realignment be included in the procedure. The different

reconstructive procedures have varying abilities to correct deformity and restore normal hallucal biomechanical function. It is essential to evaluate each patient individually and choose the best procedure to restore normal forefoot function; no single procedure is sufficient to treat the wide range of presentations of hallux valgus.

Reconstructive procedures are categorized as follows: medial eminence resection with soft-tissue realignment; osteotomy of the proximal phalanx or the proximal or distal first metatarsal; realignment and arthrodesis of the first MTP or TMT joints; and joint resection procedures. Patients with mild deformity and an incongruent joint generally respond well to a distal metatarsal osteotomy combined with a soft-tissue realignment procedure at the MTP joint. For patients with substantial lateral angulation of the distal first metatarsal joint surface, a closing wedge osteotomy can be combined with the distal metatarsal osteotomy to realign the hallux into a neutral position. When performing distal metatarsal osteotomies, it is critical not to strip the metatarsal head of its extraosseous blood supply to avoid the potential complication of metatarsal head necrosis. If a lateral release is required to correct the deformity, only minimal dissection should be carried out.

Patients with greater degrees of metatarsosesamoid subluxation or first to second intermetatarsal angles generally require a proximal procedure to realign the MTP joint. Either a TMT joint arthrodesis or a proximal metatarsal osteotomy can be considered. TMT arthrodesis stabilizes the first ray, but has the disadvantage of causing stress transfer to adjacent joints and may result in some shortening. This procedure is indicated in patients with first TMT joint hypermobility or generalized ligamentous laxity. Currently, proximal metatarsal osteotomies are more popular than TMT arthrodeses, but require soft-tissue balancing of the first MTP joint. Both crescentic and chevron osteotomies of the proximal metatarsal have been advocated. The crescentic osteotomy provides less stability but allows some rotation of the metatarsal. The chevron osteotomy is more stable and is somewhat easier to perform consistently. The goal of the chevron osteotomy is to realign the MTP joint in 3 dimensions, including restoration of normal metatarsosesamoid congruence. The lateral capsule and tendinous structures are lengthened or released and the medial capsular tissue is reefed to hold the toe in the corrected position.

Patients with hallux valgus and MTP joint arthritis can be treated with arthrodesis or resection arthroplasty. Arthrodesis generally is preferred because it facilitates hallucal weightbearing and unloads the lesser metatarsal heads. Arthrodesis also should be considered for patients with severe instability and deformity of the first MTP joint, especially if there is an underlying neuromuscular disease. For patients with limited ambulation needs who wish to avoid an arthrodesis, resection of the base of the proximal phalanx should be considered. This procedure involves minimal resection (one fourth to one third of the proximal phalanx), temporary pin fixation, and possible adjunctive soft-tissue interposition.

If valgus deviation of the hallux occurs at the interphalangeal joint, a closing wedge osteotomy of the base of the proximal phalanx can be helpful to reorient the hallux. If a patient also has symptomatic bunions, a medial eminence resection is performed.

There are many reasons for failure of hallux valgus surgery. Incomplete or overcorrection of the deformity, excessive resection of bone, excessive tightening or loosening of the ligaments, entrapment of the nerves, failure in recognizing generalized ligamentous laxity, osteonecrosis of the metatarsal head, and postoperative infection are some of the more common reasons. Arthrodesis is the most frequently used salvage procedure for failed hallux valgus surgery with residual postoperative deformity or degenerative joint disease. Surgical results appear to be improved by careful patient selection, correcting biomechanical imbalances, taking appropriate intraoperative radiographs, and limiting weightbearing after surgery.

Hallux Varus

Hallux varus, a medial deviation of the great toe, generally is caused by overcorrection after hallux valgus surgery, although in some patients the cause is congenital. In the past, iatrogenic hallux varus was associated with procedures that involved excision of the lateral sesamoid; however, with the changes in surgical approaches, this problem now occurs most commonly after proximal metatarsal osteotomy with distal soft-tissue realignment. The surgical factors that lead to an acquired hallux varus include excessive medial eminence resection, excessive tightening of the medial capsule, excessive lateral release, and excessive lateral positioning of the metatarsal head after osteotomy. The most severe problem of these is excessive medial eminence resection.

Treatment of acquired hallux varus depends on the etiology, associated disability, presence of arthritis, and degree of fixed contracture. Most mild, supple deformities are well tolerated and do not require surgery. For symptomatic passively correctable deformities, realignment of the soft tissues alone or in combination with an extensor tendon rerouting can be used. The short or long extensor hallucis tendon can be used for this purpose. If the entire extensor hallucis longus (EHL) tendon is used, an interphalangeal arthrodesis is required. A split EHL tendon transfer or an extensor hallucis brevis (EHB) tendon joint transfer avoids the need for an

interphalangeal arthrodesis. The extensor tendon is routed beneath the intermetatarsal ligament and secured to the plantar lateral aspect of the proximal phalanx to serve as a check rein to varus deviation of the hallux. Sometimes the medial sesamoid requires excision to realign the MTP joint. An MTP joint arthrodesis is indicated when hallux varus deformity is associated with MTP joint arthritis and can be the simplest solution to a hallux varus associated with malunion of the first metatarsal, although a realignment osteotomy holds the potential for restoring normal forefoot biomechanics.

Hallux Rigidus

Hallux rigidus is progressive degenerative arthritis of the first MTP joint and is characterized by painful motion, especially with dorsiflexion. The condition generally begins with a mechanical or biologic insult to the articular surface and subsequent bone formation about the dorsal, medial, and lateral aspects of the metatarsal head. Osteophyte formation may occur on the dorsal aspect of the proximal phalanx. Mechanical causes include a dorsally angulated first ray, such as a dorsal bunion, and an incongruous MTP joint.

Clinical Presentation Patients typically have pain with activity and shoe wear that is exacerbated by walking uphill or stair climbing. Physical examination demonstrates a painful dorsal prominence over the metatarsal head with increased bulk around the joint, limited dorsiflexion, and, occasionally, pain with plantarflexion resulting from an inflamed EHL tendon stretching over a dorsal osteophyte. Radiographs show arthritis with squaring-off of the first MTP joint, sclerosis, osteophyte formation, and, in advanced cases, cyst formation. A dorsal bunion from dorsiflexion of the first ray may be present as well.

Treatment The decision regarding treatment is based on the extent and nature of the disease and the patient's activity level. Nonsurgical treatment options include use of a wide toe box shoe that can accommodate the enlarged joint, a rigid sole with a rocker or roller bottom design, a full-length carbon fiber insert, and acetaminophen or nonsteroidal anti-inflammatory medication.

Surgical treatment options include cheilectomy, arthrodesis, or resection arthroplasty. Cheilectomy is the resection of proliferative bone around the metatarsal head and proximal phalanx. All the osteophytes around the metatarsal head are removed to allow approximately 70° of dorsiflexion at the time of surgery. A cheilectomy is indicated for patients who have mild to moderate arthritis of the joint. Satisfaction rates from this surgery average approximately 70% at 5-year follow-up. The failure rate increases with worsening arthritis. If 70° of dorsiflexion are not obtained, a dorsiflexion osteotomy of the proximal phalanx can be used to improve the functional joint range of motion.

MTP joint arthrodesis is indicated for severe arthritis. This procedure reliably relieves MTP joint pain at the expense of motion and requires a more involved postoperative course. A resection arthroplasty of the proximal phalanx can be considered for patients with low functional demands. However, recurrent MTP joint pain or transfer metatarsalgia may occur.

Sesamoid Disorders

Sesamoid disorders are characterized by pain localized beneath the first metatarsal head on weightbearing. Often the patient has no recollection of a specific precipitating event. Examination demonstrates tenderness to direct palpation under the metatarsal head, with restriction of motion because of pain. The examiner must differentiate sesamoid-related pain from tenosynovitis of the FHL tendon. Radiographs can be helpful in identifying acute fractures, whose sharp irregular borders differ from the smooth cortical edges of bipartite sesamoids.

Initial treatment for sesamoiditis, osteochondrosis, stress fractures, or acute fractures is immobilization. For fractures a short-leg toe-spica walking cast is recommended, followed by use of a stiff-soled shoe with a spring steel or a removable full-length carbon fiber insert, a metatarsal pad, and a neutral heel height. If these modalities fail, surgical treatment can be considered.

Patients with isolated stress fractures of the medial sesamoid and intact articular cartilage may respond well to an in situ bone grafting procedure. With articular involvement, sesamoid excision is preferred. Single sesamoid excision does not substantially decrease the power of hallucal push-off. The medial sesamoid can be approached through a medial longitudinal incision and the lateral sesamoid can be approached dorsally or plantarly. The dorsal incision avoids the potential of a painful scar and lessens the risk of injury to the lateral plantar digital nerve, but can be challenging to perform in the foot with a narrow first-to-second intermetatarsal angle. Care should be taken to avoid injury to the FHL tendon with sesamoid excision. Satisfaction rates after single sesamoid excision typically range from 80% to 90%.

Problems of the Lesser Toes

Deformities of the lesser toes are commonly associated with hallux valgus deformities and the use of constrictive footwear, although they can be caused by neuromuscular diseases, rheumatoid arthritis, nonspecific synovitis, or trauma.

With mechanical causes, the second and third toes are most commonly involved, whereas, with neurologic or generalized arthritis, all 4 lesser toes usually develop some degree of deformity.

Clinical Presentation Patients complain of painful corns or calluses, toe tip or nail pain, and difficulty wearing shoes. Metatarsalgia, especially around the central metatarsal heads, can be a prominent clinical feature. The examination should include a complete evaluation of lower extremity neuromuscular function and vascular status. Upper extremity neurologic function should be assessed for evidence of intrinsic dysfunction. Specifically, each lesser toe joint involved should be assessed for instability, flexibility, or rigidity.

Treatment The goal of nonsurgical treatment is to reduce stress to symptomatic areas. Corns should be carefully trimmed and protected with the use of pads, caps, lamb's wool, and extra-depth or longer shoes. A stiffened sole with a rocker bottom and a metatarsal pad is particularly helpful in treating metatarsalgia.

If nonsurgical methods fail, surgical options may be offered to patients with realistic long-term expectations. Correction of lesser toe deformities will not allow unlimited use of fashionable shoes. Although the surgical treatments range from simple tenotomy to toe amputation, some basic guiding principles generally apply. Fixed deformities require bony resection. Arthroplasty with hemiresection seems to have better and more predictable outcomes than arthrodesis. Removing the base of the proximal phalanx destabilizes the toe and should be used as a salvage procedure. Bony resection of the proximal aspect of the rigidly flexed joint should be done for rigid deformities of the distal and proximal interphalangeal joints. Extension deformity of the first MTP joint is treated with extensor tendon lengthening, dorsal joint capsulotomy, and collateral ligament release.

If the joint is reducible but unstable after soft-tissue release, the surgeon may consider a flexor-to-extensor tendon transfer or a plantar metatarsal condylectomy. The flexor-to-extensor tendon transfer has increased morbidity and decreases toe push-off strength, but may add intrinsic stability, especially in patients with neuromuscular disorders. The plantar condylectomy is used to increase stability by exposing raw bone to the plantar plate region during the postoperative period. This approach reduces metatarsalgia under that isolated metatarsal head, but carries the risk of transfer metatarsalgia. In some chronic situations, soft-tissue releases around the MTP joint alone do not permit joint reduction, and surgical options include resection of the distal aspect of the metatarsal head or shortening of the metatarsal. The shortening procedures are intrinsically more attractive in terms of preserving joint function; however, they must be performed with caution because of the risk of nonunion or transfer metatarsalgia. Resection should be considered a salvage procedure and should be avoided in young or active patients.

Morton's Interdigital Neuroma

Patients with interdigital neuroma usually have a history of pain in the central forefoot extending into the toes, which is relieved by removing shoes, sitting, or massaging the feet. Physical examination should include palpation of the plantar aspect of the web space immediately distal to the metatarsal heads. If symptoms are exacerbated by compressing the forefoot together with the opposite hand (Mulder's click test), the diagnosis of an interdigital neuroma should be entertained. The clinician must, however, differentiate interdigital neuroma symptoms from metatarsalgia, MTP joint problems, lesser metatarsal stress fractures, and other peripheral entrapment neuropathies. Local injection of an anesthetic with or without corticosteroid instillation around the common digital nerve is diagnostic. Because the common digital nerve innervates many of the structures around the web space, this test must be interpreted with caution.

Nonsurgical treatment includes use of loose-fitting, low-heeled shoes with soft soles. Metatarsal pads are placed proximal to the interdigital web space to spread the metatarsal heads and relieve pressure on the interdigital nerve. If these simple modifications fail, the clinician can stiffen the shoe with either spring steel or carbon fiber to reduce toe dorsiflexion and resultant mechanical irritation of the interdigital nerve. The judicious use of a local steroid injection around the interdigital nerve may give temporary or long-lasting relief. The vast majority of patients improve with nonsurgical treatment.

The indications for surgical treatment are symptoms that persist for more than 6 months, temporary relief with local anesthetic and corticosteroid injection, and failure of non-surgical modalities. Other local or general medical conditions, such as ischemia, diabetes, infection, and causalgia must be ruled out. Poor surgical results have been reported in patients with bilateral symptoms or symptoms involving more than 1 web space. These patients should undergo further evaluation for a generalized cause of forefoot pain (rheumatoid arthritis, fat pad insufficiency, fibromyalgia, etc).

The surgical approach for a primary interdigital neuroma is from the dorsal web space. The standard treatment entails excision of the interdigital nerve. Overall satisfaction rates average 80%, although recently some authors have reported similar success rates with nerve retaining neurolysis procedures and release of the intermetatarsal ligament.

Persistent symptoms after interdigital nerve resection may cause greater pain than the patient had before surgery. Recurrent symptoms may result from (1) incorrect initial web space surgery, (2) incorrect diagnosis, (3) technical problems with the initial surgery (incomplete removal, failure to divide transverse metatarsal ligament, or failure to resect the nerve proximal to the metatarsal head), or (4) recurrence of neuroma under the metatarsal head. Resection of a recurrent neuroma can be performed from either the plantar or dorsal approach. The satisfaction rates with reoperation are worse than with primary operations.

Bunionette Deformity

Patients with bunionette deformities complain of pain over the lateral process of the fifth metatarsal head and may have an inflamed bursa in this region or a varus toe deformity. These problems usually are caused by a mismatch between the patient's foot anatomy and shoes.

Shoe modifications, including the use of soft leather and a wide toe box usually relieves pain. Shoes can be stretched in this area and a pad can be placed laterally to reduce pressure along the symptomatic region. Patients with plantar symptoms may benefit from callus trimming and use of a metatarsal pad.

Surgical treatment is reserved for patients with significant pain and deformity if they have a reasonable perspective on future footwear limitations. In mild cases, a simple lateral process resection may be the most expedient and sensible approach, especially in low demand patients. With moderate deformities, a chevron distal metatarsal osteotomy with medial displacement may be used. In patients with prominent plantar symptoms, the osteotomy can be oriented such that the distal fragment slides dorsally as well as medially. In patients with more severe bunionette deformity, especially when the plantar pain is substantial, a midshaft oblique osteotomy may be considered. Complications of osteotomies include delayed union, nonunion, and malunion. Patients may develop MTP instability, a persistent lateral prominence, or transfer metatarsalgia. Because the magnitude of the complications can be substantial, patients undergoing this procedure should be carefully selected on the basis of the degree of their deformity, symptoms, and understanding of the overall surgical and postsurgical considerations.

Rheumatoid Arthritis

Approximately 16% of patients who have rheumatoid arthritis will develop initial symptoms in the foot. After 10 years with rheumatoid disease, virtually all patients have some forefoot symptoms. The MTP joints are most commonly affected. The degree of forefoot involvement ranges from occasional synovitis to massive joint destruction with rigid deformity. With MTP synovitis, the capsular tissues and ligamentous support become deficient. Over time the hallux usually pronates and adducts into a valgus position. The lesser MTP joints typically dislocate dorsally, and the toes assume flexed deformities.

Most patients with rheumatoid forefoot symptoms can be treated with orthotics and shoe modifications. Orthotics must be made with soft, shock-absorbing materials. A metatarsal pad will help unload prominent metatarsal heads. Shoes that are made out of a soft and mostly seamless leather should have extra depth and some degree of a rocker sole.

A variety of surgical strategies have been proposed for the treatment of rheumatoid forefoot problems. Initially, resection of all the metatarsal heads was used to reduce metatarsalgia. More recently, this approach has been improved with first MTP joint arthrodesis to maintain forefoot weightbearing. Although metatarsal head resection generally results in pain relief and has better reported outcomes than resection of the proximal phalangeal bases alone, some surgeons still have strong concerns about the ablative nature of this procedure. Shortening osteotomies of the lesser metatarsals have been proposed as an alternative to metatarsal head resection in the treatment of severe rheumatoid forefoot deformities.

The Diabetic Foot

Introduction
An estimated 15% of patients with diabetes mellitus will develop a foot ulcer. Furthermore, 20% of all diabetic-related hospitalizations are related to the foot. With this patient population living longer and remaining physically active, chronic complications to the foot are more evident than ever. The basic pathophysiologic processes that lead to these foot problems are unknown, but vasculopathy, neuropathy, and deformity caused by mechanical imbalance are believed to contribute. The Centers for Disease Control and Prevention (CDC) estimates that 50% of diabetic foot problems and subsequent amputations can be eliminated by educating both patients and their physicians about these physiologic problems, as well as prevention and early treatment. In the landmark Diabetes Control and Complications Trial study, it was found that the severity of diabetic complications is not related to the severity of the disease, but rather to the lack of control of blood glucose levels.

Diabetic Neuropathy
Although the importance of vasculopathy should not be ignored, most foot problems are related to loss of sensation and mechanical alterations that place the skin at risk. Diabetic neuropathy affects the sensory, motor, and autonomic pathways. Sensory neuropathy results in the loss of protective sensation, in which areas of increased mechanical stress are not perceived and may lead to skin breakdown. Numbness and paresthesias in a symmetric stocking distribution are characteristic of this form of neuropathy, which frequently presents as a nocturnal burning sensation. The sensory neuropathy can be quantified using a Semmes-Weinstein monofilament of 5.07 size. It has been demonstrated that 90% of patients perceiving this size monofilament were free of neuropathic ulceration, whereas those unable to perceive it were considered to have loss of protective sensation and to be at risk for developing neuropathic complications to the foot. More sophisticated and expensive evaluation techniques are available and include vibratory or nerve conduction velocity testing.

Motor neuropathy is characterized by intrinsic muscle atrophy that results in a motor imbalance and foot deformity. Diffuse clawtoe, often with a lesser MTP joint dislocation, is the most common deformity. The foot may assume a cavus-like posture with apparent plantarflexion of the first ray and may have associated hyperextension of the hallux. The cumulative effect is increased plantar pressure on the metatarsal heads, as well as extrinsic shoe pressure placed on the dorsum of the toes. In a large study, it was found that toe deformities are the most common causes for subsequent amputation in diabetic patients in Veteran's Administration facilities.

The autonomic nervous system is responsible for glandular control and assists in thermal regulation. Autonomic dysfunction in a diabetic person results in thick, dry, scaly skin with associated nail deformities and affects the normal hyperemic response necessary to heal wounds. In addition, the risk of bacterial invasion is increased because of the skin fissuring that occurs. The combined and ultimate effect of each of these neuropathies is that of callus formation, unperceived pressure necrosis, and eventual risk for ulceration with secondary osteomyelitis or gangrene.

Another complication in patients with diabetes is that of Charcot disease. This neuropathic osteoarthropathy results in fragmentation, destruction, and dislocation of the bones of the foot and ankle. The incidence of Charcot osteoarthropathy in this population is reported at 1% to 2.5%, with the average interval between the onset of diabetes and occurrence averaging 15 years. The process may be spontaneous or may follow trauma. Often it is occult and has been described as a sequela of surgery. Twenty-five percent of patients may develop contralateral involvement. Charcot disease does not occur with ischemia; presumably blood flow must be present to support the inflammatory process that results in bone destruction. Three clinical stages have been described. The first stage lasts 6 to 8 weeks and is characterized by an acutely swollen, warm, and erythematous foot. The second stage is subacute, characterized by gradual subsidence of swelling and warmth, and new bone formation occurs. This stage may last 6 months and is followed by the final stage in which there is completion of bone healing and resolution of the inflammatory response.

Charcot disease may occur at any level of the foot and ankle; the midfoot is the most common site of involvement, while the forefoot is the least common. Midfoot disease usually involves the tarsometatarsal joint (Fig. 8) and is characterized more by symptomatic bony prominences than instability. In contrast, Charcot disease involving the hindfoot and ankle joints is associated with progressive instability and secondary bony deformity. This neuropathic process also can involve the calcaneus as an isolated event and may be identified by neuropathic fracture through the posterior tuberosity. As a result of bony prominence or instability, there is a 74% incidence of associated mal perforans ulcerations in feet with significant deformity.

Ulcer Evaluation and Treatment

The size and depth of areas of skin breakdown or frank ulceration should be carefully observed, as well as the presence of exposed bones or tendon. Arterial flow should be assessed. If pedal pulses are absent, a vascular surgeon should be consulted. Arterial Doppler that includes absolute toe pressures or transcutaneous oxygen measurement is useful. The most widely used classification scheme for diabetic ulcers is that of Wagner, which is based on ulcer depth. Newer classification schemes grade both depth and ischemia. Common to these schemes are grade 0, intact skin but "at risk" with areas of bony prominence; grade I, superficial ulcerations; grade II, deep ulceration with exposed tendon or joint capsule; and grade III, extensive ulceration with exposed or palpable bone (implied osteomyelitis).

Treatment algorithms can be developed from these classification schemes. Identifying patients at risk for developing ulcerations and educating them on prevention and proper shoe wear can prevent 65% to 80% of ulcerations.

Grade 0 For patients who are at risk for developing an ulcer, a strict program of blood glucose control is initiated. The patient is instructed on skin and nail care and observation of plantar skin surfaces. Orthotic management includes accommodative shoe wear and relief of bony prominences. Leather devices, carefully placed padding, and shoe modifications can be used. Custom shoes are considered if the foot deformity is too severe and modifications are too extensive for an off-the-shelf shoe. Full-length, soft accommodative inserts can reduce shock and shear forces and help transfer these forces from areas of high pressure to low.

Grade I The majority of diabetic foot ulcers are not clinically infected. In regard to the ulceration, local wound care is begun with relief of mechanical pressure caused by the effects of muscle imbalance. A total contact cast is considered to be standard treatment for uncomplicated ulcerations. Should a cast be contraindicated, alternatives include a healing sandal, walker boot, or modified shoe wear.

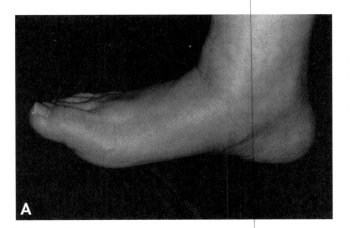
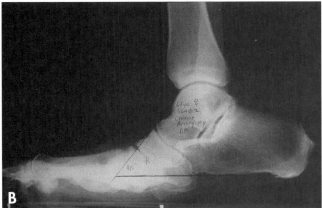

Figure 8

"Midfoot collapse" deformity in a 62-year-old woman with Charcot osteoarthropathy from diabetes. A, Clinical appearance of foot. B, Radiographic appearance.

The physician should avoid culturing superficial ulcerations because colonization overrepresents pathogens and omits anaerobes. However, the presence of mild cellulitis requires broad spectrum, oral antibiotic therapy. Patients who fail to clinically improve on this regimen, or who are allergic to penicillin, may require a fluoroquinolone or clindamycin. Limb-threatening infections require parenteral regimens that may include vancomycin, ticarcillin-clavulanate, and ampicillin-subactin.

Grade II Necrotic tissue is debrided and wound care instituted. Barring infection, total contact casts can be used. Infected ulcers are treated as above.

Grade III If bone can be probed through the ulcer there is a greater probability of contiguous osteomyelitis, the extent of which may be determined by clinical evaluation and plain radiography. Magnetic resonance imaging is more sensitive in this regard but may overestimate the extent of bone involvement. This diagnostic tool is especially helpful in determining the presence of occult abscesses if the patient does not respond to initial care. Surgical debridement may be necessary at times to remove areas of infected or necrotic bone, as well as to decompress areas of abscess formation. Broad-spectrum antibiotics are begun only if the infection is active, and metronidazole is given for anaerobic infections. If possible, renal-toxic regimens should be avoided. Should the patient fail to improve clinically, regimens may be adjusted so that they are culture-specific. Tetanus coverage should be considered for all patients. The duration of therapy depends on the extent of involvement and whether or not clean margins are obtained at the time of surgical debridement. Consultation with an infectious disease specialist may be helpful, particularly in patients with renal impairment.

Persistent or Recurrent Ulceration

Ulcers that do not heal are assessed for persistent mechanical pressure, infection, and inadequate healing potential. In addition, the nutritional status of the patient should be determined. Surgical intervention can be considered for patients with underlying bony deformity and sufficient blood supply. In general, procedures include exostectomy, realignment arthrodesis, or arthroplasty. All patients with plantar forefoot ulcers should be assessed for a heel-cord contracture, which frequently requires lengthening as an adjuvant procedure. Total contact casting should be considered postoperatively to assist with wound healing, as well as to minimize the risk of Charcot sequelae.

Preventing Ulceration Recurrence

Shoe modifications are critical in diabetic patients. A CDC study conducted in 1991 noted an 80% recurrence rate of mal perforans ulcers in patients without shoe modifications in contrast to 20% recurrence in patients with shoe modifications. The area of ulceration requires specific relief of pressure in an accommodative shoe. The shoe itself requires adequate toe-box depth, a removable insole, and a shock absorbing or crepe sole. Dense neuropathy may mandate a deerskin leather upper for further protection. The most frequent shoe modification is that of a rocker sole, which further reduces pressure and impact shock. The apex of the rocker can be placed proximal to the site of ulceration, thus alleviating significant weightbearing pressures. In addition, the rocker sole is so rigid that it will limit the motion of unstable joints.

For areas of persistent plantar bony prominence that are at risk for recurrent ulceration, an insole excavation can be placed in apposition to the prominence and filled with a low-density material such as silicone or a viscoelastic polymer. SACH material can be placed in the heel of the shoe to further absorb shock at heel-strike and protect this region of the foot. Inserts are an important part of diabetic shoe management. A customized device typically is necessary to provide adequate protection in these individuals. Devices made of multiple-density materials improve durability and can be modified to decrease or eliminate weightbearing from certain areas of the foot. Simple and inexpensive protection of the diabetic foot can be obtained through closed or open cell materials. A micropore rubber device reduces shear stress, while a closed cell polyethylene device helps to reduce impact pressure.

Maintaining a healed ulceration in the midfoot or hindfoot is often difficult, particularly if there is associated instability. In such instances, a brace can be added to the modified shoe to assist with transfer of loads from the foot to the leg. A polypropylene patellar tendon bearing (PTB) or double upright calf-lacing brace reduces loads in the foot approximately 30%. The ankle hinge is typically locked, and a rocker sole is added to the shoe.

The key to success in maintaining a healed ulcer rests on proper shoe wear, patient education, and appropriately scheduled follow-up visits (every 3 months). Ideally, the patient should possess 2 to 3 pairs of shoes and 2 pairs of inserts to interchange frequently. Patients with visual impairment and neuropathy may need assistance from visiting medical personnel to prevent ulcers.

Prescription Writing

Communication between the physician and the pedorthist or orthotist is crucial. If this communication cannot be performed in person, then a prescription provides the pedorthist or orthotist with an authorization to treat the patient and documentation for the patient's record. The prescription requires a complete diagnosis of the foot disorder that is to be treated. It should include the desired biomechanical effect, typically an accommodation of a fixed deformity or relief of prior ulceration. The type of shoe needs to be considered as well as recommendations for internal or external shoe modifications. Locations of unstable deformities and whether or not a brace is to be attached to the shoe are documented. A mnemonic for this prescription writing is PEDS (problems, effect, direction, shoe).

Cost Reimbursement of the Orthopaedic Shoe

Unfortunately, the cost of nonsurgical treatment of the diabetic foot often results in patient noncompliance. This is particularly true when modified shoe wear is prescribed, because the initial deposit for an elderly patient on a fixed income may be difficult. Often, insurance reimbursement is inconsistent. In 1994, the Therapeutic Shoe Bill was passed that provided for financial assistance for patients covered under Medicare. The bill allows for partial reimbursement of 1 pair of shoes and 3 molded inserts per year or 1 pair of custom-molded shoes and 2 pairs of inserts per year. Medicaid patients only obtain financial assistance if a brace is used and only for the shoe that is attached to the brace.

Treatment of Charcot Osteoarthropathy

The mainstay of treatment for acute Charcot foot, once diagnosed, is that of prolonged external immobilization in a total contact cast or orthosis. Orthotic treatment has improved, particularly with the development of the Charcot Restraining Orthotic Walker (CROW), a custom molded bivalved AFO that includes a rocker sole. It can be used for an extended period of treatment, and uses stump socks to manage fluctuations in swelling. Both the cast and the orthosis serve to stabilize fractured or dislocated bones while minimizing the inflammatory response. With continued protection, gradual resolution will occur as evidenced clinically by reduction of warmth or swelling. An objective means to measure improvement uses water displacement techniques. Once quiescence is achieved through prolonged immobilization, the patient may be advanced to a shoe and brace combination, which further provides joint stability and alignment, as well as relief of bony prominences.

Charcot deformities involving the forefoot, or mild stable deformities at the midfoot level, may be managed with an accommodative shoe alone. A wide-shank shoe with extra depth is attached to a double upright, calf-lacing or PTB brace with a fixed ankle joint and rigid rocker sole. The shoe should have a cushioned insert that may be customized to relieve areas of bony prominence. If necessary, plantar and midfoot prominences can be further relieved with an insole excavation filled with a low-density material. This shoe and brace combination is typically used for a period of 6 to 12 months as the neuropathic process reaches complete resolution. In the absence of significant malalignment or instability, the brace may then be removed and the patient managed in an accommodative shoe alone. Knee-high elastic compressive hose should be used in all patients with adequate vascularity.

The physician may be faced with the dilemma of determining whether an erythematous swollen foot is secondary to a Charcot process or infection. In the event of a closed skin barrier, infection in the diabetic foot is extremely rare. However, because a large number of Charcot foot deformities are associated with ulceration, the physician frequently is required to rule out the presence of cellulitis or osteomyelitis. Clinically, the inflammatory responses to Charcot and to infection are nearly indistinguishable, but infection is tender and painful while Charcot degeneration is not. Occasionally, elevation of the limb may lead to improvement in the erythematous appearance of Charcot inflammation, but not of the infection. Plain radiographs demonstrate nonspecific areas of lysis and periosteal reaction, and a magnetic resonance imaging scan fails to differentiate between marrow edema of the infected and noninfected bone. If clinical evaluation is uncertain, technetium bone scan combined with a labeled leukocyte scan appears to be the most sensitive and specific method of distinguishing between osteomyelitis and Charcot disease.

The presence of osteomyelitis in the Charcot foot mandates aggressive treatment, including removal of infected or necrotic bone, wound care, and external immobilization. A bivalved AFO is useful in this case. Studies have shown that the use of total contact casting and subsequent orthotic management is successful in 75% of all patients with type I midfoot Charcot deformities. However, complex cases remain in which bony prominences or instability will result in persistent or recurrent ulceration, as well as a foot that cannot be treated by bracing or shoe modifications.

Surgical intervention has gained recent popularity in both the acute and chronic situations. Indications for surgery in the acute setting include a severe dislocation of the tarsometatarsal joint that is unstable but manually reducible. Open reduction and primary arthrodesis may help to prevent future skin necrosis and ulceration while maintaining alignment. Surgery should be avoided if there is evidence of bone resorption or fragmentation on radiographs, because this evidence implies a subacute stage in which osteopenia is present and may preclude stable reduction and fixation. Displaced bimalleolar fractures in the neuropathic patient also demand anatomic reduction and rigid internal fixation. Postoperatively, prophylactic intravenous antibiotics are used in addition to strict evaluation, nonweightbearing, and prolonged external immobilization. This surgical intervention in the acute setting is considered prophylactic and must be weighed against the potential for significant wound complications and infection.

Surgical intervention is even more commonplace in the chronic Charcot deformity associated with symptomatic bony prominences or instability. Most commonly, bony prominences are removed via ostectomy, decompressing areas of skin breakdown. If possible, areas of ulceration are healed before surgery. However, often the ulcer will heal only if the prominence is corrected. Access to the bony prominence is typically achieved via an incision on a nonweightbearing surface of the foot. Ostectomy is most successful not only when the arthropathy is chronic, but when the deformity is rigid and stable. Although midfoot instability patterns are uncommon, when identified and associated with symptomatic bony prominence, a realignment arthrodesis should be considered. Multiple biplanar osteotomies and generous bone and joint resection are typically necessary to achieve a stable and plantigrade foot, often with the addition of an Achilles tendon lengthening. Rigid internal fixation is needed as well as prolonged immobilization. For unstable deformities in the hindfoot and ankle region that frequently lead to fixed varus or valgus malalignment and secondary bony prominences and ulceration, realignment arthrodesis is a salvage option and an alternative to amputation. Realignment is maintained with internal or external fixation, with the latter avoided if possible because of the increased risk of infection and wound problems. Internal fixation modalities include large cancellous screws or the use of an interlocked intramedullary nail from tibia to calcaneus. Long-term results of salvage have been reported to be successful in 93% of patients, with a high incidence of stable and asymptomatic pseudarthrosis. Despite success, long-term and lifetime bracing is recommended because of the risk of tibial diaphyseal stress fractures in this neuropathic patient population.

Annotated Bibliography

Hindfoot and Ankle

Chao W, Wapner KL, Lee TH, Adams J, Hecht PJ: Nonoperative management of posterior tibial tendon dysfunction. *Foot Ankle Int* 1996;17:736–741.

Fifty-three feet in 49 patients with posterior tibial tendon dysfunction were treated with orthoses. Sixty-seven percent had good or excellent results. Nonsurgical management using an orthosis was particularly useful for elderly patients with a sedentary lifestyle or for patients at high risk because of medical problems.

Dyal CM, Feder J, Deland JT, Thompson FM: Pes planus in patients with posterior tibial tendon insufficiency: Asymptomatic versus symptomatic foot. *Foot Ankle Int* 1997;18:85–88.

Bilateral weightbearing radiographs were analyzed in 43 patients with a clinical diagnosis of posterior tendon insufficiency. Strong correlation was found in the degree of severity of flatfoot deformity between the asymptomatic and symptomatic feet as well as the values used to assess pes planus. A preexisting flexible flatfoot is one of several etiologic factors in the development of posterior tibial tendon insufficiency.

Gazdag AR, Cracchiolo A III: Rupture of the posterior tibial tendon: Evaluation of injury of the spring ligament and clinical assessment of tendon transfer and ligament repair. *J Bone Joint Surg* 1997;79A:675–681.

Spring ligament injury was found in 18 of 22 patients undergoing tendon transfer for posterior tibial tendon rupture. The injury consisted of a longitudinal tear in 7 patients, a lax ligament without a tear in 7, and a complete rupture in 4. A variety of methods were used to repair the ligament.

Saltzman CL, el-Khoury GY: The hindfoot alignment view. *Foot Ankle Int* 1995;16:572–576.

A modification of Cobey's method for radiographically imaging the coronal plane alignment is described. The weightbearing line of the tibia falls within 8 mm of the lowest calcaneal point in 80% of subjects and within 15 mm of the lowest calcaneal point in 95% of subjects. The technique is reliable, with an interobserver correlation coefficient of 0.97 and should help in the evaluation of complex hindfoot malalignments.

Sands A, Harrington RM, Tencer AF, Ching RP: The kinematics of the hindfoot with lateral column lengthening and calcaneocuboid fusion for symptomatic flatfoot. *Trans Orthop Res Soc* 1997;22:273.

Calcaneocuboid fusion with the calcaneus lengthened and the foot in neutral position has no effect on hindfoot kinematics. However, fusing the foot in other orientations limits talocalcaneal and talonavicular joint motion.

Sands A, Early J, Harrington RM, Tencer AF, Ching RP, Sangeorzan BJ: Effect of variations in calcaneocuboid fusion technique on kinematics of the normal hindfoot. *Foot Ankle Int* 1998;19:19–25.

This study examined how calacaneocuboid fusion at different lengths and foot positions impacted hindfoot kinematics. Fusing the foot with the lateral column lengthened (10 mm) or shortened (5 mm) and the foot in neutral position did not change the hindfoot joint motion compared with that of the intact foot. However, fusion with the foot in plantarflexion and eversion or dorsiflexion and inversion resulted in significant decreases in motion in the talocalcaneal and talonavicular joints.

Sekiya JK, Saltzman CL: Long term follow-up of medial column fusion and tibialis anterior transposition for adolescent flatfoot deformity. *Iowa Orthop J* 1997;17:121–129.

The authors present results of 3 patients (4 feet) who had correction of adolescent flatfoot over 50 years ago. There was a high rate of painful arthrosis in the contiguous joints of the foot.

Thordarson DB, Schmotzer H, Chon J: Reconstruction with tenodesis in an adult flatfoot model: A biomechanical evaluation of four methods. *J Bone Joint Surg* 1995;77A:1557–1564.

Six fresh frozen cadaveric feet were loaded to create a flatfoot model. Each foot was then subjected to 4 reconstructions with tenodesis-peroneus longus transfer, posterior tibialis transfer, anterior tibialis transfer, Achilles tendon allograft. Each was then subjected to plantar loads.

Hallux Valgus

Easley ME, Kiebzak GM, Davis WH, Anderson RB: Prospective, randomized comparison of proximal crescentic and proximal chevron osteotomies for correction of hallux valgus deformity. *Foot Ankle Int* 1996;17:307–316.

In this prospective study of 97 feet randomized to either proximal chevron or proximal crescentic osteotomies, the outcomes were similar, but the authors thought the chevron approach was surgically simpler and more stable.

Saltzman CL, Brandser EA, Berbaum KS, et al: Reliability of standard foot radiographic measurements. *Foot Ankle Int* 1994; 15:661–665.

Error is intrinsic in all radiographic measurements. This study brings into question the use of strict radiographic guidelines when making surgical decisions.

Saltzman CL, Brandser EA, Anderson CM, Berbaum KS, Brown TD: Coronal plane rotation of the first metatarsal. *Foot Ankle Int* 1996;17:157–161.

A reliable and valid technique is presented for determining first metatarsal rotation.

Saltzman, CL, Aper RL, Brown TD: Anatomic determinants of first metatarsophalangeal flexion moments in hallux valgus. *Clin Orthop* 1997;339:261–269.

This experimental study demonstrates that the direction of flexion moments changes with hallux valgus, and distal metatarsal osteotomies alone do not restore normal biomechanics.

Talbot KD, Saltzman CL: Hallucal rotation: A method of measurement and relationship to bunion deformity. *Foot Ankle Int* 1997;18:550–556.

A reliable and valid technique is presented for determining hallucal rotation.

Tourné Y, Saragaglia D, Zattara A, et al: Hallux valgus in the elderly: Metatarsophalangeal arthrodesis of the first ray. *Foot Ankle Int* 1997;18:195–198.

This case series demonstrates predictably good fusion rates and pain relief from first MTP arthrodesis in elderly patients with severe hallux valgus deformities and degenerative changes.

Hallux Varus

Myerson MS, Komenda GA: Results of hallux varus correction using an extensor hallucis brevis tenodesis. *Foot Ankle Int* 1996; 17:21–27.

The authors used an extensor hallucis brevis tenodesis to correct 6 cases of iatrogenic hallux varus. Correction was maintained in all patients at a mean follow-up of 28 months.

Sanders AP, Snijders CJ, Linge BV: Potential for recurrence of hallux valgus after a modified Hohmann osteotomy: A biomechanical analysis. *Foot Ankle Int* 1995;16:351–356.

This article evaluates the "foot-widening effect" of active great toe flexion due to the path of the FHL tendon just lateral to the MTP joint. A significant effect persisted in a series of patients even after first metatarsal osteotomies to correct hallux valgus; it may be a factor in recurrence of the deformity.

Sesamoid Disorders

Anderson RB, McBryde AM Jr: Autogenous bone grafting of hallux sesamoid nonunions. *Foot Ankle Int* 1997;18:293–296.

In this retrospective study of 21 patients with tibial sesamoid nonunions treated with bone grafting, 19 healed and 17 returned to their preinjury level of sports and work.

Problems of the Lesser Toes

Trepman E, Yeo SJ: Nonoperative treatment of metatarsophalangeal joint synovitis. *Foot Ankle Int* 1995;16:771–777.

The authors successfully treated 12 of 13 patients with idiopathic second and third MTP synovitis with corticosteroid injections and shoe modifications. Metatarsalgia can last many months.

Morton's Interdigital Neuroma

Bennett GL, Graham CE, Mauldin DM: Morton's interdigital neuroma: A comprehensive treatment protocol. *Foot Ankle Int* 1995; 16:760–763.

A staged treatment program for Morton's neuroma, consisting of orthotics, steroid injections, and ultimate excision, was applied with a 79% success rate without surgery. Of the patients who eventually underwent excision, 96% had relief of pain.

Okafor B, Shergill G, Angel J: Treatment of Morton's neuroma by neurolysis. *Foot Ankle Int* 1997;18:284–287.

High success rates were achieved with neurolysis and release of the intermetatarsal ligament as an alternative to neurectomy.

Rheumatoid Arthritis

Hanyu T, Yamazaki H, Murasawa A, Tohyama C: Arthroplasty for rheumatoid forefoot deformities by a shortening oblique osteotomy. *Clin Orthop* 1997;338:131–138.

This is a retrospective study of 75 rheumatoid feet treated with lesser metatarsal shortening osteotomies combined with a first MTP procedure. At 6 years, 83% of patients were satisfied and 12% had recurrent, painful callosities.

Mann RA, Schakel ME II: Surgical correction of rheumatoid forefoot deformities. *Foot Ankle Int* 1995;16:1–6.

Correction of severe rheumatoid forefoot deformities was undertaken with first MTP arthrodesis and resection arthroplasties of the lesser toes. Ninety percent of the patients had a good or excellent functional result despite often severe initial deformities.

The Diabetic Foot

Early JS: Surgical intervention in diabetic neuroarthropathy of the foot, in Brodsky JW, Myerson MS (eds): *Foot and Ankle Clinics: The Diabetic Foot.* Philadelphia, PA, WB Saunders, 1997, pp 23–36.

The author presents a detailed review of Charcot deformities in the foot and ankle and surgical management options. Preoperative considerations, surgical options, and complications associated with surgery in this diabetic population are presented.

Krause JO, Brodsky JW: The natural history of type I midfoot neuropathic feet, in Brodsky JW, Myerson MS (eds): *Foot and Ankle Clinics: The Diabetic Foot.* Philadelphia, PA, WB Saunders, 1997, pp 1–22.

In this large series of 211 patients having a total of 279 neuropathic processes involving foot and ankle, midfoot neuropathic involvement (type 1) was present in 145 patients, bilateral in 35, at an average age of 52 years. Patient population was followed in regard to severity of neuropathy, extent of deformity, presence of ulceration, and treatment outcome. A depth/ischemic classification for diabetic foot lesions is also presented.

Wooldridge J, Moreno L: Evaluation of the costs to Medicare of covering therapeutic shoes for diabetic patients. *Diabetes Care* 1994;17:541–547.

A 3-year demonstration, fielded in 3 states, to evaluate the cost to Medicare of therapeutic shoes in patients with severe diabetic foot disease provided no evidence that expanding Medicare to cover therapeutic shoes would increase total Medicare cost. Although clinical effectiveness was not analyzed, it was concluded that a larger proportion of diabetic patients at risk acquired therapeutic shoes and wore them outdoors.

Classic Bibliography

Anderson RB, Davis WH: The pedorthic and orthotic care of the diabetic foot, in Brodsky JW, Myerson MS (eds): *Foot and Ankle Clinics: The Diabetic Foot.* Philadelphia, PA, WB Saunders, 1993, pp 137–151.

Bonakdar-pour A, Gaines VD: The radiology of osteomyelitis. *Orthop Clin North Am* 1983;14:21–37.

Brage M, Hansen ST, Sangeorzan BJ: Abstract: Treatment of severe posterior tibial tendon insufficiency by triple arthrodesis. Proceedings of the American Academy of Orthopaedic Surgeons 60th Annual Meeting, Rosemont, IL, American Academy of Orthopaedic Surgeons, 1993, p 196.

Brodsky JW: The diabetic foot, in Mann RA, Coughlin MJ (eds): *Surgery of the Foot and Ankle,* ed 6. St. Louis, MO, Mosby Year Book, 1993, pp 877–958.

Brodsky JW: Outpatient diagnosis and care of the diabetic foot, in Heckman JD (ed): *Instructional Course Lectures 42.* Rosemont, IL, American Academy of Orthopaedic Surgeons, 1993, pp 121–139.

Burgess EM, Matsen FA: Determining amputation levels in peripheral vascular disease. *J Bone Joint Surg* 1981;63A:1493–1497.

Carr JB, Hansen ST, Benirschke SK: Subtalar distraction boneblock fusion for late complications of os calcis fractures. *Foot Ankle* 1988;9:81–86.

Centers for Disease Control and Prevention: *Economic Aspects of Diabetes Services and Education: Selected Annotations.* Atlanta, GA, US Department of Health and Human Services, 1992.

Coughlin MJ: Treatment of bunionette deformity with longitudinal diaphyseal osteotomy with distal soft tissue repair. *Foot Ankle* 1991;11:195–203.

Craxford AD, Stevens J, Park C: Management of the deformed rheumatoid forefoot: A comparison of conservative and surgical methods. *Clin Orthop* 1982;166:121–126.

Dal Monte A, Andrisano A, Capanna R: Results of surgical treatment of idiopathic pes plano-valgus by means of Grice's operation combined with reconstruction of the glenoid (accessory plantar) ligament and anterior transposition of tibialis posterior: A review of 90 cases. *J Orthop Traumatol* 1979;5:19–34.

Deland JT, Arnoczky SP, Thompson FM: Adult acquired flatfoot deformity at the talonavicular joint: Reconstruction of the spring ligament in an in vitro model. *Foot Ankle* 1992;13:327–332.

Dwyer FC: Osteotomy of the calcaneum for pes cavus. *J Bone Joint Surg* 1959;41B:80–86.

Evans D: Relapsed club foot. *J Bone Joint Surg* 1961;43B: 722–733.

Fitzgerald JA: A review of long-term results of arthrodesis of the first metatarso-phalangeal joint. *J Bone Joint Surg* 1969;51B: 488–493.

Frey C, Jahss M, Kummer FJ: The Akin procedure: An analysis of results. *Foot Ankle* 1991;12:1–6.

Frey C, Shereff M, Greenidge N: Vascularity of the posterior tibial tendon. *J Bone Joint Surg* 1990;72A:884–888.

Giannestras NJ (ed): *Foot Disorders: Medical and Surgical Management*, ed 2. Philadelphia, PA, Lea & Febiger, 1973.

Goldner MG: The fate of the second leg in the diabetic amputee. *Diabetes* 1960;9:100–103.

Graves SC, Mann RA, Graves KO: Triple arthrodesis in older adults: Results after long-term follow-up. *J Bone Joint Surg* 1993; 75A:355–362.

Hattrup SJ, Johnson KA: Subjective results of hallux rigidus following treatment with cheilectomy. *Clin Orthop* 1988;226: 182–191.

Johnson KA, Spiegl PV: Extensor hallucis longus transfer for hallux varus deformity. *J Bone Joint Surg* 1984;66A:681–686.

Kidner FC: The prehallux (accessory scaphoid) in its relation to flat-foot. *J Bone Joint Surg* 1929;11:831–837.

Kitaoka HB, Holiday AD Jr: Lateral condylar resection for bunionette. *Clin Orthop* 1992;278:183–192.

Kitaoka HB, Holiday AD Jr, Campbell DC II: Distal chevron metatarsal osteotomy for bunionette. *Foot Ankle* 1991;12: 80–85.

Mann RA, Clanton TO: Hallux rigidus: Treatment by cheilectomy. *J Bone Joint Surg* 1988;70A:400–406.

Mann RA, Rudicel S, Graves SC: Repair of hallux valgus with a distal soft-tissue procedure and proximal metatarsal osteotomy: A long-term follow-up. *J Bone Joint Surg* 1992;74A:124–129.

Morton DJ (ed): *The Human Foot: Its Evolution, Physiology and Functional Disorders*. New York, NY, Columbia Univesity Press, 1935.

O'Doherty DP, Lowrie IG, Magnussen PA, Gregg PJ: The management of the painful first metatarsophalangeal joint in the older patient: Arthrodesis or Keller's arthroplasty? *J Bone Joint Surg* 1990;72B:839–842.

Ratcliff DA, Clyne CA, Chant AD, Webster JH: Prediction of amputation wound healing: The role of transcutaneous pO_2 assessment. *Br J Surg* 1984;71:219–222.

Raunio P, Lehtimäki M, Eerola M, Hämäläinen M, Pulkki T: Resection arthroplasty versus arthrodesis of the first metatarsophalangeal joint for hallux valgus in rheumatoid arthritis. *Rheumatol Annu Rev* 1987;11:173–178.

Sangeorzan BJ, Hansen ST Jr: Modified Lapidus procedure for hallux valgus. *Foot Ankle* 1989;9:262–266.

Sangeorzan BJ, Mosca V, Hansen ST Jr: Effect of calcaneal lengthening on relationships among the hindfoot, midfoot, and forefoot. *Foot Ankle* 1993;14:136–141.

Schauwecker DS: Osteomyelitis: Diagnosis with In-111 labeled leukocytes. *Radiology* 1989;171:141–146.

Stein M, Provan JL, Prosser R, Barrett C, Ameli FM: A statistical assessment of the dependability of transcutaneous tissue oxygen tension measurements. *J Surg Res* 1989;46:70–75.

Taylor RG: The treatment of claw toes by multiple transfers of flexor into extensor tendons. *J Bone Joint Surg* 1951;33B:539–542.

Wagner FW Jr: The diabetic foot. *Orthopedics* 1987;10:163–172.

Wagner FW Jr: Management of the diabetic-neurotrophic foot: Part II. A classification and treatment program for diabetic, neuropathic, and dysvascular foot problems, in Cooper RR (ed): American Academy of Orthopaedic Surgeons *Instructional Course Lectures XXVIII*. St. Louis, MO, CV Mosby, 1979, pp 143–165.

Wagner FW: Transcutaneous Doppler ultrasound in the prediction of healing and the selection of surgical level for dysvascular legions of the toes and forefoot. *Clin Orthop* 1979;142: 110–114.

Wang A, Weinstein D, Greenfield L, et al: MRI and diabetic foot infections. *Magn Reson Imaging* 1990;8:805–809.

Weinstein D, Wang A, Chambers R, Stewart CA, Motz HA: Evaluation of magnetic resonance imaging in the diagnosis of osteomyelitis in diabetic foot infections. *Foot Ankle* 1993;14: 18–22.

Section 5
Spine

Chapter 47
Pediatric Spine

Pediatric Spinal Deformity

Congenital Scoliosis

Congenital scoliosis is caused by structural abnormalities of the vertebrae that result in asymmetric growth. It has been classified as type I, failure of formation, and type II, failure of segmentation, although sometimes both types are found in the same spine (Fig. 1). In type I, the abnormality can be a true isolated hemivertebra, a wedged vertebra, multiple wedged vertebrae, or multiple hemivertebrae, and these can occur anywhere in the spine. The abnormality is further categorized by how the hemivertebra is segmented and positioned between vertebrae. Thus, it can be fully or partially segmented, tucked within the contour of the spine (incarcerated), or lateralized from the rest of the spine (unincarcerated). The potential growth of the hemivertebra is the key to its ability to produce deformity. Healthy-appearing disks between the hemivertebra and its neighbors implies good growth potential, and thus the fully segmented unincarcerated hemivertebra would be most likely to cause progressive deformity of the type I abnormalities. Type II abnormalities are caused by failures of segmentation between adjacent vertebrae. This failure may be unilateral, resulting in an unsegmented bar on one side, or it can be bilateral, causing a block vertebra. The unsegmented bar often is associated with rib abnormalities. The unsegmented area can involve only 2 segments or multiple segments. Also, a hemivertebra may be present on the opposite side of the spine from the unsegmented bar, and this represents the most likely scenario for curve progression. A large segment of bilaterally unsegmented vertebrae will stunt the growth of the spine.

Although congenital spinal deformities are present at birth, there is no consistent evidence that the abnormality is hereditary in most patients. Associated anomalies that

can occur with congenital scoliosis are Klippel-Feil syndrome (25%), genitourinary tract abnormalities (30%), and cardiac abnormalities (12%). Intraspinal abnormalities occur in about 15% and need to be ruled out by magnetic resonance imaging (MRI) or myelogram before surgical intervention. Plain radiographs of the spine may not be sufficient to properly classify the vertebral anomaly, and tomography, computed tomography (CT) with reconstructions, or MRI may yield that information.

Goals in the management of congenital scoliosis are to recognize progression and to eliminate asymmetric growth before the deformity becomes large. Controlled observation has shown a wide variability of behavior of the spinal anom-

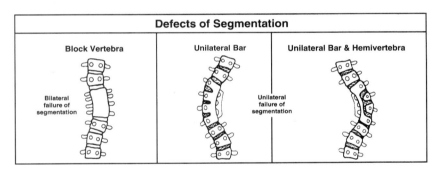

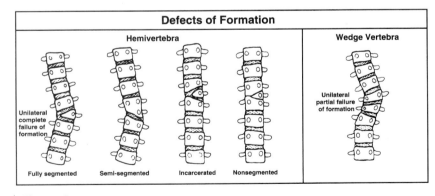

Figure 1
Congenital scoliosis: A unilateral bar with hemivertebra carries the highest risk of rapid progression. The fully segmented nonincarcerated hemivertebra grows from both the cephalad and caudal growth centers, causing progressive scoliosis. The nonsegmented hemivertebra may not be apparent clinically. (Reproduced with permission from McMaster MJ: Congenital scoliosis, in Weinstein SL (ed): *The Pediatric Spine: Principles and Practice.* New York, NY, Raven Press, 1994, pp 227–244.)

alies, sometimes defying what may have been predicted by the initial anatomic abnormality. This condition must never be allowed to relentlessly progress in the mistaken belief that doing so allows growth of the vertebrae and preservation of trunk height. This does not happen, and trunk height lost by progression of the curve can never be restored by later reconstructive surgery. Bracing of a congenital curve is ineffective (although bracing may be used for an associated compensatory noncongenital curve). Only surgery is effective in controlling progressive curves.

Surgical treatment of congenital scoliosis in growing children involves destroying all or part of the vertebral physes and fusion of the posterior elements of the same vertebrae; ie, anterior and posterior spinal fusion. The surgical treatment of congenital scoliosis in growing children can be divided into 3 broad strategies. The first is anterior and posterior spinal fusion, either in situ or with correction, with or without instrumentation. This strategy represents definitive and final control of the deformity, eliminating the possibility of "crankshafting." The crankshaft phenomenon occurs when there is continued anterior growth of the vertebrae in the presence of a solid posterior fusion, resulting in increasing rotation of the affected vertebrae, and thus presenting an increase in residual curve. This strategy does not use growth as a potential correcting force and is appropriate for both type I and type II deformities. The second option is anterior hemiepiphysiodesis and posterior hemiarthrodesis on the convex side, with or without instrumentation. This involves removal of the disks around the hemivertebrae and one half of the disk 1 or 2 levels above and below the hemivertebrae, anterior arthrodesis of these disk spaces, and posterior spinal fusion on the convex side only. (This treatment may be supplemented by a growing rod posteriorly.) This technique halts the deformity-causing growth on the convex side, while allowing whatever growth is possible on the concave side, with variable correction of the deformity over time. It is appropriate only for type I deformities. Finally, hemivertebra excision provides tremendous correction at 1 level and totally eliminates the abnormal growth. It is done most commonly at the lumbosacral junction, but can be done in the lumbar spine as well, and is usually done with instrumentation. This strategy also only applies to type I abnormalities. The more complicated strategies are associated with greater risk of neurologic complications, but may represent the most effective treatment.

Idiopathic Scoliosis

Infantile and Juvenile Idiopathic Scoliosis Classification of idiopathic scoliosis into infantile or early onset (birth to 3

years old) and juvenile or late onset (4 to 10 years old) is somewhat arbitrary. However, classic early onset scoliosis behaves quite differently than the juvenile onset form. Severe chest wall deformity and subsequent cardiopulmonary dysfunction are more likely in the early onset type. A severe curve with marked rib deformity may inhibit alveolar formation. Relentless progression of these curves leads to severe restrictive lung disease and subsequent cor pulmonale.

The classic early onset curve pattern is quite distinct, a left thoracic curve most commonly seen in boys. It can also be seen in girls, as a right-sided curve with a poor prognosis. The etiology of infantile idiopathic scoliosis is obscure, just as it is for the juvenile and adolescent onset forms; rib-chest molding and subsequent curving of the spine may play a role. Other etiologies (for all 3 forms) include intraspinal abnormalities (hydrosyringomyelia with or without the Chiari malformation) and spinal cord tethering. This can be evaluated with spinal canal imaging such as MRI. The rib-vertebra angle difference (RVAD) on plain radiographs may yield information regarding relative risk of progression (Fig. 2). In the infantile form, an RVAD > 20° is associated with significant risk of progression, and aggressive treatment is needed to control such curves. Curves with an RVAD < 20° may spontaneously regress. The use of this measure in the juvenile form is not as reliable or predictive.

Treatment of progressive infantile idiopathic scoliosis should begin early and includes initial casting to gain some

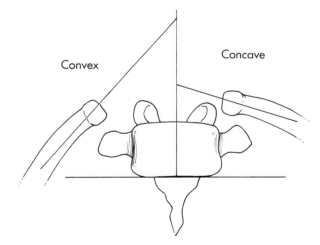

Figure 2

The rib-vertebra angle difference (RVAD) is calculated by subtracting the angle of the rib on the convex side of the curve relative to a line perpendicular to the vertebral body end plate from the angle on the concave side of the curve. (Adapted with permission from Koop SE: Infantile and juvenile idiopathic scoliosis. *Orthop Clin North Am* 1988;19:331–337.)

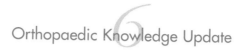
correction before brace application. This is followed by prolonged bracing. If nonsurgical treatment is ineffective, surgical treatment coupled with postoperative bracing may be needed. To gain sufficient correction and curve control, a short segment anterior spinal fusion across the apex of the curve, with or without instrumentation, is done in combination with a posteriorly growing rod, which is periodically elongated as the child grows. This treatment is continued until age 10 or 11 years, when the definitive posterior spinal fusion and instrumentation is done. This strategy is arduous and can be associated with numerous complications, particularly of the instrumentation.

Progressive juvenile idiopathic scoliosis requires appropriate bracing, initially full time. In a small percentage of these patients, curve correction is achieved and maintained even during growth. Successful bracing can be achieved in this group of patients even when the initial curve is much larger than that usually considered braceable for the adolescent form. If bracing does not control the curve, especially in younger juvenile onset patients, a growing rod construct can be used, with periodic elongation and with continued bracing. If definitive spinal fusion is indicated in older patients in this group, a posterior spinal fusion with instrumentation combined with anterior spinal fusion or an anterior spinal fusion with instrumentation is necessary to prevent crankshafting.

Adolescent Idiopathic Scoliosis

Etiology Because adolescent idiopathic scoliosis is partially familial, research is ongoing to discover the responsible gene. A number of possible causative factors have been identified, such as abnormal collagen content of the disks, fibrilin fibers in ligaments, platelet calmodulin, and equilibrium reactions. Most research points to an abnormal neuromuscular mechanism. Recent studies in chicken and bipedal rat models have shown that pinealectomy results in the development of scoliosis. Animals that received melatonin after the pinealectomy did not develop scoliosis, while those not given melatonin became scoliotic. Human research tends to support these findings.

Prevalence When a Cobb angle of 10° is the lower threshold for diagnosis of this condition, the prevalence is 25 per 1,000 population. Raising the threshold decreases the prevalence. Although prevalence is equal in girls and boys with small curves, the ratio of girls to boys increases with increasing Cobb angle (7:1 for curves > 25°).

Screening School screening has been recommended for identification and treatment of children with scoliosis. The most common method is the Adams (forward bend) test. Using a

scoliometer to measure the angle of trunk rotation (ATR) at the apex of the rib hump provides a useful number on which to base referrals and definitive diagnosis. With an ATR of 5°, only 2% of 20° curves are missed, whereas 12% are missed using an ATR of 7°. There are objections to screening because the testing is costly and because it injects large numbers of patients into the health care system. Moreover, some believe that no nonsurgical treatment can change the natural history even if the diagnosis is made.

Natural History Progression of a curve depends on its magnitude and the skeletal maturity of the patient at the time it is identified. The smaller the curve and the more advanced the skeletal maturity, the less likely it is to increase. Other predictive factors are female sex, premenarchal status, early Risser sign, and young age. Family history, sagittal alignment, trunk imbalance, and lumbosacral abnormalities are not predictive. Vertebral and trunk rotation may be predictive. The concepts of peak growth velocity and peak growth age have been found to be very useful in looking at relative risk for progression. Peak growth age, that age after which the rate of growth decreases, appears to be very reliable, not only in terms of progression, but also in the risk for crankshafting after surgical treatment. It can be applied to both girls and boys, and seems to be more reliable than menarchal status.

Clinical Evaluation Careful physical examination is needed, both to define curve characteristics and to identify other conditions that may influence diagnosis and management. This applies especially to the neurologic examination, including assessment of superficial abdominal reflexes. Certain abnormalities should trigger evaluation of the spinal canal to rule out hydrosyringomyelia and other abnormalities. Upright radiographs are essential for proper curve classification and measurement. Modern techniques minimize the radiation dose.

Nonsurgical Treatment The only effective nonsurgical treatment is bracing, which is appropriate for curves between 25° and 40° that are progressing or are likely to progress. Because remaining active growth is necessary for bracing, patients who are Risser 4 or 5 are not candidates. The Milwaukee brace should be used for thoracic curves with an apex of T8 or T9 or higher. A number of regimens have been devised (eg, part-time bracing) to make bracing more palatable; however, recent meta-analysis of a number of studies showed that full-time bracing is more effective. The Charleston bending night brace was also less effective in curves > 35° and thoracic curves, and was most useful for treating lumbar curves of 25° to 35°. Bracing must continue until the cessation of growth, after which the patient is weaned from the brace.

Surgical Treatment Many surgical strategies and instrumentation systems now exist for scoliosis treatment (Fig. 3). Their common goal is a solid fusion over the fewest vertebrae that will allow adequate correction and maintenance of coronal and sagittal balance. This can be accomplished with a posterior spinal fusion with segmental implants, with or without anterior spinal fusion, which may be needed to ensure a solid fusion, prevent crankshafting, or provide better correction. Certain thoracolumbar and lumbar curves can be corrected with instrumented anterior spinal fusion alone. Adequate bone graft, preferably autogenous, is necessary. In patients with large rib humps, appearance can be improved with thoracoplasty. The excised ribs provide excellent bone graft material.

Spinal cord monitoring (somatosensory- and/or motor-evoked potentials), the clonus test, and/or the Stagnara wake-up test should be used during spinal corrective surgery. Because recovery from spinal cord injury resulting from stretching of the cord is time dependent, early identification of the problem is essential. Although the wake-up test is the most accurate assessment of spinal cord function, it reflects only one point in time. Continuous monitoring of somatosensory and motor-evoked potentials is less likely to yield false positive or false negative findings.

Complications of Surgical Treatment Immature patients may undergo the crankshaft phenomenon, which results in increasing curve size and change in trunk balance in the presence of a solid posterior spinal fusion. Assessment of this risk includes skeletal age, peak growth age, status of the triradiate cartilages, and potential residual curve size on preoperative bending films. It can be avoided by combined anterior and posterior spinal fusion or anterior fusion with instrumentation only for appropriate curves. Spinal cord injury, pseudarthrosis, infection, and hardware failure are unlikely but definite risks of surgical treatment.

Neuromuscular Scoliosis
Scoliosis is a common deformity in many types of neuromuscular diseases, and generally is most severe in nonambulatory patients. Severe curves cause difficulties in sitting, and

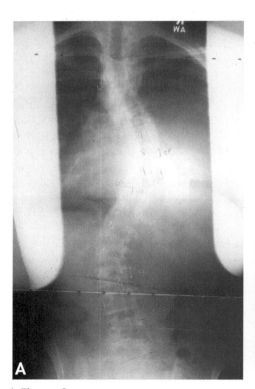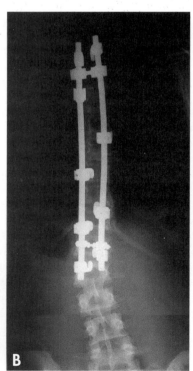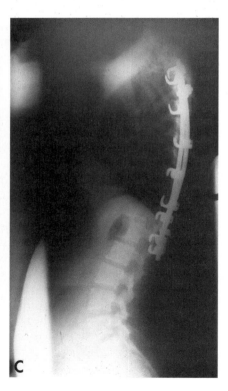

Figure 3
A, Preoperative anteroposterior (AP) radiograph shows King type II right thoracic scoliosis with compensatory lumbar scoliosis. B, Postoperative AP radiograph shows fusion and CD instrumentation of the thoracic scoliosis only, with good correction of the curves and coronal balance. C, Postoperative lateral radiograph shows good correction and maintenance of sagittal balance. (Courtesy of Howard S. An, MD)

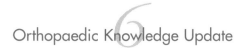
when the curves become large and stiff, improvement in posture cannot be achieved with external devices. Bracing of neuromuscular curves does not affect the natural history and is not definitive treatment. Progressive curves require surgical correction and stabilization. The goals of surgical treatment in this group of patients include a level pelvis, spinal balance in the coronal plane, and a normal sagittal contour to allow proper weight distribution during sitting. Fusion levels should extend to at least T2 superiorly and should include the pelvis in nonambulatory patients. Other important factors include segmental posterior instrumentation, adequate bone graft, the addition of an anterior fusion when indicated, and proper patient nutrition. Combining anterior and posterior fusions at the same surgery seems to be advantageous, but only when done expeditiously. Otherwise, staged procedures may be a wiser choice.

Cerebral Palsy Scoliosis is common in children with cerebral palsy, and the greater the severity of the disease, the more likely that scoliosis will develop. Although the growth spurt may cause rapid and severe progression of the curve, evidence shows that progression can occur even after skeletal maturity. Severe curves in children with cerebral palsy may have serious effects on their most basic functions, such as sitting and using their upper extremities. Any possible activities that even a child severely affected by cerebral palsy undertakes require proper sitting. Seating systems have been designed to position these children, but improvement in posture cannot occur with stiff curves. Thoracolumbosacral orthoses in immature children with supple curves will improve position and allow time for spinal growth before surgical treatment.

Indications for surgery include progressive curves > 50° in patients older than 10 years of age. Whether or not surgical treatment of scoliosis in cerebral palsy is justified in all patients meeting these criteria remains controversial. Therefore, selection of patients for surgery must be individualized, and the patient's comorbidities and overall function considered before definitely recommending surgery. Parents and other caregivers must understand the somewhat limited goal of the surgery and the fact that the children will still have cerebral palsy even after their scoliosis has been corrected. Ambulatory patients should have fusions short of the pelvis as long as the goals of surgery can be accomplished. Both anterior and posterior spinal fusion should be used if crankshafting is of concern, if the curve is severe and rigid with pelvic obliquity, and if the risk of pseudarthrosis is high. Recent reports indicate that, in nonambulatory patients, combined anterior and posterior fusion to the pelvis results in the best surgical outcomes.

Duchenne and Becker Muscular Dystrophy Progressive scoliosis develops in most patients with Duchenne and Becker muscular dystrophy. Cessation of walking usually heralds the development and progression of the scoliosis; 10° of curve progression per year can be expected once the child stops walking. This occurs with a concomitant decrease in the forced vital capacity of about 4% to 5% per year. Not every child with muscular dystrophy develops worsening scoliosis. Those with a lordotic posture tend to progress less than those with a kyphotic posture. Progressive curves in these patients interfere with proper and comfortable sitting. Bracing is not definitive treatment, may mask an increase in the curve, and may interfere with respiratory function. To allow proper sitting and improve the quality of life, posterior fusion with instrumentation should be done as soon as the curve becomes progressive, and before pulmonary function deteriorates beyond a forced vital capacity < 30% to 40%, at which point the patient is no longer a reasonable surgical candidate.

Surgical treatment should consist of a posterior spinal fusion with segmental posterior instrumentation. A number of reports indicate that ending the fusion and instrumentation short of the pelvis may be acceptable, but the presence of a significant pelvic obliquity requires extension to the pelvis. Including the pelvis in nonambulatory patients avoids having to deal with a progressive curve and pelvic obliquity in patients who are no longer surgical candidates.

Myelomeningocele The incidence of spinal deformity in myelomeningocele has been correlated with the level of the last intact posterior vertebral arch; the higher the neurologic level, the more likely a spinal deformity. These deformities can be neuromuscular, congenital (up to one third of patients have congenital vertebral anomalies in addition to the spina bifida defect), or both. Primary kyphotic deformities, some of which are the very severe congenital or angular/dysplastic type, occur in 8% to 15% of patients.

Progressive curves in myelomeningocele interfere with function and may predispose to other problems such as pressure sores over prominent insensate areas. Other factors that influence curve behavior and treatment are abnormal function of the central nervous system (eg, uncontrolled hydrocephalus), Chiari malformations, hydrosyringomyelia, and cord tethering. Clinical examination and imaging studies are necessary to evaluate these abnormalities. Bracing is ineffective in altering the natural history of these deformities, but may provide better trunk and sitting posture in young children with flexible curves until they are old enough for definitive surgery. Because the lack of posterior elements in the bifid area of the spine makes solid arthrodesis with a posterior fusion alone unlikely, surgical treatment includes anterior and posterior spinal fusion with instrumentation. Extending the fusion to the pelvis depends on the ambulatory status, magnitude of the curve, and pelvic obliquity. In selected ambulatory patients with thoracolumbar or lumbar curves, anterior spinal fusion with instrumentation alone may be the most appropriate treatment.

Brace treatment for children with severe angular/dysplastic kyphosis is not effective and can cause problems with skin breakdown over the gibbus. Selected children, who have significant deformity that interferes with sitting and/or who have skin breakdown over the apex, are candidates for vertebrectomy and/or vertebral body decancellation with or without spinal cord resection. Long segmental posterior instrumentation with special lower rod contouring is typically used. However, not all patients with this deformity are candidates for this rather complex operation, and the risk benefit ratio must be considered before recommending surgery. Short posterior instrumentation is ineffective for the long-term control of these deformities.

Kyphosis

Scheuermann's Disease There are 2 types, classic and lumbar. In classic Scheuermann's disease, abnormally increased kyphosis in the thoracic or thoracolumbar areas of the spine is associated with vertebral body wedging. Criteria for the diagnosis include wedging $\geq 5°$ at 3 adjacent vertebral body levels at the apex of the curve. Large curves cause compensatory lordotic curves above and below the deformity, which may result in a typical forward head and neck thrust in patients with classic Scheuermann's disease. With lumbar Scheuermann's disease, there is flattening of the lumbar lordosis, narrowed disk spaces, Schmorl's node formation, and irregular ossification of the vertebral end plates. Both types can cause back pain, but it is much more common in the lumbar type.

Scheuermann's disease is more common in males. No definitive etiology has been identified, although osteochondrosis, osteonecrosis of the vertebral end plates, juvenile osteoporosis, and various endocrine abnormalities have been suggested. A similarity to Blount's disease is suggested by progressive deformity accompanied by worsening vertebral body wedging. The differential diagnosis includes postural roundback, congenital type I kyphosis, skeletal dysplasias, and compression fractures. Increasing kyphosis does not seem to be associated with cardiopulmonary compromise, but low back pain associated with thoracic kyphosis may be problematic and is caused by excessive compensatory lumbar lordosis below the deformity.

Treatment is individualized. Adolescents with future spinal growth may be candidates for bracing with the Milwaukee brace. If the kyphosis is rigid, Risser casting before brace application may improve the deformity. Exercises to stretch the hamstrings and strengthen the abdominal muscles may provide symptomatic improvement. Surgical indications vary, but most agree that patients with kyphosis > 70°, progressive kyphosis, or persistent pain benefit from fusion. Lumbar Scheuermann's disease causes low back pain in older adolescents. Bracing can decrease the pain.

Congenital Kyphosis This disease has been classified as type I, failure of formation, and type II, failure of segmentation. A third type, congenital dislocation of the spine, has been recognized recently, but is uncommon. Type I is the most common spinal deformity to cause neurologic deficit. Type II does not cause neurologic deficit and has less tendency to progress. Congenital dislocation of the spine is always associated with neurologic deficit.

Treatment of congenital kyphosis is surgical. In growing children with progressive type I and II curves without neurologic deficit, posterior spinal fusion with or without instrumentation is the treatment of choice for curves < 70°. The hemiepiphysiodesis effect of the fusion results in a gradual correction of type I curves. Neurologic deficits in type I curves can be treated by either "orthopaedic decompression" (realignment of the spine) or by direct decompression of the spinal cord. Congenital dislocation of the spine usually requires direct decompression combined with appropriate anterior and posterior spinal fusion with or without instrumentation.

Neurofibromatosis

Scoliosis is common in patients with neurofibromatosis-1 (NF-1), although only 2% to 3% of all scoliosis patients have NF-1. Two curve patterns have been found: an idiopathic-like pattern and a dystrophic type with a short, sharply angulated curve often with kyphosis. In the latter type, penciling of the ribs, scalloping of the vertebral bodies, and enlargement of the neural foramina may be present. The rib penciling makes the ribs weak, and even with relatively minor trauma such ribs can fracture and displace through the foramina into the spinal canal, causing paralysis. The dystrophic type is more likely to progress.

Idiopathic-like NF curves are treated the same as other idiopathic curves. The dystrophic type does not respond well to bracing. When recognized as progressive, a dystrophic curve should undergo anterior and posterior spinal fusion with instrumentation to avoid pseudarthrosis. Kyphoscoliotic deformities also can cause paralysis in patients with NF-1. The curvature and malaligned vertebrae may cause the paralysis, but intraspinal masses may be responsible as well; therefore, preoperative evaluation of the spinal canal is necessary. "Orthopaedic" or direct spinal cord decompression in addition to an appropriate anterior and posterior fusion with instrumentation are necessary for the proper management of this severe deformity.

Kyphosis of the cervical spine is relatively common and may cause symptoms such as spinal cord dysfunction, dysphasia, and torticollis. Collapse of vertebral bodies may occur. Appropriate imaging studies are necessary to define the exact problem. Appropriate treatment includes correction of the deformity, neural element decompression, and anterior and posterior fusion with or without instrumentation, supplemented with halo brace or cast immobilization.

Cervical Spine Deformities

Klippel-Feil Syndrome Klippel-Feil syndrome is a congenital fusion of 2 or more cervical vertebrae. However, multiple levels can be involved with only 1 motion segment preserved. It frequently is associated with other anomalies such as the VATER (vetebral defects, imperforate anus, tracheoesophageal fistula, and radial and renal dysplasia) association, Goldenhar's syndrome, and Sprengel's deformity and occurs in 25% of patients with congenital thoracolumbar spine deformities.

Only 40% to 50% of patients display the classic triad of a short neck, low hairline, and decreased neck motion, but most have some degree of limited neck motion. Other symptoms include neck pain, radiculopathy, and myelopathy. These patients should be evaluated for associated genitourinary and cardiovascular abnormalities, as well as hearing loss.

These patients generally function normally throughout life, but some develop neck pain or a neurologic problem requiring stabilization and decompression or both. Those with occipitalization of C1 with a C2-3 fusion are especially prone to C1-2 instability.

Torticollis Torticollis is a head tilt with rotation. It may be congenital or acquired. Some causes of acquired torticollis include posterior fossa tumors, superior oblique eye muscle palsy, and C1-2 rotary subluxation. Congenital muscular torticollis, the most common type of torticollis, may be caused by a compartment syndrome of the sternocleidomastoid muscle. Early on, a palpable mass may be present within the muscle. It is often associated with developmental dysplasia of the hip. The longer the deformity remains uncorrected, the more likely that secondary deformities such as plagiocephaly will develop. Radiographs of the cervical spine are needed to rule out bony abnormalities. Nonsurgical treatment aims to reverse the head tilt by stretching the tight structures. If

unsuccessful, surgical treatment (either a unipolar or bipolar release of the sternocleidomastoid muscle) followed by immobilization of the head is indicated.

Back Pain in Children

Epidemiology
Back pain in children is nearly always associated with a pathologic process, and a diagnosis can be made in 84% of children. Recent studies show that over half of adolescents have back pain that can resemble adult back pain, although few seek medical attention.

Evaluation
The patient's age is an important factor. Children younger than 5 years often have infections or neoplasms, whereas adolescents are more likely to have spondylolysis or Scheuermann's kyphosis. The nature of the pain also is critical. Intermittent pain associated with activities is more likely due to spondylolysis, whereas unremitting pain and night pain are associated with tumors. Fever, weight loss, and anorexia may indicate malignancy or infection. Activities that require repetitive lumbar hyperextension, such as gymnastics, ballet, and football, predispose toward spondylolysis.

Scoliosis and trunk decompensation are often seen on physical examination with irritative spinal lesions. Lumbar lordosis may not be reversed with forward bending, and hamstring tightness is common. If spondylolysis is present, lumbar pain may be worsened by hyperextension. Clonus or an abnormal Babinski reflex indicates cord abnormalities or compression. Abdominal reflexes may be asymmetric in syringomyelia.

Anteroposterior (AP) and lateral radiographs are inspected for disk space narrowing, lytic or blastic lesions, alignment, and vertebral scalloping. If a specific area is painful, or a suspicious lesion is seen, a supine cone-down radiograph yields superior detail. The pelvis also should be examined because sacral and pelvic lesions may cause back pain. If plain radiographs are nondiagnostic and further studies are indicated, a bone scan is recommended for children with normal neurologic examinations. The bone scan is a sensitive but not specific modality, showing increased uptake with infection, fracture, and most tumors. Although scintigraphy is an excellent localization tool, CT shows bony anatomy better. Single photon emission CT (SPECT) combines the physiology of a bone scan with the localization of tomography. If the neurologic examination is abnormal, MRI is indicated. A complete blood cell count with differential and peripheral smears, and a sedimentation rate or C-reactive protein should be ordered in any child with constitutional symptoms and in young children.

Causes of Back Pain

Diskitis Infection is the most common cause of back pain in young children. Presenting complaints vary from back pain to abdominal pain to limp and refusal to walk. A history of fever and malaise is common. Physical examination reveals a loss of spinal flexibility and reluctance to bend. Neurologic findings are rare.

Radiographs are initially normal. Subtle disk space narrowing is the first abnormality to appear. End plate irregularities follow. Because the initial radiographs are usually unimpressive, the diagnosis frequently is made by bone scan, which shows increased uptake across the involved disk. MRI rarely is needed for diagnosis, but is helpful when looking for an abscess in patients with pain that is refractory to treatment.

In the past, treatment was most often orthotic management and rest alone, but recent reports describe improved outcomes with the use of antistaphylococcal antibiotics. Disk cultures are not necessary and are positive only 60% of the time. Bony destruction and soft-tissue extension are more prevalent with tuberculosis than with other infections, and tuberculous osteomyelitis tends to recur.

Scoliosis Until recently, idiopathic scoliosis was not believed to cause pain, but one report indicates that pain does occur in 33% of girls with scoliosis. Plain radiographs were most likely to identify bony pathology, which was located at the apex of the deformity or at the lumbosacral junction. If the neurologic examination was normal, MRI was not useful. Painful left thoracic curves have been linked with intraspinal pathology such as syringomyelia.

Scheuermann's Kyphosis The most common cause for thoracic back pain in adolescents is Scheuermann's kyphosis. The pain is located in the midscapular region at the apex of the kyphosis.

Spondylolysis and Spondylolisthesis Spondylolysis is the most common cause of low back pain in adolescents. Spondylolysis or spondylolisthesis was diagnosed in 47% of teens complaining of back pain in a sports medicine clinic. Repetitive lumbar hyperextension stresses the pars interarticularis, leading to fracture. The pain is activity-related and can radiate into the buttocks or legs. Physical examination may reveal flattening of lumbar lordosis and tight hamstrings. Lateral radiographs may reveal a pars defect, which is better demonstrated on oblique radiographs. Scintigraphy has been used to differentiate the prefracture and acute stages (increased uptake on SPECT scan) from the chronic stage (decreased uptake).

Treatment begins with activity modification. If the fracture is acute, use of a low profile thoracolumbosacral orthosis can relieve symptoms and encourage healing. If pain persists despite rest, bracing, and physical therapy, surgery is indicated. Controversy exists as to whether repair of the lytic defect is superior to posterolateral fusion in spondylolysis. The treatment of spondylolisthesis varies with slip severity.

Traumatic Etiologies Herniated disk disease is rare in children. Presenting complaints are back pain radiating to the leg, often after trauma. The most frequent sign on physical examination is a positive straight leg raise, with neurologic findings less common. Radiographs may show reactive scoliosis, but usually are normal. MRI shows the herniated disk most clearly. Initial treatment is conservative. In children in whom a short course of rest does not relieve pain, the best results are obtained after diskectomy. Prolonged conservative treatment is associated with persistent pain.

Slipped Vertebral Apophysis Vertebral end plate fractures usually occur in adolescent boys, with traumatic displacement of the lumbar vertebral ring apophysis into the spinal canal and associated disk protrusion. The posteroinferior rim of L4 is the most common site. Thirty-eight percent of these injuries are associated with lumbar Scheuermann's disease. Clinical symptoms of a slipped vertebral apophysis are similar to those of a herniated disk: numbness, muscle weakness, absent reflexes, and positive straight leg raises. Vertebral end plate fractures are classified into 4 types. Type I lesions are pure avulsions of the posterior cortical vertebral margin without osseous defects (pure cartilage injuries). Type II lesions have larger central fractures that include portions of the cortical and cancellous bony rim. Type III lesions are localized fractures posterior to an irregularity of the cartilage end plate. Type IV lesions span the entire length and breadth of the posterior vertebral body. This injury is difficult to see on plain radiographs. An MRI or CT scan is needed to make a definitive diagnosis. Treatment is laminotomy and removal of bone and cartilage fragments.

Inflammatory Etiologies Arthritis is a diagnosis of exclusion in children with back pain. Ankylosing spondylitis can occur in adolescents, is more common in males, and is linked with the HLA-B27 locus. Radiographs may show sclerosis, narrowing, or erosions of the sacroiliac joint. MRI is superior to scintigraphy in demonstrating the inflamed sacroiliac joint when radiographs are nondiagnostic.

Eosinophilic Granuloma This tumor can cause back pain, usually in children younger than 10 years of age. Neurologic deficits are rare. Spinal involvement is seen in 7% to 15% of patients. Lesions can be multiple or single. Radiographs show lytic lesions in the vertebral body or the "coin-on-end" appearance of vertebra plana. Differential diagnosis includes leukemia and infection. Bracing may relieve pain, and, because spontaneous resolution may occur, surgery is reserved for those with neurologic deficits. Biopsy is indicated for noncharacteristic lesions, and the presence of multiple lesions may confirm the diagnosis or provide a more accessible biopsy site if needed. The role of chemotherapy and irradiation is controversial.

Osteoid Osteoma and Osteoblastoma Osteoid osteomas occur in the posterior elements, and typically cause night pain relieved by nonsteroidal anti-inflammatory drugs (NSAIDs) in a child older than 5 years. Physical examination may reveal loss of flexibility or scoliosis. Plain radiographs usually are nondiagnostic, but CT scans identify the radiolucent nidus surrounded by sclerosis. Treatment usually is surgical, but a trial of NSAIDs is rarely successful. Percutaneous CT-guided burring of the nidus has been reported to relieve symptoms.

Forty percent of osteoblastomas occur in the spine, usually the posterior elements. Because of their larger size, they may extend into the vertebral body. Whereas osteoid osteomas do not cause neurologic symptoms, osteoblastomas often do. Scoliosis occurs in 40% of children with osteoblastomas. Treatment is surgical excision.

Aneurysmal Bone Cysts (ABCs) These cysts usually originate in the posterior elements, but if large can extend into the vertebral body. Radiographs show an expansile lytic lesion with a blown-out appearance. CT scans document the extent of the cyst and demonstrate a thin rim of surrounding bone. Treatment is curettage and bone grafting. Preoperative embolization with gelfoam decreases surgical blood loss, and definitive treatment of ABCs of the spine with repeated embolization has been described.

Malignant Tumors Leukemia is the most common malignancy that produces back pain. Back pain is the presenting complaint in 6% of children with acute lymphocytic leukemia. An elevated sedimentation rate mimics infection. Radiographic findings include osteopenia, vertebral body compression, and metaphyseal leukemic lines. Bone marrow aspiration is diagnostic.

Primary malignant tumors of the spine include osteosarcoma, Ewing's sarcoma (usually sacral), and chordoma, while neuroblastoma metastasizes to spine. The most common spinal cord tumor is astrocytoma.

Pediatric Spine Trauma

Cervical Spine

Cervical spine injuries are uncommon in children. Fewer than 1% of all fractures and only 2% of spinal fractures in children involve the cervical spine. This incidence may be low because some injuries cannot be detected clinically and are found only at autopsy.

The level at which cervical spine injuries occur in children varies with age. Occiput, C1, and C2 injuries are more common in children younger than 8 years of age. The relatively large head size compared with the trunk in small children, combined with increased ligamentous laxity, places the fulcrum of motion at the upper cervical spine and allows for greater mobility. Flexion and extension at C2-3 are 50% greater in children between the ages of 3 and 8 years than in adults. The level of greatest mobility descends with increasing age. Between the ages of 3 and 8 years, C3-4 is the most mobile segment; from ages 9 to 11, C4-5 is the most mobile segment; and from ages 12 to 15, C5-6 is the most mobile segment. The immature musculature of a child gives much less resistance to displacement forces than that of an adult, and the facet joint angles are less, which allows more horizontal displacement. The facet joint angle at C1-C2 ranges from 55° at birth to 70° by 8 years of age. In the lower cervical spine, the facet joint angle is 35° in neonates and progresses to 65° at adulthood. The relative flatness of the facet joints allows for increased mobility and forward translation of the spine in young children. By 12 years of age the subaxial cervical spine is more frequently affected, similar to adult cervical spine injuries.

Neurologic deficits are infrequent with pediatric cervical spine fractures, but tend to have a better prognosis than in adults. However, in children development of late spinal deformity after traumatic spinal cord injury is more common.

Most cervical spine injuries are caused by falls or motor vehicle accidents. Cervical spine injuries in neonates can result from birth trauma or child abuse. Neck pain, limited neck motion, torticollis, cervical muscle spasms, occipital headaches, and localized tenderness are the most frequent complaints. Often head or facial trauma is present. A child with head or facial trauma who is comatose or has an altered mental status should be thoroughly examined for a cervical spine injury. A detailed neurologic examination is difficult in a frightened child and should be repeated if necessary. Extremity weakness and neurologic deficits may be obvious or subtle. Clinical signs of a neck injury in newborns usually are absent, but unexplained hypotonia or respiratory difficulty should alert the physician to the possibility of a cervical spine injury.

Radiographs should include AP, lateral, odontoid, and oblique views of the cervical spine. Flexion and extension lateral views should be obtained only in an awake and cooperative patient. Radiographs are indicated in the emergency room if a child has neck pain or head or facial trauma associated with a motor vehicle accident. A screening lateral cervical spine radiograph can be obtained initially but should be followed by a complete cervical spine series after the patient has been stabilized, because false negative results occur in 23% to 26% of single cross-table lateral views. If a cervical spine injury is detected at 1 level, injuries at other levels should be sought; multiple level injuries occur in 24% of children with cervical spine injuries.

Radiographically, the cervical spine has developed most of its adult characteristics by 8 to 10 years of age. In younger children, normal ossification centers may be mistaken for fractures; therefore, the treating physician should be aware of the appearance and time of closure of normal ossification centers of the cervical spine. Although interpretation of radiographs of cervical spine injuries in children may be difficult, some general guidelines can be used. Physeal plates are smooth and regular, in a predictable location, and have subchondral sclerotic lines. Fractures tend to be irregular, without sclerosis, and in a location other than that of a predicted physis. An atlanto-dens interval of 4 to 4.5 mm in a child is normal because of increased ligamentous laxity and incompletely ossified cartilage. What appears to be odontoid hypoplasia on a lateral extension radiograph may actually be the anterior arch of the atlas protruding beyond the ossified portion of the dens to lie against the unossified tip of the odontoid. Signs of instability on lateral cervical radiographs are increased intraspinous distance, divergence of the articular processes, and widening of the posterior aspect of the disk space. Pseudosubluxation of C2 and C3 in flexion is an anatomic feature unique to children that can be mistaken for instability. Anterior displacement in flexion of as much as 3 mm in the upper cervical spine may be normal. The posterior cervical spinolaminar line has been described as a guide to distinguish pathologic subluxation from pseudosubluxation in children. In both flexion and extension, the anterior edges of the spinous processes of C1, C2, and C3 should line up within 1 mm of each

other. Soft-tissue injury at C1-2 should be suspected if there is a widening of more than 10 mm between the spinous processes of C1 and C2.

Soft-tissue swelling should be carefully evaluated on a lateral cervical radiograph, because it may be the only sign of a significant cervical spine injury. Interpretation of these soft-tissue spaces must be done with caution, especially in a child who is crying. Soft-tissue swelling on radiographs should be interpreted only when the patient is at rest and is breathing quietly. The retropharyngeal soft-tissue space is measured from the pharyngeal air column to the anteroinferior aspect of the base of C2; a space of > 7 mm is abnormal in both children and adults. The retrotracheal space is measured from the anteroinferior aspect of the body of C6 to the posterior tracheal wall; a space of > 14 mm in children is considered abnormal and suggests edema or hemorrhage.

Care should be taken during the emergency treatment and immobilization of a child with a suspected cervical spine injury. Commercial pediatric cervical collars do not completely immobilize the cervical spine, and tape and sand bags may be necessary in addition to a collar. Traction should be

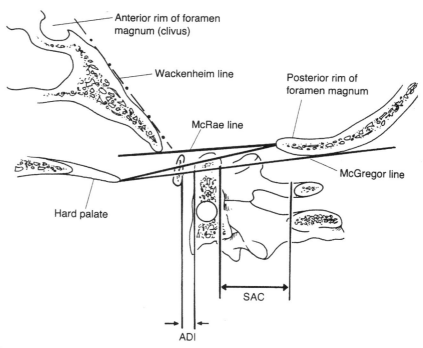

Figure 4

Wackenheim clivus-canal line. This line is drawn along the clivus into the cervical spinal canal and should pass posterior to the tip of the odontoid. ADI, atlantodens interval; SAC, space available for cord. (Adapted with permission from Menezes AH, Ryken TC: Craniovertebral junction abnormalities, in Weinstein SL (ed): *The Pediatric Spine: Principles and Practice.* New York, NY, Raven Press, 1994, pp 307–321.)

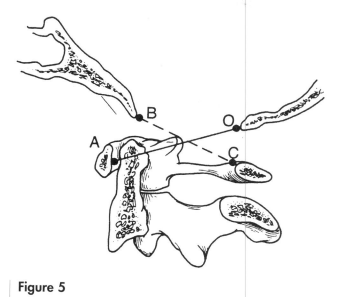

Figure 5

The Powers ratio is determined by drawing a line from the basion (B) to the posterior arch of the atlas (C) and a second line from the opisthion (O) to the anterior arch of the atlas (A). The length of the line BC is divided by the length of the line OA, producing the Powers ratio. (Adapted with permission from Lebwohl NH, Eismont FJ: Cervical spine injuries in children, in Weinstein SL (ed): *The Pediatric Spine: Principles and Practice.* New York, NY, Raven Press, 1994, pp 725–741.)

used with caution in children with suspected cervical spine injury. Children should not be placed on standard backboards. Because a small child's head is disproportionately large in comparison to the trunk, a standard backboard allows the neck to flex, which may result in kyphosis and anterior translation of the upper cervical spine in unstable fractures. Instead of the standard backboard a split mattress technique can be used to elevate the thorax 2 to 4 cm and allow the occiput and neck to maintain a normal relationship with the thorax. Alternatively, a backboard with an occipital recess can be placed in the emergency department for use with children.

An unstable cervical spine injury can be immobilized with a Minerva cast or a halo cast or vest. If a halo is applied, CT scanning may be needed to determine the thickness of the skull for safe insertion of halo pins. Multiple pins can be used (up to 10), and should be tightened to 2 to 4 in/lb. A halo should not be used in patients younger than 2 years of age because the anterior fontanels are open up to 18

months of age. Commercial halo vests do not provide a proper fit to the thorax in most children. Although the head is immobilized in the halo ring, the thorax can move, allowing displacement and distraction at the fracture site. A halo vest should be custom-fitted or a halo cast should be applied.

Atlanto-occipital Dislocation Atlanto-occipital dislocation was once thought to be a fatal injury found only at the time of autopsy; now, however, some children survive this injury. Sudden deceleration, such as occurs in motor vehicle or pedestrian-vehicle accidents, carries the head forward and causes sudden craniovertebral separation. Most of the stability at the craniovertebral junction is provided by the surrounding ligaments with very little bony stability present, making radiographic diagnosis difficult. Associated soft-tissue swelling, however, may be indicative of this injury. The Wackenheim line, Powers ratio, and occipital condyle distance can help make this diagnosis. The Wackenheim line is drawn along the clivus and should intersect tangentially the tip of the odontoid (Fig. 4). A Powers ratio (Fig. 5) > 1.0 is diagnostic of anterior occipitoatlantal dislocation. Values < 0.9 are considered normal. A distance of more than 5 mm from the occipital condyle to the C1 facet also indicates an atlanto-occipital injury (Fig. 6).

Because atlanto-occipital dislocation is a ligamentous injury, nonsurgical treatment usually is unsuccessful. Traction should be avoided because it may increase displacement. Posterior fusion is recommended and can be per-

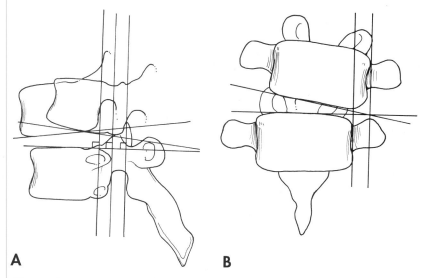

A   **B**

Figure 6

Facet condylar distance. Facet condylar distance is measured on (A) lateral radiograph and (B) anteroposterior radiograph. A facet condylar distance of more than 5 mm is considered abnormal.

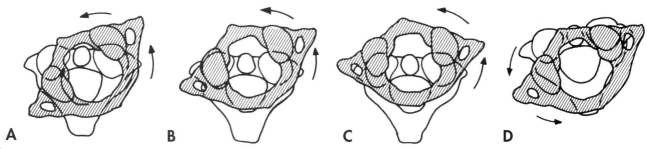

Figure 7

Fielding and Hawkins classification of rotatory displacement. A, Type I, simple rotatory displacement without anterior shift; odontoid acts as pivot. B, Type II, rotatory displacement with anterior displacement of 3 to 5 mm; lateral articular process acts as pivot. C, Type III, rotatory displacement with anterior displacement of more than 5 mm. D, Type IV, rotatory displacement with posterior displacement. (Reproduced with permission from Fielding JW, Hawkins RJ Jr: Atlanto-axial rotatory fixation [fixed rotatory subluxation of the atlanto-axial joint]. *J Bone Joint Surg* 1977;59A:37–44.)

formed in situ, with wire fixation or fixation with a contoured Luque rod and wires. If the C1-2 articulation is stable, fusion should be only from the occiput to C1 so that C1-2 motion is preserved; if stability is questionable, fusion should extend to C2.

Occipital Condylar Fracture Occipital condylar fractures are rare injuries for which CT scanning with multiplanar reconstruction usually is necessary to establish the diagnosis. Three types of occipital condylar fractures have been described: type 1, impaction fracture; type 2, basilar skull fracture extending into the condyle; and type 3, avulsion fracture, which is the only unstable type. Type 1 and 2 injuries can be treated with a cervical orthosis. Type 3 injuries require halo immobilization or occipitocervical fusion.

Atlas Fractures Atlas fractures are caused by an axial compression load to the head that is transmitted through the lateral occipital condyles to the lateral masses of C1. The ring usually breaks in more than 1 place. This fracture commonly occurs through the open synchondroses of C1 in children younger than 8 years of age and may be incomplete or a greenstick type fracture. As the lateral masses separate, the transverse atlantal ligament may be disrupted or avulsed, making the C1-C2 articulation unstable. Symptoms include muscle spasms, tenderness, head cradling, and torticollis. Diagnosis may be difficult using plain radiographs, and a CT scan is usually necessary. For stable fractures, treatment is simple collar immobilization; unstable fractures should be treated with an initial period of traction followed by halo cast or brace immobilization.

Atlantoaxial Instability In young children the synchondrosis at the base of the dens usually fails before disruption of the transverse ligament. Transverse ligament disruption, however, can occur either by rupture of the ligament or avulsion of the ligamentous attachment at the atlas. When this occurs, displacement of 4.5 mm is suggestive of atlantoaxial instability and displacement of > 5 mm in flexion is diagnostic. Reduction and posterior C1-C2 fusion followed by immobilization in a halo brace or Minerva cast are recommended.

Atlantoaxial Rotatory Subluxation Atlantoaxial rotatory subluxation can occur after minor or major trauma, but most often occurs after upper respiratory tract infections. Fielding and Hawkins classified this condition into 4 types, depending on the direction and degree of displacement (Fig. 7). Clinically the head is tilted to 1 side and rotated to the opposite side, and the sternocleidomastoid muscle usually is in spasm on the long side. Although neurologic injury is rare, there have been isolated reports of death and quadriparesis. On AP open mouth odontoid views, the lateral mass that is rotated forward appears wider and closer to the midline while the opposite lateral mass is narrower and farther away from the midline. One of the facet joints may be obscured because of apparent overlapping. On the lateral projection, a wedge-shaped lateral mass anteriorly is noted, and the posterior arches fail to superimpose, suggesting a fusion of the atlas to the occiput. Flexion and extension radiographs should be obtained to document any instability, although most are stable type I injuries. Dynamic CT scan with the head turned maximally to the right and left is the best way to confirm the diagnosis by showing loss of normal rotation between C1 and C2.

When this condition is not the result of trauma and there is no instability, simple immobilization may be all that is needed. If symptoms persist after 1 week, head halter traction is recommended. When atlantoaxial rotatory subluxation is the result of trauma, halo brace immobilization may be required to reduce and maintain the rotatory subluxation in a reduced position. Immobilization for a minimum of 4 weeks is recommended.

Odontoid Fractures This fracture resembles a physeal injury because it most commonly occurs through the synchondrosis of C2. The synchondrosis, which is located in the body of the axis and is below the level of the facet joints, is a weak area in children. By the age of 7 to 8 years, this synchondrosis closes, and the adult pattern of odontoid fracture is seen. Odontoid fractures result from falls or motor vehicle accidents. Neurologic deficits are rare. Lateral radiographs are most helpful in establishing a diagnosis. Usually anterior displacement or angulation of the odontoid occurs through the fracture site.

Treatment consists of postural reduction. An intact hinge of soft tissue or periosteum anteriorly accounts for the ease and stability of reduction. If postural reduction cannot be obtained, halo traction may be necessary. After reduction a Minerva cast or halo vest is worn for 6 weeks, followed by a soft collar for 1 to 2 weeks. Surgery rarely is indicated. Excellent long-term results can be expected without significant growth disturbances, because little growth occurs from the synchondrosis.

Failure to recognize and immobilize an odontoid fracture in childhood may be responsible for development of os odontoideum, which can lead to atlantoaxial instability. When this occurs, the os odontoideum moves forward with the atlas and the intact transverse ligament. Motion occurs through the nonunion site, decreasing the space available for the spinal cord. Treatment of os odontoideum is posterior cervical fusion.

Spondylolisthesis of C2 (Hangman's Fracture) Fracture of the pedicles of the axis, which results in a traumatic spondylolisthesis of C2, has been termed hangman's fracture. The exact mechanism of this injury in children is not known. Some authors support a hyperextension etiology while others support a flexion-distraction mechanism. Neurologic deficits are uncommon with this injury. Most fractures can be seen on lateral radiographs but are better seen on oblique views. Recommended treatment includes reduction by gentle positioning and immobilization in a halo or Minerva cast for 8 to 12 weeks. Surgery is indicated only for delayed union or an unstable nonunion.

Subaxial Cervical Spine Injuries Subaxial cervical spine injuries are more common in children older than 8 years as the cervical spine becomes more mature, and the injury patterns are similar to those in adults. The mean age at injury in 1 study was 13.6 years. The mechanism of injury usually is a flexion force to the cervical spine. Unilateral facet dislocations are treated with traction and reduction. If reduction cannot be obtained easily, open reduction is required. Complete bilateral facet dislocations, although rare, are more unstable and have a higher incidence of neurologic deficits. Treatment consists of traction and stabilization with posterior fusion. Anterior fusion rarely is recommended in pediatric patients except in the rare patient with a burst fracture and canal compromise. Anterior fusion destroys the anterior growth potential and as posterior growth continues, a kyphotic deformity results. Disk disruption requiring anterior surgery is rare in children, but should be looked for with an MRI. If a posterior fusion is required, autogenous bone graft should be used. The use of allograft is associated with a high rate of pseudarthrosis. Laminectomies do not help with neurologic recovery and should not be performed to avoid late postlaminectomy deformity. Excessive dissection should also be avoided to prevent unintentional progression of the fusion mass.

Posterior ligamentous injuries have limited potential for healing, and if instability is documented the injury should be stabilized with a posterior fusion. Unrecognized posterior ligamentous disruption in children may allow gradual displacement of one segment on the other and adaptive changes may occur in the spine, making reduction difficult.

Compression fractures are the most common subaxial cervical spine injuries in children. The mechanism of injury is axial loading in flexion with radiographic loss of vertebral body height. These usually are stable injuries unless there has been significant posterior ligamentous disruption indicated by widening of the spinous processes. When this occurs, repeat flexion and extension lateral radiographs should be obtained 2 to 4 weeks after injury to document stability. Stable compression fractures can be treated with immobilization in a cervical orthosis for 3 to 6 weeks. Children younger than 8 years of age have some ability to reconstitute vertebral body height after a compression fracture.

Injury through the vertebral end plate is unique to pediatric patients and occurs when the end plate is separated from the vertebral body, as in physeal injuries. This is similar to a Salter type I fracture in infants and young children and a type III fracture in adolescents. The inferior end plate usually is more involved than the superior end plate because the uncinate process protects the superior end plate. Radiographic identification may be difficult because the fracture may spontaneously reduce and return to normal alignment. Physeal separation may be involved in injuries with neurologic deficit but no radiographic abnormalities. These usually are unstable injuries and often require surgical stabilization.

Spinal Cord Injury Without Radiographic Abnormality (SCIWORA) SCIWORA is a condition unique to the pediatric spine. The incidence varies from 7% to 66% in children with spinal cord injuries, with the most common quoted incidence between 20% and 30%. Children younger than 8 years of age appear to have a predisposition for this injury. Although the reason for this is not known, ligamentous laxity, cervical spine hypermobility, and immature vascular supply to the spinal cord appear to be contributing factors. Theories regarding the causes of SCIWORA include traction injury to the spinal column and cord, end plate separation, transient disk herniation, and vascular compromise with infarction of the cord. The infantile spinal column can be stretched 2 inches but the spinal cord can be stretched only ¼ inch before rupturing. In most series, involvement of the cervical spine is slightly more common. Incomplete neurologic injuries have a good prognosis for recovery, while complete neurologic injuries have a poor prognosis. Younger children have a higher level of injury and more frequent and severe neurologic deficits. Delayed onset of neurologic symptoms is reported in up to 52% of patients with SCIWORA. Careful radiographic evaluation is essential to identify any unrecognized end plate fractures or potential instability patterns so as to prevent more injury to the spinal cord. The role of steroids in preventing a progressive neurologic deficit is not known.

Thoracic and Lumbar Injuries

These usually result from motor vehicle accidents or falls from heights, but in neonates they may result from child abuse. The most common injuries are compression fractures and flexion-distraction type injuries.

Hyperflexion with vertical compression is the most common mechanism of injury. Because the pediatric disk is stronger than the cancellous bone, the vertebral body fails before the disk. Multiple compression fractures are more frequent in children than single compression fractures. The compression usually is less than 20% of the vertebral body height. If compression of the vertebral body is more than 50% of the vertebral body height, the posterior elements should be evaluated for damage and possible instability that might require surgical intervention. A CT scan may be required to differentiate a compression fracture from a burst fracture. Compression fractures should be treated with rest and brace immobilization.

Flexion and Distraction Injuries (Seat Belt Injuries) Seat belt injuries generally occur in school-aged children (4 to 9 years of age) and are caused by a flexion and distraction mechanism. The seat belt slides up above the iliac crests and lies over the abdomen. With sudden deceleration, the seat belt acts as an axis for the spine to rotate around, allowing the spine to fail in tension. Approximately two thirds of patients have intra-abdominal injuries that may be life-threatening. Some abdominal injuries may not be discovered at initial examination, and signs and symptoms may be delayed because of ischemic bowel necrosis.

Four types of seat belt injuries have been described in children. Type A is a bony disruption of the posterior column, extending just into the middle column. Type B is an avulsion of the posterior elements with facet joint disruption or fracture and extension into the apophysis of the vertebral body. Type C is a posterior ligamentous disruption with a fracture line entering the vertebra close to the pars interarticularis and extending into the middle column. Type D is a posterior ligamentous disruption with a fracture line traversing the lamina and extending into the apophysis of the adjacent vertebral body. A lateral radiograph is most helpful in determining this diagnosis. In subtle injuries, widening of the posterior interspinous space is noted. MRI should be strongly considered in all children with seat belt injuries, because bony injury at one level and a disk injury at another level are possible. Disruption of the disk is uncommon, and the injury usually separates the vertebral body from the vertebral end plate.

Lap belt injuries with mostly bony involvement can be treated nonsurgically with hyperextension casting if the kyphosis is < 20°. If there is a large amount of soft-tissue damage and posterior ligamentous disruption, surgical stabilization with posterior fusion is recommended. Stabilization can be achieved with short compression rods 1 level above and 1 level below the injury site or by wire fixation in a small child.

Sacral Fractures Sacral fractures are uncommon in children and often are associated with pelvic fractures. Those that involve the sacral nerve roots may cause neurologic deficits, such as bladder, rectal, and sexual dysfunction. Denis classified sacral fractures into 3 types. Zone I injuries involve the ala and rarely cause neurologic deficits. Zone II fractures involve 1 or more of the sacral foramina, and neurologic injuries occur in 28% of patients with these fractures. Zone III injuries involve primarily the central sacral canal, and neurologic damage occurs in > 50% of patients. Decompression of the sacral nerve root in the acute phase may be necessary to improve neurologic function, followed by stabilization of the sacral fracture and associated pelvic fractures.

Fracture-Dislocations Fracture-dislocations of the spine rarely occur in children. The most common location is the thoracolumbar junction. This is an unstable injury that often causes neurologic deficits, either at the conus medullaris or nerve roots. Surgical stabilization and fusion are recommended, with instrumentation at least 2 levels above and below the injury site. Long instrumentation constructs assure increased stability and prevent subsequent paralytic deformity in patients with complete neurologic deficits.

Burst Fractures Burst fractures result from an axial compression force to the spine and are rare in children. The thoracolumbar junction and lumbar spine are most commonly involved. Burst fractures can be stable or unstable fractures, depending on the involvement of the anterior, middle, or posterior columns. CT is helpful to determine if retropulsed fragments are present. The need for surgical decompression of the spinal canal is based on the stability of the fracture and the presence of any neurologic deficits. If decompression of the spinal canal is needed, surgical stabilization and fusion should be done.

Annotated Bibliography

Pediatric Spinal Deformity

Congenital

Marks DS, Sayampanathan SR, Thompson AG, Piggott H: Long-term results of convex epiphysiodesis for congenital scoliosis. *Eur Spine J* 1995;4:296–301.

The rate of progression was reversed or slowed in 97% of hemivertebra patients following surgery after a mean follow-up of 8.8 years. Greater correction occurred in patients operated on at a younger age.

Idiopathic Scoliosis

Machida M, Dubousset J, Imamura Y, Miyashita Y, Yamada T, Kimura J: Melatonin: A possible role in pathogenesis of adolescent idiopathic scoliosis. *Spine* 1996;21:1147–1152.

Normal melatonin synthesis or metabolism may have a role in spinal growth, and the serum level of melatonin may be a predictor of curve progression.

Rowe DE, Bernstein SM, Riddick MF, Adler F, Emans JB, Gardner-Bonneau D: A meta-analysis of the efficacy of non-operative treatments for idiopathic scoliosis. *J Bone Joint Surg* 1997;79A:664–674.

This analysis demonstrated that bracing was effective in treating idiopathic scoliosis. The highest success was with the Milwaukee brace, and full-time (23 h/d) brace wear was significantly more effective than part-time bracing.

Sanders JO, Little DG, Richards BS: Prediction of the crankshaft phenomenon by peak height velocity. *Spine* 1997;22:1352–1356.

This study shows that posterior spinal fusion at or after peak growth age is not associated with crankshafting.

Neuromuscular Scoliosis

Ferguson RL, Hansen MM, Nicholas DA, Allen BL Jr: Same-day versus staged anterior-posterior spinal surgery in a neuromuscular scoliosis population: The evaluation of medical complications. *J Pediatr Orthop* 1996;16:293–303.

In 29 patients, 36 (124%) complications occurred in staged patients, whereas 14 (88%) were seen in the same-day group. Only 35% of staged patients had no complications, as opposed to 63% of same-day surgery patients.

Winter S: Preoperative assessment of the child with neuromuscular scoliosis. *Orthop Clin North Am* 1994;25:239–245.

An outline of preoperative screening tests and a discussion of common medical issues helps the surgeon prepare the child with neuromuscular scoliosis for spinal surgery.

Back Pain in Children

Blum U, Buitrago-Tellez C, Mundinger A, et al: Magnetic resonance imaging (MRI) for detection of active sacroiliitis: A prospective study comparing conventional radiography, scintigraphy, and contrast enhanced MRI. *J Rheumatol* 1996;23:2107–2115.

Gadolinium-enhanced MRI was most specific in identifying active sacroiliitis.

Burton AK, Clarke RD, McClune TD, Tillotson KM: The natural history of low back pain in adolescents. *Spine* 1996;21:2323–2328.

An episode of back pain occurs in over 50% of children by age 15 years.

650 Spine

DeLuca PF, Mason DE, Weiand R, Howard R, Bassett GS: Excision of herniated nucleus pulposus in children and adolescents. *J Pediatr Orthop* 1994;14:318–322.

Surgical diskectomy yielded superior results to prolonged conservative treatment.

Floman Y, Bar-On E, Mosheiff R, Mirovsky Y, Robin GC, Ramu N: Eosinophilic granuloma of the spine. *J Pediatr Orthop* 1997;6B:260–265.

The authors recommend observation for solitary spinal lesions.

Ginsburg GM, Bassett GS: Back pain in children and adolescents: Evaluation and differential diagnosis. *J Am Acad Orthop Surg* 1997;5:67–78.

This is a comprehensive review of the etiology and evaluation of back pain in the pediatric age group.

Grubb MR, Currier BL, Pritchard DJ, Ebersold MJ: Primary Ewing's sarcoma of the spine. *Spine* 1994;19:309–313.

The sacrum is the most frequent site of Ewing's sarcoma of the spine. Unrelenting back pain is the most common symptom, with neurologic deficits present in 58%.

Lusins JO, Elting JJ, Cicoria AD, Goldsmith SJ: SPECT evaluation of lumbar spondylolysis and spondylolisthesis. *Spine* 1994;19:608–612.

SPECT scans were positive in acute spondylolysis and negative with chronic fractures.

Meehan PL, Viroslav S, Schmitt EW Jr: Vertebral collapse in childhood leukemia. *J Pediatr Orthop* 1995;15:592–595.

Children with acute lymphoblastic leukemia may present with back pain and normal complete blood cell counts. Radiographic findings if present consist of osteopenia and compression fractures.

Micheli LJ, Wood R: Back pain in young athletes: Significant differences from adults in causes and patterns. *Arch Pediatr Adolesc Med* 1995;149:15–18.

Spondylolysis occurred in 47% of pediatric athletes with back pain. Disk disease was rare.

Ramirez N, Johnston CE, Browne RH: The prevalence of back pain in children who have idiopathic scoliosis. *J Bone Joint Surg* 1997;79A:364–368.

Back pain was present in 32% of 2,442 patients with idiopathic scoliosis. Only 9% of the patients with pain had an underlying pathologic condition. Painful left thoracic curves were predictive of pathology.

Ring D, Johnston CE II, Wenger DR: Pyogenic infectious spondylitis in children: The convergence of discitis and vertebral osteomyelitis. *J Pediatr Orthop* 1995;15:652–660.

Treatment with intravenous antibiotics led to earlier resolution of symptoms and fewer recurrences.

Pediatric Spine Trauma

Donahue DJ, Muhlbauer MS, Kaufman RA, Warner WC, Sanford RA: Childhood survival of atlantooccipital dislocation: Underdiagnosis, recognition, treatment, and review of the literature. *Pediatr Neurosurg* 1994;21:105–111.

These authors report 4 patients with atlanto-occipital dislocation who have survived. All patients were treated with an occipital cervical fusion. Two developed postoperative hydrocephalus after fusion. The literature, diagnosis, and treatment recommendations for this injury are reviewed.

Dormans JP, Criscitiello AA, Drummond DS, Davidson RS: Complications in children managed with immobilization in a halo vest. *J Bone Joint Surg* 1995;77A:1370–1373.

This is a report of complications associated with the use of halo vest immobilization in 37 patients younger than 16 years of age. Complications occurred in 68%; infections and pin loosening were the most common complications. Despite the increased frequency of problems with the use of halo immobilization in children, all patients were able to wear the halo vest until healing of the fracture or fusion occurred.

Greenwald TA, Mann DC: Pediatric seatbelt injuries: Diagnosis and treatment of lumbar flexion-distraction injuries. *Paraplegia* 1994;32:743–751.

Six seat belt injuries of the lumbar spine are reported. This article gives a good overview of the mechanism of injury, diagnosis, and surgical and nonsurgical treatment of this injury.

Hilibrand AS, Urquhart AG, Graziano GP, Hensinger RN: Acute spondylolytic spondylolisthesis: Risk of progression and neurological complications. *J Bone Joint Surg* 1995;77A:190–196.

Acute spondylolytic spondylolisthesis is described in 5 patients after major trauma. Spondylolysis or spondylolisthesis after high-energy trauma is much more unstable than after minor or repetitive trauma. This type of injury has a high propensity for significant progression and surgical stabilization usually is required.

McGrory BJ, Klassen RA: Arthrodesis of the cervical spine for fractures and dislocations in children and adolescents: A long-term follow-up study. *J Bone Joint Surg* 1994;76A:1606–1616.

These authors report long-term follow-up of 42 patients (ages 23 months to 15 years at the time of injury) who had an arthrodesis of the cervical spine for instability from trauma. Seventy-six percent had excellent results, 14% had good results, and 10% had fair results. Spontaneous extension of the fusion mass occurred in 38% of the patients. Decreased mobility of the cervical spine was seen at follow-up with an associated increase in osteoarthritic changes on radiographs.

McGrory BJ, Klassen RA, Chao EY, Staeheli JW, Weaver AL: Acute fractures and dislocations of the cervical spine in children and adolescents. *J Bone Joint Surg* 1993;75A:988–995.

This article is a review of 143 cervical spine injuries in children younger than 15 years of age. The upper cervical spine was more frequently involved in children younger than 11 years of age, and most of these injuries were ligamentous. A higher mortality rate as a result of spinal cord injury was reported in this age group. The lower cervical spine was more frequently involved in patients who were older than 11 years of age, and injury patterns were similar to adult cervical spine injuries.

Neumann P, Nordwall A, Osvalder A-L: Traumatic instability of the lumbar spine: A dynamic in vitro study of flexion-distraction injury. *Spine* 1995;20:1111–1121.

This biomechanical cadaver study simulates lap seat belt injuries. Radiographic guidelines for instability in this injury pattern are proposed.

Sponseller PD, Cass JR: Atlanto-occipital fusion for dislocation in children with neurologic preservation: A case report. *Spine* 1997;22:344–347.

These authors report 2 patients with atlanto-occipital dislocation. Both survived and neurologic function was preserved. They recommend fusion from occiput to C-1 to preserve normal rotation at C1-C2.

Voss L, Cole PA, DíAmato C: Pediatric Chance fractures from lap-belts: Unique case report of three in one accident. *J Orthop Trauma* 1996;10:421–428.

These authors report lap belt injuries in 3 patients involved in the same accident. Injury occurred from a relatively low speed accident. The article gives a good overview of classification and mechanism of injury.

Chapter 48
Adult Spine Trauma

Introduction

In the United States there are approximately 177,000 to 200,000 people living with spinal cord injuries, with around 50,000 new spinal injuries reported yearly. Of these 50,000 injuries, half are located in the cervical region, and approximately 11,000 will result in a spinal cord injury with some degree of neurologic deficit. The estimated cost for the treatment of persons with spinal cord injuries is $4 billion annually.

The average patient who incurs spine trauma is a man in his 30s. There is a bimodal age distribution, with most patients between 15 and 24 years old and a secondary age concentration in patients older than 55 years. The mechanism of injury in adults includes motor vehicle accidents (40% to 56%), falls (20% to 30%), violence such as gunshots (12% to 21%), sports (6% to 13%), and other miscellaneous causes.

Initial Management

The initial management of a patient with a spine and/or spinal cord injury begins at the scene of the accident. The ultimate outcome of a patient with a spinal injury depends on early recognition of the injury, prompt medical resuscitation, attainment of spinal stability, prevention of additional injuries, and avoidance of complications. There are 5 generally accepted stages in the initial management of a spinal trauma patient: (1) evaluation, (2) resuscitation, (3) immobilization, (4) extrication, and (5) transport.

Patient Evaluation
Evaluation of the accident patient includes a primary and a secondary survey. Following the initial ABCs of trauma care (Airway, Breathing, Circulation), a primary survey is undertaken to evaluate for life-threatening injuries as well as injury to the spinal column. The secondary survey involves a more complete head to toe examination.

Resuscitation and Oxygenation
The resuscitation stage ensures adequate oxygenation of the patient in light of a possible injury to the spinal cord. In a cadaver model, the chin lift and jaw thrust method of securing an airway decreased the available space for the spinal cord more than either nasal or oral intubation. Once an airway is established, ventilation with oxygenation is begun. Maintenance of adequate circulation also is imperative to maximize perfusion of the contused spinal cord.

Immobilization and Extrication
Proper immobilization is essential to prevent additional spinal column and/or spinal cord injury. At the accident scene, initial in-line manual traction is recommended before moving the spinal injured patient, and hard cervical collar should be applied. The collar should have a manufactured opening in the front in case an emergency cricothyroidotomy is needed. After the cervical collar is in place, the patient is moved to a firm spine board for transportation. If a helmet is involved, as in football and hockey injuries, it should not be removed until arrival at the hospital. If necessary, the face mask or cage can be removed at the accident scene to perform necessary emergency care.

Transport
The length of hospital stay and the incidence of complications, such as pressure ulcers and mortality, are significantly reduced when the patient is admitted to a spinal cord injury center. General guidelines for means of transportation are (1) an ambulance for distances < 50 miles, (2) a helicopter for distances of 51 to 150 miles or heavy traffic patterns and severe injuries, and (3) a fixed-wing aircraft for distances > 150 miles.

Hospital Management

The in-hospital trauma team continues basic and advanced life support procedures. Selected pharmacologic agents are administered. Airway patency and ventilation may now be more accurately measured by arterial blood gases and pulse oximetry.

Although hemorrhagic shock is the most common cause of hypotension in trauma patients, a patient with a spinal cord injury may be in shock without any appreciable blood loss. The term neurogenic shock describes cardiovascular instability that occurs with complete injuries to the cervical or upper thoracic spinal cord. Pathophysiologically, there is disruption of the descending sympathetic pathways, which leaves the parasympathetic innervation of the vagus nerve unchecked.

Table 1
The key muscle groups used in the ASIA motor source evaluation of a spinal cord injury patient

Level	Muscle Group
C5	Elbow flexors (biceps, brachialis)
C6	Wrist extensors (extensor carpi radialis longus and brevis)
C7	Elbow extensors (triceps)
C8	Finger flexors (flexor digitorum profundus) to the middle finger
T1	Small finger abductors (abductor digiti minimi)
L2	Hip flexors (iliopsoas)
L3	Knee extensors (quadriceps)
L4	Ankle dorsiflexors (tibialis anterior)
L5	Long toe extensors (extensor hallucis longus)
S1	Ankle plantarflexors (gastrocnemius, soleus)

Sympathetic disruption results in a generalized vasodilatation with increased vessel capacitance, decreased central venous return, and lower extremity venous stasis. Bradycardia and frequently hypotension are present in comparison to patients in hypovolemic shock who are tachycardic. The initial treatment of a patient in neurogenic shock consists of placing the patient in the Trendelenburg position with judicious administration of intravenous fluids. If blood pressure instability persists, cardiac pressors along with atropine may be used. The cardiovascular sequelae of neurogenic shock secondary to spinal cord injury may last from days to months.

Pharmacologic Therapy

Extensive research has been undertaken in the evaluation of various pharmacologic agents regarding their ability to modify or lessen the secondary injury cascade that occurs after an injury to the spinal cord. Such agents include but are not limited to corticosteroids, 21-aminosteroids, antioxidants, gangliosides, opioid antagonists, thyrotro-releasing hormone, prostacyclin analogs, and calcium channel blockers.

Several mechanisms have been proposed for the positive effect steroids have on the recovery of patients with spinal cord injuries. Steroid administration increases blood flow to the spinal cord, which increases perfusion of the white matter. Studies have shown that steroid administration impairs lipid peroxidation that occurs after an injury to the spinal cord, resulting in inhibition of cell membrane breakdown. The maintained integrity of this cellular barrier prevents the sudden intra- and extracellular ion shifts seen immediately after cell membrane impairment. Steroids also have been shown to reduce tissue edema and inflammation, promote the restoration of acid-base balance and the reestablishment of cell membrane sodium-potassium adenosine triphosphatase activity, and act as free radical scavengers.

The standard accepted steroid protocol after a spinal cord injury is the administration of high-dose methylprednisolone (30 mg/kg, given over 15 minutes, followed by 5.4 mg/kg per hour dosage over 24 hours) within 8 hours of injury. Penetrating wounds, pregnancy, age younger than 13 years, significant infection, or unstable diabetes are all relative contraindications to the use of high-dose corticosteroids. Recently, the Third National Acute Spinal Cord Injury Study (NASCIS 3) recommended that patients who receive methylprednisolone treatment within 3 hours of injury should continue the steroid administration for 24 hours, while patients with treatment beginning 3 to 8 hours after injury should continue steroid therapy for 48 hours.

Other investigational drugs, such as 21-aminosteroids (lazeroids), gangliosides, opiate receptor analogs, oxygen free-radical scavengers, calcium channel blockers, osmotic diuretics, thromboxane inhibitors, and potassium channel blockers, have shown beneficial effects on the damaged spinal cord. Future controlled prospective clinical studies will elucidate the efficacy of these agents.

Timing of Surgery

There is much controversy regarding the timing of surgery (early versus late) after a spinal cord injury in a patient with documented cord compression. Proponents of early surgical intervention believe that immediate relief of pressure from the neural elements will decrease the extent of the secondary injury cascade, such as the progression of edema, hematoma formation, and membrane destabilization, as well as avoid the negative biomechanical effects of an unstable spine. The advantages of late surgery are that the patient is generally more medically stable and able to physiologically tolerate a surgical procedure and cord swelling has been given the opportunity to subside.

History and Physical Examination

After the initial resuscitation and medical stabilization of a spinal cord injury patient, a history and physical examination are undertaken before definitive spinal management. The physical examination should begin with an inspection for the obvious stigmata of potential spinal injury, including scalp and facial lacerations and associated blunt abdominal injuries. The neurologic examination should include an evaluation of motor and cranial nerve function, sensation, rectal tone, and reflexes (Tables 1 and 2). A complete spinal cord lesion results in the absence of all sensation and voluntary movement in the S4-5 distribution. A lesion is incomplete if there is preservation of any sensation in the S4-5 distribution or if there is voluntary contraction of the anal sphincter. Prognosis for future neurologic recovery is determined by the degree and type of incomplete neurologic lesion.

The presence of a complete or incomplete lesion can only be definitely determined in the absence of spinal shock. Spinal shock implies the transient loss of all motor, sensory, and reflex function distal to the level of injury.

Classification of Spinal Cord Injury

Many different grading systems are available for describing the degree of spinal cord injury. There are impairment-based scores (Frankel Scale, ASIA scale, Yale Scale, Motor index scale) and function-based scales (Modified Barthel Index). The ASIA (American Spinal Injury Association) impairment scale, which is a modification of the Frankel scale or classification, is one of the most commonly used scales for evaluating spinal cord injury.

An incomplete spinal cord syndrome describes a constellation of neurologic findings determined by the anatomic location of tissue injury. These include a central cord syndrome, an anterior cord syndrome, a posterior cord syndrome, and the Brown-Séquard syndrome (Fig. 1). The central cord syndrome is the most common type of spinal cord injury seen. Patients with this syndrome usually have motor weakness or paralysis in the upper extremities with relative sparing in the lower extremities. Functional recovery usually is poor to fair.

In the anterior cord syndrome there is damage to the anterior two thirds of the spinal cord with sparing of the posterior third. Damage to the pyramidal tracts results in loss of motor function below the level of injury. If the spinothalamic tracts are injured there is loss of touch, pain, and temperature sensation. Because the posterior cord is undamaged, there is preservation of vibration and position sense. Functional prognosis depends on the degree of neurologic deficit (complete or incomplete) as well as the level of injury. The Brown-Séquard syndrome is a rare spinal cord injury that results in damage to half the spinal cord. This results in ipsilateral motor weakness and loss of proprioception with contralateral loss of pain and temperature sensation as well as light touch. This syndrome has an excellent prognosis for ambulation.

Table 2
Muscle grading chart

Grade	Muscle Action
0 = zero	Total paralysis
1 = trace	Visual or palpable contraction
2 = poor	Active movement, gravity eliminated
3 = fair	Active movement against gravity
4 = good	Active movement against resistance
5 = normal	Active movement against full resistance

(Reproduced with permission from Connolly P, Yuan HA: Cervical spine fractures, in White AH (ed): *Spine Care: Diagnosis and Conservative Treatment.* St. Louis, MO, Mosby, 1995.)

The posterior cord syndrome is the least common spinal cord injury. Because the posterior columns carry vibration and proprioception, this syndrome is characterized by loss of vibration sensation and positional sense. There may be sparing of crude touch because of the anterior location of the anterior spinothalamic tracts. Functional outcome in patients with posterior cord syndrome is fair.

Imaging Studies

A complete radiologic survey including an anteroposterior (AP) and lateral radiograph of the entire spine is essential so as not to miss a noncontiguous spinal injury. Various centers recommend either a 3- or 5-film cervical series in a patient in whom injury to the cervical spine is suspected. It is mandatory to examine all 7 cervical vertebrae as well as the top of the T1 vertebral body because approximately 10% of cervical spine fractures occur at the C7 level.

At present, magnetic resonance imaging (MRI) has supplanted conventional myelography with or without computed tomography (CT) as a diagnostic tool in evaluating cervical cord compression after trauma. MRI allows optimal visualization of cervical soft tissues and demonstrates intra- or extramedullary and epidural hemorrhage or the presence of intervertebral disk herniation. It has been shown using MRI that cervical disk herniations occur in 30% to 50% of cervical fracture subluxations.

Controversy exists as to the timing of MRI in patients with cervical dislocations. Proponents of prereduction MRI cite the potential for neurologic injury with further compression by a previously extruded disk fragment during spinal column

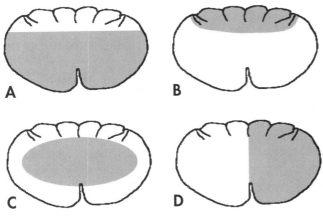

Figure 1

The four incomplete spinal cord injury syndromes: Anterior cord syndrome (A), posterior cord syndrome (B), central cord syndrome (C), and Brown-Séquard syndrome (D). (Reproduced with permission from Kasser JR (ed): *Orthopaedic Knowledge Update 5*. Rosemont, IL, American Academy of Orthopaedic Surgeons, 1996, p 582.)

manipulation (closed reduction). Many institutions have reported closed reduction of cervical dislocations without neurologic incidents before MRI evaluation in awake, alert patients with stable neurologic examinations. Recently magnetic resonance angiography has been useful in delineating the integrity of the cervical extracranial circulation after cervical trauma.

Upper Cervical Spine Injuries

Occipital Condyle Fractures

A fracture to the occipital condyles is rare, with few reported cases or series in the literature. Approximately 33% of occipital condyle fractures occur in conjunction with atlanto-occipital dislocations. Patients may complain of pain and tenderness in the suboccipital region associated with particular cranial nerve deficits. The cranial nerves susceptible to injury at this level are the IX, X, XI, and XII, with rare injury to cranial nerves VI and VII. Cervical radiographs rarely are diagnostic of occipital condyle fractures. Unenhanced CT is the imaging modality of choice for identification of these fractures.

Current classification of occipital condyle fractures divides them into 3 types. Type I is an impacted comminuted fracture of the occipital condyle with minimal or no displacement. These fractures usually are due to axial loading. The tectoral membrane and contralateral alar ligament are intact; however, the ipsilateral alar ligament may be injured. A type II fracture is a basilar skull fracture that may extend into the

foramen magnum and usually is the result of a direct blow to the occiput or upper cervical spine. The tectoral membrane and alar ligaments remain intact. Type I and II injuries are stable and can be managed in a cervical orthosis or halo vest for approximately 2.5 to 3 months until healing occurs. A type III fracture is a displaced avulsion fracture of the occipital condyle caused by shear, lateral bending, or rotary forces. These injuries are potentially unstable because of the avulsion of the ipsilateral alar ligament and require immediate halo vest application.

Atlanto-Occipital Dislocation

Survivors of atlanto-occipital injuries are extremely rare, and most patients who survive this injury have some degree of neurologic deficit. Injury commonly occurs to cranial nerves VII to X, the brain stem, the spinomedullary portion of the spinal cord, and, rarely, a unilateral vertebral or basilar artery.

Many radiographic indicators of atlanto-occipital injury exist. The degree of prevertebral soft-tissue swelling may be an indicator. Displacement of the occipital-atlantal relationship can be determined by the Wackenheim line, which is a line that normally extends from the posterior tip of the clivus tangentially to the posterior tip of the dens. The most common measurement to determine normal upper cervical anatomy is the Powers ratio, which is the ratio of the distance from the basion to the anterior border of the posterior arch of the atlas divided by the distance from the opisthion to the posterior border of the anterior arch of the atlas. The normal ratio is between 0.77 and 1.0. Values greater than 1.0 indicate anterior subluxation or displacement.

In the classification system that is most commonly used for atlanto-occipital dislocations, type I injuries have radiologic evidence of longitudinal distraction without dislocation. Type II injuries, the most common, are anterior subluxations or dislocations of the occiput on C1. Type III injuries are posterior subluxations or dislocations of the occiput on C1. The goals of treatment of these injuries are reduction, maintenance of normal alignment, and stabilization of the injured segment.

Atlas Fractures

Atlas fractures are relatively uncommon and generally result from an axial load to the head. Isolated atlas fractures occur less than 50% of the time. Neurologic injury is infrequently associated with isolated atlas fractures because of the large size of the spinal canal at this level.

Fracture stability is based on the integrity of the transverse ligament. A disruption of this ligament is suggested by a combined lateral mass spread or overhang greater than 7 mm on an open mouth odontoid view. Although many classification systems exist for atlas fractures, none give particular treatment indications because most fractures are treated nonsurgically.

Transverse ligament injuries have been classified into 2 types: type I injuries involve disruption of the midsubstance of the ligament, and type II injuries are fractures or avulsions of the transverse ligament from the atlas tubercle. Of 15 patients with type I injuries, none healed with nonsurgical treatment, whereas 17 of 23 patients (74%) with type II fractures healed without surgery. Thus, type I injuries have unpredictable healing potential and often require acute surgical stabilization. Acute type II injuries can be treated satisfactorily with external immobilization. Overall, most isolated atlas fractures can be treated conservatively.

C1-C2 Subluxation

Etiologies for atlantoaxial rotatory abnormalities are numerous: traumatic, infectious, congenital, inflammatory, tumors, and miscellaneous disease. Traumatic atlantoaxial rotatory subluxation in adults is most frequently the result of motor vehicle accidents.

Patients with this injury typically present with suboccipital pain and limited cervical rotation. The head usually is in the characteristic "cock robin" position, rotated approximately 20° in one direction and tilted 20° in the opposite direction. On an open mouth AP radiograph the C1 lateral masses are displaced relative to the odontoid. The lateral mass that rotates forward appears broader, superior, and more midline than the lateral mass that rotates posteriorly. More advanced imaging studies, such as CT, cineradiography, and MRI, can be helpful in diagnosing the presence of rotatory fixation.

Treatment depends on the type of injury, the patient's age, and the presence or absence of abnormal neurologic findings. Nonsurgical treatment with a cervical orthosis, halo vest, head-halter traction, or skeletal traction may be adequate. If reduction and stability cannot be obtained with these methods, a posterior fusion may be necessary followed by cervical orthosis or halo immobilization.

Odontoid Fractures

Odontoid fractures account for approximately 5% to 15% of all cervical spine fractures. In the most widely accepted classification system for odontoid fractures, type I fractures are rare and involve a small oblique avulsion fracture of the superior third of the odontoid. Controversy exists over the existence of this fracture type, with some suggesting that this may actually be evidence of an occult occipital-C1 dissociation. Type II fractures are the most common and occur at the junction of the dens with the body of the axis. Type III fractures extend into the body of C2. Hadley and associates described type IIA fractures, which are similar to type II fractures but with comminution of the anterior and posterior cortical frac-

ture margins. Type I fractures in the presence of occipital C1 stability usually are stable and can be treated with a cervical orthosis for approximately 3 months. Then, flexion and extension radiographs should be taken to evaluate for occult instability. Patients with nondisplaced type II fractures or displacement < 5 mm should be treated by closed skeletal traction reduction followed by halo immobilization. Relative indications for surgical stabilization of type II fractures include displacement > 5 mm, age older than 60 years, failure of a successful previous reduction, or nonunion. The surgical procedure may be posterior C1-2 arthrodesis or anterior odontoid screw fixation. Type III fractures often can be managed successfully with halo vest immobilization.

Geriatric patients represent a unique population of patients with odontoid fractures. These patients show a greater incidence of fracture nonunion than the population on a whole. Several authors have reported that acute perifracture mortality and morbidity can be decreased by early surgical stabilization in this patient subgroup.

Axis Fractures

Traumatic spondylolisthesis of the axis, also referred to as a hangman's fracture, usually is caused by a hyperextension force. Immediate death occurs in 25% to 40% of patients with these injuries. Survivors, however, usually do not have neurologic deficits because of the large size of the canal at the C2 level and the fact that a C2 pars interarticularis fracture usually results in an increase in spinal canal area.

Patients with hangman's fractures usually have nonspecific complaints of pain localized to the suboccipital region and, occasionally, a subjective sense of instability. Adequate imaging studies include plain radiographs and CT or tomograms if additional studies are deemed necessary.

The most widely accepted classification of traumatic spondylolisthesis has 3 parts. Type I injuries consist of either bilateral pars interarticularis or adjacent superior and inferior articular facet fractures. There is no resultant angulation and less than 3 mm of displacement of C2 on C3. These fractures are the result of a hyperextension force with no injury to the C3 body below. Type II fractures have significant angulation and > 3 mm of displacement. There usually is an associated wedge compression fracture to the anterosuperior aspect of the C3 vertebral body. Fractures with significant angulation and minimal displacement are classified as type IIA. These fractures have a secondary flexion component resulting in disruption of the posterior longitudinal ligament and disk space, with retained integrity of the anterior longitudinal ligament. Type III injuries are fracture dislocations of C2 on C3 with an associated pars fracture. There is severe angulation, displacement, and associated unilateral or bilat-

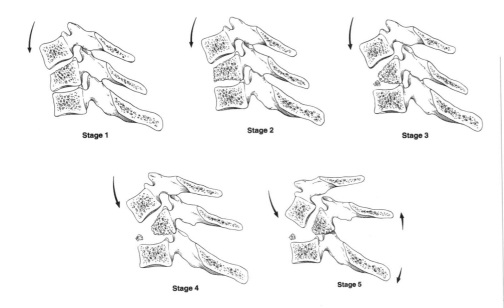

Figure 2

Allen and Ferguson classification of traumatic cervical spine injuries. Compression flexion injury. Stage 1: Blunting and rounding off of anterosuperior vertebral margin. Stage 2: Loss of anterior height and beak-like appearance anteroinferiorly. Stage 3: Fracture line from anterior surface of vertebral body extending obliquely through the subchondral plate (a fractured beak). Stage 4: Some displacement (< 3 mm) of the posteroinferior vertebral margin into the neural canal. Stage 5: Displacement (> 3 mm) of the posterior part of vertebral body. Although vertebral arch is intact, entire posterior ligamentous complex is ruptured. (Reproduced with permission from Rizzolo SJ, Cotler JM: Unstable cervical spine injuries: Specific treatment approaches. *J Am Acad Orthop Surg* 1993;1:57–66.)

eral facet dislocation. The integrity of both the anterior and posterior longitudinal ligaments is compromised.

Atypical hangman's fractures have been described in which there is fracture through the posterior cortex of the C2 body. These atypical hangman's fractures result in narrowing of the spinal canal. A 33% incidence of neurologic deficit was found in patients with atypical hangman's fractures.

Type I fractures usually can be immobilized successfully with a cervical orthosis. Type II fractures can be treated by skeletal traction reduction if necessary, followed by a rigid cervicothoracic orthosis or halo vest immobilization. The use of axial traction with type IIA injuries is contraindicated and may result in fracture fragment distraction. These injuries should be treated with cervical extension and halo immobilization. Type III injuries require surgical intervention. A bilateral C2 pars interarticularis fracture with an associated facet dislocation is extremely difficult to reduce by closed methods. These require an open reduction and stabilization of C2 on C3 with subsequent halo immobilization for treatment of the pars interarticularis fracture. If a successful closed reduction of a unilateral facet dislocation subtype can be obtained, halo immobilization alone may be adequate.

Subaxial Cervical Spine Injuries

The most widely accepted classification of subaxial cervical spine fractures is based on the mechanism of injury. A mechanistic classification provides information about the probable biomechanical deficiencies of the supporting bony and ligamentous structures and, therefore, guides treatment recommendations. The Allen and Ferguson classification system, which is based on the position of the neck at time of the injury, is divided into 6 categories or phylogenies: compression flexion (Fig. 2), vertical compression (Fig. 3), distractive flexion (Fig. 4), compression extension (Fig. 5), distractive extension (Fig. 6), and lateral flexion (Fig. 7). Each phylogeny is further subdivided into numbered stages, with the higher numbers denoting more severe injuries. The initial insult is referred to as the major injury vector, with the other contributing forces referred to as the minor injury vectors.

Compression Flexion Injuries Compression flexion injuries, which make up about 20% of subaxial cervical spine fractures, usually result from a motor vehicle or diving accident. As the continuum of force progresses with this injury mechanism, the posterior column of the cervical spine fails in distraction while the anterior column fails in compression (Fig. 2). In stage 1 and 2 injuries there is no significant disruption of the middle or posterior cervical columns with partial stability remaining in the anterior column. Rarely is there a presenting neurologic deficit in stages 1 and 2, and most patients can be treated in a cervical orthosis or halo vest for 8 to 12 weeks. Lack of immobilization may result in a late kyphotic deformity. An MRI evaluation is useful to evaluate the extent of posterior ligamentous injury in the stage 3 and 4 subtypes. These fractures can be managed effectively in a halo vest or can be treated surgically if the potential for late deformity is present.

In a stage 5 injury, the posterior ligamentous complex is completely disrupted, resulting in a significant 3-column injury to the cervical spine (Fig. 8). Often these injuries can be satisfactorily managed with an anterior corpectomy and fusion with stabilization. If marked posterior dislocation or instability is noted at the time of anterior graft placement, then a supplemental posterior fixation procedure may be necessary.

Vertical Compression Injuries Vertical compression injuries account for roughly 15% of subaxial cervical spine injuries. They usually are the result of a motor vehicle accident, diving accident, or an axial blow to the top of the head. The most common site is the C6-C7 level (Fig. 3). Patients without neurologic involvement can be treated with halo vest immobilization for 8 to 12 weeks. A vertical compression stage 3 injury is a continuum of a stage 2 injury with fragmentation and peripheral displacement of the vertebral centrum. Patients with evidence of neurologic deficit can be effectively treated with an anterior corpectomy, fusion, and stabilization procedure.

Distraction Flexion Injuries Distraction flexion injuries account for 9% to 10% of all subaxial cervical spine injuries (Fig. 4). Immediate closed reduction is recommended for most injuries of this type (Fig. 9).

Simulating distractive flexion injuries in cadavers, Ebraheim and associates calculated the average axial spinal canal areas after different degrees of anterior translation of the cephalad vertebrae on the caudal vertebral level. After 3 mm of anterior translation, the average remaining spinal canal area of the inferior vertebra was 75% for C6, 77% for C7, and 79% for T1. After 6 mm of anterior translation (50% anterior translation), the average spinal canal area decreased to 59%, 51%, and 56% for C6, C7, and T1, respectively.

Kang and associates demonstrated a significant association between the actual space available for the spinal cord at the

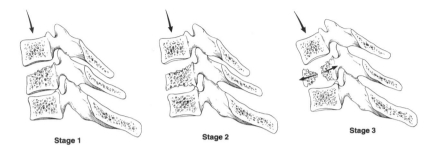

Figure 3

Allen and Ferguson classification continued. Vertical compression injury. Stage 1: Central cupping fracture of superior or inferior end plate. Stage 2: Similar to stage 1, but fracture of both end plates; any fracture of the centrum is minimal. Stage 3: Fragmentation and displacement of vertebral body. (Reproduced with permission from Rizzolo SJ, Cotler JM: Unstable cervical spine injuries: Specific treatment approaches. *J Am Acad Orthop Surg* 1993;1:5—66.)

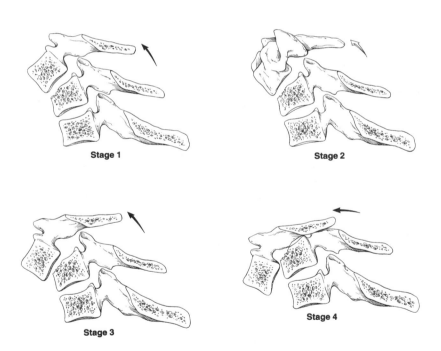

Figure 4

Allen and Ferguson classification continued. Distractive flexion injury. Stage 1: Facet subluxation in flexion and divergence of spinous processes (flexion sprain); some blunting of anterosuperior vertebral margin as in a stage 1 compression flexion injury. Stage 2: Unilateral facet dislocation; there may be some rotary spondylolisthesis. Stage 3: Bilateral facet dislocation with about 50% anterior vertebral body displacement. Facets may have completely leapfrogged over those below or may be "perched." Stage 4: Full width vertebral body displacement or completely unstable motion segment. (Reproduced with permission from Rizzolo SJ, Cotler JM: Unstable cervical spine injuries: Specific treatment approaches. *J Am Acad Orthop Surg* 1993;1:57—66.)

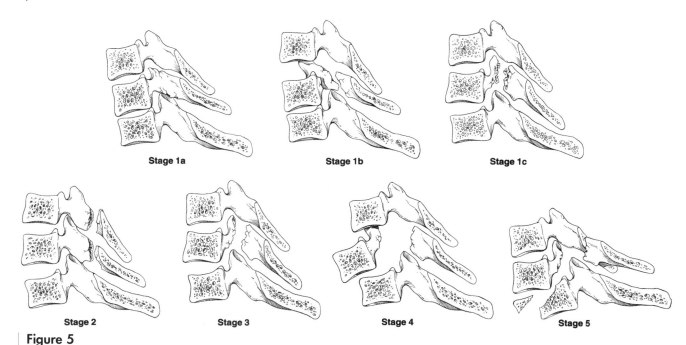

Figure 5

Allen and Ferguson classification continued. Compressive extension injury. Stage 1: Unilateral vertebral arch fracture; may be through articular process (stage 1a), pedicle (stage 1b), or lamina (stage 1c); there may be rotary spondylolisthesis of centrum. Stage 2: Bilaminar fracture, which may be at multiple contiguous levels. Stage 3: Hypothetical modes not seen clinically by authors of classification, characterized by bilateral fractures of vertebral arch (articular processes, pedicles, or laminae) and partial-width anterior vertebral body displacement. Stage 4: Partial-width anterior vertebral body displacement. Stage 5: Full-width anterior vertebral body displacement. (Reproduced with permission from Rizzolo SJ, Cotler JM: Unstable cervical spine injuries: Specific treatment approaches. *J Am Acad Orthop Surg* 1993;1:57–66.)

level of injury and the severity of the injury. They found that a sagittal canal diameter of less than 13 mm was highly associated with potential injury to the spinal cord. Patients who sustained more severe injuries (complete or incomplete spinal cord injuries) had a significantly narrower sagittal canal diameter with a smaller Pavlov ratio than patients who did not have spinal cord injuries. In contrast, in a review of 33 patients with facet fractures, subluxations, or dislocations, the authors found no correlation between the preinjury canal size and neurologic outcome, although there was a definite trend between the severity of trauma and the degree of neurologic deficit.

Usual treatment of these unstable and potentially unstable injuries is closed reduction, then posterior fusion and stabilization. If an associated herniated disk may compromise the spinal cord during this treatment, anterior diskectomy and fusion should be considered first. If reduction is obtained by this approach and anterior plating alone gives sufficient stability, the posterior approach may be avoided.

Compression Extension Injuries Compression extension injuries are most commonly the result of diving and motor

vehicle accidents (Fig. 5). The progression of injury is from the posterior to anterior vertebral spinal elements. Stages 3, 4, and 5 injuries are effectively reduced and stabilized with a posterior cervical approach and stabilization.

Distraction Extension Injuries Distraction extension injuries resulting from motor vehicle accidents and falls account for 22% of subaxial cervical spine injuries (Fig. 6). Stage 1 injuries usually are stable and can be treated effectively with halo vest immobilization. A stage 2 injury is similar to stage 1 but with injury to the posterior ligamentous complex resulting in posterior displacement of the upper vertebral body (Fig. 10). These injuries can be effectively treated with an anterior cervical decompression and fusion with application of an anterior cervical plate acting as a tension band.

Lateral Flexion Lateral flexion injuries account for approximately 20% of subaxial cervical spine injuries and usually are a result of a blow to the side of the head (Fig. 7). Stage 1 injuries are considered relatively stable and usually do not require surgical stabilization. Ligamentous failure occurs in stage 2 injuries, which usually are unstable and require surgical stabilization.

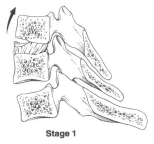 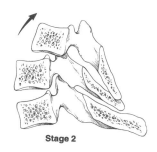

Stage 1   **Stage 2**

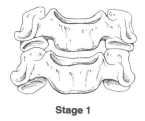 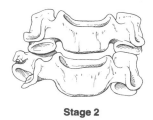

Stage 1   **Stage 2**

Figure 6

Allen and Ferguson classification continued. Distractive extension injury. Stage 1: Failure of anterior ligamentous complex. Injury may be a nondeforming transverse fracture through the centrum or widening of disk space. Stage 2: Injury may be anterior marginal avulsion fracture of centrum. Some posterior ligamentous complex failure may be revealed by posterior displacement of upper vertebra. Fracture reduces in flexion. (Reproduced with permission from Rizzolo SJ, Cotler JM: Unstable cervical spine injuries: Specific treatment approaches. *J Am Acad Orthop Surg* 1993;1:57–66.)

Figure 7

Allen and Ferguson classification continued. Lateral flexion injury. Stage 1: Asymmetric compression fracture of centrum with associated vertebral arch fracture ipsilaterally; anteroposterior film shows no displacement. Stage 2: Displacement of ipsilateral arch fracture seen on AP view. There also may be ligamentous tension failure on contralateral side with facet separation. (Reproduced with permission from Rizzolo SJ, Cotler JM: Unstable cervical spine injuries: Specific treatment approaches. *J Am Acad Orthop Surg* 1993;1:57–66.)

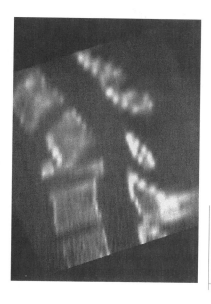

Figure 8

A sagittal computed tomography reconstruction of a high grade flexion compression injury of the C5 vertebral body.

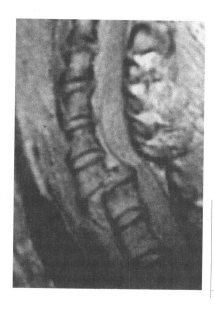

Figure 9

A sagittal magnetic resonance imaging scan of a distraction-flexion injury (bilateral facet dislocation) with an extruded disk herniation.

The magnitude of vertebral deformation at the time of trauma following a fracture or dislocation is not well understood. Chang and associates demonstrated that 2 geometric changes, canal occlusion and vertebral column shortening, occur in compressive burst injuries to the cervical spine. The resultant compressive injury to the spine and degree of spinal canal narrowing is only a fraction of the deformity noted at impact. Postinjury midsagittal canal diameter was 269% of the minimal transient canal diameter at injury, with the mean postinjury canal area representing 139% of the minimal transient area also at the time of injury.

Burner Syndrome

The burner syndrome or "stinger," which is common in contact sports such as football and rugby, is described as a temporary episode of upper extremity unilateral burning dysesthesias with motor weakness. Patients usually describe a painful sensation that radiates from their neck to their fingertips after an impact load to the neck or shoulder. The biceps, deltoid, and spinatus are the muscle groups most commonly involved. The complaint of pain usually lasts for a few seconds to minutes, but symptoms may persist for as long as a few weeks. Three different mechanisms have been proposed for this syndrome: (1) stretch or traction injury to the brachial plexus, (2) extension of the cervical spine resulting in nerve root compression within the neural foramina, and (3) a direct blow resulting in injury to the brachial plexus. The reported incidence of a burner syndrome is between 49% and 65% in college football players.

Transient Quadriplegia

The incidence of neurapraxia of the cervical spinal cord with transient quadriplegia in collegiate football players is approximately 7.3 per 10,000 athletes. The mechanism of injury is usually axial compression with a component of either hyperflexion or hyperextension. Sensory and motor abnormalities are present bilaterally, usually for approximately 10 to 15 minutes; however, some patients may have residual symptoms for up to 48 hours. Sensory disturbances vary from burning pain to loss of sensation along with motor abnormalities ranging from bilateral upper and lower extremity weakness to complete paralysis. Transient quadriplegia is associated with developmental cervical stenosis, the presence of a congenital fusion, cervical instability, and/or an intervertebral disk protrusion or herniation.

Thoracolumbar Fractures

Appropriate management of a patient with traumatic thoracic or lumbar spinal injury requires a sound understanding of anatomy, pathomechanics of injury, and the concept of stability. The principles of fracture reduction and stabilization, preservation of intact or remaining neurologic function, and early patient mobilization are paramount in the recovery from such injuries.

Spinal Stability

The concept of spinal stability has evolved from a purely anatomic description to an analysis of the mechanism of injury to schemes incorporating both anatomy and mechanism. Originally, a 2-column concept of spinal stability was described. The anterior column consisted of the vertebral body, disk, and anterior and posterior longitudinal ligaments, while the posterior column was defined as the pedicles, laminae, transverse and spinous processes, and all associated ligamentous structures (facet capsules, ligamentum flava, interspinous and supraspinous ligaments). Instability was present if the posterior column was unable to bear weight after anterior column compromise. This concept was effective in explaining the chronic instability seen in trauma; however, it was limited in applicability to acute injuries.

In 1983, Denis devised a 3-column concept of clinical and

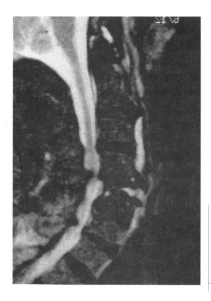

Figure 10

A sagittal magnetic resonance imaging scan of a distraction extension injury at the C4-C5 level.

biomechanical stability of thoracolumbar injuries. The anterior column is composed of the anterior two thirds of the vertebral body, disk, and anterior longitudinal ligament. The middle column consists of the posterior vertebral body, disk, and posterior longitudinal ligament. The posterior column includes the pedicles, laminae, transverse and spinous processes, and the posterior ligamentous structures. On the basis of radiographic and CT imaging, this classification divides injuries into minor and major categories. Minor injuries account for 15% of all injuries and include fractures of the transverse or spinous processes, laminae, or pars interarticularis. Major injuries are classified as 4 basic mechanisms including compression, distraction, rotation, and shear resulting in compression fractures, burst fractures, seat belt-type injuries, and fracture-dislocations. Instability is defined as structural involvement and compromise of at least 2 of the 3 spinal columns.

The middle osteoligamentous column is believed to be the key element in determining stability and has been incorporated into another classification. Fracture patterns have been described based on the integrity of the middle column and mechanism of injury. Finally, a mechanistic classification proposed to describe thoracolumbar injuries uses the force application as a means of description and treatment.

Mechanism of Injury

Several mechanisms can lead to loss of structural integrity of the spinal column, including forces such as flexion, axial compression, lateral compression, flexion combined with rotation, flexion combined with distraction, and extension that may occur in various combinations.

Flexion Injuries occurring from pure hyperflexion result in compressive failure of the anterior spinal column. The middle osteoligamentous and the posterior columns usually are intact when anterior compression is < 50% of the anterior vertebral body height. These injuries, which are more common in the thoracic spine, are considered stable. When anterior compression is > 50% of the anterior body height, the posterior column is subjected to significant tensile force and may fail, leading to an acute or delayed unstable injury pattern.

Axial Compresion Axial load applied to the spine can result in variable injury patterns based on the location of applied force (for example, thoracic versus thoracolumbar) and preexisting alignment (for example, kyphotic versus lordotic spine). When an axial load is applied to the thoracic or kyphotic spine, a flexion-type moment results, and if failure occurs it is with anterior column wedging. Axial load to the relatively straight, nonkyphotic thoracolumbar spine may result in compressive failure of the anterior bony column and middle osteoligamentous column. Fragmentation of the vertebral body and retropulsion of the posterior vertebral wall into the spinal canal may occur with increased rate and magnitude of applied force and is responsible for neurologic deficit along with the kyphotic deformity that may accompany these injuries. In addition, posterior column compressive failure may occur and manifest as articular facet fracture and/or subluxation or vertical fractures of the laminae or spinous process. Posterior element tensile failure may also occur if significant flexion force is applied to the posterior column following axial load injury, further increasing the instability of the spinal segment.

Lateral Compression A laterally-applied compression force causes injury similar to that of pure flexion. The vertebral body sustains asymmetric collapse on the side of the applied load and tensile failure of the contralateral side. This injury results in coronal plane deformity with focal scoliosis and may be unstable and progressive.

Flexion-Distraction The axis of rotation of the applied force in this type of injury pattern is located anterior to the vertebral body, usually on the anterior abdominal wall (seat belt injury). The posterior column fails under tensile load and is the initial site of injury. The injury then passes through the disk space and/or vertebral body. When the line of force passes through the bony elements alone it is referred to as a Chance fracture.

The axis of rotation may also transfer to the middle column, causing significant posterior tensile failure and anterior column compressive failure. This variant of a flexion

moment mechanism is a more extensive injury than an anterior wedge fracture and is more likely to be unstable.

Flexion-Rotation This mechanism of injury leads to failure of all 3 columns and indicates a grossly unstable injury. There may be anterior column compressive failure due to the flexion force. There also is posterior disruption of the facet articulations, capsules, and ligamentous structures. As the degree of rotation increases, shear type injury occurs through the anterior, middle, and posterior columns, leading to dislocation of the spinal segment. The fracture-dislocation may reduce spontaneously and give a false impression of the degree of instability that these injuries represent.

Extension Extension injury results in tensile failure of the anterior longitudinal ligament and anterior disk, often manifesting as avulsion fractures of the vertebral bodies. The posterior column is subjected to compressive forces and may sustain fractures of the spinous process, laminae, and, occasionally, the pedicles. These uncommon injuries usually are stable.

Decompression

The treatment of unstable fractures or fracture-dislocations of the thoracolumbar and lumbar spine with neurologic compromise remains controversial. A complete spinal cord injury often is managed by spinal stabilization to allow early patient mobilization and limit the consequences of prolonged bed rest. A complete injury is more common in the thoracic region, and neurologic outcome after decompression has not been shown to be significantly improved as compared to that after stabilization alone.

In the presence of incomplete neurologic deficits, decompression and spinal stabilization can be beneficial in terms of neurologic recovery. The exact methods of management are numerous and controversy prevails on the issue of an anterior versus posterior approach for patients with an incomplete spinal cord injury.

The spinal canal dimensions can be restored indirectly from a posterior approach by distraction instrumentation and ligamentotaxis or directly by posterior transpedicular or posterolateral decompression. Ligamentotaxis depends on an intact posterior longitudinal ligament or annular disk fibers and their bony attachments for reduction of the retropulsed fragments. An indirect posterior decompression requires that the reduction be performed within the first several days after the injury because fracture hematoma can rapidly organize, allowing the fragments to slowly gain stability. Canal clearance of 32% to 50% has been shown in various studies.

Direct canal decompression also can be accomplished from a posterior approach using a transpedicular or posterolateral technique. Both techniques are safe and can be effective in the lumbar region below the level of the conus medullaris, especially if there is a large retropulsed fragment lodged to 1 side of the canal adjacent to the pedicle. The transpedicular technique involves a unilateral laminotomy made at the level of the pedicle; the pedicle is then taken down with a high speed burr. A reversed angle curette or a special impactor is placed lateral and anterior to the dura to allow safe tamping of the retropulsed fragment. A defect should be developed in the posterior vertebral wall to allow the retropulsed fragments to be impacted into a reduced position. The cauda equina or exiting nerve roots can be gently retracted, but the spinal cord or conus should not be manipulated in this procedure. The posterolateral decompression technique frequently requires excision of the transverse process along with the pedicle. However, the decompression is then performed similarly to the technique previously described.

Each patient should be evaluated for canal clearance after posterior indirect or direct decompression. Evaluation can be done either intraoperatively or postoperatively. Ultrasound has been used for intraoperative assessment of the patency of the spinal canal. Using real-time ultrasonic images, the thecal sac and canal can be observed through a laminotomy or laminectomy without direct manipulation of the neural structures. Residual anterior compression by bone or disk material can be detected and further decompression can be done. Alternatively, postoperative evaluation of canal clearance can be done with a CT scan, including axial and sagittally-reconstructed images. Although artifact from the instrumentation can make the images difficult to interpret, the spinal canal often can be adequately demonstrated to determine the extent of decompression.

Primary anterior decompression is preferred if the retropulsed fragment is large and located in the midline in a patient with incomplete neurologic deficit or if more than 2 weeks has passed since the time of injury. Secondary anterior decompression should also be done if imaging studies show persistent canal compromise following posterior decompression in a patient with residual neurologic deficits. The surgical approach is left-sided to the thoracolumbar spine based on the ease of locating and manipulating the aorta as compared to the inferior vena cava. A thoracoabdominal approach is used for exposure of the T10 to T12 vertebrae and a retroperitoneal approach for the first lumbar vertebra or more caudal. The spine is exposed 1 level cephalad and 1 level caudad to the injured segment. The segmental vessels are ligated at the midpoint of the vertebral bodies. The disk material and end plate cartilage of the level cephalad and caudad to the damaged vertebra are removed and a subtotal corpectomy performed. To prevent inadequate canal clearance,

several key points must be remembered during anterior decompression. Initially, the patient must be properly positioned in lateral decubitus with the shoulders and pelvis stabilized so that the back is perpendicular to the floor. Maintaining the patient in the true lateral position allows proper orientation of the spinal canal. The decompression must be continued to the contralateral pedicle. This extent of the decompression can be extrapolated to the opposite side of the spinal cord or thecal sac and serve as an indication of canal patency without direct manipulation or visualization of the neural contents. The presence of a pulsating dural sac also can be a useful marker for evaluating the adequacy of canal decompression.

Management of Specific Injuries

Compression Fractures Compression fractures involve failure of the anterior column with an intact middle column. These injuries often occur in the elderly, are usually stable from the added rigidity provided by the rib cage, and require symptomatic treatment including pain control and early ambulation.

A hyperextension orthosis may be recommended on an individualized basis if the degree of compression of the anterior vertebral body is > 50% or segmental kyphosis is > 30°. These findings are suggestive of posterior ligamentous disruption and indicate a potentially unstable injury. In addition, multiple adjacent compression fractures increase the risk of delayed kyphosis and potential neurologic compromise and should be treated more aggressively.

Surgical treatment is reserved for unstable compression fractures (> 50% anterior height loss or significant kyphosis) in which progression of deformity is documented despite conservative management or neurologic stability is compromised because of the resultant deformity. In these situations CT imaging is necessary to evaluate the structure of the middle column to rule out a burst fracture component. These injuries can be treated through a posterior surgical approach with compression-type instrumentation to restore sagittal alignment. Overcompression must be avoided to prevent retropulsion of a degenerated thoracic disk.

Burst Fractures Burst fractures are defined by axial compressive failure of the anterior and middle columns and possible compressive or tensile failure of the posterior column. Although controversial, management is based on kyphotic angulation at the fracture site, the degree of canal compromise from retropulsed fragments, and the extent of neurologic involvement. These injuries are more common at the thoracolumbar junction for several reasons, including the increased mobility in this region as the shift from the rigid

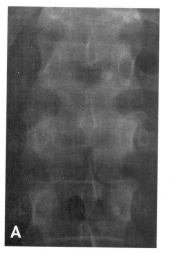

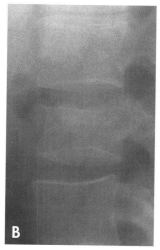

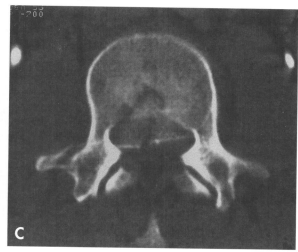

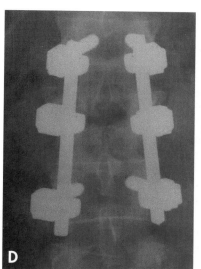

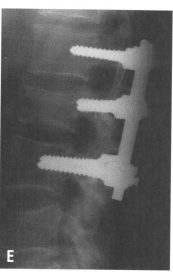

Figure 11

A, Anteroposterior lumbar radiograph of a 37-year-old man who became paraparetic with this burst fracture of L2. Collapse of the L2 vertebral body and widening of the interarticular distance as compared to the level above and below can be seen. A laminar fracture of L2 is also present. B, Lateral radiograph showing collapse of the L2 vertebral body. Note the rotation of the posterior superior corner at the level of the pedicle leading to the intracanal fragment. C, Computed tomography scan through the body of L2 at the level of the pedicles. There are large retropulsed fragments causing severe canal narrowing. D and E, At surgery, this patient initially had unilateral distraction rodding on the right side with a posterior lateral decompression performed through a laminectomy site. A pedicle screw fixation device was placed on the opposite side from the distraction rodding. The latter was subsequently removed and replaced with a rigid segmental pedicle screw and rod system. Note the restoration of lordosis on the lateral radiograph with the reduction of the posterior superior corner at L2. (Reproduced with permission from Kasser JR (ed): *Orthopaedic Knowledge Update 5*. Rosemont, IL, American Academy of Orthopaedic Surgeons, 1996, p 582.)

thoracic spine to the mobile lumbar spine creates a transition high-stress zone and the sagittal alignment assumes a relatively straight position. An axial load applied to the kyphotic thoracic spine produces a combination flexion-compression moment, but, in the lordotic lumbar spine this loading produces an extension-compression moment. In the transitional relatively straight thoracolumbar junction, axial force results in pure vertical compression affecting all 3 columns of the spinal segment (Fig. 11).

Patients who have thoracolumbar burst fractures with < 20° of segmental kyphosis and < 45% canal compromise and are neurologically intact can be treated nonsurgically with short-term bed rest followed by external fracture stabilization and patient mobilization. A customized total contact thoracolumbosacral orthosis (TLSO) or hyperextension cast is worn for 3 months with serial radiographic follow-up.

Fractures with angulation > 20° or canal compromise > 45% in neurologically intact patients may be best treated with surgical intervention to prevent progressive deformity. Stabilization can be obtained with posterior or anterior instrumentation or both. A variety of stabilization devices are available for posterior instrumentation, including Harrington distraction hook-rod and segmental stabilization implants. The concept of 3-point fixation, bending, and distraction is applied to reduce the fracture fragments and restore sagittal alignment. However, the use of distraction must be avoided when there is concomitant tensile failure of the posterior column, because distraction could actually worsen the deformity. The fixation is improved when hooks are placed 3 levels above and 2 levels below the thoracolum-

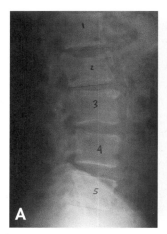
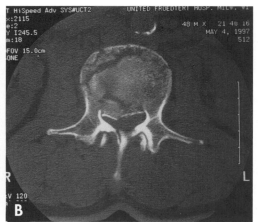

Figure 12

A, Lateral radiograph of a 48-year-old man with an L2 burst fracture and incomplete neurologic deficit. Anterior comminution and posterior superior vertebral wall retropulsion into the vertebral canal are seen. B, Computed tomography scan at level of L2 pedicles. Significant canal compromise is noted secondary to the retropulsed fragments.

bar fracture. Transpedicular implants for posterior stabilization may allow a shorter fusion construct because of the increased purchase of all 3 bony columns with these devices. Intracanal fracture fragment resorption has been shown to occur over time after posterior stabilization.

Patients with burst fractures and neurologic injury are candidates for canal decompression. Many techniques are available to effect decompression. Laminectomy without stabilization is never indicated in the presence of burst fractures because of the destabilizing effect and the lack of adequate decompression anterior to the neural structures where compression is greatest.

Anterior decompression and fusion can be performed in the neurologically compromised patient when the fracture retropulses a large midline fragment (Fig. 12) or when surgical intervention is delayed longer than 2 weeks from the injury. An anterior approach also can be used after failure of complete canal decompression by posterior techniques and residual neurologic dysfunction. Anterior decompression with complete or partial corpectomy is followed by anterior strut grafting and posterior compression instrumentation. Another option is anterior instrumentation, including various vertebral body screw-plate or rod systems, to stabilize the graft (Fig. 13).

Low lumbar fractures are relatively uncommon and are estimated to account for 4% of all spine fractures. Low lumbar burst fractures, specifically from L3 to L5, occur in a unique anatomic and biomechanical area. A significant degree of lordosis exists in the lumbar spine, and fractures in the lower levels of this area have a tendency to alter the sagittal alignment. The specific surgical indications for a low lumbar burst fracture include the presence of neurologic deficits, severe malalignment of the lumbar spine, and progression of the deformity despite nonsurgical treatment. The presence of vertical lamina fractures may indicate entrapped dural elements and require careful dissection for release. In the absence of significant angulation or collapse or neurologic compromise, bed rest followed by various types of body cast immobilization are appropriate options.

Flexion-Distraction Injuries The management of flexion-distraction injuries is determined by the degree of involvement of bone and soft tissue. When these injuries extend entirely through the bony posterior elements and into the vertebral body (Chance fracture) without disk involvement, prognosis for healing is good. Treatment involves immobilization with hyperextension casting or a total contact TLSO for 3 months, with serial radiographic evaluation to detect progressive deformity. Before immobilization is discontinued, lateral dynamic flexion-extension radiographs should be obtained to document fracture stability.

An injury that involves posterior ligamentous disruption or that extends into the disk space carries a less optimistic prognosis for healing because of the soft-tissue damage. These injuries are best treated with surgical stabilization, including posterior compression instrumentation without decompression using hooks or transpedicular instrumentation placed 1 above and below the level of injury. Preoperative evaluation of the integrity of the middle column is imperative because compression could lead to retropulsion of fracture fragments if the posterior vertebral wall is compromised.

Fracture-Dislocations Fracture-dislocations occur with high-energy trauma and from combinations of forces, and most have associated neurologic injury. The goal of treatment of these injuries is surgical stabilization to permit early patient mobilization and to limit the risk of concomitant medical problems in these polytrauma patients. Early mobilization and upright positioning have been shown to decrease overall mortality and morbidity from pulmonary dysfunction, skin problems, and deep venous thrombosis.

The posterior approach is used in most of these injuries. Posterior or anterior decompression can be done in patients with incomplete neurologic deficits, although decompression results from improvement in the gross malalignment of the

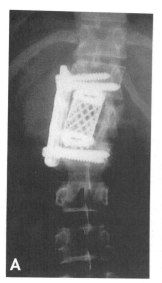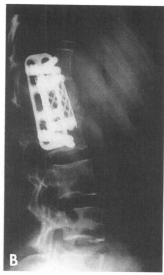

Figure 13

Anteroposterior (A) and lateral (B) radiographs following anterior decompression and stabilization of the injury in Figure 8 with anterior plate. A rib strut graft along with titanium mesh cage was utilized to reconstruct the defect from the partial corpectomy.

injury. Posterior rigid fixation maintains fracture reduction and allows early mobilization, often without the use of external bracing. Segmental fixation is used to maintain control of axial, translation, and rotational forces.

Minor Fractures Fractures of the transverse process occur from direct trauma or from violent paraspinal muscle contraction. Multiple fractures may occur and are commonly nondisplaced. Treatment of these stable fractures includes pain control, mobilization without bracing, and evaluation for associated spinal and other organ system injuries. Rarely, a displaced fracture places traction on the exiting nerve root and results in a neurapraxia. Avulsion of the L5 transverse process (Tile's sign) may indicate a fracture of the pelvis, and careful evaluation must be undertaken to identify injury to the sacroiliac region.

Spinous process avulsion fractures, common in the cervical spine, are rare in the lumbar spine. These injuries are considered stable and are treated accordingly.

Gunshot Wounds to the Spine The treatment of civilian gunshot wounds to the spine in the past has been nonsurgical to avoid potential complications of laminectomy and bullet removal. However, surgical intervention is indicated when progressive neurologic deficits develop in the presence of demonstrable neural compression from bullet, fracture frag-

ments, or hematoma. Management of gunshot wounds accompanied by perforation of the colon is a controversial subject. Studies have recommended surgical removal of the bullet, debridement, and antibiotic therapy, whereas others have exhibited the efficacy of antibiotic treatment alone. The benefits of bullet removal are minimal with complete spinal cord injury in the thoracic spine. However, bullet removal has been shown to increase nerve root recovery in thoracolumbar and lumbar injuries and is recommended in patients with incomplete neurologic loss.

Spinal canal decompression often is all that is needed because intrinsic stability is maintained in most patients. Early patient mobilization without external bracing is common in the postoperative period. Occasionally, iatrogenic instability may occur from extensive decompression and should be accompanied by concomitant fusion with or without instrumentation.

Osteoporotic Compression Fractures

Osteoporosis is a major health problem affecting more than 25 million Americans and contributing to more than 1.5 million fractures each year. The diminished bone mass and fragility of the skeletal structure may result in pathologic fractures that can occur during normal activities or with minimal trauma such as a fall. Osteoporotic fractures in the spine commonly occur in the vertebral bodies, leading to extensive comminution and collapse.

Elderly patients may have a sudden onset of severe back pain or a gradually increasing gibbus deformity. Neurologic deficits including myelopathy, radiculopathy, or cauda equina syndrome are possible presenting features. Radiographs of thoracic spine fractures demonstrate the washed-out appearance of the vertebral bodies and anterior collapse, often of several adjacent wedge-shaped vertebrae. Because the force is placed onto the anterior column in the kyphotic thoracic spine, middle column involvement is uncommon. In the lordotic lumbar spine, middle column involvement is more common, and evaluation for bone fragment retropulsion into the spinal canal is necessary.

Osteoporotic compression fractures must be differentiated from other causes of pathologic fractures. The initial evaluation should include medical workup for conditions that could lead to a bone demineralization process. Laboratory evaluation should include a complete blood count with differential; chemistry panel with calcium and phosphorus; thyroid, renal, and liver function tests; erythrocyte sedimentation rate; and a urinalysis. Patients with an unexplained compression fracture, especially males, should be evaluated for myeloma with a serum and urine protein electrophoresis. Additionally, an MRI scan may help in the differentiation of benign from malignant compression fractures. Acute benign fractures often have increased intensity of the vertebral body on T1-weighted images, suggesting fat replacement of normal marrow tissue. Some preservation of normal marrow with a smooth linear margin is often seen, and this returns to normal (intermediate signal on T1 and decreased signal on T2-weighted images) after 1 to 3 months. Acute fractures from malignant causes produce an irregular pattern of marrow replacement with decreased signal on T1 and increased signal on T2-weighted images. The pedicle, marrow, and posterior elements are involved along with paraspinal or epidural masses.

The treatment of osteoporotic compression fractures includes pain control for those with acute injuries or progressive deformity. An aerobic conditioning and back strengthening program is advised, and antiosteoporotic medications should be prescribed. Brace treatment often is limited in the elderly population because rigid devices are poorly tolerated. Hyperextension Jewett-type orthoses or soft corsets should be considered in the acute management because these are better tolerated. Surgical treatment is rare and reserved for those individuals with significant or progressive neurologic dysfunction. The poor quality of bone, including the posterior elements, limits the use of instrumentation in this population. Therefore, if decompression is indicated, it often is done through an anterior approach and with strut grafting and anterior instrumentation. Posterior instrumentation can be added and supplemented with polymethylmethacrylate as needed.

At the time of this writing, bone screws placed posteriorly into vertebral elements have been cleared for use in this specific manner by the Food and Drug Administration (FDA) to provide immobilization and stabilization as an adjunct to fusion in the treatment of the following acute and chronic instability or deformities of the thoracic, lumbar and sacral spine: degenerative spondylolisthesis with objective evidence of neurologic impairment; fracture; dislocation; scoliosis; kyphosis; spinal tumor and failed previous fusion (pseudoarthrosis). In addition, anterior vertebral body screws (cervical, thoracic, and lumbar) are Class II devices and can be used as labeled in vertebral bodies.

Annotated Bibliography

Cervical Spine Trauma

Bednar DA, Parikh J, Hummel J: Management of type II odontoid process fractures in geriatric patients: A prospective study of sequential cohorts with attention to survivorship. *J Spinal Disord* 1995;8:166–169.

The authors prospectively studied the effect of early stabilization on perioperative mortality in geriatric patients with odontoid fractures and a neurologic injury. They found that acute perifracture mortality and morbidity may be decreased by early surgical stabilization in elderly patients.

Bracken MB, Shepard MJ, Holford TR, et al: Administration of methylprednisolone for 24 or 48 hours or tirilazad mesylate for 48 hours in the treatment of acute spinal cord injury: Results of the Third National Acute Spinal Cord Injury Randomized Controlled Trial. *JAMA* 1997;277:1597–1604.

This double-blind randomized clinical trial compared the efficacy of methylprednisolone administered for 24 hours with methylprednisolone administered for 48 hours or tirilazad mesylate administered for 48 hours in patients with acute spinal cord injury.

Chang DG, Tencer AF, Ching RP, Treece B, Senft D, Anderson PA: Geometric changes in the cervical spinal canal during impact. *Spine* 1994;19:973–980.

The authors demonstrate that 2 geometric changes, canal occlusion and vertebral column shortening, occur in compressive burst injuries to the cervical spine.

Cusick JF, Yoganandan N, Pintar F, Gardon M: Cervical spine injuries from high-velocity forces: A pathoanatomic and radiologic study. *J Spinal Disord* 1996;9:1–7.

The authors analyzed 10 human cadaver cervical spines subjected to high velocity flexion-compression loads to the cranium and found multiple contiguous and noncontiguous injuries. Many specimens showed evidence of injury resulting from multiple force vectors including flexion, extension, and shear forces. It was concluded that a universal classification system was not adequate in describing the complexity of injuries to the subaxial spine and that noncontiguous injuries may not be due to similar mechanisms. In addition, the authors postulated that the presence of spondylotic changes restricted the transmission of forces distal to the area of spondylopathy.

Dickman CA, Greene KA, Sonntag VK: Injuries involving the transverse atlantal ligament: Classification and treatment guidelines based upon experience with 39 injuries. *Neurosurgery* 1996;38:44–50.

The authors classified transverse atlantal ligament injuries into 2 types. Type I injuries have unpredictable healing potential and often require acute surgical stabilization. Acute type II injuries may be treated satisfactorily with external immobilization.

Donaldson WF III, Heil BV, Donaldson VP, Silvaggio VJ: The effect of airway maneuvers on the unstable C1-C2 segment: A cadaver study. *Spine* 1997;22:1215–1218.

Using a cadaver model, the authors demonstrated that the chin lift and jaw thrust method of securing an airway caused a larger decrease in available space for the spinal cord than either nasal or oral intubation. The authors also found that nasal and oral intubation caused similar narrowing of the available space for the spinal cord.

Ebraheim NA, Xu R, Ahmad M, Heck B, Yeasting RA: The effect of anterior translation of the vertebra on the canal size in the lower cervical spine: A computer-assisted anatomic study. *J Spinal Disord* 1997;10:162–166.

Simulating distractive flexion injuries in 18 cadavers, the authors calculated the average axial spinal canal areas after different degrees of anterior translation of the cephalad vertebrae.

Kang JD, Figgie MP, Bohlman HH: Sagittal measurements of the cervical spine in subaxial fractures and dislocations: An analysis of two hundred and eighty-eight patients with and without neurological deficits. *J Bone Joint Surg* 1994;76A:1617–1628.

Using 288 patients with and without neurologic deficits, the authors demonstrated a significant association between the actual space available for the spinal cord at the level of injury and the severity of neurologic injury.

Lieberman IH, Webb JK: Cervical spine injuries in the elderly. *J Bone Joint Surg* 1994;76B:877–881.

This is a retrospective review of 41 patients over 65 years who sustained cervical trauma. Twelve of these patients had neurologic deficits and 11 died during treatment. These patients were treated with various methods: surgical stabilization, halo traction, rigid collars, and halo vests. The patients treated with bed rest or traction did not tolerate their treatment modalities well. The authors concluded that most of these injuries should have and can be treated with a rigid collar, halo vest, or surgical stabilization. Physicians treating elderly patients after a fall or minor trauma should have a high index of suspicion for cervical spine injury.

Shapiro SA: Management of unilateral locked facet of the cervical spine. *Neurosurgery* 1993;33:832–837.

This study reviewed 24 patients with a unilateral facet dislocation. Ninety-six percent of patients (23/24) were successfully stabilized with a posterior spinous process and/or facet wiring procedure. At 1-year follow-up all patients experienced improvement in their neurologic deficits. The authors concluded that a posterior decompression, if necessary, and fusion with internal fixation is the treatment of choice in the management of unilateral facet dislocations.

Thoracolumbar Fractures

An HS, Andreshak TG, Nguyen C, Williams A, Daniels D: Can we distinguish between benign versus malignant compression fractures of the spine by magnetic resonance imaging? *Spine* 1995;20:1776–1782.

The authors reviewed MRI scans of 22 patients with confirmed lesions of the thoracolumbar spine. MRI reliably distinguished benign versus malignant lesions based on anatomic distribution and enhancement characteristics and changes over time.

An HS, Vaccaro A, Cotler JM, Lin S: Low lumbar burst fractures: comparison among body cast, Harrington rod, Luque rod, and Steffee plate. *Spine* 1991;16(suppl 8):S440–S444.

The authors reviewed 31 low lumbar burst fractures and stressed the necessity for restoration and maintenance of lumbar lordosis in the management of these injuries to prevent disabling back pain.

Clohisy JC, Akbarnia BA, Bucholz RD, Burkus JK, Backer RJ: Neurologic recovery associated with anterior decompression of spine fractures at the thoracolumbar junction (T12-L1). *Spine* 1992;17(suppl 8):S325–S330.

The authors treated 22 patients with incomplete neurologic injury from thoracolumbar junction fractures. They noted that patients treated with early anterior decompression (< 48 hours) experienced improved rates of neurologic recovery including conus medullaris function.

Cuenod CA, Laredo JD, Chevret S, et al: Acute vertebral collapse due to osteoporosis or malignancy: Appearance on unenhanced andgadolinium-enhanced MR images. *Radiology* 1996;199: 541–549.

Sixty-three osteoporotic and 30 malignant vertebral collapse fractures were studied. Findings suggestive of osteoporosis were retropulsion, normal T1-signal intensity, return to normal intensity after gadolinium, and isointense on T2 images. Malignancy was suggested by epidural mass, low T1 intensity, and high intensity after gadolinium and T2 images.

Ghanayem JA, Zdeblick TA: Anterior instrumentation in the management of thoracolumbar burst fractures. *Clin Orthop* 1997; 335:89–100.

The authors describe the evolution of anterior instrumentation devices and the indications and surgical techniques for their safe and effective use.

Hamilton A, Webb JK: The role of anterior surgery for vertebral fractures with and without cord compression. *Clin Orthop* 1994;300:79–89.

The authors review the literature on the role of anterior decompression for thoracolumbar spine injuries, including the indications and timing of surgical intervention.

670　Spine

Kaneda K, Taneichi H, Abumi K, Hashimoto T, Ssatoh S, Fujiya M: Anterior decompression and stabilization with the Kaneda device for thoracolumbar burst fractures associated with neurological deficits. *J Bone Joint Surg* 1997;79A:69–83.

The authors report on 150 patients treated with single-stage anterior decompression and fusion. Ninety-five percent had at least 1 Frankel grade improvement in neurologic function, and 72% recovered complete bladder function. The fusion rate was 93%, and 86% of patients returned to their previous occupations.

Schlegel J, Bayley J, Yuan H, Fredricksen B: Timing of surgical decompression and fixation of acute spinal fractures. *J Orthop Trauma* 1996;10:323–330.

The authors retrospectively reviewed 138 patients with spinal injuries and concluded that surgical decompression and stabilization should be performed within 72 hours in multitrauma (ISS ≥ 18) and in cervical injuries with a neurologic deficit.

Sjostrom L, Karlstrom G, Pech P, Rauschning W: Indirect spinal canal decompression in burst fractures treated with pedicle screw instrumentation. *Spine* 1996;21:113–123.

The authors pospectively evaluated 67 consecutive burst fractures treated with posterior fixation and "indirect" decompression. The results showed 50% canal clearance at T12 and L1, with less improvement at L2.

Stambough JL: Posterior instrumentation for thoracolumbar trauma. *Clin Orthop* 1997;335:73–88.

The authors describe the advantages of posterior instrumentation, available devices, surgical techniques, and outcomes in the management of unstable thoracolumbar injuries.

Yazici M, Atilla B, Tepe S, Calisir A: Spinal canal remodeling in burst fractures of the thoracolumbar spine: A computerized tomographic comparison between operative and nonoperative treatment. *J Spinal Disord* 1996;9:409–413.

Eighteen patients were followed with serial CT scans for at least 18 months postinjury. The authors found that resorption of bony fragments was less favorable in the group treated without surgery.

Classic Bibliography

Allen BL Jr, Ferguson RL, Lehmann TR, O'Brien RP: A mechanistic classification of closed, indirect fractures and dislocations of the cervical spine. *Spine* 1982;7:1–27.

American Spinal Injury Association (ASIA): *Standards for Neurological and Functional Classification of Spinal Cord Injury*, rev ed. Chicago, IL, American Spinal Injury Association, 1992.

Anderson LD, DíAlonzo RT: Fractures of the odontoid process of the axis. *J Bone Joint Surg* 1974;56A:1663–1674.

Anderson PA, Montesano PX: Morphology and treatment of occipital condyle fractures. *Spine* 1988;13:731–736.

Benzel EC, Hart BL, Ball PA, Baldwin NG, Orrison WW, Espinosa MC: Magnetic resonance imaging for the evaluation of patients with occult cervical spine injury. *J Neurosurg* 1996;85:824–829.

Bohlman HH: Treatment of fractures and dislocations of the thoracic and lumbar spine. *J Bone Joint Surg* 1985;67A:165–169.

Bohlman HH, Freehafer A, Dejak J: The results of treatment of acute injuries of the upper thoracic spine with paralysis. *J Bone Joint Surg* 1985;67A:360–369.

Bracken MB, Shepard MJ, Collins WF, et al: A randomized, controlled trial of methylprednisolone or naloxone in the treatment of acute spinal-cord injury: Results of the Second National Acute Spinal Cord Injury Study. *N Engl J Med* 1990;322:1405–1411.

Bradford DS, McBride GG: Surgical management of thoracolumbar spine fractures with incomplete neurologic deficits. *Clin Orthop* 1987;218:201–216.

Cammisa FP Jr, Eismont FJ, Green BA: Dural laceration occurring with burst fractures and associated laminar fractures. *J Bone Joint Surg* 1989;71A:1044–1052.

Denis F: The three column spine and its significance in the classification of acute thoracolumbar spinal injuries. *Spine* 1983;8:817–831.

Dickson JH, Harrington PR, Erwin WD: Results of reduction and stabilization of the severely fractured thoracic and lumbar spine. *J Bone Joint Surg* 1978;60A:799–805.

Eismont FJ, Green BA, Berkowitz BM, Montalvo BM, Quencer RM, Brown MJ: The role of intraoperative ultrasonography in the treatment of thoracic and lumbar spine fractures. *Spine* 1984;9:782–787.

Ferguson RL, Allen BL Jr: A mechanistic classification of thoracolumbar spine fractures. *Clin Orthop* 1984;189:77–88.

Frankel HL, Hancock DO, Hyslop G, et al: The value of postural reduction in the initial management of closed injuries of the spine with paraplegia and tetraplegia: I. *Paraplegia* 1969;7:179–192.

Fredrickson BE, Mann KA, Yuan HA, Lubicky JP: Reduction of the intracanal fragment in experimental burst fractures. *Spine* 1988;13:267–271.

Gertzbein SD, Court-Brown CM: Flexion-distraction injuries of the lumbar spine: Mechanisms of injury and classification. *Clin Orthop* 1988;227:52–60.

Greene KA, Dickman CA, Marciano FF, Drabier J, Drayer BP, Sonntag VK: Transverse atlantal ligament disruption associated with odontoid fracture. *Spine* 1994;19:2307–2314.

Hadley MN, Browner CM, Liu SS, Sonntag VK: New subtype of acute odontoid fractures (type IIA). *Neurosurgery* 1988;22: 67–71.

Levine AM, Edwards CC: The management of traumatic spondylolisthesis of the axis. *J Bone Joint Surg* 1985;67A:217–226.

Levitz CL, Reilly PJ, Torg JS: The pathomechanics of chronic, recurrent cervical nerve root neuropraxia: The chronic burner syndrome. *Am J Sports Med* 1997;25:73–76.

McAfee PC, Bohlman HH, Yuan HA: Anterior decompression of traumatic thoracolumbar fractures with incomplete neurological deficit using a retroperitoneal approach. *J Bone Joint Surg* 1985; 67A:89–104.

Meyer SA, Schulte KR, Callaghan JJ, et al: Cervical spinal stenosis and stingers in collegiate football players. *Am J Sports Med* 1994;22:158–166.

Slucky AV, Eismont FJ: Treatment of acute injury of the cervical spine. *J Bone Joint Surg* 1994;76A:1882–1896.

Starr JK, Eismont FJ: Atypical hangman's fractures. *Spine* 1993;18:1954–1957.

Stauffer ES, An HS (eds): *Thoracolumbar Spine Fractures Without Neurological Deficit.* Rosemont, IL, American Academy of Orthopaedic Surgeons, 1993.

Torg JS, Naranja RJ Jr, Pavlov H, Galinat BJ, Warren R, Stine RA: The relationship of developmental narrowing of the cervical spinal canal to reversible and irreversible injury of the cervical spinal cord in football players. *J Bone Joint Surg* 1996; 78A:1308–1314.

Traynelis VC, Marano GD, Dunker RO, Kaufman HH: Traumatic atlanto-occipital dislocation: Case report. *J Neurosurg* 1986; 65:863–870.

Vaccaro AR, An HS, Betz RR, Cotler JM, Balderston RA: The management of acute spinal trauma: Prehospital and in-hospital emergency care, in Springfield DS (ed): *Instructional Course Lectures 46.* Rosemont, IL, American Academy of Orthopaedic Surgeons, 1997, pp 113–125.

Chapter 49
Cervical Degenerative Disk Disorders

Natural History

Cervical spondylosis is a result of disk degeneration and is present in over half of the population by the age of 50 years. Slow loss of water content, proteoglycan changes, and microfissures in the anulus fibrosus and nucleus pulposus result in an altered biomechanical environment for that motion segment. This results in chondro-osseous spur formation at the end plates adjacent to the disk or in the posterior facet joints. Either soft disk herniations or spondylotic changes can result in neck pain alone, radiculopathy syndromes from root compression, or cervical myelopathy from spinal cord compression. The natural history of the cervical radiculopathy generally is favorable, with 1 study documenting only 25% of patients having persistent or worsening symptoms. The natural history of cervical myelopathy generally is not as favorable. Based on natural history observations of Nurick, and Clarke and Robinson, a higher percentage of these patients will slowly deteriorate over time; often this deterioration is in a slow, stepwise fashion and it is believed to depend primarily on the age of the patient and the severity of the compression.

History and Physical Examination

There are 3 main diagnostic categories for patients with degenerative disorders of the cervical spine: (1) axial neck pain alone, (2) cervical radiculopathy, and (3) cervical myelopathy. Radiculopathy is caused by root compression, and patients with this problem have a history of radiating arm pain, with or without weakness and sensory complaints. Usually they have associated neck pain as well, and similar neurologic symptoms of weakness or numbness may predominate without pain, but this is rare. Many patients with cervical radiculopathy

initially have neck pain alone, often without any known antecedent trauma, but within a few days radicular arm symptoms develop. Patients with cervical myelopathy from spinal cord compression may initially note difficulty with gait and balance. They can have weakness in their upper and/or lower extremities that they perceive as difficulty working buttons or climbing stairs. Sensory complaints in the upper extremities also are common, and may be a more global numbness of the hands rather than a dermatomal pattern in radiculopathy patients. Interestingly, approximately 20% of patients with cervical myelopathy have no neck or arm pain whatsoever; this should not dissuade the physician from considering the diagnosis. Bladder and bowel function can be altered in severe cervical myelopathy, although this is a late finding when other symptoms are already established.

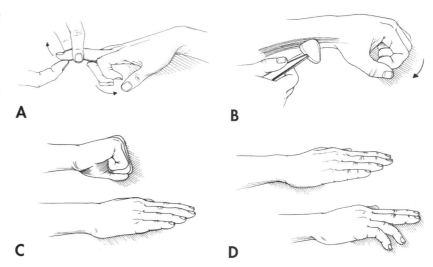

Figure 1

Physical examination findings in cervical myelopathy. A, Hoffman's reflex is elicited by suddenly extending the middle finger distal interphalangeal joint. Production of reflex finger flexion, particularly when asymmetric, is indicative of spinal cord impingement. B, Inverted radial reflex: tapping of the distal brachioradialis tendon produces spastic contraction of the finger flexors. C, Grip and release test: the patient is asked to form a fist and then to release all digits into extension, rapidly repeating the sequence. A normal patient should be able to perform this motion 20 times within a 10-second period. D, Finger escape sign: the patient is asked to hold all digits of the hand in an adducted and extended position. In cases of myelopathy, the 2 ulnar digits will fall into flexion and abduction, usually within 30 seconds. (Reproduced with permission from Simpson SM, Silveri CP: Clinical evaluation of cervical spine disorders, in An HS, Simpson JM (eds): *Surgery of the Cervical Spine.* London, England, Martin Dunitz, 1994, pp 108–109.)

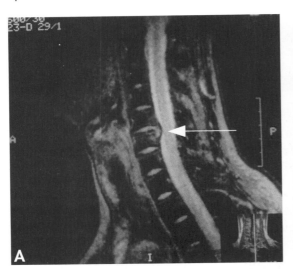
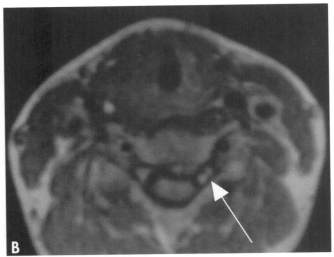

Figure 2

A, Sagittal T2-weighted image of the cervical spine shows a herniated disk at C5-6 (arrow). B, Axial T1-weighted image shows a left sided paracentral herniated disk (arrow).

Physical examination should include neck palpation, range of motion testing, and a full neurologic examination (Fig. 1). Most patients with symptomatic degenerative disk conditions have more pain with neck extension than flexion. With cord compression, however, flexion may produce a Lhermitte's sign, an electric-type shock running down the spinal column. Gait should be tested, specifically toe- and heel-walking and tandem toe-to-heel walking (walking the tightrope), looking for balance difficulty or spasticity consistent with myelopathy. Motor strength testing of the upper and lower extremities may reveal weakness consistent with unilateral root compression as in cervical radiculopathy or a more global weakness in multiple groups more typically seen with moderate to severe myelopathy. Nerve root compression is confirmed by Spurling's sign in which extension and rotation toward the symptomatic side reproduces the radicular symptoms. Sensory examination may show a dermatomal pattern consistent with radiculopathy or more generalized findings of decreased pin prick and even position-sense changes consistent with spinal cord compression. Patients with radiculopathy may or may not have hyporeflexia in the given nerve root distribution.

Myelopathy is an upper motor neuron disorder; thus hyperreflexia and other long-tract signs, such as a positive Hoffmann's clonus and/or Babinski's, may be present. The Hoffmann's reflex is positive when reflex finger and thumb flexion is elicited by sudden extension of the long finger distal interphalangeal joint (Fig. 1, A). Also, patients with spinal cord compression at C6 may exhibit a paradoxical brachioradialis reflex in which tapping the distal brachioradialis tendon elicits a diminished reflex with a reciprocal spastic contraction of the finger flexors; this is known as the inverted radial reflex (Fig. 1, B). Shimizu and associates described the scapulohumeral reflex, which is positive in > 95% of patients with high cervical cord compression. This reflex is elicited by tapping the tip of the spine of the scapula, and the test is positive if there is a brisk scapular elevation and abduction of the humerus. If there has been drop-out of anterior horn cells from cord compression, then a mixed picture of generalized hyperreflexia with absent reflexes at a given level can occur.

The history and physical examination should also be directed toward the possibility of rotator cuff tendinitis and peripheral nerve entrapment syndromes. Rotator cuff tendinitis commonly mimics acute neck pain or C4 or C5 radiculopathy. Pain with forward arm elevation and inability to sleep on the symptomatic side are more consistent with shoulder pathology. Local tenderness, a positive impingement sign, and subacromial lidocaine injection usually can establish this diagnosis. Night pain and numbness in the hand and forearm in the median nerve distribution plus positive Tinel's and Phalen's tests may identify carpal tunnel syndrome rather than cervical radiculopathy. Thoracic outlet syndrome also causes arm pain and numbness (usually in the ulnar nerve distribution because of lower trunk compression over the first rib) and should be considered in the differential diagnosis. Double crush phenomenon is frequent.

Radiographic Evaluation

Plain radiographs, especially the lateral view, best reflect the degree of cervical spondylosis. Simple measurements of the sagittal canal diameter and the sagittal vertebral body distance determine Pavlov's ratio (sagittal canal diameter divided by sagittal diameter of vertebral body); a ratio of 0.8 or less defines a congenitally narrow spinal canal, which puts the patient at a higher risk for cord compression in degenerative disk disorders. Oblique views can show foraminal encroachment from uncovertebral joint hypertrophy. Lateral flexion-extension views are helpful in identifying compensatory subluxation, which is hypermobility of motion segments 1 or 2 levels above the stiff spondylotic levels.

Magnetic resonance imaging (MRI) is the easiest and least invasive method of further evaluating these degenerative conditions. Soft tissues, such as disk herniations and the spinal cord itself, are clearly visible on MRI with good-quality imaging (Fig. 2). Often this is the only study needed for diagnosis and treatment decisions. Plain computed tomography (CT) is not recommended because accurate evaluation of cord or root compression is more difficult. Myelography and CT myelography, however, are excellent ways to look for neural compression, and indeed may give better anatomic information than MRI.

Electrodiagnosis

For most degenerative disk disorders of the cervical spine, electrodiagnostic evaluation is unnecessary. In patients with signs and symptoms of possible cervical radiculopathy, it can be helpful from a differential diagnosis standpoint. Electromyography and/or nerve conduction velocity changes can diagnose peripheral nerve entrapment, such as carpal tunnel syndrome or ulnar cubital tunnel syndrome. Electrodiagnostic evaluation is less helpful but occasionally positive in thoracic outlet syndrome. It is more useful in less common conditions that can be confusing, such as brachial neuritis or mononeuritis multiplex. For patients with neck pain alone or obvious clinical cervical myelopathy, electrodiagnostic studies generally are not indicated.

Treatment

Nonsurgical Treatment
Patients with neck pain alone or cervical radiculopathy usually can be treated with nonsurgical measures. The 3 main conservative treatment modalities for these 2 diagnostic groups are (1) immobilization in a soft cervical collar; (2) anti-inflammatory medications and, at times, oral narcotic pain medications; and (3) physical therapy modalities. The use of a soft cervical collar helps limit the patient's range of motion, which minimizes irritation of the nerve root and relieves paraspinal muscle spasms. Nonsteroidal anti-inflammatory drugs are the first choice for treatment but a short decreasing dosage of oral steroids may be useful for severe radiculopathy. Cervical traction may be helpful in young patients with soft disk herniations but is less successful in patients with spondylosis and should be used carefully in patients with narrow spinal canals. Response to these treatment modalities usually occurs over days to weeks. If no improvement is noted after 2 to 3 months of nonsurgical treatment, these medical measures have probably failed. Severe uncontrollable pain or significant motor weakness may be an indication for earlier surgical intervention.

Epidural steroids, root injections, and facet blocks are used in some centers. These are not used as often in the neck as in the lumbar spine, most likely because the anatomic structures in the neck, such as the spinal cord and the esophagus, make these injections riskier. If considered, they should be performed by an experienced individual trained in these techniques to minimize the risk of complications.

Patients with early cervical myelopathy can be followed closely on an outpatient basis if there are no substantial neurologic deficits and the cord compression is mild to moderate. In patients with gross signs of myelopathy, functional impairment, and significant cord compression, surgical intervention is recommended to prevent deterioration and promote improvement in the neurologic status. A soft cervical collar can help prevent dynamic pinching of the cord and often is used to prevent further damage while awaiting surgical scheduling.

Surgical Treatment

Indications Patients who have neck pain caused by degenerative changes alone without neurologic compression, radiculopathy, or myelopathy are typically treated nonsurgically. Some patients with neck pain alone who have diskogenic pain from significant spondylosis or disk disruption, perhaps from trauma, may benefit from anterior cervical diskectomy and fusion. Some patients have significant spinal stenosis without myelopathy or radicular symptoms, and this stenosis responds well to anterior decompression and fusion.

The largest group of patients who may benefit from surgery are those with cervical radiculopathy. Indications include patients in whom medical management has failed and those with significant neurologic deficit, particularly weakness.

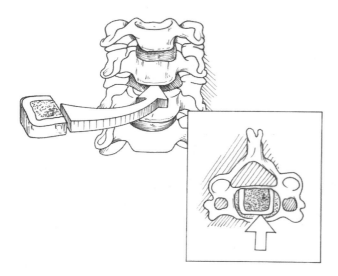

Figure 3

Anterior cervical diskectomy and fusion with insertion of tricortical iliac crest graft. (Reproduced with permission from Herkowitz HN: Surgical management of cervical radiculopathy, in Rothman RH, Simeone FA (eds): *The Spine*. Philadelphia, PA, WB Saunders, 1992, pp 597–608.)

Patients with moderate to severe cervical myelopathy are good candidates for surgical intervention to prevent neurologic deterioration and to promote neurologic as well as functional improvement. The natural history of myelopathy is not as favorable as that of radiculopathy, and nonsurgical measures are limited. The diagnosis, of course, must be confirmed with neuroradiologic imaging, which also provides a detailed map of the pathoanatomy needed for appropriate surgical decision-making.

Anterior Approach Because most of the compressive pathology in the cervical spine, such as disk herniations, spondylosis, or ossification of the posterior longitudinal ligament, is anterior to the cord, the anterior approach has become widely used for surgical treatment for these conditions. Anterior decompression allows direct observation of the pathology and direct removal of the anterior cord compression. This procedure needs to be followed by some sort of stabilization, usually with iliac or fibular grafts for arthrodesis. If the compressive pathology is limited to the disk space, then an anterior cervical diskectomy and fusion at the appropriate levels is recommended (Fig. 3). This procedure involves curettage of the disk space and removal of all disk material back to the posterior longitudinal ligament and out lateral to the uncovertebral joints. Burring of the end plates is strongly recommended to provide a raw bleeding surface of subchondral

bone to help promote fusion. Autogenous Robinson-type tricortical horseshoe grafts also are recommended over allograft or dowel-type grafts. Postoperative bracing is used, typically with a soft collar after 1-level diskectomy and fusion procedures and a 2-poster type brace after multilevel procedures.

Patients with cervical myelopathy (and occasionally those with radiculopathy) often have compressive pathology behind the vertebral bodies. This can be a soft disk that has tracked behind the body, but is more commonly associated with large osteophyte changes or ossification of the posterior longitudinal ligament. Cervical kyphosis also may contribute to compression behind the bodies. The anterior procedure needed for safe and adequate decompression in these patients is cervical corpectomy followed by strut fusion. This procedure is a subtotal vertebrectomy with a channeling out of the midportion of the vertebral body as well as the disks above and below (Fig. 4). The vertebra is removed from in between the uncovertebral joints and back to the posterior longitudinal ligament. Any ossification of the posterior longitudinal ligament should be removed as well so that the dura can reexpand, thus decompressing the cord. Multilevel corpectomies commonly are needed for patients with severe cervical spondylotic myelopathy. Iliac strut grafts usually are used for 1-level corpectomies, but fibular strut grafts are recommended for multilevel corpectomies (Fig. 4). These procedures are technically demanding in this high-risk population and require significant experience to be done safely. Use of spinal cord monitoring for most of these patients is strongly recommended.

Results In a series of 122 patients with long-term follow-up, approximately 80% had overall pain relief, and 90% had full neurologic recovery. Others have reported similar success with anterior cervical diskectomy and fusion for radiculopathy. Pain relief, motor recovery, gait improvement, and functional improvement also have been shown to be significant after adequate anterior decompression and arthrodesis procedures in patients with myelopathy. The most important prognostic factor is the severity of preoperative myelopathy. Other factors include the amount of cord compression based on cross-sectional imaging and the age of the patient.

Posterior Surgical Procedures Laminotomy/foraminotomy is an option for treatment for a lateral soft disk herniation. This procedure is most appropriate for patients with radiculopathy without significant neck pain. If there is an associated segmental kyphosis, an anterior approach is preferred. The keyhole foraminotomy does not destabilize the spine, and with appropriate surgical technique a lateral soft disk hernia-

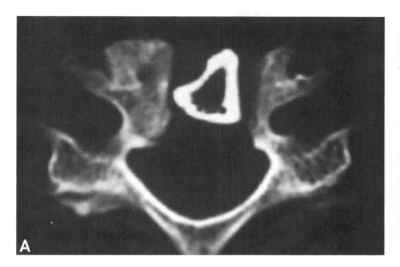

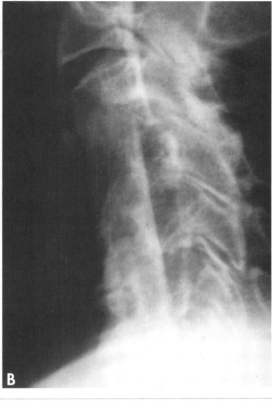

Figure 4

A, A computed tomography scan following subtotal multilevel corpectomy and fibular strut grafting. Note the decompression of the spinal canal and the fibular graft in cross section. B, A lateral radiograph of the same patient showing a healed, remodeled graft from C3 to C7.

tion fragment can be removed without the need for any stabilization procedure. This procedure also may be useful for patients with cervical spondylotic radiculopathy. Removal of the osteophyte or disk is not always necessary because adequate foraminotomy alone can decompress the nerve root.

For many years, laminectomy has been used to treat patients with cervical spondylosis and canal stenosis. Short-term neurologic recovery has typically been good with this procedure; however, longer-term follow-up has documented postlaminectomy kyphosis as a problem in some patients after multilevel laminectomies. Laminectomy plus fusion with or without lateral mass plating can avoid postlaminectomy kyphosis.

Laminoplasty was developed in the 1970s in Japan as an alternative to laminectomy for treatment of canal stenosis that typically is a result of ossification of the posterior longitudinal ligament, which is common in Asians. Laminoplasty is a canal-expanding procedure of which there are many variations. The goal is to enlarge the canal by opening up the lamina either in the midline or unilaterally in trap-door fashion (Fig. 5). This procedure gives more room in the spinal canal, thereby relieving cord compression, yet maintains bony architecture posteriorly so that the paraspinal muscula-

ture can heal to the posterior elements and help prevent late kyphosis. Because laminoplasty relies on indirect decompression of the spinal cord, relatively normal cervical lordosis is required to achieve this goal. Most patients with preoperative cervical kyphosis are best treated by anterior decompression and fusion. Laminectomy or laminoplasty generally is performed from C3 to C7 to produce posterior migration of the spinal cord.

Complications Complications can generally be divided into 4 categories: (1) approach-related, (2) intraoperative, (3) early postoperative, and (4) late postoperative. Anterior approach-related problems include esophageal injury, recurrent laryngeal nerve injury, superior laryngeal nerve injury, and stretch of the sympathetic chain resulting in a Horner's syndrome. All of these injuries are uncommon and usually recoverable. Intraoperative complications from the anterior approach include root or cord injury, vertebral artery injury, spinal fluid leaks, and graft placement problems. Posterior approaches also have a risk of neurologic injury to the spinal cord or nerve roots as well as violation of the dura. Early postoperative complications include graft dislodgment or collapse, wound infection of the surgical site or the bone graft

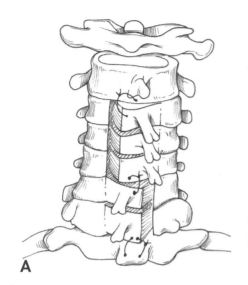

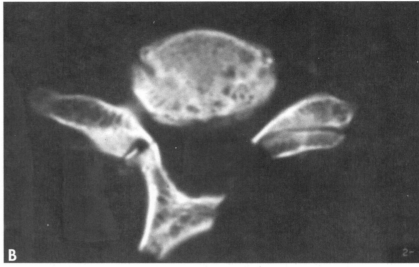

Figure 5

A, One method (Chiba University) of open-door laminoplasty. C3 through C5 are opened one way and C6 and C7, the opposite way. Sutures as shown will prevent closing down of the trap doors. B, Postoperative computed tomography scan showing 1 level of a laminoplasty. Note the trap-door opening of the lamina hinged on 1 side, with enlargement of the spinal canal.

harvest site, and hematoma formation. Late problems after anterior arthrodesis procedures include nonunion and adjacent-level disease. Multilevel posterior procedures run a risk of late instability with kyphosis or subluxation, as mentioned earlier.

Controversies

Controversy exists about the use of an anterior or posterior approach in the treatment of patients with cervical myelopathy from spondylosis or ossification of the posterior longitudinal ligament. Patients with preoperative cervical kyphosis are not believed to be candidates for posterior laminectomy or laminoplasty because the cord will stay draped over the kyphotic area, resulting in persistent anterior spinal cord compression. These patients respond best to anterior decompression, usually multilevel corpectomies depending on the pathoanatomy present, followed by strut fusion. In patients with normal lordosis and no preoperative instability, a laminectomy (or laminectomy plus facet fusion) or a laminoplasty have their proponents. Some authors prefer the anterior approach for 1- or 2-level disease and posterior procedures for 3- or more level disease. Anterior procedures seem to produce better relief of axial neck pain, yet have a small but definite risk of graft complications. Laminoplasty avoids potential graft complications, but is an indirect method of decompression, is not as reliable in relieving neck pain, and still results in some loss of motion.

The use of autograft versus allograft for anterior arthrode-

sis also remains controversial. Most authors believe autograft has a higher union rate, particularly in multilevel procedures, with a low but definite possibility of donor-site morbidity, such as wound infection or chronic pain. Anterior plating for internal fixation after anterior grafting procedures for degenerative conditions of the neck has increased in popularity over the last few years. Current use favors anterior plate fixation to increase the union rate for 3-level anterior diskectomy and fusion procedures and possibly 2-level anterior cervical diskectomy and fusion procedures (Fig. 6), although for this latter group the data is insufficient at this time. The union

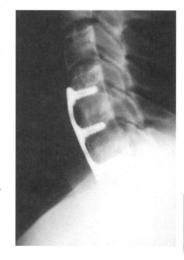

Figure 6

Anterior plating following a 2-level anterior cervical diskectomy and fusion.

Chapter 50
Thoracic Disk Herniation

Incidence

The incidence of thoracic disk herniation has been estimated to range from 1 in 10,000 to 1 in a million. Magnetic resonance imaging (MRI) has helped increase this estimate because it has identified previously unrecognized herniated thoracic disks. In studies of large numbers of people it was found that almost 40% of otherwise asymptomatic individuals had some radiographic criteria of herniated disks. All remained asymptomatic at an average follow-up of 26 months. The size of the disk herniation has not been shown to correlate with clinical symptoms.

In general, fewer than 1% of all clinically relevant disk herniations occur in the thoracic spine, and most of these are located between T8 and T12 (Fig. 1).

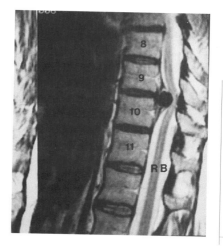

Figure 1

A sagittal magnetic resonance image demonstrates an extruded herniated disk between the T9 and T10 vertebral bodies. There is considerable stenosis of the spinal canal and resultant spinal cord compression. The patient has clinical thoracic level myelopathy on examination.

Classification

Thoracic disk herniations are classified by location and level as are herniations in other areas of the spine. They may be central, lateral, central-lateral, or, rarely, intradural. Although some correlation exists between the location and the type of disk herniation and the symptoms it produces, there are no rigid guidelines for distinction. For instance, central disk herniations typically cause myelopathy, but may cause radiating low back, radicular, pseudoradicular, or referred pain. Most lateral disk herniations cause radiculopathy or localized paraspinal pain. Although classifications can help determine treatment, the most important consideration is anterior spinal cord compression, which mandates an anterior decompressive procedure. A lateral herniation can be treated through a limited posterior approach, but the presence of posterior compression, such as an ossified ligament flavum, necessitates a laminectomy or laminoplasty.

Etiology

As in the cervical and lumbar spine, the etiologies of thoracic disk herniations are diverse and include torsion, repetitive twisting or overhead lifting activities, athletic pursuits, and activities such as sneezing or coughing that are associated

with increased Valsalva maneuvers. Some individuals report no inciting event before the onset of symptoms. Coexistent problems (hyperostotic calcification disorders, ossification of the yellow ligament, or ossification of the posterior longitudinal ligament) confound the symptoms.

Clinical Presentation

Herniated thoracic disks cause many different symptoms, including back pain alone, thoracic radiculopathy, pseudoradicular signs and symptoms (nondescript low back, radiating buttock and leg pains in the absence of definable lumbar pathology), and thoracic myelopathy. The myelopathy can vary from subtle motor and sensory changes to florid paraparesis with bowel and bladder incontinence, broad based gait, ataxia, and differential spasticity.

Most recent literature suggests that the signs and symptoms of herniated thoracic disks are nonspecific. In particular, the physical examination should evaluate for localized tenderness and sensory changes that correlate with neuroradiologic imaging. A careful lumbar spinal examination, looking for sciatic notch tenderness, the presence of femoral stretch signs, and other stigmata of lumbar radiculopathy should be made. Proximal weakness, especially of the hip flexors, should be noted. Differential spasticity, which indicates a thoracic level spinal cord lesion, is evaluated by comparing the quality and briskness of the deep tendon reflexes and clonus in the upper and lower extremities. Although other central nervous system findings could explain differential spasticity, its presence should alert the examiner to a potential thoracic level lesion. Changes in proprioception also should be investigated. Occasionally, the coexistence of demyelinating disorders with herniated thoracic disks further confounds the clinical assessment.

Demyelinating disorders, intradural neoplasms, more global central nervous system problems such as multiple sclerosis, or associated cervical lesions can cause symptoms of lower extremity dysfunction secondary to an upper motor neuron lesion. Nonspinal disorders with referred symptoms include intracardiac, pericardial, and pulmonary diseases.

Imaging Studies

MRI is the diagnostic study of choice for herniated thoracic disks. In patients who are not appropriate candidates for thoracic MRI, such as those with cardiac pacemakers or metal implants, computed tomography can be used. Both tests may be necessary when localization of the level is difficult and dystrophic calcification, such as ossification of the yellow ligament, is present.

Other studies, such as thoracic diskography, are helpful in characterizing pain response. Diskography is controversial, and the information may be somewhat inconclusive. However, in appropriate circumstances it can provide important localizing information, particularly when multilevel degenerative disk disease is present and when various gradations of severity of disk herniations are present. Central disk herniations with spinal cord compression or eccentric cord compression with predominantly nerve root compression represent diagnostic dilemmas. Thoracic diskography may prove helpful in identifying those with amplified pain syndrome and those with clear-cut focal degenerative painful thoracic disk disease. The findings of relatively painless disks associated with 1 or perhaps 2 levels of concordantly painful disks on provocative injection may provide further information to determine if anterior fusion with or without spinal canal decompression, posterior fusion, or anterior/posterior fusion is applicable because of coexistent deformity.

Nonsurgical Treatment

Nonsurgical treatment can be used in patients without progressive spinal cord signs or symptoms. A short course of limitation of activity coupled with bracing and gentle mobilization and physical therapy may be effective. Pain management could consist of nonsteroidal anti-inflammatory or narcotic medications. Selective nerve blocks can be performed to accurately localize the symptomatic disk level and to provide relief of the radicular pain. Occasionally, long-term relief is obtained with injections. Erector spinae muscle strengthening, postural awareness, and generalized aerobic conditioning are used along with physical therapy modalities.

Surgical Treatment

The only absolute indication for surgery is progressive neurologic deficit. Intractable pain, unrelenting radiculopathy, or significant pseudoradicular symptoms are relative indications for surgery.

Surgery for localized axial pain warrants caution. If the pain is well localized, and the level of pain is well correlated with imaging or diskographic abnormalities, a localized fusion can be done (Fig. 2). However, surgical results for axial pain are less predictable than for radiculopathy or myelopathy.

The treatment of thoracic deformity or instability, particularly that associated with Scheuermann's disease, requires systematic preoperative assessment to clarify the extent of surgery. If the deformity is the significant component of the clinical presentation, localized fusion will fail.

A variety of surgical approaches to decompress the spinal canal have been described, including costotransversectomy, lateral extracavitary approach, transpedicular approach, transthoracic approach, laminectomy, and thoracoscopic approach.

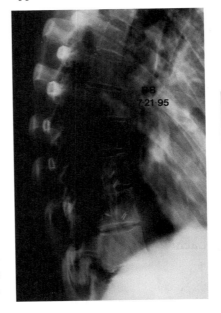

Figure 2

A postoperative lateral radiograph demonstrates the changes from a transthoracic decompression and fusion. Approximately one fourth of the inferior portion of T9 and one fourth of the superior portion of T10 were removed in addition to the disk and end plate to achieve spinal canal decompression. Multiple rib grafts were impacted into carefully created mortises for achieving a fusion.

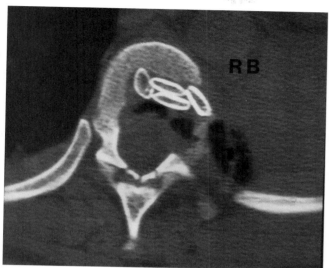

Figure 3

A postoperative computed tomography scan demonstrating a complete base of pedicle to base of pedicle decompression. The spinal canal is completely decompressed and numerous bone grafts have been inserted for fusion purposes.

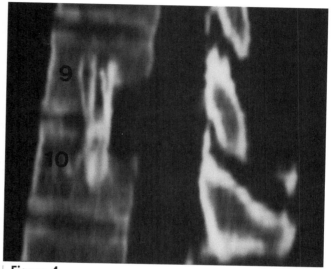

Figure 4

A sagittal reformation of the computed tomography data demonstrating the extent of vertebral body and end plate resection needed for complete canal decompression. The bone grafts are "stacked" to graft the intervertebral space as much as possible; in addition, the residual disk space anterior to the struts is debrided and grafted with morcellized bone.

Costotransversectomy or Posterolateral Extracavitary Approach

A costotransversectomy is a posterolateral approach that involves making a generous incision lateral to the spinal column. The medial portions of 2 or 3 ribs are removed, and the surgery does not violate the chest cavity itself. It provides good lateral exposure of the vertebral bodies and the lateral portion of the disk, but it has limited anterior exposure. Lateral extracavitary approach is another extrapleural approach with reasonable exposure of the anterior and lateral aspects of the vertebrae and disks.

Transpedicular Approach

The transpedicular approach is a limited excision of posterior lamina, facet joint, and pedicle, through which it provides lateral and subsequent posterolateral exposure of the spinal canal. The exposure is adequate for most lateral disk herniations. To fully decompress the spinal canal, a cavity is created within the vertebral body and the disk space lateral to the spinal cord (Fig. 3). All dissection is done laterally and anteriorly away from the spinal cord. Complications may occur because of the limitations of exposure from the back to the front approach.

Transthoracic Approach

A transthoracic approach is the standard approach for thoracic disk herniation and allows for good anterior exposure of all lateral and anterior disk herniations. It involves a par-

tial resection of the vertebral body and the disk, and is useful for a thorough side-to-side disk resection, particularly when the disk is calcified (Fig. 4). Typically, the approach is done from the right side for the upper thoracic region because of the aortic arch on the left, and the approach is done from the left for the lower thoracic region because the aorta is more tolerant to surgical manipulation than the vena cava. In terms of blood supply to the spinal cord, segmental vessel ligation generally is safe as long as it is carried out away from the intervertebral foramen. Anterior instrumentation can be used to stabilize a fusion if more stability is necessary. The instrumentation should be applied laterally away from the great vessels, and low profile instrumentation should be used. Disadvantages of thoracotomy include the need for rib resection and postoperative pain. The advantages include wide surgical exposure and safety in complete visualization of the spinal canal.

Laminectomy

Laminectomy generally is contraindicated for thoracic disk herniation because of the need for extensive cord mobilization to provide suitable exposure of the disk herniation. Laminectomy approaches to thoracic disk herniations have resulted in an unacceptably high rate of paraplegia. Therefore, unless extenuating circumstances exist, the laminectomy approach for routine thoracic disk herniations should be avoided.

Thorascopic Diskectomy

Thorascopic spinal canal decompression and fusion is evolving in its technical feasibility and, in skilled hands, can lower the overall morbidity from an anterior approach. This approach allows excellent visualization and assured spinal canal decompression. Anterior instrumentation can also be done at the same time if necessary, using specialized instrumentation. The patients clearly have less postoperative morbidity than after thoracotomy. Surgical times in early reports have been long, but this should improve with increased experience.

Wood KB, Garvey TA, Gundry C, Heithoff KB: Magnetic resonance imaging of the thoracic spine: Evaluation of asymptomatic individuals. *J Bone Joint Surg* 1995;77A:1631–1638.

This study reviewed MRI studies of the thoracic spines of 90 asymptomatic individuals to determine the prevalence of abnormal anatomic findings. Sixty-six (73%) of the 90 asymptomatic individuals had positive findings at one level or more. These findings included herniation of a disk in 33 (37%), bulging of a disk in 48 (53%), an annular tear in 52 (58%), deformation of the spinal cord in 26 (29%), and Scheuermann's end-plate irregularities or kyphosis in 34 (38%). This study underscores the importance of clinical correlation when interpreting MRI of the thoracic spine.

Annotated Bibliography

Jho HD: Endoscopic microscopic transpedicular thoracic discectomy: Technical note. *J Neurosurg* 1997;87:125–129.

In an effort to make thoracic diskectomy simple and less invasive while using direct visualization, a 70° -angled lens endoscope has been adopted to view the ventral aspect of the spinal cord dura mater during microsurgical thoracic diskectomy via a transpedicular approach. Patients with myelopathy are kept overnight in the hospital; however, those with radiculopathy are sent home on the same day as their operation.

Regan JJ, Mack JM, Picetti GD III: A technical report on video-assisted thoracoscopy in thoracic spinal surgery: Preliminary description. *Spine* 1995;20:831–837.

Video-assisted thoracoscopic surgery was performed in 12 thoracic spinal patients (herniated nucleus pulposus, infection, tumor, or spinal deformity). The results showed little postoperative pain, short intensive care unit and hospital stays, and little or no morbidity. In the short follow-up period, there was neither postthoracotomy pain syndrome nor neurologic sequelae in these patients. Time in surgery decreased dramatically as experience was gained with the procedure. Given consistently improving surgical skills, a number of thoracic spinal procedures using video-assisted thoracoscopic surgery, including thoracic diskectomy, internal rib thoracoplasty, anterior osteotomy, corpectomy, and fusion, can be performed safely with no additional surgical time or risk to the patient.

Wood KB, Blair JM, Aepple DM, et al: The natural history of asymptomatic thoracic disc hernations. *Spine* 1997;22: 525–529.

MRI was used to determine the natural history of asymptomatic thoracic disk herniations. Twenty patients with 48 asymptomatic thoracic disk hernations previously diagnosed with MRI underwent repeat MRI after a mean follow-up period of 26 months. All patients remained asymptomatic during the follow-up period. Asymptomatic disk herniations may change in size but the patients usually remain asymptomatic. There was a trend for small disk herniations either to remain unchanged or to increase in size and for large disk herniations to decrease in size.

Classic Bibliography

Blumenkopf B: Thoracic intervertebral disc hernations: Diagnostic value of magnetic resonance imaging. *Neurosurgery* 1988;23:36–40.

Bohlman HH, Zdeblick TA: Anterior excision of herniated thoracic discs. *J Bone Joint Surg* 1088;70A:1038–1047.

Brown CW, Deffer PA Jr, Akmakjian J, Donalson DH, Brugman JL: The natural history of thoracic disc hernation. *Spine* 1992;17(suppl 6):S95–S102.

Currier BL, Eismont FJ, Green BA: Transthoracic disc excision and fusion for herniated thoracic discs. *Spine* 1994;19: 323–328.

Dietze DD Jr, Fessler RG: Thoracic disc herniations. *Neurosurg Clin N Am* 1993;4:75–90.

Fidler MW, Goedhart ZD: Excision of prolapse of thoracic intervertebral disc: A transthoracic technique. *J Bone Joint Surg* 1984;66B:518–522.

Otani K, Yoshida M, Fujii E, Nakai S, Shibasaki K: Thoracic disc hernation: Surgical treatment in 23 patients. *Spine* 1988;13: 1262–1267.

Rogers MA, Crockard HA: Surgical treatment of the symptomatic herniated thoracic disk. *Clin Orthop* 1994;300:70–78.

Ross JS, Perez-Reyes N, Masaryk TJ, Bohlman H, Modic MT: Thoracic disk herniations: MR imaging. *Radiology* 1987;165: 511–515.

Schellhas KP, Pollei SR, Dorwart RH: Thoracic discography: A safe and reliable technique. *Spine* 1994;19:2103–2109.

Simpson JM, Silveri CP, Simeone FA, Balderston RA, An HS: Thoracic disc herniation. Re-evaluation of the posterior approach using a modified costotransversectomy. *Spine* 1993;18: 1872–1877.

Chapter 51
Lumbar Degenerative Disorders

Low Back Pain

Despite a wealth of research concerning risk factors, pathophysiology, prognostic indicators, and treatment methods, low back pain continues to be an epidemic, yet poorly understood, problem. The lifetime prevalence of low back pain is estimated at 50% to 80%, with 2% to 5% of people affected yearly. Low back pain is the most common cause of disability in persons younger than 45 years of age and second only to arthritis in patients 45 to 60 years of age. Although only 15% to 20% of those affected seek medical attention, the annual fiscal expenditure for health care and disability approaches $100 billion, reflecting an inappropriate amount of unwarranted medical care and wide variations in diagnosis and treatment methods.

Acute low back problems are defined as activity intolerance due to low back or back-related leg symptoms lasting less than 3 months. Most low back problems are considered nonspecific because no discernible etiology can be established by conventional diagnostic measures. Up to 97% are ascribed to soft-tissue strain or sprain, while fewer than 5% result from more serious underlying conditions. Because 90% of low back pain resolves within 1 month, an extensive workup in that time frame is not warranted. Socioeconomic and psychological issues must not be overlooked as contributing to a person's manifestation of symptoms and response to therapy.

Whereas no risk factors have been rigidly linked to the development of low back pain, weaker links exist for certain individual, biomechanical, and psychosocial qualities, including obesity, smoking, gender, heavy lifting, vibrational stresses, prolonged sitting, and job dissatisfaction. Because the management of low back pain often is initiated in a primary care setting, the future validation of potential risk factors may allow predisposed patients to adopt early preventive strategies, reducing the prevalence of this disorder.

Although recognized as a probable cause of low back pain, disk degeneration has never been scientifically correlated with the development or persistence of symptoms. Nevertheless, the identification of sinuvertebral and sympathetic nerves located in the outer layers of the anulus fibrosus has fostered a recent interest in the role of biomechanical and biochemical factors in producing both localized and referred pain. Further details on the effects of inflammatory peptides

on both disk structure and localized nerve fibers and roots are discussed in the following section on herniated disks. Inflammatory mediators also may contribute to the pain associated with facet arthrosis, a sequela of severe symptomatic disk degeneration, which resembles osteoarthritis of other major joints. Histologic and biochemical studies of arthritic facet joints reveal denuded articular cartilage demonstrating vascular ingrowth and expression of the biochemically active pain peptide, substance P.

In 1994, the Agency for Health Care Policy and Research (AHCPR) amassed a multidisciplinary panel to address existing confusion on the management of low back pain that stems from reported wide variations in diagnosis and treatment strategies. Although flawed by a deficiency of outcomes-based studies, their published *Clinical Practice Guidelines* on "Acute Low Back Pain Problems in Adults" remains a valuable science-based reference assembled from a critical review and synthesis of existing valid evidence. Recent reviews of randomized clinical trials of various conservative treatment strategies generally agree with AHCPR's recommendations, suggesting that the algorithms defined by this panel represent the most current and empiric basis on which more standardized management approaches can be based.

The initial assessment of a patient with low back pain should begin with a detailed history to define the problem's quality and duration, and to gain insight into nonphysical issues and expectations that may complicate management. The physical examination should aim to elicit neurologic deficits and possible nonspinal pathology involving the thorax, abdomen, or pelvis. Clinicians should strictly attend to signs or symptoms of nonmechanical pain that point to a more serious etiology. Findings suggestive of a tumor include constitutional symptoms, a history of cancer, and night pain. Recent bacterial infection, urinary tract manipulation, immunosuppression, or intravenous drug use should raise the suspicion of infection, including the possibility of an abscess. Fractures are suggested by a history of minor or major trauma such as from a fall or motor vehicle accident. Signs of cauda equina syndrome include bowel and bladder dysfunction, severe lower extremity neurologic deficit, saddle anesthesia, and anal sphincter laxity.

Imaging studies are obtained for findings suggestive of serious spinal pathology, evidence of tissue insult, and of specific neurologic deficit. In the last case, imaging is used only after failed conservative treatment, when surgery is being considered for a persistent loss of neurologic function. Laboratory studies such as complete blood count (CBC), erythrocyte sedimentation rate (ESR), and uric acid (UA) may be useful to rule out a tumor or infection. Bone scans also may aid in the detection of tumors, infection, or occult fractures. Neurophysiologic tests, such as electromyography and somatosensory evoked potentials, are appropriate when neurologic deficits are not clearly defined by routine assessment and imaging studies. Although these tests cannot accurately define the precise level of deficits, they are valuable for excluding distal nerve damage and myelopathy.

Barring any "red flags" in the initial assessment, the management of low back pain should aim to facilitate a return to function and prevent prolonged disability. Patient education on a likely recovery and activity modification should be combined with medications to alleviate pain. Acetaminophen and nonsteroidal anti-inflammatory drugs (NSAIDs) are recommended oral agents, whereas muscle relaxants are no longer considered effective in treating back pain. Opioids, although an optional treatment, are discouraged because of the potential for adverse side effects and dependence. Bed rest should be limited to 2 to 4 days, after which aerobic exercises are recommended for muscle strengthening and general conditioning. Prolonged bed rest promotes deconditioning and disability and should be avoided. Spinal manipulation is optional only in the first 4 weeks and is contraindicated by the presence of sciatica. Other treatment modalities, including massage, diathermy, ultrasound, cutaneous laser treatment, biofeedback, transcutaneous electrical nerve stimulation, and traction, have no proven efficacy in the treatment of low back pain.

The role of epidural steroids in the treatment of both nondiskogenic and diskogenic low back pain remains controversial, with few controlled data. The alleged benefit of epidural steroids stems from their ability to reduce inflammation around nerve roots as herniated material elicits an immune response. While evidence suggests that such inflammation contributes to the generation of low back pain, limited data preclude a definitive association between steroid injection and successful outcome. The beneficial effects of epidural steroids diminish over time, with studies reporting continued pain relief in only 7% of patients at 6 months. The AHCPR guidelines suggest a possible role for epidural steroids in delaying the need for surgical intervention by managing acute pain associated with a radiculopathy. They further recommend against epidural steroids in back pain without objective findings suggestive of nerve root compression. These recommendations are based on limited empiric

evidence, and such an absence of controlled data limits any validity in outlining specific indications for the use of this treatment. Surgery for diskogenic low back pain generally is less predictable and should be considered as a last resort.

Herniated Disk

Epidemiology, Prognosis, and Treatment Indications

Herniated disks represent a limited and defined subset of patients with low back pain whose financial impact on the health care system is a fraction of that of nonspecific cases. Determination of the prevalence of disk herniation is complicated by the finding that 20% to 35% of working-age adults have evidence of herniation by magnetic resonance imaging (MRI); however, estimates report a lifetime prevalence of 2%. A wide variability in the treatment of this disorder exists in the United States, where the incidence of surgical intervention is 160/100,000. Given the favorable prognosis for nonsurgical management, many of these operations are likely inappropriate and reflect regional differences in patient and physician expectations.

As a normal consequence of aging, intervertebral disks undergo degenerative changes, marked by dehydration of the nucleus pulposus with depletion of the proteoglycan content. Progressive fibrillation, separation, and tearing of annular fibers from prolonged axial and shear stress may result in a complete radial annular tear. Such damage to the structural integrity potentiates displacement of nuclear, annular, or end plate material beyond the margins of adjacent vertebral end plates. Disk material that remains beneath an intact outer anulus defines a constrained herniation or disk protrusion. Disk extrusion implies violation of the outer annular fibers. Depending on the integrity of the posterior longitudinal ligament (PLL), extrusions can be further classified as subligamentous and transligamentous. Separation of material from the parent disk describes a sequestered fragment. Sequestered material may penetrate the PLL or peridural membrane and come to lie in the epidural space.

Most lumbar disk herniations occur between 30 and 50 years of age and may result in back pain and pain radiating down the leg in the distribution of affected nerve roots. The pathophysiology of sciatic pain likely involves both mechanical and biochemical factors. Recent investigations have begun to clarify the role of inflammatory mediators in disk degeneration and nerve root irritation. Extruded disk material can elicit an immune response characterized by the infiltration of macrophages and secretion of various cytokines, including interleukin-1 (IL-1), IL-6, nitric oxide, and prostaglandins. Through local autocrine and paracrine mechanisms, the tissue effects of these cytokines include: (1) direct stimulation of nerve endings in the anulus, ligaments, dorsal root ganglion, spinal nerve, and dura; (2) sensitization of nociceptors in the anulus; (3) promotion of the loss of proteoglycans from nuclear material by disruption of the equilibrium between proteolytic enzymes and their natural inhibitors; and (4) neovascularization, which promotes persistence of inflammation at the site of extrusion.

Symptoms of sciatica also may relate to the local anatomy of the spinal canal and neural foramina. Stenosis of both the canal and lateral recess reduces the space that can accommodate herniated material, making mechanical compression against adjacent structures more likely. Migration of sequestered disk material into a stenotic lateral recess exacerbates the effect of stenosis on neural structures.

The natural history of lumbar disk herniation shows a favorable response to conservative treatment, even in the presence of neurologic deficit; thus, an isolated neurologic deficit without function-impairing pain does not warrant surgical intervention. Several studies have shown that most herniated disks resorb over time, particularly large and extruded herniated disks. Conservative measures should be instituted for 6 weeks before considering surgery. For patients with persistent pain and neurologic compromise unresponsive to conservative measures, surgery should not be delayed beyond 6 months because of the risks of chronic disability. Outcome studies have yet to determine the true optimal duration of conservative treatment or the type of herniation, canal location, or concomitant pathology as they relate to the efficacy of nonsurgical treatment.

The differences in outcome between surgical and nonsurgical treatment are not known because of lack of appropriate outcome studies. The reported superior benefit of surgery in the first year likely reflects the rapid relief of symptoms from decompression. Interval comparisons also report better outcomes after surgery with no difference after 10 years.

Proper patient selection for surgical treatment is fundamental to the immediate and long-term success of restoring function. Candidates for surgery should exhibit a clinical syndrome and unequivocal lesion by imaging that corresponds anatomically with a specific root level. Comorbid conditions should be weighed carefully when considering the benefits of surgery, especially systemic disorders with a known neurologic component. Diabetic peripheral neuropathy will not improve after lumbar decompression.

Although no predictors of outcome have been validated by randomized controlled trials, the decision to operate can be based on certain absolute and relative indications. Accepted absolute indications include cauda equina syndrome (Fig. 1)

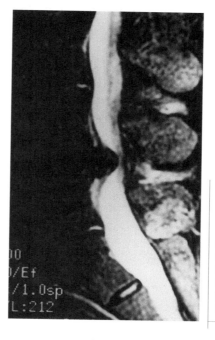

Figure 1

Midsagittal magnetic resonance image of a 54-year-old woman presenting with cauda equina syndrome. This image demonstrates a massive L4-5 disk herniation with near-complete obliteration of the spinal canal. The patient underwent immediate surgical decompression.

and rapidly progressing motor deficit. Intractable pain that does not correlate with a specific anatomic lesion is not an absolute indication. Relative indications include (1) persistent sciatica and/or neurologic deficits despite 6 weeks of conservative therapy, (2) recurrent sciatica and/or neurologic deficits, (3) significant motor deficit with positive sciatic tension signs, and (4) disk herniation into a stenotic canal.

Optimal treatment for acute motor weakness without pain remains controversial. Despite obvious neurologic impairment, the absence of debilitating symptoms favors conservative treatment modalities over surgical intervention initially. There is no evidence to suggest that surgical decompression of an inciting lesion will lead to a more timely recovery of nerve function than nonsurgical care. If the motor weakness is functionally significant and no improvement is noted over a few weeks, surgical decompression may become an option.

Preoperative Investigations

Spinal imaging studies should be used only to confirm the clinical diagnosis when surgical intervention is considered. MRI has become the test of choice for assessing degenerative or herniated disks. Diagnostic and prognostic implications are limited by the MRI finding of disk herniation in 20% to 35% and disk bulging in 56% of asymptomatic adults under age 60 years. The advantages of MRI over computed tomography (CT) include: (1) no radiation, (2) multiplanar imaging, (3) better visualization of the conus medullaris and cauda equina, and (4) information on the physicochemical degenerative changes that precede an alteration in disk contour.

Surgical Options

The goals of surgery are neural decompression and relief of symptoms without harm to surrounding tissues. Proper patient selection is the most important factor in achieving these aims. Disk removal, intended to relieve sciatica, does not restore the normal mechanics of the lumbar spine and should not be undertaken to relieve isolated back pain without evidence of a radiculopathy.

Open diskectomy through a limited laminotomy (Fig. 2) and microdiskectomy remain the gold standard procedures; 90% of properly selected patients experience successful short-term relief of symptoms. Long-term follow-up of these patients, however, reveals a progressive decline in success,

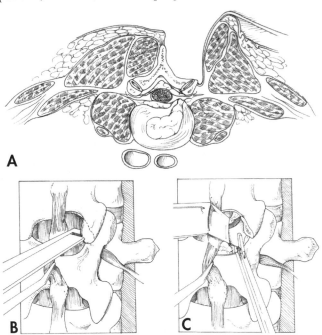

Figure 2

A, Axial view of approach for limited laminotomy-diskectomy showing herniated disk compressing exiting nerve root. Dissection and muscle elevation are limited to the interlaminar level being exposed. (Reproduced with permission from Wood EG, Hanley EN: Lumbar disc herniation and open limited discectomy: Indications, technique, and results. *Oper Tech Orthop* 1991;1:23–28.) B, Entry into the spinal canal is accomplished by removing several millimeters of the cephalad lamina using a high-speed burr. Kerrison rongeurs are used to remove the medial edge of the superior facet, thus removing any lateral recess stenosis and allowing exposure of the lateral disk space. C, Retraction of the nerve root, ligamentum flavum, and epidural fat toward the midline allows exposure to and removal of the disk herniation with pituitary rongeurs. (Reproduced with permission from Hanley EN, Delamarter RB, McCulloch JA, et al: Surgical indications and techniques, in Wiesel SW, Weinstein JN, et al (eds): *The Lumbar Spine*. Philadelphia, PA, WB Saunders, 1996.)

resulting from subsequent degenerative changes. This emphasizes the importance of postsurgical rehabilitation and proper lifelong back care by the patient.

Complications of disk surgery include retained fragments, dural tears, disk space infection, epidural hematoma, and instability. Although various reports have documented a higher infection rate with minimally invasive techniques, the probable cause of these statistics relates more to a surgeon's experience than factors inherent in the equipment and limited exposure. Routine gram-positive antimicrobial prophylaxis is recommended for all surgical patients regardless of the technique used.

Percutaneous Lumbar Diskectomy In recent years, a trend toward the application of minimally invasive techniques has evolved, including percutaneous suction diskectomy, percutaneous laser diskectomy, percutaneous arthroscopic disk decompression, and microendoscopic diskectomy. These techniques have several theoretical advantages over open procedures: (1) shorter hospital stay, (2) decreased epidural scar formation, and (3) preservation of spinal stability. These procedures are limited in the extent to which migrated and/or sequestered fragments can be retrieved or ablated, and proper patient selection is critical to their success. The approach to the L5-S1 disk space is more difficult because of limitations imposed by the iliac crest.

Percutaneous Suction Diskectomy Automated percutaneous lumbar diskectomy (APLD) uses an aspiration and rotary debridement nucleotome to create a window in the nucleus pulposus that reduces intradiskal pressure, allowing herniated material, in theory, to regress back into the confines of the disk space. The mechanism of pain relief after this procedure is unknown because postoperative imaging studies often fail to show changes in the morphology and volume of the herniation. Randomized studies comparing suction diskectomy to other forms of percutaneous lumbar diskectomy and microdiskectomy have revealed inferior results for APLD. Further, success rates based on retrospective studies have been reported as low as 45% at 55 months. Up to 12% of patients may require open diskectomy within 3 months, and the probability of success for these patients is lower compared to those undergoing an original open diskectomy.

Percutaneous Laser Diskectomy The application of laser technology to the treatment of disk herniation involves vaporizing material internal to the disk structure using thin optical fibers to direct the laser beam. The volume of material vaporized depends on the wavelength of the laser energy, and both KTP and Holmium:YAG lasers are currently approved by the U.S. Food and Drug Administration (FDA), and are available in the United States. Although laser diskectomy can desiccate the nucleus pulposus and decrease intradiskal pressure, it cannot obliterate the entire volume of a herniated mass. Only small to moderately sized, contained herniations are appropriate for this approach, and prospective studies show a success rate for relief of radiculopathy from 54% to 72%. Retrospective reviews indicate these rates diminish over time with reoperation rates as high as 35%. The inability of these procedures to treat extruded and sequestered herniations implicates improper patient selection in poorer reported success rates.

Percutaneous Arthroscopic Diskectomy Cadaveric studies have shown that a cannula with an outer diameter of 6.5 mm can be safely inserted into the "triangular working zone" without jeopardizing neighboring neural structures (Fig. 3). With improvements in access to the spinal canal and foramina, most types of herniations can be retrieved, except migrated extraligamentous disk material. Successful removal of herniated disks has been performed for sequestered, extraforaminal, foraminal, and nonmigrated extraligamentous herniations. Outcomes comparable to those of open diskectomy have been reported in the hands of experienced arthroscopic surgeons, but generalizations about the long-term success of this procedure require further outcome studies.

Microendoscopic Diskectomy Microendoscopic diskectomy (MED) combines endoscopic technology with the principles of microdiskectomy, approaching the spinal canal posteriorly through a small 15- to 16-mm incision. The principal advantage of MED over open and microdiskectomy techniques lies in minimizing damage to the paraspinal musculature by using muscle-splitting dilators. Direct visualization of herniated disk material is achieved by performing the laminotomy using an endoscope and a video monitor. Specially designed endoscopic instruments allow removal of the herniated disk in a manner similar to techniques used in traditional diskectomy procedures. As with other newer minimally invasive procedures, MED shows initial promising results in carefully selected patients and in the hands of experienced surgeons. The comparative long-term outcome, however, awaits further investigation. These minimally invasive procedures must be compared to the gold standard of limited laminotomy or microdiskectomy.

Special Situations With a Herniated Disk

Foraminal Disk Herniation Superior and lateral migration of herniated material results in compression and irritation of

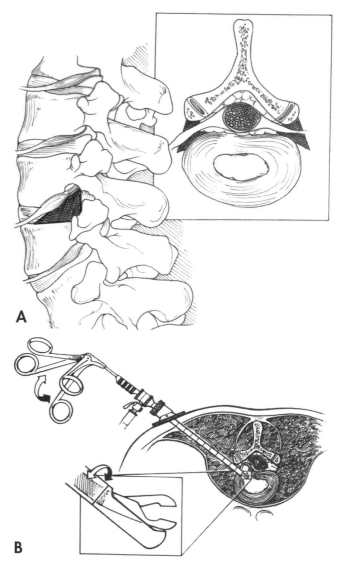

Figure 3

A, The triangular working zone for introduction of arthroscopic instruments. The boundaries include the proximal vertebral plate of the lower lumbar segment inferiorly, the proximal articular process of the lower segment posteriorly, and the spinal nerve anteriorly. B, Lateralization of the skin entry point permits medialization of the inner end of the access cannula adjacent to neural structures, allowing access to and removal of posterior and posterolateral herniations. (Reproduced with permission from Kambin PZ: *AMD System: Surgical Technique.* Memphis, TN, Smith & Nephew, 1996.)

the dorsal root ganglion, termed a foraminal or far lateral herniation (Fig. 4). These herniations, accounting for 3% to 10% of all disk herniations, typically occur in older patients (average age of 50) and from wide disk spaces rather than degenerated spaces. Most foraminal herniations occur at the

L4-5 and L3-4 levels and affect the L4 and L3 roots, respectively. This may result in anterior thigh pain and a markedly positive femoral stretch test rather than the classic symptoms of sciatica. Symptoms often are severe and unresponsive to conservative therapy. Attempts to remove herniated material through the standard interlaminar window may result in damage to the facet joint with destabilization. Hence, some clinicians have advocated an approach through the intertransverse window using Wiltse's paraspinal muscle splitting exposure. This exposure allows full view of the pathology without jeopardizing the nerve root and inferior facet.

Disk Herniation With Spondylolisthesis Herniation most commonly occurs at the level above the slip and is managed according to standard principles of decompression. Herniation at the level of a spondylolisthesis is rare and may indicate developing segmental instability. To minimize the risk of postoperative slip and back pain, disk removal should be accompanied by stabilization of the level.

Herniated Disk With Spinal Stenosis Spinal stenosis, either central or lateral, may be fully asymptomatic or only mildly symptomatic, rendering the detection of a herniated disk by routine assessment and radiographic studies difficult and often confusing. An acute increase in leg pain or weakness on conventional straight leg raising should raise suspicion of this entity. In patients with asymptomatic spinal stenosis with disk herniation, simple diskectomy with or without local canal decompression is the treatment of choice. When spinal stenosis is symptomatic before disk herniation, a wider decompression along with diskectomy is required for successful treatment.

Recurrent Disk Herniation
Initial relief of sciatica after diskectomy carries a 5% chance of recurrence and typically occurs for 1 of 3 reasons. Recurrence within 2 to 15 days of surgery usually indicates a massive sequestered fragment not detectable at the time of initial surgery. Recurrence within 3 to 12 months typically involves reinjury to the disk at the same level. Recurrence after many years often results from herniation at another level, which must be treated as a new herniation.

The main complication of recurrence at the same level is the presence of scar tissue from the previous operation. Successful treatment relies on proving the existence of compression by a herniation. Differentiating epidural fibrosis from recurrent herniation is complicated by the limited sensitivity of imaging studies in detecting herniations in the presence of scar tissue. In addition to a careful history and physical examination, contrast-enhanced MRI is useful but

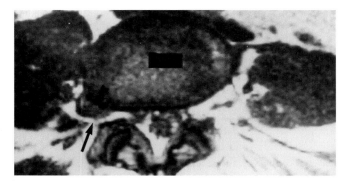

Figure 4

Axial magnetic resonance image showing a lateral herniation compressing the nerve root as it exits the neural foramen (arrow).

may show equal amounts of fibrosis in patients with and without symptoms shortly after surgery.

The decision to proceed with further surgical intervention is based on criteria similar to those for patients undergoing a first-time procedure. Failure of nonsurgical treatment, severe disabling sciatic pain, or evidence of progressing neurologic deficit should prompt the consideration of further surgical treatment. Specific findings of neurologic compromise in an anatomic distribution and radiographic evidence of compression that compliments the physical findings are fundamental to the success of reoperation. The clinical relevance of fibrosis as the only finding in patients with recurrent sciatica after surgery is poorly understood; however, most agree that the absence of evidence of compression is a contraindication to further surgery. Success rates in revision surgery decrease in relation to the number of reoperations.

Spinal Stenosis

Introduction
Spinal stenosis is defined as a narrowing of the vertebral canal, lateral recesses, and/or intervertebral foramina. The narrowing can be local, segmental, or generalized. Stenosis can be caused by bone, soft tissue, or combinations thereof; depending on location, it is divided into vertebral canal stenosis (central stenosis) and lateral stenosis.

Based on etiology, stenosis has been divided into 2 congenital-developmental groups and 6 acquired groups (Outline 1). This section deals only with the degenerative variety of stenosis, which is the most common.

Development of Degenerative Stenosis
The "degenerative cascade" is based on the analysis of autopsy specimens. This concept of the motion segment degener-

Outline 1
Classification of spinal stenosis

Congenital-developmental stenosis

  Idiopathic

  Achondroplastic

Acquired stenosis

  Degenerative

    Central portion of spinal canal

    Peripheral portion canal, lateral recesses and nerve root canals (tunnels)

    Degenerative spondylolisthesis

  Combined

    Any possible combinations of congenital-developmetal stenosis, degenerative stenosis and herniations of the nucleus pulposus

  Spondylolisthetic, spondylolytic

  Iatrogenic

    Postlaminectomy

    Postfusion (anterior and posterior)

    Postchemonucleolysis

    Posttraumatic, late changes

  Miscellaneous

    Paget disease

    Fluorosis

(Reproduced with permission from Arnoldi CC, Brodsky AE, Cauchoix J, et al: Lumbar spinal stenosis and nerve root entrapment syndrome: Definition and classification. *Clin Orthop* 1976;115:4–5.)

ating involves 3 stages (Fig. 5). Initially, dysfunction of the spinal motion segment occurs (stage 1) as a result of circumferential tears of the disk and synovitis in the facet joints. Subsequently, segmental instability (stage 2) develops when further internal disruption of the disk occurs and capsular laxity develops. From this second stage a gradual restabilization (stage 3) occurs in which spinal stenosis often develops because of enlargement of the articular processes of the facet joints, development of osteophytes on the vertebral bodies,

and hypertrophy and collapse of the ligamentum flavum. This restabilization sometimes occurs in a position where 1 vertebra has slipped forward on an adjacent vertebra. This degenerative spondylolisthesis is most common at L4-5 when L5 is hemisacralized. It is more common in women than in men, and the slippage rarely exceeds 25% to 30% of vertebral body width. Because the posterior elements are attached to the slipping vertebral body, they also move forward, causing central and foraminal stenosis (the ring-on-ring phenomenon). The risk of spondylolisthesis depends on the orientation of the facet joints. A more vertical orientation of the facet joints in the axial plane increases the risk of forward slippage and foraminal stenosis. Because degenerative spondylolisthesis is more frequent at the L4-5 level, it is primarily the L5 nerve root that is affected laterally and, because of the ring-on-ring phenomenon, these patients often have central stenosis as well.

Clinical Presentation

Spinal stenosis causes 1 of 4 clinical symptom complexes: intermittent neurogenic claudication, radiculopathy, chronic cauda equina syndrome, and atypical leg pain. The main clinical features of these 4 subgroups are listed in Table 1. Overlap is not uncommon and other clinical entities may result in similar symptom patterns.

Neurogenic claudication was initially thought to be synonymous with spinal stenosis. The patient complains of difficulty walking because of pain, weakness, or other symptoms in the legs. Occasionally these symptoms arise simply from standing up. Typically they are relieved by bending forward or sitting down. The reason for neurogenic claudication appears to be the increased demand on circulation to cauda equina nerve roots that occurs with activity as well as a change in intervertebral canal and foraminal diameters caused by changes in posture. Thus, the spinal canal and the foramina enlarge with flexion and decrease with extension. This change can be as large as 50% of the transverse area of the dural sac and can be identified on dynamic myelograms. On examination these patients present a benign picture in which straight leg raising usually is negative and neurologic deficits may be entirely absent.

Radiculopathy primarily occurs in patients who have lateral stenosis (recess or foraminal). The clinical picture may be similar to that of a herniated disk and, indeed, an asymmetric bulging of the disk may contribute considerably to the development of this syndrome. The chronic cauda equina syndrome is quite different from the acute cauda equina syndrome. Being secondary to a slowly developing spinal stenosis, it most often causes bladder dysfunction. There may be perineal and rectal pain, but other findings may be few or absent.

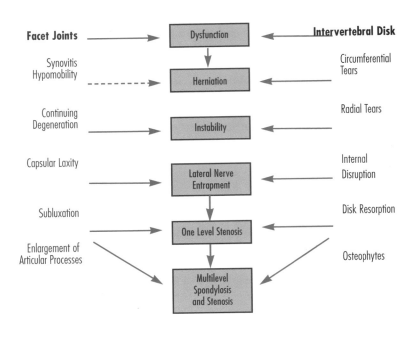

Figure 5

Development of the degenerative process, ultimately resulting in spinal stenosis. (Adapted with permission from Kirkaldy-Willis WH: *Managing Low Back Pain.* New York, NY, Churchill Livingstone, 1993.)

ferent positions, permitting diagnosis of spinal stenosis occurring with positional changes (dynamic stenosis). CT provides excellent images of the osseous structures of the spine. One disadvantage of CT is that only axial images are obtained directly. Sagittal and coronal reconstructions do not allow the same resolution. However, sagittal reconstructions of the foramena are frequently diagnostic for osteophytic encroachment of the nerve root in the foramen. MRI has emerged as the most important modality for the evaluation of lumbar spinal stenosis. MRI provides images in all planes and of the entire lumbar and lower thoracic areas. MRI images also provide important information about the soft-tissue structures that often contribute to spinal stenosis as well as any bone marrow changes that may exist. Anatomic observations from imaging studies do not necessarily equal clinical disease. A large percentage of asymptomatic individuals have MRI changes that indicate stenosis. As in many other spinal conditions, clinical correlation is very important.

Decompression in these patients is not as urgent as in patients with acute spinal stenosis and the prognosis is quite different. Decompression should be done only after a complete medical workup, and should be directed toward all elements of stenosis. Recovery is slow and often incomplete, which must be communicated to the patient. The fourth symptom, complex atypical leg pain, presents a true diagnostic challenge. Other sources of leg pain, such as hip osteoarthritis and pelvic disease, must be excluded before accepting this diagnosis, which is confirmed by the imaging studies.

Imaging Studies

The history and physical examination should suggest the possibility that stenosis is causing the back and/or leg pain. Plain film analysis of the spine is an efficient and inexpensive means of initial evaluation. In patients with degenerative spinal stenosis, it is not sufficiently specific, however, to allow treatment decisions. In earlier years, myelography was the most frequently used procedure in the evaluation of spinal stenosis. Myelograms are still being used, but now always in conjunction with CT. One advantage of myelography over other imaging methods is the ability to obtain images in dif-

Treatment

Most patients with lumbar spinal stenosis can be treated nonsurgically. The patients must be educated to understand the goal of therapy and have realistic expectations. Treatment begins with the simplest mode of therapy, such as temporary limitations of physical activities and nonsteroidal anti-inflammatory drugs (NSAIDs). If no improvement occurs over a 3- to 6-week period, a change in the type of NSAID or a trial of epidural steroid injections may be considered. These patients rarely respond to corsets or braces. However, when degenerative spondylolisthesis or degenerative scoliosis exists, this may be a worthwhile treatment alternative. Physical therapy has variable effects.

Patients who do not respond to conservative treatment are candidates for surgery. Surgery needs to be carefully planned to treat all aspects of the stenosis. All surgery includes a decompression in the form of laminectomy, lateral recess decompression (undercutting the facet joints), and foraminotomy. Foraminal stenosis is often overlooked, and it is a frequent cause of failed back syndrome. In patients with primarily radicular symptoms and pseudoclaudication, but without significant back pain, decompression may be the only surgical treatment required. Some patients, however, require decompressions that involve significant portions of the facet joints. If more than 50% of a facet joint is removed, then a fusion should accompany the decompression to prevent postoperative instability. Decompression and fusion also have been shown to produce the best results in patients with degenerative spondylolisthesis. The use of internal fixation remains controversial. Internal fixation improves the fusion rate and provides better initial stability, which may obviate the need for postoperative bracing and shorten the recovery period. Follow-up studies show that over time, many patients will again become symptomatic even after initial successful surgery. This finding suggests that the degenerative process continues, and the continuation should be explained to the patient before surgery.

Degenerative Segmental Instability

Spinal instability generally is defined as abnormal motion between 2 or more vertebra resulting in mechanical deformation of the facet joints, nerve roots, and other spinal components, but the diagnostic criteria remain controversial. In the presence of a stable psychological profile and the absence of confounding work or social factors, symptoms of clinical instability include: back giving way or slipping out, frequent acute attacks of low back pain, and difficulty with prolonged standing.

The radiographic diagnosis of segmental instability requires static and dynamic radiographs. Static radiographic criteria associated with segmental instability include retrolisthesis, traction spur, spondylolisthesis, previous total laminectomy or fusion below the affected motion segment, gas in the disk space, disk space narrowing, facet degeneration, malalignment of the spinous processes, and rotational deformity of the pedicles. Dynamic criteria, based on flexion-extension radiographs, include translational motion of 3 mm or more, or an abnormal angular displacement of at least 15° in relation to an adjacent segment (Fig. 6).

Diagnostic attempts have included the treadmill test, external segmental fixation, casts, and side bending, flexion-extension, and traction radiographs. The treadmill test involves stressing the patient walking on a flat road or incline. There appears to be correlation between the severity of pain with exercise and segmental instability. External fixation and hip spica casts have been used to immobilize the motion segment in question. Both are impractical in most situations. Flexion-extension radiographs have been helpful, but side bending and traction radiographs are of no use. None of these are absolute diagnostic indicators of degenerative instability. The

---

Table 1

Signs and symptoms in patients presenting with the four main symptom complexes of spinal stenosis

Radiculopathy	Chronic Canda Equina Syndrome*	Neurogenic Intermittent Claudication	Atypical Leg Pain
Sciatica	Urinary/bowel incontinence	Pseudoclaudication	Leg pain[†]
Low back pain	Urinary urgency/hesitancy	Low back pain	Low back pain
Motor deficit	Low back pain	Sciatica	Tingling
Sensory deficit	Sciatica	Motor deficit	
Paresthesias		Sensory deficit	
Weakness			

*The primary distinguishing symptom is listed at the top of the table.

†Leg pain that is not typical of either radicular or neurogenic claudication. Distribution is often diffuse, bizarre, and is nondermatomal.

(Reproduced with permission from Andersson GBJ, McNeill TW (eds): *Lumbar Spinal Stenosis*. St. Louis, MO, CV Mosby, 1992.)

use of radiographic, clinical, and mechanical classifications have not proven to be clinically useful.

The clinical prognosis in patients with lumbar degenerative instability depends primarily on the development of spinal canal stenosis rather than the existence or type of radiographic instability.

Segmental instability may follow decompressive procedures. Intraoperative instability is not difficult to diagnose. Biomechanical investigations have demonstrated that removal of 50% or more of both facets or removal of an entire facet will cause instability in that motion segment. Disk excision, if it involves annulotomy, may further aggravate instability when performed with other decompressive procedures.

The clinical result may be influenced by advanced age, disk space narrowing, and osteophytic formation, which will impart additional stability to a specific motion segment and reduce the need for fusion. If adequate decompression in a young patient involves removal of 50% or more of both facets or total removal of one facet at 1 or more levels, fusion should be considered.

Postfusion instability or transition syndrome is a condition that is being recognized more frequently. Postfusion instability can occur at 1 or 2 levels above or below a long-standing fusion. The most common site is directly above the fusion. The diagnosis is made by a combination of clinical symptoms and the radiographic appearance of the segment in question. Posterior translation is the most common radiographic finding, but an anterolisthesis of the superior vertebrae may also be another sign.

Factors relating to the development of postfusion instability include a relatively flat sagittal alignment in the previously fused segment with compensatory hyperextension, concen-

tration of abnormally high stresses in the motion segment above or below leading to facet degeneration, disk degeneration, and ligamentous hypertrophy. Once the diagnosis of stenosis and instability is confirmed, the treatment usually consists of adequate decompression of the segment and fusion with or without instrumentation.

Diskogenic Low Back Pain

Diskogenic back pain can be caused by numerous factors. The onset of degeneration in the disk may be explained by genetic influences, environmental stresses, and unidentified factors interacting in an unpredictable fashion. The accumulation of major and minor trauma may also lead to accelerated degeneration.

Disk degeneration or premature disk aging has been theorized to be an environmentally and genetically induced phenomenon that creates abnormal motion patterns. These patterns subject various anatomic structures to stress, which results in pain. In cases of severe symptomatic disk degeneration, facet arthroses also occurs and resembles osteoarthritis of other major joints. The arthritic joint is denuded of cartilage and demonstrates vascular ingrowth with the biochemically active pain peptide, substance P.

The disk is a complex anatomic structure with innervation by the sinuvertebral and sympathetic nerves located in the periphery of the disk and outer portions of the anulus fibrosus. Biochemical factors also play a role in the production of pain by a direct initial effect on the nerve root and then individual effects on disk structure.

There is general agreement that surgery as part of the initial treatment for acute low back pain should be limited to patients with serious spinal pathology or worsening nerve root dysfunction. If conservative management fails to result in functional recovery, other possible causes should be considered before recommending surgical treatment. Criteria that warrant consideration of surgical treatment include: (1) chronic pain of at least 6 months' duration and off of work for 4 months, (2) local tenderness with painful flexion at 20° to 30° and sitting intolerance, (3) provocative diskography and an abnormal MRI, and (4) absence of other underlying conditions.

Surgical treatment of low back pain with disk degeneration remains a controversial subject because as many as 65% of patients with diskogenic pain gradually improve over time with conservative treatment. Surgery in this subset of patients should be approached with caution and with assurance that patients have realistic expectations about the outcome. Some authors advocate fusion procedures in a select

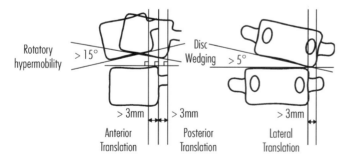

Figure 6

Criteria of instability. In the functional lateral radiographs, > 15° rotatory hypermobility, > 3-mm anterior translation, and > 3-mm posterior translation. In static anteroposterior radiographs; disk wedging > 5° and > 3-mm lateral translation. (Reproduced with permission from Aota Y, Kumano K, Hirabuyashi S: Post fusion instability at the adjacent segments after rigid pedicle screw fixation for degenerative lumbar spinal disorders. *J Spinal Disord* 1995;18:464–473.)

group of patients with persistent symptoms despite a prolonged and aggressive trial of conservative therapy lasting up to 1 year. Patients who do not meet specific criteria seldom benefit from surgical intervention, and surgery further increases the risk of complications in future procedures.

Fusion techniques include posterolateral in situ fusion, anterior interbody fusion, posterior lumbar interbody fusion, and instrumented fusion. Newer techniques include threaded titanium cages, which are inserted between adjacent end plates to provide a theoretical strut against collapse. The role of fusion, including the use of cages, remains highly controversial, with only preliminary evidence to support its use in carefully selected patients with no secondary gain. The limited role of interbody fusion in the treatment of low back pain and disk herniation is further tempered by evidence suggesting that the increased stiffness imposed by fusion constructs results in accelerated degeneration of adjacent segments. The incidence of degenerative changes in an intact adjacent segment above a solid anterior lumbar interbody fusion has been reported as 68% after 10 years, appears to increase in an age-related manner, and does not appear to be influenced by fusion length.

The reported success rate of fusions for symptomatic disk degeneration varies from 30% to 90%, although variable outcome parameters and complicating social factors mitigate the comparison of different studies. In a series of 62 patients treated with diskectomy and posterior interbody fusion, 89% of patients reported satisfactory results with a 94% fusion rate and a 92.5% return-to-work rate. Provocative diskography associated with a positive MRI scan may be a successful predictor of surgical outcome and a selection criterion for surgical candidates.

Failed Back Surgery

The causes of failed back syndrome include pseudarthrosis, recurrent herniation, residual stenosis, postfusion instability, fibrosis, and psychological factors. The decision to reoperate is difficult and should be based on multiple objective criteria. Imaging studies including diskography, MRI, and CT myelography are used. Additional diagnostic modalities include psychological testing, selective nerve blocks, and brace immobilization.

Reported success rates for revision low back surgery range from 28% to 81% for all causes. Specific factors associated with a successful outcome are listed in Outline 2. Factors associated with a poor response to revision surgery also are given in Outline 2.

> **Outline 2**
> Factors predicting outcome from repeat lumbar surgery
>
> Predictive of a good outcome
>
> Greater than 6 months' pain relief after previous surgery
>
> Leg pain worse than back pain
>
> Nerve root compression from disk or bone
>
> Contrast study correlates with clinical examination
>
> Neurologic deficit
>
> No litigation
>
> Noncompensable cause of pain
>
> Solid fusion achieved
>
> Predictive of a poor outcome
>
> Less than 6 months' pain relief
>
> Scarring, fibrosis found at surgery
>
> Radiographic evidence of arachnoiditis
>
> Poor psychological profile
>
> Litigation active
>
> Compensable cause of pain
>
> Multiple operations
>
> Substance abuse

(Reproduced with permission from Barnard T: Repeat lumbar spine surgery: Factors influencing outcome. *Spine* 1993;18:2196–2200.)

Recurrent disk herniation has a reported incidence rate of 2% to 19%. Low back pain, as a criterion of failure after diskectomy, has been reported in up to 20% of postdiskectomy patients. Factors associated with postoperative back pain are a compensable injury, 15-pack-year history of smoking, and an age greater than 40 years.

Failure of surgery for spinal stenosis may be caused by disk herniations, iatrogenic instability, degenerative instability, and residual stenosis. The failure of the first procedure for spinal stenosis has a negative impact on any additional salvage surgeries.

Pseudarthrosis after lumbar fusion has been reported in from 8% to 60% of patients. Variables related to the development of pseudarthrosis include number of levels, previous surgery, smoking, and the use of instrumentation. The treatment of this patient group is challenging. Some authors contend that a pseudarthrosis may not be the principal cause of symptoms and repair is not always necessary. This contention can make the selection of the patient for repair difficult. Pseudarthrosis can be repaired anteriorly, posteriorly, or both. The use of instrumentation generally is recommended.

In one study, 81 of 86 (94%) attempted repairs were successful in obtaining solid fusion, and most patients thought the operation was beneficial. Most were repaired posteriorly with instrumentation in 76 and bone graft without instrumentation in 5. Workers' compensation and smoking were associated with poorer outcomes. A cautious approach to pseudarthrosis repair is recommended. Intense rehabilitation, conditioning, and pain management should be attempted before undertaking a salvage procedure.

It is clear that, overall, revision surgery of the lower back has a less favorable outcome than primary surgery regardless of the diagnosis. Patient selection, as well as the type of surgical procedure, is extremely important. The best way to deal with surgical failures is to try to prevent them with the first operation.

In spite of the best performed operations and strict selection criteria, failures still occur. Most patients with chronic pain can be treated with oral medications, physiotherapy, electrostimulation, and psychological counseling. Patients with continuing radicular and low back pain in whom analgesics and pain management have failed may be helped by spinal cord stimulation. Residual low back pain, as well as radicular pain, can be treated with continuous intrathecal opioids, but experience with these devices is important to select the proper patient for implantation. Occasionally, this treatment may be an alternative to reoperation. Both spinal cord stimulation and intrathecal opioids have shown to be cost-effective by reducing the demands for medical care by failed back surgery patients.

Annotated Bibliography

Low Back Pain

Bigos SJ, et al: *Acute Low Back Problems in Adults: Assessment and Treatment. Quick Reference Guide for Clinicians No 14.* AHCPR Publication No 95-0643. Rockville, MD, Agency for Health Care Policy and Research, U.S. Department of Health and Human Services, 1994.

Based on a critical review of available literature and opinions from private sector consultants, this manual represents a science-based compilation of recommendations on the assessment and treatment of adults with acute low back pain. It provides an excellent and succinct series of empiric management algorithms and a synthesis of knowledge on the success of various conservative and surgical interventions.

van Tulder MW, Koes BW, Bouter LM: Conservative treatment of acute and chronic nonspecific low back pain: A systematic review of randomized controlled trials of the most common interventions. *Spine* 1997;22:2128–2156.

This article presents the results of an extensive meta-analysis of selected existing randomized, controlled clinical trials addressing various aspects of conservative treatment. In rating trials, this study found a need for higher quality of design, execution, and reporting of established evidence to answer many of the remaining questions regarding the management of low back pain.

Lumbar Disk Herniation

Andersson GB, Brown MD, Dvorak J, et al: Consensus summary of the diagnosis and treatment of lumbar disc herniation. *Spine* 1996;21(suppl 24):75S–78S.

This article represents a consensus of expert opinions on the problems associated with many aspects of the diagnosis and treatment of lumbar disk herniation. Further, it presents an outline of necessary future actions needed to better define the causes of these problems.

Jonsson B, Stromqvist B: Clinical characteristics of recurrent sciatica after lumbar discectomy. *Spine* 1996;21:500–505.

This prospective study addresses the difficulty in diagnosing recurrent herniation with the presence of epidural fibrosis. Results suggest that pain on coughing, reduced walking capacity, and positive straight leg raise less than 30° may help distinguish recurrence from scar formation.

Kang JD, Stefanovic-Racic M, McIntyre LA, Georgescu HI, Evans CH: Toward a biochemical understanding of human intervertebral disc degeneration and herniation: Contributions of nitric oxide, interleukins, prostaglandin E2, and matrix metallo-proteinases. *Spine* 1997;22:1065–1073.

Addressing the growing interest in biochemical changes that occur during degeneration, this study provides evidence that herniated disks are capable of increasing the production of various inflammatory mediators in response to stimulation by IL-1. In addition to concluding that diskal cells have an active metabolic capacity, this article suggests that autocrine and paracrine mechanisms play an important role in mediating the inflammatory changes that accompany degeneration.

Surgery

Grevitt MP, McLaren A, Shackleford IM, Mulholland RC: Automated percutaneous lumbar discectomy: An outcome study. *J Bone Joint Surg* 1995;77B:626–629.

This prospective study of 137 patients treated with APLD found a success rate of only 45% at 55 months of follow-up. Furthermore, 12% of patients required open laminotomy and decompression within 3 months, and one third of patients experienced worsening disability over time.

McCulloch JA: Focus issue on lumbar disc herniation: Macro- and microdiscectomy. *Spine* 1996;21(suppl 24):45S–56S.

This article is based on an extensive review and analysis of literature on open and minimally invasive surgical procedures. It summarizes the information to date on the indications and expected outcomes for each procedure.

Schaffer JL, Kambin P: Percutaneous posterolateral lumbar discectomy and decompression with a 6.9-millimeter cannula: Analysis of operative failures and complications. *J Bone Joint Surg* 1991;73A:822–831.

A prospective study of 100 patients deemed as surgical failures after having undergone percutaneous disk surgery, this paper cites 12 failed outcomes including transient sensory and motor deficits. Eleven patients required subsequent laminectomy, and all complications resolved without sequelae.

Spinal Stenosis

Fischgrund JS, Mackay M, Herkowitz HN, Brower R, Montgomery DM, Kurz LT: Degenerative lumbar spondylolisthesis with spinal stenosis: A prospective, randomized study comparing decompressive laminectomy and arthrodesis with and without spinal instrumentation. *Spine* 1997;22:2807–2812.

The influence was analyzed of transpedicular instrumentation on the surgical treatment of 67 patients with degenerative spondylolisthesis and spinal stenosis. Clinical outcome was excellent or good in 76% of the patients with instrumentation and in 85% of those without instrumentation ($p = 0.45$). Successful arthrodesis occurred in 82% of the instrumented versus 45% of the noninstrumented patients ($p = 0.0015$). Overall, successful fusion did not influence patient outcome ($p = 0.435$).

Herkowitz HN: Spine update: Degenerative lumbar spondylolisthesis. *Spine* 1995;20:1084–1090.

This article presents a detailed description of the pathophysiology, clinical presentation, and nonsurgical and surgical intervention of degenerative lumbar spondylolisthesis.

Jonsson B, Annertz M, Sjoberg C, Stromqvist B: A prospective and consecutive study of surgically treated lumbar spinal stenosis: Part II. Five-year follow-up by an independent observer. *Spine* 1997;24:2938–2944.

This prospective study followed patients with central lumbar spinal stenosis for 5 years after a laminectomy without fusion. The results deteriorated over time, and the reoperation rate was 18%.

Katz JN, Lipson SJ, Chang LC, Levine SA, Fossel AH, Liang MH: Seven- to 10-year outcome of decompressive surgery for degenerative lumbar spine disorders. *Spine* 1996;21:92–98.

This study confirms the earlier observation that results deteriorate over time. Eighty-eight patients were studied retrospectively. Twenty-three percent had undergone reoperation and 33% had severe back pain. Nevertheless, 75% were satisfied with the results of the operation.

Failed Surgery and Instability

Aota Y, Kumano K, Hirabayashi S: Postfusion instability at the adjacent segments after rigid pedicle screw fixation for degenerative lumbar spinal disorders. *J Spinal Disord* 1995;8:464–473.

Sixty-five patients who had wide laminectomy, Cotrel-Dubousset instrumentation, and fusion for lumbar degenerative disorders were reviewed radiographically. The incidence of postfusion instability was 24.6%. Instability was most common in the adjacent segment above the fusion. The most common radiographic sign was posterior translation.

Burchiel KJ, Anderson VC, Brown FD, et al: Prospective, multi-center study of spinal cord stimulation for relief of chronic back and extremity pain. *Spine* 1996;21:2786–2794.

This study confirms that spinal cord stimulation can be effective therapy for the management of chronic low back and extremity pain.

Winkelmuller M, Winkelmuller W: Long-term effects of continuous intrathecal opioid treatment in chronic pain of nonmalignant etiology. *J Neurosurg* 1996;85:458–467.

The long-term effects of continuous intrathecal opioid therapy were evaluated in 120 patients. Of the patients, 92% were happy with this therapy. The average pain reduction was 67.4% at 6 months and 58.1% at final follow-up.

Classic Bibliography

Boden SD, Davis DO, Dina TS, Patronas NJ, Wiesel SW: Abnormal magnetic-resonance scans of the lumbar spine in asymptomatic subjects: A prospective investigation. *J Bone Joint Surg* 1990;72A:403–408.

Hanley EN Jr, Shapiro DE: The development of low-back pain after excision of a lumbar disc. *J Bone Joint Surg* 1989;71A:719–721.

Herkowitz HN, Kurz LT: Degenerative lumbar spondylolisthesis with spinal stenosis: A prospective study comparing decompression with decompression and intertransverse process arthrodesis. *J Bone Joint Surg* 1991;73A:802–808.

Katz JN, Lipson SJ, Larson MG, McInnes JM, Fossel AH, Liang MH: The outcome of decompressive laminectomy for degenerative lumbar stenosis. *J Bone Joint Surg* 1991;73A:809–816.

698   Spine

Kostuik JP, Harrington I, Alexander D, Rand W, Evans D: Cauda equina syndrome and lumbar disc herniation. *J Bone Joint Surg* 1986;68A:386–391.

Sato H, Kikuchi S: The natural history of radiographic instability of the lumbar spine. *Spine* 1993;18:2075–2079.

Spengler DM, Ouellette EA, Battie M, Zeh J: Elective discectomy for herniation of a lumbar disc: Additional experience with an objective method. *J Bone Joint Surg* 1990;72A:230–237.

Waddell G, Kummel EG, Lotto WN, Graham JD, Hall H, McCulloch JA: Failed lumbar disc surgery and repeat surgery following industrial injuries. *J Bone Joint Surg* 1979;61A: 201–207.

Waddell G, McCulloch JA, Kummel E, Venner RM: Nonorganic physical signs in low-back pain. *Spine* 1980;5:117–125.

Weber H: Lumbar disc herniation: A controlled, prospective study with ten years of observation. *Spine* 1983;8:131–140.

Chapter 52
Spondylolysis and Spondylolisthesis

Spondylolysis and spondylolisthesis are relatively common in the general population, but they are generally asymptomatic and require no treatment. However, these entities do have the potential to cause problems, such as back pain, neurologic deficit, or progressive deformity.

Spondylolysis and spondylolisthesis are derived from the Greek words spondylos (spine), lysis (breakdown), and olisthanerin (to slip). Spondylolysis is the term used when there is no slippage of the vertebral body. Spondylolisthesis usually occurs at the L5-S1 level, but can occur more proximally in the lumbar spine. Isolated reports describe spondylolisthesis in the cervical or thoracic spine.

Classification and Etiology

Five different types of spondylolisthesis have been described by Wiltse: isthmic, dysplastic, degenerative, traumatic, and pathologic. Isthmic spondylolisthesis can be divided into 3 types: spondylolytic, elongated pars, and acute traumatic pars fracture. In the spondylolytic type, there is a break in the pars interarticularis caused by repetitive stress. This repeated stress may be associated with gradual healing, resulting in an elongated pars. Massive trauma also can cause an acute pars fracture. Dysplastic spondylolisthesis is associated with abnormalities of the upper sacrum or posterior arch of L5. Marchetti and Bartolozzi divided spondylolisthesis into developmental or acquired conditions (Outline 1). Developmental types are described as low dysplastic or high dysplastic. Low dysplastic spondylolisthesis is characterized by fairly normal bony anatomy with minimal slip angle. High dysplastic spondylolisthesis is associated with dysplastic changes of the sacrum, high slip angle, and hyperlordosis of the lumbar spine. Acquired types include traumatic, post-surgery, pathologic, and degenerative conditions.

Dysplastic spondylolisthesis (Wiltse classification) is more common in females, with a 2:1 female to male ratio, and it occurs in approximately 20% of patients with spondylolisthesis. Incompetency of the lumbosacral facet allows forward displacement of L5 on S1 (Fig. 1). Patients with dysplastic spondylolisthesis have deficient development of the superior facets of the upper sacrum, which contributes to the progressive slip. The pars in dysplastic spondylolisthesis may become attenuated and, occasionally, lysis may develop. Patients with dysplastic spondylolisthesis without lysis may develop significant constriction of the cauda equina with much less slippage than patients with spondylolytic spondylolisthesis. This encroachment of the cauda equina may result in significant

Outline 1
Marchetti-Bartolozzi Classification

Developmental
High dysplastic
    With lysis
    With elongation
Low dysplastic
    With lysis
    With elongation
Acquired
Traumatic
    Acute fracture
    Stress fracture
Postsurgery
    Direct surgery
    Indirect surgery
Pathologic
    Local pathology
    Systemic pathology
Degenerative
    Primary
    Secondary

lower lumbar and leg discomfort. Surgical stabilization may be required to relieve the symptoms.

The most common type of spondylolisthesis is isthmic spondylolisthesis. Rare cases have been reported in infancy. Spondylolysis or spondylolisthesis generally develops between the ages of 7 to 10 years, when the prevalence is 4%. The incidence increases to adulthood, when the general prevalence is between 4% and 6%. The male to female ratio in isthmic spondylolisthesis is 2:1.

Genetic factors play a role in the development of spondylolysis and spondylolisthesis. Defects in the pars interarticularis have a familial incidence ranging from 30% to 70%. The familial incidence is higher in dysplastic than in isthmic spondylolisthesis. In 1 series, there was a 33% incidence in relatives of patients with dysplastic spondylolisthesis and a 15% incidence in relatives of patients with isthmic spondylolisthesis. The dysplastic form has an increased incidence of sacral spina bifida.

Incidence of isthmic spondylolisthesis varies by race: African American females, 1%; African American males, 3%; white females, 2%; white males, 6%. Certain Eskimo groups have been noted to have a prevalence of over 50%.

Repetitive stress and microtrauma are believed to be the major factors in the development of the defect in the pars interarticularis. Some authors have suggested that the etiology of spondylolisthesis is related to an inherited dysplasia present in the arch, which is affected by the strain of upright stance and lumbar lordosis. Spondylolysis and spondylolisthesis are found only in humans.

Increased lumbar lordosis also may be an etiologic factor. The high rate of spondylolysis reported in Scheuermann's disease may be related to compensatory excessive lumbar lordosis, secondary to the thoracic hyperkyphosis. Athletic activities causing excessive stress in the lumbosacral spine, including gymnastics, football, and wrestling, have a known association with the development of spondylolisthesis.

Certain neuromuscular conditions, including myelodysplasia and cerebral palsy, have also been noted to be associated with an increased incidence of spondylolisthesis. In a large study of spina bifida patients, the incidence of spondylolisthesis increased with the increasing level of neurologic function, with patients who had L5-S1 level function having a 16% prevalence of spondylolisthesis. The factors believed to be important were increased lumbar lordosis, the patient's body weight, and ambulatory status. Spondylolisthesis developed only in ambulatory patients. Patients with spastic diplegia also have an increased incidence of spondylolisthesis, with a reported prevalence of 14%.

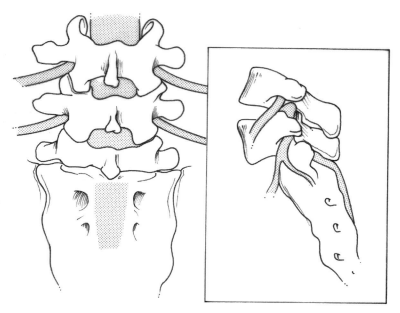 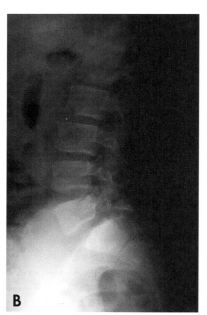

Figure 1

A, Spondylolisthesis secondary to dysplastic L5-S1 articulation. B, Lateral radiograph of a patient with grade I spondylolisthesis at L5-S1.

Clinical Findings

Spondylolisthesis often is discovered as an incidental radiographic finding because most children are asymptomatic. Symptoms usually present during the preadolescent growth spurt. It is important to rule out other organic causes for back pain, such as tumor or infection. Pain often is exacerbated by activity and may be localized to the lower lumbar spine. Occasionally, discomfort may radiate to the buttocks and posterior aspect of the thighs. True radicular symptoms are rare, and in this situation, the physician must rule out a herniated disk. Radicular symptoms may be associated with more severe spondylolistheses (grades III and IV). With a mild degree of slip, the appearance of the spine and the child's gait may be normal, although the lumbar spine may show increased lumbar lordosis. With more severe spondylolisthesis, as the patient develops lumbosacral kyphosis, he or she may develop the classic knees bent/hips flexed stance and gait. Paravertebral spasm may be present. Hamstring tightness often develops.

The mechanism causing these changes is unknown but has been hypothesized by some to be related to nerve root irritation from the pars defect. In the most severe cases, where significant lumbosacral kyphosis is present, the rib cage approaches the iliac crest. The child has an awkward gait, wide base and short stride length with limited hip flexion. The buttocks become flattened. A palpable step-off at the lumbosacral junction may develop. The torso is foreshortened; straight leg raising is limited. Above the area of lumbosacral kyphosis, hyperlordosis of the lumbar spine develops, and the torso is shifted backwards to maintain spinal balance. In addition to radicular symptoms, signs of bowel or bladder impairment may develop.

Scoliosis is infrequently associated with spondylolisthesis, particularly in those patients who are symptomatic. It may be related to muscle spasm or rotatory slippage of the spondylolisthesis. With these conditions, stabilization of the spondylolisthesis often causes the scoliosis to resolve. However, an associated true structural scoliosis may require treatment.

Radiographic Findings

In addition to anteroposterior and lateral views of the entire lumbar spine, right and left oblique views should be obtained (Fig. 2). The oblique view will illustrate the Scottish terrier with the defect in the dog's "neck," which is the defect in the pars interarticularis. Both oblique views must be taken because a unilateral defect occurs in 20% of patients.

In unilateral spondylolysis, there may be hypertrophy of the opposite pars or pedicle. If the diagnosis is questionable, computed tomography (CT) is helpful in determining the exact nature of the defect and also can help assess the status of healing during treatment. CT also may be helpful in identifying sites of neural compression. Bone scans can be helpful in detecting very early defects before they can be seen on plain films. Single photon emission CT is sensitive in detecting a stress fracture before disruption is evident on plain radiographs. Some authors suggest that immobilization at this point will result in union. In patients who are suspected of having an associated herniated disk, magnetic resonance imaging (MRI) is helpful to determine whether disk degeneration or herniation is present.

Many radiographic methods have been described to determine the severity of the spondylolisthesis, which is measured on a standing lateral radiograph. These measurements quantify the amount of translation or angulation. To determine the amount of translational displacement, the Meyerding grading system is most frequently used. No slippage is grade 0, 1% to 25% slippage is grade I, 26% to 50% is grade II, 51% to 75% is grade III, and 76% to 100% is grade IV.

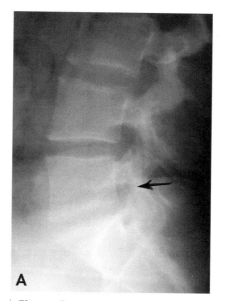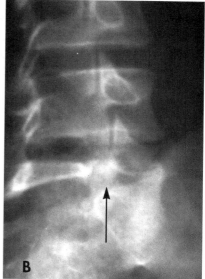

Figure 2

A, Lateral radiograph of a patient with spondylolysis shows a break at the pars interarticularis (arrow). B, Oblique radiograph shows the pars defect more clearly (arrow).

The slip angle is the measurement used to determine the amount of lumbosacral kyphosis. This is determined by drawing a line along the posterior cortex of the sacrum and measuring the angle between its perpendicular and a line drawn along the inferior border of L5. The normal angle ranges between 0° and 10°. A slip angle > 50° is associated with progression. If deformity of the inferior border of the L5 vertebral body is significant, the superior border can be used. The sacral inclination angle is the angle formed by a line perpendicular to the floor and a line along the posterior margin of the sacrum. A more vertically oriented sacrum is associated with progression. DeWald recommended a modification of the Newman system in which the amounts of L5 slip and roll are quantified by dividing the dome and the anterior surface of the sacrum into 10 equal parts. The amount of slip is measured by the distance from the posteroinferior corner of L5 and the posterosuperior corner of the sacrum. The amount of roll is measured from the anteroinferior corner of L5 to the anterosuperior corner of the sacrum (Fig. 3).

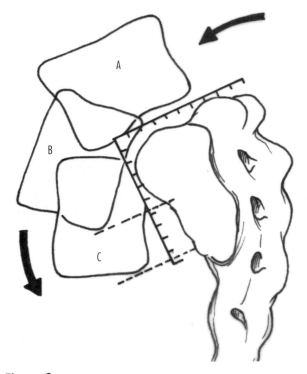

Figure 3

Forward displacement develops into lumbosacral kyphosis. Modified Newman spondylolisthesis grading system. The degree of slip is measured using 2 numbers; the first along the sacral end plate and the second along the anterior portion of the sacrum. A = 3 + 0; B = 8 + 6; C = 10 + 10. (Reproduced with permission from DeWald RL: Spondylolesthesis, in Bridwell KU, DeWald RL (eds): *Textbook of Spinal Surgery*, ed 2. Philadelphia, PA, Lippincott-Raven, 1997, p 1207.)

Natural History

Spondylolisthesis develops as a result of fatigue fracture in the pars interarticularis. The fatigue fracture may unite, leaving no evidence of spondylolysis, repetitive stress may lead these fatigue fractures to heal in an elongated position, or nonunion may develop. With bilateral pars involvement, spondylolisthesis, or forward slippage, may develop. This may be associated with disk degeneration and, very rarely, a disk herniation.

In a long-term study, the incidence of spondylolysis was 4% at 6 years of age and increased to 6% by adulthood. Spondylolisthesis developed in 13 of 19 patients (68%) when the pars defects were noted at the age of 6 years. However, in most patients, the amount of slip was mild.

A number of risk factors have been associated with progressive slippage in spondylolisthesis. As might be expected, younger patients who have significant periods of rapid growth are at risk for further slip. Females are at greater risk for progressive slip, particularly with dysplastic spondylolisthesis. Patients with excessive ligamentous laxity also are believed to have increased risk for progression of the spondylolisthesis.

Radiologic parameters have been associated with progression of spondylolisthesis. Severe slips frequently progress. Patients with slips > 50% often show continued progression as well as patients who have slip angles > 55°. Patients with slips > 50% and who are symptomatic are highly unlikely to have the symptoms resolved with nonsurgical management.

Patients who have instability at the L5-S1 level, as indicated by flexion-extension radiographs, also have increased potential for progression. Additional anatomic factors implicated in progression of the spondylolisthesis are a trapezoidal-shaped fifth lumbar vertebral body and a dome-shaped first sacral vertebra. However, a buttress of the anterior lip of the sacrum with a narrowed disk space indicates that significant progression is unlikely.

Treatment

In asymptomatic patients with Meyerding grade I or II slips, no treatment is warranted. Patients may participate in sports as tolerated. Natural history studies indicate that the likelihood of slip progression in this group is low. However, if significant progression does occur, even if the patient is asymptomatic, posterolateral fusion is recommended. Because the risk of progression is great, surgical stabilization should be done for slips > 50% whether or not the patient is symptomatic. Symptomatic patients in this group rarely respond to conservative management.

Initial treatment of a patient with symptomatic spondylolysis should be conservative. Assessment should determine the type of spondylolysis and rule out other causes for back discomfort such as disk herniation, bone or spinal cord tumors, or disk space infection.

Activity restriction with anti-inflammatory medications is the initial treatment. When pain is severe, a brace, corset, or body cast may be used. Isometric abdominal and paraspinal strengthening exercises have been reported to help relieve symptoms and also to maintain back conditioning. Stretching exercises for the tight hamstrings also have been advised to improve flexibility.

It is important to remember that at least 80% of patients with symptomatic spondylolysis or mild spondylolisthesis respond to conservative therapy and are able to return to prior activities.

In the small percentage of patients who do not respond to conservative therapy, surgical stabilization may be necessary. When activity restriction, physical therapy, and bracing have failed, fusion from the L5 transverse process to the sacral ala has been shown to reliably relieve symptoms. In fact, many patients who have a radiographically less than optimal fusion often have significant relief of symptoms. When bilateral pseudarthrosis is present, however, the symptoms often persist.

Recently, a number of reports have described a variety of techniques to directly repair the pars defect in spondylolysis or mild spondylolisthesis. These include screw fixation, hook screw fixation, pedicle screw wiring, Scott wiring, and modified Scott wiring techniques. Some authors have reported consistently good results and others have noted a significant

failure rate with these techniques. Some authors describe the best candidates for repair of the pars defect as those who have a defect between L1 and L4 with evidence of less than 1 or 2 mm of slippage. A degenerated disk on MRI may be a relative contraindication to the techniques for repairing the pars because of the possibility of continued back discomfort caused by the accompanying abnormal disk.

Surgical intervention is necessary when (1) there is a persistent back discomfort that interferes with activities of daily living and has failed conservative management, (2) there is significant progression of the slip, (3) the slip is > 50% with a slip angle of over 55°, and (4) a neurologic deficit is present that does not respond to conservative management.

Fusion in situ has been the most commonly performed surgical procedure (Fig. 4). In patients with grade I or grade II slips and slip angles < 50%, a solid fusion and relief of symptoms have been reported in 70% to 100%. Successful in situ fusion can be obtained even in patients with severe slips. For patients with slips < 50%, an L5-S1 fusion is adequate. With slips > 50%, extension of the fusion to L4 is necessary to create a satisfactory fusion and offer better mechanical advantage to prevent continued progression.

Patients with severe spondylolisthesis can have evidence of slip progression despite a radiographically solid fusion. The progression usually is noted within the first or second year after surgery, and the amount of progression generally is small. Mild nerve root irritation often resolves after spinal fusion. Removal of the loose lamina without fusion is contraindicated, because this will increase the chance of progression.

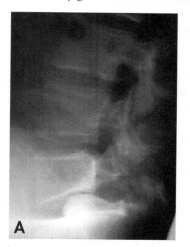 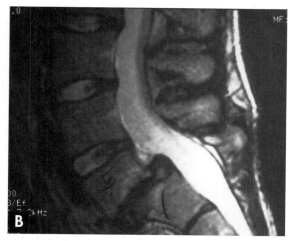 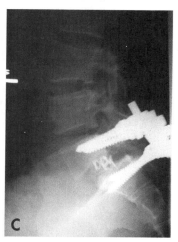

Figure 4

A, A lateral radiograph of a patient with grade II-III spondylolisthesis and lumbosacral kyphosis. B, A T2-weighted sagittal magnetic resonance image shows the spondylolisthesis and normal L4-5 disk. C, Postoperative lateral radiograph of this patient shows monosegmental fusion with stabilization. The slip angle is corrected but the slip percentage is intentionally not much changed. Stabilization was by posterior lumbar interbody fusion using Harms cages (Depuy-Motech-Acromed Inc, Cleveland, OH) and posterior ISOLA instrumentation (Depuy-Motech-Acromed Inc, Cleveland, OH).

Neurologic injury with an isolated posterolateral fusion is rare, but cauda equina syndrome has been reported after in situ fusion. Patients with dysplastic spondylolisthesis without lytic defects often develop encroachment of the spinal canal with cauda equina irritation. Surgical manipulation may result in a full-blown cauda equina syndrome. A patient with significant neurologic deficit requires decompression, which could include resection of the lamina of L5 with L5 nerve root foraminotomies and, rarely, posterosuperior sacroplasty.

Closed reduction of high-grade spondylolisthesis has been attempted in combination with posterolateral fusion techniques. Reduction methods have been used in which axial traction is applied to the spine, and direct pressure is applied to the posterior portion of the sacrum to improve the slip angle and the translation (Fig. 5). These methods are more successful in improving the slip angle than in correcting translation. Postoperatively, these patients must be kept in a pantaloon cast to prevent the lumbosacral kyphosis from recurring while the fusion matures. Some patients have a rigid lumbosacral kyphosis that cannot be corrected with traction. In these severe slips, progression has been documented to occur despite a radiographically solid fusion.

Posterior interbody arthrodesis with a fibular strut graft also has been used in patients with severe spondylolisthesis, with a satisfactory fusion rate and relief of symptoms. Potential complications include graft dislodgment, sacral

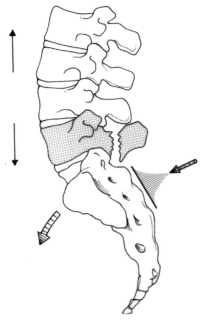

Figure 5

Forces applied for closed reduction of spondylolisthesis.

fracture, or neurovascular injury. Slotted anterior interbody fusion for spondylolisthesis has been done with tibial strut grafts or fibular dowel grafts, but this is technically challenging. These last 2 techniques are infrequently used in children.

In recent years, open reduction has become popular for the reduction of slips in patients with severe translation and high slip angles. The arguments that have been advanced are that open reduction allows improved cosmesis, restoration of trunk height, improved buttock and spine contour, more localized spine fusion, and nerve root decompression for patients who have root pain or irritation.

Some authors maintain that signs of impending cauda equina syndrome are a relative indication for open reduction. Patients with a strongly positive Lasegue's sign, diminished Achilles reflex, or early bowel or bladder dysfunction may develop cauda equina syndrome postoperatively, particularly those with dysplastic spondylolisthesis. The advantages of reduction of the spondylolisthesis include improved spinal alignment with normal body proportions. A number of techniques have been advocated for reducing the spondylolisthesis, including mechanisms using posterior distraction instrumentation, anterior/posterior resection reductions, L5 vertebrectomy, pedicle screw fixation, posterior level reduction, and a gradual instrumented reduction. Complications, however, have been frequent with significant nerve root deficits in numerous series.

Open reduction techniques that use only posterior distraction systems have proven to yield unsatisfactory results, with at best partial correction of the slip and no improvement in the slip angle. Anterior/posterior resection reductions have been used in patients with slips > 50%, but complications have been frequent, with neurologic deficits occurring in 10% to 20% of patients in some series. L5 vertebrectomy has been used primarily in patients with a spondylolisthesis that requires an L4 to sacrum fusion. This technique may gain significant correction but also has been plagued by a high incidence of neurologic deficits.

Pedicle screw fixation has become more common in the treatment of severe spondylolisthesis. The concept of a gradual instrumented reduction has been developed to restore normal anatomic alignment. Using pedicle screws and a special reduction device, corrective forces of distraction, posterior translation, and sacral flexion are gradually applied. As more experience has been gained with reduction techniques, the incidence of neurologic deficit appears to be diminishing. Although many of the neurologic deficits reported with reduction techniques are transient, some are permanent.

Reduction should be considered only by experienced spinal surgeons and only if the cosmetic deformity is severe. First, complete decompression of the thecal sac and nerve roots is mandatory. The reduction is done to restore sagittal balance, and shortening of the spinal column helps improve the slip angle without excessive tethering of the neural structures. It must be remembered that reduction creates instability and the preoperative deformity tends to recur. If reduction has been performed, stabilization must be rigid and biomechanically sound. The best method of achieving rigid fixation and stabilization is anterior interbody load-sharing graft through anterior or posterior lumbar interbody fusion, followed by posterior transpedicular compression instrumentation that acts as a tension band.

At the time of this writing, bone screws placed posteriorly into vertebral elements have been cleared for use in this specific manner by the Food and Drug Administration (FDA) to provide immobilization and stabilization as an adjunct to fusion in the treatment of the following acute and chronic instability or deformities of the thoracic, lumbar, and sacral spine: degenerative spondylolisthesis with objective evidence of neurologic impairment; fracture; dislocation; scoliosis; kyphosis; spinal tumor and failed previous fusion (pseudoarthrosis). In addition, anterior vertebral body screws (cervical, thoracic, and lumbar) are Class II devices and can be used as labeled in vertebral bodies.

Annotated Bibliography

Dreyzin V, Esses SI: A comparative analysis of spondylolysis repair. *Spine* 1994;19:1909–1914.

Two surgical techniques for repair of a pars interarticularis defect were studied: Buck wire fixation and modified Morscher-designed spondylolysis distraction hook. Of 20 patients with either a grade 0 or 1 spondylolytic spondylolisthesis, 9 had the Morscher technique, and 11 were treated with the Buck technique. The clinical outcome was poor using either technique.

Dubousset J: Treatment of spondylolysis and spondylolisthesis in children and adolescents. *Clin Orthop* 1997;337:77–85.

The author describes 17 cases treated by gradual traction and hyperextension followed by cast immobilization with an excellent fusion rate and good correction of the slip angle. When the lumbosacral angle cannot be corrected, anterior release and fusion with strut graft is performed. This correction of the slip angle allows for improved cosmesis and satisfactory clinical results.

Fabris DA, Costantini S, Nena U: Surgical treatment of severe L5-S1 spondylolisthesis in children and adolescents: Results of intraoperative reduction, posterior interbody fusion, and segmental pedicle fixation. *Spine* 1996;21:728–733.

Adolescents with severe spondylolisthesis were treated with a single stage procedure involving posterior interbody fusion with reduction and segmental fixation. This procedure allows for an 80% correction of the deformity. All patients in this series had a solid fusion with no intraoperative or postoperative complications.

Hilibrand AS, Urquhart AG, Graziano GP, Hensinger RN: Acute spondylolytic spondylolisthesis: Risk of progression and neurological complications. *J Bone Joint Surg* 1995;77A:190–196.

Four patients who sustained acute spondylolytic spondylolisthesis after major trauma were managed nonsurgically; 3 patients showed progression of the spondylolisthesis, and 1 developed a cauda equina syndrome. The authors believe that because of progression and neurologic compromise, patients with acute traumatic spondylolytic spondylolisthesis should be surgically stabilized.

Newton PO, Johnston CE II: Analysis and treatment of poor outcomes following in situ arthrodesis in adolescent spondylolisthesis. *J Pediatr Orthop* 1997;17:754–761.

Results of in situ arthrodesis for the treatment of spondylolisthesis were studied in 39 patients with an average of 4.7 years' follow-up; 82% had good or excellent results. Patients with the most severe slip angle had the greatest chance of a poor result. The outcome was correlated with the quality of the fusion mass, with the poorest results in the Lenke grade D fusion.

Petraco DM, Spivak JM, Cappadona JG, Kummer FJ, Neuwirth MG: An anatomic evaluation of L5 nerve stretch in spondylolisthesis reduction. *Spine* 1996;21:1133–1138.

The authors studied 4 embalmed human spines to quantify the change and length of L5 nerve root associated with reduction of spondylolisthesis. Initially little strain was produced in the L5 nerve root as the L5 vertebral body was reduced in high-grade slips; 71% of the total L5 nerve strain occurred during the second half of vertebral body reduction. Lumbosacral kyphosis in high-grade spondylolisthesis was believed to be protective of the L5 nerve root during attempts at reduction
.

Classic Bibliography

Bell DF, Ehrlich MG, Zaleske DJ: Brace treatment for symptomatic spondylolisthesis. *Clin Orthop* 1988;236:192–198.

Blanda J, Bethem D, Moats W, Lew M: Defects of pars interarticularis in athletes: A protocol for nonoperative treatment. *J Spinal Disord* 1993;6:406–411.

Bohlman HH, Cook SS: One-stage decompression and posterolateral and interbody fusion for lumbosacral spondyloptosis through a posterior approach: Report of two cases. *J Bone Joint Surg* 1982;64A:415–418.

Boos N, Marchesi D, Aebi M: Treatment of spondylolysis and spondylolisthesis with Cotrel-Dubousset instrumentation: A preliminary report. *J Spinal Disord* 1991;4:472–479.

Boxall D, Bradford DS, Winter RB, Moe JH: Management of severe spondylolisthesis in children and adolescents. *J Bone Joint Surg* 1979;61A:479–495.

Bradford DS, Gottfried Y: Staged salvage reconstruction of grade-IV and V spondylolisthesis. *J Bone Joint Surg* 1987; 69A:191–202.

Burkus JK, Lonstein JE, Winter RB, Denis F: Long-term evaluation of adolescents treated operatively for spondylolisthesis: A comparison of in situ arthrodesis only with in situ arthrodesis and reduction followed by immobilization in a cast. *J Bone Joint Surg* 1992;74A:693–704.

Fredrickson BE, Baker D, McHolick WJ, Yuan HA, Lubicky JP: The natural history of spondylolysis and spondylolisthesis. *J Bone Joint Surg* 1984;66A:699–707.

Freeman BL III, Donati NL: Spinal arthrodesis for severe spondylolisthesis in children and adolescents: A long-term follow-up study. *J Bone Joint Surg* 1989;71A:594–598.

Gaines RW, Nichols WK: Treatment of spondyloptosis by two stage L5 vertebrectomy and reduction of L4 onto S1. *Spine* 1985;10:680–686.

Grobler LJ, Novotny JE, Widler DG, Frymoyer JW, Pope MH: L4-5 isthmic spondylolisthesis: A biochemical analysis comparing stability in L4-5 and L5-S1 isthmic spondylolisthesis. *Spine* 1994;19:222–227.

Hambly MF, Wiltse LL: A modificataion of the Scott wiring technique. *Spine* 1994;19:354–356.

Hanley EN Jr, Levy JA: Surgical treatment of isthmic lumbosacral spondylolisthesis: Analysis of variables influencing results. *Spine* 1989;14:48–50.

Johnson JR, Kirwan EO: The long-term results of fusion in situ for severe spondylolisthesis. *J Bone Joint Surg* 1983;65B:43–46.

Jones AA, McAfee PC, Robinson RA, Zinreich SJ, Wang H: Failed arthrodesis of the spine for severe spondylolisthesis: Salvage by interbody arthrodesis. *J Bone Joint Surg* 1988;70A:25–30.

O'Brien JP, Mehdian H, Jaffray D: Reduction of severe lumbosacral spondylolisthesis: A report of 22 cases with a ten-year follow-up period. *Clin Orthop* 1994;300:64–69.

Osterman K, Schlenzka D, Poussa M, Seitsalo S, Virta L: Isthmic spondylolisthesis in symptomatic and asymptomatic subjects, epidemiology, and natural history with special reference to disk abnormality and mode of treatment. *Clin Orthop* 1993; 297:65–70.

Peek RD, Wiltse LL, Reynolds JB, Thomas JC, Guyer DW, Widell EH: In situ arthrodesis without decompression for Grade-III or IV isthemic spondylolithesis in adults who have severe sciatica. *J Bone Joint Surg* 1989;71A:62–68.

Pizzutillo PD, Mirenda W, MacEwen GD: Posterolateral fusion for spondylolithesis in adolescence. *J Pediatr Orthop* 1986; 6:311–316.

Saraste H: Long-term clinical and radiological follow-up of spondylolysis and spondylolisthesis. *J Pediatr Orthop* 1987; 7:631–638.

Scaglietti O, Frontino G, Bartolozzi P: Technique of anatomical reduction of lumbar spondylolisthesis and its surgical stabilization. *Clin Orthop* 1976;117:164–175.

Steffee AD, Sitkowski DJ: Reduction and stabilization of grade IV spondylolisthesis. *Clin Orthop* 1988;227:82–89.

Chapter 53
Adult Scoliosis

Introduction

Adult scoliosis has been defined as the presentation of a scoliosis deformity after skeletal maturity. A chronologic definition specifies the patient must be at least 21 years of age when he or she first presents for treatment of the deformity. Adult scoliosis can be further subdivided into curves that started before skeletal maturity, although the patient did not present for treatment until after skeletal maturity; or deformity that arose de novo after skeletal maturity, with the patient then presenting for evaluation and potential treatment of the condition.

The etiologies of adult scoliosis can be described as idiopathic, degenerative (de novo), congenital, paralytic, and adolescent/adult postspinal fusion, which occurs in patients who develop problems later in life.

Idiopathic Scoliosis

Idiopathic scoliosis is the most common form of adult scoliosis, with a reported prevalence of approximately 5%. In a study of 5,000 adult patients having intravenous polygrams, 3.9% had lumbar scoliosis > 10°. The 2 main symptoms in adults with scoliosis are progressive deformity and pain. These patients may notice increased waistline asymmetry, altered fitting of clothes, or progressive loss of height.

Pain is a more common complaint. The pain may be axial or radicular. Patients with thoracic scoliosis and a significant rib hump can have convex scapular pain caused by prominence and irritation of the posterior shoulder girdle. In addition, axial pain can be caused by degenerative changes that occur primarily on the concavity of curves as a result of facet arthrosis. Spinal fatigue pain can occur in the region of the scoliosis and is often vague and only fully appreciated after a successful spinal fusion when the fatigue pain subsides. Overall, spinal fatigue pain seems to be most correlated with the age of the patient and the degree of curvature.

Physical examination of these patients centers on 3 components: overall spinal alignment, mobility, and neurologic status. Coronal and sagittal alignment must be evaluated with respect to (1) shoulder balance; (2) any deviation of the plumb line, trunk shift or waistline asymmetry, suggesting

overall coronal imbalance; and (3) rib and/or lumbar prominences evaluated by an Adam's forward bend test and quantified by a scoliometer measurement. A thorough upper and lower extremity neurologic examination should be performed and, in idiopathic scoliosis, should be normal in the absence of any cervical or lumbar degenerative radiculopathies.

Diagnostic imaging of an adult with scoliosis begins with standing posteroanterior (PA) and lateral long cassette (36-inch) radiographs of the entire spinal axis. Comparison with any previously obtained spinal radiographs is important to document curve progression by comparing Cobb measurements on serial radiographs (Fig. 1). The radiographs are also examined for overall spinal balance; degenerative changes, such as facet arthropathy, bony spurring, and degenerative disk changes with loss of disk height; and any coronal and/or lateral vertebral subluxations. It is also important to evaluate the patient's regional alignment and global spinal balance in the sagittal plane. Ancillary studies, such as spinal and pelvic bone scans, lumbar spine magnetic resonance imaging (MRI), and/or computed tomography (CT) myelogram are helpful to further quantify degenerative changes and sources of radiculopathies. Although somewhat controversial, diskography can be used to determine disk morphology and also to quantify pain reproduction in the mid to lower lumbar regions to detect symptomatic disk degeneration. Baseline pulmonary function studies quantify the degree of restrictive disease that often accompanies thoracic curves, which can be quite severe in large (> 90°) curves.

It is important to counsel these patients as to the future implications of their scoliosis. Natural history studies have shown that certain idiopathic scoliosis curves progress after skeletal maturity. Curves < 30° are unlikely to progress. Progression is greatest in thoracic curves > 60°, lumbar curves > 50°, and lumbar portions of double major curves. The progression of lumbar curves is particularly problematic in those with an L5 segment at or above the intercrestal line (a "high riding" L5), significant apical rotation (Nash-Moe grade III or higher), and a right convex deformity. Although pregnancy has been implicated as a risk factor for progression, most curves that are progressive after pregnancy were noted to be progressive curves even before pregnancy. As a general rule, adult scoliosis progresses 1° to 2° per year. However, some curves do not progress at all, and some curves progress more rapidly, especially curves in the lumbar spine in patients with accelerated degenerative changes. Superimposition of degenerative changes can lead to rotatory subluxations in the mid to lower lumbar spine, most common at the L3-4 and L4-5 levels. This superimposition may produce not only degenerative instability with axial pain, but also lumbosacral radiculopathies from varying types of spinal stenosis as a result of the spinal subluxation producing central, lateral recess, or foraminal stenosis. Carefully documented follow-up (every 1 to 3 years) remains the best method for determining progression of adult idiopathic scoliosis and concomitant symptomatology.

Cardiopulmonary symptoms occur more frequently in patients with curves of > 90° to 100°. Progressive pulmonary function deterioration in these patients with large deformities may result in pulmonary hypertension and cor pulmonale. Pulmonary function tests are seldom abnormal in thoracic deformities < 60°. Although large thoracic curves are associated with decreased spinal capacity and oxygen transport, subjective dyspnea is experienced only by patients with curves of 90° to 100°. In addition to deformity in the coronal plane, loss of normal thoracic kyphosis, especially severe lordosis in the thoracic spine, is implicated in deterioration of pulmonary function. Other causes of cardiorespiratory compromise, such as smoking, asthma, chronic obstructive pulmonary disease, or occupational lung disease, should also be considered in the adult patient with scoliosis and any type of pulmonary abnormality.

Treatment

Conservative treatment, such as medication, exercise, bracing, physical therapy, and injections, should be tried first to control pain. The primary indications for considering surgery in adults with scoliosis are to halt progression of the deformity and to obtain relief of pain that is not responsive to conservative treatment. Scoliosis surgery for pain relief alone has varying degrees of success, with reports of success rates as low as 40% to 50%. It is important to try to quantify and localize the patient's pain generator(s) before undertaking a spinal fusion. Indications for surgery with respect to treating the deformity include: (1) documented progressive thoracic curves > 50° to 60°; (2) double major curves > 60°; (3) thoracic curves > 80° to 90° with diminished pulmonary function; and (4) lumbar curves with rotatory subluxations causing increased axial pain and/or spinal stenosis.

Once surgery is decided upon, the basic components of a successful surgery include a thorough arthrodesis with autogenous bone graft and a rigidly immobilized spine secured with segmental spinal instrumentation. In most adults with scoliosis, instrumentation and fusion are done through a posterior approach, although some younger adult patients with primary thoracolumbar and lumbar curve patterns can be successfully treated with anterior instrumentation and fusion alone. Many patients are best treated with a circumferential anterior and posterior fusion to optimize both correction of the deformity and fusion consolidation. Potential indications for combined fusions include a large rigid primary scoliotic curve (> 80°), a rigid kyphotic component to the deformity (> 70° kyphosis), advanced age or spinal osteoporosis, and requirement for fusion to the sacrum. Anterior fusion requires thorough diskectomies and autograft (usually rib graft from the approach) for fusion. All periapical segments should be included in the anterior fusion; for lumbar curves, as many segments as possible that will be treated posteriorly should be fused anteriorly. Consideration should be given to

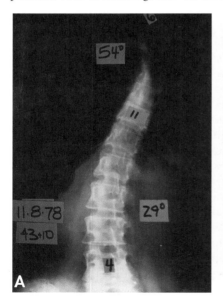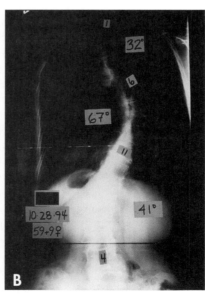

Figure 1

A, A 43-year-old patient presented for evaluation of a right thoracic deformity. The radiographs demonstrated a 54° right thoracic curve with a compensatory 29° lumbar curve. B, Sixteen years later, the patient's thoracic curve has increased 13° to 67°, and the lumbar curve 12° to 41°. The patient complained of moderate to severe thoracic pain as well as a 2-inch loss of height over the last decade.

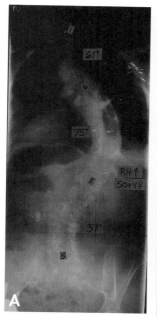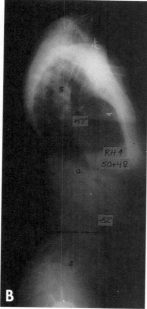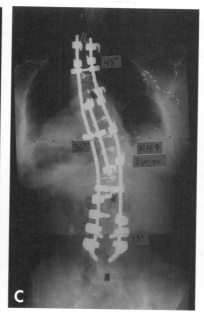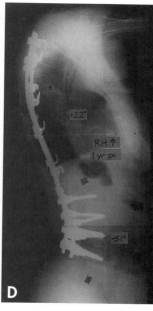

Figure 2

A, Fifty-year-old woman who presented with documented progression of a thoracic scoliosis with increasing thoracic and lumbar spinal pain. B, Her sagittal long cassette radiograph demonstrated acceptable alignment with evidence of rather severe osteopenia secondary to chronic steroid use for asthma. C, After a posterior segmental spinal instrumentation and fusion from T2 to L4 with a 3-rod technique, and multiple fixation points to distribute the corrective forces over many segments of her vertebral column, her preoperative pain was significantly improved. D, Her postoperative sagittal plane shows maintenance of her lumbar lordosis and overall favorable sagittal global alignment.

placing structural bone graft in the mid to lower lumbar disks to maintain support for lumbar lordosis and also to load share the posterior instrumentation during union.

The posterior procedure involves applying rigid segmental spinal instrumentation for the planned posterior fusion levels (Fig. 2). Fusion should extend from a neutral vertebra proximally to a (ideally) neutral, horizontal, and centered vertebra distally. Autogenous bone graft is harvested from either convex ribs (thoracoplasty) or, more commonly, the posterior iliac crest. It is important to obtain rigid immobilization of the involved segments to increase the fusion rate and depend less on external immobilization. In patients with a cosmetically unacceptable rib hump preoperatively, a convex rib thoracoplasty should be considered. However, preoperative pulmonary function should be checked, because pulmonary function appears to be decreased by rib harvest in adults, even at 2 years after the procedure.

Scoliosis surgeries in adults are much more difficult and have many more complications than similar types of deformity corrections in adolescents. Reported complication rates include neurologic deficits (< 1% to 5%), infection (0.5% to 5%), pseudarthrosis (5% to 27%), residual pain (5% to 15%), pulmonary embolism (1% to 20%), and mortality (< 1% to

5%). The reasons for these increased complication rates include (1) increased blood loss resulting from more difficult subperiosteal stripping of the posterior musculature off the spine; (2) less rigid instrumentation caused by soft or osteoporotic bone stock; (3) lower fusion rates as a result of the older age of these patients; and (4) higher peri- and postoperative medical complication rates as a result of many factors, including a longer time in surgery, a higher risk of infection, deep venous thromboses, and pulmonary sequelae. Because some complications appear to result from nutritional depletion that occurs after extensive spinal reconstructions, it is important to optimize the nutritional status of adults undergoing extensive spinal fusion. The return to a normal nutritional status usually takes longer than 6 weeks in patients with fusions of 10 levels or more. Staging circumferential fusions further deteriorates the nutritional status of these patients, and hyperalimentation between the first and second stages and after the second stage of these combined procedures may be advantageous. It probably is better to do circumferential anterior and posterior fusions on the same day under a single anesthetic if possible.

When choosing the lowest fusion level in an adult idiopathic thoracic curve, it usually is best to fuse to the stable vertebra. This is the vertebra most closely bisected by the center sacral line, which is a line bisecting the sacrum, drawn perpendicular to the horizontal line that goes across the top of the iliac crests. In the mid to lower lumbar spine, the distal level of fusion should be at a segment that is as close to neutrally rotated and horizontal and as centered on the sacrum as possible. In addition, preoperative confirmation of the absence of severe degenerative changes below the intended fusion level is important. Occasionally, fusion to the sacrum is indicated in an adult with primary lumbar scoliosis. Fusion to the sacrum should be considered for patients with fixed lumbar curves with L5 lumbosacral obliquity, patients with severe loss of coronal and/or sagittal balance, and patients with severe degenerative changes at the L4-5 and L5-S1 segments. Anterior structural grafting of these lowest disks is important to obtain and maintain as much segmental lordosis as possible and to achieve optimum sagittal global alignment when instrumenting and fusing the entire spine to the pelvis.

Degenerative (de novo) Scoliosis

Degenerative lumbar scoliosis with onset well into adult life is being identified more and more often in patients 60 years of age and older. The multifactorial etiology of these lumbar spinal deformities includes disk degeneration, facet arthropathy, ligamentous laxity, and osteoporosis. Patients have clinical symptoms of back and/or leg pain. Back pain normally is caused by degeneration of the disks and is mechanical, while leg pain usually is the result of spinal stenosis.

Initial evaluation of these patients begins with upright PA and lateral lumbar spine radiographs. More important than the actual Cobb measurement of the deformity is the presence and degree of rotatory subluxations, which occur most commonly at L3-4 and L4-5, but can occur at any level. Multilevel disk degeneration in the sagittal plane is present, with varying degrees of loss of lumbar lordosis or absolute kyphosis. The natural history of degenerative scoliosis is quite variable, with rates of annual progression ranging from 1° to 6°. The main thoracolumbar and lumbar curves can be as large as 50° to 60°, with a concomitant contralateral lumbosacral curve. Spinal stenosis with associated lower extremity claudication and/or radicular complaints is common, and a CT-myelogram provides the most accurate neuroradiographic information about these deformities.

Conservative treatment options in these patients are similar to those for adults with idiopathic scoliosis, and include physical therapy programs to strengthen, as well as maintain flexibility of, the spinal musculature and increase aerobic fitness. Surgical treatment depends on the amount of coronal deformity with vertebral rotatory subluxations, the sagittal alignment, and the presence and amount of spinal stenosis. The 3 levels of surgical treatment are decompression alone, decompression with posterior fusion and instrumentation, and decompression with anterior and posterior fusion and posterior instrumentation. Decompression alone is reserved for patients who have spinal stenosis but no major coronal or sagittal deformities and no rotatory subluxation. In addition, flexion-extension and side bending radiographs should show a minimum of detectable motion. Midline and lateral recess decompression should not destabilize the spine as long as it is not done at the apex of the curve where a rotatory subluxation exists.

Patients who require decompression with posterior fusion and instrumentation have a greater degree of spinal deformity, with mild to moderate rotatory subluxations present in regions that require a stenosis decompression. However, in the sagittal plane overall spinal alignment is acceptable without significant kyphosis. The third group of patients have more severe deformities in both the coronal and sagittal planes, with marked hypolordosis or frank kyphosis of the lumbar spine, severe stenosis, and rotatory subluxations > 5 mm. Their coronal and sagittal imbalances usually are not correctable on side bending or hyperextension lateral radiographs. For these patients, anterior diskectomy and fusion with placement of structural grafts in the disk spaces to re-create lumbar lordosis are appropriate. The placement of structural grafts with anterior distraction creates a ligamentotaxis effect that helps reduce the rotatory subluxations and also increases the cross-sectional diameter of the corresponding foramen. A posterior procedure is done next, with the appropriate stenosis decompressions, posterior instrumentation and fusion, and posterior convex compression forces applied to further lordose the spine and reduce the scoliosis. As in surgery for idiopathic scoliosis in adults, it is important to begin and end the fusion at both a neutral and stable vertebra. At times, it is acceptable to stabilize with instrumentation and fusion only those levels with rotatory subluxations that are being decompressed and to leave levels above and below uninstrumented and unfused. This procedure requires careful consideration to avoid transition syndromes or subluxations that occur in the coronal and sagittal planes either above (most common) or below a short lumbar fusion. It is important to appropriately judge the physiologic age of the patient, not just the chronologic age, as a guideline for surgical indications. The results of surgery appear to be somewhat less predictable for degenerative scoliosis than for spinal stenosis without any deformity, probably because of the increased amount of surgery required to treat degenerative scoliosis.

Adolescent and Adult Postscoliosis Fusion

The development of Harrington instrumentation was a significant advance in scoliosis surgery, improving fusion rates and considerably increasing the amount of correction. Although results in the thoracic spine were good, Harrington instrumentation extending into the mid and lower lumbar spine often produced residual problems. The most significant of these problems is a relative loss of lumbar lordosis as a result of "flattening" of the lumbar sagittal plane, producing a "flat back" syndrome. This syndrome is characterized by progressive lumbosacral pain, mild to marked forward sagittal imbalance, and progressive disk and facet degeneration below the fusion.

Long-term studies of younger individuals who have had a posterior instrumentation and fusion for scoliosis have shown no increase in disability overall, provided the distal fusion ends in the upper lumbar spine. However, when the fusion extends below L3, there is a significant tendency toward low back disability and pain, with 62% of patients fused down to L4 and 82% of patients fused down to L5 having significant complaints. Many of these patients required revision surgery to extend their fusions more distally, often to the sacrum. In addition, some of these patients required extension lumbar osteotomies to improve lordosis and, thus, global sagittal balance. Prevention of flat back syndrome appears to be an important component of managing these difficult spinal reconstructions.

At the time of this writing, bone screws placed posteriorly into vertebral elements have been cleared for use in this specific manner by the Food and Drug Administration (FDA) to provide immobilization and stabilization as an adjunct to fusion in the treatment of the following acute and chronic instability or deformities of the thoracic, lumbar and sacral spine: degenerative spondylolisthesis with objective evidence of neurological impairment; fracture; dislocation; scoliosis; kyphosis; spinal tumor and failed previous fusion (pseudoarthrosis). In addition, anterior vertebral body screws (cervical, thoracic, and lumbar) are Class II devices and can be used as labeled in vertebral bodies.

Annotated Bibliography

Albert TJ, Purtill J, Mesa J, McIntosh T, Balderston RA: Health outcome assessment before and after adult deformity surgery: A prospective study. *Spine* 1995;20:2002–2004.

Health status of 55 patients undergoing surgery for adult spinal deformity was assessed using a generic health outcome instrument before surgery and an average of 2 years following spinal reconstruction. The results demonstrated that adult scoliosis surgery significantly improved patient self-reported health assessment and function. The beneficial results did not appear to deteriorate with age or more distal vertebral levels of spinal fusion. The authors also suggested that a more highly disease-specific outcome analysis as well as generic health surveys will be required to assess the clinical outcome of adult spinal deformity surgery.

Bradford DS: Adult scoliosis, in Lonstein JE, Bradford DS, Winter RB, Ogilvie JW (eds): *Moe's Textbook of Scoliosis and Other Spinal Deformities*, ed 3. Philadelphia, PA, WB Saunders, 1995, pp 369–386.

This excellent book chapter is devoted to discussion of the management of the adult patient with spinal deformity. Specific sections of the chapter explore in detail issues of prevalence, presentation, evaluation, and treatment for these patients.

Bridwell KH: Where to stop the fusion distally in adult scoliosis: L4, L5, or the sacrum?, in Pritchard DJ (ed): *Instructional Course Lectures 45*. Rosemont, IL, American Academy of Orthopaedic Surgeons, 1996, pp 101–107.

This excellent chapter reviews multiple considerations that must be weighed and discussed with the patient before deciding on a long fusion down to the middle or distal lumbar spine. Many factors are outlined which will play a vital role in the decision and eventual outcome of such spinal reconstructions.

Grubb SA, Lipscomb HJ: Diagnostic findings in painful adult scoliosis. *Spine* 1992;17:518–527.

Diagnostic findings in a group of 55 adult patients with both scoliosis and pain were documented. Patients with degenerative onset scoliosis (49%) had myelographic defects most commonly within the primary curve, and on diskography, multiple abnormal, and not necessarily painful, disks were seen throughout the lumbar spine. Patients with idiopathic onset scoliosis (44%) had myelographic defects most commonly in a compensatory lumbar or lumbosacral curve, and all patients had at least 1 abnormal, painful disk (88% with pain reproduction). Pain-producing pathology was frequently identified in areas that would not have been included in the fusion area according to accepted rules for treatment of idiopathic scoliosis.

Grubb SA, Lipscomb HJ, Suh PB: Results of surgical treatment of painful adult scoliosis. *Spine* 1994;19:1619–1627.

Twenty-eight adults with idiopathic scoliosis and 25 with degenerative scoliosis treated with spinal fusion were followed prospectively for 2 to 7 years. Pain relief was associated with solid fusion (*p*= 0.02). Reported pain reproduction was 80% among patients with idiopathic scoliosis and 70% among patients with degenerative scoliosis. Sitting and walking tolerances were improved in patients with idiopathic scoliosis, and standing and walking were improved in patients with degenerative scoliosis.

Ogilvie JW: Adult scoliosis: Evaluation and nonsurgical treatment, in Eilert RE: *Instructional Course Lectures XLI*. Park Ridge, IL, American Academy of Orthopaedic Surgeons, 1992, pp 251–255.

This chapter states that it is incumbent on the surgeon to understand the pathology involved in painful adult spinal deformities and to have a reasonable understanding of the prognosis before attempting invasive therapy. The decision to proceed with surgical treatment is justified in many cases, but it must be based on a thorough understanding of the anticipated benefits and of the risk of serious complications.

Simmons ED Jr, Kowalski JM, Simmons EH: The results of surgical treatment for adult scoliosis. *Spine* 1993;18:718–724.

The authors found that the relative incidence of pain and progression as indications for surgery were found to vary with respect to age. In the younger groups, progression was more often the indication for surgery, and these patients also had greater deformity. The degree of pain was not found to correlate with the magnitude of the deformity. Surgical treatment can be done with a relatively low serious complication rate and good results in terms of pain relief and reasonable correction of the deformity.

Classic Bibliography

Ascani E, Bartolozzi P, Logroscino CA, et al: Natural history of untreated idiopathic scoliosis after skeletal maturity. *Spine* 1986;11:784–789.

Cordover AM, Betz RR, Clements DH, Bosacco SJ: Natural history of adolescent thoracolumbar and lumbar idiopathic scoliosis into adulthood. *J Spinal Disord* 1997;10:193–196.

Dick J, Boachie-Adjei O, Wilson M: One-stage versus two-stage anterior and posterior spinal reconstruction in adults: Comparison of outcomes including nutritional status, complication rates, hospital costs, and other factors. *Spine* 1992;17(suppl 8):S310–S316.

Edgar MA, Mehta MH: Long-term follow-up of fused and unfused idiopathic scoliosis. *J Bone Joint Surg* 1988;70B:712–716.

Fowles JV, Drummond DS, L'Ecuyer S, Roy L, Kassab MT: Untreated scoliosis in the adult. *Clin Orthop* 1978;134:212–217.

Grubb SA, Lipscomb HJ, Coonrad RW: Degenerative adult onset scoliosis. *Spine* 1988;13:241–245.

Jackson RP, Simmons EH, Stripinis D: Coronal and sagittal plane spinal deformities correlating with back pain and pulmonary function in adult idiopathic scoliosis. *Spine* 1989;14:1391–1397.

Kostuik JP: Operative treatment of idiopathic scoliosis. *J Bone Joint Surg* 1990;72A:1108–1113.

Kostuik JP: Treatment of scoliosis in the adult thoracolumbar spine with special reference to fusion to the sacrum. *Orthop Clin North Am* 1988;19:371–381.

Lenke LG, Bridwell KH, Blanke K, Baldus C: Prospective analysis of nutritional status normalization after spinal reconstructive surgery. *Spine* 1995;20:1359–1367.

Mandelbaum BR, Tolo VT, McAfee PC, Burest P: Nutritional deficiencies after staged anterior and posterior spinal reconstructive surgery. *Clin Orthop* 1988;234:5–11.

Nachemson A: Adult scoliosis and back pain. *Spine* 1979;4:513–517.

Robin GC, Span Y, Steinberg R, Makin M, Menczel J: Scoliosis in the elderly: A follow-up study. *Spine* 1982;7:355–359.

Simmons EH, Jackson RP: The management of nerve root entrapment syndromes associated with the collapsing scoliosis of idiopathic lumbar and thoracolumbar curves. *Spine* 1979;4:533–541.

Weinstein SL, Ponseti IV: Curve progression in idiopathic scoliosis. *J Bone Joint Surg* 1983;65A:447–455.

Weinstein SL, Zavala DC, Ponseti IV: Idiopathic scoliosis: Long-term follow-up and prognosis in untreated patients. *J Bone Joint Surg* 1981;63A:702–712.

Winter RB, Lonstein JE, Denis F: Pain patterns in adult scoliosis. *Orthop Clin North Am* 1988;19:339–345.

Chapter 54
Spinal Infections

The prognosis of patients with spinal infections has improved significantly in the past few decades. The mortality rate of patients with a neurologic deficit from tuberculous spondylitis is now less than 5%, down from 60% before antibiotics. Advances in radiology and surgery have allowed earlier treatment with less morbidity.

Most spinal infections occurring in developed countries are caused by pyogenic bacteria. Mycobacteria, brucella, and fungi induce a granulomatous response, and they are the organisms most often encountered in under-developed countries and in immunocompromised hosts.

Pyogenic Vertebral Osteomyelitis

Epidemiology and Etiology

The vertebrae are susceptible to hematogenous bacterial seeding, with resultant osteomyelitis. The seeding occurs via septic emboli from a remote infection, usually in the urinary tract, respiratory tract, or skin. The vertebral bodies have rich arterial anastomoses that end at the vertebral end plates. These blind loops are remnants of the vascular channels in the cartilaginous end plates in children. Bacteria are deposited in these loops and initiate the disease process. This occurs most often in elderly men and immunocompromised patients. The incidence of pyogenic vertebral osteomyelitis has been increasing in recent years. This increase likely is the result of the relative increase in population age and the greater number of immunocompromised patients. The other population groups with an increased frequency are human immunodeficiency virus (HIV)-infected patients and young intravenous drug abusers.

Historically, *Staphylococcus aureus* was the exclusive pathogen, but it now accounts for only 50% of all infections. Gram-negative bacteria and flora infections are increasing. *Pseudomonas*, *Escherichia coli*, *Enterococcus*, and *Proteus* species are most frequently identified.

Clinical Presentation

The most common complaint among patients with pyogenic vertebral osteomyelitis is back pain with an insidious onset. The pain is vague, nonspecific, and lacks dermatomal or radicular characteristics. Fever is present in about half of the patients. Other symptoms may include local spinal tenderness and marked limitation of motion. Local inflammation of surrounding muscles may result in complaints of nonspecific chest and abdominal symptoms. Less frequent clinical signs include torticollis with cervical spine involvement, hip flexion contractures with psoas inflammation, and meningeal signs.

The lumbar spine is most commonly affected (50% of cases); the thoracic spine is second in frequency, and the cervical spine is involved in fewer than 10%. A paraspinal soft-tissue component is common, whereas the presence of a frank abscess is uncommon. Neurologic findings occur in 17% of patients and are more common in the cervical spine because of the smaller space available for the spinal cord. Compression of the spinal cord or nerves occurs from impingement by bone, disk, pus, or granulation tissue. Spinal instability resulting from collapse of supporting structures may also result in compression. Systemic factors that increase the likelihood of neurologic compromise include diabetes, rheumatoid arthritis, age, and systemic corticosteroid therapy.

Diagnosis

The white blood cell count is elevated in 42% of patients. The erythrocyte sedimentation rate (ESR) is useful for screening and is increased in approximately 90% of patients with pyogenic vertebral osteomyelitis. Sensitivity is increased for the C-reactive protein (CRP). This acute phase inflammatory marker is more sensitive for infections and can be used in combination with the ESR to follow a patient's response to antibiotic treatment. A rapid decline of the ESR in the first month indicates successful treatment, but a persistently increased or even rising ESR does not necessarily indicate treatment failure. The ESR should be interpreted in conjunction with other clinical findings and CRP.

Blood cultures are positive in only 24% of patients with pyogenic vertebral osteomyelitis. The value of other positive culture results, such as a urine culture, is only for confirmation of an infection. There may be coexistent infections caused by different organisms.

Radiology

Routine radiography of the spine demonstrates pyogenic vertebral osteomyelitis when the disease has progressed sufficiently over time. This process takes 3 weeks and initially appears as disk-space narrowing followed by destructive changes of the vertebral end plates, with progression to the anterior vertebral body. Plain tomography or noncontrast computed tomography (CT) reveals the extensive bony destruction earlier. Additionally, the presence of a soft-tissue abscess identified by CT scan may help eliminate a neoplasm from the differential diagnosis. Neoplasms usually do not surround the anterior spine, as is often seen in an abscess. A neoplasm usually remains localized to the paravertebral region and does not extend beyond the vertebral body early in the disease, and the disk is not involved in most neoplasms.

Radionuclide studies are valuable as diagnostic adjuncts. Because of its poor sensitivity and accuracy (17% and 31%, respectively), the indium scan is not helpful in the diagnosis of vertebral osteomyelitis despite having a specificity of 100%. Technetium bone scans and gallium scans are the preferred imaging techniques, with sensitivity of 90% and accuracy of 85%. The gallium scan is more useful because it detects the infection earlier and may be used as an aid to follow the infection during treatment. Like the CRP, it returns to normal with resolution of the infection. The technetium scan remains active for months after resolution of the infection.

Magnetic resonance imaging (MRI) is the modality of choice in the diagnosis of pyogenic vertebral osteomyelitis (Fig. 1). With a sensitivity of 96%, a specificity of 93%, and an accuracy of 94%, MRI demonstrates pathologic changes at a time similar to the gallium scan, yet discerns greater anatomic details. T1-weighted sequences demonstrate a decrease in the signal intensity at the peridiskal region. The distinction between the disk margin and the vertebral body also is lost. On T2-weighted images, abnormal increased signal is seen in the disk and adjacent vertebral bodies. There is loss of the intranuclear cleft in the disk. The administration of gadolinium enhances the disk space, delineating the extent of a soft-tissue abscess and identifies neoplasms. MRI can be helpful during the course of treatment if the patient does not respond as expected or deteriorates neurologically. Routine follow-up MRI, however, can be misleading because the findings lag behind the clinical response and may give the impression that the disease is progressive despite clinical improvement.

Definitive diagnosis of pyogenic vertebral osteomyelitis is based on a biopsy with bacteriologic and histologic confirmation. This biopsy is not necessary in children and may not be necessary in the symptomatic adult with a positive blood culture. The biopsy can be performed by percutaneous or open techniques. The diagnostic yield of a needle biopsy depends on several factors: the core size must be sufficient to obtain an adequate specimen, and the biopsy site must be accessible and provide appropriate tissue for histologic and microbiologic analysis. Open biopsies have a lower false-negative rate than needle biopsies. The use of antibiotics before any biopsy increases the false-negative rate regardless of the technique chosen. In the case of a negative biopsy, the surgeon must determine whether the biopsy should be repeated

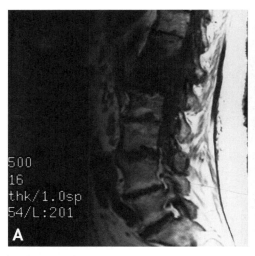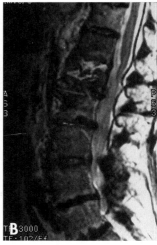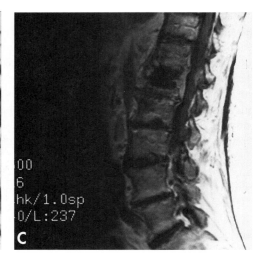

Figure 1

Magnetic resonance imaging findings in pyogenic vertebral osteomyelitis. A, On this T1-weighted sagittal sequence, the T12-L1 disk space and the entire L1 body have decreased signal and the end plates are indistinct. B, High signal is seen in the T12-L1 disk space and the L1 vertebral body on the T2-weighted sagittal sequence. C, Enhancement in the T12-L1 disk space, the L1 vertebral body, and the epidural space is seen on the postgadolinium T1-weighted sagittal sequence.

and whether the patient is to be observed or empirically treated with antibiotics. In general, a repeat biopsy, either by needle or open, is indicated.

Management

The management of pyogenic vertebral osteomyelitis is directed toward removing the focus of infection by medical or surgical means and by activating the patient's own defenses to fight infections. Medical treatment is directed toward improving nutrition, optimizing the immune system, preventing hypoxia, and controlling diabetes when present. Surgical management involves removing the focus of infection, restoring spinal stability, restoring or preventing neurologic compromise, and relieving pain. Antibiotic therapy is chosen based on the culture results and sensitivities of the organism. Initially, a broad-spectrum antibiotic is chosen for the patient in a toxic condition or the immunocompromised patient, but this is changed to one specific for the isolated bacteria. The length of treatment with parenteral antibiotics should be 6 weeks, with conversion to an oral preparation until the infection resolves.

Pain control is achieved by immobilization of the spine, initially bed rest, until acute symptoms abate. Further immobilization is based on the location of the infection. Cervical and cervicothoracic osteomyelitis are rapidly progressive and lead to instability early in the disease. Immobilization with a halo vest is preferred, but cervicothoracic orthoses may be sufficient in certain situations. For osteomyelitis in the thoracic and lumbar spine, a thoracolumbosacral orthosis is used with a chin extension for high thoracic lesions. Bracing is continued for 3 months until the infection resolves and stability is ensured.

Surgical intervention is needed when there is failure to obtain an adequate specimen or to make the diagnosis from the needle biopsy. Other indications for surgery include drainage of an abscess, decompression for neurologic deficits, correction of deformity, spinal instability, and failure of medical treatment to relieve the infection. A neurologic deficit that develops or progresses demands emergent surgical decompression. Otherwise, surgery is performed at the earliest opportunity after medical clearance of the patient.

Anterior exposure is preferred because its direct access to the pathologic area permits debridement of the abscess, vertebral body, and disk and direct decompression of the spinal canal. A kyphotic deformity, if present, often can be reduced and alignment maintained with appropriate bone graft placement. Anterior intervertebral body bone grafting is performed with autogenous tricortical iliac crest or rib graft. Fibular grafts are used when longer strut grafting is necessary. Anterior autogenous bone grafting has proved safe and effective in the face of an acute infection of the spine. With a severe kyphotic deformity or instability from major bony destruction, posterior stabilization with instrumentation may be required (Fig. 2).

Laminectomy is contraindicated for pyogenic vertebral osteomyelitis because increased spinal instability and kyphotic deformity may result. If a limited decompression is indicated for osteomyelitis that is localized to the posterolateral body or if gross purulence is expected, a costotransversectomy may be performed. This approach prevents contamination of the pleural and abdominal cavities; however, it is limited in its ability to correct deformity or to decompress the anterior epidural space.

Traumatic Etiologies

Penetrating spinal trauma may result in the development of pyogenic vertebral osteomyelitis by the direct inoculation of the disk or bone. The origin of the pathogen is the skin or a hollow viscus that the projectile has traversed, typically the colon or small bowel. The penetrating missile creates a path of devitalized tissue that serves as a culture medium for pathogens if it is not debrided adequately. Military-type weapon injuries dictate aggressive serial debridements to reduce this risk, even in the absence of visceral injury. Low-velocity civilian-type weapon wounds that have not penetrated a hollow viscus may be observed. For penetrating injuries

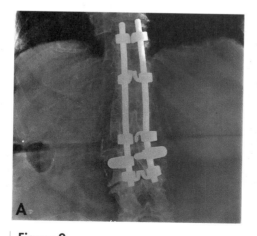
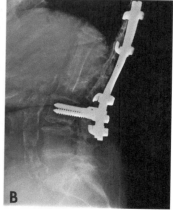

Figure 2

Posterior fusion and instrumentation stabilized the spine after anterior L1 corpectomy and T12-L2 strut graft for the patient with L1 osteomyelitis seen in Figure 1. A, Anteroposterior radiograph. B, Lateral radiograph.

of the abdomen with bowel and spine injuries, the spine does not need debridement nor do bullet fragments need removal at the initial exploration by the trauma surgeon. The patient should be covered by 5 to 7 days of appropriate parenteral antibiotics to include gram-positive, gram-negative, and anaerobic coverage. Cervical injuries that pass through the anterior portion of the neck necessitate a panendoscopic evaluation for laryngotracheal, pharyngeal, and esophageal injury. Treatment includes appropriate debridement, repair, and parenteral antibiotic coverage for 3 to 5 days. As in the thoracolumbar spine, debridement of the cervical spine has not decreased the incidence of infection.

Tuberculosis

Epidemiology

Among the granulomatous infections, tuberculosis is the classic disease in its presentation. Organisms that cause infections that appear at presentation as a granulomatous disease include the fungi, spirochetes, and bacteria of the order Actinomycetales (mycobacteria, actinomycetes, and *Nocardia*). Tuberculosis is prevalent in underdeveloped and third world countries; however, the recent resurgence in the developed world is postulated to result from the increasing population of immunocompromised patients (from acquired immunodeficiency syndrome (AIDS), chemotherapy regimens, and transplantations). The infection usually is spread to the spine via hematogenous seeding from the pulmonary or genitourinary systems, but it also may invade locally by direct extension. The spine is involved in 50% of patients with systemic tuberculosis. Neurologic involvement varies in spinal tuberculosis (10% to 47%).

Pathogenesis

Granulomatous infection of the spine has characteristics that distinguish it from a pyogenic vertebral infection. Large abscess formation is common with granulomatous infections. The disk is more resistant to infection and is preserved despite the extensive bone loss in the vertebral bodies. Because of the indolent nature of the disease, the pathologic changes occur more slowly, allowing greater deformity to develop before symptoms appear.

Vertebral destruction generally follows 1 of 3 patterns: peridiskal, anterior, and central. The peridiskal pattern of spinal tuberculosis begins in the metaphyseal region of 1 vertebra, extends to the adjacent vertebra, and resembles a pyogenic infection. The vertebral involvement may remain anterior beneath the ligament and destroy the anterior portion of consecutive vertebral bodies in a scalloping fashion, leaving the majority of the metaphysis intact. This is described as the anterior form of involvement. The central form is the most difficult to diagnose because it resembles a tumor. The infection stays contained within a single vertebral body and often leads to vertebral collapse, causing a spinal deformity.

Neurologic involvement results from compression by epidural granuloma or bone or disk protrusion into the spinal canal secondary to collapse or deformity. Risk factors for increased neurologic deficits include advanced age, cephalad level of spinal involvement, and lack of paraspinal abscess.

Diagnosis

The patient with tuberculosis appears to be chronically ill, with pain, weight loss, and malaise. Fever is intermittent. The patient with neglected disease may present with deformity and even paraplegia from the neurologic compression. The thoracic spine is involved most often, followed by the lumbar spine. The cervical spine rarely is involved in tuberculous infections.

The ESR is increased. The white blood cell count usually is not increased, although it may be slightly above normal. A tuberculin skin test is positive in patients with tuberculosis and is useful as a screening test. The physician must be wary of a negative test result in a patient suspected of having tuberculosis, and the presence of anergy caused by severe immunoincompetence must be considered. The definitive diagnostic test is a positive biopsy, with identification of the acid-fast bacilli. The mycobacteria may take up to 10 weeks to grow in culture before identification. The sensitivity may be as low as 50%. Polymerase chain reaction has been shown to aid in the rapid identification of mycobacteria. This test has a sensitivity of 94.7% and an accuracy of 92%.

Imaging studies help demonstrate the extent of the disease and presence of deformity. Nuclear imaging scans with technetium or gallium are not sensitive and have no diagnostic value. CT scans help evaluate the extent of bone destruction and are useful in planning surgery. When combined with myelography, CT can help determine whether soft tissue or bone involvement is responsible for the neurologic deficit. The imaging study of choice, as in the pyogenic infections, is MRI. The extent of bone involvement is shown as changes in the bone marrow signal of the vertebral bodies. The disks usually are preserved in tuberculosis. The use of gadolinium helps to differentiate pus from granulation tissue. A mass with enhancement only at the periphery generally is an abscess, whereas a mass that enhances completely is likely to be granulation tissue (Fig. 3).

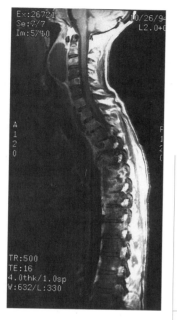

Figure 3

T1-weighted magnetic resonance imaging sequence with gadolinium in a 25-year-old man with tuberculous spondylitis. A large retropharyngeal abscess with peripheral enhancement is seen extending from the base of the skull to the inferior aspect of T9. The anterior aspect of all of the vertebral bodies is involved in a scalloped fashion and the disk spaces are preserved.

Management

The goals of treatment for spinal tuberculosis are eradication of the infection, prevention of further neurologic deterioration, and prevention or correction of spinal deformity. Antibiotic treatment should consist of a multiple-drug regimen for at least 6 to 9 months. Multiple drugs, which are used to prevent the emergence of drug resistance, include isoniazid, rifampin, pyrazinamide, streptomycin, and ethambutol.

Surgical treatment is indicated to obtain sufficient tissue for diagnosis, to debride an abscess, to decompress the spinal cord, and to correct spinal deformity. Decompression for neurologic deficits has improved the neurologic outcome (94% improved) compared with nonsurgical management alone (79% improved). Early decompression results in optimal neurologic improvement. Anterior decompression is preferred, with thorough debridement to viable bleeding bone. The decompression must extend to the posterior longitudinal ligament or dura if there is epidural compression. Spinal deformity is corrected and alignment maintained with an autogenous strut graft. Iliac crest or ribs are readily obtainable and function well in most cases. If a longer strut is needed, a fibular graft may be used.

Laminectomy has limited indications in spinal tuberculosis. Alone, it destabilizes the spine and results in rapid progression of the kyphotic deformity. When there is posterolateral vertebral involvement, laminectomy is appropriate to relieve posterior epidural compression; however, it may need to be combined with a posterior fusion. Posterior spinal fusion with instrumentation is the optimal method for maintaining spinal alignment. If anterior decompression or debridement

of an abscess is necessary, it should be performed in a staged manner with the posterior fusion. Wound closure must be meticulous and in a layered fashion. Nonabsorbable sutures should be used to prevent dehiscence because wound healing is poor. These chronically ill patients are often malnourished, compounding this problem.

The incidence of complications from surgical treatment of these patients is high, with 3% mortality. With early detection and diagnosis of tuberculosis in combination with an appropriate antibiotic regimen, the overall mortality from the disease is less than 5%, with little relapse. The fusion rate in spinal tuberculosis varies with treatment. Nonsurgical antibiotic therapy alone results in a 23% fusion rate of the involved spinal segment at 12 months. This increases to 52% at 18 months and 84% at 5 years. Surgical fusion after debridement and bone grafting (the Hong Kong procedure) changes these fusion rates to 70% at 12 months, 85% at 18 months, and 92% at 5 years. The advantages of surgical fusion are the ability to achieve correction of the deformity and maintenance of alignment.

Epidural Abscess

The incidence of epidural abscesses is increasing. Factors that may explain this increase include the increased number of spinal procedures performed, the improved diagnostic imaging capability, and the increasing number of intravenous drug abusers. The spinal procedures include surgery, injections into and around the epidural space, and diagnostic injections, such as diskography and facet or nerve root blocks.

The epidural space is seeded directly by the spinal procedure, indirectly by hematogenous seeding from a remote site, or by direct extension from a contiguous site. The susceptibility for infection increases in patients with diabetes, intravenous drug abusers, or patients who have had multiple prior surgeries or procedures. The causative organism is *S aureus* in more than 60% of patients, and gram-negative rods account for about 20%. Gram-negative infections, especially *Pseudomonas*, are commonly found in intravenous drug users.

Pathology

Epidural abscesses most often occur in the thoracic and lumbar spine. The posterior epidural space is involved in 75% of patients, with the remainder located anteriorly. The abscess typically extends over 3 to 4 spinal segments, but may involve the entire spinal column. The early phase of an epidural abscess involves an inflammatory reaction in the epidural fat, which exists most abundantly posteriorly. This inflammatory granulation tissue then progresses to suppuration, necrosis, and fibrosis. Left untreated, this destructive process may compress the thecal sac, and result in neurologic symptoms. Necrosis also may compromise the vascular supply to the spinal cord, with the devastating result of paralysis.

Clinical Presentation and Diagnosis

As in most spinal infections, the usual presenting complaint is intractable back pain. Fever and spinal tenderness usually are also present. Without treatment, back pain is often followed by radicular pain, weakness, and paralysis. The virulence of the organism and the immune defenses of the host determine the severity and aggressiveness of the disease. Long delays in diagnosis are not uncommon because of this variable presentation. Neurologic deficits develop acutely or insidiously over weeks to months. These patients often are ill-appearing and may have a toxic reaction with fever, tachycardia, hypotension, or sepsis. Laboratory evaluation with a complete blood cell count, ESR, and CRP confirms an infectious process. Radiographs help eliminate pyogenic vertebral osteomyelitis or diskitis as the source of infection. CT scanning has poor sensitivity for an epidural abscess. MRI with contrast enhancement is the diagnostic imaging modality of choice. The location and extent of the abscess are easily determined, the extent of neurologic compression is evaluated readily, and coexistent or contiguous spinal infections can be identified. The definitive diagnosis of an epidural abscess and subsequent identification of the organism must be from a biopsy of the abscess.

Management

Once the diagnosis is made, an epidural abscess is treated as a medical and surgical emergency. Untreated epidural abscesses progress relentlessly, with subsequent paralysis and possibly death. Before the advent of effective antibiotics, the mortality rate was more than 50%. Current surgical and medical treatment have drastically reduced mortality. Goals of treatment are to eradicate the infection, preserve neurologic status, and prevent the development of spinal instability.

Surgical intervention is the mainstay of treatment for the epidural abscess that has not responded to medical management. Nonsurgical management may be indicated in patients who are highly debilitated and poor surgical candidates, have extensive spinal involvement, and have complete paralysis of more than 3 days' duration. If medical management is chosen, the development of any neurologic signs or symptoms in a patient with a previously normal neurologic examination should be treated with urgent surgical abscess decompression. The surgical procedure is based on the location of the abscess.

A laminectomy over the involved levels provides direct exposure for a posterior abscess. Care must be taken during laminectomy to preserve spinal stability by leaving the facet joints intact. This is of particular concern in children, who are susceptible to development of a postlaminectomy kyphosis if an extensive decompression is performed. The use of multiple laminotomies in children may play a role in reducing this complication as long as the abscess is debrided adequately. If a concomitant vertebral osteomyelitis or diskitis is present, a combined anterior and posterior decompression may be indicated. Postoperatively the wounds are packed open or, preferably, closed over drains. Antibiotic treatment is parenteral for 2 to 4 weeks. With coexistent osteomyelitis, parenteral antibiotic therapy should be continued for 6 weeks.

Prognosis

With aggressive surgical decompression and the appropriate antibiotic regimen, patients with an epidural abscess and recent neurologic symptoms have a recovery rate of 78%. The time from neurologic deterioration to surgical decompression plays a significant role in neurologic recovery. Optimal recovery usually is attained if the patient is treated in less than 36 hours. Poor prognostic indicators for recovery of neurologic function include complete sensory paralysis, paralysis existing more than 36 hours, or the acute onset of paralysis in 12 hours. Rapid paralysis usually is secondary to spinal cord ischemia or infarction. Other factors that contribute to a poor prognosis include advanced age, diabetes, HIV, and a coexistent vertebral osteomyelitis.

Postoperative Infections of the Spine

Etiology

Infections in the postoperative period may result from inoculation during the initial procedure or hematogenous seeding of the wound. Although *S aureus* is the organism most often identified, gram-negative bacteria and mixed bacterial infections are not uncommon. Prophylactic antibiotic therapy must be given before skin incision to be effective. Postoperative spine infection occurs in about 2.5% of all surgical spine procedures. This includes rates of 0.7% for a simple lumbar diskectomy, 1.4% for a microscopic diskectomy, and 6% for fusion and instrumentation. Factors that increase the risk for postoperative infection include age, malnutrition, obesity, smoking, diabetes, immunosuppression, and prolonged preoperative hospitalization. For every week the patient is in the hospital before an operation, there is a twofold increase in the infection rate.

Other factors that increase the risk for infection include myelodysplasia, spinal dysraphism, prior spine surgery, preoperative radiation therapy, and the intraoperative use of polymethylmethacrylate. Methylmethacrylate may impair the chemotaxic and phagocytotic mechanisms of the polymorphonuclear leukocytes. The surgical time should be kept to a minimum. Tissues should be handled with care and retractors periodically released to minimize tissue ischemia and necrosis. Devitalized tissue should be debrided before closure, which is performed in a layered manner with meticulous attention to hemostasis. Drains should be used if necessary to minimize hematoma formation.

Clinical Presentation

A superficial wound infection is associated with the classic signs and symptoms of fever, warmth, erythema, tenderness, fluctuance, and possibly drainage. The superficial wound infection, by definition, must be contained above the deep fascia. If there is any compromise of this boundary, it is classified as a deep wound infection. A deep wound infection can be insidious in presentation. Complaints are limited to pain that is progressive, worse at night, and typically within several weeks of operation. Fever often is seen with a deep wound infection.

Diskitis

Diskitis usually follows a manipulation of the disk. Initially, the patient follows an expected course postoperatively, with resolution of radicular pain and improvement of incisional pain; however, the back pain returns in several weeks to months. Radicular symptoms with nerve tension signs also may return, and scoliosis may develop as a result of paraspinal muscle spasms. These signs and symptoms should alert the physician to the diagnosis of diskitis. In the presence of a developing neurologic deficit, the existence of an epidural abscess must be sought.

Laboratory tests should be done to assist in the diagnosis. The white blood cell count is usually normal, but if it is elevated this may heighten suspicion for a deep wound infection. The ESR and CRP are useful markers in the diagnosis of spinal infections. Although both markers are increased after the operation, the pattern and time course are predictable. Therefore, persistent elevated levels signal an abnormal process and should heighten suspicion of an infection. The ESR reaches a maximum by day 5 postoperatively. Although its decline is irregular, the ESR usually has returned to its baseline value by 2 weeks. The CRP is more predictable, reaching its maximal value by 3 days after the procedure and returning to normal by 2 weeks. An increased ESR or CRP value that is not declining or one that remains increased

beyond 2 weeks should be investigated. Definitive diagnosis of a deep wound infection is by a positive culture result from a biopsy sample. Initial investigation may use a blind, 4-quadrant deep wound aspiration of the surgical area after sterile surgical preparation of the skin. If suspicion exists despite a negative result of wound aspiration then open exploration with debridement is performed. Tissue samples are taken for culture from each layer explored.

Management

Postoperative diskitis should be treated in the same manner as idiopathic hematogenous diskitis discussed earlier. Postoperative wound infection should be managed with early and aggressive debridement. The debridement should proceed to bone and instrumentation with removal of all necrotic tissue. Specimens of soft tissue and bone should be sent for culture. Any loose necrotic-appearing bone graft should be removed. The instrumentation is left in place if it has not loosened or broken. The stability it provides aids the eradication of the infection. Serial debridements are performed until the wound is clean and healthy in appearance. If the wound infection is superficial in appearance, the patient does not have sepsis, and there is no fascial defect that communicates to the deep layers, a limited debridement may be performed in the operating room. However, the surgeon is encouraged to perform a detailed inspection and possibly a subfascial aspiration once the superficial space has been debrided. Often the infection still tracks deep to the fascia, and many authors advocate exploration of the spine and instrumentation. Sinus tracts, which often are not seen, allow the fascia to remain benign in appearance.

Wound care after debridement is based on the nature of the infection and the experience of the surgeon. The wound may be packed open and treated with serial debridements and dressing changes until closing by secondary intention. It may be closed primarily in delayed fashion once it is clean and granulating. Alternatively, it may be closed over large-bore drains. Particular care must be taken to obliterate all dead space and obtain hemostasis. Secure fascial closure is performed with nonabsorbable sutures. Skin closure also is with nonabsorbable sutures, often of the retention type to prevent dehiscence. If suction-irrigation drains are used, they should be used with normal saline or an antibiotic irrigation solution. Toxic systemic reaction from the irrigating antibiotic may develop, and it is necessary to monitor carefully for this complication.

Medical management of these patients should be aggressive. Patients with infection have increased metabolic demands that must be met. Nutritional supplementation often is needed to prevent the common protein deficiency that develops after surgery. Other contributory factors and comorbidities, such as diabetes, the patient's immune status, and the presence of remote secondary infections, need careful management. Patients with retained instrumentation must receive long-term follow-up because the hardware may be associated with a low-grade infection.

Annotated Bibliography

Berk RH, Yazici M, Atabey N, Ozdamar OS, Pabuccuoglu U, Alici E: Detection of mycobacterium tuberculosis in formaldehyde solution-fixed, paraffin-embedded tissue by polymerase chain reaction in Pott's disease. *Spine* 1996;21:1991–1995.

The authors demonstrate the value of the polymerase chain reaction in the diagnosis of tuberculosis infections compared with culture results and acid-fast staining, which are time consuming and have low yield.

Boachie-Adjei O, Squillante RG: Tuberculosis of the spine. *Orthop Clin North Am* 1996;27:95–103.

This review discusses the current chemotherapeutic success with treating spinal tuberculosis. The advances in imaging have allowed earlier detection of the disease. Patients who need surgical intervention are less well defined but have the propensity to develop a kyphotic deformity with neurologic consequences. Improvements in anteriorly based surgery have improved the results of treatment.

Carragee EJ: The clinical use of magnetic resonance imaging in pyogenic vertebral osteomyelitis. *Spine* 1997;22:780–785.

MRI is invaluable for early diagnosis of pyogenic vertebral osteomyelitis. Follow-up MRI scans were often misleading because the studies showed evidence of progressive disease despite clinical improvement.

Carragee EJ, Kim D, van der Vlugt T, Vittum D: The clinical use of erythrocyte sedimentation rate in pyogenic vertebral osteomyelitis. *Spine* 1997;22:2089–2093.

This is a retrospective review of 44 cases of pyogenic vertebral osteomyelitis in which the clinical use of the ESR was evaluated. In general, the ESR correlates well with response to treatment, but a persistently increased or even rising ESR does not necessarily indicate treatment failure. The ESR should be interpreted in conjunction with other clinical findings.

Currier BL: Spinal infections, in An HS (ed): *Principles and Techniques of Spine Surgery*. Baltimore, MD, Williams & Wilkins, 1998, pp 567–603.

Currier BL, Heller JG, Eismont FJ: Cervical spinal infections, in Clark CR, Ducker TB, Dvorak J, et al (eds): *The Cervical Spine*, ed 3. Philadelphia, PA, Lippincott-Raven, 1998, pp 659–690.

Levine MJ, Heller JG: Spinal infections, in Garfin SR, Vaccaro AR (eds): *Orthopaedic Knowledge Update: Spine*. Rosemont, IL, American Academy of Orthopaedic Surgeons, 1997, pp 257–271.

The above 3 chapters provide a current review of spinal infections.

Martin RJ, Yuan HA: Neurosurgical care of spinal epidural, subdural, and intramedullary abscesses and arachnoiditis. *Orthop Clin North Am* 1996;27:125–136.

Epidural abscesses are managed successfully with early diagnosis and treatment. The diagnosis, pathophysiology, and treatment of the disease are reviewed. Indications for medical treatment as well as surgical methods are discussed.

Ozuna RM, Delamarter RB: Pyogenic vertebral osteomyelitis and postsurgical disc space infections. *Orthop Clin North Am* 1996;27:87–94.

The diagnosis and treatment of hematogenous vertebral osteomyelitis and postoperative diskitis are presented. Aggressive treatment with immobilization and parenteral antibiotics usually leads to a favorable outcome. The indications for surgical interventions are for abscess, neurologic deficits, and failure to respond to the nonsurgical treatment.

Sapico FL: Microbiology and antimicrobial therapy of spinal infections. *Orthop Clin North Am* 1996;27:9–13.

This is a review of the common organisms that cause hematogenous osteomyelitis and epidural abscesses. The treatment is parenteral in high doses and can be followed clinically and with the results of the ESR. Failure to respond to medical treatment may necessitate prolonged therapy or surgical debridement.

Classic Bibliography

An HS, Vaccaro AR, Dolinskas CA, Cotler JM, Balderston RA, Bauerle WB: Differentiation between spinal tumors and infections with magnetic resonance imaging. *Spine* 1991;16(suppl 8): S334–S338.

Danner RL, Hartman BJ: Update on spinal epidural abscess: 35 cases and review of the literature. *Rev Infect Dis* 1987; 9:265–274.

Dempsey R, Rapp RP, Young B, Johnston S, Tibbs P: Prophylactic parenteral antibiotics in clean neurosurgical procedures: A review. *J Neurosurg* 1988;69:52–57.

Djukic S, Lang P, Morris J, Hoaglund F, Genant HK: The postoperative spine: Magnetic resonance imaging. *Orthop Clin North Am* 1990;21:603–624.

Eismont FJ, Bohlman HH, Soni PL, Goldberg VM, Freehafer AA: Pyogenic and fungal vertebral osteomyelitis with paralysis. J Bone Joint Surg 1983;65A:19–29.

Emery SE, Chan DP, Woodward HR: Treatment of hematogenous pyogenic vertebral osteomyelitis with anterior debridement and primary bone grafting. Spine 1989;14:284–291.

Güven O, Kumano K, Yalcin S, Karahan M, Tsuji S: A single stage posterior approach and rigid fixation for preventing kyphosis in the treatment of spinal tuberculosis. Spine 1994;19:1039–1043.

Hodgson AR, Skinsnes OK, Leong CY: The pathogenesis of Pott's paraplegia. J Bone Joint Surg 1967;49A:1147–1156.

Hodgson AR, Stock FE: Anterior spine fusion for the treatment of tuberculosis of the spine: The operative findings and results of treatment in the first one hundred cases. J Bone Joint Surg 1960;42A:295–310.

Horwitz NH, Curtin JA: Prophylactic antibiotics and wound infections following laminectomy for lumbar disc herniation: A retrospective study. J Neurosurg 1975;43:727–731.

Hsu LC, Cheng CL, Leong JC: Pott's paraplegia of late onset: The cause of compression and results after anterior decompression. J Bone Joint Surg 1988;70B:534–538.

Hsu LC, Leong JC: Tuberculosis of the lower cervical spine (C2 to C7): A report on 40 cases. J Bone Joint Surg 1984;66B:1–5.

Lifeso RM: Pyogenic spinal sepsis in adults. Spine 1990;15:1265–1271.

Lifeso RM, Weaver P, Harder EH: Tuberculous spondylitis in adults. J Bone Joint Surg 1985;67A:1405–1413.

Massie JB, Heller JG, Abitbol JJ, McPherson D, Garfin SR: Postoperative posterior spinal wound infections. Clin Orthop 1992;284:99–108.

Modic MT, Feiglin DH, Piraino DW, et al: Vertebral osteomyelitis: Assessment using MR. Radiology 1985;157:157–166.

Nussbaum ES, Rigamonti D, Standiford H, Numaguchi Y, Wolf AL, Robinson WL: Spinal epidural abscess: A report of 40 cases and review. Surg Neurol 1992;38:225–231.

Oga M, Arizono T, Takasita M, Sugioka Y: Evaluation of the risk of instrumentation as a foreign body in spinal tuberculosis: Clinical and biological study. Spine 1993;18:1890–1894.

Petty W, Spanier S, Shuster JJ, Silverthorne C: The influence of skeletal implants on incidence of infection: Experiments in a canine model. J Bone Joint Surg 1985;67A:1236–1244.

Rubin G, Michowiz SD, Ashkenasi A, Tadmor R, Rappaport ZH: Spinal epidural abscess in the pediatric age group: Case report and review of literature. Pediatr Infect Dis J 1993;12:1007–1011.

Sadato N, Numaguchi Y, Rigamonti D, et al: Spinal epidural abscess with gadolinium-enhanced MRI: Serial follow-up studies and clinical correlations. Neuroradiology 1994;36:44–48.

Sapico FL, Montgomerie JZ: Pyogenic vertebral osteomyelitis: Report of nine cases and review of the literature. Rev Infect Dis 1979;1:754–776.

Sapico FL, Montgomerie JZ: Vertebral osteomyelitis in intravenous drug abusers: Report of three cases and review of the literature. Rev Infect Dis 1980;2:196–206.

Schulitz KP, Assheuer J: Discitis after procedures on the intervertebral disc. Spine 1994;19:1172–1177.

Sixth report of the Medical Research Council Working Party on Tuberculosis of the Spine: Five-year assessments of controlled trials of ambulatory treatment, debridement and anterior spinal fusion in the management of tuberculosis of the spine: Studies in Bulawayo (Rhodesia) and in Hong Kong. J Bone Joint Surg 1978;60B:163–177.

Smith AS, Weinstein MA, Mizushima A, et al: MR imaging characteristics of tuberculous spondylitis vs vertebral osteomyelitis. Am J Roentgenol 1989;153:399–405.

Stambough JL, Beringer D: Postoperative wound infections complicating adult spine surgery. J Spinal Disord 1992;5:277–285.

Thelander U, Larsson S: Quantitation of C-reactive protein levels and erythrocyte sedimentation rate after spinal surgery. Spine 1992;17:400–404.

Wheeler D, Keiser P, Rigamonti D, Keay S: Medical management of spinal epidural abscesses: Case report and review. Clin Infect Dis 1992;15:22–27.

Chapter 55
Tumors of the Spine

Introduction

Surgical treatment can increase survival and improve quality of life for many patients with spinal column tumors. Failure to diagnosis or provide appropriate initial care can lead to premature deterioration, paralysis, and death. The goals of treatment are to (1) protect or restore neurologic function, (2) control pain, (3) maximize physical capacity, and (4) obtain local control of disease whenever possible. Aggressive surgical approaches, combined with adjuvant medical therapy, now offer improved short-term and long-term outcomes for lesions previously considered untreatable.

Diagnosis

History and Review of Symptoms

Primary spinal column tumors can arise from any of the osseous or soft tissues of the spinal column. Secondary lesions can extend directly from contiguous paraspinal structures or metastasize by lymphatic or hematogenous routes. Although certain primary tumors, such as chordoma, osteoblastoma, and plasmacytoma, show a predilection for the spinal column, metastatic disease still accounts for 98% of all spinal lesions. Adenocarcinomas of lungs, breast, prostate, kidneys, gastrointestinal tract, and thyroid are the most common metastatic lesions. In a patient with persistent back pain and a history of previous malignancy, metastatic disease should immediately be suspected.

In adults, because of the age-related increase in metastatic disease and the emergence of systemic diseases, such as myeloma and lymphoma, both primary and secondary lesions are likely to be malignant. In children and adolescents, only 30% of primary tumors are malignant. Malignant lesions, either primary or metastatic, tend to involve the vertebral body and pedicles. Tumors of the posterior elements are more typically benign.

Although almost any neoplastic process can establish skeletal metastases, certain tumors are particularly adept at reaching and surviving in the trabecular environment. Breast carcinoma accounts for 21% of all spinal metastases, pulmonary carcinoma for 14%, prostate carcinoma for 7.5%, renal or gastrointestinal carcinomas for approximately 5.0%, and thyroid carcinoma for 2.5%. If myeloma and lymphoma are counted as metastatic lesions, then breast, lung, prostate, and lymphoreticular disease account for 60% of all spinal column metastases requiring treatment. A complete review of symptoms should look for unintended weight loss, fatigue, anorexia, or anemia. Symptoms suggestive of common primary malignancies should be sought.

Back pain is the presenting complaint in 85% of patients with a spinal tumor. This common, nonspecific symptom may have characteristic features that suggest malignancy. Back pain caused by neoplasm typically is (1) progressive and unrelenting, (2) unrelieved by rest, and (3) often more severe or disturbing at night. Rapidly progressive symptoms of pain or neurologic compromise suggest a more aggressive, malignant process, whereas symptoms that progress slowly over months are typical of slow-growing or benign processes. Pain occurs when the tumor causes pathologic fracture, distortion of the periosteum and surrounding tissues, direct compression or invasion of nerve roots, segmental spinal instability, or spinal cord compression.

Leg pain often accompanies back pain. Isolated radicular symptoms may simulate a herniated nucleus pulposus. Symptoms from lumbar and sacral neoplasms tend to progress relentlessly and do not respond to rest and recumbency. Weakness rarely is the first sign of disease in patients with a spinal neoplasm; however, it may be detectable in half of all patients by the time they seek medical attention and in over 70% by the time a diagnosis is made. Symptoms of weakness may be related to neural compression or systemic disease.

Physical Examination

All pertinent systems should be examined, including the breasts, abdomen, lungs, head and neck, and rectal vault. Palpation should identify signs of lymphadenopathy in the cervical, axillary, and inguinal chains. The extremities and rib cage should be examined for areas of focal tenderness or pain. A careful motor and sensory examination should document function in all dermatomes and motor groups. Reflexes should be carefully assessed for evidence of impending myelopathy, such as hyperreflexia and clonus, and a bulbocavernosus reflex should be documented in any patient with an existing deficit.

724   Spine

Palpating the spine may reveal tenderness over the involved segment or bony prominence in areas of kyphotic collapse. Spinal deformity is uncommon; scoliosis rarely occurs as a feature of a spinal tumor, but vertebral collapse may cause kyphosis. Scoliosis caused by a tumor tends to present acutely and progress rapidly. Curves associated with osteoid osteoma and osteoblastoma typically are painful.

Laboratory Studies

Screening laboratory studies usually are carried out before more elaborate imaging studies are indicated. Complete blood cell counts, with differential and erythrocyte sedimentation rate, are sensitive indicators for systemic disease, tumor, or infection. Serum chemistries, urine and serum protein electrophoresis also should be ordered. It is now possible to measure specific antigens that reliably detect the presence of tumors; prostate specific antigen can reveal the primary lesion responsible for metastasis. Stool should be examined for occult blood, sputum for blood or cells, and urine for blood, cells, or casts.

Imaging

Plain Radiographs Plain radiographs demonstrate some abnormality in 80% to 90% of spinal neoplasms. Even if the tumor type cannot be identified, the benign or malignant nature of the lesion often is implied by the pattern of bone destruction (Fig. 1, *A* and *B*). Plain radiographs cannot distinguish benign compression fractures from metastatic disease and may not detect small tumor foci early in the disease process.

Bone Scans Because radiographs do not detect bony destruction until 30% to 50% of the trabecular bone has been demineralized or destroyed, bone scans are more sensitive for early vertebral involvement. They are not specific, however, and must be followed by more definitive imaging studies. Isolated areas of uptake are common around arthritic joints and among the ribs, but multiple "hot-spots" suggest metastatic

spread. A focal uptake in the spinal column can be used to target more specific imaging studies later. Conditions that can present a false negative bone scan include widely disseminated metastatic disease (uniformly increased uptake masks metastatic pattern) and multiple myeloma. When these con-

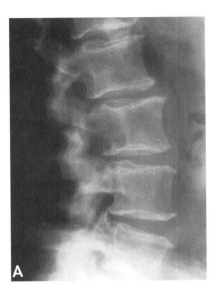
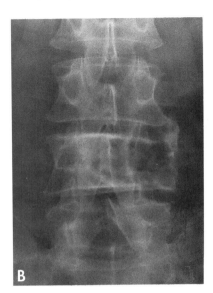
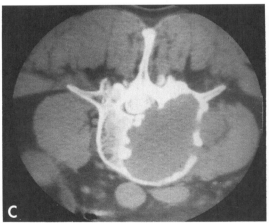
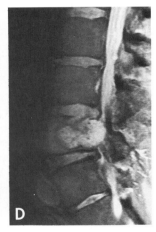

Figure 1

Plain radiographs demonstrate the location and extent of the tumor and provide information on its behavior and type. A, The lateral view shows a rarified vertebral body with a geographic pattern of bony replacement, suggestive of a slow-growing malignancy or benign, aggressive tumor type. This tumor, a chordoma, had replaced most of the vertebral body by the time the patient had sought medical attention. B, Anteroposterior radiograph shows a classic "winking owl" sign caused by destruction of the right pedicle by a fibrosarcoma. The tumor has also expanded and disrupted the lateral vertebral cortex. C, Computed tomography of patient in 1, *B* demonstrates bony destruction and expansion of the anterior and lateral vertebral cortex. D, Sagittal magnetic resonance image shows the substance of a renal cell metastasis in the L4 vertebral body, as well as a small soft-tissue extension posteriorly. Sagittal sections demonstrate multiple spinal segments at a time, and demonstrate the tumor's invasion of the neural canal. On this T2-weighted image the tumor tissue is lighter than the surrounding bone. The cauda equina is compressed.

Spinal tumors characteristically show the following MRI features: (1) convexity of the posterior vertebral cortex, (2) epidural mass, (3) low-intensity T1 signal, (4) high-intensity or inhomogenous T2 signal, and (5) gadolinium enhancement. Newer techniques can accurately differentiate tumor from hematoma, edema, and inflammation (Fig. 1, *D*). MRI directly images the spinal cord, cauda equina, and nerve roots without the aid of intrathecal contrast, can reveal invasion of paravertebral structures better than either CT or myelography, and can differentiate osteoporotic compression fractures from metastatic disease.

Myelography Previously considered the "gold standard" for spinal imaging, myelography has been largely replaced by MRI. When MRI cannot be done, myelography with postmyelogram CT may provide comparable information.

Treatment Principles

Before selecting the "best" treatment for any individual patient, the surgeon must identify any neurologic compromise, determine the patient's fitness for surgery, determine whether the lesion is primary or metastatic, and understand the local and systemic behavior of the specific tumor type. These last 2 require a tissue diagnosis (Fig. 2).

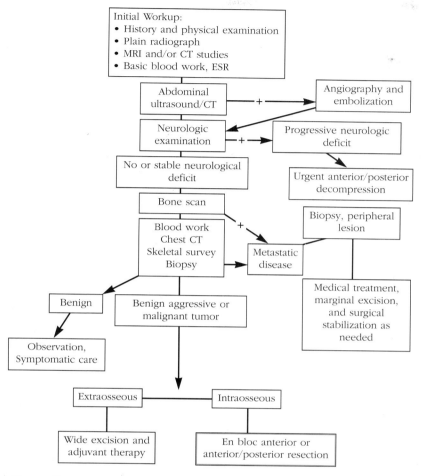

Figure 2

Algorithm for a diagnostic evaluation of spine tumors. MRI, magnetic resonance imaging; CT, computed tomography; ESR, erythrocyte sedimentation rate.

ditions are suspected, a plain radiographic skeletal survey will reveal the lesions.

Computed Tomography Once the suspected lesion is identified on plain films or bone scan, computed tomography (CT) provides excellent imaging of the bony architecture (Fig. 1, *C*). CT is the best way to study intraosseous lesions, such as osteoid osteoma. However, soft-tissue imaging is of limited value, and these studies are time-consuming and not suitable for screening large segments of the spine.

MRI Magnetic resonance imaging (MRI) provides multiplanar images of large segments of the spine and surrounding tissues and can be used to screen for disseminated disease.

Biopsy

Biopsy is necessary in undiagnosed metastatic disease and in all but a few primary lesions. Patients with a previously documented carcinoma, or with lesions that can be biopsied at a more peripheral site, usually do not require a biopsy of the spinal lesion. When the differential diagnosis is limited to lesions that are easily distinguished histologically, needle biopsy is ideal (Fig. 3). More subtle differentials usually require an open biopsy.

Fine needle aspiration or biopsy can be carried out with CT guidance and minimal risk to the patient. Because the sample obtained is small, there is a possibility of sampling nondiagnostic regions of the tumor. Needle biopsy is not adequate to differentiate cartilage tumors, osteoblastic tumors, or most

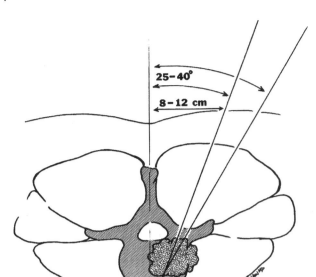

Figure 3

Approach for percutaneous biopsy. Needle biopsy of the thoracolumbar spine is performed through a posterior, percutaneous, or minimally open route. The needle is positioned 8 to 12 cm lateral of the midline at the level of the documented lesion. Advancing the needle at a 30° to 45° angle, under fluoroscopic control, the posterolateral aspect of the vertebral body is targeted. Alternatively, a small posterior exposure is made over the documented lesion, and a burr is used to take down the cortex overlying the pedicle. A Craig needle or a small curette is then passed down the pedicle to harvest larger samples of bone and tumor from the vertebral body.

Outline 1
Indications for surgery in spine tumors

Biopsy

Establish a tissue diagnosis

Decompression

Neurologic compression due to fracture or bony

impingement

Resection

Resectable primary tumor

Resectable solitary metastasis

Stabilization

Mechanical instability or pathologic fracture

Radioresistant tumor

Progression in face of or following radiotherapy

Known radioresistant tumor

spindle cell tumors, but can distinguish between infection, adenocarcinoma, and sarcoma. A Craig needle biopsy, although more invasive, is more likely to obtain diagnostic material. This large bore trephine provides a core sample that may retain a bit of the tumor architecture, and it can cut dense soft tissue as well as trabecular bone. When the biopsy is carried out through a posterior percutaneous approach or through a limited open incision, the biopsy tract can be included in the definitive resection if a primary sarcoma is discovered. If the needle procedure fails to provide diagnostic material, either because of sampling error or a difficult differential, open biopsy is recommended (Outline 1).

Incisional biopsy is carried out as the last step in tumor staging, just before or at the time of definitive resection. The incision is longitudinal; transverse incisions should be avoided. Tissues must be handled gently during the approach, and hemostasis must be meticulous. A section of tissue large enough for histologic and ultrastructural analysis, as well as immunologic staining, should be cut from the margin of the lesion using a sharp scalpel. Central sections of an aggressive tumor may be necrotic. Electrocautery should not be used on the biopsy specimen itself.

Occasionally, posterior lesions may present an opportunity for en bloc excision at the first procedure. Otherwise, a small longitudinal incision should be centered over the soft-tissue mass and an ample specimen sent for analysis before attempting the definitive procedure. Anterior lesions rarely offer a chance for a wide marginal excision without extensive reconstruction, and it is usually preferable to have a tissue diagnosis before undertaking such an aggressive procedure. There are only a few tumors (chondrosarcoma, for instance) that present so classic an image that vertebrectomy may be planned at the first operation to avoid exposing tumor tissue during resection.

Decompression

Early recognition and treatment of spinal cord compression may prevent permanent neurologic injury. Compression may be caused by the tumor's enlarging soft-tissue mass, a pathologic fracture forcing bone fragments into the canal, vertebral collapse and kyphosis, or direct metastasis or extension into the meninges or epidural space.

Patients with rapidly progressive paralysis have a poor prognosis for recovery. Between 60% and 95% of intact patients will remain ambulatory after treatment, but only 35% to 65% of paraparetic patients and less than 30% of paraplegic patients will regain ambulation after either surgical or medical treatment.

Radiotherapy is the treatment of choice for most patients with neurologic symptoms. Prostatic and lymphoreticular neoplasms are typically radiosensitive, and satisfactory local control can be gained through postoperative radiotherapy, even after an intralesional resection. Gastrointestinal and renal neoplasms, on the other hand, are often unresponsive to irradiation. Similarly, a number of primary tumor types—chondrosarcoma, chordoma—are not radiosensitive, and, consequently, neurologic compromise caused by these lesions is better treated by surgery. In certain tumor types—hemangioma, aneurysmal bone cyst—embolization of the tumor may cause shrinkage of the tumor mass, alleviating neurologic symptoms, and may trigger healing of the lesion.

Surgical decompression must be tailored to the compressive lesion, with anterior decompression for anterior tumors and posterior decompression for posterior ones. For anterior compressive lesions, laminectomy provides no incremental benefit compared to radiotherapy alone, and complications are increased. Posterior decompression, with or without radiotherapy, provides a satisfactory result (maintenance of ambulation and sphincter control) in fewer than 40% of patients with spinal cord compression. By comparison, anterior decompression provides a satisfactory outcome in 80% of these patients. In the cervical spine above the level of C3, the posterior surgical approach usually is most appropriate. Below this level, the posterior approach is limited to lesions of the dorsal elements. Lesions of the vertebral body are most successfully treated through the appropriate anterior approach.

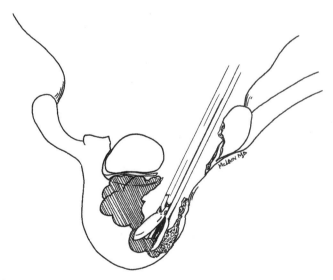

Figure 4

Posterolateral decompression. Metastatic and radiosensitive lesions may be approached through a costotransversectomy or transpedicular approach, allowing intralesional tumor removal and spinal cord decompression without formal thoracotomy.

As an alternative, lesions of the thoracic spine can be successfully approached through a posterolateral dissection (Fig. 4), using either a costotransversectomy or transpedicular technique to access the vertebral body and decompress the anterior aspect of the spinal cord. Anterior decompression through a posterolateral approach has not been universally satisfactory, because full decompression depends on adequately exposing the entire width of the anterior thecal sac. A bilateral, transpedicular approach, or unilateral video-assisted approach may allow full visualization of the volar dura and permit a complete decompression of metastatic or lymphoreticular lesions. This is an intralesional procedure, however, and is not intended to treat isolated primary malignancies.

Resection

When a primary malignant lesion can be completely resected, patient survival improves significantly. The anterior and posterior longitudinal ligaments, vertebral body, adjacent disks, and even the overlying dura can be resected to obtain local control. If necessary, 1 or more nerve roots can be sacrificed to provide a wide margin of excision. Even in metastatic lesions, a complete resection can improve survival and quality of life. The decision to attempt a wide resection in these lesions must be weighed against the risks of vascular or neurologic injury. For some patients, the most prudent approach may be to accept a marginal or intralesional resection, supplementing local treatment with adjuvant radio- or cryotherapy.

The surgical approach and resection margins are planned from the following staging system: the vertebral body is divided into 4 zones, with 3 degrees of tumor extension, intraosseous, extraosseous, and metastatic (Fig. 5). Zones 1, 2, and 3 contain the posterior elements, pedicle and transverse process, and anterior vertebral body, respectively. Zone 4 contains the posterior vertebral body and that portion of the cortex just anterior to the neural elements. To approach any lesion involving zone 4, zones 1, 2, and/or 3 must be crossed as well. Zone 4 lesions require a total vertebrectomy to obtain a clean margin.

Zone 1 lesions are approached through a midline posterior incision, basing the extent of the incision on the extent of the soft-tissue mass. Tumors of the spinous process can be removed en bloc by cutting the lamina on either side. En bloc resection of laminar tumors requires dissection laterally down 1 of the transverse processes to the level of the pedicle.

Zone 2 lesions require a posterolateral approach (Fig. 6). The laminectomy and bone resection necessary for tumor excision generally results in some degree of segmental instability, and posterior instrumentation and fusion usually are necessary.

Zone 3 lesions involve the anterior portion of the vertebral body and usually are approached anteriorly. Depending on the extent of resection, a formal reconstruction may or may not be necessary.

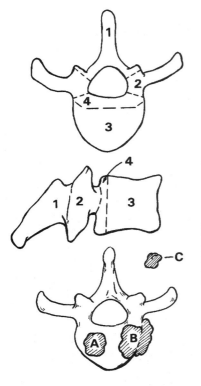

Figure 5

Tumor staging. Axial (top), and lateral (center) views of the vertebral body showing 4 zones of tumor involvement and 3 stages of progression (bottom). Stage A represents intraosseous spread; stage B, extraosseous extension; and stage C, distant metastasis.

Zone 4 lesions require a combined surgical approach if a clear margin is desired. Complete resection requires separating the posterior structures (zones 1 and 2) from the anterior structures (zones 3 and 4) at the junction between the pedicles and the vertebral body (Fig. 7). Standard treatment combines a midline posterior incision for laminectomy and stabilization, with a retroperitoneal, thoracoabdominal, or transthoracic approach to resect the vertebral body. If at least 1 pedicle is uninvolved, a wide margin is technically possible. Alternatively, the surgeon can extend the posterior dissection around the side of the vertebral body, completing the vertebrectomy piecemeal through a posterolateral resection. Irrespective of approach, complete vertebrectomy requires both anterior and posterior stabilization. This aggressive surgical approach can improve patient survival and neurologic function even when a cure cannot be obtained.

Spinal Stabilization

Rigid spinal instrumentation prevents early progressive deformity, limits pain due to segmental instability, and facilitates bone graft incorporation and fusion. The proper instrumentation system must compensate for loss of bony elements resulting from resection or laminectomy and permit postoperative imaging with CT and MRI.

Posterior distraction Harrington instrumentation still has a role in tumor reconstruction. Combined with sublaminar or spinous process wires, these inexpensive systems provide

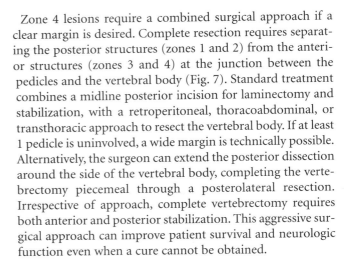

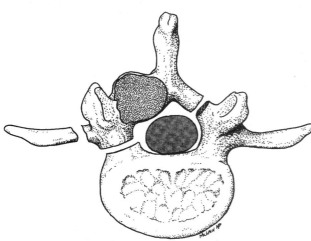

Figure 6

Resection of zone 2 lesion. Posterolateral approach allows access to uninvolved lamina on contralateral side along with uninvolved ipsilateral pedicle. A marginal margin can be obtained if the pedicle is free of tumor.

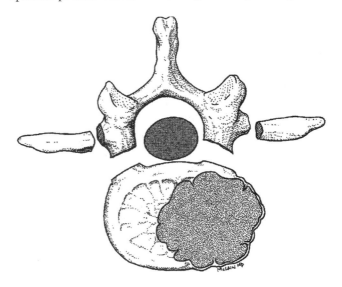

Figure 7

Resection of zone 4 lesion. En bloc excision of thoracolumbar vertebra requires posterior release, removing laminae and both pedicles, prior to en bloc resection of the vertebral body through an anterior approach.

segmental fixation to adequately stabilize compression fractures or short laminectomies in the thoracic spine. Beyond this, however, their use is limited. These systems are vulnerable to fatigue failure, particularly in tumor patients in whom perioperative irradiation and systemic disease increase the risk of delayed union and nonunion. They do not contour well to the lumbar spine, and distraction tends to flatten the normal lumbar lordosis, resulting in a painful flat-back deformity.

Luque rods, used in conjunction with sublaminar wires, provide better fixation in soft bone than the Harrington system and have been used successfully in treating degenerative and neoplastic disease of the cervical, thoracic, and lumbar spine. The system offers good stability in torsion and flexion, but cannot resist pure axial loads. The sublaminar wires are free to slide down the rod, allowing the instrumented segment to collapse under axial loading. Fixation is possible only in segments where the laminae are intact, and the risks of passing sublaminar wires must be considered.

Segmental instrumentation systems are highly versatile tools for stabilizing the spine. Instead of distracting the posterior elements to obtain reduction, these systems neutralize the overall length of the spine while either compressing or distracting the intercalary segments involved in the reconstruction. Hooks and screws placed at multiple levels distribute reduction forces and improve construct strength, while pedicle screws allow fixation of levels with no intact posterior elements. Segmental systems are widely available in titanium, improving postoperative imaging capabilities. Screw and plate constructs can be used in the upper thoracic spine to stabilize the cervicothoracic jution, to treat laminectomized segments, and to limit the bulk of instrumentation placed under thin, irradiated soft tissues (Fig. 8).

Combined with an anterior strut, screw/rod and screw/plate constructs provide superior axial, torsional, and sagittal rigidity. Using the combined approach, surgeons can often limit instrumentation to only 2 motion segments when treating lesions of the thoracolumbar spine. Unless the anterior weightbearing column is reconstructed, screws will be exposed to excessive cantilever loads and screw failure can be expected. In the absence of an intact anterior column, substantial residual motion can occur despite rigid posterior fixation or solid fusion. Untreated anterior column deficiency leads to fatigue failure of pedicle screws and eventual screw or rod breakage. Because tumor patients often are systemically ill, may have undergone regional radiation therapy, have lost muscle mass and subcutaneous fat, and have impaired healing potential, anterior reconstruction may be better tolerated than posterior instrumentation.

Depending on the situation, there are a number of reconstructive options to consider. Polymethylmethacrylate (PMMA) is resilient in compression, but because it has no potential for biologic incorporation it has a tendency to loosen and extrude over time and should only be used in patients with < 6 months life expectancy. Longitudinal

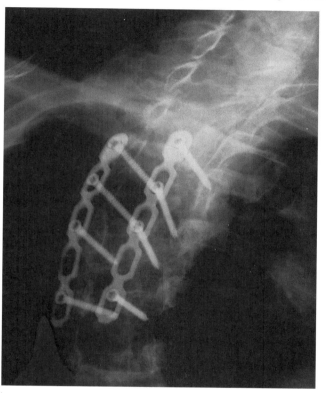

Figure 8

Screw and plate construct for upper thoracic spine. An alternative to rod and hook constructs, low-profile plates may be useful in patients with absent or incompetent posterior elements, or those with tenuous dorsal skin. (Reproduced with permission from McLain RF, Kabins MB, Weinstein J: Use of titanium fixation plates for pedicle screw fixation of the thoracic spine. *J Orthop Tech* 1993;1:55–63.)

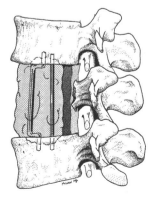

Figure 9

Reconstruction of the anterior column with polymethylmethacrylate (PMMA). To protect the neural elements from thermal injury, a broad sheet of Gelfoam is placed between the PMMA mass and the dura, and the mass is irrigated constantly with saline until it cures.

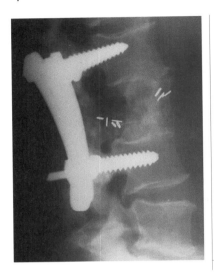

Figure 10

Anterior reconstruction with tricortical graft. Anterior superior iliac crest is harvested and contoured to fill and distract the vertebrectomy defect. Graft ends are contoured to articulate with grooves and pits fashioned in the end plates. At follow-up, end plates and graft coalesce, and trabeculae can be seen crossing the interface. This patient underwent vertebrectomy for lumbar chordoma 4 years earlier. (Reproduced with permission from McLain RF, Weinstein JN: Primary tumor of the spine. *Spine* 1987;12:843–851.)

Steinmann pins driven proximally and distally into the adjacent vertebrae may be incorporated into the PMMA mass to anchor the spacer and improve its bending resistance (Fig. 9). Harrington distraction rods or Knodt rods can be used with PMMA as well; the rod ends are countersunk into the opposing end plates, with distraction applied to restore sagittal alignment.

For patients with a longer expected survival, biologic incorporation is desirable. A tricortical strut graft or titanium cage with morcelized autograft is favored in the treatment of benign or slow-growing tumors, when a patient's survival is likely to be measured in years. Autograft struts also are used in isolated, primary malignancies, for which successful treatment will result in prolonged survival. Tricortical struts are cut from the anterior superior iliac crest so they measure 5 to 10 mm longer than the defect to be filled. The graft is keyed into the vertebral end plates to prevent displacement when the patient is mobilized (Fig. 10). A single 6.5-mm cancellous screw can be driven into the vertebral body just lateral to the graft to prevent displacement.

A titanium cage can be used to supplement either methylmethacrylate or autograft reconstructions. The cage is impacted between the vertebral end plates in the same way as the tricortical graft except that the end plates are not violated and the cage is not keyed into place. The cage is packed full of morcelized autograft if fusion is intended, and after impaction more graft is placed anterior to the cage to augment the fusion. Because the cage provides little torsional rigidity on its own, an anterior fixation system often is added to stabilize the spinal construct (Fig. 11).

Tumor Types

Metastatic Tumors

When conservative therapy fails to control metastatic disease, the physician must determine whether surgery will improve the patient's function, quality of life, or longevity. Because recurrent tumors are more difficult to treat, the surgeon should plan an adequate resection and stabilization at the first procedure.

The vertebral column is predisposed to metastatic proliferation by its vascular anatomy, architecture, and proximity to common sites of disease. The venous drainage of the spine is contiguous with pulmonary and abdominal visceral beds, allowing retrograde flow to carry cells from a variety of tumors into the vertebral body. Tumor cells that would otherwise be filtered out by the lungs or liver gain access to the

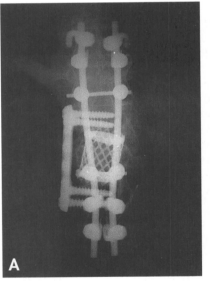
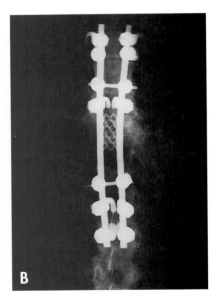

Figure 11

Anterior decompression and reconstruction. Anterior approach allows direct access to involved vertebral body. After removing retropulsed fragments and extruded tumor from in front of the thecal sac, the vertebral defect can be filled with a structural autograft, allograft, or prosthetic cage. A, Titanium cage filled with autograft bone applied through an anterior retroperitoneal approach following vertebrectomy for metastatic renal cell carcinoma. B, Titanium cage applied through a posterolateral (costotransversectomy) approach, in a patient with metastasis from colon carcinoma. (Reproduced with permission from McLain RF: Endoscopically assisted decompression for metastatic thoracic neoplasm. *Spine* 1998;23:1130–1135.)

vascular sinusoids of the vertebral body, where metastatic emboli tend to settle and implant in the trabecular end loops adjacent to the vertebral end plates. The biochemistry and hemodynamics of the vertebral red marrow provides a favorable environment for tumor cell proliferation. The vertebral trabecular bone has a rich blood supply, with few barriers to tumor growth; once implanted the tumor can grow for some time before it becomes symptomatic.

Many patients with symptomatic metastases are successfully treated with bracing and irradiation. As bony destruction becomes more advanced, surgical stabilization may be necessary. If the tumor is radiosensitive, the simplest approach is to stabilize the spine with posterior instrumentation and control tumor growth with adjuvant radiotherapy. If the tumor is not radiosensitive, or if bony destruction is advanced, an anteroposterior (AP) or posterolateral reconstruction can combine decompression and stabilization, allowing early mobilization.

In patients with neurologic involvement, decompression becomes the primary goal of surgery. If the tumor is radiosensitive, and neural progression is gradual, radiotherapy is the initial treatment of choice. If progression is rapid, unresponsive to radiotherapy, or secondary to bony, as opposed to soft-tissue, encroachment, surgical decompression through the most direct approach is indicated.

If a patient has an isolated metastasis from a tumor with potential long-term survival (breast, colon, prostate, kidney), it is reasonable to consider a combined procedure to obtain a wide excision of the lesion. The tumor is treated in the same way as a primary malignancy, with emphasis on local control.

Because of the potential for catastrophic hemorrhage, renal cell metastases must be identified before biopsy and should be approached more cautiously than other tumors. Urinalysis followed by abdominal ultrasound or CT will reveal hypernephroma before the surgeon performs a biopsy that may lead to uncontrollable bleeding. Preoperative angiography often reveals extensive neovasculature around these metastatic foci, and abnormal vessels can be embolized.

Benign Primary Tumors
With benign tumors, the surgical goals are to treat pain and to prevent local tumor expansion. Intralesional excision is adequate in tumors with limited potential for local extension and recurrence (aneurysmal bone cyst, osteoblastoma) and should be carried out through the most direct approach. Curettage and bone grafting are sufficient for most of these tumors. However, recurrence of some histologically benign lesions may prove lethal because of their location.

Osteochondroma Seven percent of osteochondromas occur in the spine, but symptomatic lesions are rare. Eighty percent of symptomatic osteochondromas occur in the cervical and upper thoracic spine. The expanding cartilage cap that usually causes spinal cord compression is best seen on MRI. Excision of the tumor, en bloc or piecemeal, provides reliable neurologic recovery with little risk of recurrence.

Osteoid Osteoma This lesion is difficult to detect among the overlying shadows of the spinal column and is most reliably localized by bone scan. It may present as a painful scoliosis. A follow-up CT targeted around the area of uptake will define the lesion. Complete excision relieves the patient's pain. Successful treatment requires accurately localizing and completely removing the tumor nidus.

Osteoblastoma Osteoblastoma is typically larger than the 2 cm osteoid osteoma from which it is histologically indistinguishable. This lesion is characterized by cortical expansion, with a thin rim of reactive bone at the tumor margin. Either excision or curettage and bone grafting provide an acceptable long-term result. Reactive scoliosis can be seen with either osteoid osteoma or osteoblastoma. Recurrence is uncommon, but if it occurs, the tumor usually can be cured by repeated resection.

Hemangioma Asymptomatic hemangiomas are common in the spine. The lesion is characterized by prominent vertical trabeculae that show up as vertical striations on plain radiographs and as a prominent stippled pattern on CT. Reports of deformity or pain associated with hemangioma are rare, and surgeons should not automatically attribute mechanical or chronic pain symptoms to these lesions. Asymptomatic hemangiomas rarely become symptomatic, and do not require follow-up. If vertebral collapse or neural compression occurs, surgical decompression and reconstruction through an anterior approach usually is successful.

Eosinophilic Granuloma This benign, self-limiting lesion is commonly seen in children younger than 10 years of age. Vertebral involvement can be associated with any of 3 syndromes: isolated eosinophilic granuloma, Hand-Schüller-Christian syndrome, and Letterer-Siwe disease. The classic radiographic presentation of vertebra plana is not pathognomonic, and a similar picture can result from either infection or Ewing's sarcoma. If uncertain, needle or trochar biopsy will establish the diagnosis. Most patients can be treated with bracing and observation. Rarely, when neurologic symptoms are present, biopsy, resection and strut grafting, and immobilization may be necessary. Radiotherapy, advocated in the past, is now reserved primarily for recurrent lesions. Recovery of neurologic function usually is excellent, and reconstitution of vertebral height is seen in most young patients.

Aneurysmal Bone Cyst Aneursymal bone cysts usually involve the posterior elements and most commonly occur in the lumbar spine. Radiographs demonstrate an expansile lesion with an osteolytic cavity, which may extend to involve 2 or even 3 adjacent vertebrae. The eggshell-thin cortex is often blown-out, with numerous strands of bone that give a typical "bubbly" appearance. Curettage is sufficient to eradicate most lesions, and recurrences, which do not tend to invade vital structures, can be treated by repeated curettage or excision.

Locally Aggressive Tumors
Locally aggressive tumors include benign lesions with a strong tendency to invade adjacent tissues and slow-growing malignancies whose local extension and tendency to recur are more dangerous than their likelihood of metastasis. These lesions require a rigorous treatment approach, seeking a clear surgical margin wherever possible. A recurrent tumor is more difficult to irradicate than a primary tumor and may become unresectable if not adequately excised initially.

Locally Aggressive Benign umors
Even though histologically benign, local extension of a giant cell tumor or osteoblastoma may lead to lethal complications if local extension is not arrested. Giant cell tumors, usually seen in the third or fourth decade of life, appear lucent on plain radiographs, with marginal sclerosis and a geographic pattern of bone destruction. These slow-growing tumors arise in the vertebral body, expanding the vertebral cortex as they grow. En bloc excision is indicated when possible. When a marginal resection is not possible, repeated curettements may be necessary to obtain a clean margin, and some authors have advocated cryotherapy or postoperative radiotherapy to ensure a clean tumor bed. Anterior/posterior vertebrectomy followed by a combined reconstruction limits the likelihood of recurrence and allows the most rapid return to function.

Primary Malignant Tumors
The principal goal of treatment is local control and cure. In the absence of neural compromise or segmental instability, the approach and resection are designed to give the best chance of an adequate margin with the least disruption of vertebral stability. The surgical procedure should be planned to ensure a clear margin. Appropriate surgical staging will dictate the optimal approach.

Dorsal (stage A) tumors require a longitudinal posterior approach, incorporating any previous biopsy wound in the incision and taking care not to enter the soft-tissue mass of the tumor surgically or with retractors or rakes. A cuff of normal muscle is excised with the tumor. Laminectomy above and below the involved level allows the involved elements to be isolated and resected by cutting through uninvolved lamina or pedicle. The tumor is removed en bloc, and the spine is stabilized with a posterior instrumentation construct.

Anterior column lesions require a combined anterior and posterior approach. The posterior elements, pedicles, and posterior anulus are released first to allow the vertebral body to be removed en bloc through an anterior approach. The spine is stabilized posteriorly with a segmental system at the time of posterior release. A transthoracic or retroperitoneal approach is used to reach the tumor from the front. The adjacent disks are excised back to the posterior longitudinal ligament, and all anterior soft tissues are removed with the body, developing a plane between the great vessels and the anterior longitudinal ligament. Any involved dura can be excised and patched with a fascial graft to improve local control. The anterior reconstruction fills the vertebrectomy defect with tricortical or fibular graft, or with a prosthetic cage. Anterior plate fixation may be used to augment overall stability.

Once mechanical instability has developed, the tumor has usually extended into the extraosseous tissues (stage B). Progressive deformity will produce pain and threaten the spinal cord. The principles of excision are not changed, but the reconstruction must also treat any deformity or residual instability associated with the tumor. Excision margins must include the extraosseous tumor extension. Adjuvant radiotherapy often is useful postoperatively when the tumor margin has not been adequate. Radiotherapy to the tumor bed may be started 2 weeks after surgery, allowing initial healing of the incisions.

If extensive collapse has occurred, a surgical margin is not possible and local control depends on adjuvant therapy. An intralesional resection of the vertebral body is sufficient to debulk the tumor and prepare the vertebrectomy site for anterior reconstruction. In radioresistant tumors, such as chondrosarcoma or chordoma, every effort should be made to obtain an adequate surgical margin.

Lesions of the sacrum present a particular therapeutic and reconstructive dilemma. Tumors involving the distal sacrum require a partial sacral amputation through a combined anterior and posterior approach, sacrificing whatever nerve roots exit the involved segment. For higher sacral lesions, more roots will need to be sacrificed. If the S2 roots can be spared bilaterally, or if S2 and S3 roots are spared on one side, bowel and bladder function should be retained. Reconstruction following sacral amputation is most challenging when one or both of the sacroiliac joints is involved.

Chordoma Chordoma is a relatively rare lesion of the axial skeleton that is found most often in the spine and sacrum. The tumor derives from notochordal nests within the skull base, sacrococcygeal region, or vertebral segments. This slow-growing tumor is characterized by relentless local progression and an aggressive tendency to recur at the surgical site. Chordomas are more histologically variable and more clinically aggressive in children than in adults. They can reach remarkable size before they are detected (Fig. 12), and patients may present with a year or more of progressive pain, sitting intolerance, and constipation. Sacrococcygeal tumors are easily detected on rectal examination.

A clean surgical margin is crucial to local control, because these lesions generally are unresponsive to radiotherapy and chemotherapy. Although only 5% of patients with spinal chordoma develop metastases, nearly 70% die of their disease as a result of local tumor extension. Biopsy is performed through a posterior approach and never through the rectal vault; violation of the rectal wall necessitates colectomy. A combined anterior and posterior excision is indicated for vertebral lesions. For sacral lesions a high sacral amputation is the procedure of choice.

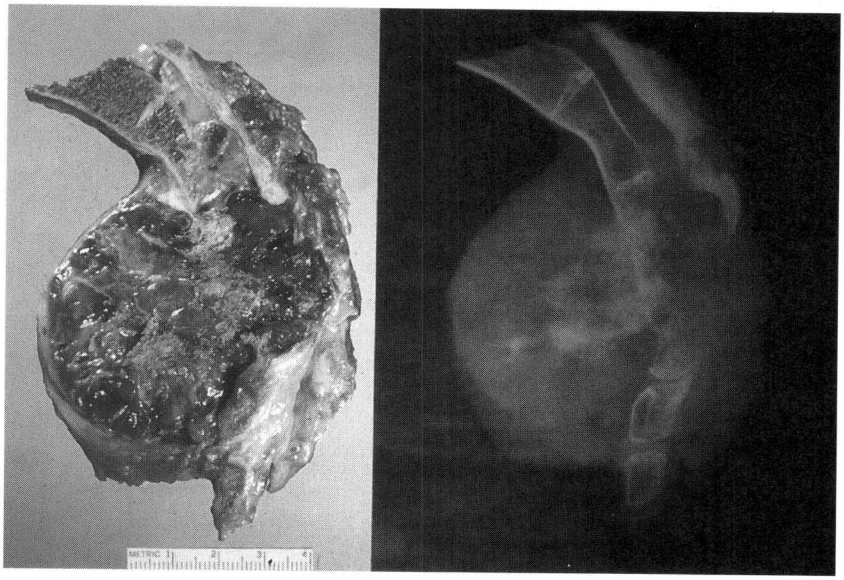

Chondrosarcoma Approximately 10% of chondrosarcomas arise in the spinal column or sacrum. Resistant to both radio- and chemotherapy, these slow-growing, locally invasive tumors are difficult to eradicate from the spinal column. Although survival may be prolonged in spite of residual disease, the ultimate prognosis for patients with spinal chondrosarcoma is poor.

Chondrosarcoma produces extensive bony destruction and a prominent soft-tissue mass stippled with flocculent calcifications. CT and MRI are crucial in determining soft-tissue extensions and the potential for surgical resection. Although long-term survival occasionally is possible with intralesional resection, a wide margin is the most reliable means of local control and cure. When a clear margin cannot be obtained, new radiotherapeutic modalities offer some hope of improved local control.

High-Grade Primary Malignancies

Patients presenting with a high-grade spinal malignancy have a poor prognosis regardless of treatment. These rapidly growing lesions rarely manifest before they have extended to the extraosseous tissues. Neurologic deficit is common and generally caused by 1 of 3 problems: a pathologic fracture, with either retropulsed bone fragments or acute kyphosis; tumor extension through the posterior vertebral cortex, with direct compression of the neural elements; or direct involvement of 1 or more nerve roots. In every case, the resection margins are likely to be contaminated, and adjuvant therapy should be considered. Nerve roots directly involved by the tumor must be resected along with the primary mass. Adherence or investment of the dura or great vessels is an ominous finding. Curettage is of no benefit in these patients. However, improved survival and function have been reported in patients in whom resection is attempted, although margins are difficult to obtain.

Figure 12

Sectioned surface of large sacral chordoma resected from a 74-year-old man with 4 years of sacral and coccygeal symptoms. Patient presented with progressive constipation. (Reproduced with permission from McLain RF, Weinstein JN: Tumors of the spine. *Semin Spine Surg* 1990;2:157–180.)

Osteosarcoma Osteosarcoma of the spine remains an ominous disease; median survival after diagnosis has ranged from 6 to 18 months, regardless of the surgical approach. Survival is comparable to that of extremity lesions when local control can be obtained surgically, but fewer than half of all spine patients obtain a complete local excision.

Spinal osteosarcoma arises in the vertebral body in 95% of cases. Radiographs reveal cortical destruction, soft-tissue calcification, and periosteal reaction, as well as vertebral collapse in some patients. There usually is a paraspinal soft-tissue mass, which may be extensive, and the tumor may encase or invade the great vessels or other contiguous structures. Intraspinal extension may result in either cord or cauda equina compression. CT and MRI are necessary to delineate tumor margins before any surgical procedure.

Aggressive treatment protocols have improved overall survival. Combining current adjuvant therapy with extensive anterior and posterior resections has improved local control, neurologic function, and survival rates.

Ewing's Sarcoma Ewing's sarcoma may be primary or metastatic to the spine. Approximately 3.5% of Ewing's lesions are thought to arise in the spinal column primarily. These tumors produce a permeative destructive pattern that can be difficult to discern on plain radiographs, and the first radiographic finding may be vertebral collapse and vertebra planum. Intraspinal extension may produce neurologic symptoms before bony involvement becomes apparent on plain radiographs. MRI demonstrates the lesion and its extensions, as well as occasional epidural metastases that do not involve bone.

Effective therapy for Ewing's sarcoma includes a program of multiagent chemotherapy and high-dose radiotherapy. Surgical treatment is indicated to decompress neurologic structures and stabilize the spinal column. Thoracic and thoracolumbar laminectomies should be instrumented to prevent kyphosis, both because the laminectomies are often extensive and because the patients are children. The prognosis generally is worse than for extremity lesions, but encouraging disease-free survival rates have been obtained using current chemotherapeutic regimens.

Solitary Plasmacytoma Solitary plasmacytoma and multiple myeloma are both B-cell lymphoproliferative diseases, but they behave in very different ways. Multiple myeloma is rapidly progressive and highly lethal, requiring supportive care for spinal disease. Solitary plasmacytoma may remain under local control for years before eventually disseminating. Although most, if not all, of these lesions will eventually degenerate into disseminated myeloma, with a rapidly lethal course, survivals of 20 years or more have been reported in solitary plasmacytomas.

Plasmacytoma is a radiosensitive tumor. Although spinal involvement in multiple myeloma is associated with a poor 1-year and almost no prolonged survival, patients with solitary plasmacytoma of the spine have a 60% 5-year survival rate. Surgical treatment is indicated to stabilize the spine and reduce mechanical pain, and to decompress neurologic elements in patients with rapidly progressive symptoms. Surgery also is warranted for patients with recurrent disease or tumors that have not responded to radiotherapy. Surgical debridement and prophylactic reconstruction, augmented by a full course of radiotherapy, may provide a prolonged disease-free survival. Postoperative follow-up with MRI and serum protein electrophoresis will provide the earliest indicators of recurrence or dissemination.

Lymphoma Lymphoma may occur as an isolated lesion or as a focal manifestation of a disseminated disease. Surgical treatment usually is an adjuvant to chemo- and radiotherapy, but local control of isolated lymphoma can be improved through adequate resection. Surgical decompression is indicated to relieve cord, cauda equina, or nerve root compression resulting from tumor extension or pathologic fracture and to stabilize damaged spinal segments.

Primary Malignancies With Metastasis

Once metastasis has occurred, the patient's survival becomes dependent on systemic therapy. Local control is still important in these stage C lesions, primarily to prevent neurologic compromise and pain, but the impetus toward aggressive resection procedures is reduced. Reconstruction of the involved segment should be sound, however, and both anterior and posterior columns should be treated to insure that late collapse, kyphosis, and pain will not occur.

Pediatric Tumors

Metastatic disease is the most common malignancy of the spine in children. Metastatic neuroblastoma accounts for nearly a third of all pediatric spinal tumors. Ewing's sarcoma is the most common primary malignancy, but still occurs more often as a metastasis than a primary lesion. Seventy percent of primary pediatric tumors are benign. Among the malignant lesions, there is a greater propensity for epidural spread as compared to tumors in the adult spine, and spinal cord compression can develop before any bony changes can be seen. MRI will show the epidural lesions well. Although survivals in metastatic disease remain limited, there is a trend toward more aggressive treatment in children as compared to adults.

Neuroblastoma This is a highly aggressive malignancy that may spread to the spine by either vascular dissemination or contiguous spread from the primary malignancy. Treated with a combination of chemotherapy, radiotherapy, and surgical excision, these tumors have a poor prognosis overall. Patients who do survive are at high risk of developing a progressive spinal deformity as a result of either rib resection or hemibody irradiation.

Leukemia Leukemia may occur as solitary or multiple vertebral lesions in a patient with systemic disease. Patients will have back pain, and some may have vertebral collapse at the time of presentation. Nonspecific complaints of muscular aches and pains, lethargy, and fatigue, as well as findings of fever or anemia, should prompt a search for the underlying disease. Radiographs may show vertebral collapse, focal lytic changes, and sclerotic geographic lesions or may be entirely normal. Bone scan also may be equivocal, but MRI will reliably demonstrate the infiltrate.

Conclusion

Improved medical and adjuvant therapy continue to enhance cancer survival in patients with both primary and metastatic disease. As patients live longer, spinal disease will pose a greater threat to independence and survival, and musculoskeletal lesions will require treatment that protects function and provides pain relief for years rather than months. Vertebrectomy, considered a radical procedure in the past, is coming to be seen as the conservative approach to tumor management in many situations. Appropriate surgical management can have an immediate and dramatic effect on patient function and survival, and should never be dismissed out of hand.

At the time of this writing, bone screws placed posteriorly into vertebral elements have been cleared for use in this specific manner by the Food and Drug Administration (FDA) to provide immobilization and stabilization as an adjunct to fusion in the treatment of the following acute and chronic instability or deformities of the thoracic, lumbar, and sacral spine: degenerative spondylolisthesis with objective evidence of neurologic impairment; fracture; dislocation; scoliosis; kyphosis; spinal tumor and failed previous fusion (pseudoarthrosis). In addition, anterior vertebral body screws (cervical, thoracic, and lumbar) are Class II devices and can be used as labeled in vertebral bodies.

Annotated Bibliography

Boriani S, Biagini R, De Iure F, et al: En bloc resections of bone tumors of the thoracolumbar spine: A preliminary report on 29 patients. *Spine* 1996;21:1927–1931.

En bloc resection is the ideal treatment for selected patients with primary malignant and aggressive benign tumors of the spine. Preoperative staging is crucial to selecting patients likely to benefit. Even when a wide margin cannot be achieved, prolonged local control is possible when surgery is combined with adjuvant radiotherapy. Of 29 patients treated, 9 failed to obtain a wide surgical margin. No local recurrence was found in any patient at a mean follow-up of 30 months.

Boriani S, Chevalley F, Weinstein JN, et al: Chordoma of the spine above the sacrum: Treatment and outcome in 21 cases. *Spine* 1996;21:1569–1577.

The authors reviewed 21 cases of chordoma of the mobile spine, demonstrating the value of appropriate oncologic and surgical staging in planning surgery and predicting outcome. Wide resection is the treatment of choice, but a marginal resection is superior to an intralesional procedure. When margins cannot be obtained, megavoltage or proton beam radiotherapy should be considered as adjuvant treatment.

Freiberg AA, Graziano GP, Loder RT, Hensinger RN: Metastatic vertebral disease in children. *J Pediatr Orthop* 1993;13: 148–153.

The authors reviewed 19 children with osseous vertebral metastases, average age 11 years at time of metastasis. Treatment consisted of chemotherapy (19), radiation therapy (12), and surgical excision (7). Nine children were alive at an average of 72 months after diagnosis. Children treated with chemotherapy, spinal radiation, and laminectomy, and who survived > 2 months, developed deformity. Spinal stabilization should be performed when laminectomy is combined with radiation and chemotherapy.

Grubb MR, Currier BL, Pritchard DJ, Ebersold MJ: Primary Ewing's sarcoma of the spine. *Spine* 1994;19:309–313.

The authors reviewed 36 patients (mean age 17 years) with primary Ewing's sarcoma of the spine. Fifty-eight percent had neurologic involvement, and 17 of 21 underwent laminectomy for decompression. Patients undergoing decompression for thoracic level lesions developed postlaminectomy kyphosis. Five-year survival was 33%, and not related to level of lesion or choice of surgical treatment.

Samson IR, Springfield DS, Suit HD, Mankin HJ: operative treatment of sacrococcygeal chordoma: A review of twenty-one cases. *J Bone Joint Surg* 1993;75A:1476–1484.

Twenty-one patients had a primary operation for sacrococcygeal chordoma. The average age at surgery was 55 years; in all patients, a posterior approach was used, even for resections at the cephalic levels of the sacrum. Sixteen patients were treated with adjuvant radiation therapy. Fifteen patients were free of disease and local recurrence at 4 years' follow-up. In 7 patients, the second sacral roots were the most caudal nerve-roots spared; 4 patients had normal bladder control and 5 had normal bowel control. Of the 4 patients in whom the most caudal nerve roots spared were the first sacral or more cephalic roots, all had impaired bladder control, 1 had impaired bowel control, and 3 required a colostomy.

Simpson AH, Porter A, Davis A, Griffin A, McLeod RS, Bell RS: Cephalad sacral resection with a combined extended ilioinguinal and posterior approach. *J Bone Joint Surg* 1995;77A:405–411.

A combined anterior and posterior approach is described for the resection of large tumors of the cephalad part of the sacrum. The anterior aspect of the sacrum is exposed through an extended ilioinguinal approach and the posterior aspect through a midline approach. This permits simultaneous exposure of the anterior, posterior, and circumferential aspects of the sacrum at the time of the osteotomy, facilitating the resection. At the time of follow-up (mean, 37 months), 10 of 11 patients were able to walk independently. The results of the study suggest that a combined extended ilioinguinal and posterior approach can be used effectively for the wide resection of a tumor arising in the cephalad part of the sacrum.

Sundaresan N, Steinberger AA, Moore F, et al: Indications and results of combined anterior-posterior approaches for spine tumor surgery. *J Neurosurg* 1996;85:438–446.

The authors analyzed 110 patients who underwent surgery for primary and metastatic spinal tumors over a 5-year period (1989-1993) at a single institution. Forty-eight patients (44%) were nonambulatory, and severe paraparesis was present in 20 patients. Major indications for anterior and posterior resection included 3-column involvement, high-grade instability, involvement of contiguous vertebral bodies, and solitary metastases. Postoperatively, 90 patients improved neurologically. The overall median survival was 16 months, with 46% of patients surviving 2 years. The majority of patients reported improvement in their quality of life at follow-up. Their findings suggest that half of all patients with spinal malignancies require combined anterior and posterior surgery for adequate tumor removal and stabilization.

Turcotte RE, Sim FH, Unni KK: Giant cell tumor of the sacrum. *Clin Orthop* 1993;291:215–221.

Twenty-six patients with giant cell tumors of the sacrum (mean age of 29 years) were treated from 1960 through 1986. A neurologic deficit was present in 88%. Twenty-one patients had radiation therapy; malignant transformation later occurred in 3. Three benign giant cell tumors metastasized to the lungs. The local recurrence rate for patients treated by curettage was 33%. Three patients died of tumor-related complications. The suggested initial treatment is complete curettage. Radiation therapy should be reserved for those with incomplete resection and local recurrence.

Classic Bibliography

Bohlman HH, Sachs BL, Carter JR, Riley L, Robinson R: Primary neoplasms of the cervical spine: Diagnosis and treatment of twenty-three patients. *J Bone Joint Surg* 1986;68A:483–494.

Gennari L, Azzarelli A, Quagliuolo V: A posterior approach for the excision of sacral chordoma. *J Bone Joint Surg* 1987;69B: 565–568.

Gilbert RW, Kim JH, Posner JB: Epidural spinal cord compression from metastatic tumor: Diagnosis and treatment. *Ann Neurol* 1978;3:40–51.

Harrington KD: Anterior decompression and stabilization of the spine as a treatment for vertebral collapse and spinal cord compression from metastatic malignancy. *Clin Orthop* 1988;233: 177–197.

Keim HA, Reina EG: Osteoid-osteoma as a cause of scoliosis. *J Bone Joint Surg* 1975;57A:159–163.

Kostuik JP, Errico TJ, Gleason TF, Errico CC: Spinal stabilization of vertebral column tumors. *Spine* 1988;13:250–256.

McLain RF, Weinstein JN: Solitary plasmacytomas of the spine: A review of 84 cases. *J Spinal Disord* 1989;2:69–74.

McLain RF, Weinstein JN: Tumors of the spine. *Semin Spine Surg* 1990;2:157–180.

Pettine KA, Klassen RA: Osteoid-osteoma and osteoblastoma of the spine. *J Bone Joint Surg* 1986;68A:354–361.

Shives TC, Dahlin DC, Sim FH, Pritchard DJ, Earle JD: Osteosarcoma of the spine. *J Bone Joint Surg* 1986;68A 660–668.

Shives TC, McLeod RA, Unni KK, Schray MF: Chondrosarcoma of the spine. *J Bone Joint Surg* 1989;71A:1158–1165.

Siegal T, Tiqva P, Siegal T: Vertebral body resection for epidural compression by malignant tumors: Results of forty-seven consecutive operative procedures. *J Bone Joint Surg* 1985;67A: 375–382.

Weinstein JN, McLain RF: Primary tumors of the spine. *Spine* 1987;12:843–851.

Chapter 56
Inflammatory Arthritis of the Spine

Adult Rheumatoid Arthritis

Rheumatoid spondylitis primarily affects the cervical spine; involvement of the thoracic and lumbar spine is unusual. Depending on the diagnostic criteria used, the prevalence of cervical spine involvement in patients with rheumatoid arthritis (RA) ranges from 25% to 80%. Abnormalities occur in this condition as a consequence of the synovitic destruction of joints, ligaments, and bone with extension of pannus into surrounding structures. Ligament laxity and rupture lead to instability or frank subluxation of the cervical spine. Compression of the spinal cord or brain stem can result from this static or dynamic subluxation or by direct pressure from synovial pannus. Cervical involvement typically begins early in the disease process, and its progression has been closely correlated with the extent of peripheral disease. In a 49-patient series in which cervical disease was correlated with peripheral disease activity, none of the subset with least erosive peripheral disease developed vertical subluxation of the odontoid, whereas 52% of the subset with more erosive disease and 88% of the subset with mutilating disease advanced to vertical subluxation. Male sex, seropositivity, and a history of corticosteroid therapy also have been correlated with more extensive cervical involvement.

Subluxations
Three deformities occur most commonly in the rheumatoid cervical spine. Atlantoaxial instability (AAI) or subluxation (AAS) is most common and has been reported to occur in up to 49% of patients. This subluxation usually is anterior, although up to 20% may be lateral, and 6.9% are reported to be posterior. AAS can be reducible, partially reducible, or fixed, and this determination is important in planning treatment. The next most common deformity in the rheumatoid spine is superior migration of the odontoid (SMO). Erosion of the occiput-C1 and C1-C2 joints leads to a decrease in the vertical distance between the brain stem and the odontoid. This condition, which occurs in up to 38% of patients with RA, also is described as cranial settling, atlantoaxial impaction, and pseudobasilar invagination. Superior migration of the odontoid can lead to direct compression of the brain stem or can cause neurologic injury by placing the cervicomedullary junction into excessive kyphosis.

The third and least common type of deformity in the rheumatoid cervical spine is subaxial subluxation. This has been found to occur in 10% to 20% of patients and often is seen at multiple levels, producing a stepladder type of deformity with associated kyphosis. Subaxial subluxation also has been reported to occur after previous upper cervical fusions. In a series of 79 patients, 36% developed subaxial subluxation an average of 2.6 years after occipitocervical fusion and 5.5% developed subaxial subluxation an average of 9 years after atlantoaxial fusion. The results of this series emphasize the need to consider extending a planned upper cervical fusion in patients with early subaxial disease.

Natural History and Clinical Manifestations

In patients with RA, a careful history is important to look for symptoms of cervical involvement. Neck pain, which is classically found at the craniocervical junction, is common and is frequently associated with occipital headaches. Ear pain, occipital neuralgia, and facial pain can be caused by compression of the greater auricular nerve, greater occipital nerve, or the trigeminal nucleus, respectively. Patients may also complain of myelopathic symptoms including weakness, loss of endurance, and gait disturbance, as well as loss of dexterity and paresthesias of the hands. Urinary retention and later incontinence are symptoms of more severe involvement. Neck motion may result in electric shock-like sensations of the torso or extremities (Lhermitte's sign). Vertebrobasilar insufficiency may occur and is usually found in patients with AAI. Symptoms can include visual disturbances, loss of equilibrium, vertigo, tinnitus, and dysphagia.

Physical examination of these patients frequently is confounded by the severity of their peripheral rheumatoid involvement. A high index of suspicion for signs of myelopathy must be maintained. The Ranawat classification of rheumatoid myelopathy has proven useful in evaluating patients, planning treatment, and examining results. Class I patients have no neural deficit, class II patients have subjective weakness with hyperreflexia and dysesthesia, and class III patients have objective weakness and long tract signs. Class III has been subdivided into IIIA for ambulatory patients and

IIIB for the patients who are no longer ambulatory. Patients with superior migration of the odontoid also may develop cranial nerve dysfunction secondary to compression of the cranial nerve nuclei in the medulla oblongata by the odontoid process.

Numerous studies have been undertaken to examine the natural history of RA involving the cervical spine. In one study, patients were divided into 3 groups based on the duration of their rheumatic disease: group I had disease for < 5 years, group II for 5 to 10 years, and group III for > 10 years. AAS was present in 3 of 21 (14%) patients in group I, 12 of 22 (55%) in group II, and 34 of 57 (60%) in group III. Several other studies also have correlated the incidence of cervical findings with the duration of rheumatic disease, and it is now well established that the longer a patient has RA the greater the likelihood of cervical disease. In another study, serial radiographs of 49 patients with RA revealed a progressive pattern of upper cervical subluxations. Patients progressed from reducible AAS to irreducible subluxation, which was then followed by SMO. The incidence of progression was closely correlated with the severity of the patient's peripheral disease. Other radiologic surveys have reported incidences of progressive cervical subluxation ranging from 43% to 80%.

Reported rates of neural impairment resulting from cervical instability have ranged from 11% to 58%. In a group of 73 patients with rheumatoid involvement of the cervical spine, 42 (57%) developed neurologic dysfunction (Ranawat class II in 11 and class III in 31). Thirty-five of the patients who developed paralysis underwent surgical treatment, thus altering the natural history. Of the 7 patients with neurologic dys-

function who were not treated surgically, either because they refused or were medically unable to have the operation, all had an increase in the severity of their paralysis. Other studies have shown that once cervical myelopathy develops, death is a common outcome if it is left untreated. Another disturbing fact is the reported incidence of sudden death caused by fatal medullary compression in patients with upper cervical instability. One postmortem study of 104 patients with RA found that 10% of the deaths resulted from fatal medullary compression. Despite all of the literature available on the natural history of rheumatoid involvement of the cervical spine, it remains impossible to predict with certainty which patients will have progression of their deformity or develop neurologic sequelae.

Radiologic Imaging

The initial radiographic assessment of patients with RA of the cervical spine should consist of plain radiographs, including lateral flexion and extension views. In a retrospective study of 113 rheumatoid patients treated with total hip or knee arthroplasty, preoperative cervical radiographs indicated cervical spine abnormalities, including AAS, SMO, and subaxial subluxation, in 61% of patients. Only 50% of the patients with radiographic abnormalities had symptoms of cervical disease. Thus, radiographs of the cervical spine should be obtained in all patients with RA because many patients with cervical involvement are asymptomatic. Several measurements can be made from plain films to help delineate the need for further evaluation and to plan treatment. The

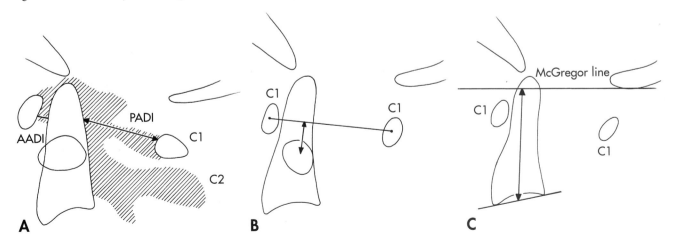

Figure 1

A, Measurement of anterior atlantodental interval (AADI) and posterior atlantodental interval (PADI). B, The Ranawat method of measurement of vertical settling. C, The Redlund-Johnell method of measurement of vertical settling. (Reproduced with permission from Monsey RD: Rheumatoid arthritis of the cervical spine. *J Am Acad Orthop Surg* 1997;5:240–248.)

most common measurements include (1) the anterior atlantodental interval (AADI), (2) the posterior atlantodental interval (PADI), (3) the subaxial canal diameter, (4) the McGregor line, (5) the Ranawat index, and (6) the Redlund-Johnell measurement (Fig. 1).

The AADI is measured on a lateral radiograph from the posterior aspect of the anterior ring of C1 to the anterior aspect of the dens. The normal value for an adult is less than 3 mm. Traditionally, the AADI has been used to follow RA patients over time, and various studies have recommended surgery for values greater than 8, 9, or 10 mm. An increasing number of studies, however, have shown that the AADI is not reliable at discriminating patients with neural deficit from those who are neurologically intact. It has also been shown that as the deformity progresses to SMO, with its associated worse neurologic prognosis, the AADI actually decreases. More recent attention has focused on the PADI, which is measured from the posterior aspect of the dens to the anterior aspect of the C1 lamina. The PADI has been shown to be a more reliable predictor of whether a patient will develop neurologic compromise. In a recent study of 73 patients with long-term follow-up, a PADI of 14 mm or less yielded a 97% sensitivity for detecting patients with paralysis, and 94% of patients with values > 14 mm had no neurologic deficit. In contrast, the same study found that the AADI did not correlate with the presence of paralysis.

SMO can be assessed with a variety of measurements. McGregor's line is drawn on the lateral view from the hard palate to the base of the occiput. Vertical settling of the occiput has been defined as migration of the odontoid more than 4.5 mm above McGregor's line. Two other useful measurements are the Ranawat index and the Redlund-Johnell values. The Ranawat index assesses pathology in the C1-2 segment and is measured on the lateral radiograph by drawing a line from the pedicles of C2 superiorly along the vertical axis of the odontoid until it intersects a line connecting the anterior and posterior arches of C1. A value < 13 mm is diagnostic of vertical settling. The Redlund-Johnell measurement assesses the entire occiput to C2 complex and when abnormal is highly correlated with severe disease and neurologic injury. Its value is determined by measuring the distance between the midpoint of the inferior margin of the body of the axis to McGregor's line. A value < 34 mm in men and < 29 mm in women is considered abnormal.

In the subaxial cervical spine, plain radiographs are useful in detecting vertebral subluxations. Traditionally, attention has focused on the percentage of vertebral slip or on the number of millimeters of listhesis of 1 vertebra on another. Slips > 20% or listhesis of 4 mm were considered significant. More recently, however, it has been shown that the sagittal

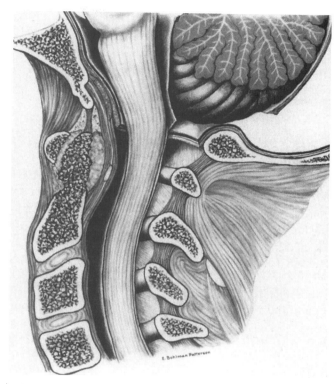

Figure 2

Illustration demonstrating anterior atlantoaxial subluxation with pannus formation around the odontoid process and osseous erosions. There is severe compression of the spinal cord between the pannus anteriorly and the arch of the atlas posteriorly. (Reproduced with permission from Boden SD, Dodge LD, Bohlman HH, Rechtine GR: Rheumatoid arthritis of the cervical spine: A long-term analysis with predictors of paralysis and recovery. *J Bone Joint Surg* 1993;75A:1282–1297.)

diameter of the subaxial canal correlates with the presence and degree of paralysis more often than does the percentage of vertebral slip. Patients with canal diameters of 13 mm or less are at higher risk of developing neurologic dysfunction.

In patients with neurologic deficits who have abnormalities on plain radiographs, a magnetic resonance imaging (MRI) scan should be obtained. MRI has provided an increased ability to view spinal cord compression, not only from bone, but also from soft-tissue pannus, which can be present in variable thickness (Fig. 2). In one study, > 3 mm of pannus was present in 22 of 34 patients studied. An MRI scan allows assessment of the degree of superior migration of the odontoid as well as measurement of the space available for the cord. Cord configuration also can be evaluated. The cervicomedullary angle is an effective measure of cord distortion. This angle is measured by drawing lines along the anterior aspects of the cervical cord and along the medulla. A normal angle is between 135° and 175°. Values < 135° are significant for vertical settling and have been correlated with myelopathy.

More recently, functional MRI scans obtained in flexion and extension have proven useful in detecting dynamic cord compression. Based on anatomic data, it has been determined that at the foramen magnum 14 mm of space is necessary to avoid neurologic compression. This space allows for the thickness of the neural elements, dura, and 1 mm of space anterior and posterior to the cord so that it is free to glide. At C1-2, 13 mm is the minimum space needed, and in the subaxial spine, 12 mm is required. These numbers are applicable to MRI measurements, but must be applied with care to measurements made on plain radiographs because of the inherent magnification present on radiographs.

Other imaging modalities that may be useful are polytomography and computed tomography (CT). Tomograms are especially useful for evaluating the degree of basilar invagination and also permit more accurate measurement of the AADI and PADI values than plain radiographs. CT scanning has been largely supplanted by MRI in evaluating the rheumatoid spine, but CT scanning does provide excellent osseous detail, and reformation into sagittal and coronal images has improved its value. CT scanning with intrathecal contrast can provide nearly the same detail as MRI scanning and is useful in patients with contraindications to MRI, such as ferromagnetic hardware in the cervical spine, claustrophobia, a cardiac pacemaker, or intracranial vascular clips.

Nonsurgical Management and Surgical Treatment

When treating patients with rheumatoid involvement of the cervical spine, several goals must be kept in mind. First, it is important to prevent the development of an irreversible neurologic deficit. The presence and severity of the preoperative neurologic deficit seems to correlate with postoperative neurologic recovery. Patients with more severe deficits tend to show less recovery and have a higher morbidity. Age, sex, and duration of paralysis before surgery have not been found to correlate with postoperative recovery. A second goal of treatment is to prevent sudden death caused by unrecognized neural compression. Studies have shown that up to 10% of deaths in patients with RA occur suddenly as a result of neurologic compression. A third goal of treatment is to avoid unnecessary surgery. Because 50% of patients with radiographic evidence of instability remain asymptomatic, it is important to avoid surgery on those patients who will remain without symptoms and not have dangerous progression of their deformity.

With the above goals in mind, a rational treatment algorithm can be designed to aid in the care of these patients. The initial evaluation of patients with RA should consist of cervical spine radiographs including lateral flexion and extension views. Patients with evidence of instability should have an MRI evaluation of their cervical spines. Patients with intractable pain and/or a clear-cut neurologic deficit should have surgical stabilization of the deformity. It is the patients with some or no pain and no neurologic deficit whose radiographs reveal instability that make up a more controversial group. To aid in planning treatment, patients can be divided on the basis of their radiographic studies into those with AAS, basilar invagination, subaxial subluxation, or some combination of the 3.

Conservative treatment of rheumatoid involvement of the spine is supportive. Because cervical involvement starts early in the course of the disease and has been correlated with systemic disease activity, early aggressive medical management is important. Cervical collars can be used for comfort, but do not protect against progressive subluxation or neurologic compromise. Although studies have shown that rigid cervical collars can partially limit AAS, the collars also prevent reduction of the deformity in extension. Rigid orthoses also are poorly tolerated in this patient population because of skin sensitivity and temporomandibular joint involvement. A crucial part of nonsurgical treatment of these patients is careful observation for gradual deterioration in function, which may indicate the development of a subtle myelopathy, and to observe for radiographic signs of impending neurologic compromise.

Surgical treatment of RA of the cervical spine often is complicated by the patient's generalized debilitated condition. These patients tend to have poor skin, poorly healing wounds, and osteopenic bone. Studies have shown that generalized bone loss occurs early in the course of RA and this bone loss correlates with systemic disease activity. Patients using steroids tend to have even lower bone mass; however, the independent effect of steroids is questionable because their use may be an indicator of more severe disease. Nutritional issues must also be addressed before surgical treatment because poor nutritional parameters have been associated with more frequent complications, including infection. Proper perioperative airway management of rheumatoid patients is critical. In one series of 128 patients, incidence of upper-airway obstruction was 14% after extubation in patients intubated without fiberoptic assistance compared with a 1% incidence in patients intubated fiberoptically.

In patients with isolated AAS and no neurologic deficit, it generally is safe to continue with observation provided the PADI is > 14 mm on plain radiographs. If, however, the PADI is ≤ 14 mm then an MRI scan should be obtained to evaluate the space available for the cord, taking into account the space occupied by synovial pannus. If the MRI scan demonstrates a cervicomedullary angle of < 135°, cord diameter in flexion of ≤ 6 mm, or space available for the cord of < 13 mm, then a posterior atlantoaxial fusion should be considered. Fusion can be accomplished using Gallie or Brooks type procedures, posterior transarticular screws, or a combination of screw and wiring. Depending on the quality of fixation, a halo device may be required postoperatively. In a study of 22 patients, fusion was obtained in 95% using only transarticular screws. If the deformity is irreducible and posterior compressive pathology is present, a C1 laminectomy with the transarticular screw technique should be considered.

In the past, if excessive retrodental pannus was producing anterior cord compression, a transoral decompression followed by a posterior cervical fusion was recommended. More recently, the need for anterior surgery has been questioned in light of new data documenting the resorption of retrodental pannus after a solid posterior fusion. One MRI study found that in 19 of 22 patients who had upper cervical fusion, a significant amount of pannus was resorbed.

Basilar invagination, with its higher surgical morbidity and poor potential for recovery, should be treated with a more aggressive surgical approach. In patients with AAS and any degree of basilar invagination, an MRI scan in flexion is recommended to evaluate the degree of spinal cord compression. Patients who have isolated and fixed basilar invagination with no symptoms and no evidence of neural compression can be treated with continued observation; however, if there is any evidence of cord compression, cervical traction should be initiated to try to achieve a reduction. If a reduction is possible, a posterior occipitocervical fusion is recommended. If reduction is not possible with traction, a C1 laminectomy or an anterior resection of the odontoid should be combined with an occipitocervical fusion. Occipitocervical fusion can be accomplished with a variety of techniques using wires, metal loops, mesh, and more recently metal plates. In one study that compared plates and screws to wiring techniques, better reduction was obtained with plating with a higher rate of neurologic improvement and lower pseudarthosis rate.

Patients with subaxial subluxation and no neurologic deficit should be followed up with plain cervical radiographs. If the subaxial canal diameter is > 14 mm, continued observation is appropriate. If the subaxial canal diameter is ≤ 14 mm, an MRI scan should be obtained to determine the true space available for the cord. If the space available for the cord is ≤ 13 mm or a significant degree of instability is present at that segment, surgical arthrodesis should be considered. In most patients, a posterior cervical fusion is the procedure of choice; however, if the subluxation is not readily reduced, anterior decompression and fusion are indicated. It is impor-

tant to realize that subaxial instability can develop after an upper cervical fusion, and patients must be followed long-term to look for this occurrence. Additionally, when upper cervical fusion is necessary and early subaxial subluxation is present, longer fusions to include the involved subaxial segment should be strongly considered.

Treatment Results and Complications

The results of treatment of the rheumatoid spine vary with the location and severity of the disease. Neurologic improvement has been reported in 27% to 100% of patients. In a recent study of 90 patients with neurologic deficits, 94.8% improved at least 1 Ranawat grade after treatment of AAS, 76% improved after treatment of combined SMO with AAS, and 94% treated for isolated subaxial subluxation improved. Pain relief can also be reliably anticipated in approximately 90% of patients. Results seem to be worse for patients with more advanced neurologic deficits preoperatively. In one study that looked exclusively at Ranawat class III patients, 58% of ambulatory patients (IIIA) attained grades I or II postoperatively whereas only 20% of nonambulatory patients (IIIB) improved to grade I or II. The nonambulatory patients also had a higher complication rate, longer hospital stay, and ultimately worse survival. Reports of other studies have indicated that, although the complication rate is higher, neurologic improvement can be expected even in class IIIB patients and surgery should be attempted. Data from one study indicated that the most important predictor of the potential for neurologic recovery after the operation was the preoperative PADI. In patients with paralysis caused by AAS, no recovery occurred if the PADI was < 10 mm and at least some recovery always occurred when the PADI was ≥ 10 mm. If basilar invagination was superimposed, neurologic recovery occurred only when the PADI was ≥ 13 mm.

Complications after surgery on the rheumatoid spine include death, infection, neurologic deterioration, wound dehiscence, nonunion, and late subaxial instability below a fused segment. Death rates following cervical surgery in rheumatoid patients have been dramatically reduced by more aggressive perioperative care. The perioperative mortality rate for most recent series is between 5% and 10%. Nonunion rates also are highly variable and nonunion is more frequent than in the general population. Meticulous surgical technique with use of redundant fixation, such as transarticular screws combined with posterior wiring procedures, appears to be useful in reducing the nonunion rates. Neurologic compromise resulting from cervical spine surgery in rheumatoid patients is uncommon. Preoperative traction to reduce subluxation, careful surgical technique, and adequate stabilization are all necessary to avoid this complication. Passage of sublaminar wires is probably the most dangerous portion of these surgical procedures and the use of intraoperative spinal cord monitoring is advised. Overall complication rates appear to be reduced with earlier surgery, as well as with optimal anesthetic and medical management.

Juvenile Rheumatoid Arthritis

Juvenile rheumatoid arthritis (JRA) is a systemic disease of childhood characterized by chronic synovitis and is often accompanied by extra-articular pathology as well. Three subsets of this disease have been identified, including monarticular, polyarticular, and systemic. Cervical spine involvement can occur in polyarticular and systemic JRA, but is rare in the monarticular variant. Cervical stiffness is the most common symptom and has been reported in 46% to 60% of patients. Radiographic changes are not as frequent as in adult RA, but can include vertebral subluxations as well as spontaneous posterior fusions, which may result in growth disturbances. These changes usually are seen in the late stages of the disease and only in children with severe involvement. Even in patients with abnormal radiographs, neck pain is uncommon and has been reported in only 2% to 17% of patients. Neurologic complications are also much less likely to develop in these patients than in adult rheumatoid patients. In one study of 92 patients treated for JRA, only 31% had cervical involvement; of these, only 2 patients developed myelopathy. Torticollis also has been reported to occur in these patients, but other sources, such as trauma and infection, must be ruled out before attributing this finding to the JRA. Surgical treatment of cervical spine involvement in JRA should be reserved for patients with severe instability or neurologic compromise. Neck stiffness, loss of lordosis, and micrognathia can make intubation difficult in these patients, and this must be kept in mind when planning any surgical procedures on a patient with JRA.

Seronegative Spondyloarthropathies

The seronegative spondyloarthropathies constitute a family of interrelated but heterogeneous chronic inflammatory conditions of unknown etiology. These diseases include ankylosing spondylitis (AS), Reiter's syndrome, psoriatic arthritis, arthritis of inflammatory bowel disease, and the undifferentiated spondyloarthropathies. The inflammations typically affect the spine, peripheral joints, and periarticular structures and produce variable extra-articular manifestations as well.

Ankylosing spondylitis is the most common of these conditions, with a prevalence rate of between 67.7 and 197 per 100,000 people in the United States. There is a strong association of AS with the class I antigen HLA-B27, which is present in 80% to 98% of affected white patients compared with only 8% of the general population. AS typically presents between ages 15 and 50 years as insidious-onset low back pain and stiffness that is worse in the morning and is mitigated by activity or a hot shower. The pain eventually localizes to the sacroiliac joints, and sacroiliac joint involvement is the radiographic hallmark of the disease. The hip and shoulders are the most commonly affected extra-axial joints and pain in these joints is the primary symptom in 15% of patients. Enthesopathy, which is inflammation at the insertion of tendons and ligaments into bone, is common and may be associated with the formation of bony spurs at these sites. Chest pain may occur as a result of involvement of the costovertebral and costotransverse joints, with an associated reduction in chest expansion. Eye disease, including acute anterior uveitis or iridocyclitis, is the most common extra-articular manifestation of AS and occurs in 25% to 30% of patients. Cardiac and pulmonary involvement are less common, but may be severe.

Spine involvement in AS usually begins with lumbar stiffness and loss of lordosis. Cervical involvement typically occurs later and results in limitation of neck motion and progressive kyphosis. Inflammation of the anulus fibrosus leads to gradual squaring of the vertebral bodies, with eventual formation of bridging syndesmophytes. Associated inflammation of the apophyseal joints and ossification of the surrounding ligaments are frequent and may eventually lead to complete bony ankylosis of the vertebral column ("bamboo spine"). Despite the ankylosed appearance on radiographs, osteoporosis of the spine also occurs and usually is not detectable with most current techniques for measuring bone mineral density because the ossification of spinal ligaments produces a falsely elevated reading. As the disease progresses over many years, the back and neck pain may actually improve, with severe deformity becoming the chief complaint.

In the lumbar spine, involvement can progress to an ankylosed kyphotic deformity that interferes with the patient's ability to see the horizon, results in compression of the abdominal viscera by the rib margin, and compromises respiration, which is highly dependent on diaphragmatic excursion. Extension osteotomies of the lumbar spine have proven very successful in these patients, with an 88.4% patient satisfaction rate reported in one recent study. Initially, these operations involved monosegmental osteotomies with or without rigid internal fixation that resulted in relative lengthening of the spine's anterior column. Vascular and neurologic complications from these procedures were not uncommon, and the mortality rate was reported to be approximately 10%. Later, polysegmental osteotomies with transpedicular fixation were used in an attempt to reduce the complication rate and to provide a more balanced correction. The drawback of these procedures was their relatively long time in surgery, the increased rate of nonunion, and the increased risk associated with multiple exposures of the dura. Moreover, many surgeons found that despite the multiple osteotomies, most of the correction was occurring at 1 or 2 levels.

More recently, the most commonly accepted osteotomy is a single level closing wedge osteotomy with transpedicular fixation (Fig. 3). This procedure avoids lengthening of the anterior column and allows a continuous view of the thecal sac and roots. The closing osteoclasis allows controlled correction with an anterior cortical hinge and 2 posterior cancellous surfaces that are rigidly fixed, allowing rapid fusion and consolidation. In a series of 22 lumbar closing wedge osteotomies, the authors reported no mortalities, no permanent neurologic complications, and 2 failures of fixation that may have been related to the construct used.

Cervical kyphosis also can progress to the point where the patient is unable to look forward because of a "chin on chest deformity." The chin-brow vertical angle, which is an intersection of a line drawn from the chin to the brow and a vertical line, is a means of quantifying a patient's overall clinical deformity and spinal balance. If the primary site of the deformity is cervical, then an osteotomy at the cervicothoracic junction can produce significant correction with improve-

ment in symptoms and function. The osteotomy typically is done between C7 and T1 because the canal is widest at this level. A halo vest is applied preoperatively after which local or general anesthesia can be used for the surgical procedure. If general anesthesia is chosen, then high-quality spinal cord monitoring becomes essential. The procedure is carried out with the patient sitting and involves removal of the posterior elements of C7, including the facet joints and lateral masses, with portions of C6 and T1 removed as needed. A controlled osteoclasis of the anterior spinal elements is done and the head is extended back to the corrected position (Fig. 4). A posterior fusion is then carried out either with or without internal fixation. If done properly this procedure can consistently allow the patient to look straight ahead and return to functional activities.

Atlantoaxial instability also can develop in AS; in one recent study it occurred in 23% of 103 patients. Routine screening cervical radiographs are recommended for any patient with AS who is scheduled for surgery.

Fractures in the osteoporotic and ankylosed cervical spine are not uncommon, even with minor trauma. Any patient complaining of new neck or back pain or change in position should be assumed to have a fracture until proven otherwise. Fractures can be difficult to detect with plain radiographs, and modalities such as CT, MRI, or bone scans may be helpful. Because bony ankylosis has turned the spine into a rigid ring, fractures of a single column cannot occur alone and, consequently, these are unstable 3-column injuries with a significant incidence of neurologic injury. Treatment should

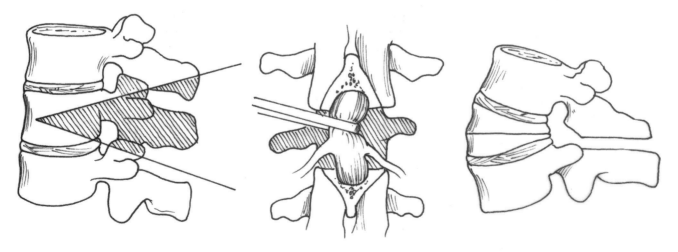

Figure 3

Closing wedge posterior osteotomy of the lumbar spine for ankylosing spondylitis. (Reproduced with permission from van Royen BJ, Slot GH: Closing-wedge posterior osteotomy for ankylosing spondylitis: Partial corporectomy and transpedicular fixation in 22 cases. *J Bone Joint Surg* 1995;77B:117–121.)

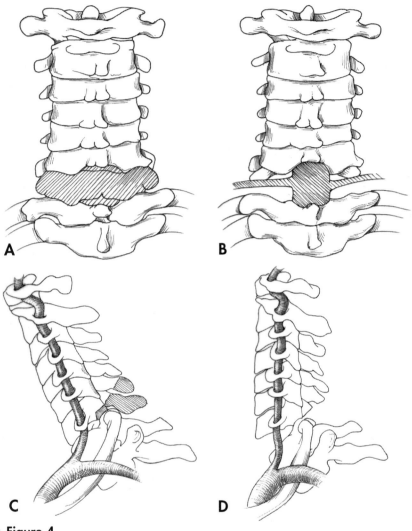

Figure 4

Extension osteotomy of the cervical spine in ankylosing spondylitis. A and B, Anteroposterior views. C and D, lateral view. (Reproduced with permission from McMaster MJ: Osteotomy of the cervical spine in ankylosing spondylitis. *J Bone Joint Surg* 1997;79B:197–203.)

with a relatively high incidence of neurologic deficit. Rigid surgical stabilization of lumbar fractures should be considered for patients with AS. In addition, symptomatic epidural hematomas occur more frequently in these patients because the spine is essentially a rigid tube with minimal capacity to expand. Another complication that can occur after thoracolumbar fractures in patients with AS is the development of spondylodiskitis. The reported incidence of spondylodiskitis ranges from 5% to 23%, and it is thought to result from a pseudarthrosis after a fracture. Patients may be asymptomatic, but usually complain of increasing pain and deformity and may also develop spinal stenosis at the level of the spondylodiskitis. Some patients treated conservatively with bed rest and/or immobilization develop a spontaneous fusion at the affected segment and become asymptomatic; however, surgical treatment should be considered for persistently symptomatic patients or those with progressive deformity.

Psoriatic arthritis and Reiter's syndrome are 2 other seronegative spondyloarthropathies that can involve the spine. Both of these conditions tend to affect the cervical spine, with a 70% incidence of radiographic involvement of the cervical spine in patients with psoriatic arthritis in one study. Spine involvement appears to be less common in Reiter's syndrome, with only a 3.4% incidence in one study. Two patterns of spinal involvement can occur in these patients. More commonly, patients develop lesions typical of AS, including ligamentous ossification and syndesmophyte formation. Some patients, however, develop inflammatory involvement more characteristic of that seen in patients with RA, including bony erosions and subluxations. Patients should be treated according to the pattern of their disease, similarly to patients with AS or RA.

consist of reduction by traction followed by halo vest immobilization. If reduction is not possible or fracture union does not occur, surgical treatment is indicated.

As in the cervical spine, fractures of the lumbar spine also can occur with trivial trauma. These also are unstable injuries

Annotated Bibliography

Boden SD: Rheumatoid arthritis of the cervical spine: Surgical decision making based on predictors of paralysis and recovery. *Spine* 1994;19:2275–2280.

This article reviews the current knowledge of predictors of paralysis and the potential for neurologic recovery in patients with RA involving the cervical spine. The primary goals are to prevent the onset of an irreversible neurologic deficit and to avoid unnecessary imaging and surgery.

Boden SD, Dodge LD, Bohlman HH, Rechtine GR: Rheumatoid arthritis of the cervical spine: A long-term analysis with predictors of paralysis and recovery. *J Bone Joint Surg* 1993;75A: 1282–1297.

The long-term results of 73 patients were carefully evaluated in this landmark study. The PADI was found to be more reliable than the AADI in predicting the risk of paralysis. A PADI and a subaxial canal diameter of ≤ 14 mm were both found to correlate with the presence of paralysis. Preoperative PADI values of ≥ 10 mm and ≥ 13 mm were shown to correlate with potential for neurologic recovery in patients with AAS and basilar invagination, respectively.

Casey AT, Crockard HA, Bland JM, Stevens J, Moskovich R, Ransford AO: Surgery on the rheumatoid cervical spine for the non-ambulant myelopathic patient: Too much, too late? *Lancet* 1996;347:1004–1007.

The authors prospectively examined the results of surgery in 134 patients, comparing preoperatively ambulatory (Ranawat IIIA) and nonambulatory (IIIB) patients. Of the ambulatory patients, 58% attained Ranawat neurologic grades I or II compared with only 20% of the nonambulatory patients ($p = 0.0001$). The nonambulatory group also fared worse in terms of postoperative complication rate, length of hospital stay, functional outcome, and ultimately, survival.

Crockard HA: Surgical management of cervical rheumatoid problems. *Spine* 1995;20:2584–2590.

This update reviews current thinking on the development of cervical spine problems and describes the histologic and macroscopic changes in RA. The various types of surgical procedures are described and outcome evaluated on the basis of the natural history of the condition.

Gough AK, Lilley J, Eyre S, Holder RL, Emery P: Generalised bone loss in patients with early rheumatoid arthritis. *Lancet* 1994;344:23–27.

Dual energy X-ray absorptiometry was performed on 148 patients with early RA and 730 normal controls. Patients with RA were found to undergo significant generalized skeletal bone loss early in the disease, and the loss was found to be associated with disease activity. Suppression of disease activity was shown to stabilize bone loss.

Grob D, Dvorak J, Panjabi MM, Antinnes JA: The role of plate and screw fixation in occipitocervical fusion in rheumatoid arthritis. *Spine* 1994;19:2545–2551.

The results of screw fixation and of wiring techniques for occipitocervical fusion were compared. The atlantodental distance could be significantly better reduced in the group with plate fixation. Neurologic improvement in the wiring group was 40% compared with 86% in the plate fixation group. Pseudarthrosis was seen in 27% of the wiring technique and in 6% in the plate and screw fixation technique.

Grob D, Wursch R, Grauer W, Sturzenegger J, Dvorak J: Atlantoaxial fusion and retrodental pannus in rheumatoid arthritis. *Spine* 1997;22:1580–1583.

Twenty-two patients with AAI and verified pannus on MRI underwent posterior fusion of the upper cervical spine. Significant pannus reduction was noted on follow-up MRI in 19 of the patients, including those whose systemic disease was active or progressing.

McMaster MJ: Osteotomy of the cervical spine in ankylosing spondylitis. *J Bone Joint Surg* 1997;79B:197–203.

Fifteen patients with severe cervical kyphosis secondary to AS were treated with extension osteotomy at C7-T1 under general anesthesia. Mean correction was 54° with all patients able to see straight ahead postoperatively. One patient developed quadraparesis and 2 others had transient unilateral palsies of C8.

Oda T, Fujiwara K, Yonenobu K, Azuma B, Ochi T: Natural course of cervical spine lesions in rheumatoid arthritis. *Spine* 1995;20:1128–1135.

This study analyzed the natural course of cervical spine involvement in RA by following serial radiographs in 49 patients. Upper cervical lesions were noted to progress to irreducible AAS and finally to SMO. Cervical disease progression was correlated with peripheral disease activity.

Stillerman CB, Wilson JA: Atlantoaxial stabilization with posterior transarticular screw fixation: Technical description and report of 22 cases. *Neurosurgery* 1993;32:948–954.

Twenty-two patients were treated with C1-2 fusion using transarticular screw fixation and bony fusion alone without associated wiring. By not using wires the authors hoped to avoid the risk of neural injury resulting from sublaminar passage and the possibility of retrodisplacement of ventral structures. Nineteen of 20 (95%) patients achieved solid fusion. There were no neurologic or vascular complications.

van Royen BJ, Slot GH: Closing-wedge posterior osteotomy for ankylosing spondylitis: Partial corporectomy and transpedicular fixation in 22 cases. *J Bone Joint Surg* 1995;77B:117–121.

The authors report the results of 22 patients with progressive kyphosis treated with lumbar closing wedge osteotomy and transpedicular fixation. Correction averaged 32° with no fatal complications. There were 2 failures of fixation and 1 patient required reoperation secondary to neural compression.

Wattenmaker I, Concepcion M, Hibberd P, Lipson S: Upper-airway obstruction and perioperative management of the airway in patients managed with posterior operations on the cervical spine for rheumatoid arthritis. *J Bone Joint Surg* 1994;76A:360–365.

The records of 128 consecutive patients who underwent posterior operations on the cervical spine for problems related to RA were reviewed. An upper-airway obstruction developed after extubation in 8 (14%) of the 58 patients who had been intubated without fiberoptic assistance compared with 1 (1%) of the 70 patients who had been intubated fiberoptically ($p = 0.02$).

Yonezawa T, Tsuji H, Matsui H, Hirano N: Subaxial lesions in rheumatoid arthritis: Radiographic factors suggestive of lower cervical myelopathy. *Spine* 1995;20:208–215.

Radiographic analysis on lateral views of the cervical spine and neurologic evaluation were carried out in 100 patients with RA. Radiographic parameters related to lower cervical myelopathy included marked destruction of spinous processes, axial shortening, and narrow spinal canal. Time-related deterioration of lower cervical myelopathy can be predicted by progressions of anterior slip, axial shortening, spinous process erosion, apophyseal joint erosion, and intervertebral disk collapse.

Zeidman SM, Ducker TB: Rheumatoid arthritis: Neuroanatomy, compression, and grading of deficits. *Spine* 1994;19:2259–2266.

The authors reviewed the relevant neuroanatomy, neurovascular anatomy, and neuropathologic lesions that interact in the rheumatoid spine. The minimum space available at the craniocervical junction for the neural structures is 13 to 14 mm, which is fairly constant. Below C2, the available space is only 12 mm. When the amount of space is reduced below this amount, there is, by definition, neural compression. The site of compression and/or repeated microcontusions will determine subsequent neurologic deficits.

Classic Bibliography

Clark CR, Goetz DD, Menezes AH: Arthrodesis of the cervical spine in rheumatoid arthritis. *J Bone Joint Surg* 1989;71A:381–392.

Collins DN, Barnes CL, FitzRandolph RL: Cervical spine instability in rheumatoid patients having total hip or knee arthroplasty. *Clin Orthop* 1991;272:127–135.

Conaty JP, Mongan ES: Cervical fusion in rheumatoid arthritis. *J Bone Joint Surg* 1981;63A:1218–1227.

Crockard HA, Calder I, Ransford AO: One-stage transoral decompression and posterior fixation in rheumatoid atlanto-axial subluxation. *J Bone Joint Surg* 1990;72B:682–685.

Dvorak J, Grob D, Baumgartner H, Gschwend N, Graver W, Larsson S: Functional evaluation of the spinal cord by magnetic resonance imaging in patients with rheumatoid arthritis and instability of upper cervical spine. *Spine* 1989;14:1057–1064.

Hensinger RN, De Vito PD, Ragsdale CG: Changes in the cervical spine in juvenile rheumatoid arthritis. *J Bone Joint Surg* 1986;68A:189–198.

Kraus DR, Peppelman WC, Agarwal AK, DeLeeuw HW, Donaldson WF III: Incidence of subaxial subluxation in patients with generalized rheumatoid arthritis who have had previous occipital cervical fusions. *Spine* 1991;16(suppl 10):S486–S489.

Lipson SJ: Cervical myelopathy and posterior atlanto-axial subluxation in patients with rheumatoid arthritis. *J Bone Joint Surg* 1985;67A:593–597.

Lipson SJ: Rheumatoid arthritis in the cervical spine. *Clin Orthop* 1989;239:121–127.

Mikulowski P, Wollheim FA, Rotmil P, Olsen I: Sudden death in rheumatoid arthritis with atlanto-axial dislocation. *Acta Med Scand* 1975;198:445–451.

Morizono Y, Sakou T, Kawaida H: Upper cervical involvement in rheumatoid arthritis. *Spine* 1987;12:721–725.

Pellicci PM, Ranawat CS, Tsairis P, Bryan WJ: A prospective study of the progression of rheumatoid arthritis of the cervical spine. *J Bone Joint Surg* 1981;63A:342–350.

Peppelman WC, Kraus DR, Donaldson WF III, Agarwal A: Cervical spine surgery in rheumatoid arthritis: Improvement of neurologic deficit after cervical spine fusion. *Spine* 1993;18:2375–2379.

Rana NA: Natural history of atlanto-axial subluxation in rheumatoid arthritis. *Spine* 1989;14:1054–1056.

Ranawat CS, O'Leary P, Pellicci P, Tsairis P, Marchisello P, Dorr L: Cervical spine fusion in rheumatoid arthritis. *J Bone Joint Surg* 1979;61A:1003–1010.

Santavirta S, Slatis P, Kankaanpaa U, Sandelin J, Laasonen E: Treatment of the cervical spine in rheumatoid arthritis *J Bone Joint Surg* 1988;70A:658–667.

Weissman BN, Aliabadi P, Weinfeld MS, Thomas WH, Sosman JL: Prognostic features of atlantoaxial subluxation in rheumatoid arthritis patients. *Radiology* 1982;144:745–751.

Zoma A, Sturrock RD, Fisher WD, Freeman PA, Hamblen DL: Surgical stabilisation of the rheumatoid cervical spine: A review of indications and results. *J Bone Joint Surg* 1987;69B:8–12.

Chapter 57
Spine Instrumentation

Cervical Spine Instrumentaion

The goals of cervical spine instrumentation are stabilization of the intended motion segments, protection of neural elements, maintenance of normal alignment of the spine, and most importantly, augmentation of the process of fusion. To this end, cervical instrumentation devices should be reasonably safe to apply and efficacious in meeting these goals.

Posterior Cervical Fixation

Posterior cervical wiring, either interspinous or sublaminar, remains the standard to which other posterior spinal fixation is compared. Rogers interspinous wiring is the least techni-cally demanding form of fixation for cervical instability. Multistrand stainless steel and titanium cables are superior to monofilament stainless steel wires in biomechanical strength and in the ability to better conform to the contour of the lamina or spinous process. Sublaminar cables or wires used at the C1-C2 level with Gallie or Brooks-Jenkins wiring techniques (Figs. 1 and 2) have good clinical results. Unfortunately, sublaminar cables and wires carry a risk of potential spinal cord injury resulting from the passage of the implants, as well as late breakage of the wire or cable. The limitation of posterior wiring is deficiency in the posterior elements as in the case of trauma, tumor, postlaminectomy, or congenital anomaly.

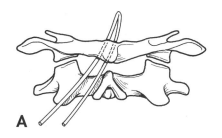 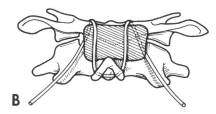 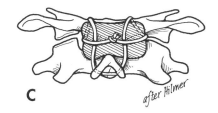

Figure 1

A modified Gallie H graft from the iliac crest over the posterior arches of C1 and C2. A, A doubled, U-shaped, 18- or 20-gauge wire is passed under the arch of C1 from inferior to superior. B, A bone block is taken from the posterior iliac crest and shaped to fit between C1 and C2 and the wires. C, The loop of the wire goes over the bone block and the spinous process of C2, and the ends of the wire are tightened around the graft between C1 and C2. (Reproduced with permission from An HS: Internal fixation of the cervical spine: Current indications and techniques. *J Am Acad Orthop Surg* 1995;3:194–206.)

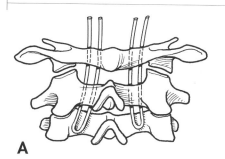 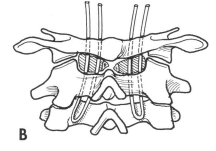 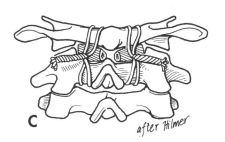

Figure 2

The Brooks-type fusion. A, Doubled, twisted 24-gauge wires are passed under the arch of C1 and then under the lamina of C2. B, Rectangular iliac-crest bone grafts (1.25 cm x 3.5 cm) are harvested and beveled to fit in the space between the arch of C1 and each lamina of the axis. C, The wires are then tightened, securing the graft. (Reproduced with permission from An HS: Internal fixation of the cervical spine: Current indications and techniques. *J Am Acad Orthop Surg* 1995;3:194–206.)

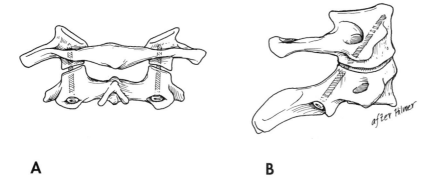

Figure 3

Magerl's technique of C1-C2 screw fixation. A, The screws are inserted by entering C2 at the inferior aspect and exiting at the posterior aspect of the upper articular process. B, The screws are placed through the facet joints into the lateral masses of C1. (Reproduced with permission from An HS: Internal fixation of the cervical spine: Current indications and techniques. *J Am Acad Orthop Surg* 1995;3:194–206.)

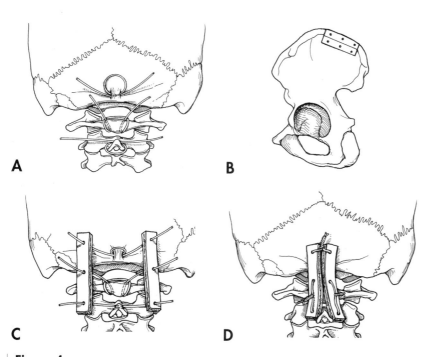

Figure 4

Werthreim and Bohlman's method of occipitocervical fusion. A, A wire is looped around the external occipital protuberance at a level 2 cm above the foramen magnum. A towel clip is then used to create a hole in the ridge, and an 18-gauge wire is passed through the hole and twisted over the ridge. A second wire loop is passed around the arch of C1 and a third is passed through and around the base of the spinous process of C2. B, The outer iliac crest is used for bone grafts. C, Drill holes are made in the bone grafts, and wires are passed through the holes. D, The wires are tightened. (Reproduced with permission from An HS: Internal fixation of the cervical spine: Current indications and techniques. *J Am Acad Orthop Surg* 1995;3:194–206.)

Transarticular Screws At the C1-C2 level, Gallie wiring was initially described as an adjunct to atlantoaxial transarticular screws; however, biomechanical and clinical studies found the wiring to add little to the overall outcome. In normal or deficient C1 or C2 posterior elements, "stand-alone" C1-C2 transarticular screws can be used (Fig. 3). When "stand-alone" screws are used, it is important to decorticate and bone graft the C1-C2 articular facets. This requires good bilateral exposure of the facet complex, which should be exposed routinely, as well as exposure of the medial border of the C2 pedicle to safely place transarticular screws. Safe placement of atlantoaxial transarticular screws also requires a clear understanding of the unique upper cervical anatomy. Some C2 pedicles cannot accommodate safe passage of a screw because of a small pedicular diameter, lack of a pedicular "medullary canal," or a vertebral artery that courses too superiorly or medially or fills the entire lateral mass. It is, therefore, mandatory that a high quality computed tomography (CT) scan of the upper cervical spine be closely scrutinized before placement of C1-C2 transarticular screws. If deficient posterior elements or anatomy precludes placement of posterior transarticular screws, C1-C2 stabilization can be gained with either (1) bilateral transarticular screws placed through lateral C1-C2 exposure, (2) occipitocervical fusion, or (3) fusion and halo immobilization.

Occipitocervical Fusion Occipitocervical fusion is rarely indicated, but when it is necessary, several techniques can provide rigid internal fixation and avoid the need for halo immobilization. The use of occipital burr holes, the passage of wires or cables between the tables of the cranium, and tightening of the cables over a bone graft (Fig. 4) or a U-shaped rod contoured to the occipitocervical junction provide adequate fixation. Unfortunately, these techniques are not rigid and sometimes require extension of fusion down to the C4 or C5 level to stabilize the upper cervical spine. More rigid fixation can be obtained with lateral mass plates and screws; with this technique only the levels intended to be fused, occiput to C2, and occasionally to C3, are instrumented (Fig. 5). Pedicle screws can be used in C2, thus gaining optimal bone purchase, and, if necessary, C1-C2 transarticular screws can be placed while incorporating the lateral mass plate. Each lateral mass plate is fixed to the cranium with 3 occipital screws placed in a paramedian position at or below the level of the superior nuchal line (SNL). Screws 8 mm long provide the best purchase of the occiput with the least chance of injury to the dura or venous sinuses. Screws at the level of the SNL can be safely placed 2 cm lateral to the midline, whereas when screws are 1 cm below the SNL, the safe zone is 1 cm lateral to the midline, and when 2 cm below the SNL, the safe zone is 0.5 cm from the midline. Complications with occipitocervical plating have been relatively few and usually are associated with hardware failure in the area of the cervical lateral masses.

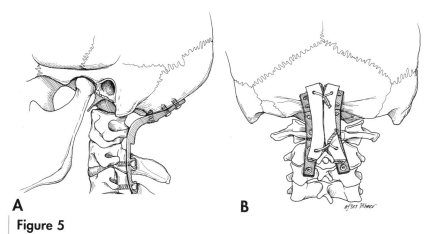

Figure 5

Roy-Camille technique of occipitocervical fixation. Lateral (A) and posterior (B) views illustrate contoured plate-and-screw fixation. (Reproduced with permission from An HS: Internal fixation of the cervical spine: Current indications and techniques. *J Am Acad Orthop Surg* 1995;3:194–206.)

Lateral Mass Plates Lateral mass plates also provide rigid internal immobilization when posterior elements are deficient in the cervical spine, whether due to fracture, previous surgery, or tumor, or when multilevel fixation is needed (Fig. 6). Vertebral artery injury resulting from screw placement is a rare clinical problem, but concern continues over the potential for nerve root injury when this technique is used with bicortical purchase of the lateral mass. Unicortical purchase of the lateral mass removes the concern of nerve root injury while sacrificing only 28% of the screw's pullout strength. The most frequent complication of posterior cervical plating is screw backout or breakage. This problem is most common at the upper and lower extremes of multilevel constructs and with unicortical purchase. Use of a rod and unicortical screw construct instead of a lateral mass plate and bicortical screw construct biomechanically increases the flexural stiffness of the fixation; however, screws still tend to fail at the extremes of the rod/screw construct. Cervical pedicle screws are recommended when C2 or C7 are incorporated, and this is most important when multiple levels are being instrumented. Otherwise, at the extreme ends of a lateral mass plate construct, bicortical purchase will gain more secure purchase of the bone, outweighing the potential risk of nerve root injury.

Cervical pedicle screw fixation has been used to treat traumatic spondylolisthesis of C2 (hangman's fracture) associated with C2-C3 dislocation. A pedicle lag screw technique can rigidly fix the fracture and avoid the need for halo immobilization. Pedicle screw fixation for lower cervical spine (C3 to C6) lateral mass fractures has been successful, but the technique is demanding, and more often than not the pedicle anatomy precludes successful placement of a screw without neurovascular injury. In anatomic studies, the lower cervical pedicles have been found to have marked variability in dimensions and projections, making screw insertion risky. Although lower cervical pedicle screw fixation is biomechanically stronger than lateral mass fixation, the technique needs to be refined before widespread use can be recommended.

Anterior Cervical Fixation

Anterior cervical plate fixation is being used more frequently (Fig. 7). Plates that allow for the placement of interlocking convergent screws gain an increased geometric purchase of the spine. These convergent-locking screws do not require bicortical purchase of the vertebral body and thus decrease or eliminate the risk of spinal cord injury. Data from biomechanical studies suggest that bicortical purchase of the vertebral body is superior to the locking plate in extension only. Because of the ease in application of these locking plates as well as the decreased risk to neurologic structures, the plates are being used for indications that have not been well substantiated. Single and 2-level anterior cervical interbody fusions for degenerative disease have established fusion rates of 85% to 95%, and no data from randomized, prospective studies have demonstrated any increase in fusion rates of 1- or 2-level fusions using anterior cervical locking plates. Some

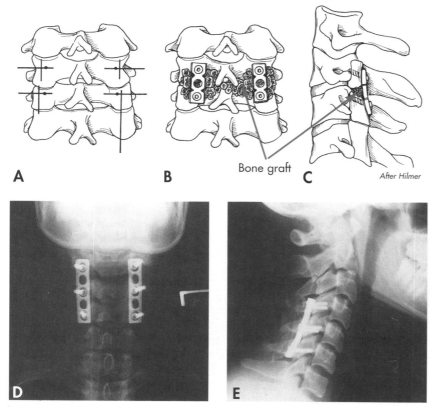

A   B   Bone graft   C   After Hilmer

D   E

Figure 6

Posterior plate-screw fixation of the cervical spine. A, The ideal drilling technique for safety of the nerve root. The starting point is 1 mm medial to the center of the lateral mass. The drill is directed 25° to 30° laterally and 15° cranially. B, Plate-screw fixation on the lateral masses of the cervical spine with bone grafts between the facet joints. C, The plates should be slightly contoured to cervical lordosis. D and E, Radiographs of a patient who underwent C4-C6 plate-screw fixation for fracture-dislocation. Anteroposterior D and lateral E views show anatomic reduction and proper screw placement and bone grafts posteriorly. (Reproduced with permission from An HS: Internal fixation of the cervical spine: Current indications and techniques. *J Am Acad Orthop Surg* 1995;3:194–206.)

Thoracolumbar Instrumentation

Thoracolumbar spinal instrumentation was originally developed and used for correction of spinal deformity. The initial instrumentation was developed by Paul Harrington and used 2 hooks on a single rod (nonsegmental system). The hooks acted as a temporary reduction system to hold the spine in the corrected position while the bony fusion occurred. Indications for use of the Harrington rod and hook system were quickly expanded to trauma and tumor surgery and to lumbar fusion surgery. Spinal instrumentation currently is used to reduce the deformity resulting from scoliosis, spondylolisthesis, and kyphosis while maintaining the spine in the corrected position during healing of the fusion and to increase the chance of successful fusion. Segmental instrumentation with multiple attachment points to the vertebrae along the same rod is preferred over nonsegmental instrumentation, which has attachments only to the upper and lower ends of the rod. Segmental instrumentation provides greater corrective capability and more stable constructs. The most rigid type of spinal constructs are achieved by a load-sharing mechanism.

The spinal implants bear most loads after posterior distraction instrumentation or anterior neutralization plating without adequate strut grafting. Anterior spinal instrumentation should always be accompanied by a load-bearing strut graft, and compression-loading on the graft further improves the stability. In some significant instabilities, anterior load-sharing graft can be combined with posterior instrumentation applied in compression, which acts as a tension band posteriorly. This construct is biomechanically superior, but it requires reconstruction of both anterior and posterior spinal columns. The choice of procedure depends on the clinical situation, the degree of instability, and the surgeon's familiarity with the techniques.

Posterior Thoracolumbar Instrumentation

Examples of nonsegmental posterior thoracolumbar hook and rod instrumentation include the Harrington rod and

authors advocate the use of plates to eliminate the use of postoperative orthoses and to speed recovery. Some recent devices offer compression or dynamic capabilities to provide a more load-sharing construct, but more clinical studies are needed.

Anterior screw placement in the odontoid for treatment of type II fractures remains technically demanding and should be left in the hands of surgeons familiar with this technique. Currently, use of a single screw to fix the odontoid fracture has clinical results similar to the use of 2 screws. The use of a double-threaded compression screw instead of a lag screw yields good clinical results.

At the time of this writing, bone screws into the vertebral body anteriorly have been fully approved by the United States Food and Drug Administration (FDA).

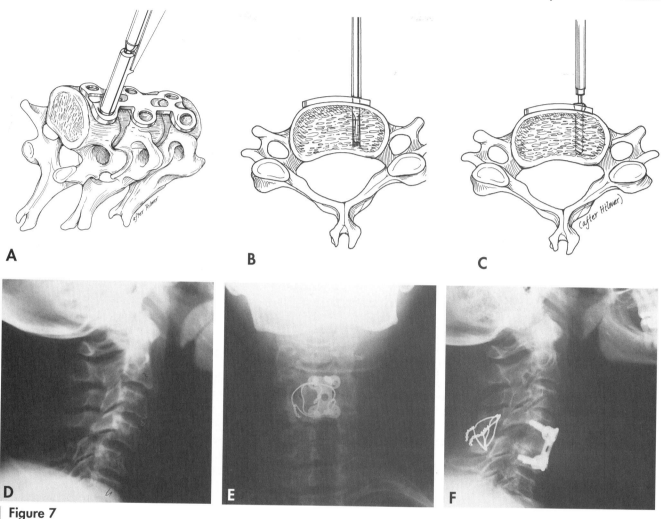

Figure 7

AO-Morscher titanium cervical plating. A, Plate of appropriate size is centered over the vertebral body. B, Drilling and tapping is done down to 16 mm. C, Screw is inserted, followed by expansion screw. D through F, Images of fracture-dislocation at C4-C5 in a quadriplegic patient. D, Lateral view was obtained before surgical treatment. Anteroposterior (E) and lateral (F) views obtained after anterior decompression, grafting, and AO-Morscher plating and posterior wiring at C4-C5 show anatomic reduction. (Posterior triple wiring was performed because the construct was unstable even after anterior plating.) (Reproduced with permission from An HS: Internal fixation of the cervical spine: Current indications and techniques. *J Am Acad Orthop Surg* 1995;3:194–206.)

Knodt rod. These instrumentation systems have little indication for use today. The Harrington instrumentation used in scoliosis provided distraction across the concavity of the curvature and elongated the spine, thereby correcting the deformity. However, when distraction was placed across the lumbar spine, it created a flat back posture and loss of a normal lumbar lordotic alignment. The 2-hook system was further advanced by using ratchet rods and sleeves to provide an anterior force on the posterior elements of the spine, thereby increasing lordosis while distracting across the spinal segment. This construct works well in lumbar burst fractures, reducing the retropulsed bony fragment and providing stability across the injured segment. Compression 2-hook constructs (nonsegmental) are indicated for distraction injuries, such as Chance fractures, or they can be placed posteriorly when there is a preemptive reconstruction of the anterior and middle columns with strut grafting.

Over the last 12 to 15 years, segmental instrumentation has been developed, first by Luque in Mexico, using multiple sublaminar wire attachments to a single rod, and then by Cotrel and Dubousset in France, using multiple hook attachments along the same rod. At present, hooks, wires, and screws are attached along the same rod for segmental distraction and compression. This type of segmental instrumentation is used for scoliotic and traumatic deformities of the lumbar spine. It is more common to use pedicle screw fixation in the lumbar spine for both degenerative disorders and deformities. Evidence that pedicle screws fail without adequate anterior column support when used for fixation of spinal fractures has decreased the use of isolated posterior short-segment pedicle instrumentation when anterior and middle column support is lost.

Biomechanical testing has demonstrated that different spinal instrumentation systems provide varying stiffness of spinal constructs. Constrained systems have a rigid link between the longitudinal member (plate or rod) and the attachment to the spine (screw or hook). Nonconstrained systems allow some motion between the longitudinal member and the attachment. Nonconstrained systems take longer to fatigue and fail because of loosening rather than by breakage of 1 of the individual members.

Hooks can be attached to the spine under or over the lamina (sub- or supralaminar, respectively), to the pedicle in the upper and mid thoracic spine, or over the transverse process in the thoracic spine in an up or downgoing fashion (Fig. 8). Pedicle screws have been placed in the lumbar spine. Pedicle screw fixation is generally more rigid than either hook or wire systems, allowing simultaneous control of all 3 columns of the spine from a posteriorly placed instrumentation member (Fig. 9). Pedicle screws have been used for the reduction and stabilization of spondylolisthesis in the lumbar spine, stabilization of motion segments in the lumbar and thoracic spine, the correction of degenerative scoliosis, and the stabilization of spinal fractures. Pedicle screw fixation is more risky and less frequently used in the thoracic spine than in the lumbar spine. Fusion rates using pedicle screw fixation are better than noninstrumented fusions.

The advantages of pedicle screw fixation are accompanied by a potential higher complication rate as well as increased operating time and blood loss. Potential complications are dural lacerations, nerve root injury, spinal cord injury, vascular damage, visceral injury, and pedicle fracture. Pedicle instrumentation has been used for spondylolisthesis, both isthmic and degenerative, reduction and fusion of lumbar scoliosis, pseudarthrosis repair, reconstruction after tumor resection, certain lumbar burst fractures, and other degenerative conditions of the lumbar spine necessitating spinal fusion. The FDA initially approved pedicle screw instrumentation only for high grade (≥ class 3) spondylolisthesis; however, it has reclassified the pedicle screws as class II devices in August 1998.

Anterior Thoracolumbar Instrumentation

Anterior thoracolumbar instrumentation was first used for correction of thoracolumbar scoliosis. This technique involved placing screws on the convexity of scoliotic curvature, performing aggressive diskectomies and annulectomies, and compressing and derotating vertebrae around the apex of the curve to correct the thoracolumbar scoliosis and save a distal level of fusion. Earlier systems consisted of a cable or threaded rod and had a higher rate of kyphosis and an increased pseudarthrosis rate than newer systems with lower profiles and solid rods. Great care must be taken to place structural graft anteriorly to impart a lordosis across the fused segment, because anterior instrumentation systems may produce kyphosis. A neutral or kyphotic sagittal alignment is a contraindication for this technique.

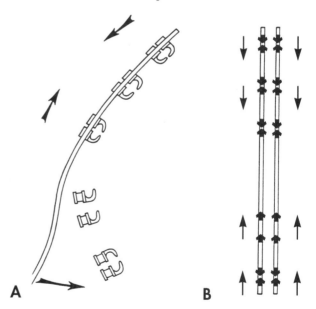

Figure 8

Posterior segmental instrumentation systems allow multiple hooks to be placed along the same rod in distraction or compression mode. The newest segmental systems allow greater corrective capabilities and increased fixation strength, thus obviating the need for excessive bracing or casting after surgery. Diagrams of posterior instrumentation for thoracic kyphosis. A, The proximal portion is cantilevered to the distal portion of the kyphus, shortening the posterior column. B, Each motion segment is compressed to further shorten the posterior column. The posterior instrumentation acts as a tension band. (Adapted with permission from An HS, Riley LH III (eds): *An Atlas of Surgery of the Spine.* London, England, Martin Dunitz, 1998, p 175.)

More recently, short-segment anterior instrumentation systems have been developed for the reconstruction of the thoracolumbar spine after trauma or tumor surgery (Fig. 10). After vertebral body resection and strut grafting, instrumentation with a rod or plate provides reduction of kyphosis, stability, and graft compression and containment. The load-sharing graft is critical for success of these anterior instrumentation systems. The graft should be sufficiently large, well placed, and loaded in compression as a load-sharing construct. The basic indications for use of anterior plate or rod reconstruction include a burst fracture after decompression with loss of the weightbearing column and reconstruction after a vertebral body resection for tumor.

These modern anterior devices, when mechanically tested, are as stable as posterior screw fixation 2 levels above and 2 levels below the injured segment. Improvements in anterior spinal instrumentation systems have resulted in better correction and maintenance, improved fusion rates, and avoidance of additional posterior procedures.

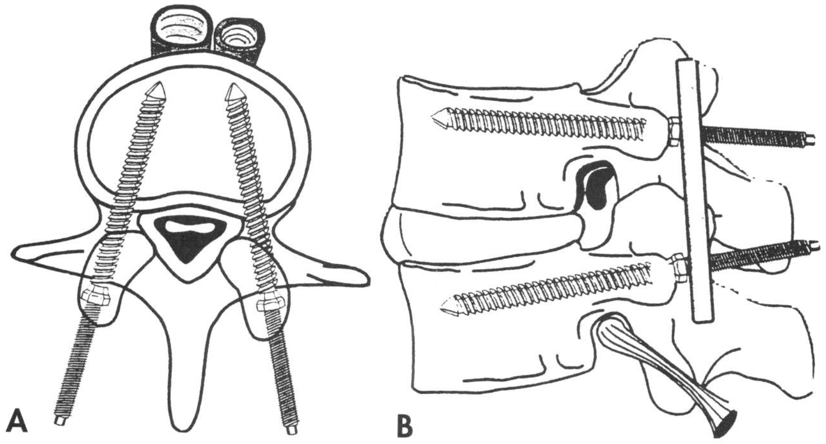

Intervertebral Fusion Cages

Hodgson first popularized the anterior approach and fusion to the thoracolumbar spine for tuberculosis in Hong Kong. Others further enhanced this technique in the lumbar spine. Lack of a strong interbody stabilization technique to be used in conjunction with lower lumbar interbody fusion has prevented the growth of this technique. The recent introduction of threaded fusion cages for intradiskal fusion of the lumbar spine has made anterior interbody fusion of the lumbar spine more popular (Fig. 11). Cages provide immediate stability in addition to disk space distraction. Testing of threaded lumbar cages has demonstrated increased stiffness in flexion and lateral bending. Additionally, pull-out strength of the threaded cages is superior to the strength needed to dislodge bone dowels or structural autograft or allograft. Stability provided by 2 cages is not significantly different than that provided by an anterior interbody fusion graft used in conjunction with posterior pedicle screw instrumentation. However, recent studies have shown that the constructs with threaded cages provide less stability in extension and in cyclic loading. Interbody cages can be placed anteriorly through a posterior lumbar interbody fusion (PLIF) technique. They also have been placed anteriorly laparoscopically or through an open minilaparotomy approach.

Figure 9

Pedicle screws can be placed segmentally in > 2 vertebrae (a form of segmental instrumentation). The screws are placed from posterior to anterior in the lumbar spine. (Reproduced with permission from Garfin SR, Vaccaro AR (eds): *Orthopaedic Knowledge Update: Spine.* Rosemont, IL, American Academy of Orthopaedic Surgeons, 1997, pp 55–61.)

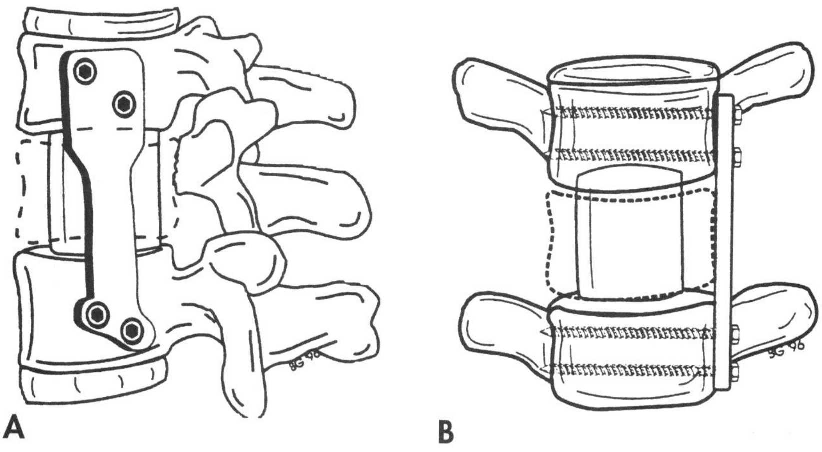

Figure 10

Anterolateral fixation of the thoracolumbar spine using a screw/bolt/plate fixation device. This device allows for graft stabilization and containment as well as compression through the graft or distraction across the bolts prior to placement of the graft and plate. (Reproduced with permission from Garfin SR, Vaccaro AR (eds): *Orthopaedic Knowledge Update: Spine.* Rosemont, IL, American Academy of Orthopaedic Surgeons, 1997, pp 55–61.)

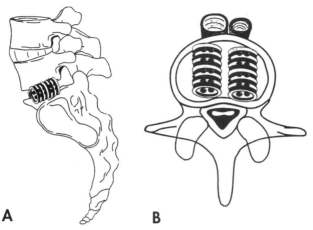

Figure 11

Various forms of intervertebral cages are being developed. The most popular cage at this point is a threaded titanium alloy. Multiple implants are available to maximize interspace distraction, bony contact, and fixation with disk space. These cages can be placed anteriorly or posteriorly, and are packed with cancellous autogenous graft prior to insertion. (Reproduced with permission from Garfin SR, Vaccaro AR (eds): *Orthopaedic Knowledge Update: Spine.* Rosemont, IL, American Academy of Orthopaedic Surgeons, 1997, pp 55–61.)

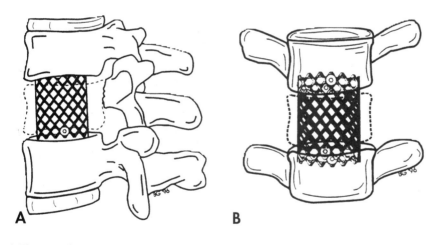

Figure 12

Following lumbar corpectomy, a cylindrical type titanium cage packed with bone graft can work to correct and prevent kyphosis and serve as an intervertebral spacer. In general, these cages necessitate load sharing with another form of fixation, either anterior or posterior instrumentation. (Reproduced with permission from Garfin SR, Vaccaro AR (eds): *Orthopaedic Knowledge Update: Spine.* Rosemont, IL, American Academy of Orthopaedic Surgeons, 1997, pp 55–61.)

placed into the cages before threading them into the interspace after preparation. Many of these devices are being placed for diskogenic low back pain, but this diagnosis must be carefully approached with regard to surgical care. The minimal indications for fusion for diskogenic low back pain are no psychosocial impediments, at least 6 months of active symptoms with failure of aggressive conservative management, and independent diskographic confirmation of pain provocation. An upright cage has been created to act as a vertebral body replacement in both the vertical and thoracolumbar spine (Fig. 12). The titanium mesh cylinders require load sharing with either an anterior plate or posterior instrumentation. These types of cages are also gaining increasing popularity when placed through a transforaminal approach for posterior interbody fusion. Although the field of spinal instrumentation is ever-evolving and new innovations are presented daily, the strict indications for surgery must not be changed or compromised. Surgeons also must realize that the operation is a fusion, and meticulous technique should be used in this regard.

Nonthreaded fusion cages have not been specifically cleared by the FDA for intraspinal implantation.

At the time of this writing, bone screws placed posteriorly into vertebral elements have been cleared for use in this specific manner by the Food and Drug Administration (FDA) to provide immobilization and stabilization as an adjunct to fusion in the treatment of the following acute and chronic instability or deformities of the thoracic, lumbar and sacral spine: degenerative spondylolisthesis with objective evidence of neurological impairment; fracture; dislocation; scoliosis; kyphosis; spinal tumor and failed previous fusion (pseudarthrosis). In addition, anterior vertebral body screws (cervical, thoracic, and lumbar) are Class II devices and can be used as labeled in vertebral bodies.

The cages create inherent stability by distraction in the interspace and tensioning of the soft tissues. They remain permanently stable once bone healing has occurred through fenestrations in the cages. Typically, cancellous autograft is

Annotated Bibliography

Cervical Spine Instrumentation

Ebraheim NA, Lu J, Biyani A, Brown JA, Yeasting RA: An anatomic study of the thickness of the occipital bone: Implications for occipitocervical instrumentation. *Spine* 1996;21: 1726–1729.

This anatomic study of cadaveric specimens establishes the appropriate areas for screw placement in the occiput.

Ebraheim N, Rollins JR Jr, Xu R, Jackson WT: Anatomic consideration of C2 pedicle screw placement. *Spine* 1996;21: 691–695.

Different techniques for placement of C2 pedicle screws are evaluated and the safest method is described.

Heller JG, Estes BT, Zaouali M, Diop A: Biomechanical study of screws in the lateral masses: Variables affecting pull-out resistance. *J Bone Joint Surg* 1996;78A:1315–1321.

This retrospective review of 78 patients who underwent posterior cervical plating describes complications involved with the technique and provides comprehensive comparison to previous studies reporting posterior cervical plating.

Heller JG, Silcox DH III, Sutterlin CE III: Complications of posterior cervical plating. *Spine* 1995;20:2442–2448.

The differences in pullout strength of unicortical versus bicortical purchase of lateral masses are demonstrated in this biomechanical cadaveric study.

Thoracolumbar Spine Instrumentation

Barr SJ, Schuette AM, Emans JB: Lumbar pedicle screws versus hooks: Results in double major curves in adolescent idiopathic scoliosis. *Spine* 1997;22:1369–1379.

Lumbar hooks (19 patients) were compared to a combination of hooks and lumbar pedicle screws (20 patients). No complications were associated with the placement of pedicle screws, and the lumbar pedicle screws appeared to offer greater lumbar curve correction, better maintenance of correction, and greater correction of the noninstrumented spine below the double major curves.

Hu SS, Bradford DS, Transfeldt EE, Cohen M: Reduction of high-grade spondylolisthesis using Edwards' instrumentation. *Spine* 1996;21:367–371.

Average slip in 16 patients improved from 89% preoperatively to 29% postoperatively. Slip angle improved from 50° to an average of 24°. Three patients (20%) suffered neurologic impairment, and 1 did not resolve; 4 patients (25%) had hardware failure. This series emphasizes the difficulty of this procedure with its inherently high complication rate when compared to fusing patients in situ without reduction.

Kaneda K, Taneichi H, Abumi K, Hashimoto T, Satoh S, Fujiya M: Anterior decompression and stabilization with the Kaneda device for thoracolumbar burst fractures associated with neurological deficits. *J Bone Joint Surg* 1997;79A:69–83.

At average follow-up of 8 years, 93% of 150 consecutive patients showed successful fusion, and all patients with a pseudarthrosis were successfully managed by posterior spinal fusion with instrumentation. Ninety-five percent of the patients improved at least 1 Frankel grade; 72% of 78 patients who were preoperatively paralyzed or had significant dysfunction of the bladder recovered completely.

Kleiner JB, Odom JA Jr, Moore MR, Wilson NA, Huffer WE: The effect of instrumentation on human spinal fusion mass. *Spine* 1995;20:90–97.

Fifty-six patients with instrumentation were compared to 12 patients who had noninstrumented fusions. Prior to reoperation, the patients had pulse dose labeling with fluorochrome. Duplicate biopsies of fusion mass and iliac crest were obtained and evaluated blindly for multiple factors. Material properties of fusion mass in instrumented spines were superior to those of noninstrumented fusion mass.

Lim TH, An HS, Hong JH, et al: Biomechanical evaluation of anterior and posterior fixations in an unstable calf spine mode. *Spine* 1997;22:261–266.

Modern anterior instrumentation systems, such as Kaneda rod and University plate, with load-sharing structural graft provided comparable stability to posterior transpedicular ISOLA rods with anterior grafting. Posterior ISOLA instrumentation alone without anterior grafting provided less rigid fixation in flexion and extension.

McLain RF, Sparling E, Benson DR: Early failure of short-segment pedicle instrumentation for thoracolumbar fractures: A preliminary report. *J Bone Joint Surg* 1993;75A:162–167.

The authors report a series of patients with lumbar burst fractures treated with short segment instrumentation. They noted a high rate of instrumentation failure when placing screws without anterior column support. All patients in the study were braced.

Ray CD: Threaded titanium cages for lumbar interbody fusions. *Spine* 1997;22:667–679.

This study presented data from the FDA multicenter investigation of the Ray threaded cage device. In 208 patients with a 2-year follow-up, the author found a 96% fusion rate with a functional outcome of 40% excellent, 25% good, 21% fair, and 14% poor results. Fewer than 1% of patients had reported complications.

Tencer AF, Hampton D, Eddy S: Biomechanical properties of threaded inserts for lumbar interbody spinal fusion. *Spine* 1995;20:2408–2414.

The authors studied the Ray threaded fusion cage in calf and human cadaveric spines to determine motion segment stiffness and laxity after implantation of the cage. They determined that the threaded cage significantly increased motion segment stiffness and decreased laxity through a distraction mechanism. They also found that this increase was not sensitive to the particular placement of the cage (front versus back of vertebral body).

Classic Bibliography

An HS, Gordin R, Renner K: Anatomic considerations for plate-screw fixation of the cervical spine. *Spine* 1991;16(suppl 10): S548–S551.

An HS, Vaccaro A, Cotler JM, Lin S: Low lumbar burst fractures: A comparison among body cast, Harrington rod, Luque rod, and Steffee plate. *Spine* 1991;16(suppl 8):S440–S444.

Anderson PA, Henley MB, Grady MS, Montesano PX, Winn HR: Posterior cervical arthrodesis with AO reconstruction plates and bone graft. *Spine* 1991;16(suppl 3):S72–S79.

Böhler J: Anterior stabilization for acute fractures and non-unions of the dens. *J Bone Joint Surg* 1982;64A:18–27.

Brooks AL, Jenkins EB: Atlanto-axial arthrodesis by the wedge compression method. *J Bone Joint Surg* 1978;60A:279–284.

Dickson JH, Harrington PR, Erwin WD: Results of reduction and stabilization of the severely fractured thoracic and lumbar spine. *J Bone Joint Surg* 1978;60A:799–805.

Ebraheim NA, An HS, Jackson WT, Brown JA: Internal fixation of the unstable cervical spine using posterior Roy-Camille plates: Preliminary report. *J Orthop Trauma* 1989;3:23–28.

Esses SI, Sachs BL, Dreyzin V: Complications associated with the technique of pedicle screw fixation: A selected survey of ABS members. *Spine* 1993;18:2231–2238.

Fielding JW, Hawkins RJ, Ratzan SA: Spine fusion for atlanto-axial instability. *J Bone Joint Surg* 1976;58A:400–407.

Grob D, Dvorak J, Panjabi M, Froehlich M, Hayak J: Posterior occipitocervical fusion: A preliminary report of a new technique. *Spine* 1991;16(suppl 3):S17–S24.

Hall JE: Dwyer instrumentation in anterior fusion of the spine. *J Bone Joint Surg* 1981;63A:1188–1190.

Hodgson AR, Stock FE: Anterior spinal fusion: A preliminary communication on the radical treatment of Pott's disease and Pott's paraplegia. *Br J Surg* 1956;44:266–275.

Magerl F, Seeman PS: Stable posterior fusion of the atlas and axis by transarticular screw fixation, in Kehr P, Weidner A (eds): *Cervical Spine.* New York, NY, Springer-Verlag, 1987, pp 322–327.

Panjabi MM: Biomechanical evaluation of spinal fixation devices: Part I. A conceptual framework. *Spine* 1988;13: 1129–1134.

Panjabi MM, Abumi K, Duranceau J, Crisco JJ: Biomechanical evaluation of spinal fixation devices: Part II. Stability provided by 8 internal fixation devices. *Spine* 1988;13:1135–1140.

Roy-Camille R, Saillant G, Berteaux D, Salgado V: Osteo-synthesis of thoraco-lumbar spine fractures with metal plates screwed through the vertebral pedicles. *Reconstr Surg Traumatol* 1976;15:2–16.

Savini R, Parisini P, Cevellati S: The surgical treatment of late instability of flexion-rotation injuries in the lower cervical spine. *Spine* 1987;12:178–182.

Smith MD, Anderson P, Grady MS: Occipitocervical arthrodesis using contoured plate fixation: An early report on versatile fixation technique. *Spine* 1993;18:1984–1990.

Wertheim SB, Bohlman HH: Occipitocervical fusion: Indications, technique, and long-term results in thirteen patients. *J Bone Joint Surg* 1987;69A:833–836.

Chapter 58
Minimally Invasive Techniques for Anterior Thoracic and Lumbar Spine Procedures

Introduction

Laparoscopy became popular in the late 1980s primarily as a result of the success of laparoscopic cholecystectomy. A vast improvement in return to work of 6.5 days after laparoscopy compared to 34 days after minilaparotomy for gallbladder disease was demonstrated in 1988. Within 3 years, 90% of cholecystectomies done in the United States used endoscopic techniques. In laparoscopy, rather than transecting abdominal musculature, narrow portals are created to access the peritoneal cavity for surgery. Consequently, postoperative pain and recovery time are reduced, leading to shortened hospital stays and earlier return to work compared to open surgery. As a direct result of the early success of laparoscopy,

the modern era of thoracoscopy or "video-assisted thoracic surgery"(VATS) began a few years later in 1990 with the addition of video to standard endoscopic techniques. In a study of patients undergoing lung biopsies, the thoracoscopic approach was associated with less pain, shorter hospital stay, decreased cost, and earlier return to work when compared to open biopsy through a thoracotomy. Anterior endoscopic spinal surgery was first described by Obenchain, who reported the first laparoscopic lumbar diskectomy. The application of thoracoscopy for diseases of the spine was initially reported by Mack and associates in 1993. More recently, several authors have reported preliminary results of laparoscopic fusion of the lumbar spine using a threaded fusion cage.

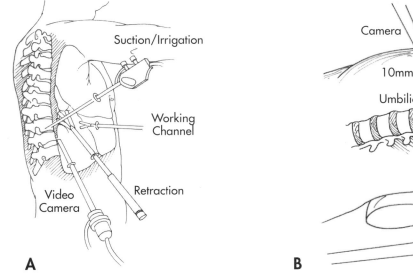

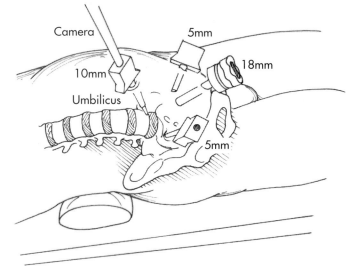

A   **B**

Figure 1

A, Instrument location for approach to T8-9 disk. Suction-irrigation and fan retractor are placed above and below working channel, which is in direct line with the disk space. A 30° angled camera is brought in from below in the midaxillary line. (Reproduced with permission from Regan JJ: Percutaneous endoscopic thoracic discectomy. *Neurosurg Clin North Am* 1996;7:87–98.)
B, Trocars are positioned at the periumbilical site for camera with two 5-mm trocars inserted lateral to the inferior epigastric arteries midway between umbilicus and pubis. An 18-mm trocar is placed above the pubis symphysis. The suprapubic trocar is placed collinear with respect to the disk to be fused. (Reproduced with permission from Regan JJ, McAfee PC, Guyer RD, Aronoff RJ: Laparoscopic fusion of the lumbar spine in a multicenter series of the first 34 consecutive patients. *Surg Laparosc Endosc* 1996;6:459–468.)

Video-Assisted Thoracic Spine Surgery

Modified long narrow instruments are passed through small skin incisions in the chest with viewing through a 10-mm diameter endoscope and high-resolution video imaging (Fig. 1). Endoscopic spinal intervention achieves the same goals as open surgery by lung deflation and optimal placement of trocar sites. The thoracic cavity allows a large working space without the need for CO_2 insufflation (Fig. 2). Potential advantages of thoracoscopy include improved view of the spine, decreased incisional pain, fewer pulmonary complications, early rehabilitation, improved cosmesis, and decreased overall cost. Possible disadvantages include the learning curve, the need for an additional surgeon, requirement of 1-lung ventilation, and difficulty of anterior endoscopic spinal fixation. Procedures that can be done with the anterior endoscopic approach include, in order of increasing difficulty, incisional biopsy, anterior release and fusion for rigid kyphosis or scoliosis, thoracoplasty, thoracic diskectomy, and corpectomy. Endoscopic anterior instrumentation of the thoracic spine after corpectomy and for deformity has been described. However, the problems of endoscopic distraction, compression, and rod rotation are not yet solved.

Preliminary results in the treatment of spinal deformity indicate that thoracoscopy is a safe and effective alternative to open thoracotomy for the treatment of certain types of pediatric and adolescent spinal deformity. Curve correction was similar between thoracoscopic and open methods. The blood loss and complication rates also were similar between the groups. However, the length of hospital stay was not reduced, and the cost of the procedure was higher for the thoracoscopy group.

Thoracoscopic techniques have been used successfully in the surgical treatment of clinically significant disk herniation from T1-2 to T12-L1 (Fig. 3). This approach allows excellent visualization of the anterior thoracic spine, which permits safe decompression of central and paracentral disk herniations. Calcified disks and large osteophytes located behind the vertebral body also can be removed once experience is gained with this technique. There is minimal resection of bone, which minimizes the likelihood of destabilization. A rib graft can be harvested using a coarse diamond-tipped burr if anterior strut graft fusion is necessary. Thoracolumbar disk herniations can be approached without taking down the diaphragm by using a fan retractor to gently depress the diaphragm and reflecting the diaphragmatic insertion on the L1 transverse process.

Thoracic vertebrectomy and reconstruction using a microsurgical endoscope have been described for the treatment of osteomyelitis, tumors, and compression fractures. This technique achieves the same amount of spinal dissection and decompression as open spinal procedures, with better visualization of the exposed dura by using the 30° angle endoscope. Thoracoscopic vertebrectomy at T3 and T4 avoids the morbidity of the transclavicular approach or high thoracotomy, which requires transection of the rhomboid muscles and mobilization of the scapula.

In a report of the first 100 anterior endoscopic spinal procedures, the most common complications of VATS spinal procedures were transient intercostal neuralgia and atelectasis. The incidence of intercostal neuralgia has been reduced by using flexible trocars.

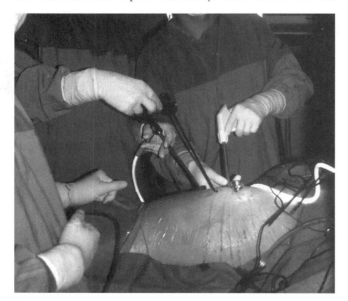

Figure 2

Surgeons maneuvering thoracoscopic instruments during video-assisted thoracic spine surgery (VATS).

Instrumented Laparoscopic Fusion of the Spine

Although the laparoscopic approach to the lumbar spine was initially described by Obenchain for the treatment of lumbar disk herniation, more enthusiasm has been generated in regard to laparoscopic anterior interbody fusion of the lumbar spine. The laparoscopic fusion procedure using the BAK (Spinetech, Inc, Minneapolis, MN) threaded interbody fusion device has recently been approved by the United States Food and Drug Administration (FDA). Patients are selected based on indications similar to those used for open techniques for lumbar interbody fusion at L4-5 and L5-S1. The primary indication for the procedure is painful disk degeneration with neuroforaminal narrowing and radiculopathy. Patients with grade I spondylolisthesis may also be considered for this procedure. The easiest level at which to access pathology through the laparoscope is L5-S1 because the bifurcation of the aorta and vena cava occurs above this disk space. The L4-5 disk can be exposed laparoscopically, but it is more difficult because of the vascular mobilization required. Most often, the left iliac artery and vein must be retracted to the right to place interbody fusion cages. Preoperative magnetic resonance imaging (MRI) is helpful in determining the level of arterial and venous bifurcation. Laparoscopic access to disks above the L4-5 level is difficult because of viscera and vascular structures, such as the inferior mesenteric artery and renal vessels. Contraindications to laparoscopy include morbid obesity, extensive peritoneal adhesions, active neoplasm or infection of the peritoneal cavity, and medical illness that would preclude surgery.

Surgical Technique

It is essential for the spine surgeon to work with a laparoscopic surgeon throughout the procedure to ensure a successful outcome. The patient is placed on a radiolucent operating table with the arms draped by the side and a roll placed under the lumbar spine to accentuate the lumbar lordosis. The table is subsequently tipped into a steep Trendelenburg position. This allows gravity to move the intestines superiorly out of the pelvis. The peritoneal cavity can be exposed using CO_2 insufflation. Four small trocar incisions are used to expose the surgical field and place instruments. The endoscope is placed through a 10-mm periumbilical trocar, two 5-mm portals are placed on either side of midline for retraction, and an 18-mm trocar is placed above the pubis to act as the delivery system for the fusion cages (Fig. 1, B). Autologous bone graft for the fusion can be harvested from the anterior iliac crest at the beginning of the procedure.

Results

Although the procedure is associated with a steep learning curve, once mastered, the technique is effective and advantageous over current approaches to lumbar fusion (Table 1).

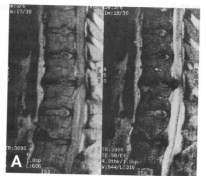
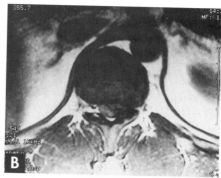
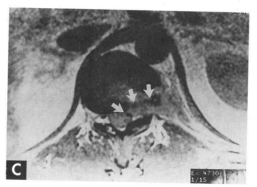
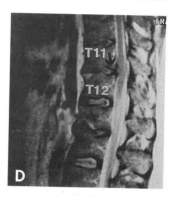

Figure 3

A 38-year-old man presented with temporary paraparesis following a waterskiing accident. Paresis partially resolved on corticosteroids but left-sided weakness, lower extremity clonus, and left thoracic radiculopathy persisted. Preoperative sagittal (A) and axial (B) magnetic resonance imaging scans demonstrate left paracentral disk herniation with free fragment at T11-12 deforming the spinal cord. Postoperative axial (C) and sagittal (D) images demonstrate successful removal of herniation and decompression of spinal cord (arrows) with minimal resection of normal disk and adjacent vertebra.

Time in surgery and hospital stay have decreased with experience, and the procedure has been demonstrated to be as safe as open anterior techniques in a large prospective multicenter trial. The rehabilitative aspects of this procedure appear to be a great improvement over traditional fusion approaches. The 10% conversion rate to open procedures, which occurs with laparoscopic fusion, is similar to conversion rates for other laparoscopic procedures. Most often this is a result of bowel adhesions, bleeding, and difficulty with access related to inexperience. The incidence of vascular injury is less than 2% in both open and laparoscopic anterior approaches, with no reports of transfusions required in the laparoscopic group. The incidence of retrograde ejaculation and intraoperative disk herniation requiring reoperation were slightly higher in the early laparoscopic series compared to open anterior fusion. However, changes in technique, most notably the elimination of monopolar cautery and the addition of endoscopic pituitary rongeurs to the instrument set, have resulted in a decline of these complications to the 1% range seen in open retroperitoneal anterior surgery.

The recent FDA approval of threaded fusion cages has stimulated interest in the open minilaparoscopy approach. A paramedian incision between 8 and 14 cm is made depending on patient size, and retroperitoneal access to the spine is gained after mobilizing the rectus abdominus. This approach has a lower incidence of retrograde ejaculation compared to transperitoneal approaches. Preliminary data suggest that experienced surgical teams devoted to the laparoscopic procedure have results similar to those of minilaparoscopy when threaded fusion cages are inserted at L5-S1. Early trends suggest a reduced length of hospitalization and a faster return to work for laparoscopic procedures.

Balloon-Assisted Endoscopic Retroperitoneal Approach to the Lumbar Spine

Laparoscopic retroperitoneal approaches to the lumbar spine have recently been described for excision of herniated disks and debridement of disk space infection from L1-2 to L4-5 (Fig. 4). This approach, initially described for laparoscopic nephrectomy, holds promise for future applications of laparoscopic approaches to the lumbar spine from L1 to L5 for anterior release, diskectomy, and lateral fusion cage insertion. The optical trocar is a recently available technology that

Table 1

Comparison of laparoscopic anterior lumbar interbody fusion with pedicle screw fixation

	Laparoscopic BAK Device (N = 13)	Pedicle Screws With PLIF (N = 11)	Pedicle Screws Without PLIF (N = 15)
Mean average operating time (hr)	2.2*	3.5	2.9
Blood loss (cc)	162*	675	408
Average hospital stay (days)	1.8*	5.1	5.0
Fusion rate	13/13	10/11	12/15
% returning to work	96*	73	76
Mean time to return to work (weeks)	11.1*	23.1	31.4

*Statistically significant results; PLIF = posterior lumbar interbody fusion.

(Reproduced with permission from Dickman CA, Sonntag VK, Russell JC: Laparoscopic approach for instrumentation and fusion of the lumbar spine. *Barrow Neurol Inst Quer* 1997;13:26–36.)

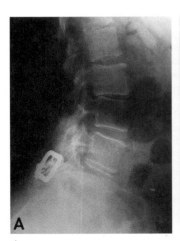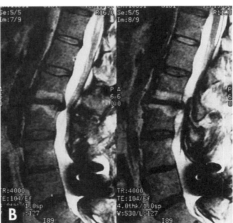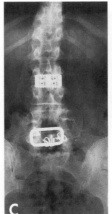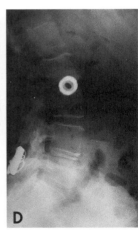

Figure 4

A 49-year-old woman with a history of L5-S1 fusion presents with mechanical back pain and left anterior thigh pain. A, Lateral radiograph demonstrates severe disk space narrowing at L2-3. B, Lateral magnetic resonance imaging scan demonstrates severe disk space narrowing with posterior disk herniation at L2-3. Modic I changes are noted in the bony end plates. C and D, AP and lateral radiographs demonstrate single 19 x 36 mm threaded fusion cage in position at L2-3. Procedure was accomplished endoscopically through a retroperitoneal approach. Disk herniation was removed through the anterior approach. Note the significant distraction of the disk space. Patient remains asymptomatic 6 months following surgery.

allows endoscopic visualization through a blunt-tipped trocar with a deployable cutting element used to dissect through the layers of the abdominal wall. Reports indicate its usefulness in providing endoscopic access to the retroperitonium. Used in combination with ballon insufflation of the retroperitonium, this approach may prove to be easier and safer than the transperitoneal approach to L4-5 and above. Laterally placed fusion cages are currently being evaluated to determine if endoscopic retroperitoneal insertion from a lateral position will provide sufficient stability for fusion to take place.

Conclusion

Minimally invasive techniques for exposing the anterior thoracic and lumbar spine show promise in reducing approach-related trauma. However, a significant learning curve is required to master these techniques. The surgical team should consist of a spinal surgeon and a thoracoscopic or laparoscopic surgeon with experience in advanced laparoscopic procedures. Complications in thoracoscopy are fewer than in thoracotomy with respect to pulmonary and post-thoracotomy syndrome. Procedures involving the spinal canal, such as thoracic diskectomy, should be approached with caution and only after experience has been gained with in vivo models, instructional courses, and clinical training. Complications of anterior lumbar spine surgery are similar for open and laparoscopic procedures with respect to vascular and neurologic injury. Laparoscopic approaches to L5-S1 have the potential for causing retrograde ejaculation in male patients.

At the time of this writing, bone screws placed posteriorly into vertebral elements have been cleared for use in this specific manner by the Food and Drug Administration (FDA) to provide immobilization and stabilization as an adjunct to fusion in the treatment of the following acute and chronic instability or deformities of the thoracic, lumbar and sacral spine: degenerative spondylolisthesis with objective evidence of neurological impairment; fracture; dislocation; scoliosis; kyphosis; spinal tumor and failed previous fusion (pseudoarthrosis). In addition, anterior vertebral body screws (cervical, thoracic, and lumbar) are Class II devices and can be used as labeled in vertebral bodies.

Annotated Bibliography

Video-Assisted Thoracic Spine Surgery

Mack MJ, Regan JJ, Bobechko WP, Acuff TE: Application of thoracoscopy for diseases of the spine. *Ann Thorac Surg* 1993; 56:736–738.

This is the first technical description of thoracoscopy in approaches to the thoracic spine for spinal abscess, herniated disk, and anterior releases for kyphoscoliosis.

McAfee PC, Regan JJ, Fedder IL, Mack MJ, Geis WP: Anterior thoracic corpectomy for spinal cord decompression performed endoscopically. *Surg Laparosc Endosc* 1995;5:339–348.

Anterior decompression using VATS and retroperitoneal approach was successful in 15 cases (8 tumors, 5 fractures, 2 infections). Mean hospitalization was 6.5 days. Ability to visualize the anterior surface of the dura was improved with a 30° angled endoscope.

Newton PO, Wenger DR, Mubarak SJ, Meyer RS: Anterior release and fusion in pediatric spinal deformity: A comparison of early outcome and cost of thoracoscopic and open thoracotomy approaches. *Spine* 1997;22:1398–1406.

The percent curve correction was similar between thoracoscopic and open methods; scoliosis 56% and 6%, respectively; kyphosis 88% and 94%, respectively. The blood loss and complications are similar in both groups. Length of hospitalization was not reduced and the cost of the open procedure is 29% less than that of the thoracoscopic approach.

Regan JJ, Ben-Yishay A, Mack MJ: Video-assisted thoracoscopic excision of herniated thoracic disc: description of technique and preliminary experience in the first 29 cases. *J Spinal Disord* 1998;11:173–191.

At 12- to 24-month follow-up, 75.8% of patients had satisfactory outcomes with relief of myelopathic and radicular symptoms. The postoperative complication rate was 13.8%; complications included excessive bleeding, atelectasis, pleural effusion, and diaphragm puncture. This procedure resulted in decreased hospitalization time, less use of postoperative narcotics, and early recovery.

Regan JJ, Mack MJ, Picetti GD III: A technical report on video-assisted thoracoscopy in thoracic spinal surgery: Preliminary description. *Spine* 1995;20:831–837.

This is a preliminary description of VATS in thoracic spinal surgery. Twelve procedures performed on patients with various pathology resulted in little postoperative pain, short intensive care unit and hospital stay, and little morbidity. No postthoracotomy pain or neurologic sequalae are reported.

Regan JJ, McAfee PC, Mack MJ (eds): *Atlas of Endoscopic Spine Surgery.* St. Louis, MO, Quality Medical Publishing, 1995.

This first comprehensive, illustrated atlas of endoscopic spinal techniques includes instrumentation, approach strategies, and step-by-step illustration of procedures.

Rosenthal D, Marquardt G, Lorenz R, Nichtweiss M: Anterior decompression and stabilization using a microsurgical endoscopic technique for metastatic tumors of the thoracic spine. *J Neurosurg* 1996;84:565–572.

The authors describe a technique for endoscopic vertebrectomy and reconstruction using a Z-plate for metastatic disease. Early results indicate adequate decompression, stabilization, and reduction of surgical morbidity can be achieved with the technique.

Laparoscopic Fusion of the Lumbar Spine

Mahvi DM, Zdeblick TA: A prospective study of laparoscopic spinal fusion: Technique and operative complications. *Ann Surg* 1996;224:85–90.

Twenty consecutive patients underwent laparoscopic anterior lumbar instrumentation using threaded cages and instruments designed for laparoscopic insertion. Three technical complications occurred in the first 4 cases requiring conversion to open surgery. The remaining 16 cases were successfully treated laparoscopically. Mean hospital stay was 1.7 days with 12 patients returning to work between 3 and 8 weeks.

McAfee PC, Regan JR, Zdeblick T, et al: The incidence of complications in endoscopic anterior thoracolumbar spinal reconstructive surgery: A prospective multicenter study comprising the first 100 consecutive cases. *Spine* 1995;20:1624–1632.

A prospective multicenter study comprising the authors' first 100 consecutive endoscopic procedures demonstrated minimal complications with no permanent iatrogenic neurologic injuries and rib deep spinal infections.

Regan JJ, McAfee PC, Guyer RD, Aronoff RJ: Laparoscopic fusion of the lumbar spine in a multicenter series of the first 34 consecutive patients. *Surg Laparosc Endosc* 1996;6:459–468.

In this first case series, 4 conversions occurred early in the series. Mean blood loss was 128 cc, surgical time 218 minutes, and hospitalization 3.6 days.

Zucherman JF, Zdeblick TA, Bailey SA, Mahvi D, Hsu KY, Kohrs D: Instrumented laparoscopic spinal fusion: Preliminary results. *Spine* 1995;20:2029–2034.

Seventeen consecutive patients underwent instrumented interbody fusion using custom-designed delivery instrumentation and "BAK" fusion cages. The procedure is associated with a long learning curve but once mastered is effective and advantageous over current approaches to lumbar fusion. Surgery time and hospital stay are expected to decrease with future instrument development and surgeon experience.

Classic Bibliography

Dickman CA, Rosenthal D, Karahalios DG, et al: Thoracic vertebrectomy and reconstruction using a microsurgical thoracoscopic approach. *Neurosurgery* 1996;38:279–293.

Gaur DD: Laparoscopic operative retroperitoneoscopy: Use of a new device. *J Urol* 1992;148:1137–1139.

Hazelrigg SR, Landreneau RJ, Boley TM, et al: The effect of muscle-sparing versus standard posterolateral thoracotomy on pulmonary function, muscle strength, and postoperative pain. *J Thorac Cardiovasc Surg* 1991;101:394–401.

Horowitz MB, Moossy JJ, Julian T, Ferson PF, Huneke K: Thoracic discectomy using video assisted thoracoscopy. *Spine* 1994;19:1082–1086.

Landreneau RJ, Dowling RD, Ferson PF: Thoracoscopic resection of a posterior mediastinal neurogenic tumor. *Chest* 1992;102:1288–1290.

Mack MJ, Regan JJ, McAfee PC, Picetti G, Ben-Yishay A, Acuff TE: video-assisted thoracic surgery for the anterior approach to the thoracic spine. *Ann Thorac Surg* 1995;59:1100–1106.

Mathews HH, Evans MT, Molligan HJ, Long BH: Laparoscopic discectomy with anterior lumbar interbody fusion: A preliminary review. *Spine* 1995;20:1797–1802.

Obenchain TG: Laparoscopic lumbar discectomy: Case report. *J Laparoendosc Surg* 1991;1:145–149.

Reddick EJ, Olsen DO: Laparoscopic laser cholecystectomy: A comparison with mini-lap cholecystectomy. *Surg Endosc* 1989;3:131–133.

Regan JJ, Yuan H, McCullen G: Minimally invasive approaches to the spine, in Springfield DS (ed): *Instructional Course Lectures 46.* Rosemont, IL, American Academy of Orthopaedic Surgeons, 1997, pp 127–141.

Rosenthal D, Rosenthal R, de Simone A: Removal of a protruded thoracic disc using microsurgical endoscopy: A new technique. *Spine* 1994;19:1087–1091.